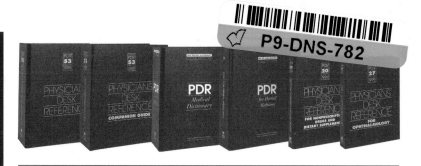

Electronic PDR Order Form

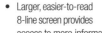

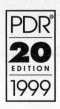

PDR®
20
EDITION
1999

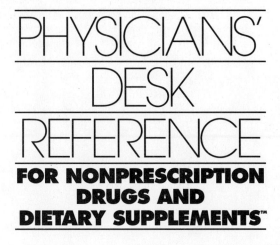

PHYSICIANS' DESK REFERENCE

FOR NONPRESCRIPTION DRUGS AND DIETARY SUPPLEMENTS™

Medical Consultant
Ronald Arky, MD, Charles S. Davidson Professor of Medicine and Master, Francis Weld Peabody Society, Harvard Medical School

---

Vice President of Directory Services: Stephen B. Greenberg

Director of Product Management: Mark A. Friedman
Associate Product Manager: Bill Shaughnessy
Business Manager: Mark S. Ritchin
Director of Sales: Dikran N. Barsamian
National Sales Manager, Pharmaceutical Sales: Anthony Sorce
National Account Manager: Don Bruccoleri
Account Managers: Marion Gray, RPh, Lawrence C. Keary, Jeffrey F. Pfohl, Suzanne E. Yarrow, RN
Electronic Sales Account Managers: Christopher N. Schmidt, Stephen M. Silverberg
National Sales Manager, Medical Economics Trade Sales: Bill Gaffney
Director of Direct Marketing: Michael Bennett
List and Production Manager: Lorraine M. Loening
Promotion Manager: Donna R. Lynn
Senior Marketing Analyst: Dina Maeder
Director, New Business Development and Professional Support Services: Mukesh Mehta, RPh

Manager, Drug Information Services: Thomas Fleming, RPh
Drug Information Specialist: Maria Deutsch, MS, RPh, CDE
Editor, Directory Services: David W. Sifton
Director of Production: Carrie Williams
Manager of Production: Kimberly H. Vivas
Senior Production Coordinator: Amy B. Brooks
Data Manager: Jeffrey D. Schaefer
Senior Format Editor: Gregory J. Westley
Index Editors: Johanna M. Mazur, Robert N. Woerner
Art Associate: Joan K. Akerlind
Senior Digital Imaging Coordinator: Shawn W. Cahill
Digital Imaging Coordinator: Frank J. McElroy, III
Electronic Publishing Designer: Robert K. Grossman
Fulfillment Managers: Stephanie DeNardi, Kenneth Siebert

Officers of Medical Economics Company: *President and Chief Executive Officer:* Curtis B. Allen; *Vice President, New Media:* L. Suzanne BeDell; *Vice President, Corporate Human Resources:* Pamela M. Bilash; *Vice President and Chief Information Officer:* Steven M. Bressler; *Vice President, Directory Services:* Stephen B. Greenberg; *Vice President, New Business Planning:* Linda G. Hope; *Executive Vice President, Healthcare Publishing and Communications:* Thomas J. Kelly; *Executive Vice President, Magazine Publishing:* Lee A. Maniscalco; *Vice President, Group Publisher:* Terrence W. Meacock; *Vice President, Business Integration:* David A. Pitler; *Vice President, Group Publisher:* Thomas C. Pizor; *Vice President, Healthcare Publishing Business Management:* Donna Santarpia; *Vice President, Magazine Business Management:* Eric Schlett; *Senior Vice President, Operations:* John R. Ware

ISBN: 1-56363-298-5

FOREWORD

Almost overnight, the way Americans tackle minor illness has undergone a stunning change. People who for decades relied almost entirely on standard antihistamines and decongestants to relieve their coughs and colds have suddenly turned to echinacea and zinc. Forsaking conventional remedies, many are combating their fatigue with ginseng, their high cholesterol levels with garlic, and their blues with St. John's Wort. Sales of herbal products are doubling every four years, and the trend continues to accelerate.

In recognition of this on-going revolution in self-care, PDR's familiar over-the-counter drug reference this year officially adopts the title *Physicians' Desk Reference for Nonprescription Drugs and Dietary Supplements™* and inaugurates a new *Dietary Supplement Information* section devoted entirely to the nutritional and natural products marketed under the Dietary Supplement Health and Education Act of 1994. Conventional remedies marketed in compliance with the Code of Federal Regulations labeling requirements for over-the-counter drugs can now be found in the section entitled *Nonprescription Drug Information*. For your convenience, products in both sections are listed in the consolidated indices at the front of the book.

Despite the wave of natural remedies now flooding the market, hundreds of medicinal herbs have yet to be commercialized. For more information on these remedies, plus an independent assessment of the most popular natural agents, PDR now offers a unique new compendium, the just-released *PDR® for Herbal Medicines™*.

Covering a total of over 600 botanicals, this important new medical reference includes detailed information on each plant's physical characteristics, chemical composition, and physiological effects, along with a summary of its accepted indications, contraindications, drug interactions, side effects, and dosage. When appropriate, symptoms and treatment of overdose are discussed as well.

Although botanical products are not officially regulated or monitored in the United States, *PDR for Herbal Medicines* provides you the closest analog to FDA-approved labeling—the findings of the German Regulatory Authority's herbal watchdog agency, Commission E—augmented with exhaustive literature reviews from the PhytoPharm U.S. Institute for Phytopharmaceuticals. These reports represent the most accurate, impartial, and reliable assessment of a botanical agent's safety and effectiveness currently available to healthcare practitioners.

Now, when patients pepper you with questions about the latest "herb du jour," *PDR for Herbal Medicines* can provide you with a rational basis for response. It tells which botanicals to encourage—and which to avoid. It clearly distinguishes between valid indications and specious claims, warns of conflicting conditions and drugs, and provides you with an exhaustive bibliography of the relevant clinical literature on each medicinal plant.

For the patients themselves, *PDR* also offers a new consumer handbook, *The PDR Family Guide to Natural Medicines and Healing Therapies*. This latest member of the popular *PDR Family Guide* series provides "patient-friendly" information on 300 herbs, 50 nutrients, and over four dozen complementary forms of therapy. Drawing on the same authoritative sources employed by *PDR for Herbal Medicines*, it sifts out documented help from baseless hype, and steers consumers towards the complementary therapies most likely to provide genuine benefits.

If you haven't already encountered a copy, you should also take a look at the new *PDR Companion Guide*, a 1,800-page reference that augments *PDR* with a total of nine unique decision-making tools:

- **Interactions Index** identifies all pharmaceuticals and foods capable of interacting with a chosen medication.

- **Food Interactions Cross-Reference** lists the drugs that may interact with a given dietary item.

- **Side Effects Index** pinpoints the pharmaceuticals associated with each of 3,600 distinct adverse reactions.

- **Indications Index** presents the full range of therapeutic options for any given diagnosis.

- **Off-Label Treatment Guide** lists medications routinely used—but never officially approved—for treatment of nearly 1,000 specific disorders.

- **Contraindications Index** lists all drugs to avoid in the presence of any given medical condition.

- **International Drug Index** names the U.S. equivalents of some 15,000 foreign medications.

- **Generic Availability Guide** shows which forms and strengths of a brand-name drug are also available generically.

- **Cost of Therapy Guide** provides a quick overview of the relative expense of the leading therapeutic options for a variety of common indications.

The PDR Companion Guide includes all drugs described in PDR, PDR for Nonprescription Drugs and Dietary Supplements, and PDR for Ophthalmology. We're certain that it will make safe, appropriate drug selection faster and easier than ever before.

With the advent of the PDR Companion Guide and PDR for Herbal Medicines, the complete roster of PDR's continually expanding library of professional medical references now includes:

- Physicians' Desk Reference®
- PDR for Nonprescription Drugs and Dietary Supplements™
- PDR for Ophthalmology®
- PDR Companion Guide™
- PDR® for Herbal Medicines™
- PDR® Medical Dictionary™
- PDR® Nurse's Handbook™
- PDR® Nurse's Dictionary™
- PDR® Atlas of Anatomy™
- PDR Supplements

PDR and its major companion volumes are also found in the PDR® Electronic Library™ on CD-ROM, now used in over 100,000 practices. This Windows-compatible disc provides users with a complete database of PDR prescribing information, electronically searchable for instant retrieval. A standard subscription includes PDR's sophisticated prescription-screening program and an extensive file of chemical structures, illustrations, and full-color product photographs. Optional enhancements include the complete contents of The Merck Manual and Stedman's Medical Dictionary. And for anyone who wants to run a fast double-check on a proposed prescription, there's the PDR® Drug Interactions, Side Effects, Indications, Contraindications System™—sophisticated software capable of automatically screening a 20-drug regimen for conflicts, then proposing alternatives for any problematic medication. The disc is available for use on individual PCs and PC networks.

Remember, too, that the contents of PDR and its main companion volumes can always be found on the Internet at www.pdr.net. And for use anywhere—on rounds or on the go—there's Pocket PDR®, a unique handheld electronic database of prescribing information that literally fits in your pocket. For more information on these or any other members of the growing family of PDR products, please call, toll-free, 1-800-232-7379 or fax 201-573-4956.

Physicians' Desk Reference for Nonprescription Drugs and Dietary Supplements is published annually by Medical Economics Company in cooperation with participating manufacturers. The function of the publisher is the compilation, organization, and distribution of product information obtained from manufacturers. Each product description has been prepared by the manufacturer, and edited and approved by the manufacturer's medical department, medical director, and/or medical consultant. During compilation of this information, the publisher has emphasized the necessity of describing products comprehensively, in order to provide all the facts necessary for sound and intelligent decision making. Descriptions seen here include all information made available by the manufacturer. Please note that descriptions of over-the-counter products marketed under the Dietary Supplement Health and Education Act of 1994 have not been evaluated by the Food and Drug Administration, and that such products are not intended to diagnose, treat, cure, or prevent any disease.

In organizing and presenting the material in Physicians' Desk Reference For Nonprescription Drugs and Dietary Supplements, the publisher does not warrant or guarantee any of the products described, or perform any independent analysis in connection with any of the product information contained herein. Physicians' Desk Reference does not assume, and expressly disclaims, any obligation to obtain and include any information other than that provided to it by the manufacturer. It should be understood that by making this material available the publisher is not advocating the use of any product described herein, nor is the publisher responsible for misuse of a product due to typographical error. Additional information on any product may be obtained from the manufacturer.

CONTENTS

MANUFACTURERS' INDEX

Listed in this index are all manufacturers that have supplied information in this edition. Each company's entry includes the address, phone, and fax number of its headquarters and regional offices, as well as contacts for inquiries, orders, and emergency information.

Products with entries in the Nonprescription Drug Information section are listed with their page numbers under the heading OTC Products Described. Products with entries in the Dietary Supplement Information section are listed with their page numbers under the

heading Dietary Supplements Described. Other OTC products and dietary supplements available from the manufacturer follow these two sections.

If an entry in the index lists multiple page numbers, the first one shown refers to the photograph of the product, the last one to its prescribing information.

- The ◆ symbol marks drugs shown in the Product Identification Guide.

- *Italic page numbers* signify partial information.

ADVOCARE INTERNATIONAL, L.L.C.   818

11431 Ferrell Street
Dallas, TX 75234
Direct Inquiries to:
Medical/Scientific Advisory Board
(972) 910-9645
FAX: (972) 831-8830

Dietary Supplements Described:
Advantin Capsules 818
Antioxidant Booster Caplets 818
BodyLean Powder.....................818
Brite-Life Caplets 818
CardiOptima Drink Mix Packets.......818
Cold Season Nutrition Booster
    Capsules...........................819
CorePlex Capsules.....................819
IntelleQ Capsules......................819
Macro-Mineral Complex Caplets......819
Metabolic Nutrition System............820
Perfect Meal...........................820
Performance Gold Caplets 820
Performance Optimizer System 820
ProMotion Capsules 821
ProBiotic Restore Capsules 821
Spark! Beverage Mix..................821
System 3-4-3 Metabolic
    Cleansing System 822

AGRO-DYNAMICS INTERNATIONAL   602

International-Bio Tech-USA
1145 Linda Vista Drive, Suite 109
San Marcos, CA 92069
Direct Inquiries to:
(800) 736-1991
FAX: (760) 471-1878

OTC Products Described:
Latero-Flora Capsules 602

AK PHARMA INC.   503, 822

P.O. Box 111
Pleasantville, NJ 08232-0111
Direct Inquiries to:
Elizabeth Klein
(609) 645-5100
FAX: (609) 645-0767
For Medical Emergencies Contact:
Alan E. Kligerman
(609) 645-5100
FAX: (609) 645-0767

Dietary Supplements Described:
◆ Prelief Tablets and Granulate 503, 822

ASTRA PHARMACEUTICALS, L.P.   503, 602

725 Chesterbrook Boulevard
Wayne, PA 19087-5677
Direct Inquiries to:
For Medical Information, Adverse Drug Experiences, and Customer Service Contact:
(800) 236-9933

OTC Products Described:
◆ Xylocaine 2.5% Ointment 503, 602

BAYER CORPORATION CONSUMER CARE DIVISION   503, 602

P.O. Box 1910
36 Columbia Road
Morristown, NJ 07962-1910

Direct Inquiries to:
Consumer Relations
(800) 331-4536
Internet: www.bayercare.com
For Medical Emergencies Contact:
Bayer Corporation
Consumer Care Division
(800) 331-4536

OTC Products Described:
◆ Aleve Tablets, Caplets and
    Gelcaps 503, 602
◆ Alka-Mints Chewable Antacid/
    Calcium Supplement
    (Spearmint and Assorted
    Flavors) 503, 603
◆ Alka-Seltzer Original
    Effervescent Antacid and
    Pain Reliever................503, 603
◆ Alka-Seltzer Cherry
    Effervescent Antacid and
    Pain Reliever................503, 603
◆ Alka-Seltzer Extra Strength
    Effervescent Antacid and
    Pain Reliever................503, 603
◆ Alka-Seltzer Gas Relief Liquid
    Softgels.....................503, 603
◆ Alka-Seltzer Gold Effervescent
    Antacid......................503, 604
◆ Alka-Seltzer Lemon Lime
    Effervescent Antacid and
    Pain Reliever................503, 603
◆ Alka-Seltzer Plus Cold &
    Cough Medicine
    Effervescent Tablets.........503, 604
◆ Alka-Seltzer Plus Cold &
    Cough Medicine Liqui-Gels...503, 605
◆ Alka-Seltzer Plus Cold & Flu
    Liqui-Gels Non-Drowsy
    Formula 503, 605

BEACH PHARMACEUTICALS   829

Division of Beach Products, Inc.
EXECUTIVE OFFICE:
5220 South Manhattan Avenue
Tampa, FL 33611
(813) 839-6565
Direct Inquiries to:
Richard Stephen Jenkins, Exec. V.P.:
(813) 839-6565
Clete Harmon, Dir. of Q.A.:
(864) 277-7282

Manufacturing and Distribution:
201 Delaware Street
Greenville, SC 29605
(800) 845-8210

BEUTLICH LP   618
PHARMACEUTICALS

1541 Shields Drive
Waukegan, IL 60085-8304
Direct Inquiries to:
(847) 473-1100
(800) 238-8542 in the U.S. and Canada
FAX: (847) 473-1122
Internet: www.beutlich.com
E-mail: fjb1541@worldnet.att.net

BLAIREX LABORATORIES,   619
INC.

3240 North Indianapolis Road
P.O. Box 2127
Columbus, IN 47202-2127
Direct Inquiries to:
Customer Service
(800) 252-4739
FAX: (812) 378-1033
For Medical Emergencies Contact:
David S. Wilson, M.D.
(800) 252-4739
FAX: (812) 378-1033

BLISTEX INC.   620

1800 Swift Drive
Oak Brook, IL 60523-1574
Direct Inquiries to:
Consumer Affairs
(800) 837-1800
For Medical Emergencies Contact:
Consumer Affairs
(800) 837-1800

Stri-Dex Antibacterial Foaming
Wash.........................**620**
Stri-Dex Clear Gel....................**620**

BLOCK DRUG COMPANY,   **506, 621**
INC.

257 Cornelison Avenue
Jersey City, NJ 07302
Direct Inquiries to:
Lori Hunt
(201) 434-3000, Ext. 1308
For Medical Emergencies Contact:
Consumer Affairs/Block
(201) 434-3000, Ext. 1308

OTC Products Described:
◆ Balmex Diaper Rash Ointment...**506, 621**
BC Powder..............................**621**
BC Allergy Sinus Cold Powder.........**621**
Arthritis Strength BC Powder..........**621**
BC Sinus Cold Powder..................**621**
Goody's Body Pain Formula
Powder.............................**622**
Goody's Extra Strength Headache
Powder.............................**622**
Goody's Extra Strength Pain
Relief Tablets.....................**622**
Goody's PM Powder....................**623**
◆ Nature's Remedy Tablets.......**506, 623**
Nytol Natural Tablets..................**623**
Nytol QuickCaps Caplets..............**624**
Maximum Strength Nytol
QuickGels Softgels.................**623**
◆ Phazyme Infant Drops..........**506, 624**
◆ Phazyme-125 Softgels..........**506, 624**
◆ Phazyme-166 Maximum
Strength Chewable Tablets ..**506, 624**
◆ Phazyme-166 Maximum
Strength Softgel Capsules...**506, 624**
Promise Sensitive Toothpaste........**625**
Sensodyne Original Flavor.............**625**
Sensodyne Cool Gel....................**625**
Sensodyne Extra Whitening...........**625**
Sensodyne Fresh Mint..................**625**
Sensodyne Tartar Control.............**625**
Sensodyne with Baking Soda.........**625**
Tegrin Dandruff Shampoo - Extra
Conditioning.......................**625**
Tegrin Dandruff Shampoo - Fresh
Herbal.............................**626**
Tegrin Skin Cream.....................**626**

Dietary Supplements Described:
Beano Liquid..........................**829**
Beano Tablets.........................**829**

BOIRON, THE WORLD LEADER   **627**
IN HOMEOPATHY

6 Campus Blvd.
Newtown Square, PA 19073
Direct Inquiries to:
Boiron Information Center
(800) 264-7661
For Medical Emergencies Contact:
Boiron Information Center
(800) 264-7661

OTC Products Described:
Oscillococcinum Pellets...............**627**

Other Products Available:
Acidil, for Heartburn
Arnica & Calendula Gel & Ointment
Arnicalm, for Bumps and Bruises
Camilia, for Baby Teething
Chestal Cough Syrup
Chestal For Children Cough Syrup
Cocyntal, for Baby Colic
Coldcalm, for Cold Symptoms
Cyclease, for Menstrual Cramps
Gasalia, for Gas
Ginsenique, for Fatigue
Homeodent Toothpaste

Natural Phases, for PMS
Optique 1 Eye Drops, for Eye Irritation
Quiétude, for Sleeplessness
Roxalia, for Sore Throat
Sabadil, for Allergies
Sedalia, for Stress
Sinusalia, for Sinus Pain
Sportenine, for Cramps and Muscle
Fatigue
Yeastaway, for Vaginal Yeast Infections

BRISTOL-MYERS   **506, 627**
PRODUCTS

A Bristol-Myers Squibb Company
345 Park Avenue
New York, NY 10154
Direct Inquiries to:
Bristol-Myers Products Division
Consumer Affairs Department
1350 Liberty Avenue
Hillside, NJ 07207
Questions or Comments:
(800) 468-7746

OTC Products Described:
Alpha Keri Moisture Rich Shower
and Bath Oil......................**627**
◆ Bufferin Analgesic Tablets.....**506, 627**
◆ Comtrex Deep Chest Cold &
Congestion Relief
Liquigels...................**506, 631**
◆ Comtrex Maximum Strength
Multi-Symptom Acute Head
Cold & Sinus Pressure
Relief Tablets..............**506, 630**
Comtrex Maximum Strength
Multi-Symptom Cold & Cough
Relief Liqui-Gels.................**628**
◆ Comtrex Maximum Strength
Multi-Symptom Cold &
Cough Relief Tablets and
Caplets....................**506, 628**
◆ Aspirin Free Excedrin Caplets
and Geltabs.................**506, 631**
◆ Excedrin Extra-Strength
Tablets, Caplets, and
Geltabs....................**506, 632**
◆ Excedrin Migraine Tablets,
Caplets, and Geltabs........**507, 633**
◆ Excedrin P.M. Tablets,
Caplets, and Geltabs........**506, 634**
◆ 4-Way Fast Acting Nasal Spray
- Regular and Mentholated
Formulas...................**506, 635**
◆ Keri Anti-Bacterial Hand Lotion ..**507, 636**
◆ Keri Lotion - Original Formula.....**507, 635**
◆ Keri Lotion - Sensitive Skin,
Fragrance Free.............**507, 635**
◆ Keri Lotion - Silky Smooth.......**507, 635**
◆ No Doz Maximum Strength
Caplets....................**507, 636**
◆ Nuprin Tablets and Caplets......**507, 636**
◆ Therapeutic Mineral Ice...............*507*
◆ Vagistat-1 Vaginal Ointment....**507, 637**

Dietary Supplements Described:
◆ Theragran-M Caplets............**507, 830**

Other Products Available:
Alpha Keri Moisture Rich Cleansing Bar
Bufferin, Arthritis Strength Caplets
Bufferin, Extra Strength Tablets
Comtrex Maximum Strength
Multi-Symptom Alergy-Sinus Day/Night
Caplets/Tablets
Comtrex Maximum Strength
Multi-Symptom Allergy-Sinus
Treatment Tablets
Comtrex Maximum Strength
Multi-Symptom Day/Night Caplets/
Tablets
Comtrex Maximum Strength
Multi-Symptom Non-Drowsy Liquigels
Fostex 10% Benzoyl Peroxide Bar

Fostex 10% Benzoyl Peroxide (Vanish) Gel
Fostex 10% Benzoyl Peroxide Wash
Fostex Medicated Cleansing Bar
Fostex Medicated Cleansing Cream
4-Way Long Lasting Nasal Spray
4-Way Nasal Moisturizing Saline Mist
KeriCort-10 Cream
Pazo Hemorrhoidal Ointment
Therapeutic Mineral Ice Exercise Formula

CARE-TECH LABORATORIES,   **637**
INC.

Over-The-Counter Pharmaceuticals
3224 South Kingshighway Boulevard
St. Louis, MO 63139
Direct Inquiries to:
Sherry L. Brereton
(314) 772-4610
FAX: (314) 772-4613
For Medical Emergencies Contact:
Customer Service
(800) 325-9681
FAX: (314) 772-4613

OTC Products Described:
Barri-Care Antimicrobial Ointment.....**637**
Care-Creme Antimicrobial Cream......**638**
Clinical Care Antimicrobial Wound
Cleanser...........................**638**
Concept Antimicrobial Dermal
Cleanser...........................**638**
Formula Magic Antimicrobial/
Anti-Fungal Powder................**638**
Humatrix Microclysmic Burn/
Wound Healing Gel................**638**
Orchid Fresh II Antimicrobial
Perineal/Ostomy Cleanser.........**638**
Satin Antimicrobial Skin Cleanser.....**638**
Techni-Care Surgical Scrub, Prep
and Wound Decontaminant........**639**

Other Products Available:
CC-500 Antibacterial Skin Cleanser for
Dialysis Patient Care
Genex Antimicrobial Rinse
Just Lotion - Highly Absorbent Aloe Vera
Glycerine Based Skin Lotion
Loving Lather Collagen Enriched Geriatric
Cleanser
Loving Lather II Antibacterial Skin
Cleanser
Loving Lotion Antibacterial Skin & Body
Lotion
Orchid Fresh Perineal/Ostomy Deodorizer
Skin Magic - Antimicrobial Body Rub &
Emollient
Soft Skin Non-greasy Bath Oil with Rich
Emollients for Severely Damaged
Dermal Tissue
Surgi-Soft Alcohol Degerming Foam
Swirlsoft Whirlpool Emollient for Dry Skin
Conditions
Tech 2000 Antimicrobial Oral Rinse (No
Alcohol, No Sodium)
Velvet Fresh Non-irritating Cornstarch
Baby Powder

CARE TECHNOLOGIES, INC.   **639**

10 Corbin Drive
Darien, CT 06820
Direct Inquiries to:
Mary Lynn M. Drake
Marketing and Sales Services Manager
(203) 655-9680
FAX: (203) 655-9682
E-mail: caretec1@aol.com
Internet: http://www.clearcare.com

OTC Products Described:
Clear Total Lice Elimination
System (Shampoo, Egg
Remover, "Nit Capturing"
Comb)............................**639**

(◆) **Shown in Product Identification Guide**   *Italic Page Number* **Indicates Brief Listing**

CARLSBAD TECHNOLOGY INC.   640
5923 Balfour Court
Carlsbad, CA 92008
For Medical and Pharmaceutical Information:
(760) 431-8284
FAX: (760) 431-7505

OTC Products Described:
YSP Aspirin Capsules..................**640**

J. R. CARLSON   830
LABORATORIES, INC.
15 College Drive
Arlington Heights, IL 60004-1985
Direct Inquiries to:
Customer Service
(847) 255-1600
FAX: (847) 255-1605
For Medical Emergencies Contact:
Customer Service
(847) 255-1600
FAX: (847) 255-1605

Dietary Supplements Described:
ACES Antioxidant Soft Gels............*830*
E-Gems Soft Gels......................*830*
Tri-B Tablets............................*831*

CHURCH & DWIGHT CO., INC.   640
469 North Harrison Street
Princeton, NJ 08543-5297
Direct Inquiries to:
Robert Coleman
(609) 497-7130
Nancy Sevinsky
(609) 683-7015
For Medical Emergencies Contact:
Hazard Information Services
(800) 228-5635
Extension 7

OTC Products Described:
Arm & Hammer Pure Baking Soda **640**

CIGARREST   640
6361 Yarrow Drive, Ste. B
Carlsbad, CA 92009
Direct Inquiries to:
Sheila Durkin
(760) 438-1935
FAX: (760) 438-3212
For Medical Emergencies Contact:
Customer Service
(800) 514-7233
FAX: (760) 438-3212

OTC Products Described:
CigArrest No Smoking Gum,
    Tablets and Lozenges **640**

COLUMBIA LABORATORIES,   641
INCORPORATED
2875 N.E. 191st Street
Suite 400
Aventura, FL 33180
Direct Inquiries to:
Columbia Laboratories, Incorporated
(800) 824-4586
FAX: (305) 933-6090
For Medical Emergencies Contact:
Columbia Laboratories, Incorporated
(305) 933-6089
FAX: (305) 933-6090

OTC Products Described:
Advantage-S Bioadhesive
    Contraceptive Gel..................**641**
Replens Vaginal Moisturizer **641**

Other Products Available:
Diasorb Suspension

Diasorb Tablets
Advanced Formula Legatrin-PM
Vaporizer in a bottle Cough Suppressant

COOKE PHARMA   507, 831
1404 Old Country Road
Belmont, CA 94002
Direct Inquiries to:
Customer Service Dept.
(888) 808-6838

Dietary Supplements Described:
◆ HeartBar........................**507, 831**

DEL PHARMACEUTICALS,   507, 642
INC.
A Subsidiary of Del Laboratories, Inc.
178 EAB Plaza
Uniondale, NY 11556
Direct Inquiries to:
Dr. Joseph A. Kanapka, Ph.D.
Sr. VP Scientific Affairs
(516) 844-2020
FAX: (516) 293-1515
For Medical Emergencies Contact:
David Grob
Director of Regulatory Affairs
(800) 952-5080

OTC Products Described:
◆ ArthriCare Arthritis Pain
    Relieving Rub **507, 642**
ArthriCare Triple Medicated
    Arthritis Pain Relieving Rub.......**642**
◆ ArthriCare Ultra Arthritis Pain
    Relieving Rub **507, 642**
◆ Baby Orajel Teething Pain
    Medicine....................**507, 642**
◆ Baby Orajel Tooth & Gum
    Cleanser **507, 642**
Orajel CoverMed Fever Blister/
    Cold Sore Treatment Cream.......**643**
◆ Orajel Mouth-Aid for Canker
    and Cold Sores **507, 643**
◆ Orajel Perioseptic Spot
    Treatment Oral Cleanser.....**507, 643**
◆ Orajel Perioseptic Super
    Cleaning Oral Rinse..........**507, 643**
◆ Orajel Sensitive Sensitive
    Teeth Toothpaste for
    Adults **507, 644**
◆ Orajel Maximum Strength
    Toothache Medication **507, 643**
Orajel PM Maximum Strength
    Toothache Medication **643**
◆ Pronto Lice Treatment **507, 644**
◆ Tanac Medicated Gel **508, 644**
◆ Tanac No Sting Liquid...........**508, 645**

Other Products Available:
Auro-Dri Ear Water-Drying Aid
Auro Ear Wax Removal Aid
Boil-Ease Pain Relieving Ointment
Dermarest DriCort Anti-Itch Creme
Dermarest Plus Gel
Detane Desensitizing Lubricant
Diaper Guard Skin Rash Ointment
Exocaine Pain Relieving Rubs
Off-Ezy Wart Remover
Baby Orajel Nighttime Formula
Orajel Denture Oral Pain Reliever
Propa pH Acne Medications
Skin Shield Liquid Bandage
Stye Ophthalmic Ointment
Triptone for Motion Sickness

EFFCON LABORATORIES,   508, 645
INC.
P.O. Box 7499
Marietta, GA 30065-1499

Direct Inquiries to:
J. Bradley Rivet
(800) 722-2428
FAX: (770) 428-6811
For Medical Emergencies Contact:
J. Bradley Rivet
(800) 722-2428
FAX: (770) 428-6811

OTC Products Described:
◆ Pin-X Pinworm Treatment **508, 645**

ENVIRODERM   645
PHARMACEUTICALS, INC.
P.O. Box 32370
Louisville, KY 40232
Direct Inquiries to:
(800) 991-3376

OTC Products Described:
Ivy Block Lotion........................**645**

FISONS CORPORATION
PRESCRIPTION PRODUCTS
(See MEDEVA PHARMACEUTICALS, INC.)

FLEMING & COMPANY   646
1600 Fenpark Dr.
Fenton, MO 63026
Direct Inquiries to:
Tom Fleming
(314) 343-8200
FAX: (314) 343-9865

OTC Products Described:
Chlor-3 Condiment.....................**646**
Impregon Concentrate.................**646**
Marblen Suspension
    Peach/Apricot **646**
Marblen Tablets.......................**646**
Nephrox Suspension **646**
Nicotinex Elixir........................**646**
Ocean Nasal Mist......................**646**
Purge Concentrate....................**646**

Dietary Supplements Described:
Magonate Liquid.......................**832**
Magonate Natal Liquid **832**
Magonate Tablets.....................**832**

GENERAL NUTRITION CORP.   832
(GNC)
300 Sixth Avenue
Pittsburgh, PA 15222
Direct Inquiries to:
Customer Resources
(888) 462-2548

Dietary Supplements Described:
Kids Multibite Plus Minerals
    Tablets............................**832**
Platinum Years Tablets **832**
Women's Pre-Natal Formula
    without Iron........................**833**

HYLAND'S INC.
(See STANDARD HOMEOPATHIC COMPANY)

JOHNSON & JOHNSON •   508, 646
MERCK CONSUMER
PHARMACEUTICALS
CO.
7050 Camp Hill Road
Fort Washington, PA 19034
Direct Inquiries to:
Consumer Affairs Department
(215) 233-7000
For Medical Emergencies Contact:
(215) 233-7000

(◆) Shown in Product Identification Guide   *Italic Page Number* **Indicates Brief Listing**

MEDEVA PHARMACEUTICALS, INC.   **680**
P.O. Box 1710
Rochester, NY 14603
Direct Inquiries to:
Customer Service Department
P.O. Box 1766
Rochester, NY 14603
(716) 274-5300
(888) 9-MEDEVA
For Emergency Medical Information Contact:
(800) 932-1950 (24 hours)
(888) 9-MEDEVA (24 hours)

MILES INC. CONSUMER HEALTHCARE PRODUCTS
(See BAYER CORPORATION CONSUMER CARE DIVISION)

MISSION PHARMACAL   **680**
COMPANY
10999 IH 10 West, Suite 1000
San Antonio, TX 78230-1355
Direct Inquiries to:
P.O. Box 786099
San Antonio, TX 78278-6099
Toll Free: (800) 292-7364
(210) 696-8400
FAX: (210) 696-6010
For Medical Emergencies Contact:
George Alexandrides
(830) 249-9822
FAX: (830) 816-2545

NATROL   **513, 841**
21411 Prairie Street
Chatsworth, CA 91311
Direct Inquiries to:
(818) 739-6000
FAX: (818) 739-6001

NICHE PHARMACEUTICALS,   **842**
INC.
200 N. Oak Street
P.O. Box 449
Roanoke, TX 76262
Direct Inquiries to:
Stephen Brandon
(817) 491-2770
FAX: (817) 491-3533

NOVARTIS CONSUMER   **513, 681**
HEALTH, INC.
560 Morris Ave.
Summit, NJ 07901-1312
Direct Product Inquiries to:
Consumer and Professional Affairs
(800) 452-0051
FAX: (800) 635-2801
Or write to the above address

(◆) **Shown in Product Identification Guide**   *Italic Page Number* **Indicates Brief Listing**

NOVOGEN, INC.   516, 844
1 Landmark Square
Stamford, CT 06901
Direct Inquiries to:
Toll-free: (877) TRINOVIN (874-6684)
FAX: (203) 327-0011
Internet: www.novogen.com
E-Mail: promensil@novogen.com

Dietary Supplements Described:

NUMARK LABORATORIES,   844
INC.
164 Northfield Avenue
Edison, NJ 08837
Direct Inquiries to:
Consumer Services
Phone: (800) 331-0221
FAX: (732) 225-0066

Dietary Supplements Described:

P & S LABORATORIES
(See STANDARD HOMEOPATHIC
COMPANY)

PARKE-DAVIS
(See WARNER-LAMBERT CONSUMER
HEALTHCARE)

THE PARTHENON COMPANY,   704
INC.
3311 West 2400 South
Salt Lake City, UT 84119

Direct Inquiries to:
(801) 972-5184
FAX: (801) 972-4734
For Medical Emergencies Contact:
Nick G. Mihalopoulos
(801) 972-5184

OTC Products Described:

PFIZER CONSUMER   516, 705
HEALTH CARE GROUP
Division of Pfizer Inc
235 E. 42nd Street
New York, NY 10017
Address Questions & Comments to:
Consumer Relations
235 E. 42nd Street
New York, NY 10017-5755
Toll Free Product Information:
(800) 723-7529
**For Medical Emergencies/Information
Contact:**
(212) 573-5656

OTC Products Described:

Other Products Available:
Hemorid Creme
Hemorid Ointment

PHARMACIA & UPJOHN   517, 713
7000 Portage Road
Kalamazoo, MI 49001
**For Medical and Pharmaceutical
Information, Including Emergencies,
Contact:**
(800) 253-8600
(616) 833-4000
Pharmaceutical Sales Areas:
Atlanta (Chamblee)
   GA 30341-2626
   (770) 452-4607
Chicago (Downers Grove)
   IL 60515
   (630) 663-9300
Cincinnati
   OH 45202
   (513) 723-1010
   (800) 543-0278
Dallas (Irving)
   TX 75039
   (972) 869-4242
Los Angeles (Simi Valley)
   CA 93065
   (805) 582-0188
Memphis (Germantown)
   TN 38183
   (901) 685-8192
New York (Valhalla)
   NY 10595
   (914) 769-5400
Philadelphia (Berwyn)
   PA 19312
   (610) 993-0100
Portland
   OR 97232
   (503) 232-2133
Distribution Centers:
Atlanta (Chamblee)
   GA 30341
   (770) 451-4822
Hartford (Enfield)
   CT 06082-4491
   (860) 741-3421
Kalamazoo
   MI 49002
   (616) 833-0099
Kansas City
   MO 64131
   (816) 361-2288
Los Angeles (Simi Valley)
   CA 93065
   (805) 582-0072

OTC Products Described:

PHARMACIA & UPJOHN—cont.

◆ NasalCrom CA Allergy
Prevention Pack..............**517, 716**
◆ PediaCare Cough-Cold
Chewable Tablets **518, 717**
◆ PediaCare Cough-Cold Liquid **518, 717**
◆ PediaCare Decongestant
Infants' Drops **518, 717**
◆ PediaCare Decongestant Plus
Cough Infants' Drops **518, 717**
◆ PediaCare Fever Drops **518, 719**
◆ PediaCare Fever Liquid **517, 719**
◆ PediaCare NightRest
Cough-Cold Liquid...........**518, 717**
◆ Rogaine Extra Strength for
Men Hair Regrowth
Treatment...................**518, 720**
◆ Rogaine for Women Hair
Regrowth Treatment **518, 723**
◆ Rogaine Regular Strength For
Men Hair Regrowth
Treatment...................**518, 721**
◆ Surfak Liqui-Gels **518, 724**

Other Products Available:
Progaine Conditioner
Progaine Shampoo (Extra Body)
Progaine Shampoo (Permed & Color
Treated)
Progaine Shampoo (2 in 1)
Unicap Capsules
Unicap Jr. Chewable Tablets
Unicap Tablets
Unicap M Tablets
Unicap T Tablets
Unicap Plus Iron Tablets
Unicap Sr. Tablets

PHARMANEX INC.   518, 845

75 West Center Street
Provo, UT 84601
Direct Inquiries to:
Customer Service
(800) 800-0260
(801) 345-1000
FAX: (801) 345-1999
For Medical Emergencies Contact:
Michael Chang, Ph.D.
Joseph Chang, Ph.D.
(800) 800-0260
(801) 345-1000

Dietary Supplements Described:
Bio St. John's Capsules **845**
◆ BioGinkgo 27/7 Extra
Strength Tablets **518, 845**
◆ Cholestin Capsules **518, 846**
CordyMax Cs-4 Capsules **847**
Tēgreen 97 Capsules **847**

PHARMATON NATURAL   518, 848
HEALTH PRODUCTS

A Division of Boehringer Ingelheim
Pharmaceuticals, Inc.
900 Ridgebury Road
Ridgefield, CT 06877
Direct Inquiries to:
Consumer Affairs
(800) 203-2916
FAX: (203) 798-5771
For Medical Emergencies Contact:
Marvin Wetter, M.D.
(203) 798-4361
FAX: (203) 798-5771

Dietary Supplements Described:
◆ Ginkoba Tablets..................**518, 848**
◆ Ginsana Capsules **518, 848**
◆ Ginsana Chewy Squares........**518, 848**
◆ Movana Tablets.................**518, 849**
◆ Venastat Supro Caps **519, 849**
◆ Vitasana Daily Dietary
Supplement **519, 849**

PHARMAVITE CORPORATION   850

15451 San Fernando Mission Blvd.
Mission Hills, CA 91345
Direct Inquiries to:
Nature's Resource Brand Group
(800) 423-2405
FAX: (818) 837-6129
For Medical Emergencies Contact:
(800) 423-2405, ext. 2281

Dietary Supplements Described:
Echinacea Herb Capsules **850**
Ginkgo Biloba Leaf Standardized
Extract Capsules..................**850**
Saw Palmetto Standardized
Extract Capsules..................**850**
St. John's Wort Herb
Standardized Extract
Capsules.........................**850**
Standardized Valerian Root
Capsules.........................**850**

Other Products Available:
Alfalfa
Astragalus
Bee Pollen
Bilberry Fruit Standardized Extract
Black Cohosh
Cascara Sagrada Bark
Cat's Claw Standardized Extract
Cayenne Pepper Fruit
Chastetree Berry
Chinese Red Panax Ginseng
Cranberry Fruit
Dong Quai Root
Echinacea-Goldenseal Combo
Echinacea Lozenge with Zinc
Evening Primrose Oil Standardized Extract
Feverfew Leaf
Garlic
Ginger Root
Ginseng Root–American, Korean &
Siberian
Goldenseal Root
Gotu Kola Root
Grape Seed Extract
Green Tea Standardized Extract
Hawthorn Berries
Kava Kava Root Standardized Extract
Licorice Root
Milk Thistle Standardized Extract
Saw Palmetto
St. John's Wort
Valerian Root

PHYTOPHARMICA   519, 851

825 Challenger Drive
Green Bay, WI 54311
Direct Inquiries to:
Doctors and Pharmacists
(800) 553-2370
Consumers
(800) 644-0799

Dietary Supplements Described:
Cellular Forte with IP-6 Capsules......**851**
◆ Esberitox Tablets **519, 851**
◆ Remifemin Tablets..............**519, 851**

PLOUGH, INC.

(See SCHERING-PLOUGH HEALTHCARE
PRODUCTS)

PROCTER & GAMBLE   519, 724

P.O. Box 5516
Cincinnati, OH 45201
Direct Inquiries to:
Charles Lambert
(800) 358-8707
For Medical Emergencies Contact:
Call Collect: (513) 558-4422

OTC Products Described:
Crest Sensitivity Protection
Toothpaste......................**724**
Metamucil Powder, Original
Texture Orange Flavor..............**725**
Metamucil Powder, Original
Texture Regular Flavor **725**
◆ Metamucil Smooth Texture
Powder, Orange Flavor **519, 725**
Metamucil Smooth Texture
Powder, Sugar-Free, Orange
Flavor **725**
Metamucil Smooth Texture
Powder, Sugar-Free, Regular
Flavor **725**
◆ Metamucil Wafers, Apple Crisp
& Cinnamon Spice Flavors...**519, 725**
Oil of Olay Complete UV
Protective Moisturizer SPF 15
Beauty Lotion/Cream-Original
and Fragrance Free **726**
◆ Pepto-Bismol Original Liquid,
Original and Cherry Tablets
& Easy-to-Swallow Caplets...**519, 726**
Pepto-Bismol Maximum Strength
Liquid **727**
Vicks 44 Cough Relief **727**
Vicks 44D Cough & Head
Congestion Relief...................**728**
Vicks 44E Cough & Chest
Congestion Relief...................**728**
Pediatric Vicks 44e Cough &
Chest Congestion Relief...........**732**
Vicks 44M Cough, Cold & Flu
Relief **729**
Pediatric Vicks 44m Cough &
Cold Relief **733**
Vicks Chloraseptic Sore Throat
Lozenges, Menthol and
Cherry Flavors **730**
Vicks Chloraseptic Sore Throat
Spray, Menthol and Cherry
Flavors **730**
Vicks Cough Drops, Menthol and
Cherry Flavors **730**
Vicks Cough Drops, Menthol and
Cherry Flavors **730**
Vicks DayQuil LiquiCaps/Liquid
Multi-Symptom Cold/Flu Relief **731**
Vicks DayQuil Sinus Pressure &
Pain Relief **731**
Children's Vicks NyQuil Cold/
Cough Relief **729**
Vicks NyQuil LiquiCaps/Liquid
Multi-Symptom Cold/Flu
Relief, Original and Cherry
Flavors **732**
Vicks Sinex Nasal Spray and Ultra
Fine Mist..........................**733**
Vicks Sinex 12-Hour Nasal Spray
and Ultra Fine Mist **734**
Vicks Vapor Inhaler **734**
Vicks VapoRub Cream **734**
Vicks VapoRub Ointment **734**
Vicks VapoSteam **734**

Dietary Supplements Described:
Metamucil Dietary Fiber
Supplement........................**851**

THE PURDUE FREDERICK   519, 735
COMPANY

100 Connecticut Avenue
Norwalk, CT 06850-3590
For Medical Information Contact:
Medical Department
(203) 853-0123

OTC Products Described:
◆ Betadine Brand First Aid
Antibiotics + Moisturizer
Ointment **519, 735**

REAL HEALTH   519, 852
LABORATORIES, INC.

1424 30th Street
San Diego, CA 92154
Direct Inquiries to:
Consumer Product Information Center
(800) 565-6656

Dietary Supplements Described:

REXALL SUNDOWN, INC.   519, 853

6111 Broken Sound Parkway NW
Boca Raton, FL 33487-2745
Direct Inquiries to:
(888) VITAHELP (848-2435)

Dietary Supplements Described:

RICHARDSON-VICKS, INC.

(See PROCTER & GAMBLE)

ROBERTS PHARMACEUTICAL   736
CORPORATION

4 Industrial Way West
Eatontown, NJ 07724-2274
Direct Inquiries to:
Customer Service Department
(732) 389-1182
(800) 828-2088
FAX: (908) 389-1014
For Medical Emergencies Contact:
Medical Services Department
(800) 992-9306

OTC Products Described:

Other Products Available:
Cheracol Cough Syrup CV
Cheracol Cough/Sore Throat Lozenges
Squibb Cod Liver Oil
Squibb Glycerin Suppositories
Squibb Mineral Oil

SCHERING CORPORATION

(See SCHERING-PLOUGH HEALTHCARE
PRODUCTS)

SCHERING-PLOUGH   519, 738
HEALTHCARE
PRODUCTS

110 Allen Road
Liberty Corner, NJ 07938
Direct Product Requests to:
(908) 604-1983
FAX: (908) 604-1776
For Medical Emergencies Contact:
Clinical Department
(908) 604-1805

OTC Products Described:

SIGMA-TAU CONSUMER   521, 854
PRODUCTS

A division of of sigma-tau Pharmaceutials,
Inc.
Gaithersburg, MD 20877
Direct Medical Inquiries to:
Toll Free: (888) 818-5448
or (301) 948-5450
FAX: (301) 948-5452
E-Mail: info@sigmatau.com
Direct Product Orders to:
Toll Free: (877) PROXEED (776-9333)
Internet: www.proxeed.com

Dietary Supplements Described:

SMITHKLINE BEECHAM   521, 748
CONSUMER
HEALTHCARE, L.P.

Unit of SmithKline Beecham Corporation
P.O. Box 1467
Pittsburgh, PA 15230
For Medical Information Contact:
(800) 245-1040 (Consumer Inquiries)
(800) 378-4055 (Healthcare Professional
Inquiries)
**Direct Healthcare Professional Sample
Requests to:**
(800) BEECHAM

OTC Products Described:

SMITHKLINE BEECHAM CONSUMER HEALTHCARE, L.P.—cont.
- ◆ Vivarin Alertness Aid Tablets **523, 767**
- ◆ Vivarin Alertness Aid Caplets....**523, 767**

Dietary Supplements Described:
- ◆ Os-Cal Chewable Tablets **522, 855**
- ◆ Os-Cal 250 + D Tablets.........**522, 856**
- ◆ Os-Cal 500 Tablets **522, 856**
- ◆ Os-Cal 500 + D Tablets.........**522, 856**

Other Products Available:
Sominex Maximum Strength Caplets Nighttime Sleep Aid
Sominex Pain Relief Formula Tablets

STANDARD HOMEOPATHIC COMPANY   **767**

210 West 131st Street
Box 61067
Los Angeles, CA 90061
Direct Inquiries to:
Jay Borneman
(800) 624-9659, Ext. 20

OTC Products Described:
Hyland's Bladder Irritation Tablets **767**
Hyland's Calms Forté Tablets **767**
Hyland's Cold Tablets with Zinc **767**
Hyland's Colic Tablets **768**
Hyland's Earache Tablets.............**768**
Hyland's Leg Cramps with Quinine Tablets.........................**768**
Hyland's Motion Sickness Tablets.....**768**
Hyland's Nerve Tonic Caplets and Tablets..........................**768**
Hyland's PMS Tablets **769**
Hyland's Poison Ivy/Oak Tablets **769**
Hyland's Teething Gel **769**
Hyland's Teething Tablets **769**
Hyland's Vaginitis Tablets **769**

SUNPOWER NUTRACEUTICAL INC.   **523, 856**

18003 Sky Park Circle
Suite G
Irvine, CA 92614
Direct Inquiries to:
(949) 833-8899

Dietary Supplements Described:
Power Arthritis Tablets.................*856*
Power Circulation Tablets..............*856*
Power Lasting Tablets *856*
Sun Beauty 1 Tablets *856*
Sun Beauty 2 Tablets.................*856*
Sun Beauty 3 Tablets.................*856*
Sun Cardio Tablets *856*
- ◆ Sun Liver Tablets *523, 856*

THOMPSON MEDICAL COMPANY, INC.   **770**

777 So. Flagler Drive
West Tower, Suite 1500
West Palm Beach, FL 33401
Direct Inquiries to:
Consumer Services
(561) 820-9900
FAX: (561) 832-2297

OTC Products Described:
Encare Vaginal Contraceptive Suppositories......................**770**
Sleepinal Night-time Sleep Aid Capsules and Softgels...........**770**

Dietary Supplements Described:
Nature's Reward Calci Complex Caplets *857*
Nature's Reward Ginkogin Caplets *857*
Nature's Reward Heart Wise Caplets *857*

Nature's Reward Prime of Life Caplets *858*

Other Products Available:
Aqua-Ban Maximum Strength Tablets
Breathe Free
Caffedrine Caplets
End Lice
Fat Inhibitor Plan Caplets
NP-27 Cream & Spray Powder
Quick Pep Tablets
Tempo
Ultra Burn Plan Caplets

TRITON CONSUMER PRODUCTS, INC.   **771**

561 West Golf Road
Arlington Heights, IL 60005
Direct Inquiries to:
Karen Shrader
(800) 942-2009
For Medical Emergencies Contact:
(800) 942-2009

OTC Products Described:
MG 217 Medicated Tar Ointment and Lotion **771**
MG 217 Medicated Tar Shampoo **771**
MG 217 Medicated Tar-Free Shampoo **771**
MG 217 Sal-Acid Ointment and Solution..........................**771**

Other Products Available:
Retre-Gel Medicated Cold Sore Gel
Skeeter Stik Insect Bite Medication

UAS LABORATORIES   **771**

5610 Rowland Road # 110
Minnetonka, MN 55343
Direct Inquiries to:
Dr. S.K. Dash
(612) 935-1707
FAX: (612) 935-1650
For Medical Emergencies Contact:
Dr. S.K. Dash
(612) 935-1707
FAX: (612) 935-1650

OTC Products Described:
DDS-Acidophilus Capsules, Tablets, and Powder **771**

UNILEVER HOME & PERSONAL CARE USA   **523, 771**

33 Benedict Place
Greenwich, CT 06830
Direct Inquiries to:
Customer Services
(800) 598-5005

OTC Products Described:
- ◆ All Free Clear with Allergen Fighter Laundry Detergent Liquid & Powder **523, 771**

UNIPATH DIAGNOSTICS COMPANY   **523, 771**

47 Hulfish Street
Suite 400
Princeton, NJ 08542
Direct Inquiries to:
(800) 321-EASY

OTC Products Described:
- ◆ ClearBlue Easy...................**523, 771**
- ◆ ClearPlan Easy...................**523, 772**

THE UPJOHN COMPANY
(See PHARMACIA & UPJOHN)

UPSHER-SMITH LABORATORIES, INC.   **772**

14905 23rd Avenue N.
Plymouth, MN 55447
Direct Inquiries to:
Professional Services
(612) 475-3023
FAX: (612) 475-3410
For Medical Emergencies Contact:
Professional Services
(612) 475-3023
(800) 654-2299
FAX: (612) 475-3410
Branch Offices:
13700 1st Avenue N.
Plymouth, MN 55441
(612) 475-3023
FAX: (612) 475-3410

OTC Products Described:
Amlactin 12% Moisturizing Lotion and Cream.........................*772*

WAKUNAGA CONSUMER PRODUCTS   **523, 858**

Subsidiary of Wakunaga Pharmaceutical Co., Ltd.
23501 Madero
Mission Viejo, CA 92691
Direct Inquiries to:
(800) 527-5200

OTC Products Described:
- ◆ Probiata Tablets **523, 858**

Dietary Supplements Described:
Ginkgo-Go Caplets....................*858*
- ◆ Kyolic Aged Garlic Extract Caplets **523, 858**

WALLACE LABORATORIES   **523, 772**

P.O. Box 1001
Half Acre Road
Cranbury, NJ 08512
Direct Inquiries to:
Wallace Laboratories
Div. of Carter-Wallace, Inc.
P.O. Box 1001
Cranbury, NJ 08512
(609) 655-6000
For Medical Information, Contact:
Generally:
Professional Services
(800) 526-3840
After Hours and Weekend Emergencies:
(609) 655-6474

OTC Products Described:
- ◆ Maltsupex Powder, Liquid, Tablets **523, 772**
Ryna Liquid **773**
- ◆ Ryna-C Liquid **524, 773**
- ◆ Ryna-CX Liquid...................**524, 773**

WARNER-LAMBERT COMPANY   **524, 775**

Consumer Health Products Group
201 Tabor Road
Morris Plains, NJ 07950 (See also Warner-Lambert Consumer Healthcare)
Direct Inquiries to:
1-(800) 223-0182
For Consumer Product Information Call:
1-(800) 524-2854 (Celestial Seasonings Soothers only)
1-(800) 223-0182

(◆) **Shown in Product Identification Guide**   *Italic Page Number* **Indicates Brief Listing**

OTC Products Described:
- Celestial Seasonings Soothers
  Herbal Throat Drops **524, 775**
- Certs Cool Mint Drops with a
  Retsyn Center................**524, 775**
- Certs Powerful Mints with
  Retsyn Crystals **524, 775**
- Halls Juniors Sugar Free
  Cough Suppressant Drops...**524, 775**
- Halls Mentho-Lyptus Cough
  Suppressant Drops **524, 775**
- Halls Plus Cough
  Suppressant/Throat Drops ..**524, 776**
- Halls Sugar Free
  Mentho-Lyptus Cough
  Suppressant Drops **524, 776**
- Halls Sugar Free Squares **776**
- Halls Vitamin C Supplement
  Drops **524, 776**

WARNER-LAMBERT **524, 776**
CONSUMER
HEALTHCARE

201 Tabor Road
Morris Plains, NJ 07950
For Product Information Call:
1-(800) 223-0182
1-(800) 378-1783 (e.p.t.)
1-(800) 337-7266 (e.p.t. – Spanish)

OTC Products Described:
- Actifed Cold & Allergy Tablets ...**524, 776**
- Anusol HC-1 Hydrocortisone
  Anti-Itch Ointment..........**524, 778**
- Anusol Hemorrhoidal Ointment..**524, 777**
- Anusol Hemorrhoidal
  Suppositories **524, 777**
- Benadryl Allergy Chewables **524, 779**
- Benadryl Allergy Kapseal
  Capsules....................**524, 778**
- Benadryl Allergy Liquid
  Medication..................**524, 780**
- Benadryl Allergy Sinus
  Headache Caplets &
  Gelcaps....................**525, 780**
- Benadryl Allergy Ultratab
  Tablets **524, 778**
- Benadryl Allergy/Cold Tablets ...**525, 778**
- Benadryl Allergy/Congestion
  Liquid Medication...........**525, 779**
- Benadryl Allergy/Congestion
  Tablets **525, 779**
- Benadryl Dye-Free Allergy
  Liquid Medication...........**525, 781**
- Benadryl Dye-Free Allergy
  Liqui-gels Softgels **525, 781**
- Benadryl Itch Relief Stick
  Extra Strength **525, 782**
- Benadryl Itch Stopping Cream
  Original Strength............**525, 782**
- Benadryl Itch Stopping Cream
  Extra Strength **525, 782**
- Benadryl Itch Stopping Gel
  Original Strength............**525, 783**
- Benadryl Itch Stopping Gel
  Extra Strength **525, 783**
- Benadryl Itch Stopping Spray
  Original Strength............**525, 782**
- Benadryl Itch Stopping Spray
  Extra Strength **525, 782**
- Benylin Adult Formula Cough
  Suppressant.................**525, 783**
- Benylin Cough
  Suppressant/Expectorant ...**525, 783**
- Benylin Multisymptom **525, 784**
- Benylin Pediatric Cough
  Suppressant.................**525, 784**
- Caladryl Clear Lotion **525, 785**
- Caladryl Cream For Kids........**525, 785**
- Caladryl Lotion................**525, 785**
- e.p.t. Pregnancy Test **526, 785**

- Listerine Antiseptic
  Mouthrinse..................**526, 786**
- Cool Mint Listerine Antiseptic
  Mouthrinse..................**526, 786**
- FreshBurst Listerine Antiseptic
  Mouthrinse..................**526, 786**
- Listermint Alcohol-Free
  Mouthrinse..................**526, 786**
- Lubriderm Advanced Therapy
  Creamy Lotion **526, 786**
- Lubriderm Bath and Shower
  Oil.........................**526, 787**
- Lubriderm Daily UV Lotion **526, 787**
- Lubriderm Dry Skin Care
  Lotion......................**526, 787**
- Lubriderm Seriously Sensitive
  Lotion......................**526, 787**
- Neosporin "Neo to Go!" *526*
- Neosporin Ointment **526, 787**
- Neosporin + Pain Relief
  Maximum Strength Cream ...**526, 788**
- Neosporin + Pain Relief
  Maximum Strength
  Ointment...................**526, 788**
- Nix Creme Rinse **526, 788**
- Polysporin Ointment **526, 789**
- Polysporin Powder **526, 789**
- Rolaids Antacid Tablets..........**527, 789**
- Sinutab Non-Drying Liquid
  Caps **527, 790**
- Sinutab Sinus Allergy
  Medication, Maximum
  Strength Formula, Tablets
  & Caplets **527, 790**
- Sinutab Sinus Medication,
  Maximum Strength
  Without Drowsiness
  Formula, Tablets & Caplets ..**527, 790**
- Sudafed 12 Hour Caplets *527*
- Sudafed 12 Hour Tablets **791**
- Sudafed 24 Hour Tablets **527, 791**
- Children's Sudafed Nasal
  Decongestant Chewables...**527, 792**
- Children's Sudafed Cold &
  Cough Liquid **527, 792**
- Children's Sudafed Nasal
  Decongestant Liquid
  Medication..................**527, 793**
- Sudafed Cold & Allergy Tablets ..**528, 793**
- Sudafed Cold & Cough Liquid
  Caps **528, 794**
- Sudafed Cold & Sinus Liquid
  Caps **527, 794**
- Sudafed Nasal Decongestant
  Tablets, 30 mg..............**527, 792**
- Sudafed Non-Drying Sinus
  Liquid Caps **528, 794**
- Sudafed Severe Cold Formula
  Caplets **527, 795**
- Sudafed Severe Cold Formula
  Tablets **527, 795**
- Sudafed Sinus Caplets **528, 795**
- Sudafed Sinus Tablets..........**528, 795**
- Tucks Premoistened
  Hemorrhoidal/Vaginal
  Pads **528, 796**
- Tucks Take-Alongs **796**
- Zantac 75 Tablets **528, 796**

Dietary Supplements Described:
- Quanterra Mental Sharpness
  Tablets **527, 859**
- Quanterra Prostate Softgels.....**527, 859**

Other Products Available:
Borofax Skin Protectant Ointment

WELLNESS INTERNATIONAL **797**
NETWORK, LTD.

5800 Democracy Drive
Plano, TX 75024

Direct Inquiries to:
Product Development
(972) 245-1097
FAX: (972) 389-3060

OTC Products Described:
Bio-Complex 5000 Gentle
  Foaming Cleanser **797**
Bio-Complex 5000 Revitalizing
  Conditioner **797**
Bio-Complex 5000 Revitalizing
  Shampoo **797**
StePHan Bio-Nutritional Daytime
  Hydrating Creme **797**
StePHan Bio-Nutritional
  Eye-Firming Concentrate..........**797**
StePHan Bio-Nutritional Nightime
  Moisture Creme **797**
StePHan Bio-Nutritional
  Refreshing Moisture Gel..........**798**
StePHan Bio-Nutritional Ultra
  Hydrating Fluid **798**

Dietary Supplements Described:
BioLean **859**
BioLean Accelerator **860**
BioLean Free **860**
BioLean LipoTrim **861**
DHEA Plus **862**
Food for Thought....................**861**
Mass Appeal........................**862**
Phyto-Vite **866**
Pro-Xtreme **863**
Satiete.............................**863**
Sleep-Tite **867**
StePHan Clarity **861**
StePHan Elasticity....................**864**
StePHan Elixir.......................**865**
StePHan Essential....................**865**
StePHan Feminine **865**
StePHan Flexibility...................**865**
StePHan Lovpil **866**
StePHan Masculine...................**866**
StePHan Protector...................**867**
StePHan Relief **867**
StePHan Tranquility..................**868**
Sure2Endure........................**868**
Winrgy **868**

WHITEHALL LABORATORIES
INC.

(See WHITEHALL-ROBINS HEALTHCARE)

WHITEHALL-ROBINS **528, 798**
HEALTHCARE

American Home Products Corporation
Five Giralda Farms
Madison, NJ 07940-0871
Direct Inquiries to:
Whitehall Consumer Product Information:
(800) 322-3129 (9-5 E.S.T.)
Robins Consumer Product Information:
(800) 762-4672 (9-5 E.S.T.)

OTC Products Described:
Advil Caplets...........................**798**
Children's Advil Oral Suspension......**799**
Advil Cold and Sinus Caplets **799**
Advil Cold and Sinus Tablets **799**
Advil Gel Caplets......................**798**
Pediatric Advil Drops..................**799**
Advil Tablets..........................**798**
Junior Strength Advil Tablets **799**
Maximum Strength Anbesol Gel **800**
Maximum Strength Anbesol Liquid **800**
Baby Anbesol Gel **800**
Axid AR Tablets.......................**800**
Dimetapp Cold & Allergy
  Chewable Tablets.................**801**
Dimetapp Cold & Allergy Quick
  Dissolve Tablets..................**801**
Dimetapp Cold & Cough
  Liqui-Gels, Maximum Strength.....**802**

J.B. WILLIAMS   **528, 810**
COMPANY, INC.
65 Harristown Road
Glen Rock, NJ 07452
Direct Inquiries to:
Consumer Affairs
(800) 254-8656
(201) 251-8100
FAX: (201) 251-8097
For Medical Emergencies Contact:
(800) 254-8656

WYETH-AYERST   **529, 812**
PHARMACEUTICALS
Division of American Home Products
Corporation
P.O. Box 8299
Philadelphia, PA 19101
Direct General Inquiries to:
(610) 688-4400
For Professional Services:
(For example: Sales representative
information, product pamphlets,
educational materials):
(800) 395-9938
For Medical Information Contact:
Medical Affairs
Day: (800) 934-5556 (8:30 AM to 4:30
PM, Eastern Standard Time, Weekdays
Only)
Night: (610) 688-4400 (Emergencies
Only; non-emergencies should wait until
the next day)
WYETH-AYERST DISTRIBUTION CENTERS
(Do not use freight addresses
for mailing orders.)

Atlanta, GA – P.O. Box 1773
Paoli, PA 19301-1773
(800) 666-7248
Freight Address:
100 Union Court
Kennesaw, GA 30144
Mail DEA order forms to:
P.O. Box 4365
Atlanta, GA 30302-4365
Chicago, IL – P.O. Box 1773
Paoli, PA 19301-1773
(800) 666-7248
Freight Address:
284 Lies Road
Carol Stream, IL 60188
Mail DEA order forms to:
P.O. Box 140
Wheaton, IL 60189-0140
Dallas, TX – P.O. Box 1773
Paoli, PA 19301-1773
(800) 666-7248
Freight Address:
11240 Petal Street
Dallas, TX 75238
Mail DEA order forms to:
P.O. Box 650231
Dallas, TX 75265-0231
Sparks, NV – P.O. Box 1773
Paoli, PA 19301-1773
(800) 666-7248
Freight Address:
1802 Brierley Way
Sparks, NV 89434
Mail DEA order forms to:
1802 Brierley Way
Sparks, NV 89434
Philadelphia, PA – P.O. Box 1773
Paoli, PA 19301-1773
(800) 666-7248
Freight Address:
31 Morehall Road
Frazer, PA 19355
Mail DEA order forms to:
P.O. Box 61
Paoli, PA 19301

YOUNGEVITY   **871**
4951 Airport Parkway
Suite 500
Dallas, TX 75001
Direct Inquiries to:
(800) 469-6864

ZILA   **529, 814**
PHARMACEUTICALS,
INC.
5227 North 7th Street
Phoenix, AZ 85014-2800
Direct Inquiries to:
Jerry Kaster
Vice President of Marketing
(602) 266-6700
Internet: www.zila.com

SECTION 2

PRODUCT NAME INDEX

This index includes all entries in the Product Information sections. Products are listed alphabetically by brand name.

If an entry in the index lists multiple page numbers, the first one shown refers to the photograph of the product, the last one to its prescribing information.

- **Bold page numbers** indicate full product information.

- *Italic page numbers* signify partial information.

Italic Page Number **Indicates Brief Listing**

Italic Page Number **Indicates Brief Listing**

SECTION 3

PRODUCT CATEGORY INDEX

This index cross-references each brand by pharmaceutical category. All fully-described products in the Product Information sections are included.

If an entry in the index lists multiple page numbers, the first one shown refers to the photograph of the product, the last one to its prescribing information.

The classification of each product is determined by the publisher in cooperation with the product's manufacturer or, when necessary, by the publisher alone.

ANTI-INFECTIVE AGENTS
(*see under:*
ANTI-INFECTIVE AGENTS, SYSTEMIC
SKIN & MUCOUS MEMBRANE AGENTS
ANTI-INFECTIVES
VAGINAL PREPARATIONS
ANTI-INFECTIVES)

ANTI-INFECTIVE AGENTS, SYSTEMIC
ANTHELMINTICS

ANTI-INFECTIVES, NON-SYSTEMIC
SCABICIDES & PEDICULICIDES
(*see also under:* **SKIN & MUCOUS MEMBRANE
AGENTS: ANTI-INFECTIVES, SCABICIDES &
PEDICULICIDES)**

ANTI-INFLAMMATORY AGENTS
(*see under:*
ANALGESICS
NONSTEROIDAL ANTI-INFLAMMATORY AGENTS
(NSAIDS)
SALICYLATES

SKIN & MUCOUS MEMBRANE AGENTS
STEROIDS & COMBINATIONS)

ANTIMYCOTICS
(*see under:*
SKIN & MUCOUS MEMBRANE AGENTS
ANTI-INFECTIVES
ANTIFUNGALS & COMBINATIONS
VAGINAL PREPARATIONS
ANTI-INFECTIVES
ANTIFUNGALS & COMBINATIONS)

ANTIPRURITICS
(*see under:*
ANTIHISTAMINES & COMBINATIONS
SKIN & MUCOUS MEMBRANE AGENTS
ANTIPRURITICS)

ANTIPYRETICS
(*see under:*
ANALGESICS
ACETAMINOPHEN & COMBINATIONS
NONSTEROIDAL ANTI-INFLAMMATORY AGENTS
(NSAIDS)
SALICYLATES)

ANTISEPTICS
(*see under:*
SKIN & MUCOUS MEMBRANE AGENTS
ANTI-INFECTIVES
MISCELLANEOUS ANTI-INFECTIVES &
COMBINATIONS)

ANTITUSSIVES
(*see under:*
RESPIRATORY AGENTS
ANTITUSSIVES)

ARTHRITIS MEDICATIONS
(*see under:*
ANALGESICS
NONSTEROIDAL ANTI-INFLAMMATORY AGENTS
(NSAIDS)
SALICYLATES
SKIN & MUCOUS MEMBRANE AGENTS
ANALGESICS & COMBINATIONS)

ARTIFICIAL TEARS
(*see under:*
OPHTHALMIC PREPARATIONS
ARTIFICIAL TEARS/LUBRICANTS & COMBINATIONS)

ASTHMA PREPARATIONS
(*see under:*
RESPIRATORY AGENTS
BRONCHODILATORS)

ASTRINGENTS
(*see under:*
SKIN & MUCOUS MEMBRANE AGENTS
ASTRINGENTS)

B

BABY PRODUCTS

BLOOD MODIFIERS
ANTIPLATELET AGENTS

BRONCHIAL DILATORS
(*see under:*
RESPIRATORY AGENTS
BRONCHODILATORS)

BURN PREPARATIONS
(*see under:*
SKIN & MUCOUS MEMBRANE AGENTS
BURN PREPARATIONS)

C

CALCIUM SUPPLEMENTS
(*see under:*
DIETARY SUPPLEMENTS
MINERALS & ELECTROLYTES
CALCIUM & COMBINATIONS)

CANKER SORE PREPARATIONS
(*see under:*
SKIN & MUCOUS MEMBRANE AGENTS
MOUTH & THROAT PRODUCTS
CANKER SORE PREPARATIONS)

CARDIOVASCULAR AGENTS
(*see under:*
BLOOD MODIFIERS
ANTIPLATELET AGENTS)

CENTRAL NERVOUS SYSTEM AGENTS
(*see under:*
ANALGESICS
CENTRAL NERVOUS SYSTEM STIMULANTS
GASTROINTESTINAL AGENTS
ANTIEMETICS
SEDATIVES & HYPNOTICS)

CENTRAL NERVOUS SYSTEM STIMULANTS
MISCELLANEOUS CENTRAL NERVOUS SYSTEM
STIMULANTS

CERUMENOLYTICS
(*see under:*
OTIC PREPARATIONS
CERUMENOLYTICS)

COLD & COUGH PREPARATIONS
(*see under:*
ANTIHISTAMINES & COMBINATIONS
NASAL PREPARATIONS
SYMPATHOMIMETICS & COMBINATIONS
RESPIRATORY AGENTS
ANTITUSSIVES
DECONGESTANTS & COMBINATIONS
DECONGESTANTS, EXPECTORANTS & COMBINATIONS
EXPECTORANTS & COMBINATIONS
MISCELLANEOUS COLD & COUGH PRODUCTS WITH
ANALGESICS
MISCELLANEOUS RESPIRATORY AGENTS

SECTION 4

ACTIVE INGREDIENTS INDEX

This index cross-references each brand by its generic ingredients. All entries in the Product Information sections are included. Under each generic heading, all fully described products are listed first, followed by those with only partial descriptions.

If an entry in the index lists multiple page numbers, the first one shown refers to the photograph of the product, the last one to its prescribing information.

- **Bold page numbers** indicate full product information.

- *Italic page numbers* signify partial information.

Classification of products under these headings has been determined in cooperation with the products' manufacturers or, if necessary, by the publisher alone.

Italic Page Number **Indicates Brief Listing**

Italic Page Number **Indicates Brief Listing**

PETROLATUM—cont.
Keri Lotion - Silky Smooth
(Bristol-Myers Products) **507, 635**
Preparation H Hemorrhoidal Cream
(Whitehall-Robins)................... **804**
Preparation H Hemorrhoidal
Ointment (Whitehall-Robins)........ **804**

PHENIRAMINE MALEATE
OcuHist Eye Allergy Relief Eye
Drops (Pfizer Consumer)...... **517, 708**

PHENOL
Vicks Chloraseptic Sore Throat
Spray, Menthol and Cherry
Flavors (Procter & Gamble)......... **730**

PHENYLEPHRINE HYDROCHLORIDE
Afrin Nasal Decongestant Children's
Pump Mist (Schering-Plough
HealthCare) **739**
Afrin Allergy Nasal Spray
(Schering-Plough
HealthCare) **519, 739**
Cerose DM (Wyeth-Ayerst)....... **529, 813**
4-Way Fast Acting Nasal Spray
- Regular and Mentholated
Formulas (Bristol-Myers
Products) **506, 635**
Neo-Synephrine Nasal Drops,
Regular and Extra Strength
(Bayer Consumer)........... **505, 616**
Neo-Synephrine Nasal Sprays,
Mild, Regular and Extra
Strength (Bayer Consumer)... **505, 616**
Preparation H Hemorrhoidal Cream
(Whitehall-Robins)................... **804**
Preparation H Hemorrhoidal
Ointment (Whitehall-Robins)........ **804**
Preparation H Hemorrhoidal
Suppositories (Whitehall-Robins)... **804**
Vicks Sinex Nasal Spray and Ultra
Fine Mist (Procter & Gamble)....... **733**

PHENYLPROPANOLAMINE
Metabolic Nutrition System
(AdvoCare) **820**

PHENYLPROPANOLAMINE BITARTRATE
Alka-Seltzer Plus Cold & Cough
Medicine Effervescent
Tablets (Bayer Consumer) **503, 604**
Alka-Seltzer Plus Cold & Flu
Medicine Effervescent
Tablets (Bayer Consumer) **503, 604**
Alka-Seltzer Plus Cold & Sinus
Medicine Effervescent
Tablets (Bayer Consumer) **503, 604**
Alka-Seltzer Plus Cold
Medicine Effervescent
Tablets (Orange, Cherry &
Original) (Bayer Consumer) ... **503, 604**
Alka-Seltzer Plus Night-Time
Cold Medicine Effervescent
Tablets (Bayer Consumer) **503, 604**

**PHENYLPROPANOLAMINE
HYDROCHLORIDE**
BC Allergy Sinus Cold Powder
(Block)............................. **621**
BC Sinus Cold Powder (Block)......... **621**
Comtrex Deep Chest Cold &
Congestion Relief Liquigels
(Bristol-Myers Products) **506, 631**
Comtrex Maximum Strength
Multi-Symptom Cold & Cough
Relief Liqui-Gels (Bristol-Myers
Products)............................ **628**
Contac Continuous Action
Nasal Decongestant/
Antihistamine 12 Hour
Capsules and Caplets
(SmithKline Beecham
Consumer) **521, 748**

Contac Severe Cold & Flu
Caplets Maximum Strength
(SmithKline Beecham
Consumer) **521, 749**
Coricidin 'D' Decongestant
Tablets (Schering-Plough
HealthCare) **520, 741**
Dimetapp Cold & Allergy Chewable
Tablets (Whitehall-Robins)......... **801**
Dimetapp Cold & Allergy Quick
Dissolve Tablets
(Whitehall-Robins)................... **801**
Dimetapp Cold & Cough Liqui-Gels,
Maximum Strength
(Whitehall-Robins)................... **802**
Dimetapp Elixir (Whitehall-Robins)..... **803**
Dimetapp DM Elixir
(Whitehall-Robins)................... **802**
Dimetapp Extentabs
(Whitehall-Robins)................... **803**
Dimetapp Liqui-Gels
(Whitehall-Robins)................... **803**
Dimetapp Tablets (Whitehall-Robins)... **803**
Robitussin-CF (Whitehall-Robins)..... **808**
Tavist•D 12-Hour Relief Caplets
(Novartis)............................ **693**
Tavist•D 12-Hour Relief
Tablets (Novartis)............ **515, 694**
Triaminic DM Syrup (Novartis).... **515, 703**
Triaminic Expectorant
(Novartis)................... **515, 698**
Triaminic Syrup (Novartis) **516, 703**
Triaminic Triaminicol Cold &
Cough (Novartis)............. **516, 703**
Triaminicin Tablets (Novartis)..... **516, 704**

PHOSPHORIC ACID
Emetrol Oral Solution
(Lemon-Mint & Cherry
Flavors) (Pharmacia &
Upjohn)..................... **517, 714**

PHYTOESTROGENS
Promensil Tablets (Novogen) **516, 844**

PIPERONYL BUTOXIDE
Clear Total Lice Elimination System
(Shampoo, Egg Remover, "Nit
Capturing" Comb) (Care
Technologies) **639**
Pronto Lice Treatment (Del) **507, 644**
Maximum Strength Rid Lice
Killing Shampoo (Pfizer
Consumer) **517, 708**

POLOXAMER 407
Baby Orajel Tooth & Gum
Cleanser (Del)................ **507, 642**

POLYCARBOPHIL
Replens Vaginal Moisturizer
(Columbia)........................... **641**

POLYETHYLENE GLYCOL
Advanced Relief Visine Eye
Drops (Pfizer Consumer)...... **517, 710**
Visine Tears Eye Drops (Pfizer
Consumer)................... **517, 712**

POLYMYXIN B SULFATE
Betadine Brand First Aid
Antibiotics + Moisturizer
Ointment (Purdue
Frederick)................... **519, 735**
Betadine Brand Plus First Aid
Antibiotics + Pain Reliever
Ointment (Purdue
Frederick)................... **519, 735**
Neosporin Ointment
(Warner-Lambert) **526, 787**
Neosporin + Pain Relief
Maximum Strength Cream
(Warner-Lambert) **526, 788**

Neosporin + Pain Relief
Maximum Strength
Ointment (Warner-Lambert)... **526, 788**
Polysporin Ointment
(Warner-Lambert) **526, 789**
Polysporin Powder
(Warner-Lambert) **526, 789**

POTASSIUM BICARBONATE
Alka-Seltzer Gold Effervescent
Antacid (Bayer Consumer) **503, 604**

POTASSIUM BITARTRATE
Ceo-Two Evacuant Suppository
(Beutlich)............................ **618**

POTASSIUM CHLORIDE
Chlor-3 Condiment (Fleming) **646**

POTASSIUM NITRATE
Crest Sensitivity Protection
Toothpaste (Procter & Gamble)..... **724**
Orajel Sensitive Sensitive
Teeth Toothpaste for Adults
(Del).......................... **507, 644**
Promise Sensitive Toothpaste
(Block).............................. **625**
Sensodyne Original Flavor (Block)...... **625**
Sensodyne Cool Gel (Block) **625**
Sensodyne Extra Whitening (Block)..... **625**
Sensodyne Fresh Mint (Block)......... **625**
Sensodyne Tartar Control (Block) **625**
Sensodyne with Baking Soda (Block) .. **625**

POVIDONE IODINE
Betadine Ointment (Purdue
Frederick)................... **519, 735**
Betadine Skin Cleanser (Purdue
Frederick)........................... **735**
Betadine Solution (Purdue
Frederick)................... **519, 735**
Massengill Medicated
Disposable Douche
(SmithKline Beecham
Consumer) **522, 757**

PRAMOXINE HYDROCHLORIDE
Anusol Hemorrhoidal Ointment
(Warner-Lambert) **524, 777**
Betadine Brand Plus First Aid
Antibiotics + Pain Reliever
Ointment (Purdue
Frederick)................... **519, 735**
Caladryl Clear Lotion
(Warner-Lambert) **525, 785**
Caladryl Cream For Kids
(Warner-Lambert) **525, 785**
Caladryl Lotion
(Warner-Lambert) **525, 785**
Neosporin + Pain Relief
Maximum Strength Cream
(Warner-Lambert) **526, 788**
Neosporin + Pain Relief
Maximum Strength
Ointment (Warner-Lambert)... **526, 788**

PSEUDOEPHEDRINE HYDROCHLORIDE
Actifed Cold & Allergy Tablets
(Warner-Lambert) **524, 776**
Advil Cold and Sinus Caplets
(Whitehall-Robins)................... **799**
Advil Cold and Sinus Tablets
(Whitehall-Robins)................... **799**
Alka-Seltzer Plus Cold & Cough
Medicine Liqui-Gels (Bayer
Consumer)................... **503, 605**
Alka-Seltzer Plus Cold & Flu
Liqui-Gels Non-Drowsy
Formula (Bayer Consumer)... **503, 605**
Alka-Seltzer Plus Cold & Sinus
Medicine Liqui-Gels (Bayer
Consumer)................... **503, 605**

Italic Page Number **Indicates Brief Listing**

COMPANION DRUG INDEX

This index provides you with a quick-reference guide to over-the-counter products that may be used, in conjunction with prescription drug therapy, to reverse drug-induced side effects, relieve symptoms of the illness itself, or treat sequelae of the initial disease. All entries are derived from the FDA-approved prescribing information published by *PDR*.

The products listed are generally considered effective for temporary symptomatic relief. Please bear in mind, however, that they may not be appropriate for sustained therapy, and that certain common side effects may be harbingers of more serious reactions. Remember, too, that each case must be approached on an individual basis. When making a recommendation, be sure to adjust for the patient's age, concurrent

medical conditions, and complete drug regimen. Consider timing as well, since simultaneous ingestion may not be recommended in all instances.

Please note that only products fully described in *Physicians' Desk Reference* and its companion volumes are included in this index. The publisher therefore cannot guarantee that all entries are totally accurate or complete. Keep in mind, too, that although a given over-the-counter product is usually an appropriate companion for an entire class of prescription medications, certain drugs within the class may be exceptions. If you have any doubt about the suitability of a particular OTC product in a given situation, be sure to check the underlying *PDR* prescribing information and the relevant medical literature.

ACUTE MOUNTAIN SICKNESS, HEADACHE SECONDARY TO —*cont.*

ALCOHOLISM, HYPOCALCEMIA SECONDARY TO

Alcoholism may be treated with disulfiram or naltrexone hydrochloride. The following products may be recommended for relief of hypocalcemia:

ALCOHOLISM, HYPOMAGNESEMIA SECONDARY TO

Alcoholism may be treated with disulfiram or naltrexone hydrochloride. The following products may be recommended for relief of hypomagnesemia:

ALCOHOLISM, VITAMINS AND MINERALS DEFICIENCY SECONDARY TO

Alcoholism may be treated with disulfiram or naltrexone hydrochloride. The following products may be recommended for relief of vitamins and minerals deficiency:

ANCYLOSTOMIASIS, IRON-DEFICIENCY ANEMIA SECONDARY TO

Ancylostomiasis may be treated with mebendazole or thiabendazole. The following products may be recommended for relief of iron-deficiency anemia:

ANEMIA, IRON-DEFICIENCY

May result from the use of chronic salicylate therapy or nonsteroidal anti-inflammatory drugs. The following products may be recommended:

ANGINA, UNSTABLE

May be treated with beta blockers, calcium channel blockers or nitrates. The following products may be recommended for relief of symptoms:

ARTHRITIS

May be treated with corticosteroids or nonsteroidal anti-inflammatory drugs. The following products may be recommended for relief of symptoms:

BRONCHITIS, CHRONIC, ACUTE EXACERBATION OF

May be treated with quinolones, sulfamethoxazole-trimethoprim, cefixime, cefpodoxime proxetil, cefprozil, ceftibuten dihydrate, cefuroxime axetil, cilastatin, clarithromycin, imipenem or loracarbef. The following products may be recommended for relief of symptoms:

BURN INFECTIONS, SEVERE, NUTRIENTS DEFICIENCY SECONDARY TO

Severe burn infections may be treated with anti-infectives. The following products may be recommended for relief of nutrients deficiency:

CANCER, NUTRIENTS DEFICIENCY SECONDARY TO

Cancer may be treated with chemotherapeutic agents. The following products may be recommended for relief of nutrients deficiency:

CANDIDIASIS, VAGINAL

May be treated with antifungal agents. The following products may be recommended for relief of symptoms:

CONGESTIVE HEART FAILURE, NUTRIENTS DEFICIENCY SECONDARY TO

Congestive heart failure may be treated with ACE inhibitors, cardiac glycosides or diuretics. The following products may be recommended for relief of nutrients deficiency:

CONSTIPATION

May result from the use of ACE inhibitors, HMG-CoA reductase inhibitors, anticholinergics, anticonvulsants, antidepressants, beta blockers, bile acid sequestrants, butyrophenones, calcium and aluminum-containing antacids, calcium channel blockers, ganglionic blockers, hematinics, monoamine oxidase inhibitors, narcotic analgesics, nonsteroidal anti-inflammatory drugs or phenothiazines. The following products may be recommended:

CYSTIC FIBROSIS, NUTRIENTS DEFICIENCY SECONDARY TO

Cystic fibrosis may be treated with dornase alfa. The following products may be recommended for relief of nutrients deficiency:

DENTAL CARIES

May be treated with fluoride preparations or vitamin and fluoride supplements. The following products may be recommended for relief of symptoms:

DIABETES MELLITUS, CONSTIPATION SECONDARY TO

Diabetes mellitus may be treated with insulins or oral hypoglycemic agents. The following products may be recommended for relief of constipation:

DIABETES MELLITUS, POORLY CONTROLLED, CANDIDAL VULVOVAGINITIS SECONDARY TO

Diabetes mellitus may be treated with insulins or oral hypoglycemic agents. The following products may be recommended for relief of candidal vulvovaginitis:

DIABETES MELLITUS, POORLY CONTROLLED, GINGIVITIS SECONDARY TO

Diabetes mellitus may be treated with insulins or oral hypoglycemic agents. The following products may be recommended for relief of gingivitis:

DIABETES MELLITUS, POORLY CONTROLLED, VITAMINS AND MINERALS DEFICIENCY SECONDARY TO

Diabetes mellitus may be treated with insulins or oral hypoglycemic agents. The following products may be recommended for relief of vitamins and minerals deficiency:

DIABETES MELLITUS, PRURITUS SECONDARY TO

Diabetes mellitus may be treated with insulins or oral hypoglycemic agents. The following products may be recommended for relief of pruritus:

DIAPER DERMATITIS

May result from the use of cefpodoxime proxetil, cefprozil, cefuroxime axetil or varicella virus vaccine live. The following products may be recommended:

DIARRHEA

May result from the use of ACE inhibitors, beta blockers, cardiac glycosides, chemotherapeutic agents, diuretics, magnesium-containing antacids, nonsteroidal anti-inflammatory drugs, potassium supplements, acarbose, alprazolam, colchicine, divalproex sodium, ethosuximide, fluoxetine hydrochloride, guanethidine monosulfate, hydralazine hydrochloride, levodopa, lithium carbonate, lithium citrate, mesna, metformin hydrochloride, misoprostol, olsalazine sodium, pancrelipase, procainamide hydrochloride, reserpine, succimer, ticlopidine hydrochloride or valproic acid. The following products may be recommended:

DIARRHEA, INFECTIOUS

May be treated with sulfamethoxazole-trimethoprim, ciprofloxacin or furazolidone. The following products may be recommended for relief of symptoms:

DRY SKIN
(see under XERODERMA)

DYSPEPSIA

May result from the use of chronic systemic corticosteroid therapy, nonsteroidal anti-inflammatory drugs, ulcerogenic medications or mexiletine hydrochloride. The following products may be recommended:

EMESIS, UNPLEASANT TASTE
SECONDARY TO

Emesis may be treated with antiemetics. The following products may be recommended for relief of unpleasant taste:

ENTEROBIASIS, PERIANAL PRURITUS
SECONDARY TO

Enterobiasis may be treated with mebendazole. The following products may be recommended for relief of perianal pruritus:

FEVER

May result from the use of immunization. The following products may be recommended:

FLATULENCE

May result from the use of nonsteroidal anti-inflammatory drugs, potassium supplements, acarbose, cisapride, guanadrel sulfate, mesalamine, metformin hydrochloride, methyldopa, octreotide acetate or ursodiol. The following products may be recommended:

FLU-LIKE SYNDROME

May result from the use of gemcitabine hydrochloride, interferon alfa-2B, recombinant, interferon alfa-N3 (human leukocyte derived), interferon beta-1B, interferon gamma-1B or succimer. The following products may be recommended:

HYPOTHYROIDISM, XERODERMA SECONDARY TO

Hypothyroidism may be treated with thyroid hormones. The following products may be recommended for relief of xeroderma:

INFECTIONS, BACTERIAL, UPPER RESPIRATORY TRACT

May be treated with amoxicillin-clavulanate, cephalosporins, doxycycline, erythromycin, macrolide antibiotics, penicillins, amoxicillin trihydrate or minocycline hydrochloride. The following products may be recommended for relief of symptoms:

PEPTIC ULCER DISEASE, IRON DEFICIENCY SECONDARY TO

Peptic ulcer disease may be treated with histamine H_2 receptor antagonists, proton pump inhibitors or sucralfate. The following products may be recommended for relief of iron deficiency:

PHARYNGITIS

May result from the use of cephalosporins, macrolide antibiotics, or penicillins. The following products may be recommended:

PHOTOSENSITIVITY REACTIONS

May result from the use of thiazides, antidepressants, antihistamines, estrogens,
nonsteroidal anti-inflammatory drugs, phenothiazines, quinolones, sulfonamides,

sulfonylurea hypoglycemic agents, tetracyclines, topical retinoids, captopril, diltiazem hydrochloride, enalapril maleate, fluorouracil, griseofulvin, labetalol hydrochloride, lisinopril, methoxsalen, methyldopa, minoxidil, nalidixic acid or nifedipine. The following products may be recommended:

PRURITUS, PERIANAL

May result from the use of broad-spectrum antibiotics. The following products may be recommended:

PSORALEN WITH UV-A LIGHT (PUVA) THERAPY

May be treated with methoxsalen. The following products may be recommended for relief of symptoms:

RENAL OSTEODYSTROPHY, HYPOCALCEMIA SECONDARY TO

Renal osteodystrophy may be treated with vitamin D sterols. The following products may be recommended for relief of hypocalcemia:

RESPIRATORY TRACT ILLNESS, INFLUENZA A VIRUS-INDUCED

May be treated with amantadine hydrochloride or rimantadine hydrochloride. The following products may be recommended for relief of symptoms:

RHINITIS, NONALLERGIC

May be treated with nasal steroids or ipratropium bromide. The following products
may be recommended for relief of symptoms:

SINUSITIS, HALITOSIS SECONDARY TO

Sinusitis may be treated with amoxicillin, amoxicillin-clavulanate, cefprozil, cefuroxime axetil, clarithromycin or loracarbef. The following products may be recommended for relief of halitosis:

SKIN IRRITATION

May result from the use of transdermal drug delivery systems. The following products may be recommended:

TASTE DISTURBANCES
May result from the use of biguanides,
acetazolamide, butorphanol tartrate, captopril, cefuroxime axetil, clarithromycin,
etidronate disodium, felbamate, flu-
nisolide, gemfibrozil, griseofulvin, interferon alfa-2B, recombinant, lithium carbonate, lithium citrate, mesna, metronida-
zole, nedocromil sodium, penicillamine,
rifampin or succimer. The following products may be recommended:

TONSILITIS, HALITOSIS SECONDARY TO
Tonsilitis may be treated with erythromycin, macrolide antibiotics, cefaclor,
cefadroxil, cefixime, cefpodoxime proxetil,
cefprozil, ceftibuten dihydrate or cefuroxime axetil. The following products may be
recommended for relief of halitosis:

TRAVELER'S DIARRHEA
(see under DIARRHEA, INFECTIOUS)

TUBERCULOSIS, NUTRIENTS
DEFICIENCY SECONDARY TO
Tuberculosis may be treated with capre-
omycin sulfate, ethambutol hydrochloride,
ethionamide, isoniazid, pyrazinamide,
rifampin or streptomycin sulfate. The following products may be recommended for
relief of nutrients deficiency:

VAGINOSIS, BACTERIAL
May be treated with sulfabenzamide/sul-
facetamide/sulfathiozole or metronida-
zole. The following products may be recommended for relief of symptoms:

VULVOVAGINITIS, CANDIDAL

May result from the use of estrogen-containing oral contraceptives, immunosuppressants or recent broad-spectrum antibiotic therapy. The following products may be recommended:

XERODERMA

May result from the use of aldesleukin, protease inhibitors, retinoids, topical acne preparations, topical corticosteroids, topical retinoids, benzoyl peroxide, clofazimine, interferon alfa-2A, recombinant, interferon alfa-2B, recombinant or pentostatin. The following products may be recommended:

XEROMYCTERIA

May result from the use of anticholinergics, antihistamines, retinoids, apraclonidine hydrochloride, clonidine, etretinate, ipratropium bromide, isotretinoin or Iodoxamide tromethamine. The following products may be recommended:

XEROSTOMIA

May result from the use of anticholinergics, antidepressants, diuretics, phenothiazines, alprazolam, bromocriptine mesylate, buspirone hydrochloride, butorphanol tartrate, clomipramine hydrochloride, clonidine, clozapine, dexfenfluramine hydrochloride, didanosine, disopyramide phosphate, etretinate, flumazenil, fluvoxamine maleate, guanfacine hydrochloride, isotretinoin, leuprolide acetate, pergolide mesylate, selegiline hydrochloride, tramadol hydrochloride or zolpidem tartrate. The following products may be recommended:

SUGAR-FREE PRODUCTS

Listed below, by therapeutic category, is a selection of drug products that contain no sugar. When recommending these products to diabetic patients, keep in mind that many may contain sorbitol, alcohol, or other sources of carbohydrates.

This list is drawn from the 1999 edition of *Drug Topics® Red Book®*. It should not be considered all-inclusive. Generics and alternate brands of some products may be available. Check product labeling for a current listing of inactive ingredients.

ANALGESICS

Children's Panadol Chewable Tablets	SKB Consumer
Children's Panadol Drops	SKB Consumer
Children's Tylenol Suspension Liquid	McNeil
Febrol	Scot-Tussin
Feverall Sprinkle Caps	Ascent Pediatrics
Infant's Tylenol Drops	McNeil
Infant's Tylenol Suspension Drops	McNeil
Tempra 1 Drops	Mead Johnson
Tempra 2 Syrup	Mead Johnson

ANTACIDS/ANTIFLATULENTS

Alka-Mints	Bayer Cons
Amphojel Suspension	Wyeth-Ayerst
Amphojel Tablets	Wyeth-Ayerst
Di-Gel Liquid	Schering-Plough
Gaviscon Liquid	SKB Consumer
Marblen Suspension	Fleming
Nephrox Suspension	Fleming
Pepto-Bismol Liquid	Procter & Gamble
Pepto-Bismol Tablets	Procter & Gamble
Riopan Plus Suspension	Whitehall-Robins
Riopan Suspension	Whitehall-Robins
Tagamet HB Tablets	SKB Consumer
Titralac Plus Liquid	3M
Titralac Plus Tablets	3M
Titralac Tablets	3M
Tums E-X Chewable Tablets	SKB Consumer
Zantac 75 Tablets	Warner-Lambert

ANTIASTHMATIC/RESPIRATORY AGENTS

Alupent Syrup	Boehringer Ingelheim
Elixophyllin-GG Liquid	Forest
Organidin NR Liquid	Wallace
Proventil Syrup	Schering
Slo-Phyllin 80 Syrup	RPR
Ventolin Syrup	Glaxo Wellcome

ANTIDIARRHEALS

Diasorb Suspension	Columbia
Donnagel Chewable Tablets	Wyeth-Ayerst
Donnagel Liquid	Wyeth-Ayerst
Pepto-Bismol Liquid	Procter & Gamble
Pepto-Bismol Tablets	Procter & Gamble

BLOOD MODIFIERS/IRON PREPARATIONS

Geritol Complete Tablets	SKB Consumer
Iberet Liquid	Abbott Laboratories
Niferex Elixir	Schwarz
Nu-Iron Elixir	Merz
Vitron-C Tablets	Novartis Consumer

CALCIUM SUPPLEMENTS

Caltrate 600 Tablets	Lederle
Posture Tablets	Self Care

CORTICOSTEROIDS

Pediapred Oral Liquid	Medeva

COUGH/COLD/ALLERGY PREPARATIONS

Cerose-DM Liquid	Wyeth-Ayerst
Codiclear DH	Schwarz
Codimal-DM Syrup	Schwarz
Diabetic Tussin DM Liquid	Health Care Products
Diabetic Tussin DM Maximum Strength Liquid	Health Care Products
Diabetic Tussin EX Liquid	Health Care Products
Diabe-Tuss DM Syrup	Paddock
Dimetane-DX Cough Syrup	Robins Pharm
Dimetapp Allergy Children's	Whitehall-Robins

Enplus-HD Syrup	Alphagen
Entuss-D Liquid	Roberts/ Hauck
Guai-CO Liquid	Alphagen
Guaifenex Liquid	Ethex
Guiatuss AC Syrup	Moore, H.L.
Hayfebrol Liquid	Scot-Tussin
Histinex D Liquid	Ethex
Histinex DM Syrup	Ethex
Histinex HC Syrup	Ethex
Histinex PV Syrup	Ethex
Hydro-Tussin HD Liquid	Ethex
Hyphen-HD Syrup	Alphagen
Iotussin HC Liquid	Iomed Labs
Nasatuss Liquid	Jones Medical
Novahistine Elixir	SKB Consumer
Organidin NR Liquid	Wallace
Poly-DM Syrup	Alphagen
Robitussin CF Syrup	Whitehall-Robins
Robitussin-DAC Syrup	Robins Pharm
Romilar AC Liquid	Scot-Tussin
Romilar DM Liquid	Scot-Tussin
Rondec DM Liquid	Dura
Rondec Syrup	Dura
Ryna-CX Liquid	Wallace
Scot-Tussin Allergy Relief Formula	Scot-Tussin
Scot-Tussin DM	Scot-Tussin
Scot-Tussin DM Cough Chasers	Scot-Tussin
Scot-Tussin Expectorant	Scot-Tussin
Scot-Tussin Original	Scot-Tussin
Scot-Tussin Senior	Scot-Tussin
S-T Forte	Scot-Tussin
S-T Forte 2	Scot-Tussin
Supress DX Pediatric	Kramer Dist
Tussafed-HC	Everett
Tussi-Organidin DM NR	Wallace
Tussi-Organidin DM-S NR	Wallace
Tussi-Organidin NR	Wallace
Tussi-Organidin-S NR	Wallace
Tussirex	Scot-Tussin
Vanex Grape Liquid	Jones Pharma
Vicodin Tuss Expectorant	Knoll Labs
Zyrtec Syrup	Pfizer U.S.P.G.

FLUORIDE PREPARATIONS

Luride Drops	Colgate Oral
Luride Lozi-Tabs	Colgate Oral
Pediaflor Drops	Ross
Phos-Flur Rinse	Colgate Oral

LAXATIVES

Citrucel Sugar Free Powder	SKB Consumer
Doxidan Capsules	Pharmacia & Upjohn
Fiberall Powder	Novartis Consumer
Fibro-XL Capsules	Key Company
Haley's MO	Bayer Cons
Hydrocil Instant Powder	Solvay
Kondremul Emulsion	Novartis Consumer
Konsyl Effervescent Powder	Konsyl
Konsyl Powder	Konsyl
Maalox Daily Fiber Therapy	Novartis Consumer
Metamucil Smooth Texture	Procter & Gamble
Surfak Capsule	Pharmacia & Upjohn

MISCELLANEOUS

Bicitra	Alza
Neutra-Phos Powder	Alza
Neutra-Phos-K Powder	Alza
Nicorette Chewing Gum 2 mg	SKB Consumer
Nicorette Chewing Gum 4 mg	SKB Consumer
Polycitra	Alza
Polycitra-K	Alza
Reglan Syrup	Robins

MOUTH/THROAT PREPARATIONS

Baby Orajel	Del
Cepacol Maximum Strength Spray	J.B. Williams
Cepastat Lozenges	SKB Consumer
Cheracol Sore Throat Spray	Roberts Pharm
Diabetic Tussin Cough Drops	Health Care Products
Fisherman's Friend	Mentholatum
Halls Juniors Sugar Free Cough Suppressant Drops	Warner-Lambert
Halls Sugar Free Cough Suppressant Drops	Warner-Lambert

N'Ice Lozenges	SKB Consumer
Nice'n Clear Lozenges	SK Beecham Cons
Optimoist Spray	Colgate Oral
Robitussin Lozenges	Whitehall-Robins
Salivart Solution	Gebauer
Tanac Liquid	Del
Throto-Ceptic Spray	S.S.S.
Vademecum Mouthwash and Gargle	Dermatone

POTASSIUM SUPPLEMENTS

Kaochlor S-F	Savage
Kaon Elixir	Savage
Kaon-Cl 20% Liquid	Savage
Kay Ciel Elixir	Forest
Kay Ciel Powder	Forest
Klor-Con Powder	Upsher-Smith
Klor-Con/25 Powder	Upsher-Smith
Klor-Con/EF Tablets	Upsher-Smith
Klorvess Effervescent Granules	Novartis
Rum K	Fleming

VITAMINS/MINERALS

Bugs Bunny Complete	Bayer Consumer
Bugs Bunny W/Extra Vitamin C	Bayer Consumer
Bugs Bunny W/Iron	Bayer Consumer
One-A-Day Essential Tablets	Bayer Consumer
One-A-Day Maximum Formula Tablets	Bayer Consumer
One-A-Day Women's Formula Tablets	Bayer Consumer
Pediavit	Advanced Nutr
Strovite Plus Caplets	Everett
Strovite Tablets	Everett
Tri-Vi-Sol Drops	Mead Johnson
Vi-Daylin ADC Drops	Ross
Vi-Daylin Drops	Ross
Vi-Daylin Plus Iron ADC Drops	Ross
Vi-Daylin Plus Iron Drops	Ross
Vi-Daylin/F ADC Drops	Ross
Vi-Daylin/F Drops	Ross
Vi-Daylin/F Plus Iron Drops	Ross
Vitafol Caplets	Everett
Vitalize Liquid	Scot-Tussin

ALCOHOL-FREE PRODUCTS

The following is a selection of alcohol-free products grouped by therapeutic category. The list is drawn from the 1999 edition of *Drug Topics® Red Book®*. It is not comprehensive. Generic and alternate brands may exist. Always check product labeling for definitive information on specific ingredients.

ANALGESICS

Children's Advil Suspension	Whitehall-Robins
Children's Motrin Suspension	McNeil Consumer
Children's Panadol Chewable Tablets	SKB
Children's Panadol Drops	SKB
Children's Tylenol Elixir	McNeil Consumer
Children's Tylenol Suspension	McNeil Consumer
Demerol Syrup	Sanofi
Infant's Tylenol Drops	McNeil Consumer
Infant's Tylenol Suspension Drops	McNeil Consumer
Liquiprin	Menley & James
PediaCare Fever Suspension	Pharmacia/ Upjohn Consumer
Tempra 1 Drops	Mead Johnson
Tempra 2 Syrup	Mead Johnson

ANTIASTHMATIC AGENTS

Alupent Syrup	Boehringer Ingelheim
Dilor G Liquid	Savage
Elixophyllin-GG Liquid	Forest
Slo-Phyllin 80 Syrup	RPR
Slo-Phyllin GG Syrup	RPR

ANTICONVULSANTS

Mysoline Suspension	Wyeth-Ayerst
Zarontin Syrup	Parke-Davis

ANTIDIARRHEALS

Diarrest Tablets	Dover
Kaodene NN Suspension	Pfeiffer
Kaopectate Advanced Formula	Pharmacia & Upjohn
Kaopectate Children's Liquid	Pharmacia & Upjohn
Pepto-Bismol Suspension	Procter & Gamble

ANTIEMETICS

Emetrol Solution	Pharmacia & Upjohn

COUGH/COLD/ALLERGY PREPARATIONS

Anamine Syrup	Merz
Anaplex HD Syrup	ECR
Atuss HD Syrup	Atley
Atuss MS Syrup	Atley
Bromanate Elixir	Alpharma USPD
Bromtapp Elixir	Hi-Tech
Bromtapp DM Elixir	Hi-Tech
Chlor-Trimeton Allergy Syrup	Schering-Plough
Codiclear DH	Schwarz
Creomulsion Complete Syrup	Creomulsion/ Lantisep
Creomulsion Cough/ Cold/Allergy Syrup	Creomulsion/ Lantisep
Creomulsion Cough Syrup	Creomulsion/ Lantisep
Creomulsion For Children Syrup	Creomulsion/ Lantisep
Diabetic Tussin Allergy Relief Liquid	Health Care Products
Diabetic Tussin Children's Liquid	Health Care Products
Diabetic Tussin DM Liquid	Health Care Products
Diabetic Tussin DM Maximum Strength Liquid	Health Care Products
Diabetic Tussin EX Liquid	Health Care Products
Diabe-Tuss DM Syrup	Paddock
Dimetapp Allergy Children's Elixir	Whitehall-Robins
Dimetapp Cold & Fever Children's Suspension	Whitehall-Robins
Dimetapp Decongestant Pediatric Drops	Whitehall-Robins
Endagen-HD Syrup	Jones Medical
Entuss-D Liquid	Roberts Pharm
Father John's Medicine Plus Drops	Oakhurst
Guaifed Syrup	Muro
Guaifenex Liquid	Ethex

Hayfebrol Liquid	Scot-Tussin
Histex Liquid	Salix Pharm
Histinex DM Syrup	Ethex
Histinex HC Syrup	Ethex
Histinex PV Syrup	Ethex
Iodal HD Liquid	Iomed Labs
Iohist DM Syrup	Iomed Labs
Iotussin HD Liquid	Iomed Labs
Kophane Elixir	Pfeiffer
Naldecon DX Capsules	Apothecon
Nasatuss Liquid	Jones Medical
Nucofed Syrup	Monarch
Organidin NR Liquid	Wallace
Pediacare Cough-Cold Drops	Pharmacia/ Upjohn Consumer
Pediacare Decongestant Infants Drops	Pharmacia/ Upjohn Consumer
Pediacare Decongestant Plus Cough Drops	Pharmacia/ Upjohn Consumer
Pediacare Nightrest Liquid	Pharmacia/ Upjohn Consumer
Pertussin CS Children's Syrup	Blairex
Phanatuss Syrup	Pharmakon
Robitussin CF Syrup	Whitehall- Robins
Robitussin Cough & Congestion Liquid	Whitehall- Robins
Robitussin DM	Whitehall- Robins
Robitussin Pediatric Cough Syrup	Whitehall- Robins
Robitussin Pediatric Drops	Whitehall- Robins
Robitussin Pediatric Night Relief Liquid	Whitehall- Robins
Robitussin PE Syrup	Whitehall- Robins
Romilar AC Liquid	Scot-Tussin
Rondec DM Drops	Dura
Rondec DM Syrup	Dura
Rondec Drops	Dura
Rondec Syrup	Dura
Scot-Tussin Allergy Relief Formula Liquid	Scot-Tussin
Scot-Tussin DM Liquid	Scot-Tussin
Scot-Tussin Expectorant	Scot-Tussin
Scot-Tussin Original Liquid	Scot-Tussin
Scot-Tussin Original Syrup	Scot-Tussin
Scot-Tussin Senior Liquid	Scot-Tussin
S-T Forte 2 Liquid	Scot-Tussin
Triaminic AM	Novartis Consumer
Triaminic AM Decongestant	Novartis Consumer

Triaminic-DM	Novartis Consumer
Triaminic Expectorant	Novartis Consumer
Triaminic Infant Decongestant Drops	Novartis Consumer
Triaminic Night Time	Novartis Consumer
Triaminic Sore Throat	Novartis Consumer
Triaminic Triaminicol Cold & Cough Liquid	Novartis Consumer
Tussafed-HC Syrup	Everett
Tussi-Organidin DM NR Liquid	Wallace
Tussi-Organidin DM-S NR Liquid	Wallace
Tussi-Organidin NR Liquid	Wallace
Tussi-Organidin-S NR Liquid	Wallace
Tussirex Liquid	Scot-Tussin
Tussirex Syrup	Scot-Tussin
Tylenol Children's Allergy-D Liquid	McNeil Consumer
Tylenol Children's Sinus Liquid	McNeil Consumer
Tylenol Cold Infants Drops	McNeil Consumer
Tylenol Flu Children's Suspension	McNeil Consumer
Vanex Grape Liquid	Jones Medical
Vanex-HD Syrup	Jones Medical
Vicks 44E Pediatric Liquid	Procter & Gamble
Vicks 44M Pediatric Liquid	Procter & Gamble
Vicks Children's NyQuil	Procter & Gamble
Vicks DayQuil Capsules	Procter & Gamble
Vicks DayQuil Liquid	Procter & Gamble
Vicks DayQuil Multi-Symptom Capsules	Procter & Gamble
Vicks DayQuil Multi-Symptom Liquid	Procter & Gamble
Vicodin Tuss Expectorant	Knoll Labs

MOUTH/THROAT PRODUCTS

Baby Gumz Gel	Lee Pharm
Baby Orajel	Del
Baby Orajel Nighttime	Del
Cheracol Sore Throat Spray	Roberts Pharm
Chloraseptic Spray/ Gargle	Procter & Gamble
Fluorinse	Oral-B
Glandosane	Kenwood
Gly-Oxide Liquid	SKB

Listermint	Warner Wellcome
Optimoist Spray	Colgate Oral
Orajel Baby Liquid	Del
Orasept Mouthwash/ Gargle	Pharmakon
Tanac Liquid	Del
Throto-Ceptic Spray	S.S.S.
Zilactin Baby Extra Strength Gel	Zila

HEMATINICS

Feostat Drops	Forest
Feostat Suspension	Forest

LAXATIVES

Agoral Emulsion	Warner Wellcome
Colace Liquid	Roberts
Kondremul Plain Liquid	Bayer
Liqui-Doss	Novartis Consumer
Milkinol Emulsion	Schwarz
Neoloid Emulsion	Kenwood
Phillips' Milk of Magnesia Liquid	Bayer
Senokot Children's Syrup	Purdue Frederick

MISCELLANEOUS

Mylicon Infants' Drops	J&J/Merck
Rum-K Liquid	Fleming

PSYCHOTROPICS

Haldol Concentrate	McNeil
Thorazine Syrup	SKB

TOPICAL PRODUCTS

Fleet Pain Relief Pads	Fleet,C.B.
Neutrogena Acne Wash	Neutrogena
Neutrogena Antiseptic Liquid	Neutrogena
Neutrogena Clear Pore	Neutrogena
Neutrogena T/Derm	Neutrogena
Neutrogena Toner	Neutrogena
Propa pH Foaming Face Wash	Del
Sea Breeze Foaming Face Wash	Bristol-Myers Prod
Stri-Dex Antibacterial Face Wash	Blistex
Dermatone Outdoor Skin Protection	Dermatone

VITAMINS

Poly-Vi-Sol Drops	Mead Johnson
Poly-Vi-Sol Drops w/Iron	Mead Johnson
Theragran Liquid	Bristol-Myers
Tri-Vi-Sol Drops	Mead Johnson
Tri-Vi-Sol Drops w/Iron	Mead Johnson
Vitafol	Everett
Vitalize SF Liquid	Scot-Tussin

LACTOSE- AND GALACTOSE-FREE PRODUCTS

The following is a selection of lactose- and galactose-free over-the-counter products. The list is drawn from the 1999 edition of *Drug Topics® Red Book®*. It is not comprehensive. Generic and alternate brands may exist. Always check product labeling for definitive information on specific ingredients.

TRADE NAME (OTC)	FORM	TRADE NAME (OTC)	FORM	TRADE NAME (RX)	FORM
Advil	Tablets	Nuprin	Tablets	Accutane	Capsules
Alka-Mints	Tablets	One-A-Day	Tablets	Actigall	Capsules
Alka-Seltzer	Effervescent Tablets	One-A-Day Antioxidant Plus	Tablets	Adalat	Capsules
Alka-Seltzer Plus	Effervescent Tablets			Aldactazide	Tablets
Alka-Seltzer Plus Liqui-Gels	Capsules	One-A-Day Garlic Softgels	Tablets	Aldactone	Tablets
Ascriptin	Tablets	One-A-Day Maximum	Tablets	Aldomet	Tablets
Aspirin Free Excedrin	Tablets	One-A-Day Men's	Tablets	Antivert	Tablets
Axid AR	Tablets	One-A-Day Women's	Tablets	Aquasol A	Capsules
Benadryl	Liquid, Tablets	Orudis KT	Tablets	Artane	Tablets
Bufferin	Tablets	Pepto-Bismol	Liquid, Tablets	Asendin	Tablets
Colace	Capsules, Syrup	Pepto-Bismol Max. Strength	Liquid, Tablets	Atrohist Pediatric	Capsules
Comtrex Multi-Symptom	Capsules, Tablets	Peri-Colace	Capsules, Syrup	Axid	Capsules
		Sinutab	Tablets	Bactrim	Tablets
Doxidan Liqui-Gels	Capsules	Sinutab Allergy	Tablets	Baycol	Tablets
Dramamine	Tablets	Sucrets Maximum Strength	Lozenges	Berocca	Tablets
Ensure	Liquid			Berocca Plus	Tablets
Excedrin Extra-Strength	Tablets	Sudafed	Tablets	Biaxin	Tablets
		Sudafed Severe Cold	Tablets	Calan SR	Tablets
Ex-lax Maximum	Tablets	Sudafed Sinus	Tablets	Carafate	Tablets
Gas-X	Liquid, Tablets	Sunkist Chewable Plus	Tablets	Cardene	Capsules
Gaviscon	Liquid, Tablets	Sunkist Complete	Tablets	Cardizem CD	Capsules
Iberet	Liquid, Tablets	Sunkist Vitamin C	Tablets	Cardizem SR	Capsules
Imodium A-D	Liquid, Tablets	Surfak	Capsules	Ceclor	Capsules
Konsyl	Powder, Tablets	Tempra	Drops, Liquid, Tablets	Ceclor CD	Tablets
Lactaid	Liquid, Tablets			Ceftin	Suspension, Tablets
Metamucil	Powder, Wafers	Titralac	Tablets	Cefzil	Suspension, Tablets
Motrin IB	Tablets	Titralac Plus	Tablets	Cipro	Tablets
Mylanta Gas Relief	Tablets	Tums	Tablets	Claritin-D	Tablets
Mylanta Gelcaps	Tablets	Tylenol	Drops, Liquid, Tablets	Clinoril	Tablets
Mylicon Infant's	Liquid			Combivir	Tablets
NoDoz Maximum	Tablets	Zantac 75	Tablets		

TRADE NAME (RX)	FORM	TRADE NAME (RX)	FORM	TRADE NAME (RX)	FORM
Covera-HS	Capsules	K-Phos Original Formula	Tablets	Rezulin	Tablets
Creon	Capsules	K-Tab	Tablets	Rifadin	Capsules
Cytotec	Tablets	Lanoxicaps	Capsules	Robaxin	Tablets
Dapsone	Tablets	Lescol	Capsules	Sectral	Capsules
Darvon-N/Darvocet-N	Tablets	Levaquin	Tablets	Serzone	Tablets
Daypro	Tablets	Levothroid	Tablets	Sinemet	Tablets
Deconsal	Tablets	Librium	Capsules	Sinemet CR	Tablets
Depakene	Capsules	LoCholest	Powder	Slo-bid	Capsules
Depakote	Tablets	LoCholest Light	Powder	Suprax	Tablets
Desoxyn	Tablets	Lomotil	Tablets	Symmetrel	Capsules
DiaBeta	Tablets	Luvox	Tablets	Tegretol/Tegretol-XR	Tablets
Diabinese	Tablets	Marax	Tablets	Tenoretic	Tablets
Diovan	Capsules	Materna	Tablets	Tenormin	Tablets
Dolobid	Tablets	Micro-K	Capsules	Tessalon	Capsules
Donnatal Extentabs	Tablets	Micronase	Tablets	Tiazac	Capsules
Donnazyme	Tablets	Minipress	Capsules	Ticlid	Tablets
Duricef	Capsules, Suspension, Tablets	Minocin	Capsules	Tofranil-PM	Capsules
E.E.S.	Suspension, Tablets	Motrin	Tablets	Toprol-XL	Tablets
Entex LA	Tablets	Mycostatin	Pastilles	Trental	Tablets
Epivir	Tablets, Solution	Natalins Rx	Tablets	Trilisate	Liquid, Tablets
EryPed	Suspension, Tablets	Niferex	Tablets	Ultrase	Capsules
Ery-Tab	Tablets	Niferex-Forte	Capsules	Uniphyl	Tablets
Esgic-Plus	Capsules, Tablets	Niferex-PN	Tablets	Valium	Tablets
Fastin	Capsules	Nolvadex	Tablets	Vibramycin Hyclate	Capsules
Fero-Folic/Iberet Folic	Tablets	Norpramin	Tablets	Vicodin	Tablets
Fero-Grad-Filmtab	Tablets	Norvasc	Tablets	Vicodin ES	Tablets
Fioricet	Tablets	Pamelor	Capsules	Vicodin HP	Tablets
Flumadine	Syrup, Tablets	Pancrease	Capsules	Vicoprofen	Tablets
Glucotrol XL	Tablets	Pancrease MT	Capsules	Vistaril	Capsules
GoLYTELY	Powder	Paxil	Capsules, Tablets	Volmax	Tablets
Grifulvin V	Suspension, Tablets	Pepcid	Suspension, Tablets	Wellbutrin	Tablets
Guaifed	Capsules	Percocet	Tablets	Wellbutrin SR	Tablets
Haldol	Tablets	Percodan	Tablets	Yocon	Tablets
Humibid	Tablets	PhosLo	Tablets	Yohimex	Tablets
Hytrin	Tablets	Placidyl	Capsules	Zantac	Capsules, Syrup, Tablets
Inderal LA	Capsules	Precose	Tablets	Zarontin	Capsules
Isoptin SR	Tablets	Prevacid	Capsules	Zebeta	Tablets
K-Dur	Tablets	Procardia	Capsules	Zestril	Tablets
K-Lor	Tablets	Procardia XL	Tablets	Ziac	Tablets
Konsyl	Powder	Prozac	Capsules	Zoloft	Tablets
K-Phos Neutral	Tablets	Quadrinal	Tablets	Zyban	Tablets
		Questran	Powder	Zyflo	Tablets
		Quinaglute	Tablets	Zymase	Capsules

PRODUCT IDENTIFICATION GUIDE

To aid in quick identification, this section provides full-color, actual-size photographs of tablets and capsules. A variety of other dosage forms and packages are shown at less than actual size. In all, the section contains a total of nearly 1,000 photos.

Products in this section are arranged alphabetically by manufacturer. In some instances, not all dosage forms and sizes are pictured. Letters or numbers representing the manufacturer's identification code are preceded by an asterisk.

For more information on any of the products in this section, please turn to the page indicated above the product's photo or check directly with the product's manufacturer.

While every effort has been made to guarantee faithful reproduction of the photos in this section, changes in size, color, and design are always a possibility. Be sure to confirm a product's identity with the manufacturer or your pharmacist.

MANUFACTURER'S INDEX

AKPHARMA INC.

AkPharma Inc.
P. 822

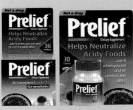

Dietary Supplement
Granulate and Tablets

Prelief®

ASTRA PHARMACEUTICALS

Astra Pharmaceuticals, L.P.
P. 602

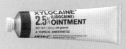

2.5% Ointment
Available in 35 gram tube

Xylocaine®
(lidocaine)

BAYER CORPORATION

Bayer Corporation
Consumer Care Division
P. 602

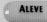

Tablets and Caplets available in
24, 50, 100 and 150 count.
Caplets also available in 200 count.
Gelcaps available in 20, 40 and 80 count.

Aleve®

Bayer Corporation
Consumer Care Division
P. 603

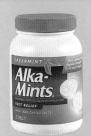

Spearmint and Assorted
Chewable Antacid and
Calcium Supplement

Alka-Mints®

Bayer Corporation
Consumer Care Division
P. 603

Original, Extra Strength,
Lemon Lime and Cherry
Effervescent Antacid and
Pain Reliever

Alka-Seltzer®

Bayer Corporation
Consumer Care Division
P. 604

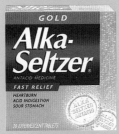

Effervescent Antacid
Aspirin Free

Alka-Seltzer® Gold

Bayer Corporation
Consumer Care Division
P. 603

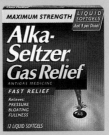

Maximum Strength Liquid Softgels

Alka-Seltzer® Gas Relief

Bayer Corporation
Consumer Care Division
P. 606

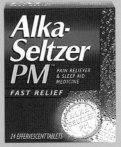

24 Effervescent Tablets

Alka-Seltzer PM®

Bayer Corporation
Consumer Care Division
P. 604

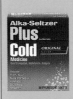

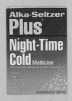

Cold, Cold & Cough,
Cold & Flu, Cold & Sinus,
and Night-Time
Effervescent Tablets

**Alka-Seltzer Plus®
Cold Medicine**

Bayer Corporation
Consumer Care Division
P. 604

Orange and Cherry Flavors

**Alka-Seltzer Plus®
Cold Medicine**

Bayer Corporation
Consumer Care Division
P. 605

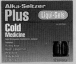

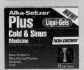

Cold, Cold & Cough, Cold & Flu,
Cold & Sinus and Night-Time.

**Alka-Seltzer Plus®
Cold Medicine Liqui-Gels®**

Bayer Corporation
Consumer Care Division
P. 611

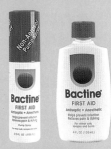

Antiseptic/Anesthetic
First Aid Spray and Liquid

Bactine®

Bayer Corporation
Consumer Care Division
P. 607

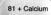
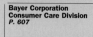
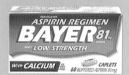

Aspirin Regimen BAYER®
81 mg with Calcium

Bayer Corporation
Consumer Care Division
P. 608

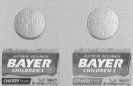

Low Strength, Chewable Aspirin
Orange and Cherry Flavors

Aspirin Regimen
BAYER® Children's

Bayer Corporation
Consumer Care Division
P. 610

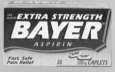
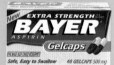
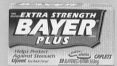
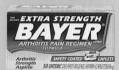
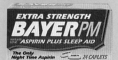

Extra Strength Caplets and Gelcaps,
Plus, Arthritis Pain Regimen and PM

Extra Strength
BAYER® Aspirin

Bayer Corporation
Consumer Care Division
P. 606

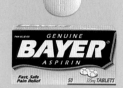
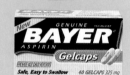
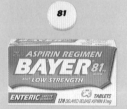
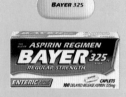

Genuine Bayer Tablets and Gelcaps,
Aspirin Regimen 81 mg,
Aspirin Regimen 325 mg

BAYER® Aspirin

Bayer Corporation
Consumer Care Division
P. 823

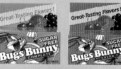

Sugar Free Children's
Chewable Vitamins
Complete, with Extra C and Plus Iron

Bugs Bunny™ Vitamins

Bayer Corporation
Consumer Care Division
P. 612

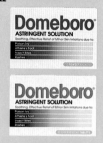

Astringent Solution
Effervescent Tablets and
Powder Packets

Domeboro®

Bayer Corporation
Consumer Care Division
P. 612

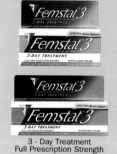

3 - Day Treatment
Full Prescription Strength

Femstat® 3

Bayer Corporation
Consumer Care Division
P. 823

Complete, Plus Extra C,
Plus Iron, Original
and Plus Calcium

Flintstones® Children's
Chewable Vitamins

Bayer Corporation
Consumer Care Division
P. 823

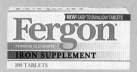

Ferrous Gluconate
Iron Supplement

Fergon®

Bayer Corporation
Consumer Care Division
P. 613

Maximum Strength
Caplets and Gelcaps

Midol® Menstrual

Bayer Corporation
Consumer Care Division
P. 613

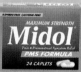

Maximum Strength
Gelcaps and Caplets

Midol® PMS

Bayer Corporation
Consumer Care Division
P. 613

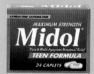

Maximum Strength Caplets

Midol® Teen

Bayer Corporation
Consumer Care Division
P. 614

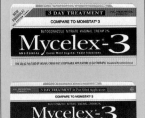

3-Day Treatment

Mycelex®-3

Bayer Corporation
Consumer Care Division
P. 615

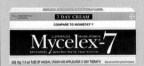

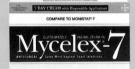

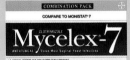

Vaginal Cream 1%
Vaginal Cream with 7
disposable applicators
Vaginal Inserts and
external vulvar cream

Mycelex®-7

Bayer Corporation
Consumer Care Division
P. 616

Nasal Decongestant
Spray and Drops
Available in Mild, Regular, Extra
Strength and Max 12-Hour Formula

Neo-Synephrine®

Bayer Corporation
Consumer Care Division
P. 825

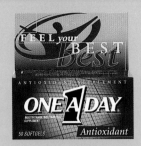

**One-A-Day®
Antioxidant Plus**

Bayer Corporation
Consumer Care Division
P. 824

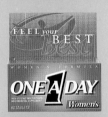

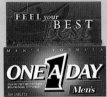

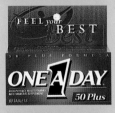

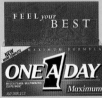

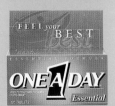

Women's, Men's, 50 Plus, Maximum
and Essential.

One-A-Day® Vitamins

Bayer Corporation
Consumer Care Division
P. 825

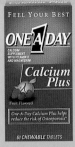

500 mg Calcium Carbonate
Plus Vitamin D and Magnesium

One-A-Day® Calcium Plus

Bayer Corporation
Consumer Care Division
P. 825

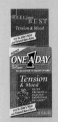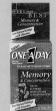

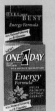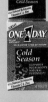

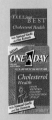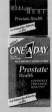

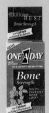

Specialized Nutritional Supplements
Tension & Mood,
Memory & Concentration,
Energy Formula, Cold Season,
Cholesterol Health, Prostate Health,
Bone Strength, Menopause Health.

One-A-Day®

Bayer Corporation
Consumer Care Division
P. 827

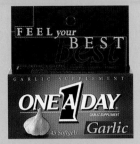

**One-A-Day®
Garlic Softgels**

Bayer Corporation
Consumer Care Division
P. 616

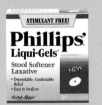

Available in 10 and 30 count Liqui-gels

Phillips'® Liqui-Gels®

Bayer Corporation
Consumer Care Division
P. 617

Available in Mint, Original,
and Cherry Flavors
4 oz, 12 oz and 26 oz Bottles

**Phillips'®
Milk of Magnesia**

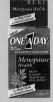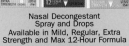

Bayer Corporation
Consumer Care Division
P. 617

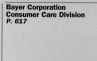

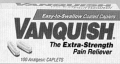

Extra-Strength Pain Formula

Vanquish®

BLOCK DRUG

Block Drug
P. 621

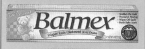

Available in 2 oz. and 4 oz. tubes
and 16 oz. jar

**Balmex®
Diaper Rash Ointment**

Block Drug
P. 623

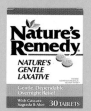

Available in packages of
15, 30 and 60 tablets.
A stimulant laxative with
natural active ingredients.

**Nature's Remedy®
Nature's Gentle Laxative**

Block Drug
P. 624

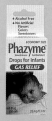

Available 1/2 oz. bottles
A liquid anti-gas that contains no
alcohol, and no artificial colors, flavors
or sweeteners.

**Phazyme® Drops
for Infants**

Block Drug
P. 624

125 mg softgels available in
packages of 12, 36, 60 and 100.
166 mg softgels available in
packages of 12, 36 and 60.
Chewable tablets available in
packages of 12 and 60.

Phazyme® Gas Relief

BRISTOL-MYERS PRODUCTS

Bristol-Myers Products
P. 635

Regular available in:
1/2 oz. and 1 oz. Atomizers
Fast Acting: 1/2 oz.
and 1 oz. Atomizers
Mentholated: 1/2 oz. Atomizer
Also available: 12 Hour
and Saline Moisturizing Mist

4-Way® Nasal Spray

Bristol-Myers Products
P. 627

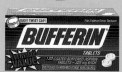

Bottles of 39, 65, 130
and 275 tablets
Also available in Arthritis Strength,
Extra Strength and
Low Dose Formulations

Bufferin®

Bristol-Myers Products
P. 628

Tablets, Caplets and
Liqui-gels available.
Also available: Allergy-Sinus
Treatment, Day/Night and
Non-Drowsy Formulations

**Comtrex® Multi-Symptom
Cold & Cough Relief**

Bristol-Myers Products
P. 631

Available in blister packages
of 24 liqui-gels

**Comtrex® Deep Chest
Cold & Congestion Relief**

Bristol-Myers Products
P. 630

Available in blister package
of 24 tablets

**Comtrex® Acute
Head Cold & Sinus
Pressure Relief**

Bristol-Myers Products
P. 634

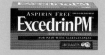

Tablets in bottles of 10
Tablets and Caplets in bottles of
24, 50 and 100
Geltabs in bottles of 24, 50 and 100

Excedrin PM®

Bristol-Myers Products
P. 631

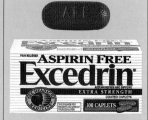

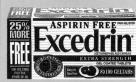

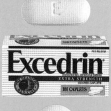

Bottles of 24, 50
and 100 caplets and geltabs

Aspirin Free Excedrin®

Bristol-Myers Products
P. 632

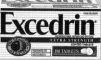

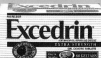

Bottles of 12, 24, 50, 100, 175
and 275, metal tins of 12 tablets
Bottles of 24, 50, 100, 175, 275
caplets and 24, 40 and 80 geltabs

Extra Strength Excedrin®

Bristol-Myers Products
P. 633

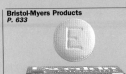
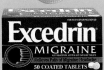
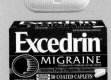

Bottles of 24, 50, 100,
175 and 275 tablets.
Bottles of 24, 50, 100
and 175 caplets.
Bottles of 24 geltabs

Excedrin® Migraine

Bristol-Myers Products
P. 636

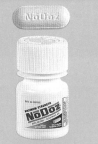

Maximum Strength
Bottles of 16, 36 and 60

No Doz®

Bristol-Myers Products
P. 636

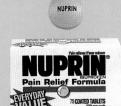

Bottles of 36, 75
and 150 tablets and caplets

Nuprin®

Bristol-Myers Products
P. 637

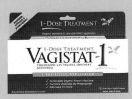

Anti-fungal Vaginal Ointment

Vagistat®-1

COOKE PHARMA

Cooke Pharma
P. 831

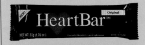
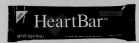

Available in Original and Cranberry

Contains L-arginine and other
important ingredients to promote
better vascular health.

HeartBar™

DEL

Del Pharmaceuticals
P. 642

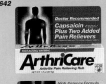

Pain Relieving Rubs

ArthriCare®

Del Pharmaceuticals
P. 643

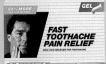
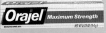
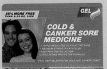

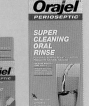

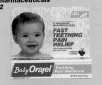

Sore Gums, Toothache Pain, and
Cold & Canker Sore Relief

Orajel®

Del Pharmaceuticals
P. 642

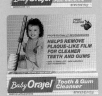

Teething Pain Medicine
Tooth & Gum Cleanser

Baby Orajel®

Bristol-Myers Products
P. 635

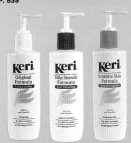

All Keri Lotions available in 2 oz.,
6 1/2 oz., 11 oz. and 15 oz.
Keri Original also available
in 20 oz. and 32 oz.

Keri® Lotion

Bristol-Myers Products
P. 830

High Potency Multivitamins
with Minerals
Available in 30 and 100 caplets

Theragran-M®

Bristol-Myers Products
P. 636

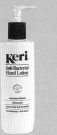

Antiseptic/Moisturizer
Clinically proven Anti-Bacterial

**Keri® Anti-Bacterial
Hand Lotion**

Bristol-Myers Products

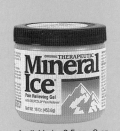

Available in: 3.5 oz., 8 oz.
and 16 oz. Pain Relieving Gel
Also available: Exercise Formula

Therapeutic Mineral Ice®

Del Pharmaceuticals
P. 644

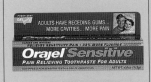

Sensitive Teeth
Toothpaste for Adults

Orajel® Sensitive™

Del Pharmaceuticals
P. 644

Maximum Strength
Lice Killing Shampoo
Household Spray

Pronto®

Del Pharmaceuticals
P. 644

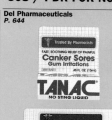

No Sting Liquid & Medicated Gel

Tanac®

EFFCON

Effcon Laboratories
P. 645

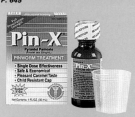

Oral Suspension 50 mg/mL
For the treatment of pinworm infections.

Pin-X®
(pyrantel pamoate)

J&J-MERCK CONSUMER

J&J-Merck Consumer
P. 647

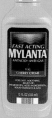

Bottles of 5, 12, 24 oz.

Fast-Acting Mylanta®

J&J-Merck Consumer
P. 647

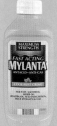

5, 12 & 24 oz. liquid

Maximum Strength Fast-Acting Mylanta®

J&J-Merck Consumer
P. 649

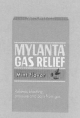

80 mg
12 & 30 tablet convenience packs, bottles of 60 and 100

Mylanta® Gas

J&J-Merck Consumer
P. 649

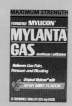

125 mg
12 & 24 tablet convenience packs

Maximum Strength Mylanta® Gas

J&J-Merck Consumer
P. 649

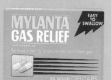

Boxes of 24 and 60 gelcaps

Mylanta® Gas Relief Gelcaps

J&J-Merck Consumer
P. 649

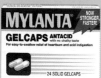

Mylanta® Gelcaps Antacid

J&J-Merck Consumer

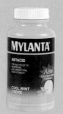

Available in Cool Mint Creme and Cherry Creme in bottles of 50 and 100 and rollpacks of 12

Mylanta® Tablets

J&J-Merck Consumer

Tablets in bottles of 35, 70 and rollpacks of 8

Mylanta® Double Strength Tablets

J&J-Merck Consumer
P. 647

4 oz. Liquid   Boxes of 24 tablets

Children's Mylanta® Upset Stomach Relief Liquid and Tablets

J&J-Merck Consumer
P. 646

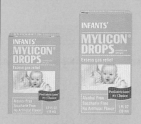

Available in 0.5 oz and 1.0 oz bottles

Infants Mylicon® Drops

J&J-Merck Consumer
P. 650

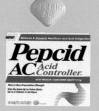

Available in 6's, 12's, 18's, 30's, 50's, 70's and 80's

Pepcid AC®

LANE LABS

Lane Labs
P. 652

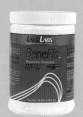

Organically Processed
100% Pure Shark Cartilage

BeneFin®

LEINER

Leiner Health Products
P. 835

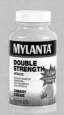

Sustained Release
300 mg Concentrate

Healthy Legs™

Leiner Health Products
P. 836

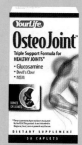

Triple Support Formula
for Healthy Joints

Osteo Joint™

LICHTWER PHARMA

Lichtwer Pharma
P. 838

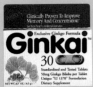

50 mg Ginkgo Biloba
Clinically Proven to Improve
Memory and Concentration

Ginkai®

Lichtwer Pharma
P. 838

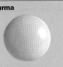

Standardized St. John's Wort Extract
To Maintain a Healthy Emotional
Balance and Well-Being

Kira®

Lichtwer Pharma
P. 839

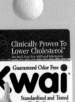

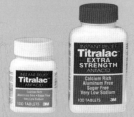

Concentrated Garlic Tablets
Clinically Proven to Lower Cholesterol

Kwai®

3M

3M
P. 653

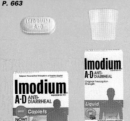

Available in: Regular Strength 40,
100, 1000 Tablets and Extra Strength
100 Tablets only

3M™ Titralac™ Antacid

3M
P. 653

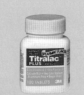

Antacid with Simethicone
Available in 100 Tablets

**3M™ Titralac™
Plus Antacid**

MATOL

Matol Botanical
P. 654

Homeopathic Nasal and Throat Spray
1 fl. oz. Spray Bottle

Biomune OSF™ Express

Matol Botanical
P. 839

Dietary Supplement
for Immune System Support
30 Capsules

Biomune OSF™ Plus

MCNEIL

McNeil Consumer Healthcare
P. 663

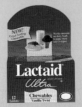

Available in 2 and 4 fl. oz. bottles
with a convenient dosage cup, and
caplets in 6's, 12's, 18's and 24's

Imodium® A-D

McNeil Consumer Healthcare
P. 663

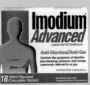

Vanilla mint chewable tablets
available in 6's, 12's, 18's and 30's

Imodium® Advanced

**Lactaid Inc. Marked By
McNeil Consumer Healthcare**
P. 839

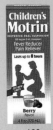

Original strength available
in bottles of 60
Extra strength available
in bottles of 24 and 50
Ultra caplets available in single serve
packets of 12 and 32 counts
Ultra chewable tablets available in
bottles of 12 and 32 counts

**Lactaid® Caplets and
Chewable Tablets**

**Lactaid Inc. Marked By
McNeil Consumer Healthcare**
P. 840

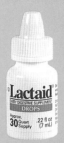

Available in 30 qt. supply

Lactaid® Drops

McNeil Consumer Healthcare
P. 654

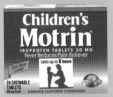

Available in Orange-Flavored
Chewable Tablets of 50 mg.
Available in blister pack of 24

**Children's Motrin®
Chewable Tablets**

McNeil Consumer Healthcare
P. 654

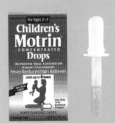

50 mg/1.25 mL
Available in 1/2 fl. oz. bottle

Children's Motrin® Drops

McNeil Consumer Healthcare
P. 654

100 mg/5 mL

**Children's Motrin®
Ibuprofen Oral
Suspension**

McNeil Consumer Healthcare
P. 664

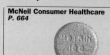

Available in Orange-Flavored
Chewable Tablets of 100 mg.
Available in blister pack of 24

Junior Strength Motrin® Chewable Tablets

McNeil Consumer Healthcare
P. 664

Available in blister packs of 24

Junior Strength Motrin® Ibuprofen Caplets

McNeil Consumer Healthcare
P. 666

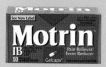

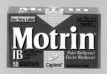

Tablets available in tamper evident
packaging of 24, 50, 100, 130, 135
and 165. Caplets available in tamper
evident packaging of 24, 50, 60, 100,
135, 165, 250 and 500. Gelcaps
available in tamper evident packaging
of 24 and 50.

Motrin® IB

McNeil Consumer Healthcare
P. 666

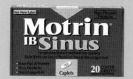

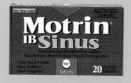

Tablets and Caplets available in blister
packs of 20's and 30's

Motrin® IB Sinus

McNeil Consumer Healthcare
P. 667

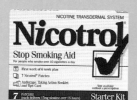

Available as Starter Kit - 7 patches,
Refill Kit - 7 and 14 patches

Nicotrol® Patch

For more detailed information on the products illustrated in this section, consult the Product Information Section or manufacturers may be contacted directly.

McNeil Consumer Healthcare
P. 668

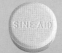

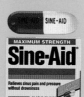

Tablets and Caplets in
blister packs of 24

Gelcaps in blister packs of 20

Maximum Strength Sine-Aid®

McNeil Consumer Healthcare
P. 655

Fruit Flavor: bottles of 30 with
child-resistant safety cap and
blister-packs of 60 and 96
Bubble Gum and Grape Flavor Bottles
of 30 with child-resistant safety cap

Children's TYLENOL® 80 mg Chewable Tablets

McNeil Consumer Healthcare
P. 655

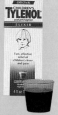

Available in cherry flavor
in 2 and 4 fl. oz. bottles with
child-resistant safety cap and
convenient dosage cup. Alcohol
Free, 80 mg. per 1/2 teaspoon

Children's TYLENOL® Elixir

McNeil Consumer Healthcare
P. 655

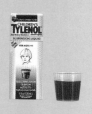

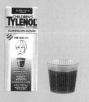

Available in Rich Cherry flavor in 2 and
4 fl. oz. bottles. Grape and Bubble
Gum Flavors in 4 fl. oz. with
child-resistant safety cap and
convenient dosage cup. Alcohol Free,
80 mg per 1/2 teaspoon

Children's TYLENOL® Suspension Liquid

McNeil Consumer Healthcare
P. 655

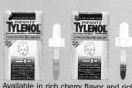

Available in rich cherry flavor and rich
grape flavor 1/2 oz. bottle with child
resistant safety cap and calibrated
dropper. Rich Grape Flavor, Alcohol
Free, 80 mg per 0.8 mL. Cherry flavor
also available in 1 oz. bottle.

Infants' TYLENOL® Concentrated Drops

McNeil Consumer Healthcare
P. 659

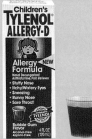

Available in Bubble Gum Flavor
in child resistant 4 fl. oz. bottles.

**Children's TYLENOL®
ALLERGY-D Liquid**

McNeil Consumer Healthcare
P. 659

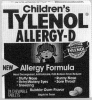

Bubble gum flavored
chewable tablets available in
blister packs of 24.

**Children's TYLENOL®
ALLERGY-D Chewable Tablets**

McNeil Consumer Healthcare
P. 659

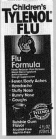

Available in Bubble Gum Flavor
in child resistant 4 fl. oz. bottles.

**Children's TYLENOL®
FLU Liquid**

McNeil Consumer Healthcare
P. 660

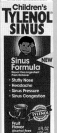
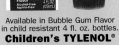

Available in Fruit Flavor in
child resistant 4 fl. oz. bottles.

**Children's TYLENOL®
SINUS Liquid**

McNeil Consumer Healthcare
P. 660

Fruit flavored chewable tablets
available in blister packs of 24.

**Children's TYLENOL®
SINUS Chewable Tablets**

McNeil Consumer Healthcare
P. 661

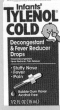

Available in 1/2 fl. oz. bottle with
child-resistant safety cap and
calibrated dropper. Bubble Gum Flavor,
Alcohol-free.

**Infant's TYLENOL® Cold
Decongestant and Fever
Reducer Concentrated Drops**

McNeil Consumer Healthcare
P. 662

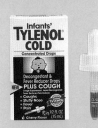

**Infants' TYLENOL® Cold
Decongestant and Fever
Reducer Concentrated
Drops Plus Cough**

McNeil Consumer Healthcare
P. 656

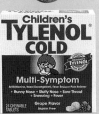

Available in blister pack of
24 chewable tablets. Grape flavor.

**Children's TYLENOL® Cold
Chewable Tablets**

McNeil Consumer Healthcare
P. 656

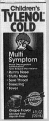

Multi-Symptom Formula
Available in 4 fl. oz. bottle with
child-resistant safety cap and
convenient dosage cup. Grape flavor.

**Children's TYLENOL®
Cold Liquid**

McNeil Consumer Healthcare
P. 657

Available in blister pack of
24 chewable tablets. Cherry flavor.

**Children's TYLENOL®
Cold Plus Cough
Chewable Tablets**

McNeil Consumer Healthcare
P. 657

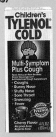
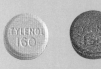

Multi-Symptom Plus Cough Formula
Available in 4 fl. oz. bottle with
child-resistant safety cap and
convenient dosage cup. Cherry flavor.

**Children's TYLENOL®
Cold Plus Cough Liquid**

McNeil Consumer Healthcare
P. 665

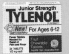

Available in Fruit Flavored and Grape
Flavored Chewable tablets of 160 mg
available in blister pack of 24

**Junior Strength
TYLENOL® Chewable Tablets**

McNeil Consumer Healthcare
P. 665

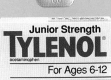

Swallowable Caplets: 160 mg
blister packs of 30

**Junior Strength
TYLENOL®**

McNeil Consumer Healthcare
P. 677

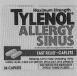

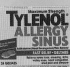

Caplets in blister packs of 24 & 48
Gelcaps in blister packs of 24 & 48
Geltabs in blister packs of 24 & 48

**Maximum Strength
TYLENOL® Allergy Sinus**

McNeil Consumer Healthcare
P. 677

Caplets available in
blister packs of 24's

**Maximum Strength
TYLENOL® Allergy Sinus
NightTime**

McNeil Consumer Healthcare
P. 677

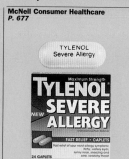

Caplets available in
blister packs of 12's and 24's

Maximum Strength
TYLENOL® Severe Allergy

McNeil Consumer Healthcare
P. 670

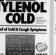
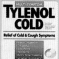

Caplets and Tablets available in
blister packs of 24

TYLENOL® Cold
Medication

McNeil Consumer Healthcare
P. 670

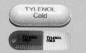
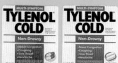

Gelcaps available in
blister packs of 24
Caplets available in
blister packs of 24
No Drowsiness Formula

TYLENOL® Cold
Medication

McNeil Consumer Healthcare
P. 672

Available in blister
packs of 12 and 24

TYLENOL® Cold Severe
Congestion

McNeil Consumer Healthcare
P. 669

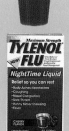
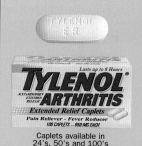

Caplets available in
24's, 50's and 100's

TYLENOL® Arthritis
Extended Relief

McNeil Consumer Healthcare
P. 673

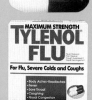
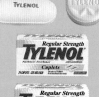

Gelcaps available in blister packs of
10's and 20's
No Drowsiness Formula

Maximum Strength
TYLENOL® Flu

McNeil Consumer Healthcare
P. 673

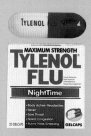

Gelcaps Available in
blister packs of 10's and 20's

Maximum Strength
TYLENOL® Flu NightTime

McNeil Consumer Healthcare
P. 673

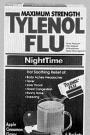
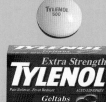

Available in cartons of 6 individual
packets. Hot Liquid Medication

Maximum Strength
TYLENOL® Flu NightTime

McNeil Consumer Healthcare
P. 673

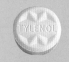

Available in 8 oz. bottles

Maximum Strength
TYLENOL® Flu
NightTime Liquid

McNeil Consumer Healthcare
P. 669

Tablets available in 24's, 50's, 100's
and 200's. Caplets available in 24's,
50's and 100's

Regular Strength
TYLENOL®

McNeil Consumer Healthcare
P. 669

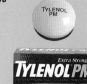
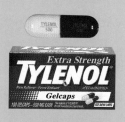

Geltabs available in tamper-resistant
bottles of 24's, 50's, 100's and 150's

Gelcaps available in tamper-resistant
bottles of 24's, 50's, 100's, 150's
and 225's and vials of 10.

Extra Strength TYLENOL®

McNeil Consumer Healthcare
P. 669

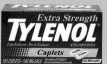
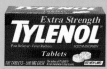

Caplets: tamper-resistant vials
of 10 and bottles of 24's, 50's,
100's, 150's and 250's

Tablets: tamper-resistant vials
of 10 and bottles of 30's,
60's, 100's and 200's

Liquid: tamper-evident
bottles of 8 fl. oz.

Extra Strength TYLENOL®

McNeil Consumer Healthcare
P. 676

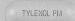

Geltabs available in tamper-resistant
bottles of 24's and 100's

Caplets available in tamper-resistant
bottles of 24's, 100's and 150's

Gelcaps available in tamper-resistant
bottles of 24

Geltabs, Caplets and Gelcaps
available in bottles of 50 for
households without children

TYLENOL® PM

McNeil Consumer Healthcare
P. 678

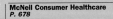
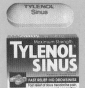
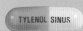

Caplets, Gelcaps, Geltabs and
Tablets in blister packs of 24 and 48

**Maximum Strength
TYLENOL® Sinus**

McNeil Consumer Healthcare
P. 678

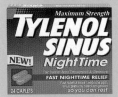

Available in blister packs of 24.

**Maximum Strength
TYLENOL® Sinus
NightTime Caplets**

NATROL

Natrol
P. 841

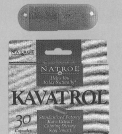

Standardized Potency Kava Extract

Kavatrol™

NOVARTIS CONSUMER HEALTH

Novartis Consumer Health, Inc.
P. 681

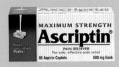
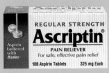
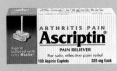

Regular Strength 100's, 160's,
225's, 500's
Maximum Strength 50's, 85's
Arthritis Pain 60's, 100's, 225's, 500's

Ascriptin®

Novartis Consumer Health, Inc.
P. 681

Adult Low Strength 120's
Regular Strength 100's

Ascriptin® enteric

Novartis Consumer Health, Inc.
P. 685

Cream 1/2 oz., 2/3 oz.
Spray Powder 3 oz., 4 oz.

Cruex®

Novartis Consumer Health, Inc.
P. 685

Spray Powder, Shake Powder,
Spray Liquid and Cream
Foot and Sneaker Spray Powder
Jock Itch Spray Powder

Desenex®

Novartis Consumer Health, Inc.
P. 686

Tablets & Suppositories

Dulcolax® Laxative

Novartis Consumer Health, Inc.
P. 688

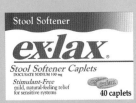

Stimulant-Free Stool
Softener Caplets

Ex•lax®

Novartis Consumer Health, Inc.
P. 687

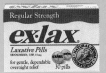

Regular Strength 8's, 30's, 60's
Maximum Relief Formula 24's, 48's
Chocolated Laxative 6's, 18's and 48's

Ex•lax®

Novartis Consumer Health, Inc.
P. 688

Extra Strength Cherry 18's, 48's
Extra Strength Peppermint 18's, 48's
(125 mg simethicone)

Gas-X®

Novartis Consumer Health, Inc.
P. 688

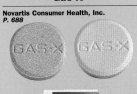

Cherry 12's, 36's
Peppermint 12's, 36's
(80 mg simethicone)

Gas-X®

Novartis Consumer Health, Inc.
P. 688

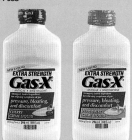

Extra Strength Cherry
and Peppermint Liquid
(50 mg per 5 mL simethicone)

Gas-X®

Novartis Consumer Health, Inc.
P. 688

Extra Strength Softgels
in packs of 10's, 30's, 50's
(125 mg simethicone)

Gas-X®

Novartis Consumer Health, Inc.
P. 690

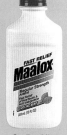

Cooling Mint
Also available in Smooth Cherry and
Refreshing Lemon
Bottles of 5 (Mint Only), 12 & 26 oz.

Maalox® Antacid

Novartis Consumer Health, Inc.
P. 690

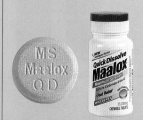

Maximum Strength Wild Berry as well
as Assorted Lemon and Wintergreen in
bottles of 35 and 65.

**Maximum Strength
Maalox® Calcium
Carbonate Antacid**

Novartis Consumer Health, Inc.
P. 689

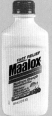

Smooth Cherry
Also available in Cooling Mint
and Refreshing Lemon
Bottles of 5 (Lemon only),
12 & 26 oz.

**Maximum Strength
Maalox® Antacid/Anti-Gas**

Novartis Consumer Health, Inc.
P. 690

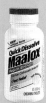

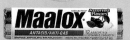

Regular Strength Lemon, as well as
Assorted, Wild Berry and Wintergreen
Flavors in bottles of 45 and 85 Tablets.
(Wild Berry not available in 85 count.
Wintergreen not available in 45 count).
Regular Strength Rollpacks available in
Lemon and Assorted Flavors.

**Maalox® Calcium
Carbonate Antacid**

Novartis Consumer Health, Inc.
P. 689

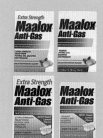

Peppermint and Sweet Lemon Flavor
Regular Strength 12's
Extra Strength 10's

Maalox® Anti-Gas

Novartis Consumer Health, Inc.
P. 691

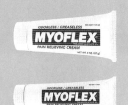

Pain Relieving Cream
Available in 2 oz. and 4 oz. tubes,
8 oz. and 16 oz. jars

Myoflex®

Novartis Consumer Health, Inc.
P. 691

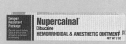

Hemorrhoidal & Anesthetic
Available in: Ointment 2 oz. & 1 oz.
Suppositories: box of 12

Nupercainal®

Novartis Consumer Health, Inc.
P. 692

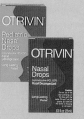

Nasal Decongestant Drops
Pediatric Drops and Nasal Spray

Otrivin®

Novartis Consumer Health, Inc.
P. 692

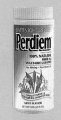

100% Natural Vegetable Laxative
250 gm and 400 gm

**Perdiem®
Overnight Relief**

Novartis Consumer Health, Inc.
P. 693

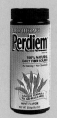

100% Natural
Daily Fiber Source
available in 250 gm

Perdiem® Fiber Therapy

Novartis Consumer Health, Inc.
P. 842

Slow Release Iron available
in 30, 60 and 90 ct.
Slow Release Iron & Folic Acid
available in 20 ct.

Slow Fe®

Novartis Consumer Health, Inc.
P. 843

Children's Multivitamins
Extra C and Complete
Vitamin C Citrus Complex
250 and 500 mg Chewable Tablets
60 mg Chewable Tablets
(11 Tablet Roll)

Sunkist®

Novartis Consumer Health, Inc.
P. 693

8's, 16's, 32's

Tavist® Allergy

Novartis Consumer Health, Inc.
P. 694

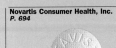

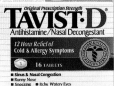

8's, 16's, 32's, 48's

Tavist•D®

Novartis Consumer Health, Inc.
P. 694

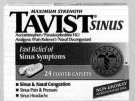

24 count

Tavist® Sinus

Novartis Consumer Health, Inc.
P. 694

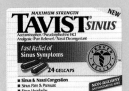

24 count

Tavist® Sinus

Novartis Consumer Health, Inc.
P. 697

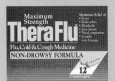

12's, 24's
Non-drowsy Flu, Cold
and Cough Caplets

TheraFlu® Maximum Strength

Novartis Consumer Health, Inc.
P. 696

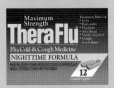

12's, 24's
Flu, Cold & Cough Medicine
Nighttime Formula

TheraFlu® Maximum Strength

Novartis Consumer Health, Inc.
P. 695

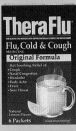

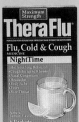

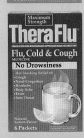

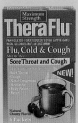

Flu, Cold & Cough Medicine
In packs of 6 and 12 count
Maximum Strength NightTime Flu,
Cold & Cough Medicine
In packs of 6 and 12 count
Maximum Strength, No Drowsiness,
and Natural Cherry Flavor
Flu, Cold & Cough Medicine
In packs of 6.

TheraFlu®

Novartis Consumer Health, Inc.
P. 695

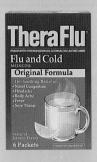

Novartis Consumer Health, Inc.

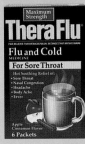

Flu and Cold Medicine
In packs of 6.
Maximum Strength Flu and
Cold Medicine for Sore Throat
In packs of 6.

TheraFlu®

Novartis Consumer Health, Inc.
P. 698

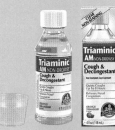

4 oz.

Triaminic® AM Cough & Decongestant

Novartis Consumer Health, Inc.
P. 698

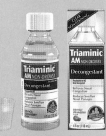

4 oz.

Triaminic® AM Decongestant

Novartis Consumer Health, Inc.
P. 703

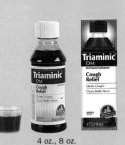

4 oz., 8 oz.

Triaminic® DM

Novartis Consumer Health, Inc.
P. 698

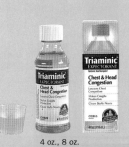

4 oz., 8 oz.

Triaminic® Expectorant

Novartis Consumer Health, Inc.
P. 699

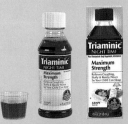

4 oz., 8 oz.

Triaminic® NightTime

Novartis Consumer Health, Inc.
P. 700

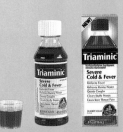

4 oz., 8 oz.

Triaminic® Severe Cold and Fever

Novartis Consumer Health, Inc.
P. 702

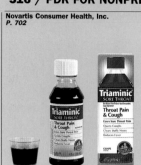

4 oz., 8 oz.

Triaminic® Sore Throat

Novartis Consumer Health, Inc.
P. 703

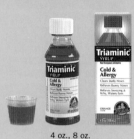

4 oz., 8 oz.

Triaminic® Syrup

Novartis Consumer Health, Inc.
P. 703

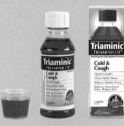

4 oz., 8 oz.

**Triaminic®
Triaminicol®**

Novartis Consumer Health, Inc.
P. 700

18 tablets
Orange Flavor

**Triaminic® Softchews®
Cold and Allergy**

Novartis Consumer Health, Inc.
P. 701

18 tablets
Cherry Flavor

**Triaminic® Softchews®
Cold and Cough**

Novartis Consumer Health, Inc.
P. 701

18 tablets
Grape Flavor

**Triaminic® Softchews®
Throat Pain and Cough**

Novartis Consumer Health, Inc.
P. 704

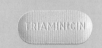
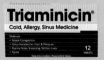

12's, 24's, 48's

Triaminicin®

Novogen
P. 844

30 Tablets
Natural plant estrogens for women
experiencing normal midlife changes.

Promensil™

Pfizer Consumer Health Care
P. 705

Arthritis Formula, Greaseless,
Original Formula, Ultra Strength
and Vanishing Scent.

BENGAY®

Pfizer Consumer Health Care
P. 705

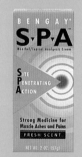

Site Penetrating Action
Fresh Scent

BENGAY® S.P.A.™

Pfizer Consumer Health Care
P. 705

Kids available in 1/2 oz.
and 1 oz. Creme
Cortizone•5 available in 1 oz.
and 2 oz. Creme and 1 oz. Ointment

Cortizone•5®

Pfizer Consumer Health Care
P. 706

Cortizone•10 available in 1/2 oz.,
1 oz., and 2 oz. Creme and 1 oz.
and 2 oz. Ointment.
Cortizone•10 Plus available in
1 oz. and 2 oz. Creme.
Cortizone•10 Quick Shot Spray
available in 1.5 oz.

Cortizone•10®

Pfizer Consumer Health Care
P. 707

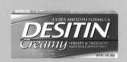
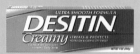

Diaper Rash Ointment

DESITIN® Creamy

Pfizer Consumer Health Care
P. 707

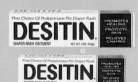

Diaper Rash Ointment

DESITIN®

Pfizer Consumer Health Care
P. 707

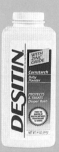

**DESITIN® Cornstarch
Baby Powder**

Pfizer Consumer Health Care
P. 708

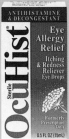

Itching and Redness
Reliever Eye Drops

OcuHist®

Pfizer Consumer Health Care
P. 708

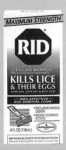

Maximum Strength Lice Killing Shampoo
Pediculicide (Lice Treatment)

RID®

Pfizer Consumer Health Care
P. 710

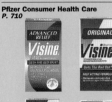

Advanced Relief, Original,
L.R. Long Lasting and
A.C. Seasonal Relief.

Visine®

Pfizer Consumer Health Care
P. 712

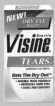

Dry Eye Relief

Visine® Tears™

Pharmacia & Upjohn
P. 713

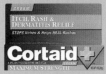

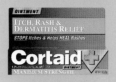

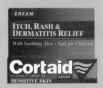

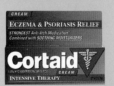

Maximum Strength (1% hydrocortisone)
is available in cream, ointment,
and FastStick™
Sensitive Skin (1/2 % hydrocortisone)
is available in cream.
Intensive Therapy (1% hydrocortisone)
is available in cream

Cortaid®

Pharmacia & Upjohn
P. 713

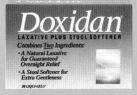

Stimulant/Stool Softener Laxative
Packages of 10, 30, 100, and
100 unit dose

Doxidan® Liqui-Gels®
(casanthranol 30 mg and docusate
sodium 100 mg)

Pharmacia & Upjohn
P. 714

Tablets, Chewables and
Children's Liquid

Dramamine®
(dimenhydrinate)

Pharmacia & Upjohn
P. 714

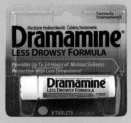

Tablets

**Dramamine® Less Drowsy
Formula**
(meclizine hydrochloride)

Pharmacia & Upjohn
P. 714

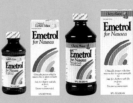

Lemon-Mint and Cherry Flavors.
Available in 4oz and 8oz sizes

Emetrol®

Pharmacia & Upjohn
P. 715

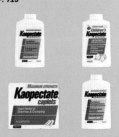

Regular, Peppermint, Children's Cherry
Flavored Liquid and Maximum
Strength Caplets

**Kaopectate®
Anti-Diarrheal**

Pharmacia & Upjohn
P. 715

Available in 3 oz. Odor Control Spray
Powder, 3.5 oz. Spray Liquid,
3 oz. Cooling Action Spray Liquid and
1/2 oz. Cream. Also available (not
shown): 3 oz. Powder, 3 oz. Spray
Powder and 1 oz. Cream

Micatin®

Pharmacia & Upjohn
P. 715

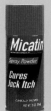

Cures Jock Itch
Available in 3 oz. Spray Powder
and 1/2 oz. Cream

Micatin®

Pharmacia & Upjohn
P. 716

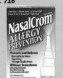

NasalCrom Nasal Spray and Children's
NasalCrom available in 100 and 200
metered sprays

**NasalCrom®
Nasal Allergy Symptom
Controller**

Pharmacia & Upjohn
P. 719

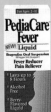

Available in 4 fl. oz. bottle with
child-resistant safety cap and
convenient doasge cup.

PediaCare® Fever Liquid

Pharmacia & Upjohn
P. 717

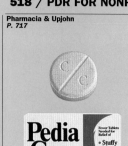

Available in 1/2 fl. oz. bottle with
child-resistant safety cap and
calibrated dropper

**PediaCare® Infants'
Decongestant Drops**

Pharmacia & Upjohn
P. 719

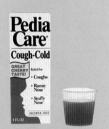

Blister Packs of 16 Chewable Tablets
Liquid available in 4 fl. oz. bottle
with child-resistant safety cap and
convenient dosage cup

PediaCare® Cough-Cold

Pharmacia & Upjohn
P. 719

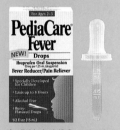

Available in 1/2 fl. oz. bottle
with child-resistant safety cap
and calibrated dropper

PediaCare® Fever Drops

Pharmacia & Upjohn
P. 717

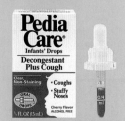

Available in 1/2 fl. oz.
bottle with child-resistant safety cap
and calibrated dropper

**PediaCare® Infants'
Drops Decongestant
Plus Cough**

Pharmacia & Upjohn
P. 717

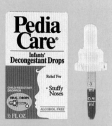

Available in 1/2 fl. oz. bottle with
child-resistant safety cap and
calibrated dropper

**PediaCare® Infants'
Decongestant Drops**

Pharmacia & Upjohn
P. 717

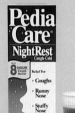

Available in 4 fl. oz. bottle with
child-resistant safety cap and
convenient dosage cup

**PediaCare® NightRest
Cough-Cold Liquid**

Pharmacia & Upjohn
P. 721

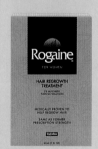

For Women

Rogaine®
(2% minoxidil)

Pharmacia & Upjohn
P. 717

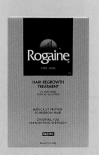

For Men
Hair Regrowth Treatment

Rogaine®
(2% minoxidil)

Pharmacia & Upjohn
P. 720

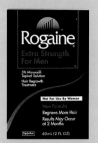

Hair Regrowth Treatment
Not For Use By Women

**Rogaine® Extra
Strength For Men**
(5% minoxidil)

Pharmacia & Upjohn
P. 724

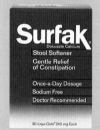

Packages of 10, 30, 100,
and 100 unit dose

**Surfak® Liqui-Gels®
Stool Softener**
(docusate calcium 240 mg)

PHARMANEX, INC.

Pharmanex, Inc.
P. 845

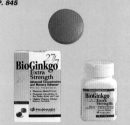

60 mg
Extra Strength Ginkgo biloba
Available in 60 ct.

BioGinkgo 27/7®

Pharmanex, Inc.
P. 846

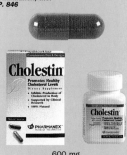

600 mg
Available in 120 ct.

Cholestin™
(Monascus purpureus Went)

PHARMATON

Pharmaton
P. 848

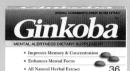

40 mg

Ginkoba™

Pharmaton
P. 848

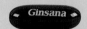
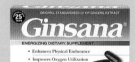

100 mg
Capsules

Ginsana®

Pharmaton
P. 848

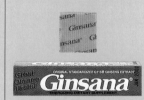

50 mg
Chewy Squares

Ginsana®

Pharmaton
P. 849

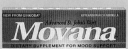

300 mg
Dietary Supplement for Mood Support

Movana™

Pharmaton
P. 849

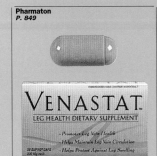

Dietary Supplement for Leg Health

Venastat™

Pharmaton
P. 849

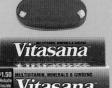

Daily Dietary Supplement

Vitasana™

PHYTOPHARMICA

PhytoPharmica
P. 851

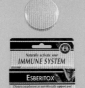

100 Tablets
Dietary supplement to nutritionally
support and stimulate the
immune system.

Esberitox™

PhytoPharmica
P. 851

60 and 120 tablets
Natural support for menopause.
Also available in Remifemin™ Plus,
with St. John's Wort.

Remifemin™

PROCTER & GAMBLE

Procter & Gamble
P. 725

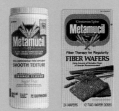

Available in 48, 72, 114 and 180
dose canisters and cartons of 30
one-dose packets.
Also available in sugar free.
Cinnamon Spice and Apple Crisp
Wafers available in 12-dose cartons.

Metamucil®

Procter & Gamble
P. 726

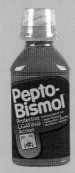

Pepto-Bismol®

PURDUE FREDERICK

The Purdue Frederick Company
P. 735

Maximum Strength Ointment

Antibiotics plus Moisturizer

Antibiotics plus Pain Reliever

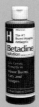

Solution

Betadine®

The Purdue Frederick Company
P. 736

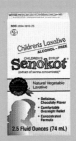

Natural Vegetable Laxative
Children's Syrup

Senokot®

The Purdue Frederick Company
P. 736

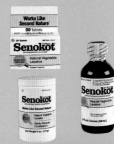

Natural Vegetable Laxative
Available in Tablets, Granules,
and Syrup.

Senokot®

The Purdue Frederick Company
P. 736

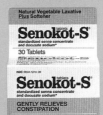

Natural Vegetable Laxative
Plus Softener

Senokot-S®

REAL HEALTH

Real Health Laboratories, Inc.
P. 852

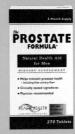

Natural Health Aid For Men
Dietary Supplement

The Prostate Formula™

Real Health Laboratories, Inc.
P. 853

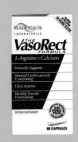

For healthy erectile and
cardiovascular function.

The VasoRect™ Formula

REXALL SUNDOWN

Rexall Sundown
P. 853

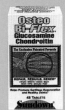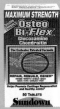

Regular and maximum strength

Osteo Bi-Flex™

SCHERING-PLOUGH

Schering-Plough HealthCare Products
P. 739

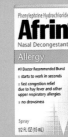

Moisturizing 4-hour formula

Afrin® Allergy

Schering-Plough HealthCare Products
P. 738

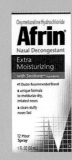

**Afrin® Extra Moisturizing
12 Hour Nasal Spray**

Schering-Plough HealthCare Products
P. 738

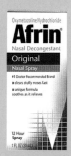

**Afrin® Original 12 Hour
Nasal Spray**

Schering-Plough HealthCare Products
P. 739

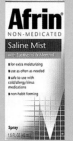

**Afrin® Saline Mist with
Eucalyptol & Menthol**

Schering-Plough HealthCare Products
P. 738

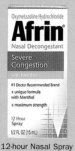

12-hour Nasal Spray

Afrin® Severe Congestion

Schering-Plough HealthCare Products
P. 738

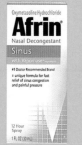

**Afrin® Sinus
12 Hour Nasal Spray**

Schering-Plough HealthCare Products
P. 740

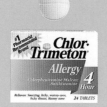

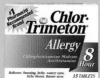

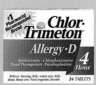

4 Hour Allergy Tablets
8 Hour Allergy Tablets
12 Hour Allergy Tablets
4 Hour Allergy Decongestant Tablets
12 Hour Allergy Decongestant Tablets

Chlor-Trimeton®

Schering-Plough HealthCare Products
P. 738

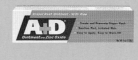

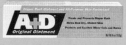

Original and with Zinc Oxide

A and D® Ointment

Schering-Plough HealthCare Products
P. 741

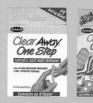

**Clear Away® One Step
Wart Removers**

Schering-Plough HealthCare Products
P. 741

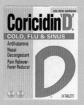

For Relief Of Cold,
Flu & Sinus Symptoms
Coricidin-D®

Schering-Plough HealthCare Products
P. 741

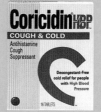

Cough and Cold Relief for people with
High Blood Pressure

Coricidin® HBP™

Schering-Plough HealthCare Products
P. 741

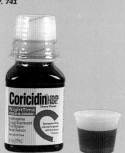

Cold and Flu Relief for people with
High Blood Pressure

Coricidin® HBP™

Schering-Plough HealthCare Products
P. 741

NightTime Cold and Cough Relief for
people with High Blood Pressure

Coricidin® HBP™

Schering-Plough HealthCare Products
P. 743

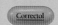

Laxative Tablets and Caplets
and Stool Softener Soft Gels

Correctol®

Schering-Plough HealthCare Products
P. 743

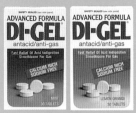

Advanced Formula

Di-Gel®

Schering-Plough HealthCare Products
P. 744

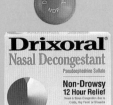

**Drixoral®
Nasal Decongestant**

Schering-Plough HealthCare Products
P. 747

Spray Powder, Spray Liquid, Spray
Deodorant Powder, Shaker Powder,
Jock Itch Spray Powder

Lotrimin® AF
(2% miconazole nitrate)

SmithKline Beecham
Consumer Healthcare, L.P.
P. 749

Multisymptom Cold & Flu Relief
Maximum Strength Formula:
Packages of 16 and 30 caplets
Non-Drowsy Formula:
Packages of 16 caplets

**Contac® Severe
Cold & Flu**

Schering-Plough HealthCare Products
P. 744

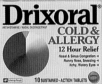

12 Hour Sustained-Action Tablets

**Drixoral®
Cold & Allergy**

Schering-Plough HealthCare Products
P. 745

**DuoFilm®/DuoPlant®
Wart Removers**

SIGMA—TAU

sigma–tau Pharmaceuticals, Inc.
P. 854

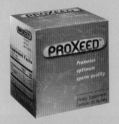

Dietary Supplement
Promotes optimum sperm quality

proXeed™

SmithKline Beecham
Consumer Healthcare, L.P.
P. 750

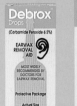
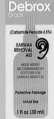

Drops
1/2 Fl. oz. 1 Fl. oz.

Debrox®

Schering-Plough HealthCare Products
P. 745

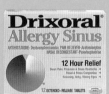

12 Hour Sustained-Action Tablets

**Drixoral®
Allergy Sinus**

Schering-Plough HealthCare Products
P. 746

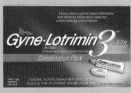

3-Day Treatment
Combination Pack

Gyne-Lotrimin®

SMITHKLINE BEECHAM

SmithKline Beecham
Consumer Healthcare, L.P.
P. 748

Fiber Therapy for Regularity
Sugar Free Orange available in:
8.6 oz. and 16.9 oz.
Regular Orange available in:
16 oz. and 30 oz. containers

Citrucel®

SmithKline Beecham
Consumer Healthcare, L.P.
P. 750

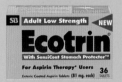

Adult Low Strength Tablets
in Bottles of 36

Ecotrin®

Schering-Plough HealthCare Products
P. 744

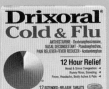

**Drixoral®
Cold & Flu**

Schering-Plough HealthCare Products
P. 747

Antifungal for Athlete's Foot
and Jock Itch

Lotrimin® AF

SmithKline Beecham
Consumer Healthcare, L.P.
P. 748

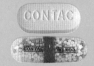
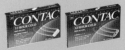

Continuous Action
Nasal Decongestant/Antihistamine
Packages of 10 and 20
Maximum Strength Caplets or
Regular Strength Capsules

Contac® 12 Hour

SmithKline Beecham
Consumer Healthcare, L.P.
P. 750

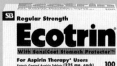

Regular Strength Tablets
in bottles of 100, 250

Ecotrin®

SmithKline Beecham
Consumer Healthcare, L.P.
P. 750

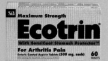

Maximum Strength Tablets
in bottles of 60, 150.

Ecotrin®

SmithKline Beecham
Consumer Healthcare, L.P.
P. 753

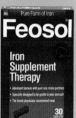

Packages of 30 caplets

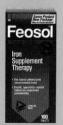

Packages of 100 tablets

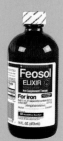

16 oz. bottle (Elixir)

Feosol®

SmithKline Beecham
Consumer Healthcare, L.P.
P. 755

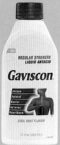

12 Fl. oz.

**Gaviscon® Regular
Strength Liquid Antacid**

SmithKline Beecham
Consumer Healthcare, L.P.
P. 754

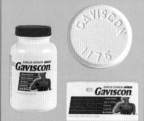

100-Tablet bottles
30-Tablet box (foil-wrapped 2s)

**Gaviscon® Regular
Strength Antacid**

SmithKline Beecham
Consumer Healthcare, L.P.
P. 755

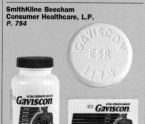

Extra Strength Formula
12 Fl. Oz.

**Gaviscon® Extra Strength
Liquid Antacid**

SmithKline Beecham
Consumer Healthcare, L.P.
P. 754

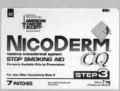

Extra Strength Formula
100-Tablet bottles
6 and 30-Tablet box
(foil-wrapped 2's)

**Gaviscon® Extra
Strength Antacid**

SmithKline Beecham
Consumer Healthcare, L.P.
P. 755

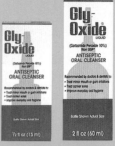

1/2 Fl. oz.   2 Fl. oz.

Gly-Oxide® Liquid

SmithKline Beecham
Consumer Healthcare, L.P.
P. 756

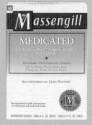

Medicated Disposable Douche
With Povidone-iodine

Available in single or twin packs

Massengill®

SmithKline Beecham
Consumer Healthcare, L.P.
P. 757

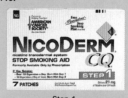

Step 1
Also available in 2 week kit

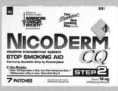

Step 2
Also available in 2 week kit

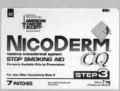

Step 3
Also available in 2 week kit

Includes User's Guide, Audio Tape and
Child Resistant Disposal Tray
Stop Smoking Aid
Nicotine Transdermal System

NicoDerm® CQ™

SmithKline Beecham
Consumer Healthcare, L.P.
P. 761

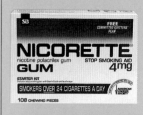

4 mg
For Smokers over 24
Cigarettes a day
Refill pack available
Stop Smoking Aid
Nicotine Polacrilex Gum

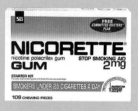

2 mg
For Smokers under 25
Cigarettes a day
Refill pack available
Stop Smoking Aid
Nicotine Polacrilex Gum

Nicorette®

SmithKline Beecham
Consumer Healthcare, L.P.
P. 855

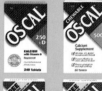

Calcium Supplement

Os-Cal®

While every effort has
been made to reproduce
products faithfully, this
section is to be consid-
ered a Quick-Reference
Identification aid.

**SmithKline Beecham
Consumer Healthcare, L.P.
P. 765**

Sore Throat Lozenges
Available in: Regular Strength
(Wild Cherry, Original Mint, Vapor
Lemon and Assorted)
Maximum Strength (Wintergreen,
Vapor Black Cherry) and
Childrens Cherry

Sucrets®

**SmithKline Beecham
Consumer Healthcare, L.P.
P. 765**

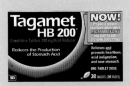

Acid Reducer
Packages of 6, 12, 18,
30, 50, 70 and 80

Tagamet HB® 200

**SmithKline Beecham
Consumer Healthcare, L.P.
P. 766**

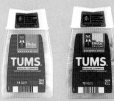

Peppermint and
Assorted Flavors

Tums®

**SmithKline Beecham
Consumer Healthcare, L.P.
P. 766**

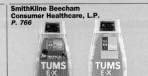
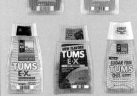

Tropical Fruit, Wintergreen,
Assorted Flavors, Assorted Berry
and SugarFree Orange Cream

Tums E-X®

**SmithKline Beecham
Consumer Healthcare, L.P.
P. 766**

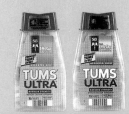

Assorted Mint and Fruit Flavors

Tums® Ultra™

**SmithKline Beecham
Consumer Healthcare, L.P.
P. 767**

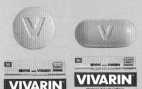

Alertness Aid with Caffeine
Available in tablets and caplets

Vivarin®

SUNPOWER

**Sunpower Nutraceutical Inc.
P. 856**

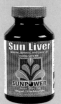

Sun Liver™

UNILEVER

**Unilever Home & Personal Care
P. 771**

Hypo-Allergenic
Free of Perfumes
Clear of Dyes

**All® Free Clear with
Allergen Fighter™**

UNIPATH

**Unipath Diagnostics Company
P. 771**

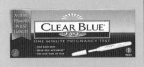

One-Step Pregnancy Test

CLEARBLUE EASY®

**Unipath Diagnostics Company
P. 772**

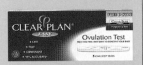

One-Step Ovulation Test

CLEARPLAN EASY®

WAKUNAGA

**Wakunaga Consumer Products
P. 858**

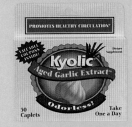

Aged Garlic Extract™

Kyolic®

**Wakunaga Consumer Products
P. 858**

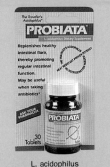

L. acidophilus

PROBIATA®

WALLACE

**Wallace Laboratories
P. 772**

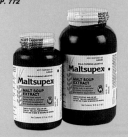

8 fl. oz. (1/2 pt) and 16 fl. oz. (1 pt)

Maltsupex® Liquid
(malt soup extract)

**Wallace Laboratories
P. 772**

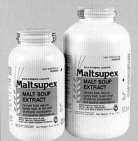

8 oz. (1/2 lb) and 16 oz. (1 lb)

Maltsupex® Powder
(malt soup extract)

**Wallace Laboratories
P. 772**

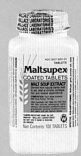

100 Tablets

Maltsupex® Tablets
(malt soup extract)

Wallace Laboratories
P. 773

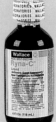

1 Pint (473 mL)
Also available: 4 fl. oz. (118 mL)

Ryna-C® Liquid
(antitussive/antihistamine/
decongestant)

Wallace Laboratories
P. 773

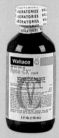

1 Pint (473 mL)
Also available: 4 fl. oz. (118 mL)

Ryna-CX® Liquid
(antitussive/decongestant/
expectorant)

WARNER-LAMBERT

Warner-Lambert Co.
P. 775

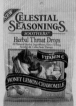

Herbal Throat Drops
Available in Golden Herbal Blend,
Honey-Lemon Chamomile, Harvest
Cherry and Herbal Orange Spice

**Celestial Seasonings®
Soothers™**

Warner-Lambert Co.
P. 775

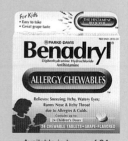

Breath drops available in Peppermint,
Freshmint and Cinnamint flavors in
slide top cartons of about 27 each.

**Certs® Cool Mint Drops
with a Retsyn® Center**

Warner-Lambert Co.
P. 775

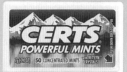

Tablets available in a credit card size
vial of 50 tablets each.

**Certs® Powerful Mints
with Retsyn® Crystals**

Warner-Lambert Co.
P. 775

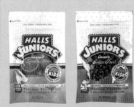

Sugar Free
Cough Suppressant Drops
Orange and Grape

Halls® Juniors Sugar Free

Warner-Lambert Co.
P. 775

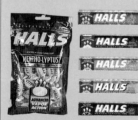

Cough Suppressant Drops
Spearmint, Mentho-Lyptus, Ice Blue,
Honey-Lemon and Cherry Flavors

Halls® Mentho-Lyptus®

Warner-Lambert Co.
P. 776

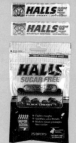

Black Cherry, Citrus Blend
and Mountain Menthol

**Halls® Sugar Free
Squares Mentho-Lyptus®**

Warner-Lambert Co.
P. 776

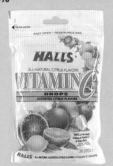

Assorted Citrus

Halls® Vitamin C Drops

Warner-Lambert Co.
P. 776

Cough Suppressant Drops with
Soothing Syrup Centers
Honey-Lemon, Mentho-Lyptus and Cherry

**Maximum Strength
Halls® Plus**

WARNER-LAMBERT

Warner-Lambert Consumer Healthcare
P. 776

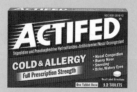

Available in boxes of 12, 24,
48 and 96 tablets

Actifed® Cold & Allergy

Warner-Lambert Consumer Healthcare
P. 777

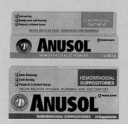

Suppositories available
in boxes of 12 and 24
Ointment available in 1 oz. tubes

Anusol®

Warner-Lambert Consumer Healthcare
P. 778

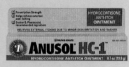

Anti-Itch Hydrocortisone Ointment
Available in 0.7 oz. tube

Anusol HC-1™

Warner-Lambert Consumer Healthcare
P. 778

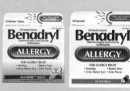

Capsules and Tablets
Available in boxes of 24 and 48
Tablets also available in
bottles of 100

Benadryl® Allergy

Warner-Lambert Consumer Healthcare
P. 780

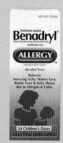

Available in 4 oz. and 8 oz. bottles

**Benadryl® Allergy
Liquid Medication**

Warner-Lambert Consumer Healthcare
P. 779

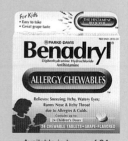

Available in boxes of 24
chewable Tablets

**Benadryl® Allergy
Chewables**

Warner-Lambert Consumer Healthcare
P. 778

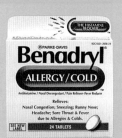

Available in boxes of 24 Tablets

**Benadryl®
Allergy/Cold**

Warner-Lambert Consumer Healthcare
P. 779

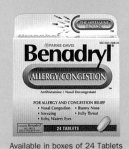

Available in boxes of 24 Tablets

**Benadryl® Allergy/
Congestion**

Warner-Lambert Consumer Healthcare
P. 779

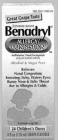

Available in 4 oz. bottles

**Benadryl® Allergy/
Congestion Liquid
Medication**

Warner-Lambert Consumer Healthcare
P. 781

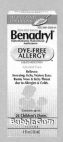

Available in 4 fl. oz. bottles

**Benadryl® Dye-Free
Allergy Liquid
Medication**

Warner-Lambert Consumer Healthcare
P. 781

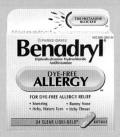

Available in Boxes of 24

**Benadryl® Dye-Free
Allergy Liqui-Gels®
Softgels**

Warner-Lambert Consumer Healthcare
P. 780

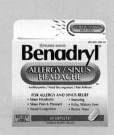

Available in boxes of 24 and 48
Caplets, box of 24 Gelcaps

**Benadryl® Allergy
Sinus Headache**

Warner-Lambert Consumer Healthcare
P. 782

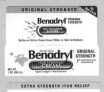

Original and Extra Strength

**Benadryl® Itch
Stopping Cream**

Warner-Lambert Consumer Healthcare
P. 782

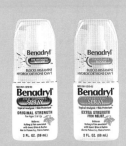

Original and Extra Strength

**Benadryl® Itch
Stopping Spray**

Warner-Lambert Consumer Healthcare
P. 782

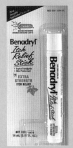

Extra Strength

**Benadryl® Itch
Relief Stick**

Warner-Lambert Consumer Healthcare
P. 783

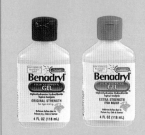

Original and Extra Strength

**Benadryl® Itch
Stopping Gel**

Warner-Lambert Consumer Healthcare
P. 783

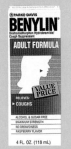

Available in 4 oz. bottles

**Benylin® Adult
Cough Suppressant**

Warner-Lambert Consumer Healthcare
P. 783

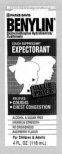

Available in 4 oz. bottles

**Benylin® Cough
Suppressant Expectorant**

Warner-Lambert Consumer Healthcare
P. 784

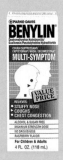

Available in 4 oz. bottles

Benylin® Multi-Symptom

Warner-Lambert Consumer Healthcare
P. 784

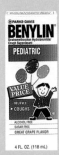

Available in 4 oz. bottles

**Benylin® Pediatric
Cough Suppressant**

Warner-Lambert Consumer Healthcare
P. 785

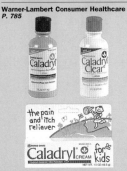

Itch Relief Plus Drying Action.
Available in Lotion, Clear Lotion
and Cream for Kids

Caladryl®

Warner-Lambert Consumer Healthcare
P. 785

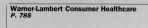
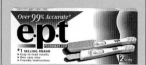

1 and 2 Pregnancy Test Kits Available
One Step. Easy to read.
Lab Accurate results.

e·p·t®

Warner-Lambert Consumer Healthcare
P. 786

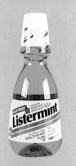

**Listermint®
Alcohol-Free Mouthwash**

Warner-Lambert Consumer Healthcare
P. 786

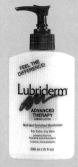

**Lubriderm® Advanced
Therapy Creamy Lotion**

Warner-Lambert Consumer Healthcare
P. 788

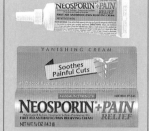

Maximum Strength Cream
Available in 1/2 oz. (14.2g) tubes

Neosporin® Plus

Warner-Lambert Consumer Healthcare
P. 786

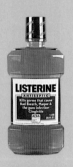

Listerine® Antiseptic

Warner-Lambert Consumer Healthcare
P. 787

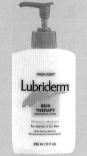

Available in Scented and
Fragrance Free

Lubriderm® Lotion

Warner-Lambert Consumer Healthcare
P. 787

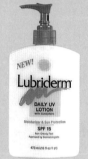

**Lubriderm® Daily UV
Lotion with Sunscreen**

Warner-Lambert Consumer Healthcare
P. 788

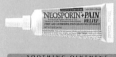
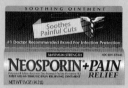

Maximum Strength Ointment
Available in 1/2 oz. (14.2g)
and 1 oz. (28.3g) tubes

Neosporin® Plus

Warner-Lambert Consumer Healthcare
P. 786

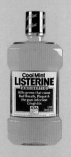

**Cool Mint
Listerine® Antiseptic**

Warner-Lambert Consumer Healthcare
P. 787

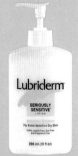

**Lubriderm® Seriously
Sensitive® Lotion**

Warner-Lambert Consumer Healthcare
P. 787

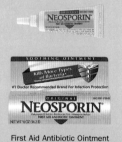

First Aid Antibiotic Ointment
Available in 1/2 oz. (14.2g) or 1 oz.
(28.3g) tubes; 1/31 oz. (0.9 g)

Neosporin®

Warner-Lambert Consumer Healthcare
P. 788

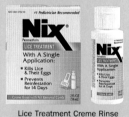

Lice Treatment Creme Rinse
2 fl. oz. (59 mL)
Also available in:
2-bottle family pack

Nix®

Warner-Lambert Consumer Healthcare
P. 786

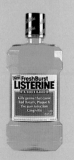

FreshBurst Listerine®

Warner-Lambert Consumer Healthcare
P. 787

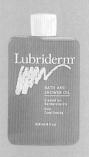

**Lubriderm® Bath &
Shower Oil**

Warner-Lambert Consumer Healthcare
P. 787

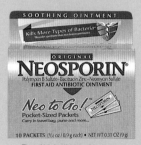

First Aid Antibiotic Ointment.
Available in Individual
Foil Packets. 0.31 oz. (9g)

Neosporin® Neo to Go!™

Warner-Lambert Consumer Healthcare
P. 789

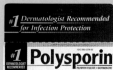

First Aid Antibiotic Powder & Ointment
Powder, 0.35 oz. (10g) Ointment,
1/2 oz. (14.2g) and 1 oz. (28.4g)

Polysporin®

Warner-Lambert Consumer Healthcare
P. 859

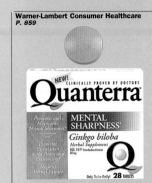

**Quanterra™
Mental Sharpness**

Warner-Lambert Consumer Healthcare
P. 859

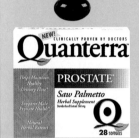

Quanterra™ Prostate

Warner-Lambert Consumer Healthcare
P. 789

Fast, Effective Relief from
Heartburn, Acid Indigestion or
Sour Stomach
Original Peppermint, Spearmint,
Cherry and Assorted Fruit Flavors
Rolaids®

Warner-Lambert Consumer Healthcare
P. 790

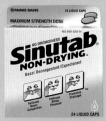

Available in Boxes of 24

**Sinutab® Non-Drying
Liquid Caps**

Warner-Lambert Consumer Healthcare
P. 790

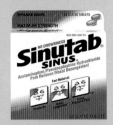

Maximum Strength
Without Drowsiness Formula
Available in 24 Caplets or Tablets

Sinutab® Sinus

Warner-Lambert Consumer Healthcare
P. 790

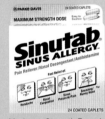

Maximum Strength Formula
Available in 24 Caplets or Tablets

Sinutab® Sinus Allergy

Warner-Lambert Consumer Healthcare
P. 794

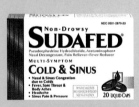

Available in boxes of
10 and 20 liquid caps

**Sudafed®
Cold and Sinus**

Warner-Lambert Consumer Healthcare
P. 792

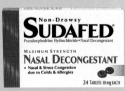

30 mg Tablets
Available in 24, 48 and 100

**Sudafed®
Nasal Decongestant**

Warner-Lambert Consumer Healthcare
P. 791

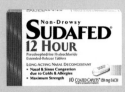

12 Hour Caplets
Available in 10 and 20 caplets

Sudafed® 12 Hour

Warner-Lambert Consumer Healthcare
P. 791

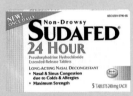

Available in boxes of 5 tablets.

Sudafed® 24 Hour

Warner-Lambert Consumer Healthcare
P. 792

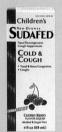

Available in 4 fl. oz. bottles

**Children's Sudafed®
Cold & Cough
Liquid Medication**

Warner-Lambert Consumer Healthcare
P. 792

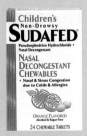

Available in boxes of
24 chewable tablets

**Children's Sudafed®
Nasal Decongestant**

Warner-Lambert Consumer Healthcare
P. 793

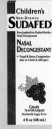

Available in 4 fl. oz. bottles

**Children's Sudafed®
Nasal Decongestant
Liquid Medication**

Warner-Lambert Consumer Healthcare
P. 795

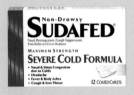

**Sudafed®
Severe Cold Formula**

Warner-Lambert Consumer Healthcare
P. 792

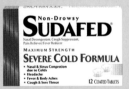

Available in 12's or 24's
caplets, 12's in tablets

**Sudafed®
Severe Cold Formula**

For more detailed infor-
mation on the products
illustrated in this section,
consult the Product
Information Section or
manufacturers may be
contacted directly.

Warner-Lambert Consumer Healthcare
P. 793

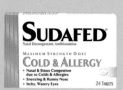

Available in boxes of 24

**Sudafed® Cold
and Allergy**

Warner-Lambert Consumer Healthcare
P. 794

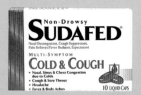

Available in 10's or 20's Liquid Caps

Sudafed® Cold & Cough

Warner-Lambert Consumer Healthcare
P. 794

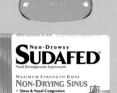

Available in 24 Liquid Caps

**Sudafed® Non-Drying
Sinus Liquid Caps**

While every effort has
been made to reproduce
products faithfully, this
section is to be consid-
ered a Quick-Reference
Identification aid.

Warner-Lambert Consumer Healthcare
P. 795

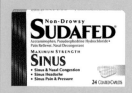

**Sudafed® Cold
and Allergy**

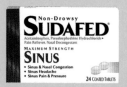

Available in 24 caplets and tablets

Sudafed® Sinus

Warner-Lambert Consumer Healthcare
P. 796

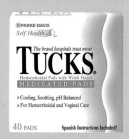

Pre-Moistened Pads
Available in 40 and 100 pad packages

Tucks®

Warner-Lambert Consumer Healthcare
P. 796

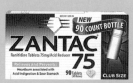

Available in boxes of
4, 10, 20, 30, 60, 80 and 90 tablets

Zantac® 75

Whitehall-Robins
P. 869

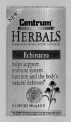

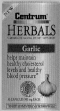

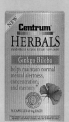

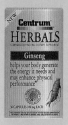

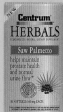

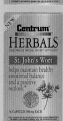

Echinacea, Garlic,
Ginkgo Biloba, Ginseng,
Saw Palmetto, St. John's Wort

Centrum® Herbals

J.B. Williams Co.
P. 810

Original and Mint Antiseptic
Mouthwash/Gargle
Available in 4, 12, 24
and 32 Fl. oz. bottles

Cepacol®

J.B. Williams Co.
P. 811

Maximum Strength Sore Throat
Lozenges
Mint and Cherry Flavors
Also Available in Regular Strength and
Sugar Free Maximum Strength
18 lozenges per pack

Cepacol®

J.B. Williams Co.
P. 811

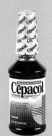
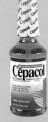

Maximum Strength Sore Throat Spray
Cool Menthol and Cherry Flavors.
4 Fl. oz. bottles

Cepacol®

J.B. Williams Co.
P. 812

Sore Throat Formula
Available in Grape and Cherry Flavors
4 oz. bottles

Children's Cepacol®

J.B. Williams Co.
P. 812

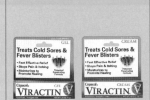

Cold Sore Treatment
Available in a gel and a cream
0.25 oz. tubes.

Cepacol® Viractin®

WYETH-AYERST

Tamper-Resistant/
Evident Packaging

Statements alerting consumers to
the specific type of Tamper-
Resistant/Evident Packaging
appear on the bottle labels and
cartons of all over-the-counter
products of Wyeth-Ayerst. This
includes plastic cap seals on bottles, individually wrapped tablets
or suppositories, and sealed
cartons. This packaging has been
developed to better
protect the consumer.

Wyeth-Ayerst Pharmaceuticals
P. 812

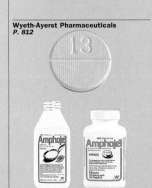

0.6 gram (10 gr.) Tablet shown above
12 Fl. oz. bottle and bottle of 100 tablets
Tablets and Suspension Antacid
Amphojel®

Wyeth-Ayerst Pharmaceuticals
P. 813

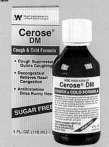

4 Fl. oz. Cough/Cold Formula
with Dextromethorphan
Also available in 1 pint bottles

Cerose® DM

Wyeth-Ayerst Pharmaceuticals
P. 813

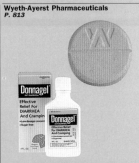

Available in bottles of 4 and 8 Fl. oz.
Chewable tablets
available in cartons of 18

Donnagel®

ZILA

Zila Pharmaceuticals, Inc.
P. 814

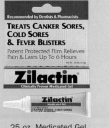

.25 oz. Medicated Gel
Unique Film Controls Pain Longer

Zilactin®

Zila Pharmaceuticals, Inc.
P. 814

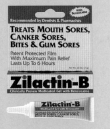

.25 oz. Medicated Gel with Benzocaine
Maximum Strength Medication

Zilactin®-B

Zila Pharmaceuticals, Inc.
P. 814

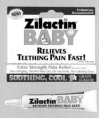

Extra Strength Pain Relief

Zilactin® Baby

NONPRESCRIPTION DRUG INFORMATION

This section presents information on nonprescription drugs, self-testing kits, and other medical products marketed for home use by consumers. It is made possible through the courtesy of the manufacturers whose products appear on the following pages. The information concerning each product has been prepared, edited, and approved by professional staff of the manufacturer.

Pharmaceutical product descriptions in this section must be in compliance with the Code of Federal Regulations labeling requirements for over-the-counter drugs. The descriptions are designed to provide all information necessary for informed use, including, when applicable, active ingredients, inactive ingredients, indications, actions, warnings, cautions, drug interactions, symptoms and treatment of oral overdosage, dosage and directions for use, professional labeling, and how supplied. In some cases, additional information has been supplied to complement the standard labeling.

In compiling this section, the publisher has emphasized the necessity of describing products comprehensively. The descriptions seen here include all information made available by the manufacturer. The publisher does not warrant or guarantee any product described here, and does not perform any independent analysis of the information provided. Inclusion of a product in this book does not represent an endorsement, and the publisher does not necessarily advocate the use of any product listed.

Agro-Dynamics International International-Bio Tech-USA

1145 LINDA VISTA DRIVE, STE. 109 SAN MARCOS, CA 92069

Direct Inquiries to:
1-800-736-1991
FAX: (760) 471-1878

LATERO-FLORA™ (Flora Balance™)

Description: Latero-Flora™ (Flora-Balance™) Is the source of a special patented strain of Bacillus laterosporus (BOD Strain) a natural occurring bacteria in spore form. Each capsule contains a minimum of 500,000 spores.

Indications and usage: Helps maintain the proper balance of intestinal flora. Candida, other yeast problems, and the use of antibiotics and chemotherapy can weaken intestinal flora balance.

Administration: Adults—One or two capsules twice daily. Children—one capsule as described above.
These statements have not been evaluated by the Food and Drug Administration. This product is not intended to diagnose, treat, cure, or prevent any disease.

How supplied:
Bottle of 30 Capsules
Bottle of 60 Capsules
Powder (To Make Liquid)—100 Gr.
Storage: Store at room temperature or refrigerate.

Astra Pharmaceuticals, L.P.

725 CHESTERBROOK BOULEVARD WAYNE, PA 19087-5677

Direct Inquiries to:
For Medical Information, Adverse Drug Experiences, and Customer Service Contact:
800-236-9933

XYLOCAINE® 2.5% Ointment (lidocaine)

For temporary relief of pain and itching due to minor burns, sunburn, minor cuts, abrasions, insect bites and minor skin irritations.
Xylocaine® 2.5% Ointment should be applied liberally over the affected areas. Use enough to provide temporary relief and reapply Xylocaine 2.5% Ointment as needed for continued relief.

Warning: Use only as directed by a physician in persistent, severe or extensive skin disorders. In case of accidental ingestion, seek professional assistance or contact a poison control center immediately.
KEEP OUT OF REACH OF CHILDREN. FOR EXTERNAL USE ONLY.
Xylocaine 2.5% Ointment is non-staining and is easily removed with water from skin or clothing.
Xylocaine 2.5% Ointment belongs in your home medicine chest and first aid kit.

Caution:: Do not use in the eyes. Not for prolonged use. If the condition for which this preparation is used persists, or if a rash or irritation develops, discontinue use and consult a physician.

How Supplied: 1.25 ounce tubes containing 2.5% lidocaine base in water soluble carbowaxes.

ASTRA®

Astra USA, Inc.   021658R02
Westborough, MA 01581   5/97
Shown in Product Identification Guide, page 503

Bayer Corporation Consumer Care Division

36 Columbia Road P.O. Box 1910 Morristown, NJ 07962-1910

Direct Inquiries to:
Consumer Relations
(800) 331-4536
www.bayercare.com

For Medical Emergency Contact:
Bayer Corporation
Consumer Care Division
(800) 331-4536

ALEVE® naproxen sodium tablets, 220 mg Pain reliever/fever reducer

ALEVE Tablets, Caplets* or Gelcaps** naproxen sodium tablets, USP

Active Ingredient
naproxen sodium
(in each tablet, caplet*, gelcap)**
220 mg (naproxen 200 mg)
Purpose
Pain reliever/fever reducer

Uses: Temporarily relieves minor aches and pains due to:
• common cold   • backache
• headache   • menstrual cramps
• toothache   • minor pain of arthritis
• muscular aches
Temporarily reduces fever

Warnings:

Allergy Alert: If, after taking a pain reliever or fever reducer, you have ever had: • hives • facial swelling • asthma • shock, do not take ALEVE. You may have a serious reaction.

Alcohol Warning: If you drink 3 or more alcoholic beverages daily, ask your doctor whether you should take ALEVE or other pain relievers. ALEVE may increase your risk of stomach bleeding.

Do not use:
• with any other pain reliever/fever reducer
• for more than 10 days for pain
• for more than 3 days for fever

Ask a doctor before use if:
• the painful area is red or swollen
• you take other drugs on a regular basis
• you are under a doctor's care for any continuing condition
• you have had serious side effects from any pain reliever

Stop using this product and ask a doctor if:
• any new or unexpected symptoms occur
• symptoms continue or worsen
• you have difficulty swallowing
• it feels like the pill is stuck in your throat
• you develop heartburn
• stomach pain occurs with use of this product or if even mild symptoms persist

If pregnant or breast-feeding, ask a health professional before use. **IT IS ESPECIALLY IMPORTANT NOT TO USE NAPROXEN SODIUM DURING THE LAST 3 MONTHS OF PREGNANCY UNLESS SPECIFICALLY DIRECTED TO DO SO BY A DOCTOR BECAUSE IT MAY CAUSE PROBLEMS IN THE UNBORN CHILD OR COMPLICATIONS DURING DELIVERY.**

Keep out of reach of children. In case of accidental overdose, seek professional assistance or contact a Poison Control Center immediately.

Dietary information (in each tablet, caplet*, gelcap**)
• sodium 20 mg

Directions: Drink a full glass of water with each dose.

Adults: • Take 1 tablet (caplet*, gelcap**) every 8 to 12 hours while symptoms persist. For the first dose you may take 2 tablets (caplets*, gelcaps**) within the first hour. The smallest effective dose should be used.

Do not take more than:
• 2 tablets (caplets*, gelcaps**) in any 8 to 12 hour period
• 3 tablets (caplets*, gelcaps**) in a 24 hour period.

Over age 65: • Do not take more than 1 tablet (caplet*, gelcap**) every 12 hours unless directed by a doctor.

Children under 12 years of age: • Do not give this product to children under 12 unless directed by a doctor.

Inactive Ingredients (Tablets/Caplets*): magnesium stearate, microcrystalline cellulose, povidone, talc, opadry YS-1-4215.

Inactive Ingredients (Gelcaps**): D&C yellow #10 lake, edetate disodium, edible ink, FD&C blue #1, FD&C yellow #6 lake, gelatin, glycerin, hydroxypropyl methylcellulose, magnesium stearate, microcrystalline cellulose, polyethylene glycol, povidone, stearic acid, talc, titanium dioxide, and triacetin.

*capsule-shaped tablet(s)

**gelatin coated capsule-shaped tablet(s)

Store at room temperature: Avoid high humidity and excessive heat 104°F (40°C).

Questions? Comments? Call 1-800-395-0689 or visit our website at www.aleve.com

Distributed by:
Bayer Corporation,
Consumer Care Division,
Morristown, NJ 07960 USA
B-RLLC

Shown in Product Identification Guide, page 503

ALKA–MINTS®
Chewable Antacid &
Calcium Supplement
Rich in Calcium

Active Ingredient: Each ALKA-MINTS Chewable Antacid tablet contains calcium carbonate 850 mg (340 mg of elemental calcium). Each tablet contains less than 5 mg sodium per tablet, and is dietarily sodium free.

Inactive Ingredients: May contain artificial colors, including FD&C yellow 6, Dioctyl sodium sulfosuccinate, flavor, hydrolyzed cereal solids, magnesium stearate, polyethylene glycol, sorbitol, sugar (compressible).

Indications: For the relief of acid indigestion, heartburn and sour stomach.

Warnings: Do not take more than 9 tablets in a 24 hour period, or use the maximum dosage of this product for more than 2 weeks, except under the advice and supervision of a physician. May cause constipation. As with any drug, if you are pregnant or nursing a baby, seek the advice of a health professional before using this product. Keep this and all drugs out of the reach of children.

Drug Interaction Precaution: Antacids may interact with certain prescription drugs. If you are presently taking a prescription drug, do not take this product without checking with your doctor or other health professional.

Directions: Chew 1 or 2 tablets every 2 hours or as directed by a physician.

How Supplied: Spearmint and Assorted flavors in bottles of 75's.

Product Identification Mark:
ALKA-MINTS embossed on each tablet.
Shown in Product Identification Guide, page 503

ALKA-SELTZER® Original
ALKA-SELTZER® Extra Strength
ALKA-SELTZER® Lemon Lime
ALKA-SELTZER® Cherry
Effervescent Antacid Pain Reliever

Active ingredients:
ALKA-SELTZER® Original:
Aspirin 325 mg, Heat Treated Sodium Bicarbonate 1916 mg, Citric acid 1000 mg.
ALKA-SELTZER® Extra Strength:
Aspirin 500 mg, Heat Treated Sodium Bicarbonate 1985 mg, Citric acid 1000 mg.
ALKA-SELTZER® Lemon Lime and Cherry:
Aspirin 325 mg, Heat Treated Sodium Bicarbonate 1700 mg, Citric acid 1000 mg.

Inactive Ingredients:
ALKA-SELTZER® Original:
none.
ALKA-SELTZER® Extra Strength:
Flavors.
ALKA-SELTZER® Lemon Lime:
Aspartame, Flavor, Tableting Aids.
ALKA-SELTZER® Cherry:
Aspartame, Flavor, Tableting Aids.
Phenylketonurics:
Each tablet contains 9 mg (Lemon Lime) or 12.3 mg (Cherry) of Phenylalanine.
Sodium Content per tablet:
Alka-Seltzer® Original: 567 mg
Alka-Seltzer® Extra Strength: 588 mg
Alka-Seltzer® Lemon Lime and Cherry: 503 mg.

Indications: For fast relief of heartburn, acid indigestion, sour stomach with headache, or body aches and pain. Also for fast relief of upset stomach with headache from overindulgence in food and drink—especially recommended for taking before bed and again on arising. Effective for pain relief alone: headache, or body and muscular aches and pains.

Directions:
Alka-Seltzer® Original, Cherry and Lemon Lime.
Adults: Dissolve 2 tablets in 4 oz. of water every 4 hours not to exceed 8 tablets in 24 hours. (60 years or older, 4 tablets in a 24-hour period).
Alka-Seltzer® Extra Strength.
Adults: Dissolve 2 tablets in 4 oz. of water every 6 hours not to exceed 7 tablets in 24 hours. (60 years or older, 4 tablets in a 24-hour period).
CAUTION: If symptoms persist or recur frequently, or if you are under treatment for ulcer, consult your doctor.

Warnings: Children and teenagers should not use this medicine for chicken pox or flu symptoms before a doctor is consulted about Reye syndrome, a rare but serious illness reported to be associated with aspirin. As with any drug, if

you are pregnant or nursing a baby, seek the advice of a health professional before using this product. **IT IS ESPECIALLY IMPORTANT NOT TO USE ASPIRIN DURING THE LAST 3 MONTHS OF PREGNANCY UNLESS SPECIFICALLY DIRECTED TO DO SO BY A DOCTOR BECAUSE IT MAY CAUSE PROBLEMS IN THE UNBORN CHILD OR COMPLICATIONS DURING DELIVERY.**
Except under the advice and supervision of a doctor. Do not take more than, ADULTS: 8 tablets (Extra Strength 7 tablets) in a 24-hour period, (60 years of age or older: 4 tablets in a 24-hour period), or use the daily maximum dosage for more than 10 days. Do not take this product if you are allergic to aspirin or have asthma, if you have bleeding problems, or if you are on a sodium restricted diet. If ringing in the ears or a loss of hearing occurs, consult a doctor before taking any more of this product.
Do not take this product for pain for more than 10 days unless directed by a doctor. If pain persists or gets worse, if new symptoms occur, or if redness or swelling is present, consult a doctor because these could be signs of a serious condition. Keep this and all drugs out of the reach of children.

Drug Interaction Precaution: Do not take this product if you are taking a prescription drug for anticoagulation (thinning the blood), diabetes, gout, or arthritis unless directed by a doctor. Antacids may interact with certain prescription drugs. If you are presently taking a prescription drug, do not take this product without checking with your doctor or other health professional.

How Supplied: Foil sealed effervescent tablets in cartons of 12's in 6 foil twin packs; 24's in 12 foil twin packs; 36's in 18 foil twin packs.
Shown in Product Identification Guide, page 503

ALKA-SELTZER GAS RELIEF ANTIGAS MEDICINE
Maximum Strength

Alka-Seltzer® Gas Relief is made with the most effective medicine available to provide fast relief in an easy to swallow, soothing liquid softgel.

Active Ingredients: Each softgel contains 125 mg of simethicone.

Inactive Ingredients: D&C Red #33, FD&C Blue #1, FD&C Red #40, Gelatin, Glycerin, Peppermint Oil, Purified Water, Sorbitol, Titanium Dioxide.

Uses: To relieve the symptoms commonly referred to as gas, such as pressure, bloating, or fullness.

Directions: Swallow one liquid softgel after meals and at bedtime or as needed. Do not exceed 4 softgels per day unless directed by a doctor. Softgels should not be chewed.

Continued on next page

Alka-Seltzer Gas—Cont.

Warning: Keep this and all drugs out of the reach of children.

To Open: Place thumb on liquid soft-gel—push down through foil. If foil has been removed or torn, do not use product.

How Supplied: Box of 12 liquid soft-gels.
Questions? Comments?
Please call 1-800-800-4793
Made in USA

Distributed by:
Bayer Corporation
Consumer Care Division
Morristown, NJ 07960 USA
Shown in Product Identification Guide, page 503

ALKA–SELTZER® GOLD
Effervescent Antacid

Does not contain aspirin.

Active Ingredients:
Each tablet contains heat treated sodium bicarbonate 958 mg, citric acid 832 mg, potassium bicarbonate 312 mg. As Effervescent Antacid in water contains principally the antacids sodium citrate and potassium citrate.

Inactive Ingredient: Tableting aid.

Indications:
For relief of heartburn, acid indigestion, or sour stomach.

Warnings: Except under the advice and supervision of a physician, do not take more than: Adults: 8 tablets in a 24-hour period (60 years of age or older: 7 tablets in a 24-hour period), Children: 4 tablets in a 24-hour period; or use the maximum dosage of this product for more than 2 weeks.

Do not use this product except under the advice and supervision of a physician if you are on a sodium restricted diet.
Keep this and all drugs out of the reach of children. As with any drug, if you are pregnant or nursing a baby, seek the advice of a health professional before using this product.

Drug Interaction Precaution: Antacids may interact with certain prescription drugs. If you are presently taking a prescription drug, do not take this product without checking with your doctor or other health professional.

Directions: Adults: Take 2 tablets fully dissolved in water every 4 hours. Children: $1/2$ the adult dosage or as directed by a doctor.

How Supplied: Boxes of 36 tablets in 18 foil twin packs.
Shown in Product Identification Guide, page 503

ALKA-SELTZER PLUS®
Cold & Cough Medicine,
ALKA-SELTZER PLUS®
Night-Time Cold Medicine,
ALKA-SELTZER PLUS®
Cold Medicine,
ALKA-SELTZER PLUS®
Cold & Sinus Medicine
ALKA-SELTZER PLUS®
Cold & Flu Medicine

Active Ingredients:
ALKA-SELTZER PLUS® Cold & Cough Medicine: Aspirin 325 mg*, Chlorpheniramine Maleate 2 mg, Phenylpropanolamine Bitartrate 20 mg, Dextromethorpan Hydrobromine 10 mg.
ALKA-SELTZER PLUS® Night-Time Cold Medicine: Aspirin 500 mg* Doxylamine Succinate 6.25 mg, Phenylpropanolamine Bitartrate 20 mg, Dextromethorpan Hydrochloride 15 mg.
ALKA-SELTZER PLUS® Cold Medicine: Aspirin 325 mg*, Phenylpropanolamine Bitartrate 20 mg, Chlorpheniramine Maleate 2 mg.
ALKA-SELTZER PLUS® Cold & Sinus Medicine: Aspirin 325 mg*, Phenylpropanolamine Bitartrate 20 mg.
*In water the aspirin is converted into its soluble ionic form, sodium acetylsalicylate.
ALKA-SELTZER PLUS® Cold & Flu Medicine: Acetaminophen 325mg, Dextromethorphan Hydrobrmoide 10 mg, Phenylpropanolamine Bitartrate 20 mg, Chlorpheniramine Maleate 2 mg.

Inactive Ingredients:
ALKA-SELTZER PLUS® Cold & Cough Medicine: Aspartame, Citric Acid, Flavor, Sodium Bicarbonate, Tableting aids.

Phenylketonurics: Contains Phenylalanine 11 mg per tablet.
ALKA-SELTZER PLUS® Night-Time Cold Medicine:
Aspartame, Citric Acid, Flavors, Sodium Bicarbonate, Tableting aids.

Phenylketonurics: Contains Phenylalanine 16 mg per tablet.
ALKA-SELTZER PLUS® Cold Medicine:
Citric Acid, Artifical and Natural Flavors, Sodium Bicarbonate. Tableting Aids (Orange & Cherry Flavors also contain Aspartame)
Phenylketonurics: Cherry contains Phenylalanine 10 mg per tablet, Orange contains Phenylalanine 14 mg per tablet.
ALKA-SELTZER® Cold & Sinus Medicine: Aspartame, Citric Acid, Flavor, Sodium Bicarbonate, Tableting aids.
PHENYLKETONURICS: Contains Phenylalanine 12 mg per tablet.
ALKA-SELTZER® Cold & Flu Medicine: Aspartame, Calcium Carbonate, Citric Acid, Croscarmellose Sodium, D&C Yellow #10, Flavor, Maltodextrin, Mannitol, Polyvinylpyrrolidone, Sodium Bicarbonate, Sodium Saccharin, Sorbitol, Starch, Stearic Acid, Tableting Aids.
Phenylketonurics: Contains Phenylalanine 11 mg per tablet.

Sodium Content per tablet
Alka-Seltzer Plus Cold & Cough 507 mg
Alka-Seltzer Plus Cold & Sinus 504 mg
Night-Time 506 mg
Alka-Seltzer Plus Cold 506 mg
Alka-Seltzer Plus Cold & Flu 111 mg

Indications: For the temporary relief of these major cold and flu symptoms: **coughing, nasal and sinus congestion, body aches and pains, runny nose, headaches, sneezing, fever, *scratchy sore throat, so you can get the rest you need.

General Directions: Adults: Dissolve 2 tablets in approximately 4 oz. of water every 4 hours. Do not exceed 8 tablets in any 24-hour period or as directed by a doctor. Children under 12 yrs of age: consult a doctor.

Warning: Children and teenagers should not use this medicine for chicken pox or flu symptoms before a doctor is consulted about Reye syndrome, a rare but serious illness reported to be associated with aspirin. Do not take this product for more than 7 days or for fever for more than 3 days unless directed by a doctor. If symptoms, including pain or fever, persist, do not improve or get worse, if new symptoms occur, or if redness or swelling is present, consult a doctor because these could be signs of a serious condition. (If sore throat is severe, persists for more than 2 days, is accompanied by fever, headache, nausea or vomiting, consult a physician promptly.)* As with any drug, if you are pregnant or nursing a baby, seek the advice of a health professional before using this product. **IT IS ESPECIALLY IMPORTANT NOT TO USE ASPIRIN DURING THE LAST 3 MONTHS OF PREGNANCY UNLESS SPECIFICALLY DIRECTED TO DO SO BY A DOCTOR BECAUSE IT MAY CAUSE PROBLEMS IN THE UNBORN CHILD OR COMPLICATIONS DURING DELIVERY.**

Do not exceed recommended dosage. If nervousness, dizziness or sleeplessness occur, discontinue use and consult a doctor. May cause excitability, especially in children. Do not take this product unless directed by a doctor if you are allergic to aspirin, have a breathing problem such as emphysema or chronic bronchitis, asthma, glaucoma, difficulty in urination due to enlargement of the prostate gland, heart disease, high blood pressure, diabetes, thyroid disease, bleeding problems or on a sodium restricted diet.

May cause marked drowsiness; alcohol, sedatives and tranquilizers may increase drowsiness effect. Avoid alcoholic beverages while taking this product. Do not take this product if you are taking sedatives or tranquilizers without first consulting your doctor. Use caution when driving a motor vehicle or operating machinery. [Do not take this product for persistent or chronic cough such as occurs with smoking, asthma, emphysema, or if cough is accompanied by excessive phlegm (mucus), unless directed by a doctor. A persistent cough may be a sign of a serious condition. If cough persists for more than 1 week, tends to recur or is accompanied by fever, rash, or persistent headache, consult a doctor.**] Keep this and all drugs out of the reach of children. In case of accidental overdose seek professional assistance or contact a Poison Control Center immediately.

Drug Interaction Precaution: Do not take this product if you are presently taking a prescription drug for anticoagulation (thinning the blood), diabetes, gout, arthritis***, or are presently taking a monoamine oxidase inhibitor (MAOI) (certain drugs for depression, psychiatric or emotional conditions, or Parkinson's disease), or for 2 weeks after stopping the MAOI drug. If you are uncertain whether your prescription drug contains an MAOI, consult a health professional before taking this product.
*Does not apply to ALKA-SELTZER PLUS Cold & Sinus Medicine.
**Applies only to ALKA-SELTZER PLUS Cold & Cough Medicine, Night-Time Cold Medicine and Cold & Flu Medicine.
***Does not apply to Alka-Seltzer Plus Cold & Flu.

How Supplied: ALKA-SELTZER PLUS Cold & Cough Medicine, and Night-Time Cold Medicine: Carton of 36 tablets in 18 foil twin packs; carton of 20 tablets in 10 foil twin packs; carton of 12 tablets in 6 foil packs.
ALKA-SELTZER PLUS Cold Medicine: Also available in the above sizes, plus carton of 48 in 24 foil twin packs.
ALKA-SELTZER PLUS Cold & Sinus: Carton of 20 tablets in 10 foil twin packs
Product Identification Mark:
Shown in Product Identification Guide, page 503

**ALKA-SELTZER PLUS®
NIGHT-TIME COLD
MEDICINE LIQUI-GELS,®**

**ALKA-SELTZER PLUS®
COLD & COUGH MEDICINE
LIQUI-GELS,®**

**ALKA-SELTZER PLUS®
COLD MEDICINE LIQUI-GELS®**

**ALKA-SELTZER PLUS®
COLD & SINUS MEDICINE
LIQUI-GELS®**

**ALKA-SELTZER PLUS®
COLD & FLU MEDICINE
LIQUI-GELS®**

Active Ingredients:
ALKA-SELTZER PLUS® NIGHT-TIME COLD MEDICINE:
Dextromethorphan Hydrobromide 10 mg, Doxylamine Succinate 6.25 mg, Pseudoephedrine HCl 30 mg, Acetaminophen 325 mg.
ALKA-SELTZER PLUS® COLD & COUGH MEDICINE:
Dextromethorphan Hydrobromide 10 mg, Chlorpheniramine Maleate 2 mg,

Pseudoephedrine HCl 30 mg, Acetaminophen 325 mg.
ALKA-SELTZER PLUS® COLD MEDICINE:
Chlorpheniramine Maleate 2 mg, Pseudoephedrine HCl 30 mg, Acetominophen 325 mg.
ALKA-SELTZER PLUS® COLD & SINUS MEDICINE: Pseudoephedrine HCl 30 mg, Acetaminophen 325 mg.
ALKA-SELTZER PLUS® COLD & FLU MEDICINE: acetaminophen 325 mg, Pseudoephedrine HCl 30 mg, Dextromethorphan Hydrobromide 10 mg.

Inactive Ingredients: Artificial Colors, Gelatin, Glycerin, Polyethylene Glycol, Potassium Acetate, Povidone, Purified Water, Sorbitol, Titanium Dioxide.

ALKA-SELTZER PLUS® COLD & SINUS MEDICINE AND COLD & FLU MEDICINE LIQUI-GELS®: FD&C Red #40, Gelatin, Glycerin, Polyethylene Glycol, Potassium Acetate, Povidone, Purified Water, Sorbitol, Titanium Dioxide.

Indications: Provides temporary relief of these major symptoms of cold and flu: *coughing, runny nose, nasal and sinus congestion, headache, body aches and pains, sneezing, fever and sore throat.
ALKA-SELTZER PLUS® COLD & SINUS MEDICINE: Provides temporary relief of these major symptoms associated with a cold and sinusitis: nasal and sinus congestion, headache, general body aches and pains, fever and sore throat.

Direction for Use: ALKA-SELTZER PLUS® COLD MEDICINE, COLD & COUGH MEDICINE, and COLD & FLU MEDICINE
ADULTS: Swallow 2 softgels with water. CHILDREN (6–12 YEARS): Swallow 1 softgel with water. Repeat every 4 hours, not to exceed 4 doses per day, or as directed by a doctor. CHILDREN (under 6 years): Consult a doctor.
ALKA-SELTZER PLUS® NIGHT-TIME COLD MEDICINE:
ADULTS: Swallow 2 softgels with water, once daily, at bedtime or as directed by a doctor. CHILDREN under 12 years of age consult a doctor.
ALKA-SELTZER PLUS® COLD & SINUS MEDICINE: ADULTS: Swallow 2 softgels with water. CHILDREN (6 to 12 years): Swallow 1 softgel with water. CHILDREN (under 6 years): Consult a doctor. Repeat every 4 hours, not to exceed 4 doses per day, or as directed by a doctor.

Warnings: Do not exceed recommended dosage. If nervousness, dizziness or sleeplessness occur, discontinue use and call a doctor. If symptoms do not improve within 7 days or are accompanied by fever, consult a doctor.
If sore throat is severe, persists for more than 2 days, is accompanied by or followed by fever, rash, headache, nausea or vomiting, consult a doctor promptly. May cause excitability especially in children.**

Do not take this product, unless directed by a doctor, if you have a breathing problem such as emphysema or chronic bronchitis***, or glaucoma, difficulty in urination due to enlargement of the prostate gland or heart disease, high blood pressure, diabetes, or thyroid disease. [May cause drowsiness; alcohol, sedatives and tranquilizers may increase drowsiness effect. Avoid alcoholic beverages while taking this product. Do not take this product if you are taking sedatives or tranquilizers without first consulting your doctor. Use caution when driving a motor vehicle or operating machinery.]*** As with any drug, if you are pregnant or nursing a baby seek the advice of a health professional before using this product. Keep this and all medication out of the reach of children. In case of accidental overdose, contact a physician or Poison Control Center immediately. Prompt medical attention is critical for adults as well as children even if you do not notice any signs or symptoms. (A persistent cough may be a sign of a serious condition. If cough persists for more than 1 week, tends to recur or is accompanied by fever, rash or persistent headache, consult a doctor. Do not take this product for persistent or chronic cough such as occurs with smoking, asthma, emphysema or if cough is accompanied by excessive phlegm (mucus) unless directed by a doctor.)****

Drug Interaction Precaution: Do not take this product if you are now taking a prescription monoamine oxidase inhibitor (MAOI) (certain drugs for depression, psychiatric or emotional conditions, or Parkinson's disease), or for 2 weeks after stopping the MAOI drug. If you are uncertain whether your prescription drug contains an MAOI, consult a health professional before taking this product.
*Does not apply to Alka-Seltzer Plus Cold Medicine.
**Does not apply to Alka-Seltzer Plus Cold & Sinus Medicine or Cold & Flu Medicine.
***Does not apply to Alka-Seltzer Plus Cold & Sinus Medicine.
****Does not apply to Alka-Seltzer Plus Cold Medicine or Cold & Sinus Medicine.

Liqui-Gels® is a trademark of R.P. Scherer Corp.

How Supplied: Carton of 12 and 20 softgels.
Shown in Product Identification Guide, page 503

**ALKA-SELTZER® PLUS Cold & Flu Liqui-Gels®
Non-Drowsy Formula**

Active Ingredients: Acetaminophen 325 mg, Pseudoephedrine Hydrochloride 30 mg, Dextromethorphan Hydrobromide 10 mg.

Inactive Ingredients: FD&C Red #40, Gelatin, Glycerin, Polyethylene Gly-

Continued on next page

Alka-Seltzer Plus Cold—Cont.

col, Potassium Acetate Povidone, Purified Water, Sorbitol, Titanium Dioxide.

Indications: Provides temporary relief of these symptoms associated with flu and common cold including: headache, body aches, fever, coughing, minor sore throat pain, nasal and sinus congestion.

Directions: ADULTS: Swallow 2 softgels with water. CHILDREN (6–12 years): Swallow 1 softgel with water. CHILDREN (under 6 years): Consult a doctor. Repeat every 4 hours, but not to exceed 4 doses per day, or as directed by a doctor.

Warnings: Do not exceed recommended dosage. If nervousness, dizziness or sleeplessness occur, discontinue use and consult a doctor. If symptoms do not improve within 7 days or are accompanied by fever, consult a doctor. A persistent cough may be a sign of a serious condition. If cough persists for more than 1 week, tends to recur or is accompanied by fever, rash, or persistent headache, consult a doctor. Do not take this product for persistent or chronic cough such as occurs with smoking, asthma, emphysema, or if cough is accompanied by excessive phlegm (mucus) unless directed by a doctor. If sore throat is severe, persists for more than 2 days, is accompanied by or followed by fever, headache, rash, nausea, or vomiting, consult a doctor promptly. Do not take this product if you have heart disease, high blood pressure, thyroid disease, diabetes or difficulty in urination due to enlargement of the prostate gland unless directed by a doctor. As with any drug, if you are pregnant or nursing a baby, seek the advice of a health professional before using this product. Keep this and all medication out of the reach of children. In case of accidental overdose, seek professional assistance or Poison Control Center immediately. Prompt medical attention is critical for adults as well as children even if you do not notice any signs or symptoms.

Drug Interaction Precaution: Do not use this product if you are now taking a prescription monoamine oxidase inhibitor (MAOI) (certain drugs for depression, psychiatric or emotional conditions, or Parkinson's disease), or for 2 weeks after stopping the MAOI drug. If you are uncertain whether your prescription drug contains an MAOI, consult a health professional before taking this product.

Liqui-Gels® is a registered trademark of R.P. Scherer Corp.

How Supplied: ALKA-SELTZER® PLUS Cold & Flu Liqui-Gels® are available in blisters of 12 and 20 count.

Shown in Product Identification Guide, page 503

ALKA-SELTZER PM™
[əl-ka sĕl-sur]
PAIN RELIEVER & SLEEP AID MEDICINE

Indications: For the temporary relief of occasional headaches and minor aches and pains with accompanying sleeplessness.

Directions: Adults: Dissolve 2 tablets in 4 oz. of water and take at bedtime, if needed, or as directed by a doctor.

Active Ingredients: Each effervescent tablet contains 325 mg aspirin and 38 mg diphenhydramine citrate.

Inactive Ingredients: Acesulfame Potassium, Aspartame, Citric acid, Flavors, Sodium bicarbonate, Tableting aids.

Warnings: Do not give to children under 12 years of age. **Children and teenagers should not use this medicine for chicken pox or flu symptoms before a doctor is consulted about Reye syndrome, a rare but serious illness reported to be associated with aspirin.** Do not take this product for pain for more than 10 days or for fever for more than 3 days unless directed by a doctor. If pain or fever persists or gets worse, if new symptoms occur, or if redness or swelling is present, consult a doctor because these could be signs of a serious condition. Do not take this product if you are allergic to aspirin or if you have asthma unless directed by a doctor. Each tablet contains 503 mg of sodium. if ringing in the ears or a loss of hearing occurs, consult a doctor before taking any more of this product. Unless directed by a doctor, do not take this product if you have ulcers or bleeding problems, or if you have stomach problems that persist or recur frequently, such as persistent stomach pain, heartburn, or upset stomach. If sleeplessness persists continuously for more than 2 weeks, consult your doctor. Insomnia may be a symptom of serious underlying medical illness. Do not take this product, unless directed by a doctor, if you have a breathing problem such as emphysema or chronic bronchitis, or if you have glaucoma or difficulty in urination due to enlargement of the prostate gland. Avoid alcoholic beverages while taking this product. Do not take this product if you are taking sedatives or tranquilizers, without first consulting your doctor. Keep this and all drugs out of the reach of children. In case of accidental overdose, seek professional assistance or contact a poison control center immediately. As with any drug, if you are pregnant or nursing a baby, seek the advice of a health professional before using this product. **IT IS ESPECIALLY IMPORTANT NOT TO USE ASPIRIN DURING THE LAST 3 MONTHS OF PREGNANCY UNLESS SPECIFICALLY DIRECTED TO DO SO BY A DOCTOR BECAUSE IT MAY CAUSE PROBLEMS IN THE UNBORN CHILD OR COMPLICATIONS DURING DELIVERY.**
Phenylketonurics: Contains Phenylalanine 4.04 mg per tablet.

Drug Interaction Precaution: Do not take this product if you are taking a prescription drug for anticoagulation (thinning the blood), diabetes, gout, or arthritis unless directed by a doctor.
Helps protect against the stomach upset aspirin users may sometimes experience.
For more information or a free sample, visit our web site at www.alka-seltzer.com

How Supplied: 24 Effervescent tablets.
Shown in Product Identification Guide, page 503

Genuine BAYER® Aspirin
Tablets, Caplets and Gelcaps

Active Ingredient: 325 mg aspirin per tablet, caplet, or gelcap, coated for easy swallowing.

Inactive Ingredients: Butylparaben, D&C Yellow #10 Gelatin, Glycerin, Hydroxypropyl Methylcellulose, Methylparaben, Propylparaben, Sodium Lauryl Sulfate, Sorbitan Trioleate, Starch, Titanium Dioxide and Triacetin.

Indications: For the temporary relief of: headache, pain and fever of colds, muscle aches and pains, menstrual pain, toothache pain, minor aches and pains of arthritis.

Directions: Adults and Children 12 years and over: One or two tablets/caplets/gelcaps with water every 4 hours, as needed, up to a maximum of 12 tablets/caplets/gelcaps per 24 hours or as directed by a doctor. Do not give to children under 12 unless directed by a doctor.

Warnings: Children and teenagers should not use this medicine for chicken pox or flu symptoms before a doctor is consulted about Reye syndrome, a rare but serious illness reported to be associated with aspirin. Do not take this product for pain for more than 10 days or for fever for more than 3 days unless directed by a doctor. If pain or fever persists or gets worse, if new symptoms occur, or if redness or swelling is present consult a doctor because these could be signs of a serious condition. Do not take this product if you are allergic to aspirin, have asthma, have stomach problems (such as heartburn, upset stomach or stomach pain) that persist or recur, gastric ulcers or bleeding problems unless directed by a doctor. If ringing in the ears or loss of hearing occurs, consult a doctor before taking any more of this product. Keep this and all drugs out of the reach of children. In case of accidental overdose, seek professional assistance or contact a poison control center immediately. As with any drug, if you are pregnant or nursing a baby, seek the advice of a health professional before using this product. **IT IS ESPECIALLY IMPORTANT NOT TO USE ASPIRIN DURING THE LAST 3 MONTHS OF PREGNANCY UNLESS SPECIFI-**

CALLY DIRECTED TO DO SO BY A DOCTOR BECAUSE IT MAY CAUSE PROBLEMS IN THE UNBORN CHILD OR COMPLICATIONS DURING DELIVERY.

Drug Interaction Precaution: Do not take this product if you are taking a prescription drug for anticoagulation (thinning the blood), diabetes, gout or arthritis unless directed by doctor.
See "Professional Labeling" listing on page 608.

How Supplied:
Genuine Bayer Aspirin 325 mg (5 grains) is supplied in pouches of 2 tablets, packs of 12 tablets, bottles of 24, 50, 100, 200, 300, and 365 tablets, bottles of 50 and 100 caplets, and bottles of 40 and 80 gelcaps.
Child-resistant safety closures on 12s, 24s, 50s, 200s, 300s, 365s tablets and 50s caplets. Bottles of 100s tablets, gelcaps and caplets available without safety closure for households without small children.
Shown in Product Identification Guide, page 504

ASPIRIN REGIMEN BAYER® 81 mg
ASPIRIN REGIMEN BAYER® 325 mg
Delayed Release Enteric Aspirin Adult Low Strength 81 mg Tablets and Regular Strength 325 mg Caplets

Enteric Coated Tablets and Caplets
The enteric coating on Aspirin Regimen Bayer is designed to allow the tablet/caplet to pass through the stomach to the intestine before it dissolves, providing protection against stomach upset.

Active Ingredient: Aspirin Regimen Bayer 81 mg — 81 mg aspirin per tablet Aspirin Regimen Bayer 325 mg — 325 mg aspirin per caplet

Inactive Ingredients:
Regular Strength 325mg—D&C Yellow #10, FD&C Yellow #6, Hydroxypropyl Methylcellulose, Iron Oxide, Methacrylic Acid Copolymer, Starch, Titanium Dioxide, Triacetin.
Adult Low Strength 81mg—Croscarmellose Sodium, D&C Yellow #10, FD&C Yellow #6, Hydroxypropyl Methylcellulose, Iron Oxides, Lactose, Methacrylic Acid, Microcrystalline Cellulose, Polysorbate 80, Sodium Lauryl Sulfate, Starch, Titanium Dioxide, Triacetin.

Indications: ASPIRIN REGIMEN BAYER® is an anti-inflammatory, analgesic, and antiplatelet agent indicated for the relief of painful discomfort and muscular aches and pains associated with conditions requiring long-term aspirin therapy, e.g., arthritis or rheumatism, and for situations where compliance with aspirin usage may be hindered by gastrointestinal side effects of non-enteric-coated or buffered aspirin. For additional **Anti-inflammatory, Antiarthritic,** and **Antiplatelet** indications,

see the **PROFESSIONAL LABELING** section on page 608. Because of its delayed action, ASPIRIN REGIMEN BAYER will not provide fast relief of headaches, fever or other symptoms needing immediate relief.

Directions: For nonprescription analgesic indications: Adults & children 12 years and older: Take one or two 325 mg caplets or four to eight 81 mg tablets every 4 hours with water.
Do not exceed 4000 mg in 24 hours. Dosage may be modified as directed by a doctor.

Warnings: Children and teenagers should not use this medicine for chicken pox or flu symptoms before a doctor is consulted about Reye Syndrome, a rare but serious illness reported to be associated with aspirin. Do not take for pain for more than 10 days or for fever for more than 3 days unless directed by a doctor. If pain or fever persists or gets worse, if new symptoms occur, or if redness or swelling is present, consult a doctor because these could be signs of a serious condition. Do not take this product if you are allergic to aspirin, have asthma, have stomach problems (such as heartburn, upset stomach or stomach pain) that persist or recur, gastric ulcers or bleeding problems unless directed by a doctor. If ringing in the ears or loss of hearing occurs, consult a doctor before taking any more of this product. Keep this and all drugs out of the reach of children. In case of accidental overdose, seek professional assistance or contact a poison control center immediately. As with any drug, if you are pregnant or nursing a baby, seek the advice of a health professional before using this product. **IT IS ESPECIALLY IMPORTANT NOT TO USE ASPIRIN DURING THE LAST 3 MONTHS OF PREGNANCY UNLESS SPECIFICALLY DIRECTED TO DO SO BY A DOCTOR BECAUSE IT MAY CAUSE PROBLEMS IN THE UNBORN CHILD OR COMPLICATIONS DURING DELIVERY.**

Drug Interaction Precaution: Do not take this product if you are taking a prescription drug for anticoagulation (thinning the blood), diabetes, gout or arthritis unless directed by a doctor.
See "Professional Labeling" listing on page 608.

Safety: The safety of enteric-coated aspirin has been demonstrated in a number of endoscopic studies comparing enteric-coated aspirin and plain aspirin, as well as buffered aspirin and "arthritis strength" doses. In these studies, endoscopies were performed in healthy volunteers either before and/or during, and/or after administration of various aspirin doses. Compared to all the other preparations, the enteric-coated aspirin produced signficantly less damage to the gastric mucosa.

Bioavailability: Dissolution of the enteric coating occurs at a neutral to basic pH and is therefore dependent on gastric

emptying into the duodenum. With continued dosing, appropriate therapeutic plasma levels are maintained.

How Supplied: ASPIRIN REGIMEN BAYER 325 mg—Regular strength 325 mg caplets in bottles of 100 with child-resistant safety closure.
ASPIRIN REGIMEN BAYER 81 mg—Adult Low Strenth 81 mg tablets in bottles of 120 with child-resistant safety closure. Also Supplied in bottles of 32 and 180 without safety closure for households without small children.
REV. 11/94
Shown in Product Identification Guide, page 504

ASPIRIN REGIMEN BAYER®
81 mg WITH CALCIUM

Each caplet provides 81 mg of aspirin and 10% (100 mg) of the Daily Value of Calcium as part of the buffered base of Calcium Carbonate.

Active Ingredient: 81 mg Aspirin per caplet in a buffered base of Calcium Carbonate (250 mg = 100 mg of elemental calcium).

Inactive Ingredients: Colloidal Silicon Dioxide, FD&C Blue #2 Lake, Hydroxypropyl Methylcellulose, Microcrystalline Cellulose, Propylene Glycol, Sodium Starch Glycolate, Starch, Titanium Dioxide, Zinc Stearate.

Indications. For the temporary relief of minor aches and pains or as recommended by your doctor.

Directions: Adults and Children 12 years and over, take 4 to 8 caplets with water every 4 hours, as needed, up to a maximum of 32 caplets per 24 hours or as directed by a doctor.

Warnings: Children and teenagers should not use this medicine for chicken pox or flu symptoms before a doctor is consulted about Reye Syndrome, a rare but serious illness reported to be associated with aspirin. Do not take for pain for more than 10 days or for fever for more than 3 days unless directed by a doctor. If pain or fever persists or gets worse, if new symptoms occur or if redness or swelling is present, consult a doctor because these could be signs of a serious condition. Do not take this product if you are allergic to aspirin, have asthma, have stomach problems (such as heartburn, upset stomach or stomach pain) that persist or recur, gastric ulcers or bleeding problems unless directed by a doctor. If ringing in the ears or loss of hearing occurs, consult a doctor before taking any more of this product. Keep this and all drugs out of the reach of children. In case of accidental overdose, seek professional assistance or contact a poison control center immediately. As with any drug, if you are pregnant or nursing a baby, seek the advice of

Continued on next page

Aspirin Regimen Bayer—Cont.

a health professional before using this product. IT IS ESPECIALLY IMPORTANT NOT TO USE ASPIRIN DURING THE LAST 3 MONTHS OF PREGNANCY UNLESS DIRECTED TO DO SO BY A DOCTOR BECAUSE IT MAY CAUSE PROBLEMS IN THE UNBORN CHILD OR COMPLICATIONS DURING DELIVERY.

Drug Interaction Precaution: Do not take this product if you are taking any prescription drug including those for anticoagulation (thinning the blood), diabetes, gout or arthritis unless directed by a doctor.

See "Professional Labeling" listing on page 608.

How Supplied: Bottles of 60 count.
Shown in Product Identification Guide, page 504

Aspirin Regimen
BAYER® Children's Chewable
81 mg Aspirin
Orange & Cherry Flavored

Active Ingredients: 81 mg Aspirin per tablet

Inactive Ingredients: Orange Flavored: Dextrose Excipient, FD&C Yellow #6, Flavor, Saccharin Sodium, Starch. Cherry Flavored: D&C Red #27 Lake, Dextrose Excipient, FD&C Red #40 Lake, Flavor, Saccharin Sodium, Starch.

Indications: For the temporary relief of minor aches, pains and headaches, and to reduce fever associated with colds, sore throats and teething.

Directions:
To be administered only under adult supervision.

Age (Years)	Weight (lbs)	Dosage
2 to under 4	32 to 35	2 tablets
4 to under 6	36 to 45	3 tablets
6 to under 9	46 to 65	4 tablets
9 to under 11	66 to 76	4–5 tablets
11 to under 12	77 to 83	4–6 tablets
Adults and Children 12 yrs and over		5–8 tablets

Repeat every four hours, while symptoms persist, up to a maximum of five doses in 24 hours or as directed by a doctor. Drink water with each dose. Children under 2 years: consult a doctor.
Ways to Administer: Tablets may be chewed, swallowed or dissolved on tongue followed with a half a glass of liquid. Tablets may also be crushed in a teaspoonful of water followed with a half a glass of liquid.

Warnings: Children and teenagers should not use this medicine for chicken pox or flu symptoms before a doctor is consulted about Reye syndrome, a rare but serious illness reported to be associated with aspirin.

Do not take for pain for more than 10 days (for adults) or 5 days (for children), and do not take for fever for more than 3 days unless directed by a doctor. If pain or fever persists or gets worse, if new symptoms occur, or if redness or swelling is present, consult a doctor because these could be signs of a serious condition. Do not give this product to children for the pain of arthritis unless directed by a doctor. If sore throat is severe, persists for more than 2 days, is accompanied or followed by fever, headache, rash, nausea, or vomiting, consult a doctor promptly. Do not take this product for at least 7 days after tonsillectomy or oral surgery unless directed by a doctor. Do not take this product if you are allergic to aspirin, have asthma, have stomach problems (such as heartburn, upset stomach or stomach pain) that persist or recur or have gastric ulcers or bleeding problems unless directed by a doctor. If ringing in the ears or loss of hearing occurs, consult a doctor before taking any more of this product.
Keep this and all drugs out of the reach of children. In case of accidental overdose, contact a doctor immediately. As with any drug, if you are pregnant or nursing a baby, seek the advice of a health professional before using this product. IT IS ESPECIALLY IMPORTANT NOT TO USE ASPIRIN DURING THE LAST 3 MONTHS OF PREGNANCY UNLESS SPECIFICALLY DIRECTED TO DO SO BY A DOCTOR BECAUSE IT MAY CAUSE PROBLEMS IN THE UNBORN CHILD OR COMPLICATIONS DURING DELIVERY.

Drug Interaction Precaution: Do not take this product if taking a prescription drug for anticoagulation (thinning the blood), diabetes, gout or arthritis unless directed by a doctor.
See "Professional labeling" listing on page 608.

How Supplied: Bottles of 36 tablets with child-resistant safety closure. Store at room temperature.
Shown in Product Identification Guide, page 504

PROFESSIONAL LABELING

Genuine Bayer Aspirin
Aspirin Regimen Bayer 325 mg
Aspirin Regimen Bayer 81 mg
Aspirin Regimen Bayer 81 mg with Calcium
Aspirin Regimen Bayer Childrens Chewable 81 mg

Professional Labeling:

INDICATIONS AND USAGE

Vascular Indications (Ischemic Stroke, TIA, Acute MI, Prevention of Recurrent MI, Unstable Angina Pectoris, and Chronic Stable Angina Pectoris): Aspirin is indicated to: (1) Reduce the combined risk of death and nonfatal stroke in patients who have had ischemic stroke or transient ischemia of the brain due to fibrin platelet emboli, (2) reduce the risk of vascular mortality in patients with a suspected acute MI, (3) reduce the combined risk of death and nonfatal MI in patients with a previous MI or unstable angina pectoris, and (4) reduce the combined risk of MI and sudden death in patients with chronic stable angina pectoris.

Revascularization Procedures (Coronary Artery Bypass Graft (CABG), Percutaneous Transluminal Coronary Angioplasty (PTCA), and Carotid Endarterectomy): Aspirin is indicated in patients who have undergone revascularization procedures (i.e., CABG, PTCA, or carotid endarterectomy) when there is a preexisting condition for which aspirin is already indicated.

Rheumatologic Disease Indications (Rheumatoid Arthritis, Juvenile Rheumatoid Arthritis, Spondyloarthropathies, Osteoarthritis, and the Arthritis and Pleurisy of Systemic Lupus Erythematosus (SLE)): Aspirin is indicated for the relief of the signs and symptoms of rheumatoid arthritis, juvenile rheumatoid arthritis, osteoarthritis, spondyloarthropathies, and arthritis and pleurisy associated with SLE.

CONTRAINDICATIONS

Allergy: Aspirin is contraindicated in patients with known allergy to nonsteroidal anti-inflammatory drug products and in patients with the syndrome of asthma, rhinitis, and nasal polyps. Aspirin may cause severe urticaria, angioedema, or bronchospasm (asthma).

Reye's Syndrome: Aspirin should not be used in children or teenagers for viral infections, with or without fever, because of the risk of Reye's syndrome with concomitant use of aspirin in certain viral illnesses.

WARNINGS

Alcohol Warning: Patients who consume three or more alcoholic drinks every day should be counseled about the bleeding risks involved with chronic, heavy alcohol use while taking aspirin.

Coagulation Abnormalities: Even low doses of aspirin can inhibit platelet function leading to an increase in bleeding time. This can adversely affect patients with inherited (hemophilia) or acquired (liver disease or vitamin K deficiency) bleeding disorders.

GI Side Effects: GI side effects include stomach pain, heartburn, nausea, vomiting, and gross GI bleeding. Although minor upper GI symptoms, such as dyspepsia, are common and can occur anytime during therapy, physicians should remain alert for signs of ulceration and bleeding, even in the absence of previous GI symptoms. Physicians should inform patients about the signs and symptoms of GI side effects and what steps to take if they occur.

Peptic Ulcer Disease: Patients with a history of active peptic ulcer disease should avoid using aspirin, which can cause gastric mucosal irritation and bleeding.

PRECAUTIONS

General

Renal Failure: Avoid aspirin in patients with severe renal failure (glomerular filtration rate less than 10 mL/minute).

Hepatic Insufficiency: Avoid aspirin in patients with severe hepatic insufficiency.

Sodium Restricted Diets: Patients with sodium-retaining states, such as congestive heart failure or renal failure, should avoid sodium-containing buffered aspirin preparations because of their high sodium content.

Laboratory Tests: Aspirin has been associated with elevated hepatic enzymes, blood urea nitrogen and serum creatinine, hyperkalemia, proteinuria, and prolonged bleeding time.

Drug Interactions

Angiotensin Converting Enzyme (ACE) Inhibitors: The hyponatremic and hypotensive effects of ACE inhibitors may be diminished by the concomitant administration of aspirin due to its indirect effect on the renin-angiotensin conversion pathway.

Acetazolamide: Concurrent use of aspirin and acetazolamide can lead to high serum concentrations of acetazolamide (and toxicity) due to competition at the renal tubule for secretion.

Anticoagulant Therapy (Heparin and Warfarin): Patients on anticoagulation therapy are at increased risk for bleeding because of drug-drug interactions and the effect on platelets. Aspirin can displace warfarin from protein binding sites, leading to prolongation of both the prothrombin time and the bleeding time. Aspirin can increase the anticoagulant activity of heparin, increasing bleeding risk.

Anticonvulsants: Salicylate can displace protein-bound phenytoin and valproic acid, leading to a decrease in the total concentration of phenytoin and an increase in serum valproic acid levels.

Beta Blockers: The hypotensive effects of beta blockers may be diminished by the concomitant administration of aspirin due to inhibition of renal prostaglandins, leading to decreased renal blood flow, and salt and fluid retention.

Diuretics: The effectiveness of diuretics in patients with underlying renal or cardiovascular disease may be diminished by the concomitant administration of aspirin due to inhibition of renal prostaglandins, leading to decreased renal blood flow and salt and fluid retention.

Methotrexate: Salicylate can inhibit renal clearance of methotrexate, leading to bone marrow toxicity, especially in the elderly or renal impaired.

Nonsteroidal Anti-inflammatory Drugs (NSAID's): The concurrent use of aspirin with other NSAID's should be avoided because this may increase bleeding or lead to decreased renal function.

Oral Hypoglycemics: Moderate doses of aspirin may increase the effectiveness of oral hypoglycemic drugs, leading to hypoglycemia.

Uricosuric Agents (Probenecid and Sulfinpyrazone): Salicylates antagonize the uricosuric action of uricosuric agents.

Carcinogenesis, Mutagenesis, Impairment of Fertility: Administration of aspirin for 68 weeks at 0.5 percent in the feed of rats was not carcinogenic. In the Ames Salmonella assay, aspirin was not mutagenic; however, aspirin did induce chromosome aberrations in cultured human fibroblasts. Aspirin inhibits ovulation in rats. (See Pregnancy.)

Pregnancy: Pregnant women should only take aspirin if clearly needed. Because of the known effects of NSAID's on the fetal cardiovascular system (closure of the ductus arteriosus), use during the third trimester of pregnancy should be avoided. Salicylate products have also been associated with alterations in maternal and neonatal hemostasis mechanisms, decreased birth weight, and with perinatal mortality.

Labor and Delivery: Aspirin should be avoided 1 week prior to and during labor and delivery because it can result in excessive blood loss at delivery. Prolonged gestation and prolonged labor due to prostaglandin inhibition have been reported.

Nursing Mothers: Nursing mothers should avoid using aspirin because salicylate is excreted in breast milk. Use of high doses may lead to rashes, platelet abnormalities, and bleeding in nursing infants.

Pediatric Use: Pediatric dosing recommendations for juvenile rheumatoid arthritis are based on well-controlled clinical studies. An initial dose of 90–130 mg/kg/day in divided doses, with an increase as needed for anti-inflammatory efficacy (target plasma salicylate levels of 150–300 <greek-m>g/mL) are effective. At high doses (i.e., plasma levels of greater than 200 mg/mL), the incidence of toxicity increases.

ADVERSE REACTIONS

Many adverse reactions due to aspirin ingestion are dose-related. The following is a list of adverse reactions that have been reported in the literature. (See Warnings.)

Body as a Whole: Fever, hypothermia, thirst.

Cardiovascular: Dysrhythmias, hypotension, tachycardia.

Central Nervous System: Agitation, cerebral edema, coma, confusion, dizziness, headache, subdural or intracranial hemorrhage, lethargy, seizures.

Fluid and Electrolyte: Dehydration, hyperkalemia, metabolic acidosis, respiratory alkalosis.

Gastrointestinal: Dyspepsia, GI bleeding, ulceration and perforation, nausea, vomiting, transient elevations of hepatic enzymes, hepatitis, Reye's Syndrome, pancreatitis.

Hematologic: Prolongation of the prothrombin time, disseminated intravascular coagulation, coagulopathy, thrombocytopenia.

Hypersensitivity: Acute anaphylaxis, angioedema, asthma, bronchospasm, laryngeal edema, urticaria.

Musculoskeletal: Rhabdomyolysis.

Metabolism: Hypoglycemia (in children), hyperglycemia.

Reproductive: Prolonged pregnancy and labor, stillbirths, lower birth weight infants, antepartum and postpartum bleeding.

Respiratory: Hyperpnea, pulmonary edema, tachypnea.

Special Senses: Hearing loss, tinnitus. Patients with high frequency hearing loss may have difficulty perceiving tinnitus. In these patients, tinnitus cannot be used as a clinical indicator of salicylism.

Urogenital: Interstitial nephritis, papillary necrosis, proteinuria, renal insufficiency and failure.

OVERDOSAGE

Salicylate toxicity may result from acute ingestion (overdose) or chronic intoxication. The early signs of salicylic overdose (salicylism), including tinnitus (ringing in the ears), occur at plasma concentrations approaching 200 <greek-m>g/mL. Plasma concentrations of aspirin above 300 <greek-m>g/mL are clearly toxic. Severe toxic effects are associated with levels above 400 <greek-m>g/mL. (See Clinical Pharmacology.) A single lethal dose of aspirin in adults is not known with certainty but death may be expected at 30 g. For real or suspected overdose, a Poison Control Center should be contacted immediately. Careful medical management is essential.

Signs and Symptoms: In acute overdose, severe acid-base and electrolyte disturbances may occur and are complicated by hyperthermia and dehydration. Respiratory alkalosis occurs early while hyperventilation is present, but is quickly followed by metabolic acidosis.

Treatment: Treatment consists primarily of supporting vital functions, increasing salicylate elimination, and correcting the acid-base disturbance. Gastric emptying and/or lavage is recommended as soon as possible after ingestion, even if the patient has vomited spontaneously. After lavage and/or emesis, administration of activated charcoal, as a slurry, is beneficial, if less than 3 hours have passed since ingestion. Charcoal adsorption should not be employed prior to emesis and lavage.

Severity of aspirin intoxication is determined by measuring the blood salicylate level. Acid-base status should be closely followed with serial blood gas and serum pH measurements. Fluid and electrolyte balance should aslo be maintained.

In severe cases, hyperthermia and hypovolemia are the major immediate threats to life. Children should be sponged with tepid water. Replacement fluid should be administered intravenously and augmented with correction of acidosis. Plasma electrolytes and pH should be monitored to promote alkaline diuresis

Continued on next page

Bayer Aspirin Prof Label—Cont.

of salicylate if renal function is normal. Infusion of glucose may be required to control hypoglycemia.

Hemodialysis and peritoneal dialysis can be performed to reduce the body drug content. In patients with renal insufficiency or in cases of life-threatening intoxication, dialysis is usually required. Exchange transfusion may be indicated in infants and young children.

DOSAGE AND ADMINISTRATION

Each dose of aspirin should be taken with a full glass of water unless patient is fluid restricted. Anti-inflammatory and analgesic dosages should be individualized. When aspirin is used in high doses, the development of tinnitus may be used as a clinical sign of elevated plasma salicylate levels except in patients with high frequency hearing loss.

Ischemic Stroke and TIA: 50–325 mg once a day. Continue therapy indefinitely.

Suspected Acute MI: The initial dose of 160–162.5 mg is administered as soon as an MI is suspected. The maintenance dose of 160–162.5 mg a day is continued for 30 days post-infarction. After 30 days, consider further therapy based on dosage and administration for prevention of recurrent MI.

Prevention of Recurrent MI: 75–325 mg once a day. Continue therapy indefinitely.

Unstable Angina Pectoris: 75–325 mg once a day. Continue therapy indefinitely.

Chronic Stable Angina Pectoris: 75–325 mg once a day. Continue therapy indefinitely.

CABG: 325 mg daily starting 6 hours post-procedure. Continue therapy for 1 year post-procedure.

PTCA: The initial dose of 325 mg should be given 2 hours presurgery. Maintenance dose is 160–325 mg daily. Continue therapy indefinitely.

Carotid Endarterectomy: Doses of 80 mg once daily to 650 mg twice daily, started presurgery, are recommended. Continue therapy indefinitely.

Rheumatoid Arthritis: The initial dose is 3 g a day in divided doses. Increase as needed for anti-inflammatory efficacy with target plasma salicylate levels of 150–300 <greek-m>g/mL. At high doses (i.e., plasma levels of greater than 200 mg/mL), the incidence of toxicity increases.

Juvenile Rheumatoid Arthritis: Initial dose is 90–130 mg/kg/day in divided doses. Increase as needed for anti-inflammatory efficacy with target plasma salicylate levels of 150–300 <greek-m>g/mL. At high doses (i.e., plasma levels of greater than 200 mg/mL), the incidence of toxicity increases.

Spondyloarthropathies: Up to 4 g per day in divided doses.

Osteoarthritis: Up to 3 g per day in divided doses.

Arthritis and Pleurisy of SLE: The initial dose is 3 g a day in divided doses.

Increase as needed for anti-inflammatory efficacy with target plasma salicylate levels of 150–300 <greek-m>g/mL. At high doses (i.e., plasma levels of greater than 200 mg/mL, the incidence of toxicity increases.

Extra Strength BAYER® Aspirin Arthritis Pain Regimen Formula
[aspirin, 500 mg]

Enteric Coated Caplets

The enteric coating on BAYER® Aspirin Arthritis Pain Regimen Formula is designed to allow the caplet to pass through the stomach to the intestine before it dissolves, providing protection against stomach upset.

Active Ingredient: 500 mg Aspirin per caplet.

Inactive Ingredients: D&C Yellow #10, FD&C Yellow #6, Hydroxypropyl Methylcellulose, Iron Oxide, Methacrylic Acid Copolymer, Starch, Titanium Dioxide, Triacetin.

Indications: For the temporary relief of minor aches and pains of arthritis or as recommended by your doctor.

Because of its delayed action, BAYER® Aspirin Arthritis Pain Regimen Formula will not provide fast relief of headaches, fever or other symptoms needing immediate relief.

Directions: Adults and Children 12 years and over, take 2 caplets with water every 6 hours, as needed, up to a maximum of 8 caplets per 24 hours. Ask your doctor about recommended dosages for other indications.

Warnings: Children and teenagers should not use this medicine for chicken pox or flu symptoms before a doctor is consulted about Reye Syndrome, a rare but serious illness reported to be associated with aspirin. Do not take for pain for more than 10 days or for fever for more than 3 days unless directed by a doctor. If pain or fever persists or gets worse, if new symptoms occur or if redness or swelling is present, consult a doctor because these could be signs of a serious condition. Do not take this product if you are allergic to aspirin, have asthma, have stomach problems (such as heartburn, upset stomach or stomach pain) that persist or recur, gastric ulcers or bleeding problems unless directed by a doctor. If ringing in the ears or loss of hearing occurs, consult a doctor before taking any more of this product. Keep this and all drugs out of the reach of children. In case of accidental overdose, seek professional assistance or contact a poison control center immediately. As with any drug, if you are pregnant or nursing a baby, seek the advice of a health professional before using this product. IT IS ESPECIALLY IMPORTANT NOT TO USE ASPIRIN DURING THE LAST 3 MONTHS OF PREGNANCY UNLESS SPECIFICALLY DIRECTED TO DO SO BY A DOCTOR BE-

CAUSE IT MAY CAUSE PROBLEMS IN THE UNBORN CHILD OR COMPLICATIONS DURING DELIVERY.

Drug Interaction Precaution: Do not take this product if you are taking a prescription drug for anticoagulation (thinning the blood), diabetes, gout or arthritis unless directed by a doctor.

How Supplied: Bottles of 50 caplets with a child-resistant safety closure.
Shown in Product Identification Guide, page 504

Extra Strength BAYER® Aspirin Caplets, Tablets and Gelcaps

Active Ingredient: Extra Strength Bayer Aspirin—Aspirin 500 mg (7.7 grains) per tablet, caplet or gelcap contains a thin, inert, coated for easier swallowing.

Inactive Ingredients: Butylparaben, FD&C Red #40, Gelatin, Glycerin, Hydroxypropyl Methylcellulose, Methylparaben, Propylparaben, Sodium Lauryl Sulfate, Sorbitan Trioleate, Starch, Titanium Dioxide and Triacetin.

Indications: Analgesic, antipyretic, anti-inflammatory. For relief of headache; painful discomfort and fever of colds; muscular aches and pains; temporary relief of minor pains of arthritis; toothache and pain following dental procedures; menstrual pain.

Directions: Adults and Children 12 years and over: Take 1 or 2 tablets/caplets/gelcaps with water every 4 to 6 hours, as needed, up to a maximum of 8 tablets/caplets/gelcaps per 24 hours or as directed by a doctor. Do not give to children under 12 unless directed by a doctor.

Warnings: Children and teenagers should not use this medicine for chicken pox or flu symptoms before a doctor is consulted about Reye Syndrome, a rare but serious illness reported to be associated with aspirin. Do not take for pain for more than 10 days or for fever for more than 3 days unless directed by a doctor. If pain or fever persists or gets worse, if new symptoms occur or if redness or swelling is present consult a doctor because these could be signs of a serious condition. Do not take this product if you are allergic to aspirin, have asthma, have stomach problems (such as heartburn, upset stomach or stomach pain) that persist or recur, gastric ulcers or bleeding problems unless directed by a doctor. If ringing in the ears or loss of hearing occurs, consult a doctor before taking any more of this product. Keep this and all drugs out of the reach of children. In case of accidental overdose, seek professional assistance or contact a poison control center immediately. As with any drug, if you are pregnant or nursing a baby, seek the advice of a health professional before using this product. **IT IS ESPECIALLY IMPOR-**

TANT NOT TO USE ASPIRIN DUR-ING THE LAST 3 MONTHS OF PREG-NANCY UNLESS SPECIFICALLY DI-RECTED TO DO SO BY A DOCTOR BECAUSE IT MAY CAUSE PROB-LEMS IN THE UNBORN CHILD OR COMPLICATIONS DURING DELIV-ERY.

Drug Interaction Precaution: Do not take this product if you are taking a prescription drug for anticoagulation (thinning the blood), diabetes, gout or arthritis unless directed by a doctor.

How Supplied: Extra Strength Bayer Aspirin 500 mg (7.7 grains) is available in bottles of 50 caplets and tablets, pouches of 2 caplets and bottles of 40 and 80 gelcaps.

Shown in Product Identification Guide, page 504

Extra Strength BAYER® PLUS
Buffered Aspirin

Active Ingredient: 500 mg Aspirin in a buffered base with Calcium Carbonate

Inactive Ingredients Colloidal Silicon Dioxide, D&C Red #7 Lake, FD&C Blue #2 Lake, FD&C Red #40 Lake, Hydroxypropyl Methylcellulose, Microcrystalline Cellulose, Propylene Glycol, Sodium Starch Glycolate, Starch, Titanium Dioxide, Zinc Stearate.

Indications: Temporary relief of: headache, pain and fever of colds, muscle aches and pains, menstrual pain, toothache pain, minor aches and pains of arthritis.

Directions: Adults and Children 12 years and over: Take 1 or 2 caplets with water every 4 to 6 hours, as needed, up to a maximum of 8 caplets per 24 hours or as directed by a doctor. Do not give to children under 12 unless directed by a doctor.

Warnings: Children and teenagers should not use this medicine for chicken pox or flu symptoms before a doctor is consulted about Reye Syndrome, a rare but serious illness reported to be associated with aspirin. Do not take for pain for more than 10 days or for fever for more than 3 days unless directed by a doctor. If pain or fever persists or gets worse, if new symptoms occur or if redness or swelling is present consult a doctor because these could be signs of a serious condition. Do not take this product if you are allergic to aspirin, have asthma, have stomach problems (such as heartburn, upset stomach or stomach pain) that persist or recur, gastric ulcers or bleeding problems unless directed by a doctor. If ringing in the ears or loss of hearing occurs, consult a doctor before taking any more of this product. Keep this and all drugs out of the reach of children. In case of accidental overdose, seek professional assistance or contact a poison control center immediately. As with any drug, if you are preg-

nant or nursing a baby, seek the advice of a health professional before using this product. **IT IS ESPECIALLY IMPOR-TANT NOT TO USE ASPIRIN DUR-ING THE LAST 3 MONTHS OF PREG-NANCY UNLESS SPECIFICALLY DI-RECTED TO DO SO BY A DOCTOR BECAUSE IT MAY CAUSE PROB-LEMS IN THE UNBORN CHILD OR COMPLICATIONS DURING DELIV-ERY.**

Drug Interaction Precaution: Do not take this product if you are taking a prescription drug for anticoagulation (thinning the blood), diabetes, gout or arthritis unless directed by a doctor.

How Supplied: Extra Strength Bayer Plus Aspirin (500 mg) —bottles of 50 caplets.

Shown in Product Identification Guide, page 504

Extra Strength BAYER® PM
Aspirin Plus Sleep Aid
[500 mg aspirin/25 mg diphenhydramine HCl]

Indications: For the temporary relief of occasional headaches and minor aches and pains with accompanying sleeplessness.

Active Ingredients: 500 mg Aspirin, 25 mg Diphenhydramine Hydrochloride per caplet.

Inactive Ingredients: Colloidal Silicon Dioxide, Dibasic Calcium Phosphate, Dibutyl Sebacate, Ethylcellulose, FD&C Blue #1 Lake, FD&C Blue #2 Lake, Hydroxypropyl Methylcellulose, Microcrystalline Cellulose, Oleic Acid, Propylene Glycol, Starch, Titanium Dioxide, Zinc Stearate.

Directions: Adults and Children 12 years of age and over, take 2 caplets with water at bedtime, if needed, or as directed by a doctor.

Warnings: Do not give to children under 12 years of age. **Children and teenagers should not use this medicine for chicken pox or flu symptoms before a doctor is consulted about Reye Syndrome, a rare but serious illness reported to be associated with aspirin.** Do not take this product for pain for more than 10 days or for fever for more than 3 days unless directed by a doctor. If pain or fever persists or gets worse, if new symptoms occur, or if redness or swelling is present, consult a doctor because these could be signs of a serious condition. Do not take this product if you are allergic to aspirin or if you have asthma unless directed by a doctor. If ringing in the ears or a loss of hearing occurs, consult a doctor before taking any more of this product. Do not take this product if you have stomach problems (such as heartburn, upset stomach, or stomach pain) that persist or recur, or if you have ulcers or bleeding problems, unless directed by a doctor. If sleepless-

ness persists continuously for more than 2 weeks, consult your doctor. Insomnia may be a symptom of serious underlying medical illness. Do not take this product, unless directed by a doctor, if you have a breathing problem such as emphysema or chronic bronchitis, or if you have glaucoma or difficulty in urination due to enlargement of the prostate gland. Avoid alcoholic beverages while taking this product. Do not take this product if you are taking sedatives or tranquilizers, without first consulting your doctor. Keep this and all drugs out of the reach of children. In case of accidental overdose, seek professional assistance or contact a poison control center immediately. As with any drug, if you are pregnant or nursing a baby, seek the advice of a health professional before using this product. IT IS ESPECIALLY IMPORTANT NOT TO USE ASPIRIN DURING THE LAST 3 MONTHS OF PREGNANCY UNLESS SPECIFICALLY DIRECTED TO DO SO BY A DOCTOR BECAUSE IT MAY CAUSE PROBLEMS IN THE UNBORN CHILD OR COMPLICATIONS DURING DELIVERY.

Drug Interaction Precaution: Do not take this product if you are taking a prescription drug for anticoagulation (thinning the blood), diabetes, gout, or arthritis unless directed by a doctor.

How Supplied: Bottles of 40 caplets with a child-resistant safety closure. Store at room temperature.

Shown in Product Identification Guide, page 504

BACTINE® Antiseptic-Anesthetic
First Aid Liquid

Product Information

Active Ingredients: Benzalkonium chloride 0.13% w/w, and lidocaine HCl 2.5% w/w.

Inactive Ingredients: Edetate disodium, fragrances, octoxynol 9, propylene glycol, purified water.

Indications: First aid to help prevent bacterial contamination or skin infection and for the temporary relief of pain and itching in minor cuts, scrapes, and burns.

Directions: For adults and children 2 years of age and older. Clean the affected area. Apply a small amount of this product on the area 1 to 3 times daily. May be covered with a sterile bandage. If bandaged, let dry first. Children under 2 years of age: consult a doctor.

Warnings: For External Use Only. Do not use in the eyes or apply over large areas of the body. In case of deep or puncture wounds, animal bites, or serious burns, consult a doctor. Stop use and consult a doctor if the condition worsens or if symptoms persist for more than seven days or clear up and occur again within a few days. Do not use for longer than one

Continued on next page

Bactine—Cont.

week unless directed by a doctor. Do not use in large quantities, particularly over raw surfaces or blistered areas. Keep this and all drugs out of the reach of children. In case of accidental ingestion, seek professional assistance or contact a Poison Control Center immediately.

Storage: Store between 15°C to 25°C (59°F to 77°F). Keep from freezing.

How Supplied: Bactine Antiseptic-Anesthetic First Aid Liquid is available as 2 oz, 4 oz, and 16 oz. liquid with child resistant closures and 3.5 oz. pump spray.

Shown in Product Identification Guide, page 503

DOMEBORO® Astringent Solution (Powder Packets)

DOMEBORO® Astringent Solution (Effervescent Tablets)

Active Ingredients: When dissolved in water and ready for use, the active ingredient is aluminum acetate resulting from the reaction of calcium acetate (938 mg) and aluminum sulfate (1191 mg) for powder packets, and calcium acetate (604 mg) and aluminum sulfate (878 mg) for the effervescent tablets. The resulting astringent solution is buffered to an acid pH.

Inactive Ingredients: DOMEBORO Astringent Solution (Powder Packets) Dextrin

DOMEBORO Astringent Solution (Effervescent Tablets) Dextrin, Polyethylene Glycol, Sodium Bicarbonate

Directions: One tablet dissolved in 12 ounces of water or one packet dissolved in 16 ounces of water makes a modified Burrow's Solution approximately equivalent to a 1:40 dilution; two packets or two tablets, a 1:20 dilution; four packets or four tablets, a 1:10 dilution. For powder packets dissolve 1 or 2 packets, or for effervescent tablets 1 or 2 tablets in water and stir the solution until fully dissolved. Do not strain or filter the solution. Can be used as a compress, wet dressing or as a soak. AS A COMPRESS OR WET DRESSING: Saturate a clean, soft, white cloth (such as a diaper or torn sheet) in the solution; gently squeeze and apply loosely to the affected area. Saturate the cloth in the solution every 15 to 30 minutes and apply to the affected area. Discard solution after each use. Repeat as often as necessary. AS A SOAK: Soak affected area in the solution for 15 to 30 minutes. Discard solution after each use. Repeat 3 times a day.

Indications: For temporary relief of minor skin irritations due to poison ivy, poison oak, poison sumac, insect bites, athlete's foot or rashes caused by soaps, detergents, cosmetics or jewelry.

Warnings: If condition worsens or symptoms persist for more than 7 days discontinue use of the product and consult a doctor. For external use only. Avoid contact with the eyes. Do not cover compress or wet dressing with plastic to prevent evaporation. Keep this and all drugs out of the reach of children. In case of accidental ingestion, seek professional assistance or contact a Poison Control Center immediately.

How Supplied: Boxes of 12 or 100 effervescent tablets or powder packets.

Shown in Product Identification Guide, page 504

FEMSTAT® 3
Antifungal Vaginal Cream with 3 Disposable Applicators

Indications: For the treatment of vaginal yeast (Candida) infection.

Active Ingredient: Butoconazole Nitrate (2%).

Inactive Ingredients: Cetyl Alcohol, Glyceryl Stearate (and) PEG-100 Stearate, Methylparaben and Propylparaben (perservatives), Mineral Oil, Polysorbate 60, Propylene Glycol, Sorbitan Monosterate, Stearyl Alcohol and Water (purified).

Femstat® 3 is the first 3-day medicine available without a prescription for the treatment of vaginal yeast (Candida) infections. Femstat 3 is clinically proven to cure most yeast infections with only 3 days of treatment. Available in convenient pre-filled or disposable applicators.

IF THIS IS THE FIRST TIME YOU HAVE HAD VAGINAL ITCH AND DISCOMFORT, CONSULT YOUR DOCTOR. IF YOU HAVE HAD A DOCTOR DIAGNOSE A VAGINAL YEAST INFECTION BEFORE AND HAVE THE SAME SYMPTOMS NOW, USE FEMSTAT 3 AS DIRECTED FOR 3 CONSECUTIVE DAYS.

Before using, read the enclosed educational pamphlet.

Directions: Fill the applicator and insert one applicatorful of cream into the vagina for 3 days in a row, preferably at bedtime. Dispose of applicator after use.

Warnings:

- Do not use if you have abdominal pain, fever, or foul-smelling discharge. Contact your doctor immediately.
- If your infection isn't gone in three days, you may have a condition other than a yeast infection or you may need to use more medication. Consult your doctor. If your symptoms return within two months or if you think you have been exposed to the human immunodeficiency virus (HIV) that causes AIDS, consult your doctor immediately. Recurring infections may be a sign of pregnancy or a serious condition, such as AIDS or diabetes.
- Do not use this product if you are pregnant or think you may be pregnant, have diabetes, a positive HIV test or AIDS. Consult Your Doctor.

- Do not rely on condoms or diaphragms to prevent sexually transmitted diseases or pregnancy while using this product. This product may damage condoms and diaphragms and may cause them to fail. Use another method of birth control to prevent pregnancy while using this product.
- Do not use tampons while using this medicine.
- Do not use in girls under 12 years of age.
- Keep this and all drugs out of the reach of children.
- For vaginal use only. Do not use in eyes or take by mouth. In case of accidental ingestion, seek professional assistance or contact a Poison Control Center immediately.

How Supplied: One 20g (0.7 oz) tube of vaginal cream and 3 disposable applicators.

Avoid excessive heat above 30°C (86°F) and avoid freezing.

Distributed by
Bayer Corporation
Consumer Care Division
Morristown, NJ 09760 USA
Consumer Questions or Comments
Call 1-800-353-3343
www.Bayercare.com

Shown in Product Identification Guide, page 504

FEMSTAT® 3
Antifungal Vaginal Cream in 3 Pre-filled Applicators

Indications: For the treatment of vaginal yeast (Candida) infection.

Active Ingredient: Butoconazole Nitrate (2%).

Inactive Ingredients: Cetyl Alcohol, Glyceryl Stearate (and) PEG-100 Stearate, Methylparaben and Propylparaben (preservatives), Mineral Oil, Polysorbate 60, Propylene Glycol, Sorbitan Monostearate, Stearyl Alcohol and Water (purified).

Femstat® 3 is the first 3-day medicine available without a prescription for the treatment of vaginal yeast (Candida) infections. Femstat 3 is clinically proven to cure most yeast infections with only 3 days of treatment. Available in convenient pre-filled or disposable applicators.

IF THIS IS THE FIRST TIME YOU HAVE HAD VAGINAL ITCH AND DISCOMFORT, CONSULT YOUR DOCTOR. IF YOU HAVE HAD A DOCTOR DIAGNOSE A VAGINAL YEAST INFECTION BEFORE AND HAVE THE SAME SYMPTOMS NOW, USE FEMSTAT 3 AS DIRECTED FOR 3 CONSECUTIVE DAYS.

Before using, read the enclosed educational pamphlet.

Directions: Insert one applicatorful of cream into the vagina for 3 days in a row, preferably at bedtime. Dispose of applicator after use.

Warnings:

- **Do not use if you have abdominal pain, fever, or foul-smelling discharge. Contact your doctor immediately.**
- **If your infection isn't gone in three days, you may have a condition other than a yeast infection or you may need to use more medication. Consult your doctor. If your symptoms return within two months or if you think you have been exposed to the human immunodeficiency virus (HIV) that causes AIDS, consult your doctor immediately. Recurring infections may be a sign of pregnancy or a serious condition, such as AIDS or diabetes.**
- **Do not use this product if you are pregnant or think you may be pregnant, have diabetes, a positive HIV test or AIDS. Consult Your Doctor.**
- **Do not rely on condoms or diaphragms to prevent sexually transmitted diseases or pregnancy while using this product. This product may damage condoms and diaphragms and may cause them to fail. Use another method of birth control to prevent pregnancy while using this product.**
- **Do not use tampons while using this medicine.**
- **Do not use in girls under 12 years of age.**
- **Keep this and all drugs out of the reach of children.**
- **For vaginal use only. Do not use in eyes or take by mouth. In case of accidental ingestion, seek professional assistance or contact a Poison Control Center immediately.**

How Supplied: Three disposable applicators pre-filled to deliver 5g vaginal cream (butoconazole nitrate 2%).
Avoid excessive heat above 30°C (86°F) and avoid freezing.
Distributed by
Bayer Corporation
Consumer Care Division
Morristown, NJ 07960 USA
Consumer Questions or Comments
Call 1-800-353-3343
www.Bayercare.com
Shown in Product Identification Guide, page 504

Maximum Strength
MIDOL® Teen
Pain & Multi-Symptom Menstrual Relief
Aspirin Free/Caffeine Free

Active Ingredients: Each caplet contains Acetaminophen 500 mg and Pamabrom 25 mg.

Inactive Ingredients: Croscarmellose Sodium, D&C Red #7 Lake, FD&C Blue #2 Lake, Hydroxypropyl Methylcellulose, Magnesium Stearate, Microcrystalline Cellulose, Starch, Titanium Dioxide and Triacetin.

Provides maximum strength relief of: cramps, bloating, water-weight gain, headaches, backaches, and muscular aches and pains.

Directions: Adults and children 12 years and over: Take 2 caplets with water. Repeat every 4 hours, as needed, up to a maximum of 8 caplets per day. Under age 12: Consult your doctor.

Warnings: Do not use for more than 10 days unless directed by a doctor. If pain persists for more than 10 days, consult a doctor immediately. Keep this and all drugs out of the reach of children. In case of accidental overdose, immediate medical attention is essential for adults as well as for children even if you do not notice any signs or symptoms. As with any drug, if you are pregnant or nursing a baby, seek the advice of a health professional before using this product.

How Supplied: Caplets-White capsule-shaped caplets available in packages of 24 caplets containing 3 blisters of 8 caplets each.
Child-resistant blisters on packages of 24 caplets.
Shown in Product Identification Guide, page 504

Maximum Strength
MIDOL® Menstrual
Pain & Multi-Symptom Menstrual Relief
Aspirin Free

Active Ingredients: Each caplet or gelcap contains Acetaminophen 500 mg, Caffeine 60 mg and Pyrilamine Maleate 15 mg.

Inactive Ingredients: Caplets—Croscarmellose Sodium, FD&C Blue #2, Hydroxypropyl Methylcellulose, Magnesium Stearate, Microcrystalline Cellulose, Pregelatinized Starch and Triacetin.
Gelcaps—Croscarmellose Sodium, D&C Red #33 Lake, EDTA Sodium, FD&C Blue #1 Lake, Gelatin, Glycerin, Hydroxypropyl Methylcellulose, Iron Oxide, Magnesium Stearate, Microcrystalline Cellulose, Starch, Stearic Acid, Titanium Dioxide, Triacetin.
Provides maximum strength relief of: cramps, bloating, water-weight gain, headaches, backaches, muscular aches and fatigue.

Directions: Adults and children 12 years and over: Take 2 caplets or gelcaps with water. Repeat every 4 hours, as needed, up to a maximum of 8 caplets or gelcaps per day. Under age 12: Consult your doctor.

Warnings: Do not use for more than 10 days unless directed by a doctor. If pain persists for more than 10 days, consult a doctor immediately. May cause drowsiness; alcohol, sedatives and tranquilizers may increase drowsiness. Avoid alcoholic beverages while taking this product. Do not take this product if you are taking sedatives or tranquilizers without first consulting your doctor. Use caution when driving or operating machinery. May cause excitability, especially in children. The recommended dose of this product contains about as much caffeine as a cup of coffee. Limit the use of caffeine-containing medications, foods, or beverages while taking this product because too much caffeine may cause nervousness, irritability, sleeplessness, and occasionally, rapid heartbeat. Do not take this product, unless directed by a doctor, if you have a breathing problem such as emphysema or chronic bronchitis or if you have glaucoma or difficulty in urination due to enlargement of the prostate gland. Keep this and all drugs out of reach of children. In case of accidental overdose, immediate medical attention is essential for adults as well as for children even if you do not notice any signs or symptoms. As with any drug, if you are pregnant or nursing a baby, seek the advice of a health professional before using this product.

How Supplied: Caplets-White capsule-shaped caplets available in packages of 24 caplets containing 3 blisters of 8 caplets each, and 8 caplet containing 1 blister of 8 caplets each. Child-resistant blisters on packages of 24 caplets.
Gelcaps—Dark/light blue capsule-shaped gelcaps available in packages of 24 gelcaps containing 3 blisters of 8 gelcaps. Child-resistant blisters on packages of 24 gelcaps.
Shown in Product Identification Guide, page 504

Maximum Strength
MIDOL® PMS
Pain & Premenstrual Symptom Relief
Aspirin Free/Caffeine Free

Active Ingredients: Each caplet or gelcap contains Acetaminophen 500 mg, Pamabrom 25 mg and Pyrilamine Maleate 15 mg.

Inactive Ingredients: Caplets—Croscarmellose Sodium, D&C Red #30, D&C Yellow #10, Hydroxypropyl Methylcellulose, Magnesium Stearate, Microcrystalline Cellulose, Pregelatinized Starch and Triacetin.
Gelcaps—Croscarmellose Sodium, D&C Red #27 Lake, EDTA Disodium, FD&C Blue #1, FD&C Red #40 Lake, Gelatin, Glycerin, Hydroxypropyl Methylcellulose, Iron Oxide, Magnesium Stearate, Microcrystalline Cellulose, Starch, Stearic Acid, Titanium Dioxide, Triacetin.
Provides maximum strength relief of: bloating, water-weight gain, cramps, headaches and backaches.

Directions: Adults and children 12 years and over: Take 2 caplets or gelcaps with water. Repeat every 4 hours, as needed, up to a maximum of 8 caplets or gelcaps per day. Under age 12: Consult your doctor.

Continued on next page

Midol PMS—Cont.

Warnings: Do not use for more than 10 days unless directed by a doctor. If pain persists for more than 10 days, consult a doctor immediately. May cause drowsiness; alcohol, sedatives and tranquilizers may increase drowsiness. Avoid alcoholic beverages while taking this product. Do not take this product if you are taking sedatives or tranquilizers without first consulting your doctor. Use caution when driving or operating machinery. May cause excitability especially in children. Do not take this product, unless directed by a doctor, if you have a breathing problem such as emphysema or chronic bronchitis or if you have glaucoma or difficulty in urination due to enlargement of the prostate gland. Keep this and all drugs out of the reach of children. In case of accidental overdose, immediate medical attention is essential for adults as well as for children even if you do not notice any signs or symptoms. As with any drug, if you are pregnant or nursing a baby, seek the advice of a health professional before using this product.

How Supplied: Caplets-White capsule-shaped caplets available in packages of 24 caplets containing 3 blisters of 8 caplets each, and 8 caplets containing 1 blister of 8 caplets each. Child-resistant blisters on packages of 24 caplets. Gelcaps—Dark/light pink capsule-shaped gelcaps available in packages of 24 gelcaps containing 3 blisters of 8 gelcaps. Child-resistant blisters on packages of 24 gelcaps.

Shown in Product Identification Guide, page 504

MYCELEX 3
ANTIFUNGAL VAGINAL CREAM WITH 3 DISPOSABLE APPLICATORS

Indications: For the treatment of vaginal yeast (Candida) infection.

Active Ingredient: Butoconazole Nitrate (2%).

Inactive Ingredients: Cetyl Alcohol, Glyceryl Stearate (and) PEG-100 Stearate, Methylparaben and Propylparaben (preservatives), Mineral Oil, Polysorbate 60, Propylene Glycol, Sorbitan Monostearate, Stearyl Alcohol and Water (purified).

Mycelex 3 is clinically proven to cure most yeast infections with only 3 days of treatment. Available with disposable applicators.

Precautions: IF THIS IS THE FIRST TIME YOU HAVE HAD VAGINAL ITCH AND DISCOMFORT, CONSULT YOUR DOCTOR. IF YOU HAVE HAD A DOCTOR DIAGNOSE A VAGINAL YEAST INFECTION BEFORE AND HAVE THE SAME SYMPTOMS NOW, USE Mycelex 3® AS DIRECTED FOR 3 CONSECUTIVE DAYS.
Before using, read the enclosed educational pamphlet.

Directions: Fill the applicator and insert one applicator full of cream into vagina for three days in a row, preferably at bedtime. Dispose of applicator after use.

Warnings:

- Do not use if you have abdominal pain, fever, or foul-smelling discharge. Contact your doctor immediately.
- If your infection isn't gone in three days, you may have a condition other than a yeast infection or you may need to use more medication. Consult your doctor. If your symptoms return within two months or if you think you have been exposed to the human immunodeficiency virus (HIV) that causes AIDS, consult your doctor immediately. Recurring infections may be a sign of pregnancy or a serious condition, such as AIDS or diabetes.
- Do not use this product if you are pregnant or think you may be pregnant, have diabetes, a positive HIV test or AIDS. Consult Your Doctor.
- Do not rely on condoms or diaphragms to prevent sexually transmitted diseases or pregnancy while using this product. This product may damage condoms and diaphragms and may cause them to fail. Use another method of birth control to prevent pregnancy while using this product.
- Do not use tampons while using this medicine.
- Do not use in girls under 12 years of age.
- Keep this and all drugs out of the reach of children.
- For vaginal use only. Do not use in eyes or take by mouth. In case of accidental ingestion, seek professional assistance or contact a Poison Control Center immediately.

Note: The active ingredient in this product (butoconazole nitrate 2%) is not the same active ingredient found in Mycelex®-7.

How Supplied: One 20g (0.7 oz) tube of vaginal cream and 3 disposable applicators.
Avoid excessive heat above 30°C (86°F) and avoid freezing.
See end panel of carton and tube crimp for lot number and expiration date.
Distributed by
Bayer Corporation
Consumer Care Division
Morristown, NJ 07960 USA
Consumer Questions or Comments
Call 1-800-800-4793
Weekdays 9am-5pm (ET)
www.Bayercare.com
Shown in Product Identification Guide, page 505

MYCELEX®-3
Antifungal Vaginal Cream in 3 Pre-filled Applicators

Indications: For the treatment of vaginal yeast (Candida) infection.

Active Ingredients: Butoconazole Nitrate (2%).

Inactive Ingredients: Cetyl Alcohol, Glyceryl Stearate (and) PEG-100 Stearate, Methylparaben and Propylparaben (preservatives), Mineral Oil, Polysorbate 60, Propylene Glycol, Sorbitan Monostearate, Stearyl Alcohol and Water (purified).
MYCELEX®-3 is clinically proven to cure most yeast infections with only 3 days of treatment. Available in convenient pre-filled or disposable applicators. IF THIS IS THE FIRST TIME YOU HAVE HAD VAGINAL ITCH AND DISCOMFORT, CONSULT YOUR DOCTOR. IF YOU HAVE HAD A DOCTOR DIAGNOSE A VAGINAL YEAST INFECTION BEFORE AND HAVE THE SAME SYMPTOMS NOW. USE MYCELEX®-3 AS DIRECTED FOR 3 CONSECUTIVE DAYS.
Before using, read the enclosed educational pamphlet.

Directions: Insert one applicatorful of cream into the vagina for 3 days in a row, preferably at bedtime. Dispose of applicator after use.

Warnings:

- Do not use if you have abdominal pain, fever, or foul-smelling discharge. Contact your doctor immediately.
- If your infection isn't gone in three days, you may have a condition other than a yeast infection or you may need to use more medication. Consult your doctor. If your symptoms return within two months or if you think you have been exposed to the human immunodeficiency virus (HIV) that causes AIDS, consult your doctor immediately. Recurring infections may be a sign of pregnancy or a serious condition, such as AIDS or diabetes.
- Do not use this product if you are pregnant or think you may be pregnant, have diabetes, a positive HIV test or AIDS. Consult Your Doctor.
- Do not rely on condoms or diaphragms to prevent sexually transmitted diseases or pregnancy while using this product. This product may damage condoms and diaphragms and may cause them to fail. Use another method of birth control to prevent pregnancy while using this product.
- Do not use tampons while using this medicine.
- Do not use in girls under 12 years of age.
- Keep this and all drugs out of the reach of children.
- For vaginal use only. Do not use in eyes or take by mouth. In case of accidental ingestion, seek professional assistance or contact a Poison Control Center immediately.

How Supplied: Three disposable applicators pre-filled to deliver 5 g vaginal cream (butoconazole nitrate 2%).

Avoid excessive heat above 30°C (86°F) and avoid freezing.
Distributed by
Bayer Corporation
Consumer Care Division
Morristown, NJ 07960 USA
Consumer Questions or Comments
Call 1-800-353-3343
www.Bayercare.com
Shown in Product Identification Guide, page 505

MYCELEX-7®
VAGINAL CREAM ANTIFUNGAL

Active Ingredient: Clotrimazole 1%

Inactive Ingredients: Benzyl alcohol, cetostearyl alcohol, cetyl esters wax, octyldodecanol, polysorbate 60, purified water, sorbitan monostearate

Indications: For treatment of vaginal yeast (Candida) infection.
Cures most vaginal yeast infections. MYCELEX®-7 Antifungal Vaginal Cream can kill the yeast that may cause vaginal infection. It is greaseless and does not stain clothes.
IF THIS IS THE **FIRST** TIME YOU HAVE HAD VAGINAL ITCH AND DISCOMFORT, CONSULT YOUR DOCTOR. IF YOU HAVE HAD A DOCTOR DIAGNOSE A VAGINAL YEAST INFECTION BEFORE AND HAVE THE SAME SYMPTOMS NOW, USE THIS CREAM AS DIRECTED FOR 7 CONSECUTIVE DAYS.

**WARNING: DO NOT USE IF YOU HAVE ABDOMINAL PAIN, FEVER, OR FOUL-SMELLING DISCHARGE. CONTACT YOUR DOCTOR IMMEDIATELY. IF YOU DO NOT IMPROVE IN 3 DAYS OR IF YOU DO NOT GET WELL IN 7 DAYS, YOU MAY HAVE A CONDITION OTHER THAN A YEAST INFECTION. CONSULT YOUR DOCTOR. If your symptoms return within two months or if you have infections that do not clear up easily with proper treatment, consult your doctor. You could be pregnant or there could be a serious underlying medical cause for your infections, including diabetes or a damaged immune system (including damage from infection with HIV-the virus that causes AIDS). (PLEASE READ PATIENT PACKAGE PAMPHLET.)
Do not use during pregnancy except under the advice and supervision of a doctor. Do not use tampons while using this medication. Keep this and all drugs out of the reach of children. In case of accidental ingestion, seek professional assistance or contact a Poison Control Center immediately. NOT FOR USE IN CHILDREN LESS THAN 12 YEARS OF AGE.**
If you have any questions about Mycelex-7 or vaginal yeast infection contact your physician.
Store at room temperature between 2° and 30°C (36° and 86°F)

Dosage and Administration: Before using, read the enclosed pamphlet.
Directions: Fill the applicator and insert one applicator full of cream into the vagina, preferably at bedtime. Repeat this procedure daily for 7 consecutive days.

How Supplied: 1.5 oz. (45g) tube and applicator. (7-Day Therapy)
Consumer Questions or Comments
Call 1-800-800-4793
8:30-5:00 EST M-F
www.Bayercare.com
Shown in Product Identification Guide, page 505

MYCELEX®-7 VAGINAL ANTIFUNGAL CREAM WITH 7 DISPOSABLE APPLICATORS
Cures Most Vaginal Yeast Infections

Active Ingredient: Clotrimazole 1%.

Inactive Ingredients: Benzyl alcohol, cetostearyl alcohol, cetyl esters wax, octyldodecanol, polysorbate 60, purified water, sorbitan monostearate.
MYCELEX®-7 Antifungal Vaginal Cream can kill the yeast that may cause vaginal infection. It is greaseless and does not stain clothes.

Indications: For treatment of vaginal yeast (Candida) infection.
IF THIS IS THE **FIRST** TIME YOU HAVE HAD VAGINAL ITCH AND DISCOMFORT, CONSULT YOUR DOCTOR. IF YOU HAVE HAD A DOCTOR DIAGNOSE A VAGINAL YEAST INFECTION BEFORE AND HAVE THE SAME SYMPTOMS NOW, USE THIS CREAM AS DIRECTED FOR 7 CONSECUTIVE DAYS.
WARNING: DO NOT USE IF YOU HAVE ABDOMINAL PAIN, FEVER, OR FOUL-SMELLING DISCHARGE. CONTACT YOUR DOCTOR IMMEDIATELY.
Before using, read the enclosed pamphlet.

Directions: Fill the applicator and insert one applicator full of cream into the vagina, preferably at bedtime. Dispose of each applicator after use. Do not flush in toilet. Repeat this procedure daily with a new applicator for 7 consecutive days.
WARNING: IF YOU DO NOT IMPROVE IN 3 DAYS OR IF YOU DO NOT GET WELL IN 7 DAYS, YOU MAY HAVE A CONDITION OTHER THAN A YEAST INFECTION. CONSULT YOUR DOCTOR. If your symptoms return within two months or if you have infections that do not clear up easily with proper treatment, consult your doctor. You could be pregnant or there could be a serious underlying medical cause for your infections, including diabetes or a damaged immune system (including damage from infection with HIV—the virus that causes AIDS). (PLEASE READ PATIENT PACKAGE PAMPHLET.)
Do not use during pregnancy except under the advice and supervision of a

doctor. Do not use tampons while using this medication. Keep this and all drugs out of the reach of children.
In case of accidental ingestion, seek professional assistance or contact a Poison Control Center immediately. NOT FOR USE IN CHILDREN LESS THAN 12 YEARS OF AGE.
If you have any questions about MYCELEX®-7 or vaginal yeast infection, contact your physician.
Store at room temperature between 2° and 30°C (36° and 86°F).

How Supplied: One 45g (1.5 oz.) tube of vaginal cream and 7 applicators (7 day therapy)
Consumer Questions or Comments
Call 1-800-800-4793
8:30–5:00 EST M–F
www.Bayercare.com
Shown in Product Identification Guide, page 505

MYCELEX®-7 Combination-Pack VAGINAL INSERTS & EXTERNAL VULVAR CREAM
• Cures Most Vaginal Yeast Infections
• Relieves Associated External Vulvar Itching and Irritation
MYCELEX®-7 Antifungal Vaginal Inserts and External Vulvar Cream can kill the yeast that may cause vaginal infection. They do not stain clothes.

Active Ingredient:
Inserts: Each insert contains 100 mg clotrimazole
Cream: Clotrimazole 1%

Inactive Ingredients:
Inserts: Corn starch, lactose, magnesium stearate, povidone
Cream: Benzyl alcohol, cetostearyl alcohol, cetyl esters wax, octyldodecanol, polysorbate 60, purified water, sorbitan monostearate

Indications: For treatment of vaginal yeast *(Candida)* infection and the relief of external vulvar itching and irritation associated with vaginal yeast infection.
IF THIS IS THE **FIRST** TIME YOU HAVE HAD VAGINAL OR VULVAR ITCH AND DISCOMFORT, CONSULT YOUR DOCTOR. IF YOU HAVE HAD A DOCTOR DIAGNOSE A VAGINAL YEAST INFECTION BEFORE AND HAVE THE SAME SYMPTOMS NOW, USE THESE INSERTS AND CREAM AS DIRECTED FOR 7 CONSECUTIVE DAYS.

Directions:
Inserts: Unwrap one insert, place it in the applicator, and use the applicator to place the insert into the vagina, preferably at bedtime. Repeat this procedure daily for 7 consecutive days to treat vaginal *(Candida)* yeast infection.
Cream: Squeeze a small amount of cream onto your finger and gently spread the cream onto the irritated area of the vulva. Use once or twice daily for

Continued on next page

Mycelex-7 Combo-Pack—Cont.

up to 7 days as needed to relieve external vulvar itching. THE CREAM SHOULD NOT BE USED FOR VULVAR ITCHING DUE TO CAUSES OTHER THAN A YEAST INFECTION.
WARNING: DO NOT USE IF YOU HAVE ABDOMINAL PAIN, FEVER, OR FOUL-SMELLING DISCHARGE. CONTACT YOUR DOCTOR IMMEDIATELY.
Before using, read the enclosed pamphlet.
IF YOU DO NOT IMPROVE IN 3 DAYS OR IF YOU DO NOT GET WELL IN 7 DAYS, YOU MAY HAVE A CONDITION OTHER THAN A YEAST INFECTION. CONSULT YOUR DOCTOR. If your symptoms return within two months or if you have infections that do not clear up easily with proper treatment, consult your doctor. You could be pregnant or there could be a serious underlying medical cause for your infections, including diabetes or a damaged immune system (including damage from infection with HIV—the virus that causes AIDS). (PLEASE READ ENCLOSED PATIENT PACKAGE PAMPHLET.)
Do not use during pregnancy except under the advice and supervision of a doctor.
Do not use tampons while using this medication.
Keep this and all drugs out of the reach of children. In case of accidental ingestion, seek professional assistance or contact a Poison Control Center immediately.
NOT FOR USE IN CHILDREN LESS THAN 12 YEARS OF AGE.
If you have any questions about MYCELEX®-7 Combination-Pack or vaginal yeast infection, contact your physician.
How Supplied: 7 vaginal inserts and applicator (7-day therapy) and one 7g (0.25 oz.) tube of external vulvar cream.
Store at room temperature between 2° and 30°C (36° and 86°F).
Consumer Questions or Comments
Call 1-800-800-4793
8:30–5:00 EST M-F
www.Bayercare.com
Shown in Product Identification Guide, page 505

NEO-SYNEPHRINE®
Mild Formula, Regular Strength, Extra Strength

Active Ingredients:
Mild Formula—0.25% phenylephrine hydrochloride
Regular Strength—0.5% phenylephrine hydrochloride
Extra Strength—1% phenylephrine hydrochloride

Inactive Ingredients: Benzalkonium Chloride and Thimerosal 0.001% as pre-

servatives, Citric Acid, Purified Water, Sodium Chloride, Sodium Citrate.

Indications: For temporary relief of nasal congestion due to cold, hay fever, or other upper respiratory allergies or association with sinusitis.

Temporary relieves stuffy nose and restores freer breathing through the nose. Helps decongest sinus openings and passages; temporary relieves sinus congestion and pressure.

Directions: For a 0.25% solution (Mild):

Adults and children 6 to under 12 years of age (with adult supervision): 2 or 3 sprays in each nostril not more often than every 4 hours. Children under 6 years of age: consult a doctor.

For a 0.5% solution (Regular):

Adults and children 12 years of age and over: 2 or 3 drops or sprays in each nostril not more often than every 4 hours. Do not give to children under 12 years of age unless directed by a doctor.

For a 1% solution (Extra):

Adults and children 12 years of age and over: 2 or 3 drops or sprays in each nostril not more often than every 4 hours. Do not give to children under 12 years of age unless directed by a doctor.

Warnings:

Do not exceed recommended dosage. This product may cause temporary discomfort such as burning, stinging, sneezing, or an increase in nasal discharge. The use of this container by more than one person may spread infection. Do not use this product for more than 3 days. Use only as directed. Frequent or prolonged use may cause nasal congestion to recur or worsen. If symptoms persist, consult a doctor. Do not use this product if you have (or give this product to a child who has) heart disease, high blood pressure, thyroid disease, diabetes, or difficulty in urination due to enlargement of the prostate gland unless directed by a doctor.

Keep this and all drugs out of the reach of children. As with any drug if you are pregnant or nursing a baby seek the advice of a health professional before using this product.

In case of accidental ingestion, seek professional assistance or contact a poison control center immediately.

Storage:

Store at room temperature. Protect from light. Do not use if solution is brown or contains a precipitate.

How Supplied: Mild Formula (0.25%) in 15 mL spray. Regular Strength (0.5%) in 15 mL drops and spray. Extra Strength (1.0%) in 15 mL drops and spray.

Shown in Product Identification Guide, page 505

NEO-SYNEPHRINE®
**12 Hour
(nasal spray)
12 Hour Extra Moisturizing
(nasal spray)**

Active Ingredient: Oxymetazoline Hydrochloride 0.05%.

Inactive Ingredients: Benzalkonium Chloride and Phenylmercuric Acetate 0.002% as preservatives, Glycerin (Extra Moisturizing), Glycine, Purified Water, Sorbitol and may also contain Sodium Chloride.

Indications: For temporary relief of nasal congestion due to a cold, hay fever, or other upper respiratory allergies or associated with sinusitis. Temporarily relieves stuffy nose and restores freer breathing through the nose. Helps decongest sinus openings and passages; temporarily relieves sinus congestion and pressure.

Directions: Adults and children 6 to under 12 years of age (with adult supervision): 2 or 3 sprays in each nostril not more often than every 10 to 12 hours. Do not exceed 2 doses in any 24-hour period. Children under 6 years of age: consult a doctor.

Warnings: Do not exceed recommended dosage. This product may cause temporary discomfort such as burning, stinging, sneezing, or an increase in nasal discharge. The use of the container by more than one person may spread infection. Do not use this product for more than 3 days. Use only as directed. Frequent or prolonged use may cause nasal congestion to recur or worsen. If symptoms persist, consult a doctor. Do not use this product if you have (or give this product to a child who has) heart disease, high blood pressure, thyroid disease, diabetes, or difficulty in urination due to enlargement of the prostate gland unless directed by a doctor.
Keep this and all drugs out of the reach of children. In case of accidental ingestion, seek professional assistance or contact a Poison Control Center immediately. As with any drug, if you are pregnant or nursing a baby, seek the advice of a health professional before using this product.
Storage:
Store at room temperature. Protect from light. Do not use if solution is brown or contains a precipitate.

How Supplied: *Nasal Spray 12 Hour* — plastic squeeze bottles of 15 ml ($^{1}/_{2}$ fl. oz.); *12 Hour Extra Moisturizing Nasal Spray* — 15 ml ($^{1}/_{2}$ fl. oz).
Shown in Product Identification Guide, page 505

PHILLIPS'® LIQUI-GELS®
Stool Softener Laxative

Active Ingredients (Per Liqui-Gel): Docusate Sodium (100 mg)

Inactive Ingredients: FD&C Blue #2 Aluminum Lake, Gelatin, Glycerin, Methylparaben, Polyethylene Glycol 400, Propylene Glycol, Propylparaben, Sorbitol, Titanium Dioxide.

Phillips' Liqui-Gels are a very low sodium product. Each Liqui-Gel contains 5.2 mg of sodium.

Indications: For the relief of occasional constipation (irregularity). This product generally produces bowel movement within 12 to 72 hours after the first dose.

Action: Phillips'® Milk of Magnesia has provided stimulant-free relief of constipation for over 125 years. Now Phillips' offers stimulant-free Liqui-Gels®. Easy-to-swallow Phillips' Liqui-Gels provide effective relief of occasional constipation and contain the #1 doctor recommended stool softening ingredient. Unlike some other laxatives, *Phillips' Liqui-Gels do not contain the harsh stimulants that can cause pain and cramping.* They work gently by drawing water into the stool making it more comfortable to pass. As with any laxative, your dose should be adjusted within the label directions to meet your own body's needs. Many people find 2 Liqui-Gels to be an effective starting adult dosage. *Phillips' Effective Relief Without Harsh Stimulants.*

Directions: Take Phillips' Liqui-Gels with a full glass (8 oz) of water. Adults and Children 12 years and older: Take 1 to 3 Liqui-Gels daily. Children 2 to under 12 years of age: Take 1 Liqui-Gel daily. Children under 2 years of age: Consult a doctor.

Drug Interaction Precaution: Do not take this product if you are presently taking mineral oil, unless directed by a doctor.

Warnings: Do not use laxative products when abdominal pain, nausea or vomiting are present unless directed by a doctor. If you have noticed a sudden change in bowel habits that persists over a period of 2 weeks, consult a doctor before using a laxative. Laxative products should not be used for a period longer than 1 week, unless directed by a doctor. Rectal bleeding or failure to have a bowel movement after use of a laxative may indicate a serious condition. Discontinue use and consult your doctor. As with any drug, if you are pregnant or nursing a baby, seek the advice of a health professional before using this product. **KEEP THIS AND ALL DRUGS OUT OF THE REACH OF CHILDREN.** In case of accidental overdose, seek professional assistance or contact a poison control center immediately.

Liqui-Gels is a registered trademark of R.P. Scherer Corp.

STORAGE: Store at controlled room temperature (59°–86°F) in a dry place.

How Supplied: Blister packs of 10, 30 and 50 Liqui-Gels.

Shown in Product Identification Guide, page 505

PHILLIPS'® MILK OF MAGNESIA
Laxative/Antacid

Active Ingredient: Magnesium Hydroxide - 400 mg per teaspoon (5 ml).

Inactive Ingredients: *Original Formula* - Purified Water. *Mint Formula* - Flavor, Mineral Oil, Purified Water, Saccharin Sodium. *Cherry Formula* - Carboxymethylcellulose Sodium, Citric Acid, D & C Red #28, Flavor, Glycerine, Microcrystalline Cellulose, Propylene Glycol, Purified Water, Sorbitol, Sugar Xanthan Gum.

Indications: AS A LAXATIVE—To relieve occasional constipation (irregularity). This product generally produces bowel movement in $1/2$ to 6 hours.

AS AN ANTACID—To relieve acid indigestion, sour stomach and heartburn.

Directions: For Laxative Use - Adults and Children 12 years & older: 2–4 tablespoonsful at bedtime or upon arising, followed by a full glass (8 oz.) of liquid. Children 6–11 years: 1–2 tablespoonsful, followed by a full glass (8 oz.) of liquid. Children 2–5 years: 1–3 teaspoonsful, followed by a full glass (8 oz.) of liquid. Children under 2 years: Consult a doctor. SHAKE WELL BEFORE USING. DO NOT USE DOSAGE CUP FOR CHILDREN UNDER 12.

Directions: For Antacid Use - Do not use dosage cup. Adults and Children 12 years & older: 1–3 teaspoonful with a little water, up to four times a day or as directed by a doctor. SHAKE WELL BEFORE USING.

Drug Interaction Precaution: Antacids may interact with certain prescription drugs. If you are presently taking a prescription drug, do not take this product without checking with your doctor or other health professional.

Laxative Warnings: Do not take any laxative if abdominal pain, nausea, vomiting or kidney disease are present unless directed by a doctor. If you have noticed a sudden change in bowel habits persisting for over 2 weeks, consult a doctor before using a laxative. Laxative products should not be used for a period longer than 1 week, unless directed by a doctor. Rectal bleeding or failure to have a bowel movement after use of a laxative may indicate a serious condition. Discontinue use and consult your doctor.

Phillips' Milk of Magnesia is a saline laxative.

Antacid Warnings: Do not take more than the maximum recommended daily dosage in a 24 hour period (See Directions), or use the maximum dosage of this product for than two weeks, or use this product if you have a kidney disease, except under the advice and supervision of a doctor. May have laxative effect.

As with any drug, if you are pregnant or nursing a baby, seek the advice of a health professional before using this product. Keep this and all drugs out of the reach of children. In case of accidental overdose, seek professional assistance or contact a poison control center immediately.

Storage: Keep tightly closed and avoid freezing. This product does not need to be refrigerated.

How Supplied: Phillips' Milk of Magnesia is available in Original, Mint, and Cherry formulas and comes in 4 oz., 12 oz., and 26 oz. bottles. Also available in chewable tablets and concentrated liquid formulas.

Shown in Product Identification Guide, page 505

VANQUISH®
Extra Strength Pain Reliever
Analgesic Caplets

Vanquish Caplets, the extra-strength pain formula with two buffers, is specially shaped for easy swallowing.

Active Ingredients: 227 mg Aspirin, 194 mg Acetaminophen and 33 mg Caffeine per caplet, in a formulation buffered with Aluminum Hydroxide and Magnesium Hydroxide.

Inactive Ingredients: Hydroxypropyl Methylcellulose, Microcrystalline Cellulose, Silicon Dioxide, Starch, Titanium Dioxide, Zinc Stearate. May also contain FD&C Blue #2 Lake, Polyethylene Glycol, Polysorbate 80, Potassium Sorbate, Triacetin, Xanthan Gum.

Store at room temperature.

Indications: Fast, safe, temporary relief of minor aches and pains associated with headaches, colds and flu, backaches, muscle aches, menstrual pain and minor pain of arthritis.

Directions: Adults (12 years and over), take 2 caplets with water every 4 hours, as needed, up to a maximum of 12 caplets in 24 hours or as directed by a doctor. **Children under 12 years,** consult a doctor.

Warnings: Children and teenagers should not use this medicine for chicken pox or flu symptoms before a doctor is consulted about Reye Syndrome, a rare but serious illness reported to be associated with aspirin. Do not take for pain for more than 10 days or for fever for more than 3 days unless directed by a doctor. If pain or fever persists or gets worse, if new symptoms occur or if redness or swelling is present, consult a doctor because these could be signs of a serious condition. Do not take this product if you are allergic to aspirin, have asthma, have stomach problems (such as heartburn, upset stomach or stomach pain) that persist or recur or if you have gastric ulcers or bleeding problems unless directed by a doctor. If ringing in the ears or loss of hearing occurs, consult a doctor before taking any more of this product. Keep

Continued on next page

Vanquish—Cont.

this and all drugs out of the reach of children. In case of accidental overdose, immediate medical attention is essential for adults as well as for children even if you do not notice any signs or symptoms. As with any drug, if you are pregnant or nursing a baby, seek the advice of a health professional before using this product. **IT IS ESPECIALLY IMPORTANT NOT TO USE ASPIRIN DURING THE LAST 3 MONTHS OF PREGNANCY UNLESS SPECIFICALLY DIRECTED TO DO SO BY A DOCTOR BECAUSE IT MAY CAUSE PROBLEMS IN THE UNBORN CHILD OR COMPLICATIONS DURING DELIVERY.**

Drug Interaction Precaution: Do not take this product if you are taking a prescription drug for anticoagulation (thinning of the blood), diabetes, gout, or arthritis unless directed by a doctor.

How Supplied: Bottles of 60 and 100 analgesic caplets.

Shown in Product Identification Guide, page 506

Beutlich LP Pharmaceuticals

**1541 SHIELDS DRIVE
WAUKEGAN, IL 60085-8304**

Direct Inquiries to:
847-473-1100
800-238-8542 in US & Canada
FAX 847–473-1122
www.beutlich.com
e-mail fjb1541@worldnet.att.net

CEO–TWO® EVACUANT SUPPOSITORY

NDC #00283-0763-09

Composition: Each adult rectal suppository contains sodium bicarbonate and potassium bitartrate in a water soluble polyethylene glycol base.

Actions: CEO-TWO suppositories are easy to use, effective and predictable. They will not disturb the homeostasis of the bowel. They are gentle and will not irritate the bowel which often would result in a secondary urge to defecate. CEO-TWO will not cause cramping. CEO-TWO suppositories combine with the natural moisture in the bowel to gently release approximately 175 cc's of carbon dioxide. The slowly released CO_2 distends the rectal ampulla thus stimulating peristalsis. The emollient base allows for easy insertion and lubricates the bowel wall to facilitate passage of feces. Defecation generally occurs within 10 to 30 minutes after insertion of the suppository.

Indications: CEO-TWO is indicated for the relief of constipation in adolescents through geriatrics. It is used effectively in bowel training and maintenance programs. It will provide predictable results prior to lower endoscopic procedures as well as pre and post operative or pre and post partum bowel emptying. CEO-TWO should be used whenever the last 25 cm of the bowel must be evacuated.

Administration and Dosage: One or two suppositories can be used as needed. Moisten CEO-TWO with warm water before inserting. Patient should retain as long as possible. Dosage can be repeated in 4–6 hours if necessary.

Contraindications: As with other enemas or laxatives.

Warnings: Do not use CEO-TWO when abdominal pain, nausea or vomiting are present unless directed by a physician.

How Supplied: In packages of 10, white opaque suppositories. Keep in cool, dry place.
DO NOT REFRIGERATE

HURRICAINE® TOPICAL ANESTHETIC

Composition: HURRICAINE contains 20% benzocaine in a flavored, water soluble polyethylene glycol base.

Action and Indications: HURRICAINE is a topical anesthetic that provides rapid anesthesia on all accessible mucous membrane in 15 to 30 seconds, short duration of 15 minutes, has virtually no systemic absorption, and tastes good. Hurricaine is used as a lubricant and topical anesthetic to facilitate passage of fiberoptic gastroscopes, laryngoscopes, proctoscopes and sigmoidoscopes. In addition, Hurricaine is effective in suppressing the pharyngeal and tracheal gag reflex during the placement of nasogastric tubes. Hurricaine is used to control pain and discomfort during certain gynecological procedures such as IUD insertion, vaginal speculum placement, and as a preinjection anesthesia prior to LEEP procedures and paracervical blocks. Hurricaine is also effective for the temporary relief of pain due to sore throat, stomatitis and mucositis. It is also effective in controlling various types of pain associated with dental procedures and the temporary relief of minor mouth irritations, canker sores and irritation to the mouth and gums caused by dentures or orthodontic appliances.

Contraindications: Patients with a known hypersensitivity to benzocaine should not use HURRICAINE. True allergic reactions are rare.

Adverse Reactions: Methemoglobinemia has been reported following the use of benzocaine on extremely rare occasions. Intravenous methylene blue is the specific therapy for this condition.

**Cautions: DO NOT USE IN THE EYES.
NOT FOR INJECTION.
KEEP THIS AND ALL DRUGS OUT OF THE REACH OF CHILDREN.**

Packaging Available
GEL
1 oz. Jar Fresh Mint NDC #00283-0998-31
1 oz. Jar Wild Cherry NDC #00283-0871-31
1 oz. Jar Pina Colada NDC #00283-0886-31
1 oz. Jar Watermelon NDC #00283-0293-31
1/6 oz. Tube Wild Cherry NDC #00283-0871-75
1/6 oz. Tube Watermelon NDC #00283-0293-75
LIQUID
1 fl. oz. Jar Wild Cherry NDC #00283-0569-31
1 fl. oz. Jar Pina Colada NDC #00283-1886-31
1/6 oz. Tube Wild Cherry NDC #00283-0569-75
.25 ml Dry Handle Swab Wild Cherry 100 Each Per Box NDC #00283-0693-01
.25 ml Dry Handle Swab Wild Cherry 6 Each Per Travel Pack NDC #00283-0693-36
SPRAY
2 oz. Aerosol Wild Cherry NDC #00283-0679-02
SPRAY KIT
2 oz. Aerosol Wild Cherry NDC #00283-0183-02 with 200 Disposable Extension Tubes

---

PERIDIN-C®

Composition: Each orange colored tablet contains 2 popular antioxidants; Vitamin C and Bioflavonoids.
Ascorbic Acid 200 mg.
Hesperidin Complex 150 mg.
Hesperidin Methyl Chalcone 50 mg. F.D. & C. #6.

Dosage: 1 tablet daily or as directed.

How Supplied: In bottles of:
100 tablets NDC #00283-0597-01
500 tablets NDC #00283-0597-05

UNKNOWN DRUG?
Consult the
Product Identification Guide
(Gray Pages)
for full-color photos of
leading over-the-counter
medications

Blairex Laboratories, Inc.

3240 NORTH INDIANAPOLIS
ROAD
P.O. BOX 2127
COLUMBUS, IN 47202-2127

Direct Inquiries to:
Customer Service
(800) 252-4739
FAX (812) 378-1033

For Medical Emergency Contact:
David S. Wilson, M.D.
(800) 252-4739
FAX (812) 378-1033

BRONCHO SALINE®
**0.9% Sodium Chloride Aerosol
for the dilution of bronchodilator
inhalation solutions. Sterile
normal saline for diluting
bronchodilator solutions
for oral inhalation.**

Description: Broncho Saline® is for
patients using bronchodilator solutions
for oral inhalation that require dilution
with sterile normal saline solution. Broncho Saline is a sterile liquid solution consisting of 0.9% sodium chloride for oral
inhalation with a pH of 4.5 to 7.5. Not to
be used for injection.

How Supplied: Broncho Saline®
comes in 90cc (mL) (NDC 50486-078-22)
and 240cc (mL) (NDC 50486-078-23)
Pressurized Containers.
Store between 15–25°C (59–77°F). Keep
out of reach of children. See WARN-
INGS.

NASAL MOIST®
Sodium Chloride 0.65%

Description: Isotonic saline solution
buffered with sodium bicarbonate. Preserved with Benzyl alcohol.

Actions and Uses: Use for dry nasal
membranes caused by chronic sinusitis,
allergy, asthma, dry air, and oxygen therapy. May be used as often as needed.

Directions: Squeeze twice into each
nostril as needed.

How Supplied: 45 mL (1.5 oz.) plastic
squeeze bottle with drop capability,
(NDC 50486-027-01) 15 mL (.5 oz.) plastic squeeze bottle with drop capability
(NDC 50486-027-05) and 15 mL (.5 oz.)
fine mist metered pump (NDC 50486-
027-55).

NASAL MOIST® GEL

Description: Nasal Moist Gel with
aloe vera is designed to relieve dryness
and soreness caused by nasal cannula or
BiPAP/CPAP use. Non-petroleum based,
Nasal Moist Gel treats dry nasal passages caused by chronic sinusitis, allergies, asthma, common colds and dry air.

Directions: Apply in and around your
nose to relieve dryness and soreness. Use
as often as needed.

How Supplied: 1 oz. (28.5g) flip-top
tube (NDC 50486-027-35)

PERTUSSIN® DM EXTRA STRENGTH
Cough Suppressant

Description: Each 5mL (one teaspoon-
ful) contains:
Dextromethorphan Hydrobromide,
USP 15mg

Inactive Ingredients: Carmel, Carboxymethylcellulose Sodium, Citric Acid,
D&C Red No. 33, Flavor, Sorbic Acid,
Sorbitol, Sugar, Purified Water. Contains
4% alcohol.

Indications: Temporarily relieves
cough due to minor throat and bronchial
irritation associated with the common
cold.

Warnings: A persistent cough may be
a sign of a serious condition. If cough persists more than 1 week, tends to recur, or
is accompanied by a fever, rash, or persistent headache, consult a doctor. Do not
take this product for persistent or
chronic cough such as occurs with smoking, asthma, chronic bronchitis, emphysema, or if cough is accompanied by excessive phlegm (mucus) unless directed
by a doctor. As with any drug, if you are
pregnant or nursing a baby, seek the advise of a health professional before using
this product.
KEEP THIS AND ALL DRUGS OUT OF
THE REACH OF CHILDREN, IN CASE
OF ACCIDENTAL OVERDOSE, SEEK
PROFESSIONAL ASSISTANCE OR
CONTACT A POISON CONTROL CEN-
TER IMMEDIATELY.

Drug Interaction Precaution: Do
not use this product if you are taking a
prescription drug containing a monoamine oxidase inhibitor (MAOI) (certain
drugs for depression or psychiatric or
emotional conditions or Parkinson's disease), without first consulting your doctor. If you are uncertain whether your
prescription drug contains an MAOI,
consult a health professional before taking this product.

Directions: Adults and children 12
years of age and older: 2 teaspoonfuls every 6–8 hours as needed. Not to exceed 8
teaspoonfuls in 24 hours. Children 6 to
under 12 years of age: One teaspoonful
every 6–8 hours as needed. Not to exceed
4 teaspoonfuls in 24 hours. Do not administer to children under 6 years of age:
Consult a doctor.

How Supplied: Available in shatter-
resistant bottles of 4 fl. oz. (NDC 50486-
048-20).

PERTUSSIN® CS CHILDREN'S STRENGTH
Cough Suppressant

Description: Each 5mL (one teaspoon-
ful) contains:
Dextromethorphan Hydrobromide,
USP 3.5mg

Inactive Ingredients: Citric Acid, Colors, Flavor, Sorbic Acid, Sorbitol, Sucrose, Purified Water. Alcohol-free.

Indications: Temporarily relieves
cough due to minor throat and bronchial
irritation associated with the common
cold.

Warnings: A persistent cough may be
a sign of a serious condition. If cough persists more than 1 week, tends to recur, or
is accompanied by a fever, rash, or persistent headache, consult a doctor. Do not
take this product for persistent or
chronic cough such as occurs with smoking, asthma, chronic bronchitis, emphysema, or if cough is accompanied by excessive phlegm (mucus) unless directed
by a doctor. As with any drug, if you are
pregnant or nursing a baby, seek the advise of a health professional before using
this product.
KEEP THIS AND ALL DRUGS OUT OF
THE REACH OF CHILDREN, IN CASE
OF ACCIDENTAL OVERDOSE, SEEK
PROFESSIONAL ASSISTANCE OR
CONTACT A POISON CONTROL CEN-
TER IMMEDIATELY.

Drug Interaction Precaution: Do
not give this product to a child who is
taking a prescription drug containing a
monoamine oxidase inhibitor (MAOI)
(certain drugs for depression or psychiatric or emotional conditions or Parkinson's disease), without first consulting
the child's doctor. If you are uncertain
whether your child's prescription drug
contains an MAOI, consult a health professional before giving this product.

Directions: Children 2 to under 6
years of age: 1 teaspoonful. Children 6 to
under 12 years of age: 2 teaspoonfuls.
Adults and children 12 years of age and
older: 4 teaspoonfuls. Repeat every 4
hours as needed. Do not exceed 6 doses in
a 24 hour period. Children under 2 years
of age: Consult a doctor.

How Supplied: Available in shatter-
resistant bottles of 4 fl. oz. (NDC 50486-
048-40).

Blistex Inc.
1800 SWIFT DRIVE
OAK BROOK, IL 60523-1574

Direct Stri-Dex Inquiries To:
Consumer Affairs
1-800-837-1800

For Medical Emergency Contact:
Consumer Affairs
1-800-837-1800

STRI-DEX® Acne Medicated Regular Strength Pads
STRI-DEX® Acne Medicated Maximum Strength Pads
STRI-DEX® Acne Medicated Sensitive Skin Pads
STRI-DEX® Acne Medicated Super Scrub Pads

Indications: For the treatment and prevention of acne. Reduces the number of acne pimples and blackheads, and allows the skin to heal. Helps prevent new acne pimples from forming.

Directions: Cleanse the skin thoroughly. Use the pad to wipe the entire affected area. Repeat with a clean pad as necessary to remove remaining traces of dirt. Use one to three times daily. Because excessive drying of the skin may occur, start with one application daily, then gradually increase to two or three times daily if needed or as directed by a doctor.

Warnings: FOR EXTERNAL USE ONLY. Using other topical acne medications at the same time or immediately following use of this product may increase dryness or irritation of the skin. If this occurs, only one medication should be used unless directed by a doctor. Persons who are sensitive to or have a known allergy to salicylic acid should not use this medication. If irritation or excessive dryness and/or peeling occurs, reduce frequency of use or dosage. If excessive itching, dryness, redness or swelling occurs, discontinue use. If these symptoms persist, consult a doctor promptly. Keep away from eyes, lips, and other mucous membranes. Keep this and all drugs out of the reach of children. In case of accidental ingestion, seek professional assistance or contact a Poison Control Center immediately. Store at room temperature. Flammable. Keep away from extreme heat or flame.

Active Ingredients:
STRI-DEX® Acne Medicated Regular Strength Pads:
Salicylic Acid 0.5%
STRI-DEX® Acne Medicated Maximum Strength Pads:
Salicylic Acid 2%
STRI-DEX® Acne Medicated Sensitive Skin Pads:
Salicylic Acid 0.5%
STRI-DEX® Acne Medicated Super Scrub Pads:
Salicylic Acid 2%

Inactive Ingredients:
STRI-DEX® Acne Medicated Regular Strength Pads:
Citric Acid, Fragrance, Menthol, Purified Water, SD Alcohol 28%, Simethicone Emulsion, Sodium Carbonate, Sodium Dodecylbenzenesulfonate, Sodium Xylenesulfonate.
STRI-DEX® Acne Medicated Maximum Strength Pads:
Ammonium Xylensulfonate, Citric Acid, Fragrance, Menthol, Purified Water, SD Alcohol 44%, Simethicone Emulsion, Sodium Carbonate, Sodium Dodecylbenzenesulfonate.
STRI-DEX® Acne Medicated Sensitive Skin Pads:
Aloe Vera Gel, Citric Acid, Fragrance, Menthol, Purified Water, SD Alcohol 28%, Simethicone Emulsion, Sodium Carbonate, Sodium Dodecylbenzenesulfonate, Sodium Xylenesulfonate.
STRI-DEX® Acne Medicated Super Scrub Pads:
Ammonium Xylenesulfonate, Citric Acid, Fragrance, Menthol, Purified Water, SD Alcohol 54%, Simethicone Emulsion, Sodium Carbonate, Sodium Dodecylbenzenesulfonate, Sodium Lauroyl Sarcosinate.

How Supplied:
STRI-DEX® Regular Strength Pads: jar of 55 pads
STRI-DEX® Maximum Strength Pads: jar of 32, 55 or 90 pads
STRI-DEX® Sensitive Skin Pads: jar of 55 or 90 pads
STRI-DEX® Super Scrub Pads: jar of 55 pads

STRI-DEX® ANTIBACTERIAL CLEANSING BAR (With Triclosan)

Indications: Antibacterial Soap.

Directions: Use STRI-DEX® Antibacterial Cleansing Bar in place of your ordinary soap. For best results use three times daily. Work up an abundant lather with warm water and massage into the skin. Rinse thoroughly and pat dry with a towel.
Use STRI-DEX® Antibacterial Cleansing Bar for facial cleansing as well as in the bath.

Warning: Do not use this product on infants under six months of age. For external use only. Do not get in eyes.

Active Ingredient: Triclosan 1%.

Inactive Ingredients: Acetylated Lanolin Alcohol, Bentonite, Cetyl Acetate, D&C Orange #4, D&C Yellow #10, Glycerin, Pentasodium Pentetate, Potassium Cyclocarboxypropyloleate, Sodium Cocoate and/or Sodium Palm Kernelate, Sodium Tallowate, Sucrose, Tetrasodium Etidronate, Water.

How Supplied: NET WT. 3.5 OZ. (99.2g).

STRI-DEX® Antibacterial Foaming Wash

Active Ingredient: Triclosan 1%

Purpose: Anti-bacterial

Indications: Facial cleansing & elimination of problem-causing bacteria.

Warnings: When using this product: • Use externally only. • Avoid contact with eyes. If contact occurs, immediately flush with water. KEEP OUT OF REACH OF CHILDREN. In case of accidental ingestion seek professional assistance or contact a Poison Control Center immediately.

Directions: Wet face. Dispense a small amount of foam (1 1/2 pumps or about 1.2 grams) into hand. When dispensing, hold bottle in upright position, or with nozzle angled down. Do not dispense with nozzle angled up. Spread on face. Rinse off with water. May be used daily. Do not use this product on infants under 6 months of age.

Also Contains: Aloe Barbadensis Gel, Calendula Officinalis Extract, Chamomile Extract, Cocamidopropyl Betaine, D&C Green #5, D&C Violet #2, Dimethicone Copolyol, Disodium Cocoyl Glutamate and Sodium Cocoyl Glutamate, Glycerin, Menthol, PEG-75 Meadow Foam Oil, Peppermint Oil, Propylene Glycol (and) Diazolidinyl Urea (and) Methylparaben (and) Propylparaben, Purified Water, Simethicone, Sodium Lauroyl Sarcosinate, Spearmint Oil, Sodium PCA, and Witch Hazel Extract.

How Supplied: Pump bottle—NET WT. 6 oz. (177 mL)
©1998 Blistex Inc., Oak Brook, IL 60523 Printed in U.S.A. #71251R.1.

STRI-DEX® Clear Gel

Indications: For the treatment of acne. Reduces the number of blackheads and allows the skin to heal. Helps prevent new acne pimples from forming.

Directions: Clean the skin thoroughly before use. Apply a thin layer to acne pimple areas of face, neck and body 1 to 3 times daily. Because excessive drying of the skin may occur, start with one application daily, then gradually increase to two or three times daily if needed or as directed by a doctor. If bothersome dryness or peeling occurs, reduce application to once a day or every other day.

Warnings: FOR EXTERNAL USE ONLY. Using other topical acne medications at the same time or immediately following use of this product may increase dryness or irritation of the skin. If this occurs, only one medication should be used unless directed by a doctor. Persons who are sensitive to or have a known allergy to salicylic acid should not use this medication. If excessive itching, dryness, redness or swelling occurs, discontinue use. If these symptoms persist, consult a doctor promptly. Keep away from eyes, lips and other mucous membranes. Keep this and all drugs out of the reach of children. In case of accidental ingestion, seek professional assistance or contact a Poison Control Center immediately.

Active Ingredient: Salicylic Acid 2%.

Inactive Ingredients: Purified Water, SD Alcohol 40–2, PVM/MA Decadiene Cross Polymer, Sodium Borate, Sodium Hydroxide, DMDM Hydantoin 55%, Tetrasodium EDTA Dihydrate, Citric Acid Anhydrous.

How Supplied: Tube – NET WT. 1 oz.

Block Drug Company, Inc.
257 CORNELISON AVENUE
JERSEY CITY, NJ 07302

Direct Inquiries to:
Lori Hunt
(201) 434-3000 Ext. 1308

For Medical Emergencies Contact:
Consumer Affairs/Block
(201) 434-3000 Ext. 1308

BALMEX®
Diaper Rash Ointment (Zinc Oxide)
With Aloe & Vitamin E

Description: Balmex® Diaper Rash Ointment with Aloe & Vitamin E contains Zinc Oxide (11.3%) in a unique formulation including Peruvian Balsam suitable for topical application for the treatment and prevention of diaper rash.

Indications and Uses: Balmex helps treat and prevent diaper rash while it moisturizes and nourishes the skin. The zinc oxide based formulation provides a protective barrier on the skin against the natural causes of irritation. Balmex spreads on smooth and wipes off the baby easily, without causing irritation to the affected area. Balmex tactile properties promote compliance amongst mothers, and clinical studies have demonstrated that Balmex is effective in treating diaper rash.

Directions: Change wet and soiled diapers promptly, cleanse the diaper area, and allow to dry. Apply ointment liberally as often as necessary, with each diaper change, especially at bedtime or anytime when exposure to wet diapers may be prolonged.

Warnings: Avoid contact with the eyes. For external use only. If condition worsens or does not improve within 7 days, contact a physician. Keep out of reach of children. If swallowed, get medical help right away.

Active Ingredient: Zinc Oxide (11.3%).

Inactive Ingredients: Aloe Vera Gel, Balsan (Specially Purified Balsam Peru), Beeswax, Benzoic Acid, Dimethicone, Methylparaben, Mineral Oil, Propylparaben, Purified Water, Sodium Borate, Tocopheryl (Vitamin E Acetate).

How Supplied: 2 oz. (57g.) and 4 oz. (113g.) tubes and 16 oz. (454g.) jar.
Shown in Product Identification Guide, page 506

BC® POWDER
ARTHRITIS STRENGTH BC® POWDER
BC® COLD POWDER LINE

Description: BC® POWDER: Active Ingredients: Each powder contains Aspirin 650 mg, Salicylamide 195 mg and Caffeine 33.3 mg. Inactive Ingredients: Dioctylsodium Sulfosuccinate, Fumaric Acid, Lactose and Potassium Chloride. ARTHRITIS STRENGTH BC® POWDER: Active Ingredients: Each powder contains Aspirin 742 mg, Salicylamide 222 mg and Caffeine 38 mg. Inactive Ingredients: Dioctylsodium Sulfosuccinate, Fumaric Acid, Lactose and Potassium Chloride.
BC® ALLERGY SINUS COLD POWDER
Active Ingredients: Aspirin 650 mg, Phenylpropanolamine Hydrochloride 25 mg, and Chlorpheniramine Maleate 4 mg per powder. Inactive Ingredients: Fumaric Acid, Glycine, Lactose, Potassium Chloride, Silica, Sodium Lauryl Sulfate.
BC® SINUS COLD POWDER. Active Ingredients: Aspirin 650 mg and Phenylpropanolamine Hydrochloride 25 mg per powder. Inactive Ingredients: Fumaric Acid, Glycine, Lactose, Potassium Chloride, Silica, Sodium Lauryl Sulfate.

Indications: BC Powder is for relief of simple headache; for temporary relief of minor arthritic pain, neuralgia, neuritis and sciatica; for relief of muscular aches, discomfort and fever of colds; and for relief of normal menstrual pain and pain of tooth extraction.
Arthritis Strength BC Powder is specially formulated to fight occasional minor pain and inflammation of arthritis. Like Original Formula BC, Arthritis Strength BC provides fast temporary relief of minor arthritis pain and inflammation, neuralgia, neuritis and sciatica; relief of muscular aches, discomfort and fever of colds; and pain of tooth extraction.
BC Allergy Sinus Cold Powder is for relief of multiple symptoms such as body aches, fever, nasal congestion, sneezing, running nose, and watery itchy eyes associated with allergy and sinus attacks and the onset of colds. BC Sinus Cold Powder is for relief of such symptoms as body aches, fever, and nasal congestion.

BC Powder®, Arthritis
Strength BC® Powder:

WARNINGS: Children and teenagers should not use this medicine for
chicken pox or flu symptoms before a doctor is consulted about Reye Syndrome, a rare but serious illness reported to be associated with aspirin. Keep this and all medicines out of children's reach. In case of accidental overdose, contact a physician or poison control center immediately.
As with any drug, if you are pregnant or nursing a baby seek the advice of a health professional before using this product.
IT IS ESPECIALLY IMPORTANT NOT TO USE ASPIRIN DURING THE LAST 3 MONTHS OF PREGNANCY UNLESS SPECIFICALLY DIRECTED TO DO SO BY A DOCTOR BECAUSE IT MAY CAUSE PROBLEMS IN THE UNBORN CHILD OR COMPLICATIONS DURING DELIVERY.

Alcohol Warning: If you consume 3 or more alcoholic drinks every day, ask your doctor whether you should take aspirin or other pain relievers/fever reducers. Aspirin may cause stomach bleeding.
This product contains aspirin and should not be taken by individuals who are sensitive to aspirin. If pain persists for more than 10 days, or redness is present, consult a physician immediately.
BC Cold Powder Line:

Warnings: Children and teenagers should not use BC for chicken pox or flu symptoms before a doctor is consulted about Reye Syndrome, a rare but serious illness reported to be associated with aspirin. Keep BC and all medicines out of children's reach. In case of accidental overdose, contact a physician or poison control center immediately.
As with any drug, if you are pregnant or nursing a baby seek the advice of a health professional before using BC.

Alcohol Warning: If you consume 3 or more alcoholic drinks every day, ask your doctor whether you should take aspirin or other pain relievers/fever reducers. Aspirin may cause stomach bleeding.
IT IS ESPECIALLY IMPORTANT NOT TO USE ASPIRIN DURING THE LAST 3 MONTHS OF PREGNANCY UNLESS SPECIFICALLY DIRECTED TO DO SO BY A DOCTOR BECAUSE IT MAY CAUSE PROBLEMS IN THE UNBORN CHILD OR COMPLICATIONS DURING DELIVERY.
Nervousness, dizziness or sleeplessness may occur if recommended dosage is exceeded. If symptoms do not improve within 7 days, or are accompanied by fever that lasts more than 3 days, or if new symptoms occur, consult a physician before continuing use. Do not take BC if you are sensitive to aspirin, or have heart disease, high blood pressure, thyroid disease, diabetes, asthma, glaucoma, emphysema, chronic pulmonary disease, shortness of breath, difficulty in breathing or difficulty in urination due to enlargement of the prostate gland, or

Continued on next page

BC Powders—Cont.

if you are presently taking a prescription antihypertensive or antidepressant drug containing a monoamine oxidase inhibitor unless directed by a doctor. BC Allergy Sinus Cold Powder with antihistamine may cause drowsiness. Avoid alcoholic beverages when taking this product because it may increase drowsiness. Use caution when driving a motor vehicle or operating machinery. May cause excitability, especially in children.

Overdosage: In case of accidental overdosage, contact a physician or poison control center immediately.

Dosage and Administration: BC® Powder, Arthritis Strength BC® Powder, BC® Cold Powder Line:
Place one powder on tongue and follow with liquid. If you prefer, stir powder into glass of water or other liquid. May be used every three to four hours, (every 4 hours for BC® Cold Powder Line) up to 4 powders each 24 hours. For children under 12, consult a physician.

How Supplied: BC Powder: Available in tamper resistant overwrapped envelopes of 2 or 6 powders, as well as tamper resistant boxes of 24 and 50 powders.
Arthritis Strength BC Powder: Available in tamper resistant over wrapped envelopes of 6 powders, and tamper resistant overwrapped boxes of 24 and 50 powders.
BC Cold Powder Line:
Available in tamper-resistant over-wrapped envelopes of 6 powders, as well as tamper-resistant boxes of 12 powders.

GOODY'S
Body Pain Formula Powder

Indications: FOR TEMPORARY RELIEF OF MINOR BODY ACHES & PAINS DUE TO MUSCULAR ACHES, ARTHRITIS & HEADACHES.

Directions: Adults: Place one powder on tongue and follow with liquid, or stir powder into a glass of water or other liquid. May be repeated in 4 to 6 hours. Do not take more than 4 powders in any 24-hour period. Children under 12 years of age: Consult a doctor.

Warnings: Children and teenagers should not use this medicine for chicken pox or flu symptoms before a doctor is consulted about Reye Syndrome, a rare but serious illness reported to be associated with aspirin. As with any drug, if you are pregnant, or nursing a baby, seek the advice of a health professional before using this product.
IT IS ESPECIALLY IMPORTANT NOT TO USE ASPIRIN DURING THE LAST 3 MONTHS OF PREGNANCY UNLESS SPECIFICALLY DIRECTED TO DO SO BY A DOCTOR BECAUSE IT MAY CAUSE PROBLEMS IN THE UNBORN CHILD OR COMPLICATIONS DURING DELIVERY.

Alcohol Warning: If you consume 3 or more alcoholic drinks every day, ask your doctor whether you should take acetaminophen and aspirin or other pain relievers/fever reducers. Acetaminophen and aspirin may cause liver damage and stomach bleeding.
Keep this and all medicines out of the reach of children. In case of accidental overdose, contact a doctor or poison control center immediately.
This product contains aspirin and should not be taken by individuals who are sensitive to aspirin. If pain persists for more than 10 days, or redness is present, consult a physician immediately.

Active ingredients: Each powder contains: 500 mg. aspirin and 325 mg. acetaminophen.

Inactive Ingredients: Each powder contains: Lactose and Potassium Chloride.
DIST. BY: GOODY'S PHARMACEUTICALS
Memphis, TN 38113

GOODY'S®
Extra Strength Headache Powder

Indications: For Temporary Relief of Minor Aches & Pains Due to Headaches, Arthritis, Colds & Fever

Directions: Adults: Place one powder on tongue and follow with liquid or stir powder into a glass of water or other liquid. May be repeated in 4 to 6 hours. Do not take more than 4 powders in any 24-hour period. Children under 12 years of age: Consult a doctor.

Warnings: Children and teenagers should not use this medicine for chicken pox or flu symptoms before a doctor is consulted about Reye Syndrome, a rare but serious illness reported to be associated with aspirin. As with any drug, if you are pregnant, or nursing a baby, seek the advice of a health professional before using this product.
IT IS ESPECIALLY IMPORTANT NOT TO USE ASPIRIN DURING THE LAST 3 MONTHS OF PREGNANCY UNLESS SPECIFICALLY DIRECTED TO DO SO BY A DOCTOR BECAUSE IT MAY CAUSE PROBLEMS IN THE UNBORN CHILD OR COMPLICATIONS DURING DELIVERY.
Alcohol Warning: If you consume 3 or more alcoholic drinks every day, ask your doctor whether you should take acetaminophen and aspirin or other pain relievers/fever reducers. Acetaminophen and aspirin may cause liver damage and stomach bleeding. **Keep this and all medicines out of the reach of children. In case of accidental overdose, contact a doctor or poison control center immediately.**
This product contains aspirin and should not be taken by individuals who are sensitive to aspirin. If pain persists for more than 10 days or redness is present, consult a physician immediately.

Active Ingredients: Each Powder contains 520 mg. aspirin in combination with 260 mg. acetaminophen and 32.5 mg. caffeine.

Inactive Ingredients: Lactose and Potassium Chloride.
Dist. By: GOODY'S PHARMACEUTICALS
Memphis, TN 38113

GOODY'S®
Extra Strength Pain Relief Tablets

Indications: Goody's EXTRA STRENGTH tablets are a specially developed pain reliever that provide fast & effective temporary relief from minor aches & pain due to headaches, arthritis, colds or "flu," muscle strain, backache & menstrual discomfort. It is recommended for temporary relief of toothaches and to reduce fever.

Dosage: Adults: Two tablets with water or other liquid. May be repeated in 4 to 6 hours. Do not take more than 8 tablets in any 24-hour period. Children under 12 years of age: Consult a doctor.

Warnings: Children and teenagers should not use this medicine for chicken pox or flu symptoms before a doctor is consulted about Reye Syndrome, a rare but serious illness reported to be associated with aspirin. As with any drug, if you are pregnant, or nursing a baby, seek the advice of a health professional before using this product. IT IS ESPECIALLY IMPORTANT NOT TO USE ASPIRIN DURING THE LAST 3 MONTHS OF PREGNANCY UNLESS SPECIFICALLY DIRECTED TO DO SO BY A DOCTOR BECAUSE IT MAY CAUSE PROBLEMS IN THE UNBORN CHILD OR COMPLICATIONS DURING DELIVERY. **Alcohol Warning:** If you consume 3 or more alcoholic drinks every day, ask your doctor whether you should take acetaminophen and aspirin or other pain relievers/fever reducers. Acetaminophen and aspirin may cause liver damage and stomach bleeding. **Keep this and all medicines out of the reach of children. In case of accidental overdose, contact a doctor or poison control center immediately.** This product contains aspirin and should not be taken by individuals who are sensitive to aspirin. If pain persists for more than 10 days, or redness is present, consult a physician immediately.

Active Ingredients: Each tablet contains 260 mg. aspirin in combination with 130 mg. acetaminophen and 16.25 mg. caffeine. **Inactive Ingredients:** Corn Starch, Crospovidone, Povidone, Pregelatinized Starch and Stearic Acid.
Dist. By: GOODY'S PHARMACEUTICALS
Memphis, TN 38113

GOODY'S PM® POWDER
For Pain with Sleeplessness

Indications: For temporary relief of occasional headaches and minor aches and pains with accompanying sleeplessness.

Directions: Adults and children 12 years of age and older: One dose (2 powders). Take both powders at bedtime, if needed, or as directed by a doctor. Place powders on tongue and follow with liquid. If you prefer, stir powders into glass of water or other liquid.

Warnings: KEEP THIS AND ALL MEDICINES OUT OF THE REACH OF CHILDREN. IN CASE OF ACCIDENTAL OVERDOSE, CONTACT A DOCTOR OR POISON CONTROL CENTER IMMEDIATELY. PROMPT MEDICAL ATTENTION IS CRITICAL FOR ADULTS AS WELL AS FOR CHILDREN EVEN IF YOU DO NOT NOTICE ANY SIGNS OR SYMPTOMS.

As with any drug, if you are pregnant or nursing a baby, seek the advice of a health professional before using this product. Do not give this product to children under 12 years of age. Do not use for more than 10 days or for fever for more than 3 days unless directed by a doctor. Consult your doctor if symptoms persist or get worse or new ones occur. If sleeplessness persists continuously for more than 2 weeks consult your doctor. Insomnia may be a symptom of serious underlying medical illness. Do not take this product, unless directed by a doctor, if you have a breathing problem such as emphysema or chronic bronchitis or if you have glaucoma or difficulty in urination due to enlargement of the prostate gland. **Do Not Use** with any other product containing diphenhydramine, including one applied topically. Avoid alcoholic beverages while taking this product. Do not use this product if you are taking sedatives or tranquilizers without first consulting your doctor. **Alcohol Warning:** If you consume 3 or more alcoholic drinks every day, ask your doctor whether you should take acetaminophen or other pain relievers/fever reducers. Acetaminophen may cause liver damage.

Caution: This product will cause drowsiness. Do not drive a motor vehicle or operate machinery after use.

Active Ingredients: Each powder contains 500 mg. Acetaminophen and 38 mg. Diphenhydramine Citrate.

Inactive Ingredients: Citric Acid, Docusate Sodium, Fumaric Acid, Glycine, Lactose, Magnesium Stearate, Potassium Chloride, Silica Gel, Sodium Citrate Dihydrate.
Dist. by: Goody's Pharmaceuticals, Memphis, TN 38113

NATURE'S REMEDY®
Nature's Gentle Laxative

Description: Nature's Remedy® is a stimulant laxative with two natural active ingredients, Cascara Sagrada and Aloe, that gently stimulate the body's natural function.

Indications: For relief of occasional constipation. Nature's Remedy tablets generally produce bowel movement in 6 to 12 hours.

Directions: Adults and children 15 years of age and over: Swallow 2 tablets daily along with a full glass of water. **Children 8 to 15 years of age:** 1 tablet daily along with a full glass of water, or as directed by a physician; **Children under 8 years of age:** Consult a physician.

Warnings: Keep this and all drugs out of the reach of children. Do not use laxative products when abdominal pain, nausea, or vomiting are present unless directed by a doctor. If you have noticed a sudden change in bowel habits that persists over a period of 2 weeks, consult a doctor before using a laxative. Laxative products should not be used for a period longer than 1 week unless directed by a doctor. Rectal bleeding or failure to have a bowel movement after use of a laxative may indicate a serious condition. Discontinue use and consult your doctor. In case of accidental overdose, seek professional assistance or contact a Poison Control Center immediately. As with any drug, if you are pregnant or nursing a baby, seek the advice of a health professional before using this product.

Store at room temperature, avoid excessive heat (greater than 100°F) or high humidity.

Active Ingredients: Each tablet contains Cascara Sagrada 150 mg, and Aloe 100 mg.

Inactive Ingredients: Calcium Stearate FD&C Blue #2, FD&C Yellow #6, Hydroxypropyl Cellulose, Hydroxypropyl Methylcellulose, Lactose, Microcrystalline Cellulose, Polyethylene Glycol, Titanium Dioxide.

How Supplied: Beige, film-coated tablets with foil-backed blister packaging in boxes of 15, 30 and 60.

Shown in Product Identification Guide, page 506

Maximum Strength
NYTOL® QUICKGELS® SOFTGELS

Indications: For relief of occasional sleeplessness.

Directions: Adults and children 12 years of age and over: oral dosage is one softgel (50 mg) at bedtime if needed, or as directed by a doctor.

Warnings: Do not give to children under 12 years of age. If sleeplessness persists continuously for more than two weeks, consult your doctor. Insomnia may be a symptom of serious underlying medical illness. **Do not take this product, unless directed by a doctor, if** you have a breathing problem such as emphysema or chronic bronchitis, or if you have glaucoma or difficulty in urination due to enlargement of the prostate gland. Do not use with any other product containing diphenhydramine, including one applied topically. Avoid alcoholic beverages while taking this product. Do not take this product if you are taking sedatives or tranquilizers, without first consulting your doctor. In case of accidental overdose, seek professional assistance or contact a Poison Control Center immediately. As with any drug, if you are pregnant or nursing a baby, seek the advice of a health professional before using this product. Keep this and all drugs out of the reach of children.

Drug Interactions: Alcohol and other drugs which cause CNS depression will heighten the depressant effect of this product. Monoamine oxidase (MAO) inhibitors will prolong and intensify the anticholinergic effects of antihistamines.

Symptoms and Treatment of Oral Overdosage: In adults overdose may cause CNS depression resulting in hypnosis and coma. In children CNS hyperexcitability may follow sedation; the stimulant phase may bring tremor, delirium and convulsions. Gastrointestinal reactions may include dry mouth, appetite loss, nausea and/or vomiting. Respiratory distress and cardiovascular complications (hypotension) may be evident. Treatment includes inducing emesis and controlling symptoms.

Active Ingredient: Diphenhydramine Hydrochloride 50 mg per softgel.

Inactive Ingredients: Edible Ink, Gelatin, Glycerin, Polyethylene Glycol, Purified Water, Sorbitol.

How Supplied: Available in packages of 8 and 16 softgels.

NYTOL® NATURAL
Homeopathic Nighttime Sleep-Aid

Active Ingredients: Each tablet contains equal parts of Ignatia amara 3X (St. Ignatius' Bean); Aconitum radix 6X (Aconite Root).

Inactive Ingredients: Lactose, Magnesium Stearate.

Indications: Temporary relief of occasional sleeplessness.

Warnings: Do not give to children under 12 years of age. If sleeplessness persists continuously for more than two weeks, consult your doctor. Insomnia may be a symptom of serious underlying medical illness. As with any drug, if you are pregnant or nursing a baby, seek the advice of a health care professional before using this product. In case of accidental overdose, seek professional assistance or contact a poison control center immediately. Keep this and all medica-

Continued on next page

Nytol Natural—Cont.

tions out of the reach of children. Avoid alcoholic beverages while taking this product. Do not take this product if you are taking sedatives or tranquilizers without first consulting your doctor.

Dosage and Administration: Adults and children 12 years of age and over: Chew 2–3 tablets ½ hour before bedtime if needed, or as directed by a doctor.

How Supplied: Available in tamper resistant packages of 16 and 32 tablets.

NYTOL® QUICK CAPS® CAPLETS

Indications: For relief of occasional sleeplessness.

Directions: Adults and children 12 years of age and over: oral dosage is 2 caplets (50 mg) at bedtime if needed, or as directed by a doctor.

Warnings: Do not give to children under 12 years of age. If sleeplessness persists continuously for more than two weeks, consult your doctor. Insomnia may be a symptom of serious underlying medical illness. **Do not take this product, unless directed by a doctor, if you have a breathing problem such as emphysema or chronic bronchitis, or if you have glaucoma or difficulty in urination due to enlargement of the prostate gland. Do not use** with any other product containing diphenhydramine, including one applied topically. Avoid alcoholic beverages while taking this product. Do not take this product if you are taking sedatives or tranquilizers, without first consulting your doctor. In case of accidental overdose, seek professional assistance or contact a Poison Control Center immediately. As with any drug, if you are pregnant or nursing a baby, seek the advice of a health professional before using this product. Keep this and all drugs out of the reach of children.

Drug Interactions: Alcohol and other drugs which cause CNS depression will heighten the depressant effect of this product. Monoamine oxidase (MAO) inhibitors will prolong and intensify the anticholinergic effects of antihistamines.

Symptoms and Treatment of Oral Overdosage: In adults, overdose may cause CNS depression resulting in hypnosis and coma. In children, CNS hyperexcitability may follow sedation; the stimulant phase may bring tremor, delirium and convulsions. Gastrointestinal reactions may include dry mouth, appetite loss, nausea and/or vomiting. Respiratory distress and cardiovascular complications (hypotension) may be evident. Treatment includes inducing emesis and controlling symptoms.

Active Ingredient: Diphenydramine Hydrochloride 25 mg per caplet.

Inactive Ingredients: Corn Starch, Lactose, Microcrystalline Cellulose, Silica, Stearic Acid.

How supplied: Available in tamper-evident packages of 16, 32 and 72 caplets.

PHAZYME®-125
[*fay-zime*]
Softgels

Description: A blue, easy to swallow softgel, containing simethicone, an antiflatulent to alleviate or relieve the symptoms referred to as gas. It has no known side effects or drug interactions.

Active Ingredient: Each softgel contains simethicone 125 mg.

Actions: Simethicone minimizes gas formation and relieves gas entrapment in both the stomach and the lower G.I. tract. This action combats the distress due to gastrointestinal gas.

Indication: Relieves bloating, pressure or fullness commonly referred to as gas.

Warnings: Keep this and all drugs out of the reach of children. If condition persists, consult your physician.
Store at room temperature 59°–86°F (15–30°C).

Inactive Ingredients: FD&C Blue No. 1, gelatin, glycerin, soybean oil, titanium dioxide, white edible ink.

Dosage: Directions: Swallow one or two Softgels as needed after meals. Do not exceed four Softgels per day except under the advice and supervision of a physician.

How Supplied: Blue Softgel capsule imprinted PZ 125, 12 count, 36 count and 60 count and 100 count bottles.

Shown in Product Identification Guide, page 506

PHAZYME® INFANT DROPS
[*fay-zime*]

Description: Contains simethicone in a natural, orange flavor, an antiflatulent to alleviate or relieve the symptoms referred to as gas. It has no known side effects or drug interactions.

Active Ingredient: Each 0.6 ml contains simethicone, 40 mg.
Inactive Ingredients: Carbomer 974P, citric acid, flavor (natural orange), hydroxypropyl methylcellulose, PEG-8 stearate, sodium benzoate, sodium citrate, water and other ingredients.

Actions: Simethicone minimizes gas formation and relieves gas entrapment in both the stomach and the lower G.I. tract. This action combats the distress due to gastrointestinal gas.

Indication: To relieve symptoms referred to as gas.

Warnings: Keep this and all drugs out of the reach of children. If condition persists, consult your physician.

Store at room temperature 59°–86°F (15°–30°C)

Dosage/Administration: Shake well before using.
Infants (under 2 years): 0.3 ml four times daily after meals and at bedtime. Do not take more than six times per day except under the advice and supervision of a physician. Can also be mixed with liquids for easier administration.
Children (2 to 12 years): 0.6 ml four times daily after meals and at bedtime. Do not take more than six times per day except under the advice and supervision of a physician.
Adults: 1.2 ml (take two 0.6 ml doses) four times daily after meals and at bedtime. Do not take more than six times per day except under the advice and supervision of a physician.

How Supplied: Dropper bottles of 15 mL (0.5 fl oz).

Shown in Product Identification Guide, page 505

Maximum Strength
PHAZYME®–166 Chewable Tablets
[*fayzime*]

Description: Phazyme Chewables contains simethicone in a single, fresh mint tasting chewable tablet. It has no known side effects or drug interactions.

Active Ingredient: Each tablet contains simethicone 166 mg.

Inactive Ingredients: Citric acid, D&C Yellow #10, dextrates, FD&C Blue #1, peppermint flavor, sorbitol, starch, sucrose, talc, tribasic calcium phosphate.

Actions: Simethicone minimizes gas formation and relieves gas entrapment in both the stomach and the lower G.I. tract. This action combats the distress due to gastrointestinal gas.

Indication: Relieves bloating, pressure or fullness commonly referred to as gas.

Warnings: Keep this and all drugs out of the reach of children. If condition persists, consult your physician.
Store at room temperature 59°–86° F (15°–30° C).

Dosage: Directions: One or two tablets chewed thoroughly, as needed after meals. Do not exceed three tablets per day except under the advice and supervision of a physician.

How Supplied: White, bevel-edged tablets with green speckles and imprinted with "Phazyme 166" in 12 count and 60 count.

Shown in Product Identification Guide, page 506

Maximum Strength
PHAZYME®–166 Softgel Capsules
[*fayzime*]

Description: A red, easy to swallow softgel, containing simethicone an antiflatulant to alleviate or relieve the symptoms referred to as gas. It has no known side effects or drug interactions.

Active Ingredient: Each capsule contains simethicone, 166 mg.

Inactive Ingredients: FD&C Red No. 40, gelatin, glycerin, and white edible ink.

Actions: Simethicone minimizes gas formation and relieves gas entrapment in both the stomach and the lower G.I. tract. This action combats the distress due to gastrointestinal gas.

Indication: Relieves bloating, pressure or fullness commonly referred to as gas.

Warnings: Keep this and all drugs out of the reach of children. If condition persists, consult your physician.
Store at room temperature 59°–86° F (15°–30° C).

Dosage: Directions: Swallow one or two Softgels as needed after meals. Do not exceed three Softgels per day except under the advice and supervision of a physician.

How Supplied: Red softgel capsule imprinted Phazyme 166 mg (PZ 166) in 12 count, 36 count and 60 count bottle.
Shown in Product Identification Guide, page 506

PROMISE® SENSITIVE TOOTHPASTE
Anticavity Toothpaste for Sensitive Teeth

Active Ingredients: Potassium Nitrate (5%) and Sodium Monofluorophosphate (0.16% w/v fluorideion) in a pleasantly mint-flavored dentifrice.

Inactive Ingredients: D&C Yellow #10, Dicalcium Phosphate, Dicalcium Phosphate Dihydrate, FD&C Blue #1, Flavor, Glycerin, Hydroxyethylcellulose, Methylparaben, Propylparaben, Silica, Sodium Saccharin, Sodium Lauryl Sulfate, Sorbitol, Water.
Promise contains Potassium Nitrate for relief of dentinal hypersensitivity resulting from the exposure of tooth dentin due to periodontal surgery, cervical (gumline) erosion, abrasion or recession which causes pain on contact with hot, cold, or tactile stimuli. Promise also contains Sodium Monofluorophosphate for cavity prevention.

Indications: Promise builds increasing protection against painful sensitivity of the teeth to cold, heat, acids, sweets or contact and aids in the prevention of dental cavities.

Actions: Promise significantly reduces tooth hypersensitivity, with response to therapy evident after two weeks of use. Controlled double-blind clinical studies provide substantial evidence of the safety and effectiveness of Promise. The current theory on mechanism of action is that the potassium nitrate in Promise has an effect on neural transmission, interrupting

the signal which would result in the sensation of pain. Sodium Monofluorophosphate protects the tooth surfaces to prevent cavities.

Warning: Sensitive teeth may indicate a serious problem that may need prompt care by a dentist. See your dentist if the problem persists or worsens. Do not use this product longer than 4 weeks unless recommended by a dentist or physician. **Keep this and all drugs out of the reach of children. If you accidentally swallow more than used for brushing seek professional assistance or contact a Poison Control Center immediately.**

Directions: Adults and children 12 years of age and older:
Apply at least a 1-inch strip of the product onto a soft bristle toothbrush. Brush teeth thoroughly for at least 1 minute twice a day (morning and evening) or as recommended by a dentist or doctor.
Make sure to brush all sensitive areas of the teeth. Children under 12 years of age: Consult a dentist or physician.

How Supplied: Promise Sensitive is supplied in a 3.0 oz. (85 g) tube.

SENSODYNE® FRESH MINT
SENSODYNE® COOL GEL
SENSODYNE® WITH BAKING SODA
SENSODYNE® TARTAR CONTROL
SENSODYNE® ORIGINAL FLAVOR
SENSODYNE® EXTRA WHITENING
Anticavity toothpaste for sensitive teeth

Active Ingredients: 5% Potassium Nitrate and 0.15% Sodium Monofluorophosphate (Extra Whitening) or Sodium Fluoride (Fresh Mint, 0.15%; Baking Soda, 0.15%; Cool Gel, 0.13%; Tartar Control, 0.13%; Original Flavor, 0.13%) in a pleasantly mint-flavored dentifrice. Sensodyne Fresh Mint, Sensodyne Cool Gel, Sensodyne with Baking Soda, Sensodyne Tartar Control, Sensodyne Original Flavor and Sensodyne Extra Whitening contain fluoride for cavity prevention and Potassium Nitrate for relief of dentinal hypersensitivity resulting from the exposure of tooth dentin due to periodontal surgery, cervical (gum line) erosion, abrasion or recession which causes pain on contact with hot, cold, or tactile stimuli.

Inactive Ingredients: Baking Soda: Flavor, Glycerin, Hydrated Silica, Hydroxyethylcellulose, Methylparaben, Propylparaben, Silica, Sodium Bicarbonate, Sodium Lauryl Sulfate, Sodium Saccharin, Titanium Dioxide, Water.
Extra Whitening: Calcium Peroxide, Flavor, Glycerin, Hydrated Silica, PEG-12, PEG-75, Silica, Sodium Carbonate, Sodium Lauryl Sulfate, Sodium Saccharin, Titanium Dioxide, Water.
Tartar Control: Cellulose Gum, Cocamidopropyl Betaine, Flavor, Glycerin,

Hydrated Silica, Silica, Sodium Bicarbonate, Sodium Saccharin, Tetrapotassium Pyrophosphate, Titanium Dioxide, Water.
Cool Gel: Cellulose Gum, FD&C Blue #1, Flavor, Glycerin, Hydrated Silica, Silica, Sodium Methyl Cocoyl Taurate, Sodium Saccharin, Sorbitol, Trisodium Phosphate, Water.
Fresh Mint: D&C Yellow #10, FD&C Blue #1, Flavor, Glycerin, Hydrated Silica, Sodium Lauryl Sulfate, Sodium Saccharin, Sorbitol, Titanium Dioxide, Trisodium Phosphate, Water, Xanthan Gum.
Original Flavor: Cellulose Gum, D&C Red No. 28, Glycerin, Hydrated Silica, Peppermint Oil, Silica, Sodium Methyl Cocoyl Taurate, Sodium Saccharin, Sorbitol, Titanium Dioxide, Trisodium Phosphate, Water.

Actions: All Sensodyne Formulas significantly reduce tooth hypersensitivity, with response to therapy evident after two weeks of use. Controlled double-blind clinical studies provide substantial evidence of the safety and effectiveness of Potassium Nitrate. The current theory on mechanism of action is that potassium nitrate has an effect on neural transmission, interrupting the signal which would result in the sensation of pain. Fluorides are anticariogenic, forming fluoroapatite in the outer surface of the dental enamel which is resistant to acids and caries.

Warnings: Sensitive teeth may indicate a serious problem that may need prompt care by a dentist. See your dentist if the problem persists or worsens. Do not use this product longer than 4 weeks unless recommended by a dentist or physician. Keep this and all drugs out of the reach of children. If you accidentally swallow more than used for brushing, seek professional assistance or contact a Poison Control Center immediately.

Dosage and Administration: Adults and children 12 years of age and older: Apply a 1-inch strip of the product onto a soft bristle toothbrush. Brush teeth thoroughly for at least 1 minute twice a day (morning and evening) or as recommended by a dentist or physician. Make sure to brush all sensitive areas of the teeth. Children under 12 years of age: consult a dentist or physician.

How Supplied: All Sensodyne formulas (except Sensodyne Cool Gel) are supplied in 2.1 oz. (60g), 4.0 oz. (113g) and 6.0 oz. (170g) tubes. Sensodyne Cool Gel is supplied in 4.0 oz. only.

TEGRIN® DANDRUFF SHAMPOO – EXTRA CONDITIONING

Description: Tegrin® Dandruff Shampoo contains 7% Coal Tar Solution, USP, equivalent to 1.1% coal tar, in a pleasantly scented, high-foaming, cleansing shampoo base with emollients, conditioners and other formula components.

Continued on next page

Tegrin—Cont.

Indications: Tegrin® Dandruff Shampoo controls the flaking and itching of the scalp associated with dandruff, seborrheic dermatitis, and psoriasis.

Directions: Shake well. Wet hair. Lather, rinse, repeat. For best results use at least twice a week or as directed by a doctor.

Warnings: For external use only. Avoid contact with eyes. If contact occurs, rinse eyes thoroughly with water. If condition worsens or does not improve after regular use of this product as directed, consult a doctor. Use caution in exposing skin to sunlight after applying this product. It may increase tendency to sunburn for up to 24 hours after application. Do not use for prolonged periods without consulting a doctor. Do not use this product with other forms of psoriasis therapy, such as ultraviolet radiation or prescription drugs, unless directed by a doctor. Keep out of reach of children. In case of accidental ingestion, seek professional assistance or contact a Poison Control Center immediately.

Active Ingredient: 7% Coal Tar Solution, USP, Equivalent to 1.1% Coal Tar. Coal Tar is obtained in the destructive distillation of bituminous coal and is a highly effective agent for controlling the flaking and itching of the scalp associated with dandruff, seborrheic dermatitis, and psoriasis. The action of coal tar is believed to be keratolytic, antiseptic, antipruritic, and astringent. The coal tar solution used in Tegrin® Dandruff Shampoo is prepared in such a way as to reduce the pitch and other irritant components found in crude coal tar without reduction in therapeutic potency.

Coal Tar Solution has been used clinically for many years as a remedy for dandruff and for scaling associated with scalp disorders such as seborrhea and psoriasis. Its mechanism of action has not been fully established, but it is believed to retard the rate of turnover of epidermal cells with regular use. A number of clinical studies have demonstrated the performance attributes of Tegrin® Dandruff Shampoo against dandruff and seborrheic dermatitis. In addition to relieving the above symptoms, Tegrin® Dandruff Shampoo, used regularly, maintains scalp and hair cleanliness and leaves the hair lustrous and manageable.

Inactive Ingredients for:
Tegrin® Dandruff Shampoo – Extra Conditioning

Alcohol (7.0%), Ammonium Lauryl Sulfate, Citric Acid, FD&C Blue #1, Fragrance, Glycol Stearate (and) Sodium Laureth Sulfate (and) Hexylene Glycol, Guar Hydroxypropyltrimonium Chloride, Hydroxypropyl Methylcellulose, Lauramide DEA, Methylparaben, Propylparaben, Sodium Lauryl Sulfate, Water.

How supplied: Tegrin® Dandruff Shampoo is available in Extra Conditioning and Fresh Herbal formulas and supplied in 7 fl. oz. (207 ml) plastic bottles.

TEGRIN® DANDRUFF SHAMPOO–FRESH HERBAL

Description: Tegrin® Dandruff Shampoo contains 7% Coal Tar Solution, USP, equivalent to 1.1% coal tar, in a pleasantly scented, high-foaming, cleansing shampoo base with emollients, conditioners and other formula components.

Indications: Tegrin® Dandruff Shampoo controls the flaking and itching of the scalp associated with dandruff, seborrheic dermatitis, and psoriasis.

Directions: Shake well. Wet hair. Lather, rinse, repeat. For best results use at least twice a week or as directed by a doctor.

Warnings: For external use only. Avoid contact with eyes. If contact occurs, rinse eyes thoroughly with water. If condition worsens or does not improve after regular use of the product as directed, consult a doctor. Use caution in exposing skin to sunlight after applying this product. It may increase tendency to sunburn for up to 24 hours after application. Do not use for prolonged period without consulting a doctor. Do not use this product with other forms of psoriasis therapy, such as ultraviolet radiation or prescription drugs, unless directed by a doctor. Keep out of reach of children. In case of accidental ingestion, seek professional assistance or contact a Poison Control Center immediately.

Active Ingredient: 7% Coal Tar Solution, USP, Equivalent to 1.1% Coal Tar. Coal Tar is obtained in the destructive distillation of bituminous coal and is a highly effective agent for controlling the flaking and itching of the scalp associated with dandruff, seborrheic dermatitis and psoriasis. The action of coal tar is believed to be keratolytic, antiseptic, antipruritic, and astringent. The coal tar solution used in Tegrin® Dandruff Shampoo is prepared in such a way as to reduce the pitch and other irritant components found in crude coal tar without reduction in therapeutic potency.

Coal Tar Solution has been used clinically for many years as a remedy for dandruff and for scaling associated with scalp disorders such as seborrhea and psoriasis. Its mechanism of action has not been fully established, but it is believed to retard the rate of turnover of epidermal cells with regular use. A number of clinical studies have demonstrated the performance attributes of Tegrin® Dandruff Shampoo against dandruff and seborrheic dermatitis. In addition to relieving the above symptoms, Tegrin®

Dandruff Shampoo, used regularly, maintains scalp and hair cleanliness and leaves the hair lustrous and manageable.

Inactive Ingredients For:
Tegrin® Dandruff Shampoo–Fresh Herbal

Alcohol (7.0%), Citric Acid, Cocamide DEA, FD&C Blue #1, Fragrance, Glycol Stearate, (and) Sodium Laureth Sulfate (and) Hexylene Glycol, Hydroxypropyl Methylcellulose, Methylparaben, Propylparaben, Sodium Lauryl Sulfate, Water.

How Supplied: Tegrin® Dandruff Shampoo is available in Extra Conditioning and Fresh Herbal formulas and supplied in 7 fl. oz. (207 ml) plastic bottles.

TEGRIN® SKIN CREAM FOR PSORIASIS

Description: Tegrin® Skin Cream for Psoriasis contains 5% Coal Tar Solution, USP, equivalent to 0.8% Coal Tar and alcohol of 4.7%.

Indications: For relief of itching, flaking and irritation of the skin associated with psoriasis and seborrheic dermatitis.

Directions: Apply to affected areas one to four times daily or as directed by a doctor.

Warnings: For external use only. Avoid contact with eyes. If contact occurs, rinse eyes thoroughly with water. If condition worsens or does not improve after regular use of this product as directed, consult a doctor. Use caution in exposing skin to sunlight after applying this product. It may increase tendency to sunburn for up to 24 hours after application. Do not use for prolonged periods without consulting a doctor. Do not use this product with other forms of psoriasis therapy, such as ultra-violet radiation or prescription drugs, unless directed by a doctor. If the condition covers a large area of the body, consult your doctor before using this product. Keep out of reach of children. In case of accidental ingestion, seek professional assistance or contact a Poison Control Center immediately.

Active Ingredient: 5% Coal Tar Solution, USP, equivalent to 0.8% Coal Tar.

Inactive Ingredients: Acetylated Lanolin Alcohol, Alcohol (4.7%), Carbomer-934P, Ceteth 2, Cetyl Alcohol, 5-Chloro-2-Methyl-4-Isothiazolin-3-One (and) 2-Methyl-4-Isothiazolin-3-One, D&C Red 28, Fragrance, Glyceryl Tribehenate, Laneth-16, Laureth 23, Methyl Gluceth 20, Mineral Oil, Mineral Oil (and) Lanolin Alcohol (and) Octyldodecanol, Petrolatum, Potassium Hydroxide, Stearyl Alcohol, Titanium Dioxide, Water.

How Supplied: Tegrin® Skin Cream for Psoriasis is available in a 2 oz (57g) tube.

Boiron
**6 CAMPUS BLVD.
NEWTOWN SQUARE, PA 19073**

Direct Inquiries and Medical Emergencies:
Boiron Information Center
(800)264-7661

OSCILLOCOCCINUM®
[oh-sill'o-cox-see'num']

Active Ingredients: Anas barbariae hepatis et cordis extractum 200CK. *Made according to the Homeopathic Pharmacopeia of the United States.*

Inactive Ingredients: sucrose, lactose.

Use: For temporary relief of symptoms of flu such as fever, chills, body aches and pains.

Directions: (Adults and children 2 years of age and older):
Take 1 dose at the onset of symptoms.
Repeat for 2 more doses at 6 hour intervals.
Allow the pellets to dissolve in the mouth, at least 15 minutes before or after meals.

Warnings: Do not use if the label sealing the cap is broken.
Ask a doctor before use in children under 2 years of age.
Stop using this product and consult a doctor if symptoms persist for more than 3 days or worsen.
As with any drug, if pregnant or nursing a baby, ask a health professional before use.
Keep this and all medication out of reach of children.
Diabetics: this product contains sugar.

How Supplied: White pellets in unit dose containers of 0.04 oz. (1 gram) each. Supplied in boxes of 3 unit doses or 6 unit doses.
NDC #0220-9280-32 (3 doses) and NDC #0220-9280-33 (6 doses)
Made in France

Bristol-Myers Products
**(A Bristol-Myers Squibb Company)
345 PARK AVENUE
NEW YORK, NY 10154**

Direct Inquiries to:
Bristol-Myers Products Division
Consumer Affairs Department
1350 Liberty Avenue
Hillside, NJ 07207
Questions or Comments?
1-(800) 468-7746

ALPHA KERI®
Moisture Rich Shower and Bath Oil

Composition: Contains mineral oil, PEG-4 dilaurate, lanolin oil, fragrance, benzophenone-3, D&C green 6, Benzophenone-3.

Indications: ALPHA KERI is a water-dispersible oil that lubricates and softens dry skin. ALPHA KERI Moisture Rich Body Oil is an all-over skin moisturizer that is valuable as an aid for dry skin and mild skin irritations.
How to Use: ALPHA KERI *should always be used with water, either added to water or rubbed on to wet skin.* Because of its inherent cleansing properties it is not necessary to use soap when ALPHA KERI is being used.
For external use only.
Label directions should be followed for use in shower, bath and cleansing.

Precaution: The patient should be warned to guard against slipping in tub or shower.

How Supplied: 4 fl. oz., 8 fl. oz., and 16 fl. oz., plastic bottles.
Also available: Alpha Keri Bar 4 oz.

BUFFERIN®
[bŭf'fĕr-ĭn]
Analgesic

Composition:
Active Ingredient: Aspirin 325 mg in a formulation buffered with Calcium Carbonate, Magnesium Oxide and Magnesium Carbonate.
Other Ingredients: Benzoic Acid, Citric Acid, Corn Starch, FD&C Blue No. 1, Hydroxypropyl Methylcellulose, Magnesium Stearate, Mineral Oil, Polysorbate 20, Povidone, Propylene Glycol, Simethicone Emulsion, Sodium Phosphate, Sorbitan Monolaurate, Titanium Dioxide. May also contain: Carnauba Wax, Zinc Stearate.

Indications: For fast temporary relief of headaches, minor arthritis pain and inflammation, muscle aches, pain and fever of colds, menstrual pain and toothaches.

Directions: Adults and chldren 12 years of age and over: 2 tablets with water every 4 hours while symptoms persist, not to exceed 12 tablets in 24 hours, or as directed by a doctor. Children under 12 years of age: Consult a doctor.
Alcohol Warning: If you consume 3 or more alcoholic drinks every day, ask your doctor whether you should take aspirin or other pain relievers/fever reducers. Aspirin may cause stomach bleeding.

Warnings: Children and teenagers should not use this medicine for chicken pox or flu symptoms before a doctor is consulted about Reye syndrome, a rare but serious illness reported to be associated with aspirin. Keep this and all drugs out of the reach of children. In case of accidental overdose, seek professional

assistance or contact a poison control center immediately. As with any drug, if you are pregnant or nursing a baby, seek the advice of a health professional before using this product. **IT IS ESPECIALLY IMPORTANT NOT TO USE ASPIRIN DURING THE LAST 3 MONTHS OF PREGNANCY UNLESS SPECIFICALLY DIRECTED TO DO SO BY A DOCTOR BECAUSE IT MAY CAUSE PROBLEMS IN THE UNBORN CHILD OR COMPLICATIONS DURING DELIVERY.** Do not take this product for pain for more than 10 days or for fever for more than 3 days unless directed by a doctor. If pain or fever persists or gets worse, if new symptoms occur, or if redness or swelling is present, consult a doctor because these could be signs of a serious condition. Do not take this product if you are allergic to aspirin, have asthma, have stomach problems (such as heartburn, upset stomach or stomach pain) that persist or recur, or if you have ulcers or bleeding problems, unless directed by a doctor. If ringing in the ears or loss of hearing occurs, consult a doctor before taking or giving any more of this product.

Drug Interaction Precaution: Do not take this product if you are taking a prescription drug for anticoagulation (thinning of blood), diabetes, gout or arthritis unless directed by a doctor.

How Supplied: BUFFERIN is supplied as:
Coated circular white tablet with letter "B" debossed on one surface.
Supplied in bottles of 39's, 65's, 130's and 275's.
All consumer sizes have child resistant closures except 130's tablets which are sizes recommended for households without young children. Store at room temperature.
Also available:
Bufferin Low Dose (81 mg) Enteric formulation,
Arthritis Strength and Extra Strength formulations.

Professional Labeling

1. BUFFERIN® FOR RECURRENT TRANSIENT ISCHEMIC ATTACKS

Indication: For reducing the risk of recurrent transient ischemic attacks (TIA's) or stroke in men who have had transient ischemia of the brain due to fibrin platelet emboli. There is inadequate evidence that aspirin or buffered aspirin is effective in reducing TIA's in women at the recommended dosage. There is no evidence that aspirin or buffered aspirin is of benefit in the treatment of completed strokes in men or women.

Clinical Trials: The indication is supported by the results of a Canadian study (1) in which 585 patients with threatened stroke were followed in a randomized clinical trial for an average of 26 months to determine whether aspirin or

Continued on next page

Bufferin—Cont.

sulfinpyrazone, singly or in combination, was superior to placebo in preventing transient ischemic attacks, stroke, or death. The study showed that, although sulfinpyrazone had no statistically significant effect, aspirin reduced the risk of continuing transient ischemic attacks, stroke, or death by 19 percent and reduced the risk of stroke or death by 31 percent. Another aspirin study carried out in the United States with 178 patients, showed a statistically significant number of "favorable outcomes," including reduced transient ischemic attacks, stroke, and death (2).

Precautions: Patients presenting with signs and symptoms of TIA's should have a complete medical and neurologic evaluation. Consideration should be given to other disorders that resemble TIA's. Attention should be given to risk factors: it is important to evaluate and treat, if appropriate, other diseases associated with TIA's and stroke, such as hypertension and diabetes.

Concurrent administration of absorbable antacids at therapeutic doses may increase the clearance of salicylates in some individuals. The concurrent administration of nonabsorbable antacids may alter the rate of absorption of aspirin, thereby resulting in a decreased acetylsalicylic acid/salicylate ratio in plasma. The clinical significance of these decreases in available aspirin is unknown.

Aspirin at dosages of 1,000 milligrams per day has been associated with small increases in blood pressure, blood urea nitrogen, and serum uric acid levels. It is recommended that patients placed on long-term aspirin treatment be seen at regular intervals to assess changes in these measurements.

Adverse Reactions: At dosages of 1,000 milligrams or higher of aspirin per day, gastrointestinal side effects include stomach pain, heartburn, nausea and/or vomiting, as well as increased rates of gross gastrointestinal bleeding.

Dosage and Administration: Adult oral dosage for men is 1,300 milligrams a day, in divided doses of 650 milligrams twice a day or 325 milligrams four times a day.

References:
(1) The Canadian Cooperative Study Group. "A Randomized Trial of Aspirin and Sulfinpyrazone in Threatened Stroke," *New England Journal of Medicine*, 299:53–59, 1978.
(2) Fields, W.S., et al., "Controlled Trial of Aspirin in Cerebral Ischemia," *Stroke* 8:301–316, 1977.

2. BUFFERIN® FOR MYOCARDIAL INFARCTION

Indication: Aspirin is indicated to reduce the risk of death and/or nonfatal myocardial infarction in patients with a previous infarction or unstable angina pectoris.

Clinical Trials: The indication is supported by the results of six, large, randomized multicenter, placebo-controlled studies[1-7] involving 10,816, predominantly male, post-myocardial infarction (MI) patients and one randomized placebo-controlled study of 1,266 men with unstable angina. Therapy with aspirin was begun at intervals after the onset of acute MI varying from less than 3 days to more than 5 years and continued for periods of from less than one year to four years. In the unstable angina study, treatment was started within 1 month after the onset of unstable angina and continued for 12 weeks and complicating conditions such as congestive heart failure were not included in the study.

Aspirin therapy in MI patients was associated with about a 20 percent reduction in the risk of subsequent death and/or nonfatal reinfarction, a median absolute decrease of 3 percent from the 12 to 22 percent event rates in the placebo groups. In the aspirin-treated unstable angina patients the reduction in risk was about 50 percent, a reduction in the event rate of 5% from the 10% rate in the placebo group over the 12 weeks of the study.

Daily dosage of aspirin in the post-myocardial infarction studies was 300 mg. in one study and 900 and 1500 mg. in five studies. A dose of 325 mg. was used in the study of unstable angina.

Adverse Reactions: Gastrointestinal Reactions: Doses of 1000 mg. per day of aspirin caused gastrointestinal symptoms and bleeding that in some cases were clinically significant. In the largest post-infarction study (The Aspirin Myocardial Infarction Study (AMIS) with 4,500 people), the percentage incidences of gastrointestinal symptoms for the aspirin (1000 mg. of a standard, solid-tablet formulation) and placebo-treated subjects, respectively, were: stomach pain (14.5%; 4.4%); heartburn (11.9%; 4.8%); nausea and/or vomiting (7.6%; 2.1%); hospitalization for gastrointestinal disorder (4.8%; 3.5%). In the AMIS and other trials, aspirin treated patients had increased rates of gross gastrointestinal bleeding. Symptoms and signs of gastrointestinal irritation were not significantly increased in subjects treated for unstable angina with buffered aspirin in solution.

Cardiovascular and Biochemical:
In the AMIS trial, the dosage of 1000 mg. per day of aspirin was associated with small increases in systolic blood pressure (BP) (average 1.5 to 2.1 mm) and diastolic BP (0.5 to 0.6 mm), depending upon whether maximal or last available readings were used. Blood urea nitrogen and uric acid levels were also increased, but by less than 1.0 mg%.

Subjects with marked hypertension or renal insufficiency had been excluded from the trial so that the clinical importance of these observations for such subjects or for any subjects treated over more prolonged periods is not known. It is recommended that patients placed on long-term aspirin treatment, even at doses of 300 mg. per day, be seen at regular intervals to assess changes in these measurements.

Administration and Dosage: Although most of the studies used dosages exceeding 300 mg., two trials used only 300 mg. and pharmacologic data indicate that this dose inhibits platelet function fully. Therefore, 300 mg. or a conventional 325 mg. aspirin dose is a reasonable, routine dose that would minimize gastrointestinal adverse reactions.

References: 1. Elwood P.C., et al., "A Randomized Controlled Trial of Acetylsalicylic Acid in the Secondary Prevention of Mortality from Myocardial Infarction," *British Medical Journal,* 1:436–440, 1974. 2. The Coronary Drug Project Research Group, "Aspirin in Coronary Heart Disease," *Journal of Chronic Disease,* 29:625–642, 1976. 3. Breddin K, et al., "Secondary Prevention of Myocardial Infarction; Comparison of Acetylsalicylic Acid Phenprocoumon and Placebo," *Thromb. Haemost.,* 41:225–236, 1979. 4. Aspirin Myocardial Infarction Study Research Group, "A Randomized, Controlled Trial of Aspirin in Persons Recovered from Myocardial Infarction," *Journal American Medical Association,* 243:661–669, 1980. 5. Elwood P.C., and Sweetnam, P.M., "Aspirin and Secondary Mortality after Myocardial Infarction," *Lancet,* pp. 1313–1315, December 22–29, 1979. 6. The Persantine-Aspirin Reinfarction Study Research Group. "Persantine and Aspirin in Coronary Heart Disease," *Circulation* 62;449–460, 1980. 7. Lewis H.D., et al., "Protective Effects of Aspirin Against Acute Myocardial Infarction and Death in Men with Unstable Angina, Results of a Veterans Administration Cooperative Study," *New England Journal of Medicine,* 309;396–403, 1983.

Shown in Product Identification Guide, page 506

COMTREX® Maximum Strength
[cŏm 'trĕx]
Multi-Symptom Cold & Cough Relief

Composition: Each tablet, caplet, liquigel and fluidounce (30 ml.) contains:
[See table at bottom of next page]

Indications: For the temporary relief of the following symptoms associated with the common cold and flu: minor aches, pains, headache, muscular aches, sore throat pain, and fever; cough; nasal congestion; runny nose and sneezing.

Directions:
Tablets or Caplets: Adults and children 12 years of age and over: 2 tablets or caplets every 6 hours while symptoms persist, not to exceed 8 tablets or caplets in 24 hours, or as directed by a doctor. Children under 12 years of age: Consult a doctor.
Liqui-Gel: Adults and children 12 years of age and over: 2 liqui-gels every 6 hours, while symptoms persist, not to ex-

ceed 8 liqui-gels in 24 hours, or as directed by a doctor. Children under 12 years of age: consult a doctor.

Liquid: Adults and children 12 years of age and over: One fluidounce using dosage cup provided or 2 tablespoonfuls every 6 hours while symptoms persist, not to exceed 4 doses in 24 hours or as directed by your doctor. Children under 12 years of age: consult a doctor.

Alcohol Warning: If you consume 3 or more alcoholic drinks every day, ask your doctor whether you should take acetaminophen or other pain relievers/fever reducers. Acetaminophen may cause liver damage.

Warnings: Keep this and all drugs out of the reach of children. In case of accidental overdose, seek professional assistance or contact a poison control center immediately. Prompt medical attention is critical for adults as well as children even if you do not notice any signs or symptoms. As with any drug, if you are pregnant or nursing a baby, seek the advice of a health professional before using this product. Do not take this product for more than 7 days. A persistent cough may be a sign of a serious condition. If cough persists for more than 7 days, tends to recur, or is accompanied by rash, persistent headache, fever that lasts for more than 3 days, or if new symptoms occur, consult a doctor. If sore throat is severe, persists for more than 2 days, is accompanied or followed by fever, headache, rash, nausea, or vomiting, consult a doctor promptly. Do not take this product for persistent or chronic cough such as occurs with smoking, asthma, emphysema, or if cough is accompanied by excessive phlegm (mucus) unless directed by a doctor. **Do not exceed recommended dosage.** If nervousness, dizziness, or sleeplessness occur, discontinue use and consult a doctor. If symptoms do not improve within 7 days or are accompanied by fever, consult a doctor. Do not take this product unless directed by a doctor, if you have a breathing problem such as emphysema or chronic bronchitis, heart disease, high blood pressure, thyroid disease, diabetes, glaucoma, or difficulty in urination due to enlargement of the prostate gland. May cause excitability especially in children. May cause marked drowsiness; alcohol, sedatives, and tranquilizers may increase the drowsiness effect. Avoid alcoholic beverages while taking this product. Do not take this product if you are taking sedatives or tranquilizers, without first consulting your doctor. Use caution when driving a motor vehicle or operating machinery. If you generally consume 3 or more alcohol-containing drinks per day, you should consult your physician for advice on when and how you should take COMTREX and other pain relievers.

Drug Interaction Precaution: Do not use this product if you are now taking a prescription monoamine oxidase inhibitor (MAOI) (certain drugs for depression, psychiatric or emotional conditions, or Parkinson's disease), or for 2 weeks after stopping the MAOI drug. If you are uncertain whether your prescription drug contains an MAOI, consult a health professional before taking this product.

Overdose:
Acetylcysteine As An Antidote For Acetaminophen Overdose
Acetaminophen is rapidly absorbed from the upper gastrointestinal tract with peak plasma levels occurring between 30 and 60 minutes after therapeutic doses and usually within 4 hours following an overdose. The parent compound, which is nontoxic, is extensively metabolized in the liver to form principally the sulfate and glucuronide conjugates which are also nontoxic and are rapidly excreted in the urine. A small fraction of an ingested dose is metabolized in the liver by the cytochrome P-450 mixed function oxidase enzyme system to form a reactive, potentially toxic, intermediate metabolite which preferentially conjugates with hepatic glutathione to form the nontoxic cysteine and mercapturic acid derivatives which are then excreted by the kidney. Therapeutic doses of acetaminophen do not saturate the glucuronide and sulfate conjugation pathways and do not result in the formation of sufficient reactive metabolite to deplete glutathione stores. However, following ingestion of a large overdose (150 mg/kg or greater) the glucuronide and sulfate conjugation pathways are saturated resulting in a larger fraction of the drug being metabolized via the P-450 pathway. The increased formation of reactive metabolite may deplete the hepatic stores of glutathione with subsequent binding of the metabolite to protein molecules within the hepatocyte resulting in cellular necrosis. Acetylcysteine has been shown to reduce the extent of liver injury following acetaminophen overdose.

Early symptoms following a potentially hepatotoxic overdose may include: nausea, vomiting, diaphoresis and general malaise. Clinical and laboratory evidence of hepatic toxicity may not be apparent until 48 to 72 hours postingestion. In most adults and adolescents, regardless of the quantity of acetaminophen reported to have been in-

Continued on next page

	COMTREX Per Tablet or Caplet	COMTREX Liquid-Gel per Liqui-Gel	COMTREX Liquid* Per Fl. Ounce
Acetaminophen:	500 mg.	500 mg.	1000 mg.
Pseudoephedrine HCl:	30 mg.	—	60 mg.
Phenylpropanolamine HCl:	—	12.5 mg.	—
Chlorpheniramine Maleate:	2 mg.	2 mg.	4 mg.
Dextromethorphan HBr:	15 mg.	15 mg.	30 mg.

Tablet/Caplet
Benzoic Acid
Corn Starch
D&C Yellow No. 10Lake
FD&C Red No. 40 Lake
Hydroxypropyl Methylcellulose
Magnesium Stearate
Methylparaben
Mineral Oil
Polysorbate 20
Povidone
Propylene Glycol
Propylparaben
Simethicone Emulsion
Sorbitan Monolaurate
Stearic Acid
Titanium Dioxide
May also contain:
Carnauba wax
D&C Yellow No. 10
FD&C Red No. 40

Liqui-Gels
D&C Yellow No. 10
FD&C Red No. 40
Gelatin
Glycerin
Polyethylene Glycol
Povidone
Propylene Glycol
Silicon Dioxide
Sorbitol
Titanium Dioxide
Water

Liquid
Alcohol (10% by volume)
Benzoic acid
D&C Yellow No. 10
FD&C Blue No. 1
FD&C Red No. 40
Flavors
Glycerin
Polyethylene Glycol
Povidone
Saccharin Sodium
Sodium Citrate
Sucrose
Water

*contains 15 mg sodium per fluid ounce (30 ml)

Comtrex—Cont.

gested, administer acetylcysteine immediately. Acetylcysteine therapy should be initiated and continued for a full course of therapy. Its effectiveness depends on early administration, with benefit seen principally in patients treated within 16 hours of the overdose.

If acetaminophen plasma assay capability is not available, and the estimated acetaminophen ingestion exceeds 150 mg/kg., acetylcysteine therapy should be initiated and continued for a full course of therapy.

For full prescribing information, refer to the acetylcysteine package insert. Do not await the results of assays for acetaminophen level before initiating treatment with acetylcysteine. The following additional procedures are recommended: The stomach should be emptied promptly by lavage or by induction of emesis with syrup of ipecac.

A serum acetaminophen assay should be obtained as early as possible, but no sooner than four hours following ingestion. Liver function studies should be obtained initially and repeated at 24-hour intervals.

For additional emergency information call your regional poison center or toll-free (1-800-525-6115) to the Rocky Mountain Poison Center for assistance in diagnosis and for directions in the use of acetylcysteine as an antidote.

How Supplied:

COMTREX® is supplied as:
Coated yellow tablet with letters "Cx" debossed on one surface.
Supplied in Blister packages of 24's
Coated yellow caplet with "Cx" debossed on one side.
Supplied in Blister packages of 24's
Yellow Liqui-Gel with "COMTREX LG" printed in red on one side.
Supplied in Blister packages of 24's
Clear Red Cherry Flavored liquid:
Supplied in 6 oz. plastic bottles.
Store caplets, tablets and liquid at room temperature.
Store liqui-gels below 86° F. (30° C.). Keep from freezing.
Other COMTREX products also available: Acute Head Cold & Sinus Pressure Relief, Deep Chest Cold and Congestion Relief, Allergy Sinus Treatment, Day/Night and Non-Drowsy formulations.

Shown in Product Identification Guide, page 506

COMTREX® MAXIMUM STRENGTH

[cŏm-trĕx]
Multisymptom Acute Head Cold & Sinus Pressure Relief

Composition: Each tablet contains:

	per tablet
acetaminophen	500 mg
brompheniramine maleate	2 mg
pseudoephedrine hydrochloride	30 mg

Other Ingredients: Benzoic Acid, Carnauba Wax, Corn Starch, Croscar-

mellose Sodium, FD&C Red No. 40 Lake, Hydroxypropyl Methylcellulose, Magnesium Stearate, Methylparaben, Microcrystalline Cellulose, Polyethylene Glycol, Polysorbate 80, Propylparaben, Stearic Acid, Titanium Dioxide.

Indications: For the temporary relief of the following symptoms associated with the common cold and flu: minor aches, pains, headache, muscular aches, sore throat pain, and fever; nasal congestion, and sinus pressure; runny nose and sneezing.

Directions: Adults and children 12 years of age and over: 2 tablets every 6 hours, while symptoms persist, not to exceed 8 tablets in 24 hours, or as directed by your doctor. Children under 12 years of age: consult a doctor.

Alcohol Warning: If you consume 3 or more alcoholic drinks every day, ask your doctor whether you should take acetaminophen or other pain relievers/fever reducers. Acetaminophen may cause liver damage.

Warnings: Keep this and all drugs out of the reach of children. In case of accidental overdose, seek professional assistance or contact a poison control center immediately. Prompt medical attention is critical for adults as well as children even if you do not notice any signs or symptoms. As with any drug, if you are pregnant or nursing a baby, seek the advice of a health professional before using this product. Do not take this product for more than 7 days. If symptoms do not improve or are accompanied by fever that lasts for more than 3 days, or if new symptoms occur, consult a doctor. If sore throat is severe, persists for more than 2 days, is accompanied or followed by fever, headache, rash, nausea, or vomiting, consult a doctor promptly. **Do not exceed recommended dosage.** If nervousness, dizziness, or sleeplessness occur, discontinue use and consult a doctor. If symptoms do not improve within 7 days or are accompanied by fever, consult a doctor. Do not take this product, unless directed by a doctor, if you have a breathing problem such as emphysema or chronic bronchitis, heart disease, high blood pressure, thyroid disease, diabetes, glaucoma, or difficulty in urination due to enlargement of the prostate gland. May cause excitability especially in children. May cause drowsiness; alcohol, sedatives, and tranquilizers may increase the drowsiness effect. Avoid alcoholic beverages while taking this product. Do not take this product if you are taking sedatives or tranquilizers, without first consulting your doctor. Use caution when driving a motor vehicle or operating machinery. If you generally consume 3 or more alcohol-containing drinks per day, you should consult your physician for advice on when and how you should take COMTREX and other pain relievers.

Drug Interaction Precaution: Do not use this product if you are now taking a prescription monoamine oxidase inhibitor (MAOI) (certain drugs for depression,

psychiatric or emotional conditions, or Parkinson's disease), or for 2 weeks after stopping the MAOI drug. If you are uncertain whether your prescription drug contains an MAOI, consult a health professional before taking this product.

Overdose:

Acetylcysteine As An Antidote For Acetaminophen Overdose

Acetaminophen is rapidly absorbed from the upper gastrointestinal tract with peak plasma levels occurring between 30 and 60 minutes after therapeutic doses and usually within 4 hours following an overdose. The parent compound, which is nontoxic, is extensively metabolized in the liver to form principally the sulfate and glucuronide conjugates which are also nontoxic and are rapidly excreted in the urine. A small fraction of an ingested dose is metabolized in the liver by the cytochrome P-450 mixed function oxidase enzyme system to form a reactive, potentially toxic, intermediate metabolite which preferentially conjugates with hepatic glutathione to form the nontoxic cysteine and mercapturic acid derivatives which are then excreted by the kidney. Therapeutic doses of acetaminophen do not saturate the glucuronide and sulfate conjugation pathways and do not result in the formation of sufficient reactive metabolite to deplete glutathione stores. However, following ingestion of a large overdose (150 mg/kg or greater) the glucuronide and sulfate conjugation pathways are saturated resulting in a larger fraction of the drug being metabolized via the P-450 pathway. The increased formation of reactive metabolite may deplete the hepatic stores of glutathione with subsequent binding of the metabolite to protein molecules within the hepatocyte resulting in cellular necrosis. Acetylcysteine has been shown to reduce the extent of liver injury following acetaminophen overdose.

Early symptoms following a potentially hepatotoxic overdose may include: nausea, vomiting, diaphoresis and general malaise. Clinical and laboratory evidence of hepatic toxicity may not be apparent until 48 to 72 hours postingestion. In most adults and adolescents, regardless of the quantity of acetaminophen reported to have been ingested, administer acetylcysteine immediately. Acetylcysteine therapy should be initiated and continued for a full course of therapy. Its effectiveness depends on early administration, with benefit seen principally in patients treated within 16 hours of the overdose.

If acetaminophen plasma assay capability is not available, and the estimated acetaminonphen ingestion exceeds 150 mg/kg., acetylcysteine therapy should be initiated and continued for a full course of therapy.

For full prescribing information, refer to the acetylcysteine package insert. Do not await the results of assays for acetaminophen level before initiating treatment with acetylcysteine. The following additional procedures are recommended: The stomach should be emptied promptly by lavage or by induction of emesis with syrup of ipecac.

A serum acetaminophen assay should be obtained as early as possible, but no sooner than four hours following ingestion. Liver function studies should be obtained initially and repeated at 24-hour intervals.

For additional emergency information call your regional poison center or toll-free (1-800-525-6115) to the Rocky Mountain Poison Center for assistance in diagnosis and for directions in the use of acetylcysteine as an antidote.

How Supplied:
Round, red coated tablets with "AHC" debossed on one side.
Other Comtrex products also available: Deep Chest Cold & Congestion Relief, Allergy Sinus Treatment, Day/Night and Non-Drowsy Formulations.

Shown in Product Identification Guide, page 506

COMTREX®
DEEP CHEST COLD
& Congestion Relief

Composition: Each liquigel contains: Acetaminophen 325 mg, Guaifenesin 200 mg, Phenylpropanolamine Hydrochloride 12.5 mg, and Dextromethorphan Hydrobromide 10 mg.
Other ingredients: FD&C Red No. 40, Gelatin, Glycerin, Polyethylene Glycol, Povidone, Propylene Glycol, Silicon Dioxide, Sorbitol, Titanium Dioxide, Water.

Indications: For the temporary relief of the following symptoms associated with the common cold and flu: minor aches, pains, headache, muscular aches, sore throat, and fever; cough; and nasal congestion. Helps loosen phlegm (mucus) and thin bronchial secretions to drain bronchial tubes and make coughs more productive.

Directions: Adults and children 12 years of age and over: 2 liquigels every 4 hours, while symptoms persist, not to exceed 12 liquigels in 24 hours, or as directed by your doctor. Children under 12 years of age: consult a doctor.

Alcohol Warning: If you consume 3 or more alcoholic drinks every day, ask your doctor whether you should take acetaminophen or other pain relievers/fever reducers. Acetaminophen may cause liver damage.

Warnings: Keep this and all drugs out of the reach of children. In case of accidental overdose, seek professional assistance or contact a poison control center immediately. Prompt medical attention is critical for adults as well as for children even if you do not notice any signs or symptoms. As with any drug, if you are pregnant or nursing a baby, seek the advice of a health professional before using this product. Do not take this product for more than 7 days or for fever for more than 3 days unless directed by a doctor. If

pain or fever persists or gets worse, if new symptoms occur, consult a doctor. A persistent cough may be a sign of a serious condition. If cough persists for more than 1 week, tends to recur, or is accompanied by fever, rash, or persistent headache, consult a doctor. Do not take this product for persistent or chronic cough such as occurs with smoking, asthma, chronic bronchitis, emphysema, or where cough is accompanied by excessive phlegm (mucus) unless directed by a doctor. If sore throat is severe, persists for more than 2 days, is accompanied or followed by fever, headache, rash, nausea, or vomiting, consult a doctor promptly. **Do not exceed recommended dosage.** If nervousness, dizziness, or sleeplessness occur, discontinue use and consult a doctor. If symptoms do not improve within 7 days or are accompanied by fever, consult a doctor. Do not take this product if you have heart disease, high blood pressure, thyroid disease, diabetes, or difficulty in urination due to enlargement of the prostate gland unless directed by a doctor. If you generally consume 3 or more alcohol-containing drinks per day, you should consult your physician for advice on when and how you should take COMTREX and other pain relievers.

Drug Interaction Precaution: Do not use this product if you are now taking a prescription monoamine oxidase inhibitor (MAOI) (certain drugs for depression, psychiatric or emotional conditions, or Parkinson's disease), or for 2 weeks after stopping the MAOI drug. If you are uncertain whether your prescription drug contains an MAOI, consult a health professional before taking this product.

Overdose: Acetylcysteine As an Antidote For Acetaminphen Overdose
Acetaminophen is rapidly absorbed from the upper gastrointestinal tract with peak plasma levels occurring between 30 and 60 minutes after therapeutic doses and usually within 4 hours following an overdose. The parent compound, which is nontoxic, is extensively metabolized in the liver to form principally the sulfate and glucuronide conjugates which are also nontoxic and are rapidly excreted in the urine. A small fraction of an ingested dose is metabolized in the liver by the cytochrome P-450 mixed function oxidase enzyme system to form a reactive, potentially toxic, intermediate metabolite which preferentially conjugates with hepatic glutathione to form the nontoxic cysteine and mercapturic acid derivatives which are then excreted by the kidney. Therapeutic doses of acetaminophen do not saturate the glucuronide and sulfate conjugation pathways and do not result in the formation of sufficient reactive metabolite to deplete glutathione stores. However, following ingestion of a large overdose (150 mg/kg or greater) the glucuronide and sulfate conjugation pathways are saturated resulting in a larger fraction of the drug being metabolized via the P-450 pathway. The in-

creased formation of reactive metabolite may deplete the hepatic stores of glutathione with subsequent binding of the metabolite to protein molecules within the hepatocyte resulting in cellular necrosis. Acetylcysteine has been shown to reduce the extent of liver injury following acetaminophen overdose. Early symptoms following a potentially hepatotoxic overdose may include: nausea, vomiting, diaphoresis and general malaise. Clinical and laboratory evidence of hepatic toxicity may not be apparent until 48 to 72 hours postingestion. In most adults and adolescents, regardless of the quantity of acetaminophen reported to have been ingested, administer acetylcysteine immediately. Acetylcysteine therapy should be initiated and continued for a full course of therapy. Its effectiveness depends on early administration, with benefit seen principally in patients treated within 16 hours of the overdose.

If acetaminophen plasma assay capability is not available, and the estimated acetaminophen ingestion exceeds 150 mg/kg., acetylcysteine therapy should be initiated and continued for a full course of therapy.

For full prescribing information, refer to the acetylcysteine package insert. Do not await the results of assays for acetaminophen level before initiating treatment with acetylcysteine. The following additional procedures are recommended: The stomach should be emptied promptly by lavage or by induction of emesis with syrup of ipecac. A serum acetaminophen assay should be obtained as early as possible, but no sooner than four hours following ingestion. Liver function studies should be obtained initially and repeated at 24-hour intervals.

For additional emergency information call your regional poison center or toll-free (1-800-525-6115) to the Rocky Mountain Poison Center for assistance in diagnosis and for directions in the use of acetylcysteine as an antidote.

How Supplied: Red Oval shaped liquigel printed with "Comtrex CC" in white supplied in bottles of 24's.
Other Comtrex products also available: Acute Head Cold and Sinus Pressure Relief, Allergy Sinus Treatment, Day/Night and Non-Drowsy Formulation's.

Shown in Product Identification Guide, page 506

Aspirin Free EXCEDRIN®

Composition: Each caplet and geltab contains Acetaminophen 500 mg. and Caffeine 65 mg. Other Ingredients: (caplet) Benzoic Acid, Carnauba Wax, Corn starch, D&C Red No. 27 Lake, D&C Yellow No. 10 Lake, FD&C Blue No. 1 Lake, Hydroxypropyl methylcellulose, Magnesium stearate, Methylparaben, Microcrystalline Cellulose, Mineral Oil, Poly-

Continued on next page

Excedrin Aspirin Free—Cont.

sorbate 20, Povidone, Propylene Glycol, Propylparaben, Simethicone Emulsion, Sorbitan Monolaurate, Stearic Acid, Titanium Dioxide.

May also contain: Croscarmellose sodium, FD&C Red No. 40, Saccharin sodium, Sodium starch glycolate

Other Ingredients: (geltab) Benzoic Acid, Corn Starch, FD&C Blue No. 1, FD&C Red No. 40, FD&C Yellow No. 6, Gelatin, Glycerin, Hydroxypropyl methylcellulose, Magnesium stearate, Methylparaben, Microcrystalline cellulose, Mineral oil, Polysorbate 20, Povidone, Propylene glycol, Propylparaben, Simethicone emulsion, Sorbitan monolaurate, Stearic acid, Titanium dioxide.

May also contain: Croscarmellose sodium, Sodium starch glycolate

Indications: For temporary relief of the minor pain of headache, sinusitis, colds, muscular aches, menstrual discomfort, toothaches and arthritis pain.

Directions: Adults: 2 caplets or geltabs every 6 hours while symptoms persist, not to exceed 8 caplets or geltabs in 24 hours, or as directed by a doctor. Children under 12 years of age: Consult a doctor.

Alcohol Warning: If you consume 3 or more alcoholic drinks every day, ask your doctor whether you should take acetaminophen or other pain relievers/fever reducers. Acetaminophen may cause liver damage.

Warnings: Keep this and all drugs out of the reach of children. In case of accidental overdose, seek professional assistance or contact a poison control center immediately. Prompt medical attention is critical for adults as well as for children even if you do not notice any signs or symptoms. As with any drug, if you are pregnant or nursing a baby, seek the advice of a health professional before using this product. Do not take this product for pain for more than 10 days or for fever for more than 3 days unless directed by a doctor. If pain or fever persists or gets worse, if new symptoms occur, of if redness or swelling is present, consult a doctor because these could be signs of a serious condition. Consult a dentist promptly for toothache. If you generally consume 3 or more alcohol-containing drinks per day, you should consult your physician for advice on when and how you should take Aspirin Free Excedrin and other pain relievers.

Overdose: Acetylcysteine As An Antidote For Acetaminophen Overdose

Acetaminophen is rapidly absorbed from the upper gastrointestinal tract with peak plasma levels occurring between 30 and 60 minutes after therapeutic doses and usually within 4 hours following an overdose. The parent compound, which is nontoxic, is extensively metabolized in the liver to form principally the sulfate and glucuronide conjugates which are also nontoxic and are rapidly excreted in the urine. A small fraction of an ingested dose is metabolized in the liver by the cytochrome P-450 mixed function oxidase enzyme system to form a reactive, potentially toxic, intermediate metabolite which preferentially conjugates with hepatic glutathione to form the nontoxic cysteine and mercapturic acid derivatives which are then excreted by the kidney. Therapeutic doses of acetaminophen do not saturate the glucuronide and sulfate conjugation pathways and do not result in the formation of sufficient reactive metabolite to deplete glutathione stores. However, following ingestion of a large overdose (150 mg/kg or greater) the glucuronide and sulfate conjugation pathways are saturated resulting in a larger fraction of the drug being metabolized via the P-450 pathway. The increased formation of reactive metabolite may deplete the hepatic stores of glutathione with subsequent binding of the metabolite to protein molecules within the hepatocyte resulting in cellular necrosis. Acetylcysteine has been shown to reduce the extent of liver injury following acetaminophen overdose. Early symptoms following a potentially hepatotoxic overdose may include: nausea, vomiting, diaphoresis and general malaise. Clinical and laboratory evidence of hepatic toxicity may not be apparent until 48 to 72 hours postingestion. In most adults and adolescents, regardless of the quantity of acetaminophen reported to have been ingested, administer acetylcysteine immediately. Acetylcysteine therapy should be initiated and continued for a full course of therapy. Its effectiveness depends on early administration, with benefit seen principally in patients treated within 16 hours of the overdose.

If acetaminophen plasma assay capability is not available, and the estimated acetaminophen ingestion exceeds 150 mg/kg, acetylcysteine therapy should be initiated and continued for a full course of therapy.

For full prescribing information, refer to the acetylcysteine package insert. Do not await the results of assays for acetaminophen level before initiating treatment with acetylcysteine. The following additional procedures are recommended: The stomach should be emptied promptly by lavage or by induction of emesis with syrup of ipecac. A serum acetaminophen assay should be obtained as early as possible, but no sooner than four hours following ingestion. Liver function studies should be obtained initially and repeated at 24-hour intervals.

For additional emergency information call your regional poison center or toll-free (1-800-525-6115) to the Rocky Mountain Poison Center for assistance in diagnosis and for directions in the use of acetylcysteine as an antidote.

How Supplied: Aspirin Free EXCEDRIN® is supplied as: Coated red caplets with AFE debossed on one side supplied in bottles of 24's, 50's, 100's.

Easy to swallow red geltabs with "AF Excedrin" printed in white on one side supplied in bottles of 20's, 40's, 80's. Store at room temperature.

Shown in Product Identification Guide, page 506

EXCEDRIN® Extra-Strength Analgesic
[ĕx "cĕd 'rĭn]

Composition: Each tablet, caplet, or geltab contains Acetaminophen 250 mg.; Aspirin 250 mg.; and Caffeine 65 mg.

Other Ingredients: (tablet, caplet) Benzoic acid, Hydroxypropylcellulose, Hydroxypropyl methylcellulose, Microcrystalline Cellulose, Mineral Oil, Polysorbate 20, Povidone, Propylene Glycol, Simethicone Emulsion, Sorbitan Monolaurate, Stearic Acid.

Tablets and caplets may also contain: Carnauba wax, FD&C Blue No. 1, Saccharin Sodium, Titanium Dioxide

Other Ingredients: (geltab) Benzoic Acid, D&C Yellow #10 Lake, Disodium EDTA, FD&C Blue #1 Lake, FD&C Red # 40 Lake, Ferric Oxide, Gelatin, Glycerin, Hydroxypropylcellulose, Hydroxypropyl Methylcellulose, Maltitol Solution, Microcrystalline Cellulose, Mineral Oil, Pepsin, Polysorbate 20, Povidone, Propylene Glycol, Propyl Gallate, Simethicone Emulsion, Sorbitan Monolaurate, Stearic Acid, Titanium Dioxide.

Indications: For temporary relief of the pain of headache, sinusitis, colds, muscular aches, menstrual discomfort, toothache and minor arthritis pain.

Alcohol Warning: If you consume 3 or more alcoholic drinks every day, ask your doctor whether you should take acetaminophen and aspirin or other pain relievers/fever reducers. Acetaminophen and aspirin may cause liver damage and stomach bleeding.

Warnings: Children and teenagers should not use this medicine for chicken pox or flu symptoms before a doctor is consulted about Reye syndrome, a rare but serious illness reported to be associated with aspirin. Keep this and all drugs out of the reach of children. In case of accidental overdose, seek professional assistance or contact a physician or poison control center immediately. Prompt medical attention is critical for adults as well as for children even if you do not notice any signs or symptoms. As with any drug, if you are pregnant or nursing a baby, seek the advice of a health professional before using this product. **IT IS ESPECIALLY IMPORTANT NOT TO USE ASPIRIN DURING THE LAST 3 MONTHS OF PREGNANCY UNLESS SPECIFICALLY DIRECTED TO DO SO BY A DOCTOR BECAUSE IT MAY CAUSE PROBLEMS IN THE UNBORN CHILD OR COMPLICATIONS DURING DELIVERY.** Do not take this product for pain for more than 10 days or for fever for more than 3 days unless directed by a doctor. If pain or fever persists or gets worse, if new symptoms occur, or if redness or swelling is present, consult a doctor because these could be signs of a serious condition. Consult a dentist promptly for toothache. Do not take this product if you are allergic to aspirin, have asthma, have stomach problems (such as heartburn, upset stomach or stomach pain) that persist or recur, or if you have ulcers or bleeding problems, unless directed by a doctor. If ringing in the ears or loss of hearing occurs, consult a doctor before taking any more of this product.

Drug Interaction Precaution: Do not take this product if you are taking a prescription drug for anticoagulation (thinning of blood), diabetes, gout or arthritis unless directed by a doctor.

Directions: Adults: 2 tablets, caplets or geltabs with water every 6 hours while symptoms persist, not to exceed 8 tablets, caplets or geltabs in 24 hours, or as directed by a doctor. Children under 12 years of age: Consult a doctor.

Overdose: Acetylcysteine As An Antidote For Acetaminophen Overdose

Acetaminophen is rapidly absorbed from the upper gastrointestinal tract with peak plasma levels occurring between 30 and 60 minutes after therapeutic doses and usually within 4 hours following an overdose. The parent compound, which is nontoxic, is extensively metabolized in the liver to form principally the sulfate and glucuronide conjugates which are also nontoxic and are rapidly excreted in the urine. A small fraction of an ingested dose is metabolized in the liver by the cytochrome P-450 mixed function oxidase enzyme system to form a reactive, potentially toxic, intermediate metabolite which preferentially conjugates with hepatic glutathione to form the nontoxic cysteine and mercapturic acid derivatives which are then excreted by the kidney. Therapeutic doses of acetaminophen do not saturate the glucuronide and sulfate conjugation pathways and do not result in the formation of sufficient reactive metabolite to deplete glutathione stores. However, following ingestion of a large overdose (150 mg/kg or greater) the glucuronide and sulfate conjugation pathways are saturated resulting in a larger fraction of the drug being metabolized via the P-450 pathway. The increased formation of reactive metabolite may deplete the hepatic stores of glutathione with subsequent binding of the metabolite to protein molecules within the hepatocyte resulting in cellular necrosis. Acetylcysteine has been shown to reduce the extent of liver injury following acetaminophen overdose. Early symptoms following a potentially hepatotoxic overdose may include: nausea, vomiting, diaphoresis and general malaise. Clinical and laboratory evidence of hepatic toxicity may not be apparent until 48 to 72 hours postingestion. In most adults and adolescents, regardless of the quantity of acetaminophen reported to

have been ingested, administer acetylcysteine immediately. Acetylcysteine therapy should be initiated and continued for a full course of therapy. Its effectiveness depends on early administration, with benefit seen principally in patients treated within 16 hours of the overdose.

If acetaminophen plasma assay capability is not available, and the estimated acetaminophen ingestion exceeds 150 mg/kg, acetylcysteine therapy should be initiated and continued for a full course of therapy.

For full prescribing information, refer to the acetylcysteine package insert. Do not await the results of assays for acetaminophen level before initiating treatment with acetylcysteine. The following additional procedures are recommended: The stomach should be emptied promptly by lavage or by induction of emesis with syrup of ipecac. A serum acetaminophen assay should be obtained as early as possible, but no sooner than four hours following ingestion. Liver function studies should be obtained initially and repeated at 24-hour intervals.

For additional emergency information call your regional poison center or toll-free (1-800-525-6115) to the Rocky Mountain Poison Center for assistance in diagnosis and for directions in the use of acetylcysteine as an antidote.

How Supplied: Extra Strength EXCEDRIN® is supplied as:
Coated white circular tablet with letter "E" debossed on one side. Supplied in bottles of 12's, 24's, 50's, 100's, 175's, 275's and metal tins of 12's.
Coated white caplets with "E" debossed on one side. Supplied in bottles of 24's, 50's, 100's, 175's, 275's.
Gel-coated round geltabs–green on one side, white on the other, printed with black "E" on one side. Supplied in bottles of 20's, 40's, 80's.
Store at room temperature.
Shown in Product Identification Guide, page 506

EXCEDRIN® MIGRAINE
Pain Reliever/Pain Reliever Aid

Active Ingredients: Each tablet, caplet or geltab contains Acetaminophen 250mg, Aspirin 250mg and Caffeine 65mg.

Inactive Ingredients: (tablet and caplet) benzoic acid, carnauba wax, hydroxypropylcellulose, hydroxypropyl methylcellulose, microcrystalline cellulose, mineral oil, polysorbate 20, povidone, propylene glycol, stearic acid, simethicone emulsion, sorbitan monolaurate. May also contain: FD&C blue no. 1, titanium dioxide.

Inactive Ingredients: (geltab) Benzoic Acid, D&C Yellow #10 Lake, Disodium EDTA, FD&C Blue #1 Lake, FD&C Red #40 Lake, Ferric Oxide, Gelatin, Glycerin, Hydroxypropylcellulose, Hydroxypropyl Methylcellulose, Maltitol

Solution, Microcrystalline Cellulose, Mineral Oil, Pepsin, Polysorbate 20, Povidone, Propylene Glycol, Propyl Gallate, Simethicone Emulsion, Sorbitan Monolaurate, Stearic Acid, Titanium Dioxide.

Use: for the temporary relief of mild to moderate pain associated with migraine headache.
Alcohol Warning: If you consume 3 or more alcoholic drinks every day, ask your doctor whether you should take acetaminophen and aspirin or other pain relievers/fever reducers. Acetaminophen and aspirin may cause liver damage and stomach bleeding.

Warnings: Children and teenagers should not use this medicine for chicken pox, or flu symptoms, before a doctor is consulted about Reye syndrome, a rare but serious illness reported to be associated with aspirin.
Allergy Alert: If after taking a pain reliever or fever reducer, you have ever had hives, facial swelling, asthma or shock, do not take Excedrin Migraine. You may have a serious reaction.
Caffeine: The recommended dose of this product contains about as much caffeine as a cup of coffee. Limit the use of caffeine-containing medications, foods, or beverages while taking this product because too much caffeine may cause nervousness, irritability, sleeplessness, and, occasionally, rapid heart beat.
Ask a Doctor Before Use If You Have:
the worst headache of your life; fever and stiff neck; bleeding problems; ulcers; asthma; liver disease; renal disease; stomach problems such as heartburn, upset stomach, or stomach pain that do not go away or recur; daily headaches; headaches beginning after or are caused by head injury, exertion, coughing or bending; experienced your first headache after the age of 50; migraine headaches so severe as to require bed rest; vomiting with your migraine headache
Ask a Doctor Before Use If You Are: taking a prescription drug for anticoagulation (thinning of the blood), diabetes, gout or arthritis
Stop Using This Product and See a Doctor If:
migraine headache pain worsens or continues for more than 48 hours; new or unexpected symptoms occur; ringing of the ears or loss of hearing occurs.
As with any drug, if you are pregnant or nursing a baby, seek the advice of a health professional before using this product. **IT IS ESPECIALLY IMPORTANT NOT TO USE ASPIRIN DURING THE LAST 3 MONTHS OF PREGNANCY UNLESS SPECIFICALLY DIRECTED TO DO SO BY A DOCTOR BECAUSE IT MAY CAUSE PROBLEMS IN THE UNBORN CHILD OR COMPLICATIONS DURING DELIVERY. Keep this and all drugs out of the reach of children.** In case of accidental overdose, seek professional assistance or contact a Poison Control Center immediately. Prompt medical attention

Continued on next page

634/BRISTOL-MYERS

Excedrin Migraine—Cont.

is critical for adults as well as for children even if you do not notice any signs or symptoms.

Directions: Adults and children over 12 years: 2 tablets, caplets or geltabs with a full glass of water every 6 hours while symptoms persist, not to exceed 8 tablets, caplets or geltabs in 24 hours, or as directed by a doctor. Do not take for more than 48 hours for the pain of migraine. Children: Do not give to children under 12 unless directed by a doctor.

Overdose:

Acetylcysteine As An Antidote For Acetaminophen Overdose

Acetaminophen is rapidly absorbed from the upper gastrointestinal tract with peak plasma levels occurring between 30 and 60 minutes after therapeutic doses and usually within 4 hours following an overdose. The parent compound, which is nontoxic, is extensively metabolized in the liver to form principally the sulfate and glucuronide conjugates which are also nontoxic and are rapidly excreted in the urine. A small fraction of an ingested dose is metabolized in the liver by the cytochrome P-450 mixed function oxidase enzyme system to form a reactive, potentially toxic, intermediate metabolite which preferentially conjugates with hepatic glutathione to form the nontoxic cysteine and mercapturic acid derivatives which are then excreted by the kidney. Therapeutic doses of acetaminophen do not saturate the glucuronide and sulfate conjugation pathways and do not result in the formation of sufficient reactive metabolite to deplete glutathione stores. However, following ingestion of a large overdose (150 mg/kg or greater) the glucuronide and sulfate conjugation pathways are saturated resulting in a larger fraction of the drug being metabolized via the P-450 pathway. The increased formation of reactive metabolite may deplete the hepatic stores of glutathione with subsequent binding of the metabolite to protein molecules within the hepatocyte resulting in cellular necrosis. Acetylcysteine has been shown to reduce the extent of liver injury following acetaminophen overdose. Early symptoms following a potentially hepatotoxic overdose may include: nausea, vomiting, diaphoresis and general malaise. Clinical and laboratory evidence of hepatic toxicity may not be apparent until 48 to 72 hours postingestion. In most adults and adolescents, regardless of the quantity of acetaminophen reported to have been ingested, administer acetylcysteine immediately. Acetylcysteine therapy should be initiated and continued for a full course of therapy. Its effectiveness depends on early administration, with benefit seen principally in patients treated within 16 hours of the overdose. If acetaminophen plasma assay capability is not available, and the estimated acetaminophen ingestion ex-

ceeds 150 mg/kg., acetylcysteine therapy should be initiated and continued for a full course of therapy.

For full prescription information, refer to the acetylcysteine package insert. Do not await the results of assays for acetaminophen level before initiating treatment with acetylcysteine. The following additional procedures are recommended: The stomach should be emptied promptly by lavage or by induction of emesis with syrup of ipecac. A serum acetaminophen assay should be obtained as early as possible, but no sooner than four hours following ingestion. Liver function studies should be obtained initially and repeated at 24-hour intervals. For additional emergency information call your regional poison center or toll-free (1-800-525-6115) to the Rocky Mountain Poison and Drug Center for assistance in diagnosis and for directions in the use of acetylcysteine as an antidote.

How Supplied: EXCEDRIN® MIGRAINE is supplied as:
Coated white circular tablets or coated white caplets with letter "E" debossed on one side. Supplied in bottles of 24's, 50's, 100's, 175's. 275's (tablets) are available in club store packages. Coated round geltabs–green on one side, white on the other, printed with black "E" on one side. Supplied in bottles of 24's.
Store at controlled room temperature: 20–25°C (68–77°F).

Shown in Product Identification Guide, page 507

EXCEDRIN P.M.®
[ĕx "cĕd 'rĭn]
Analgesic Sleeping Aid

Composition: Each tablet, caplet or geltab contains:

	EXCEDRIN®PM Per Tablet or Caplet
Acetaminophen	500 mg.
Diphenhydramine Citrate:	38 mg.

Other Ingredients:
(Tablet or Caplet)
benzoic acid
carnauba wax
corn starch
D&C yellow no. 10
D&C yellow no. 10 aluminum lake
FD&C blue no. 1
FD&C blue no. 1 aluminum lake
hydroxypropyl methylcellulose
magnesium stearate
methylparaben
pregelatinized starch
propylene glycol
propylparaben
simethicone emulsion
stearic acid
titanium dioxide
May also contain:
mineral oil
polysorbate 20
povidone
sodium citrate
sorbitan monolaurate

	EXCEDRIN®PM Per Geltab
Acetaminophen	500 mg.
Diphenhydramine Citrate	38 mg.

Other Ingredients:
(Geltab)
Benzoic Acid
Corn starch
D&C Red No. 33 Lake
D&C Yellow No. 10
D&C Yellow No. 10 Lake
Edetate Disodium
Fd&C Blue No. 1
Fd&C Blue No. 1 Lake
Gelatin
Glycerin
Hydroxypropyl Methylcellulose
Magnesium Stearate
Methylparaben
Mineral Oil
Polysorbate 20
Povidone
Pregelatinized Starch
Propylene Glycol
Propylparaben
Simethicone Emulsion
Sorbitan Monolaurate
Stearic Acid
Titanium Dioxide

Indications: For temporary relief of occasional headaches and minor aches and pains with accompanying sleeplessness.

Alcohol Warning: If you consume 3 or more alcoholic drinks every day, ask your doctor whether you should take acetaminophen or other pain relievers/fever reducers. Acetaminophen may cause liver damage.

Warnings: Keep this and all drugs out of the reach of children. In case of accidental overdose, seek professional assistance or contact a poison control center immediately. Prompt medical attention is critical for adults as well as for children even if you do not notice any signs or symptoms. As with any drug, if you are pregnant or nursing a baby, seek the advice of a health professional before using this product. Do not give to children under 12 years of age or use for more than 10 days unless directed by a doctor. If symptoms persist or get worse, if new ones occur, or if sleeplessness persists continuously for more than 2 weeks, consult your doctor. Insomnia may be a symptom of serious underlying medical illness. Do not take this product, unless directed by a doctor, if you have a breathing problem such as emphysema or chronic bronchitis, or if you have glaucoma or difficulty in urination due to enlargement of the prostate gland. Avoid alcoholic beverages while taking this product. Do not take this product if you are taking sedatives or tranquilizers, without first consulting your doctor. If you generally consume 3 or more alcohol-containing drinks per day, you should consult your physician for advice on when and how you should take Excedrin PM and other pain relievers.

Directions:
Adults and children 12 years of age and over: 2 tablets, caplets, or geltabs at bedtime if needed or as directed by a doctor.

Overdose: Acetylcysteine As An Antidote For Acetaminophen Overdose

Acetaminophen is rapidly absorbed from the upper gastrointestinal tract with peak plasma levels occurring between 30 and 60 minutes after therapeutic doses and usually within 4 hours following an overdose. The parent compound, which is nontoxic, is extensively metabolized in the liver to form principally the sulfate and glucuronide conjugates which are also nontoxic and are rapidly excreted in the urine. A small fraction of an ingested dose is metabolized in the liver by the cytochrome P-450 mixed function oxidase enzyme system to form a reactive, potentially toxic, intermediate metabolite which preferentially conjugates with hepatic glutathione to form the nontoxic cysteine and mercapturic acid derivatives which are then excreted by the kidney. Therapeutic doses of acetaminophen do not saturate the glucuronide and sulfate conjugation pathways and do not result in the formation of sufficient reactive metabolite to deplete glutathione stores. However, following ingestion of a large overdose (150 mg/kg or greater) the glucuronide and sulfate conjugation pathways are saturated resulting in a larger fraction of the drug being metabolized via the P-450 pathway. The increased formation of reactive metabolite may deplete the hepatic stores of glutathione with subsequent binding of the metabolite to protein molecules within the hepatocyte resulting in cellular necrosis. Acetylcysteine has been shown to reduce the extent of liver injury following acetaminophen overdose. Early symptoms following a potentially hepatotoxic overdose may include: nausea, vomiting, diaphoresis and general malaise. Clinical and laboratory evidence of hepatic toxicity may not be apparent until 48 to 72 hours postingestion. In most adults and adolescents, regardless of the quantity of acetaminophen reported to have been ingested, administer acetylcysteine immediately. Acetylcysteine therapy should be initiated and continued for a full course of therapy. Its effectiveness depends on early administration, with benefit seen principally in patients treated within 16 hours of the overdose.

If acetaminophen plasma assay capability is not available, and the estimated acetaminophen ingestion exceeds 150 mg/kg, acetylcysteine therapy should be initiated and continued for a full course of therapy.

For full prescribing information, refer to the package insert. Do not await the results of assays for acetaminophen level before initiating treatment with acetylcysteine. The following additional procedures are recommended: The stomach should be emptied promptly by lavage or by induction of emesis with syrup of ip-

ecac. A serum acetaminophen assay should be obtained as early as possible, but no sooner than four hours following ingestion. Liver function studies should be obtained initially and repeated at 24-hour intervals.

For additional emergency information call your regional poison center or toll-free (1-800-525-6115) to the Rocky Mountain Poison Center for assistance in diagnosis and for directions in the use of acetylcysteine as an antidote.

For overdose treatment information, consult a regional poison control center.

How Supplied: EXCEDRIN P.M.® is supplied as:
Light blue circular coated tablets with "PM" debossed on one side. Supplied in bottles of 10's, 24's, 50's, 100's, 150's.
Light blue coated caplet with "PM" debossed on one side. Supplied in bottles of 24's, 50's, 100's.
Gel coated-light blue and white geltabs with "PM" printed in black on one side. Supplied in bottles of 24's, 50's, 100's.
Store at room temperature.
Shown in Product Identification Guide, page 506

4-WAY Fast Acting Nasal Spray
Regular and Mentholated formulas

Composition:

Active ingredient:
Phenylephrine hydrochloride 1.0%,

Inactive ingredients (regular formula):
benzalkonium chloride, boric acid, sodium borate, water

Inactive ingredients (mentholated formula):
benzalkonium chloride, boric acid, camphor, eucalyptol, menthol, polysorbate 80, sodium borate, water

Indications
For the temporary relief of nasal congestion due to the common cold, hay fever or other upper respiratory allergies, or associated with sinusitis.

Directions:
Adults and children 12 years of age and older: 2 or 3 sprays in each nostril not more than every 4 hours. Do not give to children under 12 years of age unless directed by a doctor.

Use Instructions:
With head in a normal, upright position, put atomizer tip into nostril. Squeeze bottle with firm, quick pressure while inhaling. Wipe nozzle clean after each use.

Warnings:
Keep out of reach of children. If swallowed, get medical help or contact a poison control center right away. **Do not exceed recommended dosage.** This product may cause temporary discomfort such as burning, stinging, sneezing, or an increase in nasal discharge. The use of this container by more than one person may spread infections. Do not use this product for more than 3 days. Use

only as directed. Frequent or prolonged use may cause nasal congestion to recur or worsen. If symptoms persist, consult a doctor. Do not use this product if you have heart disease, high blood pressure, thyroid disease, diabetes, or difficulty in urination due to enlargement of the prostate gland unless directed by a doctor.
Note: Container is filled to proper level for best spray action.
Store at room temperature.

How Supplied:
Regular formula:
$1/2$ fluid ounce, and 1 fluid ounce size.
Mentholated formula:
$1/2$ fluid ounce.
Store at room temperature.
Also available: 4-way 12 hour and 4-way Saline Moisturizing Mist formulations.
Shown in Product Identification Guide, page 506

KERI LOTION
Skin Lubricant—Moisturizer

Available in 3 formulations:
KERI Original, Silky Smooth and Sensitive Skin

KERI Original Formula, Long Lasting Therapeutic Dry Skin Lotion: A highly emollient formula for patients who prefer a heavy formula.

Composition: Water, mineral oil, propylene glycol, PEG-40 stearate, glyceryl stearate/PEG-100 stearate, PEG-4 dilaurate, laureth-4, lanolin oil, methyl paraben, carbomer, propylparaben, fragrance triethanolamine, dioctyl sodium sulfosuccinate, quaternium-15.

Direction: For best results, apply daily to hands and body. Use after bath/shower or whenever skin feels dry or rough.
FOR EXTERNAL USE ONLY.

KERI Silky Smooth Vitamin E Enriched Formula: Fast absorbing, light therapeutic levels.

Composition: Water, petrolatum, glycerin, dimethicone, steareth-2, cetyl alcohol, benzyl alcohol, laureth-23, magnesium aluminum silicate, tocopheryl acetate or tocopheryl linoleate, carbomer, fragrance, sodium hydroxide, disodium EDTA, quaternium-15.

Directions: Apply liberally after bathing, before bed or whenever skin feels dry. Use daily on hands, arms, legs, or anywhere skin feels dry for softer, smoother, healthier-looking skin. For external use only.

KERI Sensitive Skin, Hypo-Allergenic and Fragrance-Free formula: For patients with sensitive skin.

Composition: Water, petrolatum, glycerin, dimethicone, steareth-2, cetyl alcohol, benzyl alcohol, laureth-23, magnesium aluminum silicate, tocopheryl ace-

Continued on next page

Keri—Cont.

tate or tocopheryl linoleate, carbomer, sodium hydroxide, disodium EDTA, quaternium-15.

Directions: Apply liberally after bathing, before bed or whenever skin feels dry. Use daily on hands, arms, legs, or anywhere skin feels dry for softer, smoother, healthier-looking skin. For external use only.

How Supplied: All KERI Lotions available in: 2 oz., 6½ oz., 11 oz. and 15 oz. bottles. KERI Original also available in 20 oz. and 32 oz. bottles.

Shown in Product Identification Guide, page 507

KERI® Anti-Bacterial Hand Lotion
Antiseptic/Moisturizer

Keri Anti-Bacterial Hand Lotion is a light, Vitamin E-enriched, emollient formula that restores lost moisture to dry skin to leave your hands feeling soft and smooth, without feeling greasy. Plus it kills germs with a clinically proven anti-bacterial ingredient.

Dermatologist tested for gentleness.

Indication: To help reduce bacteria that potentially can cause disease. Recommended for repeated use.

Directions: Dispense Keri Anti-Bacterial Hand Lotion into one hand. Apply to both hands and rub into the skin until dry.

Warnings: Keep out of the reach of children. For external use only. Do not use in the eyes. Discontinue use if irritation or redness develop. If condition persists for more than 72 hours, consult a doctor.

Active Ingredient: Triclosan.

Other Ingredients: Water, Glycerin, Hydrogenated Polyisobutene, Mineral Oil, Stearic Acid, Cetyl Alcohol, Tocopheryl Acetate, Dimethicone, Petrolatum, PEG-5 Soy Sterol, Dimethicone Copolyol, Cyclomethicone, Glyceryl Stearate, Triethanolamine, PEG-100 Stearate, Carbomer, Phenoxyethanol, Magnesium Aluminum Silicate, Disodium EDTA, Methylparaben, Propylparaben, Diazolidinyl Urea, Titanium Dioxide, Fragrance.

How Supplied: 2 oz, 6 1/2 oz, 11 oz and 20 oz.
Store at room temperature.
Questions or Comments? Call 1-800-468-7746
DISTR. BY: BRISTOL-MYERS SQUIBB CO.,
© 1996, NY, NY 10154 Made in USA
Shown in Product Identification Guide, page 507

NO DOZ® Maximum Strength Caplets

Composition: Each caplet contains 200 mg. Caffeine. Other ingredients: Benzoic Acid, Corn Starch, FD&C Blue No. 1, Flavors, Hydroxypropyl Methylcellulose, Microcrystalline Cellulose, Propylene Glycol, Simethicone Emulsion, Stearic Acid, Sucrose, Titanium Dioxide. May also contain: Carnauba Wax, Mineral Oil, Polysorbate 20, Povidone, Sorbitan Monolaurate.

Indications: Helps restore mental alertness or wakefulness when experiencing fatigue or drowsiness.

Directions: Adults: one-half to one caplet not more often than every 3 to 4 hours.

Warnings: KEEP THIS AND ALL OTHER MEDICATIONS OUT OF THE REACH OF CHILDREN. IN CASE OF ACCIDENTAL OVERDOSE, SEEK PROFESSIONAL ASSISTANCE OR CONTACT A POISON CONTROL CENTER IMMEDIATELY. As with any drug, if you are pregnant or nursing a baby, seek the advice of a health professional before using this product. Do not give to children under 12 years of age. For occasional use only. Not intended for use as a substitute for sleep. If fatigue or drowsiness persists or continues to occur, consult a doctor. The recommended dose of this product contains about as much caffeine as a cup of coffee. Limit the use of caffeine-containing medications, foods, or beverages while taking this product because too much caffeine may cause nervousness, irritability, sleeplessness and, occasionally, rapid heart beat.

How Supplied: NO DOZ® Maximum Strength is supplied as: White coated caplets with "NO DOZ" debossed on one side. The opposite side is scored.
Supplied in bottles of 16's, 36's, 60's.
Store at room temperature.
Shown in Product Identification Guide, page 507

NUPRIN®
(ibuprofen)
Analgesic

Warnings:
Allergy Alert: ibuprofen may cause a severe allergic reaction which may include:
• hives • facial swelling • asthma (wheezing) • shock
Do not use if you have ever had an allergic reaction to any other pain reliever/ fever reducer.
Stop use and ask a doctor if an allergic reaction occurs. Seek medical help right away.

Composition: Each tablet or caplet contains ibuprofen USP, 200 mg. **Other Ingredients:** Carnauba wax, cornstarch, D&C Yellow No. 10, FD&C Yellow No. 6, hydroxypropyl methylcellulose, propylene glycol, silicon dioxide, stearic acid, titanium dioxide.

Indications: For the temporary relief of minor aches and pains associated with the common cold, headache, toothache, muscular aches, backache, for the minor pain of arthritis, for the pain of menstrual cramps and for reduction of fever.
Alcohol Warning: If you consume 3 or more alcoholic drinks every day, ask your doctor whether you should take ibuprofen or other pain relievers/fever reducers. Ibuprofen may cause stomach bleeding.

Warnings: Do not take for pain for more than 10 days or for fever for more than 3 days unless directed by a doctor. If pain or fever persists or gets worse, if new symptoms occur, or if the painful area is red or swollen, consult a doctor. These could be signs of serious illness. If you are under a doctor's care for any serious condition, consult a doctor before taking this product. As with aspirin and acetaminophen, if you have any condition which requires you to take prescription drugs or if you have had any problems or serious side effects from taking any non-prescription pain reliever, do not take NUPRIN without first discussing it with your doctor. If you experience any symptoms which are unusual or seem unrelated to the condition for which you took ibuprofen, consult a doctor before taking any more of it. Although ibuprofen is indicated for the same conditions as aspirin and acetaminophen, it should not be taken with them except under a doctor's direction. Do not combine this product with any other ibuprofen-containing product. As with any drug, if you are pregnant or nursing a baby, seek the advice of a health professional before using this product. IT IS ESPECIALLY IMPORTANT NOT TO USE IBUPROFEN DURING THE LAST 3 MONTHS OF PREGNANCY UNLESS SPECIFICALLY DIRECTED TO DO SO BY A DOCTOR BECAUSE IT MAY CAUSE PROBLEMS IN THE UNBORN CHILD OR COMPLICATIONS DURING DELIVERY. Keep this and all drugs out of the reach of children. In case of accidental overdose, seek professional assistance or contact a poison control center immediately.

Caution: Store at room temperature. Avoid excessive heat 40°C (104°F).

Directions: Adults: Take 1 tablet or caplet every 4 to 6 hours while symptoms persist. If pain or fever does not respond to 1 tablet or caplet, 2 tablets or caplets may be used but do not exceed 6 tablets or caplets in 24 hours, unless directed by a doctor. The smallest effective dose should be used. Take with food or milk if occasional and mild heartburn, upset stomach, or stomach pain occurs with use. Consult a doctor if these symptoms are more than mild or if they persist. Children: Do not give this product to children under 12 except under the advice and supervision of a doctor.

Overdose: For overdose treatment information, consult a regional poison control center.

How Supplied:
NUPRIN® is supplied as:
Golden yellow round tablets with "NUPRIN" printed in black on one side.

Golden yellow caplets with "NUPRIN" printed in black on one side.
Supplied in bottles of 36's, 75's, 150's. All sizes packaged in child resistant closures households without young children.
Store at room temperature. Avoid excessive heat 40°C. (104°F.).
Distributed by Bristol-Myers Company
Shown in Product Identification Guide, page 507

VAGISTAT®–1
vaginal ointment
(tioconazole 6.5%)

Description: VAGISTAT-1 (tioconazole 6.5%) is a single dose treatment for recurrent vaginal yeast infections which is now available over-the-counter.

Composition: VAGISTAT-1 (tioconazole 6.5%) is formulated in a base of white petrolatum and magnesium aluminum silicate with butylated hydroxyanisole (BHA) added as a preservative. Each applicatorful of VAGISTAT-1 provides approximately 4.6 grams of ointment containing 300 mg of tioconazole.

Indications: VAGISTAT-1 is indicated for the treatment of recurrent vaginal yeast infections previously diagnosed by a physician. If this is the first time vaginal itch and discomfort have been present, a doctor should be consulted. If you have had a doctor diagnose a vaginal yeast infection before and have the same symptoms now, use this ointment as directed.
Studies have shown that women taking oral contraceptives have cure rates similar to those not taking such agents when treated with VAGISTAT-1.
Safety and effectiveness in pregnant and diabetic patients have not been established.

Contraindications: VAGISTAT-1 is contraindicated in individuals who have been shown to be sensitive to imidazole antifungal agents or to other components of the ointment.

Precautions:
Pregnancy
There are no adequate and well-controlled studies in pregnant women. VAGISTAT-1 (tioconazole 6.5%) should be used during pregnancy only if the physician believes the potential benefit justifies the potential risk to the fetus.
Nursing Mothers:
It is not known whether this drug is excreted in human milk. Because many drugs are excreted in human milk, nursing should be temporarily discontinued while VAGISTAT-1 is administered.
Pediatric Use:
Safety and effectiveness in children have not been established.

Warnings:
- Do not use if you have abdominal pain, fever (higher than 100 °F orally), chills, nausea, vomiting, diarrhea, or foul-smelling discharge. Contact your doctor immediately.

- If your symptoms do not improve in 3 days or if you still have symptoms after 7 days, consult your doctor. Your doctor may recommend other treatment, or you may have a condition other than a yeast infection.
- If your symptoms return within 2 months or if you think you have been exposed to the human immunodeficiency virus (HIV) that causes AIDS, consult your doctor immediately. Recurring yeast infections may be a sign of pregnancy or a serious condition, such as AIDS or diabetes.
- Do not use if you are pregnant or think you may be pregnant, have diabetes, a positive HIV test, or AIDS. Consult your doctor.
- Do not use tampons while using this medicine. Use sanitary napkins instead.
- Do not rely on condoms or diaphragms to prevent sexually transmitted diseases or pregnancy while using VAGISTAT-1. This product may damage condoms and diaphragms and may cause them to fail. You should wait 3 days after treatment to resume using condoms or your diaphragm.
- Do not use in girls under 12 years of age.
- Keep this and all drugs out of the reach of children.
- VAGISTAT-1 is for vaginal use only. Do not use in eyes or take by mouth. In case of accidental ingestion, seek professional assistance or contact a Poison Control Center immediately.

Side Effects: The incidence of adverse reactions to VAGISTAT-1 is based on clinical trials involving 1000 patients. Burning and itching were the most frequent side effects occurring in approximately 6% and 5% of patients, respectively. In most instances these did not interfere with the course of therapy.
There were occasional reports (less than 1%) of other side effects including irritation, discharge, vulvar swelling, vaginal pain, dysuria, (pain on urination), nocturia, (nighttime urination), dyspareunia, (painful intercourse), dryness of vaginal secretions, desquamation, (peeling skin), and burning sensation.
In two clinical trials involving 1060 patients which supported the Rx to OTC switch, the most frequently reported side effects were vaginitis (5%), headache (5%), infection (3%), and abdominal pain (2%). There were also occasional reports (less than 2%) of pharyngitis, rhinitis, vulvovaginal disorder, rash and dysuria.

Dosage And Administration: Insert one applicatorful intravaginally. Remove prefilled applicator and plunger from foil packet. Hold blue capped end of applicator and push tip of plunger into base of applicator. Remove the blue cap with a pull twist action. Insert applicatorful intravaginally while lying on your back with knees bent. Push plunger into applicator until it will go no further. Withdraw applicator and plunger and dispose of in wastebasket. Administration of VAGISTAT-1 just prior to bedtime is recommended.

How Supplied: VAGISTAT-1 is supplied in a ready-to-use, prefilled, single-dose vaginal applicator. Each applicator-

ful will deliver approximately 4.6 grams of VAGISTAT-1 containing 65 mg of tioconazole per gram of ointment.
Store at controlled room temperature 15°–30°C (59°–86°F).
Shown in Product Identification Guide, page 507

Care-Tech®
Laboratories, Inc.
Over-The-Counter Pharmaceuticals
3224 SOUTH KINGSHIGHWAY BOULEVARD
ST. LOUIS, MO 63139

Direct Inquiries to:
Sherry L. Brereton
(314) 772-4610
FAX: (314) 772-4613

For Medical Emergencies Contact:
Customer Service
(800) 325-9681
FAX: (314) 772-4613

BARRI–CARE®
ANTIMICROBIAL OINTMENT

Composition: Active Ingredient: Chloroxylenol .8%
Inactive Ingredients: Petrolatum, Water, Paraffin, Propylene Glycol, Milk Protein, Cod Liver Oil, Aloe Vera Gel, Fragrance, Potassium Hydroxide, Methyl Paraben, Propyl Paraben, Vitamin A & D_3, (E) dl Alpha-Tocopheryl Acetate, (E) dl-Alpha-Tocopherol, D&C Yellow #11 and D&C Red #17.

Actions and Uses: Topical, antimicrobial for prevention and treatment of bacterial infection. Formulated for diabetic feet, topical staph infection and immune compromised patient care. For use around edges of chronic wounds to halt additional breakdown, trac sites, I.V. sites. Proven antimicrobial action against E. coli, MRSA, S. aureus and Pseudomonas aeruginosa. Protects perineal area of the incontinent patient from painful skin rashes and relieves irritation around stoma sites. Utilize on Grades I–IV pressure ulcers to halt skin breakdown. Can be used also on minor burns. Will not melt under feverish conditions. No Contra-indications. Three year shelf life.

Precautions: External Use Only. Non-Toxic. Avoid eye contact.—Ointment-base.

Directions: Cleanse affected area with Satin thoroughly. Apply ointment topically to affected area. Reapply 2–3 times daily or as directed by physician.

How Supplied: 1 ounce tubes, 4 oz. tubes, 8 oz. jar. NDC #46706-206

Continued on next page

CARE-CREME® ANTIMICROBIAL CREAM

Composition: Active Ingredient: Chloroxylenol .8%
Inactive Ingredients: Water, Cetyl Alcohol, Lanolin Oil, Cod Liver Oil, Sodium Laureth Sulfate, Triethanolamine, Propylene Glycol, Petrolatum, Lanolin Alcohol, Methyl Gluceth 20 Distearate, Beeswax, Citric Acid, Methyl Paraben, Fragrance, Propyl Paraben, Vitamins A, D₃ and E-dl Alpha-Tocopherol.

Actions and Uses: Vitamin enriched broad spectrum topical, antimicrobial cream for treatment of atopic dermatitis, psoriasis, severe itching, staph infections. Transdermal, antimicrobial action on gram-negative, gram-positive, yeast and fungi. Extremely effective on oncology radiation burns. Use at first sign of reddened skin or initial breakdown. Vitamin and oil enriched to promote skin integrity. Contains no metallic ions. Provides moisture and vitamin enriched wound therapy.

Precautions: Non-toxic, External Use Only. Avoid use around eye area. No Contra-indications. Three year shelf life.

Directions: Cleanse affected area with Satin and gently massage Care Creme into skin until completely absorbed or as directed by physician. Apply 3–4 times daily or as needed.

How Supplied: 1 ounce tubes, 4 oz. tubes, 9 oz. jar. NDC #46706-205

CLINICAL CARE® ANTIMICROBIAL WOUND CLEANSER

Composition: Active Ingredient: Benzethonium Chloride .1%
Inactive Ingredients: Water, Amphoteric 2, Aloe Vera Gel, DMDM Hydantoin, Citric Acid.

Actions and Uses: Clinical Care is an antimicrobial, emulsifying solution which aids in removing debris and particulate matter from open, dermal wounds. Clinical Care inhibits the growth of pathogenic organisms. Proven effective at eliminating S. aureus, P. aeruginosa, S. typhimurium, Aspergillus, E. coli, MRSA, S. pyogenes and K. pneumonia. Will not produce dermal irritation.

Precautions: External Use Only. Non-Toxic. No contra-indicators.

Directions: Spray affected area as necessary to debride. Use sterile gauze to gently remove debris and necrotic tissue at dermal surface.

How Supplied: 4 oz. spray, 12 oz. spray

CONCEPT® ANTIMICROBIAL DERMAL CLEANSER

Composition: Active Ingredient: Chloroxylenol .5%
Inactive Ingredients: Water, Amphoteric 9, Polysorbate 20, PEG-150 Distearate, Cocamide DEA, Cocoyl Sarcosine, Fragrance, D&C Green #5.

Actions and Uses: Concept is a geriatric shampoo and body wash for patients with delicate tissue or for use on infants to prevent infection and cross-contamination. Concept is non-eye irritating and eliminates bacteria on the skin. Excellent for replenishing moisture in dry, flaky dermal tissues and eliminating body odors. Safe for use on infants to address rashing or atopic dermatitis. Excellent for use on HIV and oncology patients to reduce topical infection.

Precautions: External Use Only. Non-Toxic. No Contra-indications.

Directions: Use in normal manner of bathing and shampooing. Rinse thoroughly.

How Supplied: 8 oz., Gallons NDC #46706-112

FORMULA MAGIC® ANTIMICROBIAL/ANTI-FUNGAL POWDER

Composition: Active Ingredient: Benzethonium Chloride .1%
Inactive Ingredients: Talc, Mineral Oil, Magnesium Carbonate, Fragrance, DMDM Hydantoin.

Actions and Uses: Broad spectrum antimicrobial/antifungal talc base powder for treatment of diabetic feet and limbs. Aids in preventing excoriation, friction chafing and eliminating odor. Antibacterial action proven effective at 99.9% inhibition where Formula Magic is applied. Excellent for use on diabetic patients, feet and under breasts to relieve redness and skin irritation caused by excessive moisture and resulting bacterial growth.

Precautions: Non-irritating to skin, non-toxic, slightly irritating to eyes.

Directions: Apply liberally to body and rub gently into skin.

How Supplied: 4 oz. and 12 oz. NDC #46706-202

HUMATRIX® MICROCLYSMIC GEL
Burn/Wound Healing Gel for Tissue Trauma

Composition: Water, Propylene Glycol, Glycerine, Hydrolyzed Collagen, Citric Acid, Carbomer, Triethanolamine, Chondroitin Sulfate, Preservatives.

Actions and Uses: Provides endothermic and biomimetic properties to cool traumatized tissue and aid in the homeostasis of healing. HUMATRIX® provides the ultimate moisturization for burns, autograft procedures, radiation irritation, glycolic acid peel irritation, mechanical injuries, laser treatment, and chronic wound therapy. Humatrix is almost pure protein in content and aids in rapid cellular regeneration. Reduces surface temperature of tissue 12–15° within 3 minutes of application.

Precautions: External use only. Nontoxic. No contra-indications.

Directions: Cleanse the area with Techni-Care® Surgical Scrub, Prep. and Wound Cleanser, Rinse thoroughly with Clinical Care® Antimicrobial Wound Cleanser. Do not pat dry. Apply a layer of HUMATRIX® Microclysmic Gel approximately 2–4mm. thick. Cover the wound with a non-occlusive dressing. Re-apply at every dressing change to maintain a moist wound environment.

How Supplied: 8.5 oz. Spray Bottle, 4 oz. tubes, NDC# 46706-440-03

ORCHID FRESH II® ANTIMICROBIAL PERINEAL/OSTOMY CLEANSER
Perineal/Ostomy Cleanser

Composition: Active Ingredient: Benzethonium Chloride .1%
Inactive Ingredients: Water, Amphoteric 2, DMDM Hydantoin, Fragrance, Citric Acid.

Actions and Uses: Orchid Fresh II is an amphoteric, topical antimicrobial cleansing solution which gently cleans and emulsifies feces and urine on the incontinent patient. Use also on stoma sites and ostomy bags to deodorize and eliminate odor. Broad spectrum antimicrobial action on Pseudomonas, E. coli, Staphylococcus aureus, MRSA, etc. Orchid Fresh II will aid in reducing skin breakdown or tears. Significantly reduces UTI infection in the incontinent, geriatric patient.

Precautions: External Use Only, Non-Toxic—Non-Dermal Irritating No Contra-indications.

Directions: Spray topically and remove feces and urine with warm, moist washcloth. Spray directly on peristomal skin areas, clean gently and pat dry. Utilize Care Creme on reddened skin areas.

How Supplied: 4 oz., 8 oz., 16 oz. and Gallons NDC #46706-115

SATIN® ANTIMICROBIAL SKIN CLEANSER

Composition: Active Ingredient: Chloroxylenol .8%
Inactive Ingredients: Water, Sodium Laureth Sulfate, Cocamidopropyl Betaine, PEG-8, Cocamide DEA, Glycol Stearate, Lanolin Oil, Tetrasodium EDTA, D&C Yellow #10.

Actions and Uses: Satin has been specially formulated for use on sensitive or aging dermal tissue, atopic dermatitis and psoriasis. Effective in eliminating gram-positive and gram-negative pathogens such as E. coli, S. aureus, Pseudomonas, etc. Contains emollients to replenish natural oils and proteins. Satin also eliminates skin odor and dry, itchy skin. Three year shelf life.

Precautions: No contra-indicators. External use only. Non-Toxic.

Directions: Use daily during shower, bath or regular cleansing or as directed by physician.

How Supplied: 4 oz., 8 oz., 12 oz. 16 oz., 1 Gallon NDC #46706-101

TECHNI–CARE® SURGICAL SCRUB, Prep and Wound Decontaminant

Composition: Active Ingredients: Chloroxylenol 3%, Cocamidopropyl PG-Dimonium Chloride Phosphate 3% Inactive Ingredients: Water, Sodium Lauryl Sulfate, Cocamide DEA, Propylene Glycol, Cocamidopropyl Betaine, Citric Acid, Tetrasodium EDTA, Aloe Vera Gel, Hydrolyzed Animal Protein, D&C Yellow #10.

Actions and Uses: Techni-Care represents entirerly new technology in a broad-spectrum, topical, antiseptic microbicide for skin degerming. 99.99% Bacterial reduction in 30 second contact usage. Techni-Care may be used for disinfection of wounds, for pre-op and post-op along with surgical scrub applications. Non-staining and non-irritating to dermal tissue. Techni-Care conditions dermal tissue and phospholipid promotes a more rapid rate of cellular regeneration. Use for treatment of acute, chronic wounds in replacement of topical, antibiotic therapy. New U.S. Patent.

Precautions: Non-Toxic, Non-Irritating, External Use Only. Can be used safely around ears and eyes or as directed by a physician. No Contra-indications.

Directions: Apply, lather and rinse well. For pre-op, apply and let dry, no rinsing required. Three year shelf life.

How Supplied: 20 mL packets, 4 oz., 8 oz., 12 oz., 16 oz., 32 oz., Gallons and peel paks, Roll-on Prep NDC #46706–222

IF YOU SUSPECT AN INTERACTION. . .
The 1,800-page *PDR Companion Guide*™ can help. Use the order form in the front of this book.

Care Technologies, Inc.
10 CORBIN DRIVE
DARIEN, CT 06820

Direct Inquiries to:

Mary Lynn M. Drake
Marketing and Sales Services Manager
(203) 655-9680
FAX: (203) 655-9682
E-mail: caretec1@aol.com
http://www.clearcare.com

CLEAR® Total Lice Elimination System
CLEAR® Lice Killing Shampoo
CLEAR® Lice Egg Remover
CLEAR® Nit Capturing Comb

PRODUCT OVERVIEW

Key Facts: Clear® Total Lice Elimination System offers the only 2-step treatment product comprised of pediculicide and enzymatic lice egg remover with "nit capturing" comb. Clear Lice Killing Shampoo kills lice and some eggs (up to 30% of eggs survive lice killing products) with a full strength pyrethrum extract shampoo. It is effective against head, body, and pubic (crab) lice. Clear Lice Egg Remover is a patented, natural enzyme gel in a tube with special, fine-toothed "nit capturing" comb. Together they make the difficult job of lice egg removal faster and easier so that children can return to school sooner.

Major Uses: Clear® Total Lice Elimination System is used to treat head lice infestations as quickly as possible and allow children to return to school sooner. A second treatment with Clear Lice Killing Shampoo must be done in 7–10 days to kill any newly hatched lice, also followed by lice egg removal is required to ensure complete effectiveness.

Safety Information: Clear Lice Killing Shampoo should be used with caution by individuals sensitive to ragweed. This product is intended for external use only. It is harmful if swallowed. Keep this and all drugs out of reach of children. In case of accidental ingestion, seek professional assistance or contact a Poison Control Center immediately.

Clear Lice Egg Remover contains no harsh chemicals and is safe for use at any time. It is not a treatment product and needs to be used in conjunction with a lice killing product to ensure elimination and prevent re-infestation. Clear Lice Egg Remover is for external use only. If it does get into the eye, gently flush with water.

PRESCRIBING INFORMATION
CLEAR® Total Lice Elimination System
2 oz. NDC# 62653-210-02
4 oz. NDC# 62653-210-04

Description: Clear® Lice Killing Shampoo contains a liquid pediculicide whose active ingredient for each fluid ounce is pyrethrum extract (0.33%) with piperonyl butoxide (4.0%). Inert ingredients (95.67%) are: benzyl alcohol, isoparagginic petroleum solvent, and water.

Action: Clear® Lice Killing Shampoo kills head lice (Pediculus humanus capitis), body lice (Pediculus humanus humanus), pubic (crab) lice (Pthirus pubis) and some eggs (up to 30% of eggs survive lice killing products). The pyrethrum extract acts as a contact poison affecting the nervous system, resulting in paralysis and death. The efficacy of the pyrethrum extract is rinsed out after treatment leaving no appreciable residue. In addition, the pyrethrum molecules are not readily absorbed through the skin. Any minute amounts which are absorbed, are rapidly metabolized and eliminated from the body with no ill effects. Because up to 30% of head lice eggs survive lice killing products, egg removal is required to prevent re-infestation. Clear Lice Egg Remover makes hair-combing easier and egg removal faster.

Indications: For the treatment of head, body and pubic (crab) lice.

Dosage and Administration: Apply to affected area until all the hair is thoroughly wet with product. Allow product to remain on area for 10 minutes, but not longer. Add sufficient warm water to form a lather and shampoo with the lather as usual. Rinse hair thoroughly. Use regular comb to remove tangles. Apply Clear Lice Egg Remover enzyme gel to wet hair at scalp. Thoroughly cover entire scalp area and lightly massage. Wait at least three minutes before combing. Use Clear "nit capturing" comb to remove eggs. (Follow detailed instructions in the package insert). A second treatment with Clear Lice Killing Shampoo must be done in 7–10 days to kill any newly hatched lice. This treatment followed by lice egg removal is required to ensure complete effectiveness. As there is no immunity to lice, daily inspections and continued personal care will help prevent reinfestation.
The following additional steps are important to minimize opportunities for environmental reinfestation: disinfect all personal clothing, bed linen and bath linen items by machine washing in hot water and drying, using the hot cycle of the dryer, for at least 20 minutes. Personal clothing and bedding that cannot be washed may be dry-cleaned, sealed in plastic bags for a period of two weeks or thoroughly vacuumed. Personal combs and brushes may be disinfected by soaking in hot water (above 130°F) for 5 to 10 minutes. Thorough vacuuming of rooms inhabited by infected persons is recommended.

Continued on next page

Clear Lice System—Cont.

Warnings: Clear® Lice Killing Shampoo should be used with caution by individuals sensitive to ragweed. This product is intended for external use only. It is harmful if swallowed. Do not use near the eye or permit contact with mucous membranes, as irritation may occur. Keep out of eyes when rinsing hair. Adults and children: Close eyes tightly and do not open eyes until product is rinsed out. Also, protect children's eyes with washcloth, towel or other suitable material or by a similar method. If product gets into eyes, immediately flush with water. As with any drug, if you are pregnant or nursing a baby, seek the advice of a health professional before using this product.

Keep this and all drugs out of the reach of children. In case of accidental shampoo ingestion, seek professional assistance or contact a Poison Control Center immediately. If skin irritation or infection is present or develops, discontinue use and consult your doctor. Consult a doctor if lice infestation of eyebrows exists.

Carlsbad Technology Inc.

**5923 BALFOUR COURT
CARLSBAD, CA 92008**

For Medical and Pharmaceutical Information Including Emergencies:
(760) 431-8284
FAX: (760) 431-7505

YSP™ ASPIRIN
**Adult low strength aspirin
81 mg, Delayed release enteric
coated pellet aspirin capsule**

Active Ingredients: Each capsule contains 81 mg of aspirin. YSP™ Aspirin contains the same low strength as aspirin tablets, but in pellet filled capsules. YSP™ Aspirin is designed for long term heart maintenance. The enteric coated pellets provide protection against upset stomach and side effects in the small intestine due to high local concentrations.

Indications: For temporary relief of minor aches and pains or as recommended by your doctor.

Directions: Adults: Take 4 to 8 capsules with water every 4 hours, as needed, up to a maximum of 48 capsules per 24 hours or as directed by a doctor.

Warnings: Keep out of reach of children and see label for more detailed information.

Drug Interaction Precaution: Do not take this product if you are taking a prescription drug for anticoagulation (thinning of the blood), diabetes, gout, or arthritis unless directed by a doctor.

How Supplied: One bottle contains 120 capsules.

Church & Dwight Co., Inc.

**469 N. HARRISON STREET
PRINCETON, NJ 08543-5297**

Direct Inquiries to:
Robert Coleman
(609) 497-7130
Nancy Sevinsky
(609) 683-7015

For Medical Emergencies Contact:
Hazard Information Services
(800) 228-5635
Extension 7

ARM & HAMMER®
Pure Baking Soda

Active Ingredient: Sodium Bicarbonate U.S.P.

Indications: For alleviation of acid indigestion, also known as heartburn or sour stomach. Not a remedy for other types of stomach complaints such as nausea, stomachache, abdominal cramps, gas pains, or stomach distention caused by overeating and/or overdrinking. In the latter case, one should not ingest solids, liquids or antacid but rather refrain from all physical activity and—if uncomfortable—call a physician.

Actions: ARM & HAMMER® Pure Baking Soda provides fast-acting, effective neutralization of stomach acids. Each level $1/2$ teaspoon dose will neutralize 20.9 mEq of acid.

Warnings: Except under the advice and supervision of a physician: (1) do not administer to children under five years of age, (2) do not take more than eight level $1/2$ teaspoons per person up to 60 years old or four level $1/2$ teaspoons per person 60 years or older in a 24-hour period, (3) do not use this product if you are on a sodium restricted diet, (4) do not use the maximum dose for more than two weeks.

Stomach Warning: To avoid serious injury, do not take until powder is completely dissolved. It is very important not to take this product when overly full from food or drink. Consult a physician if severe stomach pain occurs after taking this product.

Drug Interaction Precaution: Antacids may interact with certain prescription drugs. If you are presently taking a prescription drug, do not take this product without checking with your physician or other health professional.

Dosage and Administration: Level $1/2$ teaspoon in $1/2$ glass (4 fl. oz.) of water every two hours up to maximum dosage or as directed by a physician. Accurately measure level $1/2$ teaspoon. Each level $1/2$ teaspoon contains 20.9 mEq (.476 gm) sodium.

How Supplied: Available in 8 oz., 16 oz., 32 oz., 64 oz., and 160 oz. boxes.

CigArrest

**6361 YARROW DRIVE, STE. B
CARLSBAD, CA 92009**

Direct Inquiries to:
Sheila Durkin
(760) 438-1935
FAX: (760) 438-3212

Medical Emergency Contact:
Customer Service
(800) 514-7233
FAX: (760) 438-3212

CIGARREST® No Smoking Gum, Tablets and Lozenges

Smoking and nicotine dependence is a complex addiction. Your stop smoking success requires not only your personal motivation, but also support to help you feel comfortable while you're trying to quit.

CigArrest® Natural Homeopathic No-Smoking Gum, Tablets and Lozenges *offer a safe treatment alternative for smoking cessation. As with all homeopathic treatments, symptom relief is attained through stimulation of the natural healing process.*

Smokers - When you can't smoke, choose not to, or want to cut down.

No Smoking Permitted - CigArrest® is the smoker's choice for restricted smoking situations and to help cut down on cigarette or tobacco use.

Ex-Smokers - Curbs the urge to smoke and helps you stay smoke-free no matter how you stopped.

Stay Smoke-Free - CigArrest® is the ex-smoker's choice to curb the periodic urge to smoke.

Indication: CigArrest® Homeopathic No-Smoking Gum, CigArrest® Homeopathic No-Smoking Tablets and CigArrest® Homeopathic No-Smoking Lozenges reduce the cravings for cigarette and tobacco products, relieve irritability and nervous tension and help detoxify.

Dosage: For Adults and Teens (13–19 years old): CigArrest® Homeopathic No-Smoking Gum - Chew one piece every 1–2 hours or as needed whenever the desire for cigarettes or tobacco occurs.

Not recommended for children under 13 years of age.

CigArrest® Homeopathic No-Smoking Tablets - Chew tablet slightly and allow to dissolve in a clean mouth. Take one tablet at least 3 times a day or as needed whenever the desire for cigarettes or tobacco occurs.

Not recommended for children under 13 years of age.

CigArrest® Homeopathic No-Smoking Lozenges - Allow lozenge to dissolve in a clean mouth. Take one lozenge every 1–2 hours or as needed whenever the desire for cigarettes or tobacco occurs.

Not recommended for children under 13 years of age.

For Best Results: Don't eat or drink for 15 minutes before using **CigArrest®**. Stop the use of tobacco products completely or reduce their use and gradually discontinue.

Warning: If symptoms persist or change, discontinue use and consult a doctor. If you experience mouth, teeth or jaw problems, discontinue use. As with any drug, if you are pregnant or nursing a baby, seek the advice of a health care professional before using this product. **Keep this and all medicines out of the reach of children.**

Active Ingredients: CigArrest® Homeopathic No-Smoking Gum, Tablets and Lozenges: *Lobelia inflata 6X, 12X, 30X, Cinchona officinalis 6X, Daphne indica 6X, Plantago major 6X, Calcarea phosphorica 12X, Nux vomica 12X*

Inactive Ingredients: CigArrest® Homeopathic No-Smoking Gum: *Sorbitol, Gum Base, Maltitol Syrup, Glycerin, Peppermint Flavor, Titanium Dioxide, Menthol, Aspertame*, Acesulfame Potassium. Phenylketonurics: Contains phenylalanine 1.5 mg per piece*
CigArrest® Homeopathic No-Smoking Tablets: *Lactose*
CigArrest® Homeopathic No-Smoking Lozenges: *Glucose, Stearic Acid, Croscarmellose Sodium, Magnesium Stearate, and Natural Mint Flavor.*

How Supplied: CigArrest® Homeopathic No-Smoking Gum: Mint-flavored coated squares. Blister packed and perforated for your safety and convenience. Available in 120 count starter kit with support program and 2, 6, 12, 24, & 60 count refills. NDC 61693-051-10, 20, 30, 40, 50, 60
CigArrest® Homeopathic No-Smoking Tablets: Blister packed for your safety and convenience. Available in 30 and 90 count blister packs. NDC 61693-050-31, 91
CigArrest® Homeopathic No-Smoking Lozenges: Blister packed for your safety and convenience. Available in 24 count blister packs. NDC 61693-052-24
CigArrest®
Distributed by:
Bancroft Pharmaceuticals
PO Box 4444 -Carlsbad, CA 92018
www.cigarrest.com
Questions or comments?
Please call: (800) 778-2283
Weekdays 12:00pm - 8:00pm EST

EDUCATIONAL MATERIALS

THE CIGARREST® APPROACH TO SMOKING CESSATION
The CigArrest® Program has been helping people stop smoking for 15 years. The Program can help you recognize and understand the physical as well as the strong psychological component of nicotine addiction. It has been designed to help you overcome the dual addictions associated with smoking using a two-step approach.
1. CigArrest® No-Smoking Gum, Tablets and Lozenges help to address the unpleasant physical discomfort of quitting as nicotine is flushed from your body. The natural, gentle action of the No-Smoking Tablets, Gum and Lozenges stimulate the body's natural defense system.
2. The CigArrest Behavior Modification Plan helps you understand and overcome your psychological dependence on smoking. It will help you address the habits and behaviors that trigger your urge to smoke.
What you need to supply is COMMITT-MENT—to the CigArrest Program and to becoming a permanent non-smoker.
If you're serious about quitting, CigArrest can help!

Columbia Laboratories, Incorporated

2875 N.E. 191st STREET, SUITE 400
AVENTURA, FL 33180

Direct Inquiries to:
Columbia Laboratories, Incorporated
(800) 824-4586
Fax (305) 933-6090

ADVANTAGE-S™
Bioadhesive Contraceptive Gel
[əd- 'vant-ij es]
(nonoxynol-9, 3.5%)

Description: Advantage-S combines patented, bioadhesive technology with the most widely used spermicide available without a prescription-Nonoxynol-9. Providing immediate, effective contraceptive protection, Advantage-S is formulated for sensitivity and contains no hormones. Unlike other products, Advantage-S will not run or leak and, there is nothing to remove. The bioadhesive properties allow the formulation to adhere to the cervix. Advantage-S is safe to use with latex condoms or diaphragms adding an extra measure of protection.

Directions: Advantage-S can be inserted up to one hour prior to each act of intercourse. One applicatorful of Advantage-S is adequate for one act of intercourse only. An additional applicatorful is required each time intercourse is repeated. Douching or bathing is not rec-

ommended after using Advantage-S. However, if desired for cleansing purposes, wait at least six hours following last intercourse to allow for full spermicidal activity. For use with a diaphragm, please follow the instructions of the individual contraceptive device.

Storage: Store at room temperature (15–30°C or 59–86°F). Avoid exposure to extreme heat or cold.

Cautions: Keep out of reach of children. In case of accidental ingestion, call a poison control center, emergency medical facility or a doctor.

Active Ingredient: Nonoxynol-9 (3.5% w/w)

Inactive Ingredients: Purified Water, Glycerin, Mineral Oil, Polycarbophil, Hydrogenated Palm Oil Glyceride, Carbomer 934P, Methylparaben, Sorbic Acid, and Sodium Hydroxide added to adjust pH.

Action: Spermicidal

Indication: Prevention of pregnancy.

Precautions: When a pregnancy is medically advised against, your contraceptive program should be prescribed by your physician. Advantage-S provides a high degree of contraceptive protection. No product, however, can provide an absolute guarantee against becoming pregnant.

Adverse Reactions: The following side effects have been reported: Occasional burning and/or irritation of the vagina or penis. If this occurs, discontinue use and consult your physician. In a few women, a slight discharge may be noted.

Questions: Please call 1-800-824-4586.

How Supplied: Advantage-S is available in boxes containing 3 or 6 pre-filled, disposable applicators and in a 30g (20 applications) tube with a reusable applicator. Each applicator delivers 1.5g. NDCs: 55056-1492-1; 55056-1492-2; 55056-1492-3.

REPLENS®
Vaginal Moisturizer
[ree 'plenz]

Ingredients: Purified Water, Glycerin, Mineral Oil, Polycarbophil, Hydrogenated Palm Oil Glyceride, Carbomer 934P, Methylparaben, Sorbic Acid, and Sodium Hydroxide added to adjust pH.

Description: Replens relieves the discomfort of vaginal dryness for days with a single application. Replens non-hormonal, vaginal moisturizer provides natural feeling moisture to continuously hydrate vaginal tissue. Replens is non-staining, fragrance free, non-greasy, non-irritating and estrogen-free.

Continued on next page

Replens—Cont.

Action: When used as directed, Replens provides long-lasting relief from the discomfort of vaginal dryness by providing continuous hydration to the vaginal tissue.

Warnings: Keep out of the reach of children. Replens is not a contraceptive. Does not contain spermicide. If vaginal irritation occurs, discontinue use.

Usage: Use as needed. One single application approximately once every 2 to 3 days is recommended.

How Supplied: Replens is available in boxes containing 3 or 8 pre-filled, disposable applicators and in a 35g (14 applications) tube with a reusable applicator. Each applicator delivers 2.5g.

Storage: Store at room temperature (15–30°C or 59–86°F). Avoid exposure to extreme heat or cold.

Del Pharmaceuticals, Inc.

**A Subsidiary of Del Laboratories, Inc.
178 EAB Plaza
Uniondale, NY 11556**

Direct Inquiries to:
Dr. Joseph A. Kanapka, Ph.D.,
Sr. VP Scientific Affairs
(516) 844-2020
FAX: (516) 293-1515

For Medical Emergencies Contact:
Serap Ozelkan, Director
David Grob, Director
of Regulatory Affairs
1-800-952-5080

ARTHRICARE®
Arthritis Pain Relieving Rubs

Description: ArthriCare® Multi-Action Capsaicin 0.025% provides temporary relief of minor aches and pains of muscles and joints associated with arthritis, simple back pain, sprains and strains. This unique formulation contains Capsicum Oleoresin (containing Capsaicin 0.025%), a strong, penetrating pain blocker not commonly found in other rubs. In addition, it has two added fast-acting pain relievers to ease stiffness of muscles and joints.

ArthriCare® Triple Medicated is specially formulated with three fast acting pain relievers. It's strong medicine that penetrates deep. You don't have to rub it in; just apply gently. ArthriCare Triple-Medicated provides temporary relief of minor aches and pains of muscles and joints associated with arthritis, simple backache, sprains and strains. Perfect for nighttime use.

ArthriCare® Ultra™ is a triple strength capsaicin* 0.075% formulation *plus* menthol. This fast-acting arthritis rub contains the doctor recommended ingredient, Capsaicin, for the relief of minor aches and pains associated with arthritis, simple backache, sprains and strains. The product should be used 3–4 times daily for maximum effectiveness. *as capsicum oleoresin.

ArthriCare® Hand & Body Lotion is the first and only product of its kind that provides fast-acting/long-lasting arthritis pain relief plus moisturizers for softer, smoother skin. The new advanced formula combines the proven arthritis pain relief ingredient, capsaicin 0.025% (with Capsicum Oleoresin containing capsaicin 0.025%), with the moisturizing benefits of Alpha Hydroxy and Aloe Vera.

Active Ingredients: ArthriCare® Multi-Action Menthol USP 1.25%, Methyl Nicotinate 0.25%, Capsicum Oleoresin (containing Capsaicin 0.025%). **ArthriCare® Triple Medicated** Methyl Salicylate 30%, Menthol 1.25%, Methyl Nicotinate 0.25%.
ArthriCare® Ultra™ Menthol USP 2.0%, Capsicum Oleoresin (Containing Capsaicin 0.075%).
ArthriCare® Hand & Body Lotion Capsicum Oleoresin (Containing Capsaicin 0.025%).

Inactive Ingredients: ArthriCare® Multi-Action Aloe Vera Gel, Carbomer, Cetyl Alcohol (and) Cetearyl Glucoside, Decyl Glucoside, methylparaben, Propylene Glycol, Propylparaben, Titanium Dioxide.
ArthriCare® Triple Medicated Carbomer 940, Dioctyl Sodium Sulfosuccinate, FD&C Blue No. 1, Glycerin, Isopropyl Alcohol, Polysorbate 60, Propylene Gycol, Purified Water.
ArthriCare® Ultra™ Aloe Vera Gel, Carbomer, Cetyl Alcohol, DMDM Hydantoin, Emulsifying Wax, Glyceryl Stearate SE, Isocetyl Alcohol, Myristyl Propionate, Propylparaben, Purified Water, Stearyl Alcohol.
ArthriCare® Hand & Body Lotion Allantoin, Aloe Vera Gel, Caprylic/Capric Triglyceride, Carbomer, Cetyl Alcohol, Dimethicone, Fragrance, Methylparaben, Mixed Fruit Acid Complex (Citric Acid, Green Tea Extract, Lactic Acid, Malic Acid), PEG-20 Glyceryl Laurate, PEG-30 Glyceryl Laurate, Propylparaben, Purified Water, Quaternium-15, Sodium Citrate, Stearyl Alcohol, Titanium Dioxide.

Directions: Adults and children 2 years of age and older: Apply to affected area not more than 3 to 4 times daily. Children under 2 years of age: Consult a physician. Read package insert before using.

Warnings: For external use only. Avoid contact with the eyes. If condition worsens, or if symptoms persist for more than 7 days or clear up and occur again within a few days, discontinue use of this product and consult a physician. Do not apply to wounds or damaged skin. Do not bandage tightly. Avoid contact with mucous membranes, broken or irritated skin. Do not use with a heating pad, or immediately before or after taking a shower or bath. As part of its warming action, temporary redness may occur Keep this and all drugs out of the reach of children. In case of accidental ingestion, seek professional assistance or contact a Poison Control Center immediately. Store at room temperature 15–30 C (59–86 F).

Shown in Product Identification Guide, page 507

BABY ORAJEL®
Teething Pain Medicine

Description: Baby Orajel with fast-acting benzocaine (7.5%) relieves teething pain within one minute. It's pleasant tasting and contains no alcohol.

Active Ingredient: Benzocaine 7.5%
Purpose: Pain Reliever

Use: For the temporary relief of sore gums due to teething in infants and children 4 months of age and older.

Directions: Wash hands. Cut open tip of tube on score mark. Use your fingertip or cotton applicator to apply a small pea-size amount of Baby Orajel. Apply to affected area not more than four times daily or as directed by a dentist or physician. For infants under 4 months of age, there is no recommended dosage or treatment except under the advice and supervision of a dentist or physician.

Warnings:
- Do not use if tube tip is cut prior to opening.
- Do not use this product for more than 7 days unless directed by a dentist or physician. If sore mouth symptoms do not improve in 7 days; if irritation, pain or redness persists or worsens; or if swelling, rash or fever develops, see your dentist or physician promptly.
- Do not exceed recommended dosage.
- Do not use this product if you have a history of allergy to local anesthetics such as procaine, butacaine, benzocaine, or other "caine" anesthetics.
- Fever and nasal congestion are not symptoms of teething and may indicate the presence of infection. If these symptoms persist, consult your physician.

Keep this and all drugs out of the reach of children. In case of accidental overdose or allergic reaction, seek professional assistance or contact a Poison Control Center immediately.

Inactive Ingredients: FD&C Red No. 40, Flavor, Glycerin, Polyethylene Glycols, Purified Water, Sodium Saccharin, Sorbic Acid, Sorbitol.

How Supplied: Available in 0.33 Oz. (9.4g) tube.

Shown in Product Identification Guide, page 507

BABY ORAJEL® TOOTH & GUM CLEANSER

Description: Baby Orajel Tooth & Gum Cleanser is specifically designed for children under four. It's safe to swallow, non-foaming, fluoride-free and abrasive-free. It contains Microdent® to help remove plaque-like film and fight plaque build-up. Available in Fruit and Peaches 'n Cream flavors.

Active Ingredients: Microdent® (Poloxamer 407 2.0%, Simethicone 0.12%.)
Microdent is a patented plaque-fighter.
Purpose: Removes plaque-like film.

Use: Helps remove plaque-like film for cleaner teeth and gums.

Warnings: Keep out of the reach of children. Do not use if tube tip is cut prior to opening.

Directions: Wash hands. Cut open tip of tube on score mark. Apply a small amount to your finger, a gauze pad or a baby toothbrush. Gently wipe or brush your child's teeth and gums to remove food and plaque-like film. For best results, use in the morning and at bedtime.

Inactive Ingredients: Carboxymethylcellulose Sodium, Citric Acid, Flavor, Glycerin, Methylparaben, Potassium Sorbate, Propylene Glycol, Propylparaben, Purified Water, Sodium Saccharin, Sorbitol.

How Supplied: Available in 0.5 Oz. (14.2 g) tube. Available in assorted flavors.
Shown in Product Identification Guide, page 507

ORAJEL® Maximum Strength
[ōr 'ah-jel]
Toothache Medicine

Descriptions: Maximum Strength Orajel with 20% benzocaine provides immediate, long lasting toothache pain relief.
Orajel P.M. is the first nighttime toothache pain relief medicine. This long-lasting paste is formulated to stay in place for extended duration of relief.

Active Ingredient: Benzocaine 20%.

Inactive Ingredients: Flavor, Polyethylene Glycols, Sodium Saccharin, Sorbic Acid.
Orajel PM Cellulose Gum, Gelatin, Menthol, Methyl Salicylate, Pectin, Plasticized Hydrocarbon Gel, Polyethylene Glycol, Sodium Saccharin.

Indications: Maximum Strength Orajel and Orajel P.M. are formulated to provide fast, long lasting relief from daytime and nighttime toothache pain.

Actions: Benzocaine is a topical, local anesthetic commonly used for pain, discomfort, or pruritis associated with wounds, mucous membranes and skin irritation.

Warning: Keep this and all drugs out of the reach of children. Do not use if tube tip is cut prior to opening. Do not use this product if you have a history of allergy to local anesthetics such as pro-

caine, butacaine, benzocaine or other "caine" anesthetics. In case of accidental overdose or allergic reaction, seek professional assistance or contact a Poison Control Center immediately.

Precaution: This preparation is intended for use in cases of toothache only as a temporary expedient until a dentist can be consulted. Do not use continuously.

Directions: Remove cap. Cut open tip of tube at score mark. Squeeze a small quantity of Maximum Strength Orajel directly into cavity and around gum surrounding the teeth. Firmly squeeze a one inch strip of Orajel P.M. onto a finger or cotton swab. Apply it to affected cavity and around the gum surrounding the teeth.

How Supplied: Gel in two sizes—.18 oz (5.3 g) and .33 oz (9.4 g) tubes.
Cream in .25 oz (7.0 g) tube.
Shown in Product Identification Guide, page 507

ORAJEL® COVERMED®
Fever Blister/
Cold Sore Treatment Cream

Description: Orajel CoverMed conceals unsightly cold sores or fever blisters for hours as it protects and relieves pain.

Active Ingredients: Dyclonine Hydrochloride 1.0%
Allantoin 0.5%

Action: Pain reliever, moisturizer and skin protectant

Use: For the temporary relief of pain and itching associated with fever blisters and cold sores. Relieves dryness and softens cold sores and fever blisters.

Directions: Remove cap and cut open tip of tube on score mark. Adults and children 2 years of age and older: Apply to fever blisters/cold sores not more than 3 to 4 times daily. Children under 2 years of age: Consult a physician.

Warnings:
• Do not use if tube tip is cut prior to opening.
• For external use only.
• Avoid contact with the eyes.
• If condition worsens, or if symptoms persist for more than 7 days or clear up and occur again within a few days, discontinue use of this product and consult a physician.
Keep this and all drugs out of the reach of children. In case of accidental overdose, seek professional assistance or contact a Poison Control Center immediately.

Inactive Ingredients: Beeswax, Citric Acid, Colloidal Silicone Dioxide, Flavor, Iron Oxides, Lanolin, Petrolatum, Propylene Glycol, Purified Water, PVP/Hexadecene Copolymer, Titanium Dioxide.

How Supplied: Cream in 0.18 Oz. (5.3 g) tube.

ORAJEL® Mouth-Aid®
[ōr 'ah-jel]
Cold/Canker Sore Medicine

Description: Orajel Mouth-Aid is a unique triple-acting medication which provides fast relief from painful minor mouth and lip sores. It has a protective formula that stays on the sore.

Active Ingredients: Benzocaine 20%, Benzalkonium Chloride 0.02%, Zinc Chloride 0.1%.

Inactive Ingredients: Allantoin, Carbomer, Edetate Disodium, Peppermint Oil, Polyethylene Glycol, Polysorbate 60, Propyl Gallate, Propylene Glycol, Purified Water, Povidone, Sodium Saccharin, Sorbic Acid, Stearyl Alcohol.

Indications: For the temporary relief of pain associated with canker sores, cold sores, fever blisters and minor irritation or injury of the mouth and gums.

Actions: Benzocaine is a topical, local anesthetic commonly used for pain, discomfort, or pruritis associated with wounds, mucous membranes and skin irritations. Benzalkonium chloride is a rapidly acting surface disinfectant. Zinc chloride provides an astringent effect.

Warnings: Do not use this product for more than 7 days unless directed by a dentist or physician. If sore mouth symptoms do not improve in 7 days; if irritation, pain, or redness persists or worsens; or if swelling, rash or fever develops, see your dentist or physician promptly. Do not exceed recommended dosage. Do not use this product if you have a history of allergy to local anesthetics such as procaine, butacaine, benzocaine or other "caine" anesthetics. Keep this and all drugs out of the reach of children. In case of accidental overdose or allergic reaction, seek professional assistance or contact a Poison Control Center immediately. Do not use if tube tip is cut prior to opening.

Precaution: If condition persists, discontinue use and consult your physician or dentist. Not for prolonged use.

Directions: Cut open tip of tube on score mark. Adults and children 2 years and older: Apply to the affected area. Use up to 4 times daily or as directed by a dentist or physician. Children under 12 years of age should be supervised in the use of the product. Children under 2 years of age: Consult a dentist or physician.

How Supplied: Gel in 2 sizes—a $1/3$ oz (9.45 g) tube and a $3/16$ oz (5.3 g) tube.
Shown in Product Identification Guide, page 507

ORAJEL® PERIOSEPTIC®

Description: Orajel® Perioseptic® Spot Treatment Oral Cleanser and Ora-

Continued on next page

Orajel Perioseptic—Cont.

jel® Periospetic® Super Cleaning Oral Rinse are oral wound cleansers that use the debriding action of peroxide to cleanse sore mouths and gums due to denture irritation, canker sores, dental procedures, accidental injuries, and gum irritation. They both have a fresh minty taste, and can supplement your regular mouthwash routine.

Active Ingredients: Spot Treatment Oral Cleanser—Carbamide peroxide 15% (maximum strength) in anhydrous glycerin. Super Cleaning Oral Rinse—Hydrogen peroxide 1.5%.

Inactive Ingredients: Spot Treatment Oral Cleanser—Citric acid, Edetate disodium, Flavor, Methylparaben, Propylene glycol, Purified water, Sodium chloride, Sodium saccharin. Super Cleaning Oral Rinse—Edetate disodium, Ethyl alcohol (4% v/v), FD&C Blue No. 1, Methyl salicylate, Methylparaben, Phosphoric acid, Poloxamer 338, Purified water, Sodium saccharin, Sorbitol.

Indications: For temporary use in cleansing minor wounds or minor gum inflammation resulting from minor dental procedures, dentures, orthodontic appliances, accidental injury, canker sores, or other irritations of the mouth or gums.

Warning: Do not use this product for more than 7 days unless directed by a dentist or doctor. If sore mouth symptoms do not improve in 7 days; if irritation, pain, or redness persists or worsens, or if swelling, rash, or fever develops, see your dentist or doctor promptly. Cap bottle tightly. Keep away from heat and direct sunlight. Do not swallow.

Dosage and Administration: Adults and children 2 years of age and older: Apply several drops of Spot Treatment Oral Cleanser directly to the affected area of the mouth with cotton swab or applicator, or swish around Super Cleaning Oral Rinse in the mouth over the affected area. Allow the medication to remain in place at least 1 minute and then spit out. Use up to 4 times daily after meals and at bedtime or as directed by a dentist or doctor. Children under 12 years of age should be supervised in the use of this product. Children under 2 years of age: Consult a dentist or doctor.

How Supplied: Spot Treatment Oral Cleanser—.42 fl. oz (11.8 ml) bottle with applicator. Super Cleaning Oral Rinse—8 fl oz (236 ml) bottle.

Shown in Product Identification Guide, page 507

ORAJEL SENSITIVE™
[ŏr 'ah-jel]
SENSITIVE TEETH TOOTHPASTE FOR ADULTS

Description: As we age, our gums start to recede, exposing the root of the tooth. In fact, 8 out of every 10 older adults have some gum recession. This can make teeth more sensitive to hot and cold because more of the tooth is exposed. It is also the primary reason why over half of older adults will develop new cavities at the gumline.

That is why Orajel, a leader in oral pain relief, offers **Orajel Sensitive Pain Relieving Toothpaste**... the first and only sensitive teeth toothpaste specially formulated to meet the special needs of adults with receding gums.

Orajel works two ways: (1) Nothing is better than Orajel Sensitive at providing pain relief of sensitive teeth; and (2) Orajel Sensitive has 33% more fluoride than *other sensitive teeth toothpastes* to aid in the prevention of cavities.

Active Ingredients:
— POTASSIUM NITRATE 5%
— SODIUM MONOFLUOROPHOSPHATE (0.20% W/V FLUORIDE ION).

Uses: To aid in the prevention of dental cavities. Helps reduce painful sensitivity of the teeth to cold, heat, acids, sweets, or contact. Builds increasing protection against painful sensitivity of the teeth to cold, heat, acids, sweets, or contact.

Directions:
— Adults and children 12 years of age and older: Apply at least a 1-inch strip of the product onto a soft bristle toothbrush.
— Brush teeth thoroughly for at least 1 minute twice a day (morning and evening) or as recommended by a dentist or doctor.
— Make sure to brush all sensitive areas of the teeth.
— Children under 12 years of age: Consult a dentist or doctor.

Warnings:
— Sensitive teeth may indicate a serious problem that may need prompt care by a dentist.
— See your dentist if the problem persists or worsens.
— Do not use this product longer than 4 weeks unless recommended by a dentist or doctor.
— Keep out of the reach of children under 6 years of age.
— If you accidentally swallow more than used for brushing, seek professional assistance or contact a Poison Control Center immediately.

Inactive Ingredients: FD&C Blue No. 1, Flavor, Glycerin, Hydrated Silica, Sodium Lauroyl Sarcosinate, Sodium Lauryl Sulfate, Sodium Saccharin, Sorbitol, Water, Xanthan Gum.

How Supplied: Available in trial size 0.85 oz., 2.3 oz. and 4.0 oz. tubes

Questions: Call us at 1-800-952-5080 or visit our website at http://www.orajel.com

Shown in Product Identification Guide, page 507

PRONTO® Lice Treatment

Description: Pronto Lice Killing Shampoo contains the maximum strength of pyrethrum extract and piperonyl butoxide. It kills lice and their eggs without leaving a lasting pesticide residue.

Active Ingredients: Piperonyl Butoxide 4%, Pyrethrum Extract 0.33%

Inactive Ingredients: Ammonium Laureth Sulfate, Benzyl Alcohol, BHT, Decyl Alcohol, Disodium EDTA, Fragrance, Isopropyl Alcohol, Glycerin, PEG-14M, Poloxamer 183, Purified Water

Indications: For the treatment of head, pubic (crab), and body lice.

Actions: Pronto contains the maximum strength of pyrethrum extract and piperonyl butoxide. Pyrethrum extract acts directly on the nervous system of insects and piperonyl butoxide enhances the neurotoxic effect of pyrethrum extract by inhibiting the oxidative breakdown of pyrethrum extract by the insect's detoxification system. This results in a longer amount of time which the pyrethrum extract may exert its toxic effect on the insect.

Warnings: Use with caution on persons allergic to ragweed. For external use only. Do not use near the eyes or permit contact with mucous membranes, such as inside the nose, mouth, or vagina, as irritation may occur. Keep out of eyes when rinsing hair. Adults and children: Close eyes tightly and do not open eyes until product is rinsed out. Also, protect children's eyes with washcloth, towel or other suitable material, or by similar method. If product gets into the eyes, immediately flush with water. If skin irritation or infection is present or develops, discontinue use and consult a doctor. Consult a doctor if infestation of eyebrows or eyelashes occurs. Keep out of reach of children. In case of accidental ingestion, seek professional assistance or contact a Poison Control Center immediately. Wash thoroughly with soap and water after handling. Do not exceed two applications within 24 hours.

Directions: Shake well. Apply to affected area until all the hair is thoroughly wet with product. Allow product to remain on area for 10 minutes but no longer. Add sufficient warm water to form a lather and shampoo as usual. Rinse thoroughly. A fine-toothed comb or a special lice/nit-removing comb may be used to help remove dead lice or their eggs (nits) from hair. A second treatment must be done in 7 to 10 days to kill any newly hatched lice. Handy applicator gloves are provided for your convenience in applying the shampoo to avoid contact with lice.

How Supplied: 2 fl. oz. (59 ml) and 4 fl. oz. (118 ml) plastic bottles.

Shown in Product Identification Guide, page 507

TANAC® Medicated Gel Fever Blister/Cold Sore Treatment

Description: Tanac Medicated Gel treats cold sores with a unique, long lasting maximum strength pain reliever, Dyclonine Hydrochloride (1.0%). It also protects lip sores while it treats them.

Active Ingredients: Dyclonine Hydrochloride 1.0%, Allantoin 0.5%.

Inactive Ingredients: Citric Acid, Flavor, Hydroxylated Lanolin, Petrolatum, Propylene Glycol, Purified Water, PVP/Hexadecene Copolymer, Yellow Wax.

Indications: For the temporary relief of pain and itching associated with fever blisters and cold sores. Relieves dryness and softens cold sores and fever blisters.

Warnings: DO NOT USE IF TIP IS CUT PRIOR TO OPENING. For external use only. Avoid contact with the eyes. If condition worsens, or if symptoms persist for more than 7 days or clear up and occur again within a few days, discontinue use of this product and consult a physician. Keep this and all other drugs out of reach of children. In case of accidental ingestion, seek professional assistance, or contact a Poison Control Center immediately.

Dosage and Administration: Cut open tip of tube on score mark. Adults and children 2 years of age and older: Apply to fever blisters/cold sores not more than 3 to 4 times daily. Children under 2 years of age: consult a physician.

How Supplied: Available in $^1/_3$ oz. (9.45g) plastic tube.
Shown in Product Identification Guide, page 508

**TANAC® No Sting Liquid
Canker Sore Medicine**

Description: **Tanac Liquid** provides fast, soothing relief from painful canker sores and gum irritations because it contains an effective anesthetic plus an antiseptic. It's alcohol-free so it doesn't sting.

Active Ingredients: Benzocaine 10%, Benzalkonium Chloride 0.12%.

Inactive Ingredients: Flavor, Polyethylene Glycol 400, Propylene Glycol, Purified Water, Sodium Saccharin, Tannic Acid.

Indications: For temporary relief of pain from mouth sores, canker sores, fever blisters and gum irritations.

Warnings: If the condition for which this preparation is used persists or if a rash or irritation develops, discontinue use and consult a physician. Use as indicated but not for more than 5 consecutive days. Not for prolonged use. Avoid getting into eyes. Do not use if you have a history of allergy to local anesthetics such as procaine, butacaine, benzocaine, or other "caine" anesthetics. KEEP THIS AND ALL DRUGS OUT OF THE REACH OF CHILDREN. In case of accidental overdose or allergic reaction, seek

professional assistance or contact a Poison Control Center immediately. Do not use if imprinted bottle cap safety seal is broken or missing prior to opening.

Dosage and Administration: Apply with cotton or cotton swab to affected area not more than 3 to 4 times daily.

How Supplied: Available in 0.45 fl. oz. (13 ml) glass bottle.
Shown in Product Identification Guide, page 508

Effcon™ Laboratories, Inc.
**P.O. BOX 7499
MARIETTA, GA 30065-1499**

Address inquiries to:
Brad Rivet
(800-722-2428)
Fax: (770-428-6811)

For Medical Emergency Contact:
Brad Rivet
(800-722-2428)
Fax: (770-428-6811)

**PIN-X®
Pinworm Treatment**

Description: Each 1 mL of liquid for oral administration contains:
Pyrantel base .... 50 mg
(as Pyrantel Pamoate)

Indication: For the treatment of pinworms.

Warnings: Keep this and all drugs out of the reach of children. In case of accidental overdose, seek professional assistance or contact a poison control center immediately.
If you are pregnant or have liver disease, do not take this product unless directed by a doctor.

Directions for Use: Adults and children 2 years to under 12 years of age: oral dosage is a single dose of 5 milligrams of pyrantel base per pound, or 11 milligrams per kilogram, of body weight not to exceed 1 gram. Dosage information is summarized on the following dosing schedule:

Weight		Dosage
		(taken as a single dose)
25 to 37 lbs.	=	$^1/_2$ tsp.
38 to 62 lbs.	=	1 tsp.
63 to 87 lbs.	=	$1^1/_2$ tsp.
88 to 112 lbs.	=	2 tsp.
113 to 137 lbs.	=	$2^1/_2$ tsp.
138 to 162 lbs.	=	3 tsp. (1 tbsp.)
163 to 187 lbs.	=	$3^1/_2$ tsp.
188 lbs. & over	=	4 tsp.

SHAKE WELL BEFORE USING

How Supplied: Pin-X is supplied as a tan to yellowish, caramel-flavored suspension which contains 50 mg of pyrantel base (as pyrantel pamoate) per mL, in bottles of 30 mL (1 fl oz). NDC 55806-024-10

Store at controlled room temperature 15°–30°C (59°–86°F).

Manufactured by:
Effcon™ Laboratories Inc.
Marietta, GA 30065-1499
Manufactured by:
PROMETIC PHARMA, INC.
MONTREAL, QUEBEC
Rev. 1/89
Code 587A00
Shown in Product Identification Guide, page 508

EnviroDerm Pharmaceuticals, Inc.
**P.O. BOX 32370
LOUISVILLE, KY 40232**

Direct Inquiries to:
800-991-3376

IVY BLOCK®

Skin protectant to help prevent poison ivy, poison oak or poison sumac rash when applied BEFORE contact.

Active Ingredient: Bentoquatam 5%

Inactive Ingredients: SDA 40 denatured alcohol (25% by weight), diisopropyl adipate, bentonite, benzyl alcohol, methylparaben, purified water.

Directions: For maximum protection, avoid contact with poison ivy, oak, and sumac. Shake bottle before each use. Apply at least 15 minutes before possible contact with plants. Rub enough lotion on exposed skin to leave smooth wet film. A visible coating indicates where skin is protected. Apply every four hours for continued protection or sooner if needed to maintain coating. May be removed with soap and water.

Warnings: For external use only. Do not use on children under 6 years of age, unless directed by a doctor, if you are allergic to any ingredients, or if you already have a rash from poison ivy, poison oak, or poison sumac. Avoid contact with eyes. If contact occurs, flush with water for at least 20 minutes. In case of accidental ingestion, seek professional assistance or contact a Poison Control Center immediately.

How Supplied: Ivy Block lotion 4 fl. oz. (120 ml) bottle

Fleming & Company
1600 FENPARK DR.
FENTON, MO 63026

Direct Inquiries to:
Tom Fleming
(314) 343-8200
FAX (314) 343-9865

CHLOR-3
Medicinal Condiment

Active Ingredients: A troika of sodium chloride (50% 24.3 mEq/half tsp. iodized); potassium chloride (30% 11.5 mEq/half tsp.); magnesium chloride (20% 5.6 mEq/half tsp.).

Indications: The first medicinal condiment to restore needed K^+ & Mg^{++} lost during diuresis, at the expense of Na^+. To restore electrolytes lost by overcooking foods, or to add to diets that lack green vegetables, bananas, etc. And to replace conventional salting of foods in culinary and gourmet arts.

Symptoms and Treatment of Oral Overdosage: Hyperkalemia and hypermagnesemia are not end-stage results of usage.

How Supplied: In 8-oz plastic shaker, tamper-evident bottles.

IMPREGON Concentrate

Active Ingredient: Tetrachlorosalicylanilide 2%

Indications: Diaper Rash Relief, 'Staph' control, Mold inhibitor.

Actions: This is a bacteriostatic/fungistatic agent for home usage and hospital usage.

Warnings: Impregon should not be exposed to direct sunlight for long periods after applications.

Precaution: Addition of bleach prior to diaper treatment negates application effects.

Dosage and Administration: One capful (5ml) per gallon of water to impregnate diapers in the diaper pail. Dilutions for many home areas accompany the full package.

Note: For disposable-type diapers, add one teaspoonful to 8 oz of water to a 'Windex-type' sprayer. Spray middle half area of diapers until damp, and allow to dry before using, to prevent rashes.

How Supplied: Four ounce amber plastic bottles.

MARBLEN Suspension and Tablet

Composition: A modified 'Sippy Powder' antacid containing magnesium and calcium carbonates.

Action and Uses: The peach/apricot (pink) antacid suspension is sugar-free and neutralizes 18 mEq acid per teaspoonful with a low sodium content of 18mg per fl. oz. Each pink tablet consumes 18.0 mEq acid.

Administration and Dosage: One teaspoonful rather than a tablespoonful or one tablet to reduce patient cost by $^2/_3$.

How Supplied: Plastic pints and bottles of 100 and 1000.

NEPHROX SUSPENSION
(aluminum hydroxide)
Antacid Suspension

Composition: A watermelon flavored aluminum hydroxide (320mg as gel)/ mineral oil (10% by volume) antacid per teaspoonful.

Action and Uses: A sugar-free/saccharin-free pink suspension containing no magnesium and low sodium (19mg/ oz). Extremely palatable and especially indicated in renal patients. Each teaspoon consumes 9 mEq acid.

Administration and Dosage: Two teaspoonfuls or as directed by a physician.

Caution: To be taken only at bedtime. Do not use at any other time or administer to infants, expectant women, and nursing mothers except upon the advice of a physician as this product contains mineral oil.

How Supplied: Plastic pints and gallons.

NICOTINEX Elixir
nicotinic acid

Composition: Contains niacin 50 mg./ tsp. in a sherry wine base (amber color).

Action and Uses: Produces flushing when tablets fail. To increase micro-circulation of inner-ear in Meniere's, tinnitus and labyrinthine syndromes. For 'cold hands & feet', and as a vehicle for additives.

Administration and Dosage: One or two teaspoonsful on fasting stomach.

Side Effects: Patients should be warned of dermal flush. Ulcer and gout patients may be affected by 10% alcoholic content.

Contraindications: Severe hypotension and hemorrhage.

How Supplied: Plastic pints and gallons.

OCEAN MIST
(buffered saline)

Composition: A 0.65% special saline made isotonic by a dual preservative system and buffering excipients prevent nasal irritation.

Action and Uses: Rhinitis medicamentosa, rhinitis sicca and atrophic rhinitis. For patients 'hooked on nose drops' and glaucoma patients on diuretics having dry nasal capillaries. OCEAN may also be used as a mist or drop.

Administration and Dosage: One or two squeezes in each nostril P.R.N.

Supplied: Plastic 45cc spray bottles and pints.

PURGE
(flavored castor oil)

Composition: Contains 95% castor oil (USP) in a sweetened lemon flavored base that completely masks the odor and taste of the oil.

Indications: Preparation of the bowel for x-ray, surgery and proctological procedures, IVPs, and constipation.

Dosage: Infants—1–2 teaspoonfuls. Children—adjust between infant and adult dose. Adult—2–4 tablespoonfuls.

Precaution: Not indicated when nausea, vomiting, abdominal pain or symptoms of appendicitis occur. Pregnancy, use only on advice of physician.

Supplied: Plastic 1 oz. & 2 oz. bottles.

Hyland's Inc.

See Standard Homeopathic Company

Johnson & Johnson • MERCK
Consumer Pharmaceuticals Co.
7050 CAMP HILL ROAD
FORT WASHINGTON, PA 19034

Direct Inquiries to:
Consumer Affairs Department
Fort Washington, PA 19034
(215) 233-7000
For Medical Information Contact:
In Emergencies:
(215) 233-7000

INFANTS' MYLICON® Drops
[*my 'li-con*]
Antiflatulent

Ingredients: Each 0.6 mL of drops contains: Active: simethicone, 40 mg. Inactive: carbomer 934P, citric acid, flavors, hydroxypropyl methylcellulose, purified water, Red 3, saccharin calcium, sodium benzoate, sodium citrate.

Indications: For relief of the symptoms of excess gas in the digestive tract. Such gas is frequently caused by excessive swallowing of air or by eating foods that disagree. The defoaming action of INFANTS' MYLICON® Drops relieves flatulence by dispersing and preventing the formation of mucus-surrounded gas pockets in the gastrointestinal tract. INFANTS' MYLICON® Drops act in the stomach and intestines to change the surface tension of gas bubbles enabling them to coalesce, thereby freeing and eliminating the gas more easily by belching or passing flatus.

Directions: Infants (under 2 years): 0.3 ml four times daily after meals and at bedtime, or as directed by a physician. The dosage can also be mixed with 1 oz of cool water, infant formula or other suitable liquids to ease administration. Adults and children: 0.6 ml four times daily, after meals and at bedtime, or as directed by a physician.

Warnings: Do not exceed 12 doses per day except under the advice and supervision of a physician. Keep this and all drugs out of the reach of chldren.

How Supplied: INFANTS' MYLICON® Drops are available in bottles of 15 ml (0.5 fl oz) and 30 ml (1.0 fl oz) original pink, pleasant tasting liquid and non-staining formula. NDC 16837-630; 16837-911.

Shown in Product Identification Guide, page 508

CHILDREN'S MYLANTA®
UPSET STOMACH RELIEF
CALCIUM CARBONATE/ANTACID
LIQUID AND TABLETS

Description: Children's Mylanta is a specially formulated antacid to quickly and effectively relieve the upset stomach kids sometime experience.

Active Ingredients: Each tablet or 5 ml teaspoonful contains 400 mg of calcium carbonate.

Inactive Ingredients: Tablets: Citric acid, confectioner's sugar, D&C Red #27, flavors, magnesium stearate, sorbitol, starch.
Liquid: Butylparaben, cellulose, flavor propylparaben, purified water, D&C Red #22, D&C Red #28, simethicone, sodium saccharin, sorbitol, xanthan gum, may contain tartaric acid.

Acid Neutralizing Capacity:

Tablet	Liquid
8 mEq	8 mEq

Indications: For the relief of acid indigestion, sour stomach, or heartburn and upset stomach associated with these conditions, or overindulgence in food and drink.

Directions: Find the right dose on the chart below. If possible use weight as your dosing guide; otherwise use age. Repeat dosing as needed. DO NOT USE MORE THAN THREE TIMES PER DAY.

WEIGHT (LB)	AGE (YR)	TABLET	LIQUID (TSP)
Under 24	Under 2	Consult	Physician
24–47	2–5	1	1
48–95	6–11	2	2

Warnings: Keep this and all drugs out of the reach of children. Do not take more than 3 tablets or 3 teaspoonfuls (2–5 years) or 6 tablets or 6 teaspoonfuls (6–11 years) in a 24-hour period, or use the maximum dosage of this product for more than two weeks, except under the advice and supervision of a physician.

Drug Interaction Precaution: Antacids may interact with certain prescription drugs. If your child is presently taking a prescription drug, do not give this product without checking with your physician or other health professional.

How Supplied: Children's Mylanta Upset Stomach Relief is supplied as a liquid and chewable tablets in bubble gum flavor.
NDC 16837-810   Bubble Gum tablets
NDC 16837-820   Bubble Gum liquid
Shown in Product Identification Guide, page 508

FAST-ACTING MYLANTA®
AND MAXIMUM-STRENGTH
FAST-ACTING MYLANTA®
[my-lan'ta]
Aluminum, Magnesium and Simethicone
Liquid
Antacid/Anti-Gas

Description: Fast-acting MYLANTA® and Maximum Strength Fast-Acting MYLANTA® are well-balanced, pleasant-tasting, antacid/anti-gas medications that provide consistent, effective relief of symptoms associated with gastric hyperacidity and excess gas. Non-constipating and very low sodium Fast-Acting MYLANTA® and Maximum Strength Fast-Acting MYLANTA® contain two proven antacids, aluminum hydroxide and magnesium hydroxide, plus simethicone for gas relief.

Active Ingredients: Each 5 mL teaspoon contains:

	MYLANTA®	MYLANTA® Double Strength
Aluminum Hydroxide	200 mg	400 mg
Magnesium Hydroxide	200 mg	400 mg
Simethicone	20 mg	40 mg

Inactive Ingredients: LIQUIDS: Butylparaben, carboxymethylcellulose sodium, flavors, hydroxypropyl methylcellulose, microcrystalline cellulose, propylparaben, purified water, saccharin sodium, and sorbitol.

Sodium Content: Each 5 mL teaspoon contains the following amount of sodium:

	MYLANTA®	MYLANTA® Double Strength
Liquid	0.68 mg (0.03 mEq)	1.14 mg (0.05 mEq)

Acid Neutralizing Capacity
Two teaspoonfuls have the following acid neutralizing capacity:

	Fast Acting MYLANTA®	Maximum Strength Fast Acting MYLANTA®
Liquid	25.4 mEq	50.8 mEq

Indications: Fast-Acting MYLANTA® and Maximum Strength Fast-Acting MYLANTA® are indicated for the relief of acid indigestion, heartburn, sour stomach, and symptoms of gas and upset stomach associated with those conditions. Fast-Acting MYLANTA® and Maximum Strength Fast-Acting MYLANTA® are also indicated as antacids for the symptomatic relief of hyperacidity associated with the diagnosis of peptic ulcer, gastritis, peptic esophagitis, heartburn and hiatal hernia and as antiflatulents to alleviate the symptoms of mucus-entrapped gas, including postoperative gas pain.

Advantages: Fast-Acting MYLANTA and Maximum Strength Fast-Acting MYLANTA are homogenized for a smooth, creamy taste. The choice of three pleasant-tasting liquid flavors and the non-constipating formula encourage patient acceptance, thereby minimizing the skipping of prescribed doses. Fast-Acting MYLANTA and Maximum Strength Fast-Acting MYLANTA are also available in tablets, and both the liquid and tablet forms are very low in sodium. Fast-Acting MYLANTA and Maximum Strength Fast-Acting MYLANTA provide consistent relief in patients suffering from distress associated with hyperacidity, mucus-entrapped gas, or swallowed air.

Directions: Liquid: Shake well. 2-4 teaspoonfuls between meals and at bedtime, or as directed by a physician.

Warnings: Keep this and all drugs out of the reach of children. Do not take more than 24 tsps of Fast-Acting MYLANTA® or 12 tsps of Maximum Strength Fast-Acting MYLANTA® in a 24-hour period or use the maximum dose of this product for more than two weeks, except under the advice and supervison of a physician. Do not use this product if you have kidney disease.
Prolonged use of aluminum-containing antacids in patients with renal failure may result in or worsen dialysis osteomalacia. Elevated tissue aluminum levels contribute to the development of the dialysis encephalopathy and osteomalacia syndromes. Small amounts of aluminum are absorbed from the gastrointestinal tract and renal excretion of aluminum is impaired in renal failure. Aluminum is not well removed by dialysis because it is bound to albumin and transferrin, which do not cross dialysis membranes. As a result, aluminum is deposited in bone, and dialysis osteomalacia may develop when large amounts of aluminum are ingested orally by patients with impaired renal function.

Continued on next page

Fast-Acting Mylanta Liq.—Cont.

Aluminum forms insoluble complexes with phosphate in the gastrointestinal tract, thus decreasing phosphate absorption. Prolonged use of aluminum-containing antacids by normophosphatemic patients may result in hypophosphatemia if phosphate intake is not adequate. In its more severe forms, hypophosphatemia can lead to anorexia, malaise, muscle weakness, and osteomalacia.

Drug Interaction Precaution: Antacids may interact with certain prescription drugs. If you are presently taking a prescription drug, do not take this product without checking with your physician or other health professional.

How Supplied: Fast-Acting MYLANTA® and Maximum Strength Fast-Acting MYLANTA® are available as white liquid suspensions in pleasant-tasting flavors, Original, Cherry Creme and Cool Mint Creme. Liquids are supplied in bottles of 5 oz, 12 oz, and 24 oz. Also available for hospital use in liquid unit dose bottles of 1 oz and bottles of 5 oz.

MYLANTA®
NDC 16837-610 ORIGINAL LIQUID
NDC 16837-629 COOL MINT CREME LIQUID
NDC 16837-621 CHERRY CREME LIQUID
NDC 16837-817 Lemon Twist Liquid
MYLANTA® Maximum Strength
NDC 16837-652 ORIGINAL LIQUID
NDC 16837-624 COOL MINT CREME LIQUID
NDC 16837-622 CHERRY CREME LIQUID
NDC 16837-818 Lemon Twist Liquid

Professional Labeling

Indications: Stress-induced upper gastrointestinal hemorrhage: Maximum Strength Fast-Acting MYLANTA® is indicated for the prevention of stress-induced upper gastrointestinal hemorrhage. Hyperacidic conditions: As an antacid, for the symptomatic relief of hyperacidity associated with the diagnosis of peptic ulcer and other gastrointestinal conditions where a high degree of acid neutralization is desired.

Directions: Prevention of stress-induced upper gastrointestinal hemorrhage: 1) Aspirate stomach via nasogastric tube* and record pH. 2) Instill 10 mL of Maximum Strength Fast-Acting MYLANTA® followed by 30 mL of water via nasogastric tube. Clamp tube. 3) Wait one hour. Aspirate stomach and record pH. 4a) If pH equals or exceeds 4.0, apply drainage or intermittent suction for one hour, then repeat the cycle. 4b) If pH is less than 4.0, instill double (20 mL) Maximum Strength Fast-Acting MYLANTA® followed by 30 mL of water. Clamp tube. 5) Wait one hour. If pH equals or exceeds 4.0, see number 7, if pH is still less than 4.0, instill double (40 mL) Maximum Strength Fast-Acting MYLANTA® followed by 30 mL of water. Clamp tube. 6) Wait one hour. If pH equals or exceeds 4.0, see number 7. If pH is still less than 4.0, instill double (80 mL)† Maximum Strength Fast-Acting MYLANTA® followed by 30 mL of water. 7) Drain for one hour and repeat cycle with the effective dosage of Maximum Strength Fast-Acting MYLANTA®.
*If nasogastric tube is not in place, administer 20 mL of Maximum Strength Fast-Acting MYLANTA® orally q2h.
†In a recent clinical study[1] 20 mL of Maximum Strength Fast-Acting MYLANTA®, q2h, was sufficient in more than 85 percent of the patients. No patient studied required more than 80 mL of Maximum Strength Fast-Acting MYLANTA® q2h.
In hyperacid states for symptomatic relief: One or two teaspoonfuls as needed between meals and at bedtime or as directed by a physician. Higher dosage regimens may be employed under the direct supervision of a physician in the treatment of active peptic ulcer disease.

Precautions: Aluminum-magnesium hydroxide containing antacids should be used with caution in patients with renal impairment.

Adverse Effects: Occasional regurgitation and mild diarrhea have been reported with the dosage recommended for the prevention of stress-induced upper gastrointestinal hemorrhage.

References: 1. Zinner MJ, Zuidema GD, Smigh PL, Mignosa M: The prevention of upper gastrointestinal tract bleeding in patients in an intensive care unit. *Surg Gynecol Obster* 153:214–220, 1981. 2. Lucas CE, Sugawa C, Riddle J, et al.: Natural history and surgical dilemma of "stress" gastric bleeding. *Arch Surg* 102:266–273, 1971. 3. Hastings PR, Skillman JJ, Bushnell LS, Silen W: Antacid titration in the prevention of acute gastrointestinal bleeding: a controlled, randomized trial in 100 critically ill patients. *N Engl J Med* 298:1042–1045, 1978. 4. Day SB, MacMillan BG, Altemeier WA: *Curling's Ulcer, An Experience of Nature.* Springfield, IL, Charles C Thomas Co., 1972, p. 205. 5. Skillman JJ, Bushnell LS, Goldman H, Silen W: Respiratory failure, hypotension, sepsis, and jaundice. A clinical syndrome associated with lethal hemorrhage from acute stress ulceration of the stomach. *Am J Surg* 117:523–530, 1969. 6. Priebe HJ, Skillman J, Bushnell LS, et al. Antacid versus cimetidine in preventing acute gastrointestinal bleeding. *N Engl J Med* 302:426–430, 1980. 7. Silen W: The prevention and management of stress ulcers. *Hosp Pract* 15:93–97, 1980. 8. Herrmann V, Kaminski DL: Evaluation of intragastric pH in acutely ill patients. *Arch Surg* 114:511–514, 1979. 9. Martin LF, Staloch DK, Simonowitz DA, et al.: Failure of cimetidine prophylaxis in the critically ill. *Arch Surg* 114:492–496, 1979. 10. Zinner MJ, Turtinen L, Gurll NJ, Reynolds DG: The effect of metiamide on gastric mucosal injury in rat restraint. *Clin Res* 23:484A, 1975. 11. Zinner M, Turtinen BA, Gurll NJ: The role of acid and ischemia in production of stress ulcers during canine hemorrhagic shock. *Surgery* 77:807–816, 1975. 12. Winans CS: Prevention and treatment of stress ulcer bleeding: Antacids or cimetidine? *Drug Ther Bull* (hospital) 12:37–45, 1981.

Shown in Product Identification Guide, page 508

FAST-ACTING MYLANTA AND MAXIMUM STRENGTH FAST ACTING MYLANTA
[mylan 'ta]
Calcium Carbonate and Magnesium Hydroxide Tablets
Antacid

Description: Fast-Acting MYLANTA and Maximum Strength Fast-Acting MYLANTA are well balanced, pleasant tasting antacid medications that provide consistent, effective relief of symptoms associated with gastric hyperacidity. Non-constipating and very low in sodium, Fast-Acting MYLANTA and Maximum Strength Fast-Acting MYLANTA contain two proven antacids, calcium carbonate and magnesium hydroxide.

Active Ingredients
Each tablet contains:

	Fast-Acting MYLANTA	Maximum Strength Fast-Acting MYLANTA
Calcium Carbonate	350mg	700mg
Magnesium Hydroxide	150mg	300mg

Inactive Ingredients
Citric acid, confectioner's sugar, flavors, magnesium stearate, sorbitol, FD&C Blue 1 or D&C Yellow 10 or D&C Red 27

Sodium Content
Each chewable tablet contains the following amount of sodium:

Fast-Acting MYLANTA	Maximum Strength Fast-Acting MYLANTA
0.3mg	0.6mg

Acid Neutralizing Capacity
Two chewable tablets have the following acid neutralizing capacity:

Fast-Acting MYLANTA	Maximum Strength Fast-Acting MYLANTA
24.0mEq	48.0mEq

Indications: Fast-Acting MYLANTA and Maximum Strength Fast-Acting MYLANTA are indicated for the relief of heartburn, acid indigestion, sour stomach and upset stomach associated with these conditions. Fast-Acting MYLANTA and Maximum Strength Fast-Acting MYLANTA are also indicated as antacids for the symptomatic relief of hyperacidity associated with the diagnosis of peptic ulcer, gastritis, peptic esophagitis, heartburn and hiatal hernia.

Directions: Thoroughly chew 2–4 tablets between meals, at bedtime or as directed by a physician.

Warnings: Keep this and all drugs out of the reach of children. Do not take more than 16 tablets of Fast-Acting MYLANTA or 8 tablets of MYLANTA Maximum Strength Fast-Acting in a 24-hour period, or use the maximum dosage for more than two weeks. Do not use this product if you have kidney disease, except under the advise and supervision of a physician.

Drug Interaction Precaution: Antacids may interact with certain prescription drugs. If you are presently taking a prescription drug, do not take this product without checking with your physician or other health professional.

How Supplied: Fast-Acting MYLANTA is available as a green Cool Mint Creme chewable tablet. Maximum Strength Fast-Acting MYLANTA is available as a green Cool Mint Creme Chewable tablet and pink Cherry Creme chewable tablet.
Fast-Acting Mylanta
NDC 16837-848 Cool Mint Creme
Maximum Strength Fast-Acting MYLANTA
NDC 16837-869 Cherry Creme
NDC 16837-849 Cool Mint Creme
Shown in Product Identification Guide, page 508

FAST ACTING MYLANTA SUPREME ANTACID LIQUID

Description: Fast acting Mylanta Supreme is a revolutionary liquid antacid that works fast and tastes great. It has a fresh smooth taste and texture that goes down easy and doesn't leave that chalky aftertaste. Plus, Mylanta Supreme is rich in calcium.
Active Ingredients: Each 5 ml teaspoon contains:
    Calcium carbonate 400 mg
    Magnesium hydroxide 135 mg
Inactive Ingredients: Flavors, hydroxyethyl cellulose, purified water, simethicone, sodium saccharin, sorbitol, xanthan gum, may also contain D&C Yellow #10 and FD&C Blue #1.
Sodium Content: Each 5 ml teaspoon contains 0.7 mg of sodium.
ACID NEUTRALIZING CAPACITY: Two teaspoonfuls provide 25.2 MEq of acid neutralizing capacity.

Indications: Mylanta Supreme is indicated for the relief of heartburn, acid indigestion, sour stomach, upset stomach associated with these conditions and overindulgence in food and drink.

Directions: Shake Well. Take 2–4 teaspoonfuls between meals, at bedtime, or as directed by a physician.

Warnings: Keep this and all drugs out of the reach of children. Do not take more than 20 teaspoonfuls in a 24-hour period, or use the maximum dosage for more than two weeks, or use this product if

you have kidney disease except under the advice and supervision of a physician.

Drug Interaction Precaution: Antacids may interact with certain prescription drugs. If you are presently taking a prescription drug, do not take this product without checking with your physician or other health professional.

How Supplied: Fast Acting Mylanta Supreme is available as white liquid suspensions in cherry, lemon and mint flavors in 12 oz and 24 oz bottles.
    NDC 16837-825 Cherry
    NDC 16837-831 Lemon
    NDC 16837-819 Mint

MYLANTA® GAS Relief Tablets
Maximum Strength MYLANTA® GAS Relief Tablets
MYLANTA® Gas Relief Gelcaps
[*My-lan '-ta*]
Antiflatulent

Active Ingredients: Each chewable tablet contains:

	Simethicone
MYLANTA® GAS Relief Maximum Strength	80 mg
MYLANTA® GAS Relief	125 mg
MYLANTA® GAS Relief Gelcaps	62.5 mg

Inactive Ingredients: TABLETS: Dextrates, flavor, sorbitol, stearic acid, tricalcium phosphate. Cherry: Red 7. GELCAPS: Benzyl alcohol, butylparaben, castor oil, croscarmellose sodium, D&C Red 28, D&C Yellow 10, dextrose, dibasic calcium phosphate dihydrate, edetate calcium disodium, FD&C Blue 1, FD&C Red 28, gelatin, hydroxypropyl methylcellulose, maltodextrin, methylparaben, microcrystalline cellulose, propylene glycol, propylparaben, silicon dioxide, sodium lauryl sulfate, sodium propionate, sorbitol, stearic acid, titanium dioxide, tribasic calcium phosphate.

Indications: For relief of the symptoms of excess gas in the digestive tract. Such gas is frequently caused by excessive swallowing of air or by eating foods that disagree. MYLANTA® GAS Relief Gelcaps, MYLANTA® GAS Relief, and Maximum Strength MYLANTA® GAS Relief Tablets are high capacity antiflatulents for adjunctive treatment of many conditions in which the retention of gas may be a problem, such as the following: air swallowing, postoperative gaseous distention, peptic ulcer, spastic or irritable colon, diverticulosis. If condition persists, consult your physician. MYLANTA® GAS Relief Gelcap, MYLANTA® GAS Relief, and Maximum Strength MYLANTA® GAS Relief Tablets have a defoaming action that relieves flatulence by dispersing and preventing the formation of mucus-surrounded gas pockets in the

gastrointestinal tract. MYLANTA® GAS Relief Gelcaps, MYLANTA® GAS Relief, and Maximum Strength MYLANTA® GAS Relief Tablets act in the stomach and intestines to change the surface tension of gas bubbles enabling them to coalesce, thereby freeing and eliminating the gas more easily by belching or passing flatus.

Directions:
MYLANTA® GAS Relief Tablets
One tablet four times daily after meals and at bedtime. May also be taken as needed up to six tablets daily or as directed by a physician.
Maximum Strength MYLANTA® GAS Relief Tablets
One tablet four times daily after meals and at bedtime or as directed by a physician.
TABLETS SHOULD BE CHEWED THOROUGHLY
MYLANTA® GAS Relief Gelcaps
Swallow 2-4 gelcaps as needed after meals and at bedtime. Do not exceed 8 gelcaps per day unless directed by a physician.

Warnings: Keep this and all drugs out of the reach of children.

How Supplied: MYLANTA® GAS Relief Tablets are available as white (mint) or pink (cherry) scored, chewable tablets identified "MYL GAS 80." Mint flavor is available in bottles of 60 and 100 tablets and individually wrapped 12 and 30 tablet packages. Cherry flavor is available in packages of 12 individually wrapped tablets. Mint NDC 16837-858. Cherry NDC 16837-859.
Maximum Strength MYLANTA® GAS Relief Tablets are available as white, scored, chewable tablets identified "MYL GAS 125" in individually wrapped 12 and 24 tablet packages and economical 48 tablet bottles. NDC 16837-455.
MYLANTA® Gas Relief Gelcaps are available as blue and yellow gelcaps identified as 'MYLANTA GAS' in individually wrapped 24 tablet packages. NDC 16837–626.
Shown in Product Identification Guide, page 508

MYLANTA® GELCAPS
[*my-lan 'ta*]
Antacid

Description: MYLANTA® GELCAPS are an easy-to-swallow, non-chalky alternative to liquid and tablet antacids. The gelcaps contain two antacid ingredients, calcium carbonate, and magnesium hydroxide, have no chalky taste, are low in sodium and provide fast, effective acid pain relief.

Ingredients: Each gelcap contains:
Active: Calcium Carbonate 550 mg and Magnesium Hydroxide 125 mg.
Inactive: Benzyl Alcohol, Butylparaben, Castor Oil, Crospovidone, D&C Red

Continued on next page

Mylanta Gelcaps—Cont.

#28, D&C Yellow 10, Disodium Calcium Edetate, FD&C Blue 1, FD&C Red #40, Gelatin, Hydroxypropyl Cellulose, Magnesium Stearate, Methylparaben, Microcrystalline Cellulose, Propylparaben, Sodium Lauryl Sulfate, Sodium Propionate, Starch, Titanium Dioxide. May also contain propylene glycol.

Sodium Content: MYLANTA® GELCAPS contain a very low amount of sodium per daily dose. Typical value is 2.5 mg (.1087 mEq) sodium per gelcap.

Acid Neutralizing Capacity: Two MYLANTA® GELCAPS have an acid neutralizing capacity of 23.0 mEq.

Indications: For the relief of acid indigestion, heartburn, sour stomach and upset stomach associated with these symptoms.

Advantages: MYLANTA® GELCAPS are easy to swallow, provide fast, effective relief, eliminate antacid taste and are low in sodium. Convenience of dosage in the unique gelcap form can promote patient compliance.

Directions: 2–4 gelcaps as needed or as directed by a physician.

Warnings: Keep this and all other drugs out of the reach of children. Do not take more than 12 gelcaps in a 24-hour period or use the maximum dosage for more than two weeks or use if you have kidney disease, except under the advice and supervision of a physician.

Drug Interaction Precaution: Antacids may interact with certain prescription drugs. If you are presently taking a prescription drug, do not take this product without checking with your physician or other health professional.

How Supplied: MYLANTA® GELCAPS are available as a blue and white gelcap in convenient blister packs in boxes of 24 solid gelcaps or in bottles of 50 and 100 solid gelcaps.
NDC 16837-850   1/93
Shown in Product Identification Guide, page 508

PEPCID AC®
TABLETS

Description:
ACTIVE INGREDIENT: Famotidine 10 mg per tablet.
INACTIVE INGREDIENTS: Hydroxypropyl cellulose, hydroxypropyl methylcellulose, red iron oxide, magnesium stearate, microcrystalline cellulose, starch, talc, titanium dioxide.

Product Benefits:
• **1 tablet** relieves heartburn and acid indigestion.
• Pepcid AC prevents heartburn and acid indigestion brought on by consuming food and beverages.
It contains famotidine, a prescription-proven medicine.

The ingredient in PEPCID AC, famotidine, has been prescribed by doctors for years to treat millions of patients safely and effectively. The active ingredient in PEPCID AC has been taken safely with many frequently prescribed medications.

Action: It is normal for the stomach to produce acid, especially after consuming food and beverages. However, acid in the wrong place (the esophagus), or too much acid, can cause burning pain and discomfort that interfere with everyday activities.

• **Heartburn—Caused by acid in the esophagus**

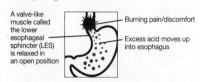

A valve-like muscle called the lower esophageal sphincter (LES) is relaxed in an open position

Burning pain/discomfort

Excess acid moves up into esophagus

In clinical studies, PEPCID AC was significantly better than placebo pills in relieving and preventing heartburn.

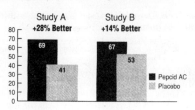

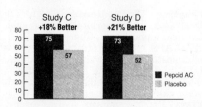

Uses:
• **For Relief** of heartburn, associated with acid indigestion, and sour stomach;
• **For Prevention** of heartburn associated with acid indigestion and sour stomach brought on by consuming food and beverages.

Tips for Managing Heartburn
• Do not lie flat or bend over soon after eating.
• Do not eat late at night, or just before bedtime.
• Avoid food or drinks that are more likely to cause heartburn, such as rich, spicy, fatty, and fried foods, chocolate, caffeine, alcohol, and even some fruits and vegetables.
• Eat slowly and do not eat big meals.
• If you are overweight, lose weight.
• If you smoke, quit smoking.
• Raise the head of your bed.
• Wear loose fitting clothing around your stomach.

Warnings:
Allergy Warning: Do not use if you are allergic to Pepcid AC (famotidine) or other acid reducers.
• Do not take the maximum daily dosage for more than 2 weeks continuously except under the advice and supervision of a doctor.

• Do not use with other acid reducers.
• If you have trouble swallowing, or persistent abdominal pain, see your doctor promptly. You may have a serious condition that may need different treatment.
• As with any drug, if you are pregnant or nursing a baby, seek the advice of a health professional before using this product.
• Keep this and all drugs out of the reach of children.
• In case of accidental overdose, seek professional assistance or contact a poison control center immediately.

Caution:
Heartburn and acid indigestion are common, but you should see your doctor promptly if:
• You have trouble swallowing or persistent abdominal pain. You may have a serious condition that may need different treatment.
• You have used the maximum dosage every day for two weeks continuously.
Important: As with any drug, if you are pregnant or nursing a baby, seek the advice of a health professional before using this product. This product should not be given to children under 12 years old, unless directed by a doctor. Keep this and all drugs out of the reach of children. In case of accidental overdose, seek professional assistance or contact a poison control center immediately.

Directions:
• To relieve symptoms, swallow 1 tablet with a glass of water.
• To prevent symptoms, swallow 1 tablet with a glass of water at any time from 15 to 60 minutes before eating food or drinking beverages that cause heartburn.
• Can be used up to twice daily (up to 2 tablets in 24 hours).
• This product should not be given to children under 12 years old unless directed by a doctor.

How Supplied:
Pepcid AC any time from 15 to is available as a rose-colored tablet identified as 'PEPCID AC'.
Pepcid AC is available in blister packs in boxes of 6, 12, 18, 30, 50, and 80 tablets.
NDC 16837-872
• Read the directions and warnings before use.
• Keep the carton. It contains important information.
Store at temperatures up to 30°C (86°F). Protect from moisture.
DO NOT USE IF THE INDIVIDUAL BLISTER UNIT IS OPEN OR BROKEN.
Shown in Product Identification Guide, page 508

Konsyl Pharmaceuticals, Inc.

4200 S. HULEN
FORT WORTH, TX 76109

Direct Inquiries to:
Bill Steiber
(817) 763-8011, Ext. 23
FAX: (817) 731-9389
Direct Healthcare Professional Sample Requests To:
(800) 356-6795 or www.konsyl.com

KONSYL® EASY MIX POWDER
(psyllium hydrophilic mucilloid)
Sugar Free, Sugar Substitute Free
6.0 grams of psyllium per heaping teaspoon dose.

Description: Konsyl Easy Mix is a bulk-forming natural therapeutic fiber for restoring and maintaining regularity. Konsyl Easy Mix contains 100% psyllium hydrophilic mucilloid, a highly efficient dietary fiber derived from the husk of the psyllium seed. Konsyl Easy Mix contains no chemical stimulants and is non-addictive. Each dose contains 6.0 grams of psyllium compared to 3.4 grams of psyllium in most other products.

Inactive Ingredients: Maltodextrin. Each 6.3 gram dose provides 3 calories. Konsyl Easy Mix has a very low sodium content. Since Konsyl Easy Mix is sugar free, it is excellent for diabetics who require a bowel normalizer.

Actions: Konsyl Easy Mix provides bulk that promotes normal elimination. The product is uniform, instantly miscible, palatable, and non-irritative in the gastrointestinal tract.

Indications: Konsyl Easy Mix is indicated in the management of chronic constipation, irritable bowel syndrome, as adjunctive therapy in the constipation of diverticular disease, bowel management of patients with hemorroids, and for constipation during pregnancy, convalescence, and senility. Konsyl Easy Mix is also indicated for other indications as prescribed by a physician.

NOTE: Konsyl Easy Mix is an excellent source of soluble fiber. Diets low in saturated fat and cholesterol that include 7 grams of soluble fiber per day from psyllium husk, as in Konsyl, may reduce the risk of heart disease by lowering cholesterol. One adult dose of Konsyl has 5 grams of soluble dietary fiber.

Contraindications: Intestinal obstruction, fecal impaction.

Warnings: KEEP THIS AND ALL DRUGS OUT OF THE REACH OF CHILDREN. TAKING THIS PRODUCT WITHOUT ADEQUATE FLUID MAY CAUSE IT TO SWELL AND BLOCK YOUR THROAT OR ESOPHAGUS AND MAY CAUSE CHOKING. DO NOT TAKE THIS PRODUCT IF YOU HAVE DIFFICULTY IN SWALLOWING. IF YOU EXPERIENCE CHEST PAIN, VOMITING, OR DIFFICULTY IN SWALLOWING OR BREATHING AFTER TAKING THIS PRODUCT, SEEK IMMEDIATE MEDICAL ATTENTION.

Precautions: May cause allergic reaction in people sensitive to inhaled or ingested psyllium powder.

Dosage And Administration:
MIX THIS PRODUCT (CHILD OR ADULT DOSE) WITH AT LEAST 8 OUNCES (A FULL GLASS) OF WATER OR OTHER FLUID. TAKING THIS PRODUCT WITHOUT ENOUGH LIQUID MAY CAUSE CHOKING. SEE WARNINGS.
ADULTS: Place one heaping teaspoonful (6.3 grams) into an empty glass. Add 8 oz. of fruit juice, cool water or your favorite beverage. Stir briskly for 3–5 seconds. Drink promptly. If mixture thickens, add more liquid and stir. Follow with additional beverage to aid product action. Konsyl Easy Mix can be taken one to three times daily, depending on need and response. Konsyl Easy Mix generally produces results within 12–72 hours. Take Konsyl Easy Mix at any convenient time, morning or evening; before or after meals. When taking Konsyl Easy Mix, one should drink several 8 oz. glasses of fluid a day to aid product action.
CHILDREN: (6–12 years old) Use 1/2 adult dose in 8 oz. of liquid, 1–3 times daily. Children under six years, consult a physician.
New Users: Easy Does It. Medical research shows that higher fiber intake is important for good digestive health. To help the body adjust and avoid minor gas and bloating sometimes associated with high fiber intake, it may be necessary to take one half dose over several days and then slowly increase the dosage over several days. Always follow with 8 oz. of liquid.

How Supplied: Konsyl Easy Mix is a Powder in container of 7 oz. (200 gram).
Is This Product OTC? YES

KONSYL® POWDER
(psyllium hydrophilic mucilloid)
Sugar Free, Sugar Substitute Free.
6.0 grams of psyllium per TEASPOON

Description: Konsyl is a bulk-forming natural therapeutic fiber for restoring and maintaining regularity. Konsyl contains 100% psyllium hydrophilic mucilloid, a highly efficient dietary fiber derived from the husk of the psyllium seed. Konsyl contains no chemical stimulants and is non-addictive. Each dose contains 6.0 grams of psyllium compared to 3.4 grams of psyllium in most other products.

Inactive Ingredients: None. Each 6 gram dose provides 3 calories. Konsyl has a very low sodium content. Since Konsyl is sugar free, it is excellent for diabetics who require a bowel normalizer.

Actions: See Konsyl Easy Mix

Indications: See Konsyl Easy Mix
NOTE: See Konsyl Easy Mix

Contraindications: See Konsyl Easy Mix

Warnings: See Konsyl Easy Mix

Precautions: See Konsyl Easy Mix

Dosage and Administration:
MIX THIS PRODUCT (CHILD OR ADULT DOSE) WITH AT LEAST 8 OUNCES (A FULL GLASS) OF WATER OR OTHER FLUID. TAKING THIS PRODUCT WITHOUT ENOUGH LIQUID MAY CAUSE CHOKING. SEE WARNINGS.
ADULTS: Place one rounded teaspoonful (6.0 grams) into a dry shaker cup or container that can be closed. Add 8 oz. of juice, cold water or your favorite beverage, preferably fruit juice. Shake, don't stir, for 3–5 seconds. Drink promptly. If mixture thickens, add more liquid and shake. Follow with an 8 oz. glass of juice or water to aid product action. Konsyl can be taken one to three times daily, depending on need and response. Konsyl generally produces results within 12–72 hours. Take Konsyl at any convenient time, morning or evening; before or after meals. When taking Konsyl, one should drink several 8 oz. glasses of water a day to aid product action.
CHILDREN: (6–12 years old) Use $1/2$ adult dose in 8 oz. of liquid, 1–3 times daily.
Children under six years, consult a physician.

New Users: Easy Does It. Medical research shows that higher fiber intake is important for good digestive health. To help the body adjust and avoid minor gas and bloating sometimes associated with high fiber intake, it may be necessary to take one half dose over several days and then slowly increase the dosage over several days. Always follow with 8 oz. of liquid.

How Supplied: Powder, containers of 10.6 oz. (300 g), 15.9 oz. (450 g) and 30 single dose (6.0 g) packets.

Is this product OTC? Yes.

KONSYL FOR KIDS
2.0 grams of psyllium per TEASPOON
BULK-FORMING LAXATIVE

Specially Formulated
For Ages 6–12 Years
Directions for Use: Mix this product (child or adult dose) with at least 8 ounces (a full glass) of water or other fluid. Taking this product without enough liquid may cause choking. See warnings.

Continued on next page

Konsyl for Kids—Cont.

1. Put one rounded **teaspoonful** into an empty glass. Add 8 oz. of cool water.
2. Stir briskly for 3–5 seconds.
3. Drink promptly. If mixture thickens, add more water and stir. Follow with additional liquid to aid product action.

Dosage: Children 6 to under 12 years of age: One rounded teaspoonful 1 to 3 times daily. Children under 6 years of age: Consult a doctor. Adults (age 12 and over) wishing to try Konsyl for Kids may take two rounded teaspoonfuls per dose. Ask your doctor or pharmacist for more information about other Konsyl products.

Indications: For relief of occasional constipation (irregularity). Konsyl for Kids generally produces bowel movement in 12 to 72 hours. Konsyl for Kids is also useful for the treatment of disorders other than constipation. Ask your doctor for more information. Konsyl for Kids is non habit-forming.

Each Rounded Teaspoonful Contains:
Active Ingredients: Psyllium Hydrophilic Mucilloid 2.0 grams.
Inactive Ingredients: Sucrose, citric acid, flavor, FD&C Red #40.
Calories: Approximately 20 per 7 g dose.

Warnings: See Konsyl description for Warnings.

How Supplied: Powder 280 g/10 oz
OTC: Yes

KONSYL® Fiber Tablets
(Calcium Polycarbophil 625mg)

Description: KONSYL Fiber Tablets is a bulk forming fiber laxative for restoring and maintaining regularity. Promotes normal function of the bowel by increasing bulk volume and water content of stool. KONSYL Fiber Tablets contain 625 mg calcium polycarbophil equivalent to 500 mg polycarbophil.

Inactive Ingredients: Calcium Carbonate, Hydroxypropyl Methylcellulose, Microcrystalline Cellulose, Powdered Cellulose, Polyplasdone, Croscarmellose Sodium, Colloidal Silicone Dioxide, Caramel Color, Magnesium Stearate.

Actions: KONSYL Fiber Tablets provide bulk that promotes normal elimination. KONSYL Fiber Tablets provide convenience of a bulk forming laxative in a tablet form. The product is easy-to-swallow and water and non-irritative in the gastrointestinal tract.

Indications: See Konsyl description for Indications

Contraindications: See Konsyl description for Contraindications

Warnings: See Konsyl description for Warnings

Interaction Precaution: Contains calcium. If you are taking any form of tetracycline antibiotic, this product should

be taken at least 1 hour before or 2 hours after you have taken the antibiotic. Store at controlled room temperature 59°–86°F (15°–30°C). Protect from moisture.

Dosage and Administration: TAKE THIS PRODUCT (CHILD OR ADULT DOSE) WITH AT LEAST 8 OUNCES (A FULL GLASS) OF WATER OR OTHER FLUID. TAKING THIS PRODUCT WITHOUT ENOUGH LIQUID MAY CAUSE CHOKING. SEE WARNINGS. **ADULTS:** 2 TABLETS 1 TO 4 TIMES A DAY. **CHILDREN** (6 TO 12 YEARS OLD): 1 TABLET 1 TO 3 TIMES A DAY. CHILDREN UNDER 6 YEARS CONSULT A PHYSICIAN. DOSAGE WILL VARY ACCORDING TO DIET, EXERCISE, PREVIOUS LAXATIVE USE OR SEVERITY OF CONSTIPATION. THE RECOMMENDED ADULT STARTING DOSE IS 2 TO 4 TABLETS DAILY. MAY BE INCREASED UP TO 8 TABLETS DAILY. KONSYL FIBER TABLETS GENERALLY PRODUCE RESULTS WITHIN 12–72 HOURS.

How Supplied: Tablets, containers of 90 tablets.
Is this product OTC? Yes

EDUCATIONAL MATERIAL

Patient Education Brochures available to Physicians on the Subjects of:
  I.B.S.
  Hemorrhoids
  Fiber Facts
  Constipation
  Diverticular Disease
  Konsyl For Kids

Lane Labs
ALLENDALE, NJ 07401

Direct Inquiries to:
800-526-3005

BENEFIN™
Organically Processed
100% Shark Cartilage

BeneFin is processed using Lane Labs' exclusive "organic" technology and is superior to conventionally processed shark cartilage brands:
• **30% more cartilage protein, gram for gram (44% by weight).**
• **Processed without chemicals for full potency**
• **Fresh, clean taste and smell**
Consult a health care professional first if you are pregnant or nursing, recovering from surgery or have a heart/circulatory condition.
DO NOT USE IF SEAL IS BROKEN OR MISSING.
To maintain proper bone and join function: Take 4 grams (2/3 scoop) stirred into a glass of water or juice.

For the benefit of additional cartilage protein and calcium: Take 6 grams (1 scoop) stirred into a glass of water or juice daily or as directed by a health professional.

NUTRITIONAL FACTS – Typical Analysis
(Daily Dietary Use) 2/3 scoop (4 grams)
Servings Per Container Approx. 76
Calories 12   Calories From Fat 0
INGREDIENTS: Contains 100% pure shark cartilage with no flavors or additives.
Keep out of reach of children.
Store at room temperature.
Shown in Product Identification Guide, page 508

Lavoptik Company, Inc.
661 WESTERN AVENUE N.
ST. PAUL, MN 55103

Direct Inquiries to:
661 Western Avenue North
St. Paul, MN 55103-1694
(651) 489-1351

For Medical Emergencies Contact:
B. C. Brainard
(651) 489-1351
FAX: (651) 489-0760

LAVOPTIK® Eye Cups

Description: Device—Sterile disposable eye cups.

How Supplied: Individually bagged eye cups are packed 12 per box, NDC 10651-01004.

LAVOPTIK® Eye Wash

Description: Isotonic LAVOPTIK Eye Wash is a buffered solution designed to help physically remove contaminants from the surface of the eye and lids. Formulated to buffer contaminants toward the safe range and help restore normal salts and water ratios in the tears.

Contents: Each 100 ml
Sodium Chloride   0.49 gram
Sodium Biphosphate   0.40 gram
Sodium Phosphate   0.45 gram
Preservative Agent
  Benzalkonium Chloride   0.005 gram

Precautions: If you experience severe eye pain, headache, rapid change in vision (side or straight ahead); sudden appearance of floating objects, acute redness of the eyes, pain on exposure to light or double vision consult a physician at once. If symptoms persist or worsen after use of this product, consult a physician. If solution changes color or becomes cloudy do not use. Keep this and all medicines out of reach of children. Keep container tightly closed. Do not use if safety seal is broken at time of purchase.

Administration: <u>6 ounce size with Eye Cup.</u>
Rinse cup with clean water immediately before and after each use, avoid contamination of rim and inside surfaces of cup. Apply cup, half-filled with LAVOPTIK Eye Wash tightly to the eye. Tilt head backward. Open eyelids wide, rotate eyeball and blink several times to insure thorough washing. Discard washings. Repeat other eye. Tightly cap bottle.
<u>32 ounce size.</u>
Break seal as you remove cap and pour directly on contaminated area.

How Supplied: 6 ounce bottle with eyecup, NDC 10651-01040.
32 ounce bottle, NDC 10651-01019.

Lederle Consumer Health

A Division of Whitehall-Robins Healthcare
FIVE GIRALDA FARMS
MADISON, NJ 07940

Direct Inquiries to:
Lederle Consumer Product Information
(800) 282-8805

FIBERCON®
[fĭ-bĕr-cŏn]
Calcium Polycarbophil
Bulk-Forming Fiber Laxative

Indications: Helps restore and maintain regularity and relieve constipation. The product generally produces bowel movement in 12 to 72 hours.

Directions: FIBERCON® works naturally so continued use for one to three days is normally required to produce full benefit. FIBERCON dosage may vary according to diet, exercise, previous laxative use or severity of constipation. **TAKE THIS PRODUCT ACCORDING TO THE DOSAGE CHART WITH A FULL GLASS (8 OUNCES) OF LIQUID. TAKING THIS PRODUCT WITHOUT ENOUGH LIQUID MAY CAUSE CHOKING. SEE WARNINGS.**
Do not take more than the maximum daily dose.
[See table above]

Warnings: Do not use laxative products when abdominal pain, nausea or vomiting are present unless directed by a doctor. If you have noticed a sudden change in bowel habits that persists over a period of 2 weeks, consult a doctor before using a laxative. Laxative products should not be used for a period longer than 1 week unless directed by a doctor. Rectal bleeding or failure to have a bowel movement after use of a laxative may indicate a serious condition. Discontinue use and consult your doctor. **TAKING THIS PRODUCT WITHOUT ADEQUATE FLUID MAY CAUSE IT TO SWELL AND BLOCK YOUR THROAT**

Age	Recommended Dose	Daily Maximum
Adults & Children over 12	2 caplets once a day	Up to 4 times a day*
Children (6 to 12 years)	1 caplet once a day	Up to 4 times a day*
Children under 6 years	Consult a physician	

*Refer to directions

OR ESOPHAGUS AND MAY CAUSE CHOKING. **DO NOT TAKE THIS PRODUCT IF YOU HAVE DIFFICULTY IN SWALLOWING. IF YOU EXPERIENCE CHEST PAIN, VOMITING, OR DIFFICULTY IN SWALLOWING OR BREATHING AFTER TAKING THIS PRODUCT, SEEK IMMEDIATE MEDICAL ATTENTION.** Keep this and all medicines out of the reach of children. In case of accidental overdose, seek professional assistance or contact a poison control center immediately.

Interaction Precaution: Contains calcium. If you are taking any form of tetracycline antibiotic, FIBERCON should be taken at least 1 hour before or 2 hours after you have taken the antibiotic.

Ingredients: Each caplet contains 625 mg calcium polycarbophil equivalent to 500 mg polycarbophil.

Inactive Ingredients: Calcium Carbonate, Caramel, Crospovidone, Hydroxypropyl Methylcellulose, Magnesium Stearate, Microcrystalline Cellulose, Mineral Oil, Povidone, Silica Gel and Sodium Lauryl Sulfate.
Store At Controlled Room Temperature 15–30° C (59–86°F).
Protect Contents From Moisture.
TAMPER RESISTANT FEATURE: Bottle sealed with printed foil under cap or in plastic blister with foil backing. Do not accept if foil barrier or plastic blister is broken.

How Supplied: Film-coated caplets, scored, engraved LL and F66.
Package of 36 caplets.
Bottles of 60 caplets.
Bottle of 90 caplets.
LEDERLE CONSUMER HEALTH DIVISION

3M
BUILDING 304-1-01
ST PAUL, MN 55144-1000

Direct Inquiries to:
Customer Service
(800) 537-2191

For Medical Emergencies Contact:
(651) 733-2882 (answered 24 hrs.)

Sales and Ordering or Returns:
(800) 832-2189

3M™ TITRALAC™ ANTACID AND TITRALAC™ EXTRA STRENGTH ANTACID
[T ĭ ' tră lăc]

Active Ingredients: Calcium Carbonate: *Regular:* 420mg./tablet (168 mg. elemental calcium). *Extra Strength:* 750mg/tablet (300 mg. elemental calcium).

Inactive Ingredients: Glycine, Magnesium Stearate, Saccharin, Spearmint Oil, Starch.

Indications: A spearmint flavored non-chalky antacid tablet which quickly relieves heartburn, sour stomach, acid indigestion and upset stomach associated with these symptoms.

Dosage and Administration: *Regular:* Two tablets every two or three hours as symptoms occur or as directed by a physician. Tablets can be chewed, swallowed or allowed to melt in the mouth. *Extra Strength:* One or two tablets every two or three hours as symptoms occur or as directed by a physician. Tablets can be chewed or allowed to melt in the mouth.

Warnings: *Regular:* Do not take more than 19 tablets in a 24-hour period or use maximum dosage for more than two weeks, except under the advise and supervision of a physician. *Extra Strength:* Do not take more than ten tablets in a 24-hour period or use maximum dosage for more than two weeks, except under the advice and supervision of a physician. **Keep this and all medication out of the reach of children**

Drug Interaction Precaution: Antacids may interact with certain prescription drugs. If you are presently taking a prescription drug, do not take this product without checking with your physician or other health professional.

Dietary Information: Titralac antacid tablets are sugar and aluminum free and have a very low sodium content (1.1 mg/tablet).

How Supplied: *Regular:* Available in bottles of 40, 100, 1000 tablets. *Extra Strength:* Available in bottles of 100 tablets.
Shown in Product Identification Guide, page 509

3M™ TITRALAC™ PLUS ANTACID
[T ĭ 'tră lăc]

Active Ingredients: Calcium Carbonate: 420 mg/tablet (168 mg elemental calcium), Simethicone: 21 mg/tablet.

Continued on next page

3M Titralac Plus—Cont.

Inactive Ingredients: Glycine, Magnesium Stearate, Saccharin, Spearmint Oil, Starch. May also contain Croscarmellose Sodium.

Indications: A spearmint flavored non-chalky antacid which quickly relieves heartburn, sour stomach, acid indigestion, and accompanying gas often associated with these symptoms.

Dosage and Administration: Two tablets every two or three hours as symptoms occur or as directed by a physician. Tablets can be chewed, swallowed or allowed to melt in the mouth.

Warnings: Do not take more than 19 tablets in a 24-hour period or use maximum dosage for more than two weeks, except under the advice and supervision of a physician. **Keep this and all medication out of the reach of children.**

Drug Interaction Precaution: Antacids may interact with certain prescription drugs. If you are presently taking a prescription drug, do not take this product without checking with your physician or other health professional.

Dietary Information: Tablets are sugar and aluminum free and have a very low sodium content, 1.1 mg/tablet.

How Supplied: Available in bottles of 100 tablets.
Shown in Product Identification Guide, page 509

Matol Botanical International, Ltd.

1111, 46th AVENUE
LACHINE, QUEBEC
CANADA H8T 3C5

Direct Inquiries to:
Ph: (800) 363-3890
website: www.matol.com

BIOMUNE OSF EXPRESS
Homeopathic nasal and throat spray for the relief of the symptoms associated with the common cold, influenza, sinusitis, otitis media and similar conditions

Active Ingredients: Silicea Compound – Silicea (Quartz) 22X, Argentum Nitricum 21X, Atropa Belladonna ex herba 15X.

Inactive Ingredients: Filtered water, proprietary extract of whey permeate, 2-deoxy-d-glucose, eucalyptus oil, disodium EDTA, thimerosal, benzalkonium chloride, sodium hydroxide.

Indications: For the relief of symptoms of the common cold, influenza, sinusitis, otitis media and similar conditions.

Directions: For children 3 years to adult. One to two sprays in each nostril every four to six hours during acute symptoms and two to three times per day with chronic symptoms. Shake well before using.

Warning: Do not use if the imprinted seal is broken or missing. If symptoms persist for more than five days or worsen, contact a licensed health professional. As with any drug, if you are pregnant or nursing a baby, seek the advice of a licensed health care professional before using the product. Keep this and all medication out of the reach of children. Store at room temperature.

How Supplied: Biomune OSF Express comes in 1 fluid ounce in spray bottle.

Clinical Study: *The Use of Matol Biomune OSF Express, a Homeopathic Medicine, in the Prevention and Treatment of Recurrent Otitis Media* by **Jesse A. Stoff, MD.** Abstract: The study using Matol Biomune OSF Express, a homeopathic medicine with the active ingredient Silicea Compound, as compared to pharmaceutical intervention, was carried out with twenty-six (26) children with a history of recurrent acute otitis media (RAOM).
Discussion: The use of the product was shown to be safe, rapid and effective and is indicated as a clear alternative to pharmaceutical intervention for the treatment of upper respiratory infection and recurrent otitis media in young children.
Shown in Product Identification Guide, page 509

McNeil Consumer Healthcare

Division of McNeil-PPC, Inc.
FORT WASHINGTON, PA 19034

Direct Inquiries to:
Consumer Affairs Department
Fort Washington, PA 19034
(215) 233-7000

Children's MOTRIN®
Ibuprofen Oral Suspension, Concentrated Drops and Chewable Tablets

Description: *Children's MOTRIN® Ibuprofen Oral Suspension* and *Children's MOTRIN® Concentrated Drops* are alcohol-free, berry-flavored suspension especially developed for children. Each 5 mL (teaspoon) of *Children's MOTRIN® Ibuprofen Oral Suspension* contains ibuprofen 100 mg. Each 1.25 mL (dropperful) of *Children's MOTRIN® Concentrated Drops* contains ibuprofen 50 mg. Each *Children's MOTRIN® Ibuprofen Chewable Tablet* contains 50 mg of ibuprofen in an orange-flavored chewable tablet.

Uses: *Children's MOTRIN® Ibuprofen Oral Suspension, Children's MOTRIN® Concentrated Drops and Children's MOTRIN® Ibuprofen Chewable Tablets* are indicated for temporary reduction of fever and relief of minor aches and pains due to colds, flu, sore throat, headaches and toothaches. One dose lasts 6–8 hours.

Directions: Repeat dose every 6–8 hours, if needed. Do not use more than 4 times a day. If possible, use weight to dose; otherwise use age. If stomach upset occurs while taking this product, give with food or milk. *Children's MOTRIN® Ibuprofen Oral Suspension:* Shake well before using. Only use enclosed measuring cup for accurate dosing. Replace original bottle cap to maintain child resistance. 2–3 years (24–35 lbs): 1 tsp; 4–5 years (36–47 lbs): $1^1/_2$ tsp; 6–8 years (48–59 lbs): 2 tsp; 9–10 years (60–71 lbs): $2^1/_2$ tsp; 11 years (72–95 lbs): 3 tsp. Under 2 years (under 24 lbs), consult a physician. *Children's MOTRIN® Concentrated Drops:* Shake well before using. Only use enclosed dropper; fill to prescribed level and dispense liquid slowly into child's mouth, toward inner cheek. 2–3 years (24–35 lbs): 2 dropperfuls (2 × 1.25 mL). Under 2 years (under 24 lbs), consult a physician. *Children's MOTRIN® Ibuprofen Chewable Tablets:* 4–5 years (36–47 lbs): 3 tablets; 6–8 years (48–59 lbs): 4 tablets; 9–10 years (60–71 lbs): 5 tablets; 11 years (72–95 lbs): 6 tablets. Under 4 years (under 36 lbs), consult a physician.

Warnings:
Allergy Alert: ibuprofen may cause a severe allergic reaction which may include: hives, facial swelling, asthma (wheezing), shock.

Do not use if you have ever had an allergic reaction to any other pain reliever/fever reducer.

Stop use and ask a doctor if an allergic reaction occurs. Seek medical help right away.

CALL YOUR DOCTOR IF:
- Your child is under a doctor's care for any serious condition or is taking any other drug.
- Your child has problems or serious side effects from taking fever reducers or pain relievers.
- Your child does not get any relief within first day (24 hours) of treatment, or pain or fever gets worse.
- Stomach upset gets worse or lasts.
- Redness or swelling is present in the painful area.
- Sore throat is severe, lasts for more than 2 days or occurs with fever, headache, rash, nausea or vomiting.
- Any new symptoms appear.

DO NOT USE:
- With any other product that contains ibuprofen, or other pain reliever/fever reducer, unless directed by a doctor.
- For more than **3 days** for fever or pain unless directed by a doctor.
- For stomach pain unless directed by a doctor.
- If your child is dehydrated (significant fluid loss) due to continued vomiting, diarrhea or lack of fluid intake.

IMPORTANT:
Do not exceed recommended dose. Taking more than the recommended dose (overdose) may not provide more relief and could cause serious health problems. **Keep this and all drugs out of the reach of children. In case of accidental overdose, seek professional assistance or contact a poison control center immediately.**
NOTE: In addition to the above:
Children's MOTRIN® Ibuprofen Oral Suspension:
• If plastic carton wrap or bottle wrap imprinted "Safety Seal®", is broken or missing.
Children's MOTRIN® Concentrated Drops:
• If plastic bottle wrap imprinted with "Safety Seal®" and "Use With Enclosed Dropper Only" is broken or missing.
Children's MOTRIN® Ibuprofen Chewable Tablets:
• If blister unit is broken or open.
WHEN USING THIS PRODUCT:
• Mouth or throat burning may occur; give with water or food.
• Phenylketonurics: Contains phenylalanine 3 mg per tablet.

PROFESSIONAL INFORMATION
Overdosage Information: The *toxicity of ibuprofen overdose* is dependent upon the amount of drug ingested and the time elapsed since ingestion, though individual response may vary, which makes it necessary to evaluate each case individually. Although uncommon, serious toxicity and death have been reported in the medical literature with ibuprofen overdosage. The most frequently reported symptoms of ibuprofen overdose include abdominal pain, nausea, vomiting, lethargy and drowsiness. Other central nervous system symptoms include headache, tinnitus, CNS depression and seizures. Metabolic acidosis, coma, acute renal failure and apnea (primarily in very young children) may rarely occur. Cardiovascular toxicity, including hypotension, bradycardia, tachycardia and atrial fibrillation, also have been reported.
The *treatment of acute ibuprofen overdose* is primarily supportive. Management of hypotension, acidosis and gastrointestinal bleeding may be necessary. In cases of acute overdose, the stomach should be emptied through ipecac-induced emesis or lavage. Emesis is most effective if initiated within 30 minutes of ingestion. Orally administered activated charcoal may help in reducing the absorption and reabsorption of ibuprofen. In children, the estimated amount of ibuprofen ingested per body weight may be helpful to predict the potential for development of toxicity although each case must be evaluated. Ingestion of less than 100 mg/kg is unlikely to produce toxicity. Children ingesting 100 to 200 mg/kg may be managed with induced emesis and a minimal observation time of four hours. Children ingesting 200 to 400 mg/kg of ibuprofen should have immediate gastric emptying and at least four hours observation in a health care facility. Children ingesting greater than 400 mg/kg require immediate medical referral, careful observation and appropriate supportive therapy. Ipecac-induced emesis is not recommended in overdoses greater than 400 mg/kg because of the risk of convulsions and the potential for aspiration of gastric contents.
In adult patients the history of the dose reportedly ingested does not appear to be predictive of toxicity. The need for referral and follow-up must be judged by the circumstances at the time of the overdose ingestion. Symptomatic adults should be admitted to a health care facility for observation.

INACTIVE INGREDIENTS
Children's MOTRIN® Ibuprofen Oral Suspension: Citric acid, cornstarch, D&C Yellow #10, FD&C Red #40, artificial flavors, glycerin, polysorbate 80, purified water, sodium benzoate, sucrose, xanthan gum.
Children's MOTRIN® Concentrated Drops: Citric acid, cornstarch, FD&C Red #40, artificial flavors, glycerin, polysorbate 80, purified water, sodium benzoate, sorbitol, sucrose, xanthan gum.
Children's MOTRIN® Ibuprofen Chewable Tablets: Aspartame, citric acid, FD&C Yellow #6, natural and artificial flavors, hydroxyethyl cellulose, hydroxypropyl methylcellulose, magnesium stearate, mannitol, microcrystalline cellulose, povidone, sodium lauryl sulfate, sodium starch glycolate.

How Supplied: *Children's MOTRIN® Ibuprofen Oral Suspension:* Orange colored liquid in tamper-evident bottles of 2 and 4 fl. oz.
Children's MOTRIN® Concentrated Drops: Pink colored liquid in 1/2 fl. oz. bottles.
Children's MOTRIN® Ibuprofen Chewable Tablets: Orange colored tablets available in 24 count blister pack.
Store at room temperature 15°-30°C (59°-86°F).
Shown in Product Identification Guide, page 509

Children's TYLENOL®
acetaminophen
Soft-Chew Chewable Tablets, Elixir, and
Suspension Liquid

Infants' TYLENOL®
acetaminophen
Concentrated Drops

Description: *Infants' TYLENOL® Grape Concentrated Drops* are stable, alcohol-free, grape-flavored and purple in color. *Infants' TYLENOL® Cherry Concentrated Drops* are stable, alcohol-free, cherry-flavored and red in color. Each 0.8 mL (one calibrated dropperful) contains 80 mg acetaminophen. *Children's TYLENOL® Elixir* is stable and alcohol-free, cherry-flavored, and red in color. *Children's TYLENOL® Suspension Liquid* is stable, alcohol-free, cherry-flavored, and red in color, or bubble gum flavored, and pink in color or grape flavored and purple in color. Each 5 mL (one teaspoonful) contains 160 mg acetaminophen. Each *Children's TYLENOL® Soft-Chew Chewable Tablet* contains 80 mg acetaminophen in a grape, bubble gum, or fruit flavor.

Actions: Acetaminophen is a clinically proven analgesic/antipyretic. Acetaminophen produces analgesia by elevation of the pain threshold and antipyresis through action on the hypothalamic heat regulating center. Acetaminophen is equal to aspirin in analgesic and antipyretic effectiveness and it is unlikely to produce many of the side effects associated with aspirin and aspirin containing products.

Uses: *Children's TYLENOL® Soft-Chew Chewable Tablets, Elixir, Suspension Liquid* and *Infants' TYLENOL® Concentrated Drops:* For the reduction of fever. For the temporary relief of minor aches and pains associated with a cold, flu, headache, sore throat, immunizations, toothache.

Precautions: If a rare sensitivity reaction occurs, the drug should be stopped.
Directions: Chew tablets before swallowing. All dosages may be repeated every 4 hours, if needed. Do not use more than 5 times a day. Under 2 years (under 24 lbs), consult a physician. *Children's TYLENOL Soft-Chew Chewable Tablets* are not the same concentration as Junior Strength Tylenol Chewable Tablets or Caplets. For accurate dosing follow dosing instructions on label. 2–3 years (24–35 lbs): 2 tablets; 4–5 years (36–47 lbs): 3 tablets; 6–8 years (48–59 lbs): 4 tablets; 9–10 years (60–71 lbs): 5 tablets; 11 years (72–95 lbs): 6 tablets.
Children's TYLENOL® Elixir & Suspension Liquid: Children's Tylenol® Liquids are **less** concentrated than Infants' Tylenol® Concentrated Drops. For accurate dosing follow dosing instructions on label. This product has been specially designed for use with the enclosed measuring cup. Use only enclosed measuring cup to dose this product. Do not use any other dosing device. 2–3 years (24–35 lbs): 1 teaspoonful; 4–5 years (36–47 lbs): 1 1/2 teaspoonfuls; 6–8 years (48–59 lbs): 2 teaspoonfuls; 9–10 years (60–71 lbs): 2 1/2 teaspoonfuls; 11 years (72–95 lbs): 3 teaspoonfuls. *Infants' TYLENOL® Concentrated Drops:* Infants' Tylenol® Drops are **more** concentrated than Children's Tylenol® Liquids. For accurate dosing follow dosing instructions on label. This product has been specially designed for use only with enclosed dropper. Do not use any other dosing device with this product. 2–3 years (24–35 lbs): 2 dropperfuls (2 × 0.8 mL).
Professional Dosage Schedule: *Children's TYLENOL® Elixir & Suspension Liquid:* Children's Tylenol® Liquids are **less** concentrated than Infants' Tylenol® Concentrated Drops. For accurate dosing follow dosing instructions on label. This product has been specially designed for use with the enclosed measuring cup.

Continued on next page

Children's Tylenol—Cont.

Use only enclosed measuring cup to dose this product. Do not use any other dosing device. 4–11 months (12–17 lbs): $^{1}/_{2}$ teaspoonful; 12–23 months (18–23 lbs): $^{3}/_{4}$ teaspoonful. *Infants' TYLENOL® Concentrated Drops:* Infants' Tylenol® Drops are **more** concentrated than Children's Tylenol® Liquids. For accurate dosing follow dosing instructions on label. This product has been specially designed for use only with enclosed dropper. Do not use any other dosing device with this product. 0–3 months (6–11 lbs): 0.4 mL; 4–11 months (12–17 lbs): 0.8 mL; 12–23 months (18–23 lbs): 1.2 mL. All dosages may be repeated every 4 hours, if needed. Do not use more than 5 times a day.

Warnings: *Children's TYLENOL® Soft-Chew Chewable Tablets, Elixir, Suspension Liquid and Infants' TYLENOL® Concentrated Drops:*
Do Not Use:
• with any other products containing acetaminophen.
• for more than 3 days for fever unless directed by a doctor.
• for more than 5 days for pain unless directed by a doctor.
Stop Using This Product and Ask a Doctor if:
• symptoms do not improve.
• new symptoms occur.
• pain or fever persists or gets worse.
• redness or swelling is present.
• sore throat is severe, lasts for more than 2 days or occurs with fever, headache, rash, nausea or vomiting.
Do not exceed recommended dose. Taking more than the recommended dose (overdose) may not provide more relief and could cause serious health problems. Keep this and all drugs out of the reach of children. In case of accidental overdose, contact a physician or poison control center immediately. Prompt medical attention is critical even if you do not notice any signs or symptoms.
NOTE: In addition to the above:
Infants' TYLENOL® Concentrated Drops: Do not use if plastic carton wrap or bottle wrap imprinted "Safety Seal®" is broken or missing.
Children's TYLENOL® Elixir and Suspension Liquid: Do not use if plastic carton wrap, bottle wrap, or foil inner seal imprinted "Safety Seal®" is broken or missing. Not a USP elixir.
Children's TYLENOL® Soft-Chew Chewable Tablets: Do not use if carton is opened or if neck wrap or foil inner seal imprinted "Safety Seal®" is broken or missing. Phenylketonurics: grape contains phenylalanine 5 mg per tablet, bubble gum contains 6 mg per tablet, fruit contains 6 mg per tablet.

PROFESSIONAL INFORMATION
Overdosage Information: Acetaminophen in massive overdosage may cause hepatic toxicity in some patients. In adults and adolescents, hepatic toxicity has rarely been reported following ingestion of acute overdoses of less than 7.5 to 10 grams. Fatalities are infrequent (less

than 3–4% of untreated cases) and have rarely been reported with overdoses of less than 15 grams. In children, an acute overdosage of less than 150 mg/kg has not been associated with hepatic toxicity. Early symptoms following a potentially hepatotoxic overdose may include: nausea, vomiting, diaphoresis and general malaise. Clinical and laboratory evidence of hepatic toxicity may not be apparent until 48 to 72 hours postingestion.

In adults and adolescents, regardless of the quantity of acetaminophen reported to have been ingested, administer acetylcysteine immediately if 24 hours or less have elapsed from the reported time of ingestion. For full prescribing information, refer to the acetylcysteine package insert. Do not await results of assays for acetaminophen levels before initiating treatment with acetylcysteine. The following additional procedures are recommended: Promptly initiate gastric decontamination of the stomach. A plasma acetaminophen assay should be obtained as early as possible, but no sooner than four hours following ingestion. If plasma level falls above the lower treatment line on the acetaminophen overdose nomogram, acetylcysteine therapy should be continued. Liver function studies should be obtained initially and repeated at 24-hour intervals.

Serious toxicity or fatalities are extremely infrequent in children, possibly due to differences in the way they metabolize acetaminophen. In children, the maximum potential amount ingested can be more easily estimated. If more than 150 mg/kg or an unknown amount was ingested, obtain a plasma acetaminophen level. The plasma acetaminophen level should be obtained as soon as possible, but no sooner than 4 hours following ingestion. If plasma level falls above the lower treatment line on the acetaminophen overdose nomogram, the acetylcysteine therapy should be initiated and continued for a full course of therapy. If plasma acetaminophen assay capability is not available, and the estimated acetaminophen ingestion exceeds 150 mg/kg, acetylcysteine therapy should be initiated and continued for a full course of therapy.

For additional emergency information, call your regional poison center or call the Rocky Mountain Poison Center toll free, (1-800-525-6115).

Inactive Ingredients: *Children's TYLENOL® Soft-Chew Fruit Flavored Chewable Tablets:* Aspartame, Cellulose, Corn Starch, D&C Red #7 Flavors, Magnesium Stearate, and Mannitol. May contain Ethylcellulose or Cellulose Acetate and Povidone.

Children's TYLENOL® Soft-Chew Grape Flavored Chewable Tablets: Aspartame, Cellulose, Citric Acid, Corn Starch, FD&C Blue #1, D&C Red #7, D&C Red #30, Flavors, Magnesium Stearate, and Mannitol. May contain Ethylcellulose or Cellulose Acetate and Povidone.

Children's TYLENOL® Soft-Chew Bubble Gum Flavored Chewable Tablets: Aspartame, Cellulose, Corn Starch, D&C Red #7, Flavors, Magnesium Stearate, and Mannitol. May contain Ethylcellulose or Cellulose Acetate and Povidone.

Children's TYLENOL® Elixir: Benzoic Acid, Citric Acid, Flavors, Glycerin, Polyethylene Glycol, Propylene Glycol, Sodium Benzoate, Sorbitol, Sucrose, Purified Water, Red #33, Red #40.

Children's TYLENOL® Suspension Liquid: Butylparaben, Cellulose, Citric Acid, Corn Syrup, Flavors, Glycerin, Propylene Glycol, Purified Water, Sodium Benzoate, Sorbitol, Xanthan Gum. In addition to the above ingredients cherry flavored suspension contains FD&C Red #40, bubble gum flavored suspension contains D&C Red #33, and FD&C Red #40, and grape flavored suspension contains D&C Blue #1 and D&C Red #33.

Infants' TYLENOL® Cherry Concentrated Drops: Butylparaben, Cellulose, Citric Acid, Corn Syrup, Flavors, Glycerin, Propylene Glycol, Purified Water, Sodium Benzoate, Sorbitol, Xanthan Gum, FD&C Red #40.

Infants' TYLENOL® Grape Concentrated Drops: Butylparaben, Cellulose, Citric Acid, Corn Syrup, Flavors, Glycerin, Propylene Glycol, Purified Water, Sodium Benzoate, Sorbitol, Xanthan Gum, D&C Red #33, and FD&C Blue #1.

How Supplied: Soft-Chew Chewable Tablets (pink colored fruit, purple colored grape, pink colored bubble gum, scored, imprinted "TY80"): Bottles of 30 and also blister packaged 60's and 96's. (fruit). **Elixir** (cherry colored red): bottles of 2 and 4 fl. oz. **Suspension liquid** (cherry colored red): bottles of 2 and 4 fl. oz. (bubble gum flavored colored pink and grape flavored colored purple): bottle of 4 fl. oz. **Concentrated drops** (grape colored purple): bottles of $^{1}/_{2}$ oz (15 mL) (cherry colored red): bottles of $^{1}/_{2}$ oz and 1 oz, each with calibrated plastic dropper. All packages listed above have child-resistant safety caps or blisters.
Shown in Product Identification Guide, page 510

Children's TYLENOL® COLD
Multi Symptom Chewable Tablets and Liquid

Description: Each *Children's TYLENOL® COLD Multi Symptom Chewable Grape-Flavored Tablet* contains acetaminophen 80 mg, chlorpheniramine maleate 0.5 mg and pseudoephedrine hydrochloride 7.5 mg. *Children's TYLENOL® COLD Multi Symptom Liquid* is grape flavored and contains no alcohol. Each teaspoon (5 mL) contains acetaminophen 160 mg, chlorpheniramine maleate 1 mg, and pseudoephedrine hydrochloride 15 mg.

Actions: *Children's TYLENOL® COLD Multi Symptom Chewable Tablets and*

Liquid combine the analgesic-antipyretic acetaminophen with the decongestant pseudoephedrine hydrochloride and the antihistamine chlorpheniramine maleate to help relieve nasal congestion, dry runny noses and prevent sneezing as well as to relieve the fever, aches, pains and general discomfort associated with colds and upper respiratory infections. Acetaminophen is equal to aspirin in analgesic and antipyretic effectiveness and it is unlikely to produce the side effects often associated with aspirin or aspirin-containing products.

Uses: For temporary relief of these cold symptoms: nasal congestion, runny nose, sore throat, sneezing, minor aches and pains, headaches and fever.

Precautions: If a rare sensitivity reaction occurs, the drug should be stopped.

Directions: All doses may be repeated every 4–6 hours, if needed. Do not use more than 4 times in 24 hours. Under 6 years (under 48 lbs), consult a physician. *Children's TYLENOL® COLD Chewable Tablets:* 6–11 years (48–95 lbs): 4 tablets. *Children's TYLENOL® COLD Liquid Formula:* An AccuDose™ measuring cup is provided and marked for accurate dosing. 6–11 years (48–95 lbs): 2 teaspoonfuls.

Professional Dosage Schedule: *Children's TYLENOL® COLD Chewable Tablets:* 2–5 years (24–47 lbs): 2 tablets. *Children's TYLENOL® COLD Liquid:* 2–5 years (24–47 lbs): 1 teaspoonful. All doses may be repeated every 4–6 hours, if needed. Do not use more than 4 times in 24 hours.

Warnings: Do not take for pain for more than 5 days or for fever for more than 3 days unless directed by a doctor. If pain or fever persists, or gets worse, if new symptoms occur, or if redness or swelling is present, consult a doctor because these could be signs of a serious condition. If sore throat is severe, persists for more than 2 days, is accompanied or followed by fever, headache, rash, nausea, or vomiting, consult a doctor promptly. **Do not exceed recommended dosage.** If nervousness, dizziness, or sleeplessness occur, discontinue use and consult a doctor. May cause excitability especially in children. Do not give this product to children who have a breathing problem such as chronic bronchitis, or who have glaucoma, heart disease, high blood pressure, thyroid disease, or diabetes without first consulting the child's doctor. May cause drowsiness. Sedatives and tranquilizers may increase the drowsiness effect. Do not give this product to children who are taking sedatives or tranquilizers, without first consulting the child's doctor. **Do not exceed recommended dose.** Taking more than the recommended dose (overdose) may not provide more relief and could cause serious health problems. Keep this and all drugs out of the reach of children. In case of accidental overdose, contact a doctor or poison control center immediately. Prompt medical at-

tention is critical even if you do not notice any signs or symptoms. Do not use with other products containing acetaminophen.

NOTE: In addition to the above: *Children's TYLENOL® COLD Chewable Tablets:* DO NOT USE IF CARTON IS OPENED OR IF BLISTER UNIT IS BROKEN. Phenylketonurics: contains phenylalanine 6 mg per tablet. *Children's TYLENOL® COLD Liquid:* DO NOT USE IF PLASTIC CARTON WRAP, BOTTLE WRAP OR FOIL IMPRINTED "SAFETY SEAL®" IS BROKEN OR MISSING.

Drug Interaction Precaution: Do not give this product to a child who is taking a prescription monamine omidase inhibitor (MAOI) (certain drugs for depression, psychiatric or emotional conditions), or for 2 weeks after stopping the MAOI drug. If you are uncertain whether your child's prescription drug contains an MAOI, consult a health professional before giving this product.

PROFESSIONAL INFORMATION

Overdosage Information: Acetaminophen in massive overdosage may cause hepatic toxicity in some patients. In adults and adolescents, hepatic toxicity has rarely been reported following ingestion of acute overdoses of less than 7.5 to 10 grams. Fatalities are infrequent (less than 3–4% of untreated cases) and have rarely been reported with overdoses of less than 15 grams. In children, an acute overdosage of less than 150 mg/kg has not been associated with hepatic toxicity. Early symptoms following a potentially hepatotoxic overdose may include: nausea, vomiting, diaphoresis and general malaise. Clinical and laboratory evidence of hepatic toxicity may not be apparent until 48 to 72 hours postingestion.

In adults and adolescents, regardless of the quantity of acetaminophen reported to have been ingested, administer acetylcysteine immediately if 24 hours or less have elapsed from the reported time of ingestion. For full prescribing information, refer to the acetylcysteine package insert. Do not await the results of assays for acetaminophen levels before initiating treatment with acetylcysteine. The following additional procedures are recommended: Promptly initiate gastric decontamination of the stomach. A plasma acetaminophen assay should be obtained as early as possible, but no sooner than four hours following ingestion. If plasma level falls above the lower treatment line on the acetaminophen overdose nomogram, acetylcysteine therapy should be continued. Liver function studies should be obtained initially and repeated at 24-hour intervals.

Serious toxicity or fatalities are extremely infrequent in children, possibly due to differences in the way they metabolize acetaminophen. In children, the maximum potential amount ingested can be more easily estimated. If more than 150 mg/kg or an unknown amount

was ingested, obtain a plasma acetaminophen level. The plasma acetaminophen level should be obtained as soon as possible, but no sooner than 4 hours following ingestion. If plasma level falls above the lower treatment line on the acetaminophen overdose nomogram, the acetylcysteine therapy should be initiated and continued for a full course of therapy. If plasma acetaminophen assay capability is not available, and the estimated acetaminophen ingestion exceeds 150 mg/kg, acetylcysteine therapy should be initiated and continued for a full course of therapy.

For additional emergency information, call your regional poison center or call the Rocky Mountain Poison Center toll-free, (1-800-525-6115).

Chlorpheniramine toxicity should be treated as you would an antihistamine/anticholinergic overdose and is likely to be present within a few hours after acute ingestion.

Symptoms from pseudoephedrine overdose consist most often of mild anxiety, tachycardia and/or mild hypertension. Symptoms usually appear within 4 to 8 hours of ingestion and are transient, usually requiring no treatment.

Inactive Ingredients: Chewable Tablets: Aspartame, Basic Polymethacrylate, Cellulose Acetate, Citric Acid, D&C Red #7, FD&C Blue #1, Flavors, Hydroxypropyl Methylcellulose, Magnesium Stearate, Mannitol, and Microcrystalline Cellulose.

Liquid: Benzoic Acid, Citric Acid, FD&C Blue #1, FD&C Red #40, Flavors, Glycerin, Malic Acid, Polyethylene Glycol, Propylene Glycol, Purified Water, Sodium Benzoate, Sorbitol, and Sucrose.

How Supplied: Chewable Tablets (colored purple, scored, imprinted "Tylenol Cold") on one side and "TC" on opposite side—Blisters of 24. **Liquid Formula**—bottles (colored purple) of 4 fl. oz.

Shown in Product Identification Guide, page 511

**Children's TYLENOL®
COLD Multi Symptom
PLUS COUGH Chewable Tablets and
Liquid**

Description: Each *Children's TYLENOL® COLD Multi Symptom Plus Cough Cherry-Flavored Tablet* contains: acetaminophen 80 mg, chlorpheniramine maleate 0.5 mg, dextromethorphan hydrobromide 2.5 mg, and pseudoephedrine hydrochloride 7.5 mg.
Children's TYLENOL® COLD Multi Symptom Plus Cough Liquid is cherry flavored and contains no alcohol. Each teaspoon (5 mL) contains acetaminophen 160 mg, chlorpheniramine maleate 1 mg, dextromethorphan hydrobromide 5 mg and pseudoephedrine hydrochloride 15 mg.

Continued on next page

Children's Tylenol Cold—Cont.

Actions: *Children's TYLENOL® COLD Multi Symptom Plus Cough Chewable Tablets* and *Liquid* combines the analgesic-antipyretic acetaminophen with the decongestant pseudoephedrine hydrochloride, the cough suppressant dextromethorphan hydrobromide, and the antihistamine chlorpheniramine maleate to help relieve coughs, nasal congestion, and sore throat, dry runny noses, and prevent sneezing as well as to relieve the fever, aches, pains and general discomfort associated with colds and upper respiratory infections.
Acetaminophen is equal to aspirin in analgesic and antipyretic effectiveness and it is unlikely to produce the side effects often associated with aspirin or aspirin-containing products.

Uses: For the temporary relief of these cold symptoms: minor aches and pains, headaches, sore throat, nasal congestion, runny nose, coughs, sneezing and fever.

Precaution: If a rare sensitivity reaction occurs, the drug should be stopped.

Directions: All doses may be repeated every 4–6 hours, if needed. Do not use more than 4 times in 24 hours. Under 6 years (under 48 lbs), consult a doctor. *Children's TYLENOL® COLD Plus Cough Chewable Tablets:* 6–11 years (48–95 lbs): 4 tablets. *Children's TYLENOL® COLD Plus Cough Liquid:* An AccuDose™ measuring cup is provided and marked for accurate dosing, 6–11 years (48–95 lbs): 2 teaspoonfuls. Professional Dosage Schedule: *Children's TYLENOL® COLD Plus Cough Chewable Tablets:* 2–5 years (24–47 lbs): 2 tablets. *Children's TYLENOL® COLD Plus Cough Liquid:* 2–5 years (24–47 lbs): 1 teaspoonful. All doses may be repeated every 4–6 hours, if needed. Do not use more than 4 times in 24 hours.

Warnings: Do not take for pain for more than 5 days or for fever for more than 3 days unless directed by a doctor. If pain or fever persists, or gets worse, if new symptoms occur, or if redness or swelling is present, consult a doctor because these could be signs of a serious condition. If sore throat is severe, persists for more than 2 days, is accompanied or followed by fever, headache, rash, nausea or vomiting, consult a doctor promptly. **Do not exceed recommended dosage.** If nervousness, dizziness, or sleeplessness occur, discontinue use and consult a doctor. May cause excitability especially in children. Do not give this product to children who have a breathing problem such as chronic bronchitis, or who have glaucoma, heart disease, high blood pressure, thyroid disease, or diabetes, without first consulting the child's doctor. May cause drowsiness. Sedatives and tranquilizers may increase the drowsiness effect. Do not give this product to children who are taking sedatives or tranquilizers without first consulting the child's doctor. A persistent cough may be a sign of a serious condition. If cough persists for more than 1 week, tends to recur, or is accompanied by fever, rash or persistent headache, consult a doctor. Do not give this product for persistent or chronic cough such as occurs with asthma or if cough is accompanied by excessive phlegm (mucus) unless directed by a doctor. **Do not exceed recommended dose.** Taking more than the recommended dose (overdose) may not provide more relief and could cause serious health problems. Keep this and all drugs out of the reach of children. In case of accidental overdose, contact a doctor or poison control center immediately. Prompt medical attention is critical even if you do not notice any signs or symptoms. Do not use with other products containing acetaminophen.
NOTE: In addition to the above:
Chewable Tablets: DO NOT USE IF CARTON IS OPENED OR IF BLISTER UNIT IS BROKEN. Phenylketonurics: contains phenylalanine 4 mg per tablet.
Liquid: DO NOT USE IF PLASTIC CARTON WRAP, BOTTLE WRAP, OR FOIL INNER SEAL IMPRINTED "SAFETY SEAL®" IS BROKEN OR MISSING.

Drug Interaction Precaution: Do not give this product to a child who is taking a prescription monoamine oxidase inhibitor (MAOI) (certain drugs for depression, psychiatric or emotional conditions), or for 2 weeks after stopping the MAOI drug. If you are uncertain whether your child's prescription drug contains an MAOI, consult a health professional before giving this product.

PROFESSIONAL INFORMATION

Overdosage Information: Acetaminophen in massive overdosage may cause hepatic toxicity in some patients. In adults and adolescents, hepatic toxicity has rarely been reported following ingestion of acute overdoses of less than 7.5 to 10 grams. Fatalities are infrequent (less than 3–4% of untreated cases) and have rarely been reported with overdoses of less than 15 grams. In children, an acute overdosage of less than 150 mg/kg has not been associated with hepatic toxicity. Early symptoms following a potentially hepatotoxic overdose may include: nausea, vomiting, diaphoresis and general malaise. Clinical and laboratory evidence of hepatic toxicity may not be apparent until 48 to 72 hours postingestion.
In adults and adolescents, regardless of the quantity of acetaminophen reported to have been ingested, administer acetylcysteine immediately if 24 hours or less have elapsed from the reported time of ingestion. For full prescribing information, refer to the acetylcysteine package insert. Do not await the results of assays for plasma acetaminophen levels before initiating treatment with acetylcysteine. The following additional procedures are recommended: Promptly initiate gastric decontamination of the stomach. A plasma acetaminophen assay should be obtained as early as possible, but no sooner than four hours following ingestion. If plasma level falls above the lower treatment line on the acetaminophen overdose nomogram, acetylcysteine therapy should be continued. Liver function studies should be obtained initially and repeated at 24-hour intervals.

Serious toxicity or fatalities are extremely infrequent in children, possibly due to differences in the way they metabolize acetaminophen. In children, the maximum potential amount ingested can be more easily estimated. If more than 150 mg/kg or an unknown amount was ingested, obtain a plasma acetaminophen level. The plasma acetaminophen level should be obtained as soon as possible, but no sooner than 4 hours following the ingestion. If plasma level falls above the lower treatment line on the acetaminophen overdose nomogram, the acetylcysteine therapy should be initiated and continued for a full course of therapy. If plasma acetaminophen assay capability is not available, and the estimated acetaminophen ingestion exceeds 150 mg/kg, acetylcysteine therapy should be initiated and continued for a full course of therapy.

For additional emergency information, call your regional poison center or call the Rocky Mountain Poison Center toll-free, (1-800-525-6115).

Chlorpheniramine toxicity should be treated as you would an antihistamine/anticholinergic overdose and is likely to be present within a few hours after acute ingestion.

Symptoms from pseudoephedrine overdose consist most often of mild anxiety, tachycardia and/or mild hypertension. Symptoms usually appear within 4 to 8 hours of ingestion and are transient, usually requiring no treatment.

Acute dextromethorphan overdose usually does not result in serious signs and symptoms unless massive amounts have been ingested. Signs and symptoms of a substantial overdose may include nausea and vomiting, visual disturbances, CNS disturbances, and urinary retention.

Inactive Ingredients: Chewable Tablets: Aspartame, Basic Polymethacrylate, Cellulose Acetate, Flavors, Hydroxypropyl Methylcellulose, Magnesium Stearate, Mannitol, and Microcrystalline Cellulose.

Liquid: Citric Acid, Corn Syrup, D&C Red #33, FD&C Red #40, Flavors, Polyethylene Glycol, Propylene Glycol, Purified Water, Sodium Benzoate, Sodium Carboxymethylcellulose, and Sorbitol.

How Supplied: Chewable Tablets (colored pink, imprinted "TYLENOL C/C" on one side and "TC/C" on the opposite side)—Blisters of 24.

Liquid Formula—(red colored) bottles of 4 fl. oz.

Shown in Product Identification Guide, page 511

Children's TYLENOL® ALLERGY-D Chewable Tablets and Liquid

Description: *Children's TYLENOL® ALLERGY-D Chewable Tablets* are bubble gum flavored and each tablet contains acetaminophen 80 mg, diphenhydramine HCl 6.25 mg and pseudoephedrine HCl 7.5 mg. *Children's TYLENOL® ALLERGY-D Liquid* is bubble gum flavored and contains no alcohol or aspirin. Each teaspoon (5 mL) contains acetaminophen 160 mg, diphenhydramine HCl 12.5 mg and pseudoephedrine HCl 15 mg.

Actions: *Children's TYLENOL® ALLERGY-D Liquid* and **Chewable Tablets** combine the analgesic-antipyretic acetaminophen with the antihistamine diphenhydramine hydrochloride and the decongestant pseudoephedrine hydrochloride to provide fast, effective, temporary relief of all your child's symptoms associated with hay fever and other respiratory allergies including sneezing, sore throat, itchy throat, itchy/watery eyes, runny nose, stuffy nose and nasal congestion. Acetaminophen is equal to aspirin in analgesic and antipyretic effectiveness and it is unlikely to produce the side effects often associated with aspirin or aspirin-containing products.

Uses: For the reduction of fever. For the temporary relief of these hay fever and other upper respiratory allergy symptoms: sneezing, itchy/watery eyes, nasal congestion, sore throat, runny nose, itchy throat and stuffy nose.

Directions: All doses may be repeated every 4-6 hours, if needed. Do not use more than 4 times in 24 hours. Under 6 years (under 48 lbs), consult a physician. An AccuDose™ measuring cup is provided for accurate dosing. *Children's TYLENOL® ALLERGY-D Chewable Tablets:* 6-11 years (48–95 lbs): 4 tablets. *Children's TYLENOL® ALLERGY-D Liquid:* 6-11 years (48–95 lbs): 2 teaspoonfuls.

Warnings: Do not take for pain for more than 5 days or for fever for more than 3 days unless directed by a doctor. If pain or fever persists, or gets worse, if new symptoms occur, or if redness or swelling is present, consult a doctor because these could be signs of a serious condition. If sore throat is severe, persists for more than 2 days, is accompanied or followed by fever, headache, rash, nausea or vomiting, consult a doctor promptly. **Do not exceed recommended dosage.** If nervousness, dizziness or sleeplessness occur, discontinue use and consult a doctor. May cause excitability especially in children. Do not give this product to children who have a breathing problem such as chronic bronchitis, or who have glaucoma, heart disease, high blood pressure, thyroid disease, or diabetes without first consulting the child's doctor. May cause marked drowsiness; sedatives and tranquilizers may increase the drowsiness effect. Do not give this product to children who are taking sedatives or tranquilizers without first consulting the child's doctor. **Do not exceed recommended dose.** Taking more than the recommended dose (overdose) may not provide more relief and could cause serious health problems. Keep this and all drugs out of the reach of children. In case of accidental overdose, contact a doctor or poison control center immediately. Prompt medical attention is critical for adults as well as for children even if you do not notice any signs or symptoms. Do not use with other products containing acetaminophen.

NOTE: In addition to the above:
Children's TYLENOL® ALLERGY-D Chewable Tablets: DO NOT USE IF CARTON IS OPENED OR IF BLISTER UNIT IS BROKEN. Phenylketonurics: Contains Phenylalanine 5.4 mg per tablet.
Children's TYLENOL® ALLERGY-D Liquid: DO NOT USE IF PLASTIC CARTON WRAP, BOTTLE WRAP, OR FOIL INNER SEAL IMPRINTED "SAFETY SEAL®" IS BROKEN OR MISSING.

Drug Interaction Precautions: Do not give this product to a child who is taking a prescription monoamine oxidase inhibitor (MAOI) (certain drugs for depression, psychiatric or emotional conditions), or for 2 weeks after stopping the MAOI drug. If you are uncertain whether your child's prescription drug contains an MAOI, consult a health professional before giving this product.

PROFESSIONAL INFORMATION

Overdosage Information: Acetaminophen in massive overdosage may cause hepatic toxicity in some patients. In adults and adolescents, hepatic toxicity has rarely been reported following ingestion of acute overdosage of less than 7.5 to 10 grams. Fatalities are infrequent (less than 3–4% of untreated cases) and have rarely been reported with overdoses of less than 15 grams. In children, an acute overdosage of less than 150 mg/kg has not been associated with hepatic toxicity.

Early symptoms following a potentially hepatotoxic overdose may include: nausea, vomiting, diaphoresis and general malaise. Clinical and laboratory evidence of hepatic toxicity may not be apparent until 48 to 72 hours postingestion. In adults and adolescents, regardless of the quantity of acetaminophen reported to have been ingested, administer acetylcysteine immediately if 24 hours or less have elapsed from the reported time of ingestion. For full prescribing information, refer to the acetylcysteine package insert. Do not await the results of assays for acetaminophen levels before initiating treatment with acetylcysteine. The following additional procedures are recommended: Promptly initiate gastric decontamination of the stomach. A plasma acetaminophen assay should be obtained as early as possible, but no sooner than four hours following ingestion. If plasma level falls above the lower treatment line on the acetaminophen overdose nomogram, acetylcysteine therapy should be continued. Liver function studies should be obtained initially and repeated at 24–hour intervals. Serious toxicity or fatalities are extremely infrequent in children, possibly due to differences in the way they metabolize acetaminophen. In children, the maximum potential amount ingested can be more easily estimated. If more than 150 mg/kg or an unknown amount was ingested, obtain a plasma acetaminophen level. The plasma acetaminophen level should be obtained as soon as possible, but no sooner than 4 hours following ingestion. If plasma level falls above the lower treatment line on the acetaminophen overdose nomogram, the acetylcysteine therapy should be initiated and continued for a full course of therapy. If plasma acetaminophen assay capability is not available, and the estimated acetaminophen ingestion exceeds 150 mg/kg, acetylcysteine therapy should be initiated and continued for a full course of therapy.

For additional emergency information, call your regional poison center or call the Rocky Mountain Poison Center toll-free (1–800–525–6115).

Diphenhydramine toxicity should be treated as you would an antihistamine/anticholinergic overdose and is likely to be present within a few hours after acute ingestion.

Symptoms from pseudoephedrine overdose consist most often of mild anxiety, tachycardia and/or mild hypertension. Symptoms usually appear within 4 to 8 hours of ingestion and are transient usually requiring no treatment.

Inactive Ingredients: Tablets: Aspartame, Cellulose, Cellulose Acetate, Flavors, Magnesium Stearate, Mannitol, Polymethacrylate, Povidone and Red #7. **Liquid:** Benzoic Acid, Citric Acid, Corn Syrup, D&C Red #33, FD&C Red #40, Flavors, Polyethylene Glycol, Propylene Glycol, Purified Water, Sodium Benzoate, and Sorbitol.

How Supplied: Tablets: Pink colored chewable tablets in blister packs of 24. **Liquid:** Pinkish-red colored liquid in child resistant bottles 4 fl. oz.

Shown in Product Identification Guide, page 511

Children's TYLENOL® FLU Liquid

Description: *Children's TYLENOL® FLU Liquid* is bubble-gum flavored and contains no alcohol or aspirin. Each teaspoon (5 mL) contains acetaminophen 160 mg, chlorpheniramine maleate 1 mg, dextromethorphan HBr 7.5 mg and pseudoephedrine HCl 15 mg.

Actions: *Children's TYLENOL® FLU Liquid* combines the analgesic-antipyretic acetaminophen with the deconges-

Continued on next page

Children's Tylenol Flu—Cont.

tant pseudoephedrine hydrochloride, the cough suppressant dextromethorphan hydrobromide and the antihistamine chlorpheniramine maleate to provide fast, effective, temporary relief of all your child's symptoms associated with flu including fever, body aches, headache, stuffy nose, runny nose, sore throat and coughs.

Acetaminophen is equal to aspirin in analgesic and antipyretic effectiveness and it is unlikely to produce the side effects often associated with aspirin or aspirin-containing products.

Uses: For the temporary relief of these cold or flu symptoms: fever, minor aches and pains, headaches, sore throat, nasal congestion, runny nose and coughs.

Directions: All doses may be repeated every 6–8 hours, if needed. Do not use more than 4 times in 24 hours. Under 6 years (under 48 lbs), consult a physician. An AccuDose™ measuring cup is provided for accurate dosing. *Children's TYLENOL® FLU Liquid.* 6–11 years (48–95 lbs): 2 teaspoonfuls.
Professional Dosage Schedule: 2-5 years (24–47 lbs): 1 teaspoonful. All doses may be repeated every 6–8 hours, if needed. Do not use more than 4 times in 24 hours.

Warnings: DO NOT USE IF PLASTIC CARTON WRAP, BOTTLE WRAP, OR FOIL INNER SEAL IMPRINTED "SAFETY SEAL"® IS BROKEN OR MISSING. Do not take for pain for more than 5 days or for fever for more than 3 days unless directed by a doctor. If pain or fever persists, or gets worse, if new symptoms occur, or if redness or swelling is present, consult a doctor because these could be signs of a serious condition. If sore throat is severe, persists for more than 2 days, is accompanied or followed by fever, headache, rash, nausea or vomiting, consult a doctor promptly. **Do not exceed recommended dosage.** If nervousness, dizziness or sleeplessness occur, discontinue use and consult a doctor. May cause excitability especially in children. Do not give this product to children who have a breathing problem such as chronic bronchitis, or who have glaucoma, heart disease, high blood pressure, thyroid disease or diabetes without first consulting the child's doctor. May cause drowsiness. Sedatives and tranquilizers may increase the drowsiness effect. Do not give this product to children who are taking sedatives or tranquilizers without first consulting the child's doctor. A persistent cough may be a sign of a serious condition. If cough persists for more than 1 week, tends to recur, or is accompanied by fever, rash, or persistent headache, consult a doctor. Do not give this product for persistent or chronic cough such as occurs with asthma or if cough is accompanied by excessive phlegm (mucus) unless directed by a doctor. **Do not exceed recommended dose.** Taking more than the recommended dose (overdose)

may not provide more relief and could cause serious health problems. Keep this and all drugs out of the reach of children. In case of accidental overdose, contact a doctor or poison control center immediately. Prompt medical attention is critical even if you do not notice any signs or symptoms. Do not use with other products containing acetaminophen.

Drug Interaction Precaution: Do not give this product to a child who is taking a prescription monoamine oxidase inhibitor (MAOI) (certain drugs for depression, psychiatric or emotional conditions) or for 2 weeks after stopping the MAOI drug. If you are uncertain whether your child's prescription drug contains an MAOI, consult a health professional before giving this product.

PROFESSIONAL INFORMATION

Overdosage Information: Acetaminophen in massive overdosage may cause hepatic toxicity in some patients. In adults and adolescents, hepatic toxicity has rarely been reported following ingestion of acute overdoses of less than 7.5 to 10 grams. Fatalities are infrequent (less than 3–4% of untreated cases) and have rarely been reported with overdoses of less than 15 grams. In children, an acute overdosage of less than 150 mg/kg has not been associated with hepatic toxicity.

Early symptoms following a potentially hepatotoxic overdose may include: nausea, vomiting, diaphoresis and general malaise. Clinical and laboratory evidence of hepatic toxicity may not be apparent until 48 to 72 hours postingestion.

In adults and adolescents, regardless of the quantity of acetaminophen reported to have been ingested, administer acetylcysteine immediately if 24 hours or less have elapsed from the reported time of ingestion. For full prescribing information, refer to the acetylcysteine package insert. Do not await the results of assays for plasma acetaminophen levels before initiating treatment with acetylcysteine. The following additional procedures are recommended: Promptly initiate gastric decontamination of the stomach. A plasma acetaminophen assay should be obtained as early as possible, but no sooner than four hours following ingestion. If plasma level falls above the lower treatment line on the acetaminophen overdose nomogram, acetylcysteine therapy should be continued. Liver function studies should be obtained initially and repeated at 24–hour intervals.

Serious toxicity or fatalities are extremely infrequent in children, possibly due to differences in the way they metabolize acetaminophen. In children, the maximum potential amount ingested can be more easily estimated. If more than 150 mg/kg or an unknown amount was ingested, obtain a plasma acetaminophen level. The plasma acetaminophen level should be obtained as soon as possible, but no sooner than 4 hours following ingestion. If plasma level falls above the lower treatment line on the ac-

etaminophen overdose nomogram, the acetylcysteine therapy should be initiated and continued for a full course of therapy. If plasma acetaminophen assay capability is not available, and the estimated acetaminophen ingestion exceeds 150 mg/kg, acetylcysteine therapy should be initiated and continued for a full course of therapy.

For additional emergency information, call your regional poison center or call the Rocky Mountain Poison Center toll-free, (1-800-525-6115).

Chlorpheniramine toxicity should be treated as you would an antihistamine/anticholinergic overdose and is likely to be present within a few hours after acute ingestion.

Symptoms from pseudoephedrine overdose consist most often of mild anxiety, tachycardia, and/or mild hypertension. Symptoms usually appear within 4 to 8 hours of ingestion and are transient, usually requiring no treatment.

Acute dextromethorphan overdose usually does not result in serious signs and symptoms unless massive amounts have been ingested. Signs and symptoms of a substantial overdose may include nausea and vomiting, visual disturbances, CNS disturbances, and urinary retention.

Inactive Ingredients: Citric Acid, Corn Syrup, D&C Red #33, FD&C Red #40 Flavors, Polyethylene Glycol, Propylene Glycol, Purified Water, Sodium Benzoate, Sodium Carboxymethylcellulose and Sorbitol.

How Supplied: Pinkish-red colored liquid in child resistant bottles of 4 fl. oz.

Shown in Product Identification Guide, page 511

Children's TYLENOL®
SINUS Chewable Tablets and Liquid

Description: *Children's TYLENOL® SINUS Chewable Tablets* are fruit flavored and each tablet contains acetaminophen 80 mg and pseudoephedrine HCl 7.5 mg. *Children's TYLENOL® SINUS Liquid* is fruit flavored and contains no alcohol or aspirin. Each teaspoon (5 mL) contains acetaminophen 160 mg and pseudoephedrine HCl 15 mg.

Actions: *Children's TYLENOL® SINUS Chewable Tablets and Liquid* combine the analgesic-antipyretic acetaminophen with the decongestant pseudoephedrine hydrochloride to provide fast, effective, temporary relief of all your child's sinus symptoms including stuffy nose, sinus headache, sinus pressure, sinus pain, and nasal congestion. Acetaminophen is equal to aspirin in analgesic and antipyretic effectiveness and is unlikely to produce the side effects often associated with aspirin or aspirin-containing products.

Indications: For the reduction of fever. For the temporary relief of minor aches, pains and headaches, sinus congestion, stuffy nose and sinus pressure.

Directions: All doses may be repeated every 4–6 hours, if needed. Do not use more than 4 times in 24 hours. Under 2 years (under 24 lbs), consult a physician. An AccuDose™ measuring cup is provided for accurate dosing. *Children's TYLENOL® SINUS Chewable Tablets:* 2–5 years (24–47 lbs) 2 tablets; 6–11 years (48–95 lbs): 4 tablets. *Children's TYLENOL® SINUS Liquid:* 2–5 years (24–47 lbs): 1 teaspoonful; 6–11 years (48–95 lbs): 2 teaspoonfuls.

Warnings: Do not take for pain for more than 5 days or for fever for more than 3 days unless directed by a doctor. If pain or fever persists, or gets worse, if new symptoms occur, or if redness or swelling is present, consult a doctor because these could be signs of a serious condition. **Do not exceed recommended dosage.** If nervousness, dizziness or sleeplessness occur, discontinue use and consult a doctor. Do not give this product to a child who has heart disease, high blood pressure, thyroid disease, or diabetes without first consulting the child's doctor. **Do not exceed recommended dose.** Taking more than the recommended dose (overdose) may not provide more relief and could cause serious health problems. Keep this and all drugs out of the reach of children. In case of accidental overdose, contact a doctor or poison control center immediately. Prompt medical attention is critical for adults as for children even if you do not notice any signs or symptoms. Do not use with other products containing acetaminophen.

NOTE: In addition to the above:
Children's TYLENOL® SINUS Chewable Tablets: DO NOT USE IF CARTON IS OPENED OR IF BLISTER UNIT IS BROKEN. Phenylketonurics: contains phenylalanine 5.4 mg per tablet.
Children's TYLENOL® SINUS Liquid: DO NOT USE IF PLASTIC CARTON WRAP, BOTTLE WRAP, OR FOIL INNER SEAL IMPRINTED "SAFETY SEAL®" IS BROKEN OR MISSING.

Drug Interaction Precaution: Do not give this product to a child who is taking a prescription monoamine oxidase inhibitor (MAOI) (certain drugs for depression, psychiatric or emotional conditions), or for 2 weeks after stopping the MAOI drug. If you are uncertain whether your child's prescription drug contains an MAOI, consult a health professional before giving this product.

PROFESSIONAL INFORMATION
Overdosage Information: Acetaminophen in massive overdosage may cause hepatic toxicity in some patients. In adults and adolescents, hepatic toxicity has rarely been reported following ingestion of acute overdosage of less than 7.5 to 10 grams. Fatalities are infrequent (less than 3–4% of untreated cases) and have rarely been reported with overdoses of less than 15 grams. In children an acute overdosage of less than 150 mg/kg

has not been associated with hepatic toxicity.

Early symptoms following a potentially hepatotoxic overdose may include: nausea, vomiting, diaphoresis and general malaise. Clinical and laboratory evidence of hepatic toxicity may not be apparent until 48 to 72 hours postingestion. In adults and adolescents, regardless of the quantity of acetaminophen reported to have been ingested, administer acetylcysteine immediately if 24 hours or less have elapsed from the reported time of ingestion. For full prescribing information, refer to the acetylcysteine package insert. Do not await the results of assays for acetaminophen levels before initiating treatment with acetylcysteine. The following additional procedures are recommended: Promptly initiate gastric decontamination of the stomach. A plasma acetaminophen assay should be obtained as early as possible, but no sooner than 4 hours following ingestion. If plasma level falls above the lower treatment line on the acetaminophen overdose nomogram, acetylcysteine therapy should be continued. Liver function studies should be obtained initially and repeated at 24–hour intervals. Serious toxicity or fatalities are extremely infrequent in children, possibly due to differences in the way they metabolize acetaminophen. In children, the maximal potential amount ingested can be more easily estimated. If more than 150 mg/kg or an unknown amount was ingested, obtain a plasma acetaminophen level. The plasma acetaminophen level should be obtained as soon as possible, but no sooner than 4 hours following ingestion. If plasma level falls above the lower treatment line on the acetaminophen overdose nomogram, the acetylcysteine therapy should be initiated and continued for a full course of therapy. If plasma acetaminophen assay capability is not available, and the estimated acetaminophen ingestion exceeds 150 mg/kg, acetylcysteine therapy should be initiated and continued for a full course of therapy.

For additional emergency information, call your regional poison center or call the Rocky Mountain Poison Center toll-free, (1–800–525–6115).

Symptoms from pseudoephedrine overdose consist most often of mild anxiety, tachycardia and/or mild hypertension. Symptoms usually appear within 4 to 8 hours of ingestion and are transient, usually requiring no treatment.

Inactive Ingredients: Tablets: Aspartame, Cellulose, Cellulose Acetate, Citric Acid, Flavor, Magnesium Stearate, Mannitol, Polymethacrylate, Povidone, and Red #7.
Liquid: Acesulfame Potassium, Benzoic Acid, Citric Acid, Corn Syrup, D&C Red #33, FD&C Red #40, Flavors, Polyethylene Glycol, Propylene Glycol, Purified Water, Sodium Benzoate, and Sorbitol.

How Supplied: Tablets: Pink colored tablets in blister packs of 24.

Liquid: Red colored liquid in child resistant bottles 4 fl oz.
Shown in Product Identification Guide, page 511

Infants' TYLENOL® COLD
Decongestant & Fever Reducer
Concentrated Drops

Description: *Infants' TYLENOL® COLD Decongestant & Fever Reducer Concentrated Drops* are alcohol-free, bubble gum flavored and red in color. Each 1.6 mL (2 dropperfuls) contains acetaminophen 160 mg and pseudoephedrine HCl 15 mg.

Actions: Acetaminophen is a clinically proven analgesic/antipyretic.
Acetaminophen produces analgesia by elevation of the pain threshold and antipyresis through action on the hypothalamic heat regulating center. Acetaminophen is equal to aspirin in analgesic and antipyretic effectiveness and it is unlikely to produce many of the side effects associated with aspirin and aspirin containing products. Pseudoephedrine hydrochloride is a sympathomimetic amine which provides temporary relief of nasal congestion.

Uses: For the reduction of fever. For the temporary relief of these cold symptoms: minor aches and pains, headaches and nasal congestion.

Precautions: If a rare sensitivity reaction occurs, the drug should be stopped.

Directions: Infants' TYLENOL® Cold Drops are more concentrated than Children's TYLENOL® Cold Liquid Products. For accurate dosing follow the dosing instructions on the label.
All dosages may be repeated every 4–6 hours, if needed. Do not use more than 4 times in 24 hours. Under 2 years (under 24 lbs), consult a physician. A calibrated dropper is provided for accurate dosing. Attention: This product has been specially designed for use only with the enclosed dropper. Do not use any other dosing device with this product.
Infants' TYLENOL® COLD Decongestant & Fever Reducer Concentrated Drops: 2–3 years (24–35 lbs): 2 dropperfuls (2 ×0.8 mL).
Professional Dosage Schedule: 0–3 months (6-11 lbs): 0.4 mL; 4–11 months (12–17 lbs): 0.8 mL; 12–23 months (18–23 lbs); 1.2 mL. All dosages may be repeated every 4–6 hours, if needed. Do not use more than 4 times in 24 hours.

Warnings: Do not use if plastic carton wrap or bottle wrap imprinted "safety seal®" is broken or missing. Do not take for pain for more than 5 days or for fever for more than 3 days unless directed by a doctor. If pain or fever persists or gets worse, if new symptoms occur, or if redness or swelling is present, consult a doctor because these could be signs of a serious condition. **Do not exceed recom-**

Continued on next page

Infants' Tylenol Cold—Cont.

mended dosage. If nervousness, dizziness or sleeplessness occur, discontinue use and consult a doctor. Do not give this product to children who have heart disease, high blood pressure, thyroid disease, or diabetes. **Do not exceed recommended dose.** Taking more than the recommended dose (overdose) may not provide more relief and could cause serious health problems. Keep this and all drugs out of the reach of children. In case of accidental overdose, contact a doctor or poison control center immediately. Prompt medical attention is critical even if you do not notice any signs or symptoms. Do not use with other products containing acetaminophen.

Drug Interaction Precaution: Do not give this product to a child who is taking a prescription monoamine oxidase inhibitor (MAOI) (certain drugs for depression, psychiatric or emotional conditions), or for 2 weeks after stopping the MAOI drug. If you are uncertain whether your child's prescription drug contains an MAOI, consult a health professional before giving this product.

PROFESSIONAL INFORMATION

Overdosage Information: Acetaminophen in massive overdosage may cause hepatic toxicity in some patients. In adults and adolescents, hepatic toxicity has rarely been reported following ingestion of acute overdoses of less than 7.5 to 10 grams. Fatalities are infrequent (less than 3–4% of untreated cases) and have rarely been reported with overdoses of less than 15 grams. In children, an acute overdosage of less than 150 mg/kg has not been associated with hepatic toxicity.

Early symptoms following a potentially hepatotoxic overdose may include: nausea, vomiting, diaphoresis and general malaise. Clinical and laboratory evidence of hepatic toxicity may not be apparent until 48 to 72 hours postingestion. In adults and adolescents, regardless of the quantity of acetaminophen reported to have been ingested, administer acetylcysteine immediately if 24 hours or less have elapsed from the reported time of ingestion. For full prescribing information, refer to the acetylcysteine package insert. Do not await results of assays for plasma acetaminophen levels before initiating treatment with acetylcysteine. The following additional procedures are recommended: Promptly initiate gastric decontamination of the stomach. A plasma acetaminophen assay should be obtained as early as possible, but no sooner than four hours following ingestion. If plasma level falls above the lower treatment line on the acetaminophen overdose nomogram, acetylcysteine therapy should be continued. Liver function studies should be obtained initially and repeated at 24-hour intervals.

Serious toxicity or fatalities are extremely infrequent in children, possibly due to differences in the way they metab-

olize acetaminophen. In children, the maximum potential amount ingested can be more easily estimated. If more than 150 mg/kg or an unknown amount was ingested, obtain a plasma acetaminophen level. The plasma acetaminophen level should be obtained as soon as possible, but no sooner than 4 hours following ingestion. If plasma level falls above the lower treatment line on the acetaminophen overdose nomogram, the acetylcysteine therapy should be initiated and continued for a full course of therapy. If plasma acetaminophen assay capability is not available, and the estimated acetaminophen ingestion exceeds 150 mg/kg, acetylcysteine therapy should be initiated and continued for a full course of therapy.

For additional emergency information, call your regional poison center or call the Rocky Mountain Poison Center toll-free, (1-800-525-6115).

Symptoms from pseudoephedrine overdose consist most often of mild anxiety, tachycardia and/or mild hypertension. Symptoms usually appear within 4 to 8 hours of ingestion and are transient, usually requiring no treatment.

Inactive Ingredients: Citric Acid, Corn Syrup, Flavors, Polyethylene Glycol, Propylene Glycol, Purified Water, Red #40, Saccharin and Sodium Benzoate.

How Supplied: Red-colored drops in bottles of $\frac{1}{2}$ fl. oz.

Shown in Product Identification Guide, page 511

INFANTS' TYLENOL® COLD
Decongestant and Fever Reducer Concentrated Drops
PLUS COUGH

Description: Infants' TYLENOL® COLD Decongestant, & Fever Reducer Concentrated Drops *PLUS COUGH* are alcohol-free, cherry flavored and red in color. Each 1.6 mL (2 dropperfuls) contains acetaminophen 160 mg, pseudoephedrine HCl 15 mg, and dextromethorphan HBr 5 mg.

Actions: Acetaminophen is a clinically proven analgesic/antipyretic. Acetaminophen produces analgesia by elevation of the pain threshold and antipyresis through action on the hypothalamic heat regulating center. Acetaminophen is equal to aspirin in analgesic and antipyretic effectiveness and it is unlikely to produce many of the side effects associated with aspirin and aspirin containing products. Pseudoephedrine Hydrochloride is a sympathomimetic amine which provides temporary relief of nasal congestion. Dextromethorphan hydrobromide is a cough suppressant which helps relieve coughs.

Uses: For the reduction of fever. For the temporary relief of these cold symptoms: coughs, sore throat, nasal congestion, headaches and minor aches and pains.

Precautions: If a rare sensitivity reaction occurs, the drug should be stopped.

Directions: Infants' TYLENOL® Cold Drops are more concentrated than Children's TYLENOL® Cold Liquid Products. For accurate dosing, follow the dosing instructions on the label. All dosages may be repeated every 4–6 hours, if needed. Do not use more than 4 times in 24 hours. Under 2 years (under 24 lbs), consult a physician. A calibrated dropper is provided for accurate dosing. Attention: This product has been specially designed for use only with the enclosed dropper. Do not use any other dosing device with this product.

Infants' TYLENOL® COLD Decongestant, & Fever Reducer Concentrated Drops *PLUS COUGH*: 2–3 years (24–35 lbs) 2 dropperfuls (2 x 0.8 mL).

Warnings: Do not use if plastic carton wrap or bottle wrap imprinted "Safety Seal®" is broken or missing. Do not take for pain for more than 5 days or for fever for more than 3 days unless directed by a doctor. If pain or fever persists, or gets worse, if new symptoms occur, or if redness or swelling is present, consult a doctor because these could be signs of a serious condition. If sore throat is severe, persists for more than 2 days, is accompanied or followed by fever, headache, rash, nausea, or vomiting, consult a doctor promptly. **Do not exceed recommended dosage.** If nervousness, dizziness or sleeplessness occur, discontinue use and consult a doctor. Do not give this product to children who have heart disease, high blood pressure, thyroid disease, or diabetes without first consulting the child's doctor. A persistent cough may be a sign of a serious condition. If cough persists for more than 1 week, tends to recur or is accompanied by fever, rash or persistent headache, consult a doctor. Do not give this product for persistent or chronic cough such as occurs with asthma or if cough is accompanied by excessive phlegm (mucus) unless directed by a doctor. **Do not exceed recommended dose.** Taking more than the recommended dose (overdose) may not provide more relief and could cause serious health problems. Keep this and all drugs out of the reach of children. In case of accidental overdose, contact a doctor or poison control center immediately. Prompt medical attention is critical even if you do not notice any signs or symptoms. Do not use with other products containing acetaminophen.

Drug Interaction Precaution: Do not give this product to a child who is taking a prescription monoamine oxidase inhibitor (MAOI) (certain drugs for depression, psychiatric or emotional conditions), or for 2 weeks after stopping the MAOI drug. If you are uncertain whether your child's prescription drug contains an MAOI, consult a health professional before giving this product.

PROFESSIONAL INFORMATION

Overdosage Information: Acetaminophen in massive overdosage may cause hepatic toxicity in some patients. In adults and adolescents, hepatic toxicity has rarely been reported following ingestion of acute overdoses of less than 7.5 to 10 grams. Fatalities are infrequent (less than 3–4% of untreated cases) and have rarely been reported with overdoses of less than 15 grams. In children, an acute overdosage of less than 150 mg/kg has not been associated with hepatic toxicity. Early symptoms following a potentially hepatotoxic overdose may include: nausea, vomiting, diaphoresis and general malaise. Clinical and laboratory evidence of hepatic toxicity may not be apparent until 48 to 72 hours postingestion. In adults and adolescents, regardless of the quantity of acetaminophen reported to have been ingested, administer acetylcysteine immediately if 24 hours or less have elapsed from the reported time of ingestion. For full prescribing information, refer to the acetylcysteine package insert. Do not await results of assays for plasma acetaminophen levels before initiating treatment with acetylcysteine. The following additional procedures are recommended: Promptly initiate gastric decontamination of the stomach. A plasma acetaminophen assay should be obtained as early as possible, but no sooner than four hours following ingestion. If plasma level falls above the lower treatment line on the acetaminophen overdose nomogram, acetylcysteine therapy should be continued. Liver function studies should be obtained initially and repeated at 24-hour intervals.

Serious toxicity or fatalities are extremely infrequent in children, possibly due to differences in the way they metabolize acetaminophen. In children, the maximum potential amount ingested can be more easily estimated. If more than 150 mg/kg or an unknown amount was ingested, obtain a plasma acetaminophen level. The plasma acetaminophen level should be obtained as soon as possible, but no sooner than 4 hours following ingestion. If plasma level falls above the lower treatment line on the acetaminphen overdose nomogram, the acetylcysteine therapy should be initiated and continued for a full course of therapy. If plasma acetaminophen assay capability is not available, and the estimated acetaminophen ingestion exceeds 150 mg/kg, acetylcysteine therapy should be initiated and continued for a full course of therapy.

For additional emergency information, call your regional poison center or call the Rocky Mountain Poison Center toll-free, (1-800-525-6115).

Symptoms from pseudoephedrine overdose consist most often of mild anxiety, tachycardia and/or mild hypertension. Symptoms usually appear within 4 to 8 hours of ingestion and are transient, usually requiring no treatment.

Acute dextromethorphan overdose usually does not result in serious signs and symptoms unless massive amounts have been ingested. Signs and symptoms of a substantial overdose may include nau-

sea and vomiting, visual disturbances, CNS distutbances and urinary retention.

Inactive Ingredients: Acesulfame Potassium, Citric Acid, Corn Syrup, Flavors, Polyethylene Glycol, Propylene Glycol, Purified Water, Red #40, Sodium Benzoate.

How Supplied: Red-colored drops in bottles of ½ fl. oz.

Shown in Product Identification Guide, page 511

IMODIUM® A–D
(loperamide hydrochloride)

Description: Each 5 mL (teaspoon) of **IMODIUM® A-D** liquid contains loperamide hydrochloride 1 mg. **IMODIUM® A-D** liquid is stable, cherry-mint flavored, and clear in color.
Each caplet of **IMODIUM® A-D** contains 2 mg of loperamide and is scored and colored green.

Actions: **IMODIUM® A-D** contains a clinically proven antidiarrheal medication. Loperamide HCl acts by slowing intestinal motility and by affecting water and electrolyte movement through the bowel.

Indications: **IMODIUM® A-D** is indicated for the control and symptomatic relief of acute nonspecific diarrhea, including Travelers' Diarrhea.

Directions: Adults and children 12 years of age and older: Take four teaspoonfuls or two caplets after first loose bowel movement. If needed, take two teaspoonfuls or one caplet after each subsequent loose bowel movement. Do not exceed eight teaspoonfuls or four caplets in any 24 hour period, unless directed by a physician.
Children 9–11 years old (60–95 lbs.): Two teaspoonfuls or one caplet after first loose bowel movement, followed by one teaspoonful or one-half caplet after each subsequent loose bowel movement. Do not exceed six teaspoonfuls or three caplets a day.
Children 6–8 years old (48–59 lbs.): Two teaspoonfuls or one caplet after first loose bowel movement, followed by one teaspoonful or one-half caplet after each subsequent loose bowel movement. Do not exceed four teaspoonfuls or two caplets a day.
Professional Dosage Schedule for children 2–5 years old (24–47 lbs): One teaspoon after first loose bowel movement, followed by one after each subsequent loose bowel movement. Do not exceed three teaspoonfuls a day.

Warnings: KEEP THIS AND ALL DRUGS OUT OF THE REACH OF CHILDREN. Do not use for more than two days unless directed by a physician. DO NOT USE IF DIARRHEA IS ACCOMPANIED BY HIGH FEVER (GREATER THAN 101°F), OR IF BLOOD OR MUCUS IS PRESENT IN

THE STOOL, OR IF YOU HAVE HAD A RASH OR OTHER ALLERGIC REACTION TO LOPERAMIDE HCl. If you are taking antibiotics or have a history of liver disease, consult a physician before using this product. As with any drug, if you are pregnant or nursing a baby, seek the advice of a health professional before using this product. In case of accidental overdose, seek professional assistance or contact a poison control center immediately.

PROFESSIONAL INFORMATION
Overdosage Information: Overdosage of loperamide HCl in man may result in constipation, CNS depression and nausea. A slurry of activated charcoal administered promptly after ingestion of loperamide hydrochloride can reduce the amount of drug which is absorbed. If vomiting occurs spontaneously upon ingestion, a slurry of 100 grams of activated charcoal should be administered orally as soon as fluids can be retained. If vomiting has not occurred, and CNS depression is evident, gastric lavage should be performed followed by administration of 100 gms of the activated charcoal slurry through the gastric tube. In the event of overdosage, patients should be monitored for signs of CNS depression for at least 24 hours. Children may be more sensitive to central nervous system effects than adults. If CNS depression is observed, naloxone may be administered. If responsive to naloxone, vital signs must be monitored carefully for recurrence of symptoms of drug overdose for at least 24 hours after the last dose of naloxone.

Inactive Ingredients: **Liquid:** Benzoic acid, citric acid, flavors, glycerin, propylene glycol, purified water, sodium benzoate, sorbitol, sucrose, contains 0.5% alcohol.
Caplets: Dibasic calcium phosphate, magnesium stearate, microcrystalline cellulose, colloidal silicon dioxide, FD&C Blue #1 and D&C Yellow #10.

How Supplied: Liquid: Cherry-mint flavored liquid (clear) 2 fl. oz., and 4 fl. oz. tamper evident bottles with child resistant safety caps and special dosage cups.
Caplets: Green scored caplets in 6's and 12's, 18's and 24's blister packaging which is tamper evident and child resistant.

Shown in Product Identification Guide, page 509

IMODIUM® ADVANCED
Chewable Tablets
(loperamide HCl/simethicone)

Description: Each chewable tablet of *Imodium® Advanced* contains loperamide HCl 2 mg/simethicone 125 mg.

Actions: *Imodium® Advanced* combines original prescription strength Imo-

Continued on next page

Imodium Advanced—Cont.

dium® to control the symptoms of diarrhea plus simethicone to relieve bloating, pressure and cramps commonly referred to as gas.

Loperamide HCl acts by slowing intestinal motility and by affecting water and electrolyte movement through the bowel. Simethicone acts in the stomach and intestines by altering the surface tension of gas bubbles enabling them to coalesce, thereby freeing and eliminating the gas more easily by belching or passing flatus.

Indications: *Imodium® Advanced* is indicated for the control of symptoms of diarrhea plus bloating, pressure, and cramps commonly referred to as gas.

Directions: Chew the first dose and take with water after the first loose stool. If needed, chew the next dose and take with water after the next loose stool. Drink plenty of clear liquids to prevent dehydration.

Adults aged 12 years and older: Chew 2 tablets and take with water after the first loose stool. If needed, chew 1 tablet and take with water after the next loose stool. Do not exceed 4 tablets a day.

Children 9-11 years (60-95 lbs): Chew 1 tablet and take with water after the first loose stool. If needed, chew 1/2 tablet and take with water after the next loose stool. Do not exceed 3 tablets a day.

Children 6-8 years (48-59 lbs): Chew 1 tablet and take with water after the first loose stool. If needed, chew 1/2 tablet and take with water after the next loose stool. Do not exceed 2 tablets a day.

Children under 6 years old (up to 47 lbs): Consult a physician. Not intended for use in children under 6 years old.

Warnings:
Do Not Use if:
- You have a high fever (over 101° F)
- Blood or mucus is in your stool
- You have had a rash or other allergic reaction to Loperamide HCl

Do Not Use Without Asking A Doctor:
- For more than 2 days
- If you are taking antibiotics
- If you have a history of liver disease

As with any drug, If you are pregnant or nursing a baby, seek the advice of a health professional before using this product.
- **Keep this and all drugs out of the reach of children.**
- In case of accidental overdose, seek professional assistance or call a poison control center immediately.

Store at 15–30°C (59–86°F).

PROFESSIONAL INFORMATION

Overdosage Information: Overdosage of loperamide HCl in man may result in constipation, CNS depression and nausea. A slurry of activated charcoal administered promptly after ingestion of loperamide hydrochloride can reduce the amount of drug which is absorbed. If vomiting occurs spontaneously upon ingestion, a slurry of 100 grams of activated charcoal should be administered orally as soon as fluids can be retained. If

vomiting has not occurred, and CNS depression is evident, gastric lavage should be performed followed by administration of 100 gms of the activated charcoal slurry through the gastric tube. In the event of overdosage, patients should be monitored for signs of CNS depression for at least 24 hours. Children may be more sensitive to central nervous system effects than adults. If CNS depression is observed, naloxone may be administered. If responsive to naloxone, vital signs must be monitored carefully for recurrence of symptoms of drug overdose for at least 24 hours after the last dose of naloxone. No treatment is necessary for the simethicone ingestion in this circumstance.

Inactive Ingredients: cellulose acetate, corn starch, dextrates, flavors, microcrystalline cellulose, polymethacrylates, saccharin sodium, sorbitol, stearic acid, sucrose, tribasic calcium phosphate, FD&C Blue No.1, D&C Yellow No.10

How Supplied: Vanilla mint chewable tablets in 6's, 12's, 18's, 30's, 36's and 42's blister packaging which is tamper evident and child resistant. Each Imodium® Advanced tablet is round, light green in color and has "IMODIUM" embossed on one side and "2/125" on the other side.

Shown in Product Identification Guide, page 509

Junior Strength MOTRIN® Ibuprofen Caplets and Chewable Tablets

Description: Each *Junior Strength MOTRIN® Ibuprofen Caplet or Chewable Tablet* contains 100 mg ibuprofen in an easy-to-swallow caplet (capsule shaped tablet) or orange-flavored chewable tablet.

Uses: *Junior Strength MOTRIN® Ibuprofen Caplets and Junior Strength MOTRIN® Ibuprofen Chewable Tablets* are indicated for temporary reduction of fever and relief of minor aches and pains due to colds, flu, sore throat, headaches and toothaches.

Directions: Repeat dose every 6–8 hours if needed. Do not use more than 4 times a day. Under 6 (under 48 lbs), consult a physician. If possible, use weight to dose; otherwise use age. If stomach upset occurs while taking this product, give with food or milk.

Junior Strength MOTRIN® Ibuprofen Caplets and Chewable Tablets: 6–8 years (48–59 lbs): 2 caplets or tablets; 9–10 years (60–71 lbs): 2 1/2 caplets or tablets; 11 years (72–95 lbs): 3 caplets or tablets.

Warnings:
Allergy Alert: ibuprofen may cause a severe allergic reaction which may include: hives, facial swelling, asthma (wheezing), shock.
Do not use if you have ever had an allergic reaction to any other pain reliever/fever reducer.

Stop use and ask a doctor if an allergic reaction occurs. Seek medical help right away.

CALL YOUR DOCTOR IF:
- Your child is under a doctor's care for any serious condition or is taking any other drug.
- Your child has problems or serious side effects from taking fever reducers or pain relievers.
- Your child does not get any relief within first day (24 hours) of treatment, or pain or fever gets worse.
- Stomach upset gets worse or lasts.
- Redness or swelling is present in the painful area.
- Sore throat is severe, lasts for more than 2 days or occurs with fever, headache, rash, nausea or vomiting.
- Any new symptoms appear.

DO NOT USE:
- With any other product that contains ibuprofen, or any other pain reliever/fever reducer, unless directed by a doctor.
- For more than **3 days** for fever or pain unless directed by a doctor.
- For stomach pain unless directed by a doctor.
- If your child is dehydrated (significant fluid loss) due to continued vomiting, diarrhea or lack of fluid intake.
- **If blister unit is broken or open.**

IMPORTANT:
Do not exceed recommended dose. Taking more than the recommended dose (overdose) may not provide more relief and could cause serious health problems. **Keep this and all drugs out of the reach of children. In case of accidental overdose, seek professional assistance or contact a poison control center immediately.**

NOTE: In addition to the above:
Junior Strength MOTRIN® Ibuprofen Chewable Tablets: Phenylketonurics: **Contains phenylalanine 6 mg per tablet.**

WHEN USING THIS PRODUCT:
- Mouth or throat burning may occur; give with water or food.

PROFESSIONAL INFORMATION

Overdosage Information: The *toxicity of ibuprofen overdose* is dependent upon the amount of drug ingested and the time elapsed since ingestion, though individual response may vary, which makes it necessary to evaluate each case individually. Although uncommon, serious toxicity and death have been reported in the medical literature with ibuprofen overdosage. The most frequently reported symptoms of ibuprofen overdose include abdominal pain, nausea, vomiting, lethargy and drowsiness. Other central nervous system symptoms include headache, tinnitus, CNS depression and seizures. Metabolic acidosis, coma, acute renal failure and apnea (primarily in very young children) may rarely occur. Cardiovascular toxicity, including hypotension, bradycardia, tachycardia and atrial fibrillation, also have been reported.

The *treatment of acute ibuprofen overdose* is primarily supportive. Management of hypotension, acidosis and gastrointestinal bleeding may be necessary. In cases of acute overdose, the stomach should be emptied through ipecac-induced emesis or lavage. Emesis is most effective if initiated within 30 minutes of ingestion. Orally administered activated charcoal may help in reducing the absorption and reabsorption of ibuprofen. In children, the estimated amount of ibuprofen ingested per body weight may be helpful to predict the potential for development of toxicity although each case must be evaluated. Ingestion of less than 100 mg/kg is unlikely to produce toxicity. Children ingesting 100 to 200 mg/kg may be managed with induced emesis and a minimal observation time of four hours. Children ingesting 200 to 400 mg/kg of ibuprofen should have immediate gastric emptying and at least four hours observation in a health care facility. Children ingesting greater than 400 mg/kg require immediate medical referral, careful observation and appropriate supportive therapy. Ipecac-induced emesis is not recommended in overdoses greater than 400 mg/kg because of the risk for convulsions and the potential for aspiration of gastric contents.

In adult patients the history of the dose reportedly ingested does not appear to be predictive of toxicity. The need for referral and follow-up must be judged by the circumstances at the time of the overdose ingestion. Symptomatic adults should be admitted to a health care facility for observation.

Inactive Ingredients: *Junior Strength MOTRIN® Ibuprofen Caplets:* Carnauba wax, colloidal silicon dioxide, cornstarch, D&C Yellow #10, FD&C Yellow #6, hydroxypropyl methylcellulose, microcrystalline cellulose, polydextrose, polyethylene glycol, propylene glycol, sodium starch glycolate, titanium dioxide, triacetin.

Junior Strength MOTRIN® Ibuprofen Chewable Tablets: Aspartame, citric acid, FD&C Yellow # 6, natural and artificial flavors, hydroxyethyl cellulose, hydroxypropyl methylcellulose, magnesium stearate, mannitol, microcrystalline cellulose, povidone, sodium lauryl sulfate, sodium starch glycolate.

How Supplied: *Junior Strength MOTRIN® Ibuprofen Caplets:* (white, imprinted "M 100" in orange) in blister packs of 24

Junior Strength MOTRIN® Ibuprofen Chewable Tablets: Orange-colored, round tablets available in blister packs of 24.

Store at room temperature 15°–30°C (59°–86°F).

Shown in Product Identification Guide, page 510

Junior Strength TYLENOL®
acetaminophen
Coated Caplets and Chewable Tablets

Description: Each *Junior Strength TYLENOL® Coated Caplet or Chewable Tablet* contains 160 mg acetaminophen

in a small, coated, capsule shaped tablet or grape or fruit flavored chewable tablet.

Actions: Acetaminophen is a clinically proven analgesic/antipyretic. Acetaminophen produces analgesia by elevation of the pain threshold and antipyresis through action on the hypothalamic heat-regulating center. Acetaminophen is equal to aspirin in analgesic and antipyretic effectiveness and it is unlikely to produce many of the side effects associated with aspirin and aspirin-containing products.

Uses: *Junior Strength TYLENOL® Caplets* are designed for easy swallowability in older children and young adults. Both *Junior Strength TYLENOL® Caplets and Junior Strength TYLENOL® Chewable Tablets* provide fast, effective temporary relief of minor aches and pains associated with a cold, flu, headache, muscle aches, sprains, overexertion and for the reduction of fever.

Precautions: If a rare sensitivity reaction occurs, the drug should be stopped.

Directions: Caplets should be taken with liquid. Chewable tablets should be well chewed. All dosages may be repeated every 4 hours, if needed. Do not use more than 5 times a day. Under 6 years (under 48 lbs), consult a physician. *Junior Strength TYLENOL® Caplets and Chewable Tablets:* 6–8 years (48–59 lbs): 2 caplets or tablets; 9–10 years (60–71 lbs): 2 1/2 caplets or tablets; 11 years (72–95 lbs): 3 caplets or tablets; 12 years (96 lbs and over): 4 caplets or tablets.

Warnings: Do not use if carton is opened or if blister unit is broken.
Do Not Use:
• with any other products containing acetaminophen.
• for more than 3 days for fever unless directed by a doctor.
• for more than 5 days for pain unless directed by a doctor.
Stop Using This Product and Ask a Doctor If:
• symptoms do not improve.
• new symptoms occur.
• pain or fever persists or gets worse.
• redness or swelling is present.
Do not exceed recommended dose. Taking more than the recommended dose (overdose) may not provide more relief and could cause serious health problems. Keep this and all drugs out of the reach of children. In case of accidental overdose, contact a physician or poison control center immediately. Prompt medical attention is critical even if you do not notice any signs or symptoms.
NOTE: In addition to the above: The Grape and Fruit Flavored Chewable Tablet packages state: Phenylketonurics: Contains phenylalanine 6 mg per tablet. The caplet package states: Not for children who have difficulty swallowing tablets.

PROFESSIONAL INFORMATION

Overdosage Information: Acetaminophen in massive overdosage may cause

hepatic toxicity in some patients. In adults and adolescents, hepatic toxicity has rarely been reported following ingestion of acute overdosage of less than 7.5 to 10 grams. Fatalities are infrequent (less than 3–4% of untreated cases) and have rarely been reported with overdoses of less than 15 grams. In children, an acute overdosage of less than 150 mg/kg has not been associated with hepatic toxicity.

Early symptoms following a potentially hepatotoxic overdose may include: nausea, vomiting, diaphoresis and general malaise. Clinical and laboratory evidence of hepatic toxicity may not be apparent until 48 to 72 hours postingestion.

In adults and adolescents, regardless of the quantity of acetaminophen reported to have been ingested, administer acetylcysteine immediately if 24 hours or less have elapsed from the reported time of ingestion. For full prescribing information, refer to the acetylcysteine package insert. Do not await the results of assays for acetaminophen levels before initiating treatment with acetylcysteine. The following additional procedures are recommended: Promptly initiate gastric decontamination of the stomach. A plasma acetaminophen assay should be obtained as early as possible, but no sooner than four hours following ingestion. If plasma level falls above the lower treatment line on the acetaminophen overdose nomogram, acetylcysteine therapy should be continued. Liver function studies should be obtained initially and repeated at 24-hour intervals.

Serious toxicity or fatalities are extremely infrequent in children, possibly due to differences in the way they metabolize acetaminophen. In children, the maximum potential amount ingested can be more easily estimated. If more than 150 mg/kg or an unknown amount was ingested, obtain a plasma acetaminophen level. The plasma acetaminophen level should be obtained as soon as possible, but no sooner than 4 hours following ingestion. If plasma level falls above the lower treatment line on the acetaminophen overdose nomogram, the acetylcysteine therapy should be initiated and continued for a full course of therapy. If plasma acetaminophen assay capability is not available, and the estimated acetaminophen ingestion exceeds 150 mg/kg, acetylcysteine therapy should be initiated and continued for a full course of therapy.

For additional emergency information, call your regional poison center or call the Rocky Mountain Poison Center toll-free, (1-800-525-6115).

Inactive Ingredients: Junior Strength Caplets: Cellulose, Corn Starch, Ethylcellulose, Magnesium Stearate, Sodium Lauryl Sulfate, and Sodium Starch Glycolate.
Junior Strength Fruit Flavored Chewable Tablets: Aspartame, Cellulose, Cit-

Continued on next page

Junior Strength Tylenol—Cont.

ric Acid, Corn Starch, D&C Red #7, Flavors, Magnesium Stearate, and Mannitol. May contain Ethylcellulose or Cellulose Acetate and Povidone.

Junior Strength Grape Flavored Chewable Tablets: Aspartame, Cellulose, Citric Acid, Corn Starch, D&C Red #7, D&C Red #30, FD&C Blue #1, Flavors, Magnesium Stearate and Mannitol. May contain Ethylcellulose or Cellulose Acetate and Povidone.

How Supplied: Coated Caplets, (colored white, coated, scored, imprinted "TYLENOL 160") Package of 30.
Chewable Tablets (colored purple or pink, imprinted "TYLENOL 160") Package of 24. All packages are safety sealed and use child resistant blister packaging.
Shown in Product Identification Guide, page 511

MOTRIN® IB Pain Reliever Tablets, Caplets and Gelcaps

Description: Each *Motrin® IB Pain Reliever Tablet, Caplet and Gelcap* contains ibuprofen 200 mg.

Indications: *Motrin® IB Pain Reliever Tablets, Caplets and Gelcaps* are indicated for the temporary relief of headache, muscular aches, the minor pain of arthritis, toothache, backache, minor aches and pains associated with the common cold, the pain of menstrual cramps, and for reduction of fever.

Directions: Adults: Take 1 tablet, caplet or gelcap every 4 to 6 hours while symptoms persist. If pain or fever does not respond to 1 tablet, caplet or gelcap, 2 tablets, caplets or gelcaps may be used, but do not exceed 6 tablets, caplets or gelcaps in 24 hours, unless directed by a doctor. The smallest effective dose should be used. Take with food or milk if occasional and mild heartburn, upset stomach or stomach pain occurs with use. Consult a doctor if these symptoms are more than mild or if they persist. **Children:** Do not give this product to children under 12 except under the advice and supervision of a doctor.

Warnings: Do not take for pain for more than 10 days or for fever for more than 3 days unless directed by a doctor. If pain or fever persists or gets worse, if new symptoms occur, or if the painful area is red or swollen, consult a doctor. These could be signs of a serious illness. If you are under a doctor's care for any serious condition, consult a doctor before taking this product. As with aspirin and acetaminophen, if you have any condition which requires you to take prescription drugs, or if you have had any problems or serious side effects from taking any non-prescription pain reliever, do not take Motrin® IB without first discussing it with your doctor. If you experience any symptoms which are unusual or seem unrelated to the condition for which you took ibuprofen, consult a doctor before taking any more of it. Although ibuprofen is indicated for the same conditions as aspirin and acetaminophen, it should not be taken with them except under a doctor's direction. Do not combine this product with any other ibuprofen-containing product. **Do not exceed recommended dose.** Keep this and all drugs out of the reach of children. In case of accidental overdose, seek professional assistance or contact a poison control center immediately. As with any drug, if you are pregnant or nursing a baby, seek the advice of a health professional before using this product. IT IS ESPECIALLY IMPORTANT NOT TO USE IBUPROFEN DURING THE LAST 3 MONTHS OF PREGNANCY UNLESS SPECIFICALLY DIRECTED TO DO SO BY A DOCTOR BECAUSE IT MAY CAUSE PROBLEMS IN THE UNBORN CHILD OR COMPLICATIONS DURING DELIVERY.
Allergy Alert: ibuprofen may cause a severe allergic reaction which may include: hives, facial swelling, asthma (wheezing), shock.
Do not use: if you have ever had an allergic reaction to any other pain reliever/fever reducer.
Stop use and ask a doctor if an allergic reaction occurs. Seek medical help right away.

Alcohol Warning: If you consume 3 or more alcoholic drinks every day, ask your doctor whether you should take ibuprofen or other pain relievers/fever reducers. Ibuprofen may cause stomach bleeding.

PROFESSIONAL INFORMATION

Overdosage Information: The *toxicity of ibuprofen overdose* is dependent upon the amount of drug ingested and the time elapsed since ingestion, though individual response may vary, which makes it necessary to evaluate each case individually. Although uncommon, serious toxicity and death have been reported in the medical literature with ibuprofen overdosage. The most frequently reported symptoms of ibuprofen overdose include abdominal pain, nausea, vomiting, lethargy and drowsiness. Other central nervous system symptoms include headache, tinnitus, CNS depression and seizures. Metabolic acidosis, coma, acute renal failure and apnea (primarily in very young children) may rarely occur. Cardiovascular toxicity, including hypotension, bradycardia, tachycardia and atrial fibrillation, also have been reported.
The *treatment of acute ibuprofen overdose* is primarily supportive. Management of hypotension, acidosis and gastrointestinal bleeding may be necessary. In cases of acute overdose, the stomach should be emptied through ipecac-induced emesis or lavage. Emesis is most effective if initiated within 30 minutes of ingestion. Orally administered activated charcoal may help in reducing the absorption and reabsorption of ibuprofen. In children, the estimated amount of ibuprofen ingested per body weight may be helpful to predict the potential for development of toxicity although each case must be evaluated. Ingestion of less than 100 mg/kg is unlikely to produce toxicity. Children ingesting 100 to 200 mg/kg may be managed with induced emesis and a minimal observation time of four hours. Children ingesting 200 to 400 mg/kg of ibuprofen should have immediate gastric emptying and at least four hours observation in a health care facility. Children ingesting greater than 400 mg/kg require immediate medical referral, careful observation and appropriate supportive therapy. Ipecac-induced emesis is not recommended in overdoses greater than 400 mg/kg because of the risk of convulsions and the potential for aspiration of gastric contents.
In adult patients the history of the dose reportedly ingested does not appear to be predictive of toxicity. The need for referral and follow-up must be judged by the circumstances at the time of the overdose ingestion. Symptomatic adults should be admitted to a health care facility for observation.

Inactive Ingredients: Tablets and Caplets: Carnauba wax, cornstarch, hydroxypropyl methylcellulose, iron oxide black, pregelatanized starch, propylene glycol, silicon dioxide, stearic acid, titanium dioxide.
Gelcaps: Benzyl alcohol, butylparaben, butyl alcohol, castor oil, colloidal silicon dioxide, cornstarch, edetate calcium disodium, FDC Yellow No. 6, gelatin, hydroxypropyl methylcellulose, iron oxide black, magnesium stearate, methylparaben, microcrystalline cellulose, povidone, pregelatinized starch, propylene glycol, propylparaben, SDA 3A alcohol, sodium lauryl sulfate, sodium propionate, sodium starch glycolate, starch and titanium dioxide.

How Supplied: Tablets: (white, printed "Motrin IB" in black) in tamper evident packaging of 24, 50, 100, 130, 135, and 165.
Caplets: (white, printed "Motrin IB" in black) in tamper evident packaging of 24, 50, 60, 100, 130, 135, 165, 250 and 500.
Gelcaps: (colored orange and white, printed "Motrin IB" in black) in tamper evident packaging of 24 and 50.
Shown in Product Identification Guide, page 510

MOTRIN® IB SINUS Pain Reliever/ Fever Reducer/Nasal Decongestant Tablets and Caplets

Description: Each *Motrin® IB Sinus Tablet and Caplet* contains ibuprofen 200 mg and pseudoephedrine HCl 30 mg
Indications: *Motrin® IB Sinus Tablets and Caplets* are indicated for the

temporary relief of symptoms associated with sinusitis, the common cold or flu including nasal congestion, headache, body aches, pains and fever.

Directions: *Adults and children 12 years of age and older:* Take 1 tablet or caplet every 4 to 6 hours while symptoms persist. If symptoms do not respond to 1 tablet or caplet, 2 tablets or caplets may be used but do not exceed 6 tablets or caplets in 24 hours, unless directed by a doctor. The smallest effective dose should be used. Take with food or milk if occasional and mild heartburn, upset stomach, or stomach pain occurs with use. Consult a doctor if these symptoms are more than mild or if they persist. *Children:* Do not give this product to children under 12 years of age except under the advice and supervision of a doctor.

Warnings: Do not take for more than 7 days. If symptoms do not improve or are accompanied by fever that persists for more than 3 days, or if new symptoms occur, consult a doctor. These could be signs of a serious illness. As with aspirin and acetaminophen, if you have any condition which requires you to take prescription drugs or if you have had any problems or serious side effects from taking any non-prescription pain reliever, do not take this product without first discussing it with your doctor. IF YOU EXPERIENCE ANY SYMPTOMS WHICH ARE UNUSUAL OR SEEM UNRELATED TO THE CONDITION FOR WHICH YOU TOOK THIS PRODUCT CONSULT A DOCTOR BEFORE TAKING ANY MORE OF IT. If you are under a doctor's care for any serious condition, consult a doctor before taking this product. **Do not exceed recommended dosage.** If nervousness, dizziness, or sleeplessness occur, discontinue use and consult a doctor. Do not take this product if you have heart disease, high blood pressure, thyroid disease, diabetes, or difficulty in urination due to enlargement of the prostate gland, unless directed by a doctor. Do not combine this product with other non-prescription pain relievers. Do not combine this product with any other ibuprofen-containing product. Keep this and all drugs out of the reach of children. In case of accidental overdose, seek professional assistance or contact a poison control center immediately.

As with any drug, if you are pregnant or nursing a baby, seek the advice of a health professional before using this product. IT IS ESPECIALLY IMPORTANT NOT TO USE THIS PRODUCT DURING THE LAST 3 MONTHS OF PREGNANCY UNLESS SPECIFICALLY DIRECTED TO DO SO BY A DOCTOR BECAUSE IT MAY CAUSE PROBLEMS IN THE UNBORN CHILD OR COMPLICATIONS DURING DELIVERY.

Allergy Alert: ibuprofen may cause a severe allergic reaction which may include: hives, facial swelling, asthma (wheezing), shock.

Do not use if you have ever had an allergic reaction to any other pain reliever/fever reducer.

Stop use and ask a doctor if an allergic reaction occurs. Seek medical help right away.

Store at room temperature, 15–30°C (59–86°F).

Alcohol Warning: If you consume 3 or more alcoholic drinks every day, ask your doctor whether you should take ibuprofen or other pain relievers/fever reducers. Ibuprofen may cause stomach bleeding.

Drug Interaction Precaution: Do not use this product if you are now taking a prescription monoamine oxidase inhibitor (MAOI) (certain drugs for depression, psychiatric or emotional conditions, or Parkinson's disease), or for 2 weeks after stopping the MAOI drug. If you are uncertain whether your drug contains an MAOI, consult a health professional before taking this product.

PROFESSIONAL INFORMATION

Overdosage Information: The *toxicity of ibuprofen overdose* is dependent upon the amount of drug ingested and the time elapsed since ingestion, though individual response may vary, which makes it necessary to evaluate each case individually. Although uncommon, serious toxicity and death have been reported in the medical literature with ibuprofen overdosage. The most frequently reported symptoms of ibuprofen overdose include abdominal pain, nausea, vomiting, lethargy and drowsiness. Other central nervous system symptoms include headache, tinnitus, CNS depression and seizures. Metabolic acidosis, coma, acute renal failure and apnea (primarily in very young children) may rarely occur. Cardiovascular toxicity, including hypotension, bradycardia, tachycardia and atrial fibrillation, also have been reported.

The *treatment of acute ibuprofen overdose* is primarily supportive. Management of hypotension, acidosis and gastrointestinal bleeding may be necessary. In cases of acute overdose, the stomach should be emptied through ipecac-induced emesis or lavage. Emesis is most effective if initiated within 30 minutes of ingestion. Orally administered activated charcoal may help in reducing the absorption and reabsorption of ibuprofen. In children, the estimated amount of ibuprofen ingested per body weight may be helpful to predict the potential for development of toxicity although each case must be evaluated. Ingestion of less than 100 mg/kg is unlikely to produce toxicity. Children ingesting 100 to 200 mg/kg may be managed with induced emesis and a minimal observation time of four hours. Children ingesting 200 to 400 mg/kg of ibuprofen should have immediate gastric emptying and at least four hours observation in a health care facility. Children ingesting greater than 400 mg/kg require immediate medical referral, careful observation and appropriate supportive therapy. Ipecac-induced emesis is not recommended in overdoses greater than 400 mg/kg because of the risk of convulsions and the potential for aspiration of gastric contents.

In adult patients the history of the dose reportedly ingested does not appear to be predictive of toxicity. The need for referral and follow-up must be judged by the circumstances at the time of the overdose ingestion. Symptomatic adults should be admitted to a health care facility for observation.

Symptoms from pseudoephedrine overdose consist most often of mild anxiety, tachycardia and/or hypertension. Symptoms usually appear within 4 to 8 hours of ingestion and are transient, usually requiring no treatment.

Inactive Ingredients: **Tablets and Caplets:** Cellulose, Corn Starch, FD&C Red #40 Aluminum Lake, Glyceryl Triacetate, Hydroxypropyl Methylcellulose, Silicon Dioxide, Sodium Lauryl Sulfate, Sodium Starch Glycolate, Stearic Acid, Titanium Dioxide.

How Supplied: Tablets: (white, printed "Motrin IB Sinus" in orange) in blister packs of 20 and 30.
Caplets: (white, printed "Motrin IB Sinus" in orange) in blister packs of 20 and 30.

Shown in Product Identification Guide, page 510

NICOTROL®
NICOTINE TRANSDERMAL SYSTEM

Description: **NICOTROL®** (nicotine transdermal system) is a multilayered, rectangular, thin film laminated unit containing nicotine as the active ingredient. **NICOTROL®** Patch provides systemic delivery of 15 mg of nicotine over 16 hours.

Actions: **NICOTROL®** (nicotine transdermal system) Patch helps smokers quit by reducing nicotine withdrawal symptoms. Many **NICOTROL®** Patch users will be able to stop smoking for a few days but often will start smoking again. Most smokers have to try to quit several times before they completely stop.

Your own chances of quitting smoking depend on how much you want to quit, how strongly you are addicted to nicotine and how closely you follow a quitting program like the PATHWAYS TO CHANGE® Program that comes with the **NICOTROL®** Patch.

If you find you cannot stop or if you start smoking again after using **NICOTROL®** Patch, please talk to a health care professional who can help you find a program that may work better for you. Remember that breaking this addiction doesn't happen overnight.

Because the **NICOTROL®** Patch provides some nicotine, the **NICOTROL®** Patch will help you stop smoking by reducing nicotine withdrawal symptoms such as nicotine cravings, nervousness and irritability.

Indications: **NICOTROL®** Patch is indicated as a stop smoking aid to reduce

Continued on next page

Nicotrol—Cont.

withdrawal symptoms, including nicotine craving, associated with quitting smoking. **NICOTROL®** Patch is for people who smoke over 10 cigarettes a day.

Directions:
- Stop smoking completely when you begin using the **NICOTROL®** Patch.
- Refer to enclosed patient information leaflet before using this product.
- Use one **NICOTROL®** Patch every day for six weeks. Remove backing from the patch and immediately press onto clean dry hairless skin. Hold for ten seconds. Wash hands.
- The **NICOTROL®** Patch should be worn during awake hours and removed prior to sleep.

For Best Results In Quitting Smoking:
1. Firmly commit to quitting smoking.
2. Use enclosed support materials.
3. Use the **NICOTROL®** Patches for six weeks.
4. Stop using **NICOTROL®** Patches at the end of week six. If you still feel the need for **NICOTROL®** Patches talk to your doctor.

Warnings:
- Keep this and all medication out of reach of children and pets. Even used patches have enough nicotine to poison children and pets. Be sure to fold sticky ends together and throw away out of reach of children and pets. In case of accidental overdose, seek professional assistance or contact a poison control center immediately.
- Nicotine can increase your baby's heart rate. First try to stop smoking without the nicotine patch. As with any drug, if you are pregnant or nursing a baby, seek the advice of a health professional before using this product.
- Do not smoke even when you are not wearing the patch. The nicotine in your skin will still be entering your bloodstream for several hours after you take the patch off.
- If you forget to remove the patch at bedtime you may have vivid dreams or other sleep disruptions.

Do Not Use if You:
- Continue to smoke, chew tobacco, use snuff, or use a nicotine gum or other nicotine containing products.

Ask Your Doctor Before Use if You:
- Are under 18 years of age.
- Have heart disease, recent heart attack or irregular heartbeat. Nicotine can increase your heart rate.
- Have high blood pressure not controlled with medication.
Nicotine can increase blood pressure.
- Take prescription medicine for depression or asthma.
Your prescription dose may need to be adjusted.
- Are allergic to adhesive tape or have skin problems, because you are more likely to get rashes.

Stop Use and See Your Doctor if You Have:
- Skin redness caused by the patch that does not go away after four days, or if your skin swells or you get a rash.
- Irregular heartbeat or palpitations.
- Symptoms of nicotine overdose such as nausea, vomiting, dizziness, weakness and rapid heartbeat.

Inactive Ingredients: Non-woven polyester, pigmented aluminized polyester, polybutene, polyisobutylenes, siliconized polyester.

How Supplied: Starter Kit-7, Refill Kit-7. DO NOT USE IF POUCH IS DAMAGED OR OPEN. Do not Store above 86°F (30°C)
- **Not for sale to those under 18 years of age.**
- **Proof of age required.**
- **Not for sale in vending machines or from any source where proof of age cannot be verified.**
Shown in Product Identification Guide, page 510

Maximum Strength SINE-AID® Sinus Medication Gelcaps, Caplets and Tablets

Description: Each **Maximum Strength SINE-AID® Gelcap, Caplet** or **Tablet** contains acetaminophen 500 mg and pseudoephedrine HCl 30 mg.

Actions: Maximum Strength SINE-AID® Gelcaps, Caplets and **Tablets** contain a clinically proven analgesic-antipyretic and a decongestant. Maximum allowable non-prescription levels of acetaminophen and pseudoephedrine provide temporary relief of sinus congestion and pain. Acetaminophen is equal to aspirin in analgesic and antipyretic effectiveness and it is unlikely to produce many of the side effects associated with aspirin and aspirin-containing products. Acetaminophen produces analgesia by elevation of the pain threshold and antipyresis through action on the hypothalamic heat-regulating center. Pseudoephedrine hydrochloride is a sympathomimetic amine that promotes sinus cavity drainage by reducing nasopharyngeal mucosal congestion.

Indications: Maximum Strength SINE-AID® Gelcaps, Caplets and **Tablets** provide effective symptomatic relief from sinus headache pain and congestion. **SINE-AID®** is particularly well-suited in patients with aspirin allergy, hemostatic disturbances (including anticoagulant therapy), and bleeding diatheses (e.g. hemophilia) and upper gastrointestinal disease (e.g. ulcer, gastritis, hiatus hernia).

Precautions: If a rare sensitivity occurs, the drug should be discontinued. Although pseudoephedrine is virtually without pressor effect in normotensive patients, it should be used with caution in hypertensives.

Directions: Adults & children 12 years of age and older: Take two every 4–6 hours as needed. Do not take more than 8 in 24 hours, or as directed by a doctor. **Children under 12 years of age:** Do not use this product in children under 12 years of age. This will provide more than the recommended dose (overdose) and could cause serious health problems.

Warnings: Do not use if carton is open or if blister unit is broken.
Do not take for pain for more than 7 days or for fever for more than 3 days unless directed by a doctor. If pain or fever persists, or gets worse, if new symptoms occur, or if redness or swelling is present, consult a doctor because these could be signs of a serious condition. **Do not exceed recommended dosage.** If nervousness, dizziness or sleeplessness occur, discontinue use and consult a doctor. Do not take this product if you have heart disease, high blood pressure, thyroid disease, diabetes or difficulty in urination due to enlargement of the prostate gland unless directed by a doctor.
As with any drug, if you are pregnant or nursing a baby, seek the advice of a health professional before using this product. Keep this and all drugs out of the reach of children. In case of accidental overdose, contact a doctor or poison control center immediately. Prompt medical attention is critical for adults as well as for children even if you do not notice any signs or symptoms. Do not use with other products containing acetaminophen.

Alcohol Warning: If you consume 3 or more alcoholic drinks every day, ask your doctor whether you should take acetaminophen or other pain relievers/fever reducers. Acetaminophen may cause liver damage.

Drug Interaction Precaution: Do not use this product if you are now taking a prescription monoamine oxidase inhibitor (MAOI) (certain drugs for depression, psychiatric or emotional conditions, or Parkinson's disease), or for 2 weeks after stopping the MAOI drug. If you are uncertain whether your prescription drug contains an MAOI, consult a health professional before taking this product.

PROFESSIONAL INFORMATION

Overdosage Information: Acetaminophen in massive overdosage may cause hepatic toxicity in some patients. In adults and adolescents, hepatic toxicity has rarely been reported following ingestion of acute overdoses of less than 7.5 to 10 grams. Fatalities are infrequent (less than 3–4% of untreated cases) and have rarely been reported with overdoses of less than 15 grams. In children, an acute overdosage of less than 150 mg/kg has not been associated with hepatic toxicity. Early symptoms following a potentially hepatotoxic overdose may include: nausea, vomiting, diaphoresis and general malaise. Clinical and laboratory evidence of hepatic toxicity may not be apparent until 48 to 72 hours postingestion.
In adults and adolescents, regardless of the quantity of acetaminophen reported to have been ingested, administer acetylcysteine immediately if 24 hours or less have elapsed from the reported time of ingestion. For full prescribing information, refer to the acetylcysteine package insert. Do not await results of assays for plasma acetaminophen levels before initiating treatment with acetylcysteine.

The following additional procedures are recommended: Promptly initiate gastric decontamination of the stomach. A plasma acetaminophen assay should be obtained as early as possible, but no sooner than four hours following ingestion. If plasma level falls above the lower treatment line on the acetaminophen overdose nomogram, acetylcysteine therapy should be continued. Liver function studies should be obtained initially and repeated at 24-hour intervals.

Serious toxicity or fatalities are extremely infrequent in children, possibly due to differences in the way they metabolize acetaminophen. In children, the maximum potential amount ingested can be more easily estimated. If more than 150 mg/kg or an unknown amount was ingested, obtain a plasma acetaminophen level. The plasma acetaminophen level should be obtained as soon as possible, but no sooner than 4 hours following ingestion. If plasma level falls above the lower treatment line on the acetaminophen overdose nomogram, the acetylcysteine therapy should be initiated and continued for a full course of therapy. If plasma acetaminophen assay capability is not available, and the estimated acetaminophen ingestion exceeds 150 mg/kg, acetylcysteine therapy should be initiated and continued for a full course of therapy.

For additional emergency information, call your regional poison center or call the Rocky Mountain Poison Center toll-free, (1-800-525-6115).

Symptoms from pseudoephedrine overdose consist most often of mild anxiety, tachycardia and/or mild hypertension. Symptoms usually appear within 4 to 8 hours of ingestion and are transient, usually requiring no treatment.

Alcohol Information: Chronic heavy alcohol abusers may be at increased risk of liver toxicity from excessive acetaminophen use, although reports of this event are rare. Reports usually involve cases of severe chronic alcoholics and the dosages of acetaminophen most often exceed recommended doses and often involve substantial overdose. Professionals should alert their patients who regularly consume large amounts of alcohol not to exceed recommended doses of acetaminophen.

Inactive Ingredients: Gelcaps: Benzyl Alcohol, Butylparaben, Castor Oil, Cellulose, Corn Starch, Edetate Calcium Disodium, Gelatin, Hydroxypropyl Methylcellulose, Iron Oxide Black, Magnesium Stearate, Methylparaben, Propylparaben, Sodium Lauryl Sulfate, Sodium Propionate, Sodium Starch Glycolate, Titanium Dioxide, FD&C Red #40.
Caplets: Cellulose, Corn Starch, Hydroxypropyl Methylcellulose, Magnesium Stearate, Polyethylene Glycol, Sodium Starch Glycolate, Titanium Dioxide, Blue #1 and Red #40.
Tablets: Cellulose, Corn Starch, Magnesium Stearate and Sodium Starch Glycolate.

How Supplied: Gelcaps (colored red and white imprinted "SINE-AID")—blister package of 20.
Caplets (colored white imprinted "Maximum SINE-AID")—blister package of 24.
Tablets (colored white embossed "SINE-AID")—blister package of 24.
Shown in Product Identification Guide, page 510

Extra Strength
TYLENOL® acetaminophen
Gelcaps, Geltabs, Caplets, Tablets
Extra Strength
TYLENOL® acetaminophen
Adult Liquid Pain Reliever
Regular Strength
TYLENOL® acetaminophen
Caplets and Tablets

TYLENOL® Arthritis Extended Relief
Caplets
acetaminophen extended release
Caplets

Product information for all dosage forms of Adult TYLENOL acetaminophen have been combined under this heading.

Description: Each *Extra Strength TYLENOL® Gelcap, Geltab, Caplet, or Tablet* contains acetaminophen 500 mg. Each 15 mL ($^1/_2$ fl oz or one tablespoonful) of *Extra Strength TYLENOL® acetaminophen Adult Liquid Pain Reliever* contains 500 mg acetaminophen (alcohol 7%).
Each *Regular Strength TYLENOL® Caplet or Tablet* contains acetaminophen 325 mg.
Each *TYLENOL® Arthritis Extended Relief Caplet* contains acetaminophen 650 mg.

Actions: Acetaminophen is a clinically proven analgesic and antipyretic. Acetaminophen produces analgesia by elevation of the pain threshold and antipyresis through action on the hypothalamic heat-regulating center. Acetaminophen is equal to aspirin in analgesic and antipyretic effectiveness and it is unlikely to produce many of the side effects associated with aspirin and aspirin-containing products.
Tylenol Arthritis Extended Relief uses a unique, patented bilayer caplet. The first layer dissolves quickly to provide prompt relief while the second layer is time released to provide up to 8 hours of relief.

Uses: For the temporary relief of minor aches and pains associated with headache, muscular aches, backache, minor arthritis pain, common cold, toothache, menstrual cramps and for the reduction of fever.

Directions: *Extra Strength TYLENOL® Gelcaps, Geltabs, Caplets, or Tablets:* **Adults and children 12 years of age and older:** Take two gelcaps, geltabs, caplets, or tablets every 4 to 6 hours as needed. Do not take more than 8 gelcaps, geltabs, caplets or tablets in 24 hours, or as directed by a doctor. **Children under 12 years:** Do not use this adult Extra Strength product in children under 12 years of age. This will provide more than the recommended dose (overdose) of TYLENOL® and could cause serious health problems.
Extra Strength TYLENOL® Adult Liquid Pain Reliever: **Adults and children 12 years of age and older:** Take 2 Tablespoons (tbsp.) in dose cup provided every 4 to 6 hours as needed. Do not take more than 8 Tablespoons in 24 hours, or as directed by a doctor. **Children under 12 years:** Do not use this adult Extra Strength product in children under 12 years of age. This will provide more than the recommended dose (overdose) of TYLENOL® and could cause serious health problems.
Regular Strength TYLENOL® Caplets or Tablets: **Adults and Children 12 years of Age and Older:** Take two caplets or tablets every 4 to 6 hours as needed. Do not take more than 12 caplets or tablets in 24 hours, or as directed by a doctor. Children 6–11 years of age. Take 1 caplet or tablet every 4 to 6 hours as needed. Do not take more than 5 caplets or tablets in 24 hours. **Children under 6 years of age:** Do not use this adult Regular Strength product in children under 6 years of age. This will provide more than the recommended dose (overdose) of TYLENOL® and could cause serious health problems.
TYLENOL® Arthritis Extended Relief Caplets: **Adults and Children 12 years of Age and Older:** Take two caplets every 8 hours, not to exceed 6 caplets in any 24-hour period. TAKE TWO CAPLETS WITH WATER, SWALLOW EACH CAPLET WHOLE. DO NOT CRUSH, CHEW, OR DISSOLVE THE CAPLET. Not for use in children under 12 years of age.

Precautions: If a rare sensitivity reaction occurs, the drug should be discontinued.

Warnings: Extra Strength TYLENOL® Gelcaps, Geltabs, Caplets, or Tablets, Extra Strength TYLENOL® Adult Liquid Pain Reliever, Regular Strength TYLENOL® Caplets or Tablets: Do not use if carton is opened or red neck wrap or foil seal imprinted with "SAFETY SEAL®" is broken.
Do not Use:
• with any other product containing acetaminophen
• for more than 10 days for pain unless directed by a doctor.
• for more than 3 days for fever unless directed by a doctor.
Stop Using and Ask a Doctor if:
• symptoms do not improve
• new symptoms occur
• pain or fever persists or gets worse
• redness or swelling is present
Do not exceed recommended dose. Keep this and all drugs out of the reach of children. In case of accidental over-

Continued on next page

Tylenol—Cont.

dose, contact a physician or poison control center immediately. Prompt medical attention is critical for adults as well as for children even if you do not notice any signs or symptoms. As with any drug, if you are pregnant or nursing a baby, seek the advice of a health professional before using this product.

TYLENOL® Arthritis Extended Relief Caplets: Do not use if carton is open or red neck wrap or foil inner seal imprinted with "Safety Seal®" is broken. Do not take for pain for more than 10 days or for fever for more than 3 days unless directed by a physician. If pain or fever persists, or gets worse, if new symptoms occur, or if redness or swelling is present, consult a physician because these could be signs of a serious condition. As with any drug, if you are pregnant or nursing a baby, seek the advice of a health professional before using this product. Keep this and all drugs out of the reach of children. In case of accidental overdose, contact a physician or poison control center immediately. Prompt medical attention is critical for adults as well as for children even if you do not notice any signs or symptoms. Do not use with other products containing acetaminophen.

Alcohol Warning: *Extra Strength TYLENOL® Gelcaps, Geltabs, Caplets and Tablets, Extra Strength TYLENOL® Adult Liquid Pain Reliever, Regular Strength TYLENOL® Caplets and Tablets and TYLENOL® Arthritis Extended Relief Caplets:* If you consume 3 or more alcoholic drinks every day, ask your doctor whether you should take acetaminophen or other pain relievers/fever reducers. Acetaminophen may cause liver damage.

PROFESSIONAL INFORMATION

Overdosage Information: Acetaminophen in massive overdosage may cause hepatic toxicity in some patients. In adults and adolescents, hepatic toxicity has rarely been reported following ingestion of acute overdoses of less than 7.5 to 10 grams. Fatalities are infrequent (less than 3–4% of untreated cases) and have rarely been reported with overdoses of less than 15 grams. In children, an acute overdosage of less than 150 mg/kg has not been associated with hepatic toxicity. Early symptoms following a potentially hepatotoxic overdose may include: nausea, vomiting, diaphoresis and general malaise. Clinical and laboratory evidence of hepatic toxicity may not be apparent until 48 to 72 hours postingestion. In adults and adolescents, regardless of the quantity of acetaminophen reported to have been ingested, administer acetylcysteine immediately if 24 hours or less have elapsed from the reported time of ingestion. For full prescribing information, refer to the acetylcysteine package insert. Do not await results of assays for plasma acetaminophen levels before initiating treatment with acetylcysteine. The fol-

lowing additional procedures are recommended: Promptly initiate gastric decontamination of the stomach. A plasma acetaminophen assay should be obtained as early as possible, but no sooner than four hours following ingestion. If an acetaminophen extended release product is involved, it may be appropriate to obtain an additional plasma acetaminophen level 4–6 hours following the initial plasma acetaminophen level. If either plasma level falls above the lower treatment line on the acetaminophen overdose nomogram, acetylcysteine therapy should be continued. Liver function studies should be obtained initially and repeated at 24-hour intervals.

Serious toxicity or fatalities are extremely infrequent in children, possibly due to differences in the way they metabolize acetaminophen. In children, the maximum potential amount ingested can be more easily estimated. If more than 150 mg/kg or an unknown amount was ingested, obtain a plasma acetaminophen level. The plasma acetaminophen level should be obtained as soon as possible, but no sooner than 4 hours following ingestion. If an acetaminophen *extended release* product is involved, it may be appropriate to obtain an additional plasma acetaminophen level 4–6 hours following the initial plasma acetaminophen level. If either plasma level falls above the lower treatment line on the acetaminophen overdose nomogram, the acetylcysteine therapy should be initiated and continued for a full course of therapy. If plasma acetaminophen assay capability is not available, and the estimated acetaminophen ingestion exceeds 150 mg/kg, acetylcysteine therapy should be initiated and continued for a full course of therapy.

For additional emergency information, call your regional poison center or call the Rocky Mountain Poison Center toll-free, (1-800-525-6115).

Alcohol Information: Chronic heavy alcohol abusers may be at increased risk of liver toxicity from excessive acetaminophen use, although reports of this event are rare. Reports usually involve cases of severe chronic alcoholics and the dosages of acetaminophen most often exceed recommended doses and often involve substantial overdose. Professionals should alert their patients who regularly consume large amounts of alcohol not to exceed recommended doses of acetaminophen.

Inactive Ingredients: *Extra Strength TYLENOL®:* **Tablets:** Magnesium Stearate, Cellulose, Sodium Starch Glycolate and Starch. **Caplets:** Cellulose, Cornstarch, Hydroxypropyl Methylcellulose, Magnesium Stearate, Polyethylene Glycol, Sodium Starch Glycolate, and Red #40. **Gelcaps:** Benzyl Alcohol, Butylparaben, Castor Oil, Cellulose, Edetate Calcium Disodium, Gelatin, Hydroxypropyl Methylcellulose, Magnesium Stearate, Methylparaben, Propylparaben, Sodium Lauryl Sulfate, Sodium Propionate, Sodium Starch Glycolate, Starch, Tita-

nium Dioxide, Blue #1 and #2, Red #40, and Yellow #10. **Geltabs:** Benzyl Alcohol, Butylparaben, Castor Oil, Cellulose, Corn Starch, Edetate Calcium Disodium, Gelatin, Hydroxypropyl Methylcellulose, Magnesium Stearate, Methylparaben, Propylparaben, Sodium Lauryl Sulfate, Sodium Propionate, Sodium Starch Glycolate, Titanium Dioxide, Blue #1 and #2, Red #40, and Yellow #10.

Extra Strength TYLENOL® Adult Liquid Pain Reliever: Alcohol (7%), Citric Acid, Flavors, Glycerin, Polyethylene Glycol, Purified Water, Sodium Benzoate, Sorbitol, Sucrose, Yellow #6 (Sunset Yellow), Yellow #10 and Blue #1.

Regular Strength TYLENOL®: **Tablets:** Magnesium Stearate, Cellulose, Sodium Starch Glycolate and Starch. **Caplets:** Cellulose, Hydroxypropyl Methylcellulose, Magnesium Stearate, Polyethylene Glycol, Sodium Starch Glycolate, Starch and Red #40.

TYLENOL® Arthritis Extended Relief Caplets: Corn Starch, Hydroxyethyl Cellulose, Hydroxypropyl Methylcellulose, Magnesium Stearate, Microcrystalline Cellulose, Povidone, Powdered Cellulose, Pregelatinized Starch, Sodium Starch Glycolate, Titanium Dioxide, Triacetin.

How Supplied: *Extra Strength TYLENOL®:* **Tablets** (colored white, imprinted "TYLENOL" and "500")—vials of 10, and tamper-evident bottles of 30, 60, 100, and 200. **Caplets** (colored white, imprinted "TYLENOL 500 mg")—vials of 10, 10 blister packs, and tamper-evident bottles of 24, 50, 100, 175, and 250. **Gelcaps** (colored yellow and red, imprinted "Tylenol 500") vials of 10 and tamper-evident bottles of 24, 50, 100, and 225. **Geltabs** (colored yellow and red, imprinted "Tylenol 500") tamper-evident bottles of 24, 50, and 100.

Extra Strength TYLENOL® Adult Liquid Pain Reliever: Mint-flavored liquid (colored green) 8 fl. oz. tamper-evident bottle with child resistant safety cap and special dosage cup.

Regular Strength TYLENOL®: **Tablets** (colored white, scored, imprinted "TYLENOL" and "325")—tamper-evident bottles of 24, 50, 100 and 200. **Caplets** (colored white, "TYLENOL 325")—tamper-evident bottles of 24, 50, 100.

TYLENOL® Arthritis Extended Relief Caplets: (colored white, engraved "TYLENOL ER") tamper-evident bottles of 24, 50, and 100's.

Shown in Product Identification Guide, page 512

TYLENOL® COLD ® Medication
No Drowsiness Formula
Caplets and Gelcaps

Multi-Symptom Formula
TYLENOL® COLD Medication
Tablets and Caplets

Product information for all dosage forms of TYLENOL COLD have been combined under this heading.

Description: Each *TYLENOL® COLD Medication No Drowsiness Formula Caplet and Gelcap* contains acetaminophen 325 mg, pseudoephedrine HCl 30 mg, and dextromethorphan HBr 15 mg. Each *Multi-Symptom Formula TYLENOL® COLD Tablet or Caplet* contains acetaminophen 325 mg, chlorpheniramine maleate 2 mg, pseudoephedrine HCl 30 mg, and dextromethorphan HBr 15 mg.

Actions: *TYLENOL® COLD Medication No Drowsiness Formula* contains a clinically proven analgesic-antipyretic, decongestant and cough suppressant. Acetaminophen produces analgesia by elevation of the pain threshold and antipyresis through action on the hypothalamic heat-regulating center. Acetaminophen is equal to aspirin in analgesic and antipyretic effectiveness and it is unlikely to produce many of the side effects associated with aspirin and aspirin-containing products. Pseudoephedrine is a sympathomimetic amine which provides temporary relief of nasal congestion. Dextromethorphan is a cough suppressant which provides temporary relief of coughs due to minor throat irritations that may occur with the common cold. *Multi-Symptom Formula TYLENOL® COLD Medication* contains, in addition to the above ingredients, an antihistamine. Chlorpheniramine is an antihistamine which helps provide temporary relief of runny nose, sneezing and watery and itchy eyes.

Indications: *TYLENOL® COLD Medication No Drowsiness Formula* provides effective temporary symptom relief of nasal congestion, coughing, sore throat, headaches, body aches and fever. *Multi-Symptom Formula TYLENOL® COLD Medication* provides effective temporary symptom relief of nasal congestion, runny nose, sneezing, watery and itchy eyes, coughing, sore throat, headaches, body aches and fever.

Directions: *TYLENOL® COLD No Drowsiness Formula and Multi-Symptom Formula TYLENOL® COLD Medication:* **Adults and children 12 years of age and older:** Take two every 6 hours. Do not take more than 8 in 24 hours, or as directed by a doctor. **Children 6–11 years of age:** Take one every 6 hours. Do not take more than 4 in 24 hours, or as directed by a doctor. **Children under 6 years of age:** Do not use this product in children under 6 years of age. This will provide more than the recommended dose (overdose) and could cause serious health problems.

Precautions: *TYLENOL® COLD Medication No Drowsiness Formula and Multi-Symptom Formula TYLENOL® COLD Medication:* If a rare sensitivity reaction occurs, the drug should be stopped. Although pseudoephedrine is virtually without pressor effect in normotensive patients, it should be used with caution in hypertensives.

Warnings: *TYLENOL® COLD Medication No Drowsiness Formula:* Do not use if carton is opened or if a blister unit is broken. Do not take for pain for more than 7 days or for fever for more than 3 days unless directed by a doctor. If pain or fever persists, or gets worse, if new symptoms occur, or if redness or swelling is present, consult a doctor because these could be signs of a serious condition. If sore throat is severe, persists for more than 2 days, is accompanied or followed by fever, headache, rash, nausea or vomiting, consult a doctor promptly. A persistent cough may be a sign of a serious condition. If cough persists for more than 1 week, tends to recur or is accompanied by fever, rash or persistent headache, consult a doctor. Do not take this product for persistent or chronic cough such as occurs with smoking, asthma, emphysema or if cough is accompanied by excessive phlegm (mucus) unless directed by a doctor. **Do not exceed recommended dosage** If nervousness, dizziness or sleeplessness, occur, discontinue use and consult a doctor. Do not take this product if you have heart disease, high blood pressure, thyroid disease, diabetes or difficulty in urination due to enlargement of the prostate gland unless directed by a doctor. As with any drug, if you are pregnant or nursing a baby, seek the advice of a health professional before using this product. Keep this and all drugs out of the reach of children. In case of accidental overdose, contact a doctor or poison control center immediately. Prompt medical attention is critical for adults as well as for children even if you do not notice any signs or symptoms. Do not use with other products containing acetaminophen.

Multi-Symptom Formula TYLENOL® COLD Medication: **Do not use if carton is opened or if a blister unit is broken** Do not take for pain for more than 7 days or for fever for more than 3 days unless directed by a doctor. If pain or fever persists, or gets worse, if new symptoms occur, or if redness or swelling is present, consult a doctor because these could be signs of a serious condition. If sore throat is severe, persists for more than 2 days, is accompanied or followed by fever, headache, rash, nausea or vomiting, consult a doctor promptly. A persistent cough may be a sign of a serious condition. If cough persists for more than 1 week, tends to recur or is accompanied by fever, rash or persistent headache, consult a doctor. Do not take this product for persistent or chronic cough such as occurs with smoking, asthma, emphysema or if cough is accompanied by excessive phlegm (mucus) unless directed by a doctor. **Do not exceed recommended dosage.** If nervousness, dizziness or sleeplessness occur, discontinue use and consult a doctor. May cause excitability especially in children. Do not take this product unless directed by a doctor, if you have a breathing problem such as emphysema or chronic bronchitis, or if you have glaucoma or difficulty in urination due to enlargement of the prostate gland. Do not take this product if you have heart disease, high blood pressure, thyroid disease or diabetes unless directed by a doctor. May cause drowsiness; alcohol, sedatives and tranquilizers may increase the drowsiness effect. Avoid alcoholic beverages while taking this product. Do not take this product if you are taking sedatives or tranquilizers without first consulting your doctor. Use caution when driving a motor vehicle or operating machinery. As with any drug, if you are pregnant or nursing a baby, seek the advice of a health professional before using this product. Keep this and all drugs out of the reach of children. In case of accidental overdose, contact a doctor or poison control center immediately. Prompt medical attention is critical for adults as well as for children even if you do not notice any signs or symptoms. Do not use with other products containing acetaminophen.

Alcohol Warning: *TYLENOL® COLD Medication No Drowsiness Formula and Multi-Symptom Formula TYLENOL® COLD Medication:* If you consume 3 or more alcoholic drinks every day, ask your doctor whether you should take acetaminophen or other pain relievers/fever reducers. Acetaminophen may cause liver damage.

Drug Interaction Precaution: *TYLENOL® COLD Medication No Drowsiness Formula and Multi-Symptom Formula TYLENOL® COLD Medication:* Do not use this product if you are now taking a prescription monoamine oxidase inhibitor (MAOI) (certain drugs for depression, psychiatric or emotional conditions, or Parkinson's disease), or for 2 weeks after stopping the MAOI drug. If you are uncertain whether your prescription drug contains an MAOI, consult a health professional before taking this product.

PROFESSIONAL INFORMATION

Overdosage Information: *TYLENOL® COLD Medication No Drowsiness Formula and Multi-Symptom Formula TYLENOL® COLD Medication:* Acetaminophen in massive overdosage may cause hepatic toxicity in some patients. In adults and adolescents, hepatic toxicity has rarely been reported following ingestion of acute overdoses of less than 7.5 to 10 grams. Fatalities are infrequent (less than 3–4% of untreated cases) and have rarely been reported with overdoses of less than 15 grams. In children, an acute overdosage of less than 150 mg/kg has not been associated with hepatic toxicity.

Early symptoms following a potentially hepatotoxic overdose may include: nausea, vomiting, diaphoresis and general malaise. Clinical and laboratory evidence of hepatic toxicity may not be apparent until 48 to 72 hours postingestion. In adults and adolescents, regardless of the quantity of acetaminophen reported to have been ingested, administer acetylcysteine immediately if 24

Continued on next page

Tylenol Cold—Cont.

hours or less have elapsed from the reported time of ingestion. For full prescribing information, refer to the acetylcysteine package insert. Do not await results of assays for plasma acetaminophen levels before initiating treatment with acetylcysteine. The following additional procedures are recommended: Promptly initiate gastric decontamination of the stomach. A plasma acetaminophen assay should be obtained as early as possible, but no sooner than four hours following ingestion. If plasma level falls above the lower treatment line on the acetaminophen overdose nomogram, acetylcysteine therapy should be continued. Liver function studies should be obtained initially and repeated at 24-hour intervals.

Serious toxicity or fatalities are extremely infrequent in children, possibly due to differences in the way they metabolize acetaminophen. In children, the maximum potential amount ingested can be more easily estimated. If more than 150 mg/kg or an unknown amount was ingested, obtain a plasma acetaminophen level. The plasma acetaminophen level should be obtained as soon as possible, but no sooner than 4 hours following ingestion. If plasma level falls above the lower treatment line on the acetaminophen overdose nomogram, the acetylcysteine therapy should be initiated and continued for a full course of therapy. If plasma acetaminophen assay capability is not available, and the estimated acetaminophen ingestion exceeds 150 mg/kg, acetylcysteine therapy should be initiated and continued for a full course of therapy.

For additional emergency information, call your regional poison center or call the Rocky Mountain Poison Center toll-free, (1-800-525-6115).

Symptoms from pseudoephedrine overdose consist most often of mild anxiety, tachycardia and/or mild hypertension. Symptoms usually appear within 4 to 8 hours of ingestion and are transient, usually requiring no treatment.

Acute dextromethorphan overdose usually does not result in serious signs and symptoms unless massive amounts have been ingested. Signs and symptoms of a substantial overdose may include nausea and vomiting, visual disturbances, CNS disturbances, and urinary retention.

Chlorpheniramine toxicity should be treated as you would an antihistamine/anticholinergic overdose and is likely to be present within a few hours after acute ingestion.

Alcohol Information: *TYLENOL® COLD Medication No Drowsiness Formula and Multi-symptom Formula TYLENOL® COLD Medication:* Chronic heavy alcohol abusers may be at increased risk of liver toxicity from excessive acetaminophen use, although reports of this event are rare. Reports usually involve cases of severe chronic alcoholics and the dosages of acetaminophen most often exceed recommended doses and often involve substantial overdose. Professionals should alert their patients who regularly consume large amounts of alcohol not to exceed recommended doses of acetaminophen.

Inactive Ingredients: *TYLENOL® COLD No Drowsiness Formula:* **Caplets:** Cellulose, Corn Starch, Glyceryl Triacetate, Hydroxypropyl Methylcellulose, Iron Oxide Black, Magnesium Stearate, Sodium Starch Glycolate, Titanium Dioxide, Blue #1 and Yellow #10. **Gelcaps:** Benzyl Alcohol, Butylparaben, Castor Oil, Cellulose, Corn Starch, Edetate Calcium Disodium, Gelatin, Hydroxypropyl Methylcellulose, Magnesium Stearate, Methylparaben, Propylparaben, Sodium Propionate, Sodium Lauryl Sulfate, Sodium Starch Glycolate, Titanium Dioxide, Red #40 and Yellow #10.

Multi-Symptom Formula TYLENOL® COLD Medication: **Tablets:** Cellulose, Corn starch, Magnesium Stearate, Sodium Starch Glycolate Yellow #6 and Yellow #10. **Caplets:** Cellulose, Corn Starch, Glyceryl Triacetate, Hydroxypropyl Methylcellulose, Iron Oxide Black, Magnesium Stearate, Sodium Starch Glycolate, Titanium Dioxide, Blue #1 and Yellow #6 and #10.

How Supplied: *TYLENOL® COLD No Drowsiness Formula:* **Caplets** (colored white, imprinted "TYLENOL COLD") blister packs of 24. **Gelcaps** (colored red and tan, imprinted "TYLENOL COLD") blister packs of 24.

Multi-Symptom Formula TYLENOL® COLD Medication: **Tablets** (colored yellow, imprinted "TYLENOL Cold") blister packs of 24. **Caplets** (light yellow, imprinted "TYLENOL Cold") blister packs of 24.

Shown in Product Identification Guide, page 512

MULTI-SYMPTOM TYLENOL® COLD SEVERE CONGESTION

Description: EACH CAPLET contains acetaminophen 325 mg, dextromethorphan HBr 15 mg, guaifenesin 200 mg and pseudoephedrine HCl 30 mg.

Actions: Multi-Symptom *TYLENOL® COLD SEVERE CONGESTION Caplets* contains a clinically proven analgesic-antipyretic, decongestant, expectorant and cough suppressant. Acetaminophen produces analgesia by elevation of the pain threshold and antipyresis through action on the hypothalamic heat-regulating center. Acetaminophen is equal to aspirin in analgesic and antipyretic effectiveness and is unlikely to produce many of the side effects associated with aspirin and aspirin-containing products. Pseudoephedrine is a sympathomimetic amine which provides temporary relief of nasal congestion. Guaifenesin is an expectorant which helps loosen phlegm (mucus) and thin bronchial secretions to make coughs more productive. Dextromethorphan is a cough suppressant which provides temporary relief of coughs due to minor throat irritations that may occur with the common cold.

Indications: Multi-Symptom *TYLENOL® COLD SEVERE CONGESTION Caplets* provide temporary symptom relief without drowsiness of nasal congestion, chest congestion, coughing, sore throat, headaches, body aches and fever.

Directions: Adults and children 12 years of age and older: Take 2 caplets every 6–8 hours. Do not take more than 8 caplets in 24 hours, or as directed by a doctor. **Children 6–11 years of age:** Take 1 caplet every 6–8 hours. Do not take more than 4 caplets in 24 hours, or as directed by a doctor. **Children under 6 years of age:** Do not use this product in children under 6 years of age. This will provide more than the recommended dose (overdose) and could cause serious health problems.

Precautions: If a rare sensitivity reaction occurs, the drug should be discontinued. Although pseudoephedrine is virtually without pressor effect in normotensive patients, it should be used with caution in hypertensives.

Warnings: DO NOT USE IF CARTON IS OPENED OR IF A BLISTER UNIT IS BROKEN. Do not take for pain for more than 7 days or for fever for more than 3 days unless directed by a doctor. If pain or fever persists, or gets worse, if new symptoms occur, or if redness or swelling is present, consult a doctor because these could be signs of a serious condition. If sore throat is severe, persists for more than 2 days, is accompanied or followed by fever, headache, rash, nausea or vomiting, consult a doctor promptly. A persistent cough may be a sign of a serious condition. If cough persists for more than 1 week, tends to recur or is accompanied by fever, rash or persistent headache, consult a doctor. Do not take this product for persistent or chronic cough such as occurs with smoking, asthma, emphysema or if cough is accompanied by excessive phlegm (mucus) unless directed by a doctor. **Do not exceed recommended dosage.** If nervousness, dizziness, or sleeplessness occur, discontinue use and consult a doctor. Do not take this product if you have heart disease, high blood pressure, thyroid disease, diabetes or difficulty in urination due to enlargement of the prostate gland unless directed by a doctor. As with any drug, if you are pregnant or nursing a baby, seek the advice of a health professional before using this product. Keep this and all drugs out of the reach of children. In case of accidental overdose, contact a doctor or poison control center immediately. Prompt medical attention is critical for adults as well as for children even if you do not notice any signs or symptoms. Do not use with other products containing acetaminophen.

Alcohol Warning: If you consume 3 or more alcoholic drinks every day, ask your doctor whether you should take acetaminophen or other pain relievers/fever reducers. Acetaminophen may cause liver damage.

Drug Interaction Precaution: Do not use this product if you are now taking a prescription monoamine oxidase inhibitor (MAOI) (certain drugs for depression, psychiatric or emotional conditions, or Parkinson's disease), or for 2 weeks after stoppping the MAOI drug. If you are uncertain whether your prescription drug contains an MAOI, consult a health professional before taking this product.

PROFESSIONAL INFORMATION

Overdosage Information: Acetaminophen in massive overdosage may cause hepatic toxicity in some patients. In adults and adolescents, hepatic toxicity has rarely been reported following ingestion of acute overdoses of less than 7.5 to 10 grams. Fatalities are infrequent (less than 3–4% of untreated cases) and have rarely been reported with overdoses of less than 15 grams. In children, an acute overdosage of less than 150 mg/kg has not been associated with hepatic toxicity. Early symptoms following a potentially hepatotoxic overdose may include: nausea, vomiting, diaphoresis and general malaise. Clinical and laboratory evidence of hepatic toxicity may not be apparent until 48 to 72 hours postingestion. In adults and adolescents, regardless of the quantity of acetaminophen reported to have been ingested, administer acetylcysteine immediately if 24 hours or less have elapsed from the reported time of ingestion. For full prescribing information, refer to the acetylcysteine package insert. Do not await results of assays for plasma acetaminophen levels before initiating treatment with acetylcysteine. The following additional procedures are recommended: Promptly initiate gastric decontamination of the stomach. A plasma acetaminophen assay should be obtained as early as possible, but no sooner than four hours following ingestion. If plasma level falls above the lower treatment line on the acetaminophen overdose nomogram, acetylcysteine therapy should be continued. Liver function studies should be obtained initially and repeated at 24-hour intervals.

Serious toxicity or fatalities are extremely infrequent in children, possibly due to differences in the way they metabolize acetaminophen. In children, the maximum potential amount ingested can be more easily estimated. If more than 150 mg/kg or an unknown amount was ingested, obtain a plasma acetaminophen level. The plasma acetaminophen level should be obtained as soon as possible, but no sooner than 4 hours following ingestion. If plasma level falls above the lower treatment line on the acetaminophen overdose nomogram, the acetylcysteine therapy should be initiated and continued for a full course of therapy. If plasma acetaminophen assay capability is not available, and the estimated acetaminophen ingestion exceeds 150 mg/kg, acetylcysteine therapy should be initiated and continued for a full course of therapy.

For additional emergency information, call your regional poison center or call the Rocky Mountain Poison Center toll-free, (1-800-525-6115).

Symptoms from pseudoephedrine overdose consist most often of mild anxiety, tachycardia and/or mild hypertension. Symptoms usually appear within 4 to 8 hours of ingestion and are transient, usually requiring no treatment.

Acute dextromethorphan overdose usually does not result in serious signs and symptoms unless massive amounts have been ingested. Signs and symptoms of a substantial overdose may include nausea and vomiting, visual disturbance, CNS disturbances, and urinary retention.

Chlorpheniramine toxicity should be treated as you would an antihistamine/anticholinergic overdose and is likely to be present within a few hours after acute ingestion. Guaifenesin should be treated as a non-toxic ingestion.

Alcohol Information: Chronic heavy alcohol abusers may be at increased risk of liver toxicity from excessive acetaminophen use, although reports of this event are rare. Reports usually involve cases of severe chronic alcoholics and the dosages of acetaminophen most often exceed recommended doses and often involve substantial overdose. Professionals should alert their patients who regularly consume large amounts of alcohol not to exceed recommended doses of acetaminophen.

Inactive Ingredients: Carnauba Wax, Cellulose, Colloidal Silicon Dioxide, Corn Starch, Hydroxypropyl Methylcellulose, Iron Oxide, Povidone, Pregelatinized Starch, Propylene Glycol, Sodium Starch Glycolate, Stearic Acid, Titanium Dioxide, Triacetin, Blue #1, Yellow #6 and Yellow #10.

How Supplied: Caplets (colored buttery-tan, with green imprinted "TYLENOL COLD SC") in blister packs of 12 and 24.

©McN-PPC, Inc. '96   8702830

Shown in Product Identification Guide, page 512

**Maximum Strength
TYLENOL® FLU Medication
No Drowsiness Formula Gelcaps**

**Maximum Strength
TYLENOL® FLU NightTime
Medication Gelcaps**

**Maximum Strength
TYLENOL® FLU NightTime
Hot Medication Packets**

**Maximum Strength
TYLENOL® FLU NightTime
Liquid**

Product information for all dosage forms of TYLENOL FLU have been combined under this heading.

Description: Each *Maximum Strength TYLENOL® FLU Medication No Drowsiness Formula Gelcap* contains acetaminophen 500 mg, dextromethorphan hydrobromide 15 mg and pseudoephedrine hydrochloride 30 mg. Each *Maximum Strength TYLENOL® FLU NightTime Medication Gelcap* contains acetaminophen 500 mg, diphenhydramine hydrochloride 25 mg and pseudoephedrine hydrochloride 30 mg. Each packet of *Maximum Strength TYLENOL FLU NightTime Hot Medication* contains acetaminophen 1000 mg, diphenhydramine hydrochloride 50 mg and pseudoephedrine hydrochloride 60 mg. *Maximum Strength TYLENOL® FLU NightTime Liquid:* Each 30 mL (2 tablespoonsful) contains acetaminophen 1000 mg, dextromethorphan HBr 30 mg, doxylamine succinate 12.5 mg, and pseudoephedrine HCl 60 mg.

Actions: *Maximum Strength TYLENOL® FLU Medication No Drowsiness Formula* contains a clinically proven analgesic-antipyretic, decongestant and cough suppressant. Acetaminophen produces analgesia by elevation of the pain threshold and antipyresis through action on the hypothalamic heat-regulating center. Acetaminophen is equal to aspirin in analgesic and antipyretic effectiveness and it is unlikely to produce many of the side effects associated with aspirin and aspirin-containing products. Pseudoephedrine hydrochloride is a sympathomimetic amine which provides temporary relief of nasal congestion. Dextromethorphan is a cough suppressant which provides temporary relief of coughs due to minor throat irritations that may occur with the common cold.

Maximum Strength TYLENOL® FLU NightTime Medication and *Maximum Strength TYLENOL® FLU NightTime Hot Medication* contains the same clinically proven analgesic-antipyretic and decongestant as Maximum Strength TYLENOL FLU Medication No Drowsiness Formula along with an antihistamine. Diphenhydramine is an antihistamine which helps provide temporary relief of runny nose and sneezing. *Maximum Strength TYLENOL® FLU NightTime Liquid* contains the same clinically proven analgesic-antipyretic, decongestant and cough suppressant as Maximum Strength TYLENOL FLU Medication No Drowsiness Formula along with an antihistamine. Doxylamine succinate is an antihistamine which helps provide temporary relief of runny nose and sneezing.

Indications: *Maximum Strength TYLENOL® FLU Medication No Drowsiness Formula* provides temporary symptom relief without drowsiness of body aches, headaches, fever, sore throat, coughing and nasal congestion.

Maximum Strength TYLENOL® FLU NightTime Medication and *Maximum Strength TYLENOL® FLU NightTime Hot Medication* provide temporary

Continued on next page

Tylenol Flu—Cont.

symptom relief so you can rest of body aches, headaches, fever, sore throat, nasal congestion, and runny nose/sneezing *Maximum Strength TYLENOL® FLU NightTime Liquid:* for the temporary relief of: body aches and headache, coughing, nasal congestion, sore throat, runny nose/sneezing, and for the reduction of fever.

Directions: *Maximum Strength TYLENOL® FLU Medication No Drowsiness Formula:* **Adults and children 12 years of age and older:** Take 2 gelcaps every 6 hours. Do not take more than 8 gelcaps in 24 hours, or as directed by a doctor. **Children under 12 years of age:** Do not use this adult product in children under 12 years of age. This will provide more than the recommended dose (overdose) and could cause serious health problems.
Maximum Strength TYLENOL® FLU NightTime Medication: **Adults and children 12 years of age and older:** Take 2 gelcaps at bedtime. May repeat every 6 hours. Do not take more than 8 gelcaps in 24 hours, or as directed by a doctor. **Children under 12 years of age:** Do not use this adult product in children under 12 years of age. This will provide more than the recommended dose (overdose) and could cause serious health problems.
Maximum Strength TYLENOL® FLU NightTime Hot Medication: **Adults (12 years and older):** Dissolve one packet in 6 oz. cup of hot water. Sip while hot. Sweeten to taste, if desired. May repeat every 6 hours, not to exceed 4 doses in 24 hours. **Children under 12 years of age:** Do not use this adult product in children under 12 years of age. This will provide more than the recommended dose (overdose) and could cause serious health problems.
Maximum Strength TYLENOL® FLU NightTime Liquid: **Adults and children 12 years of age and older:** Take 2 Tablespoons (tbsp) in dose cup provided. May repeat every 6 hours. Do not use more than 4 times in 24 hours or as directed by a doctor. **Children under 12 years:** Do not use this adult product in children under 12 years of age. This will provide more than the recommended dose (overdose) and could cause serious health problems.

Precautions: *Maximum Strength TYLENOL® FLU Medication No Drowsiness Formula, Maximum Strength TYLENOL® FLU NightTime Medication, and Maximum Strength TYLENOL® FLU NightTime Hot Medication:* If a rare sensitivity reaction occurs, the drug should be stopped. Although pseudoephedrine is virtually without pressor effect in normotensive patients, it should be used with caution in hypertensives.

Warnings: *Maximum Strength TYLENOL® FLU Medication No Drowsiness Formula:* **Do not use if carton is opened or if a blister unit is broken.** Do not take for pain for more than 7 days

or for fever for more than 3 days unless directed by a doctor. If pain or fever persists, or gets worse, if new symptoms occur, or if redness or swelling is present, consult a doctor because these could be signs of a serious condition. If sore throat is severe, persists for more than 2 days, is accompanied or followed by fever, headache, rash, nausea or vomiting, consult a doctor promptly. A persistent cough may be a sign of a serious condition. If cough persists for more than 1 week, tends to recur or is accompanied by fever, rash or persistent headache, consult a doctor. Do not take this product for persistent or chronic cough such as occurs with smoking, asthma, emphysema or if cough is accompanied by excessive phlegm (mucus) unless directed by a doctor. **Do not exceed recommended dosage.** If nervousness, dizziness or sleeplessness occur, discontinue use and consult a doctor. Do not take this product if you have heart disease, high blood pressure, thyroid disease, diabetes, or difficulty in urination due to enlargement of the prostate gland unless directed by a doctor.
As with any drug, if you are pregnant or nursing a baby, seek the advice of a health professional before using this product. Keep this and all drugs out of the reach of children. In case of accidental overdose, contact a doctor or poison control center immediately. Prompt medical attention is critical for adults as well as for children even if you do not notice any signs or symptoms. Do not use with other products containing acetaminophen.
Maximum Strength TYLENOL® FLU NightTime Medication Gelcaps: **Do not use if carton is opened or if a blister unit is broken.** Do not take for pain for more than 7 days or for fever for more than 3 days unless directed by a doctor. If pain or fever persists, or gets worse, if new symptoms occur, or if redness or swelling is present, consult a doctor because these could be signs of a serious condition. If sore throat is severe, persists for more than 2 days, is accompanied by fever, headache, rash, nausea or vomiting, consult a doctor promptly. **Do not exceed recommended dosage.** If nervousness, dizziness, or sleeplessness occur, discontinue use and consult a doctor. May cause excitability, especially in children. Do not take this product, unless directed by a doctor, if you have a breathing problem such as emphysema or chronic bronchitis, or if you have glaucoma or difficulty in urination due to enlargement of the prostate gland. Do not take this product if you have heart disease, high blood pressure, thyroid disease, or diabetes unless directed by a doctor. May cause marked drowsiness; alcohol, sedatives and tranquilizers may increase the drowsiness effect. Avoid alcoholic beverages while taking this product. Do not take this product if you are taking sedatives or tranquilizers without first consulting your doctor. Use caution when driving a motor vehicle or operating machinery.

As with any drug, if you are pregnant or nursing a baby, seek the advice of a health professional before using this product. Keep this and all drugs out of the reach of children. In case of accidental overdose, contact a doctor or poison control center immediately. Prompt medical attention is critical for adults as well as for children even if you do not notice any signs or symptoms. Do not use with other products containing acetaminophen.
Maximum Strength TYLENOL® FLU NightTime Hot Medication: **Do not use if carton is opened or if foil packet is torn or broken.** Do not take for pain for more than 7 days or for fever for more than 3 days unless directed by a doctor. If pain or fever persists, or gets worse, if new symptoms occur, or if redness or swelling is present, consult a doctor because these could be signs of a serious condition. If sore throat is severe, persists for more than 2 days, is accompanied or followed by fever, headache, rash, nausea or vomiting, consult a doctor promptly. **Do not exceed recommended dosage.** If nervousness, dizziness, or sleeplessness occur, discontinue use and consult a doctor. May cause excitability especially in children. Do not take this product, unless directed by a doctor, if you have a breathing problem such as emphysema or chronic bronchitis, or if you have glaucoma or difficulty in urination due to enlargement of the prostate gland. Do not take this product if you have heart disease, high blood pressure, thyroid disease or diabetes unless directed by a doctor. May cause marked drowsiness; alcohol, sedatives and tranquilizers may increase the drowsiness effect. Avoid alcoholic beverages while taking this product. Do not take this product if you are taking sedatives or tranquilizers without first consulting your doctor. Use caution when driving a motor vehicle or operating machinery.
As with any drug, if you are pregnant or nursing a baby, seek the advice of a health professional before using this product. Keep this and all drugs out of the reach of children. In case of accidental overdose, contact a doctor or poison control center immediately. Prompt medical attention is critical for adults as well as for children even if you do not notice any signs or symptoms. Do not use with other products containing acetaminophen.
PHENYLKETONURICS: CONTAINS PHENYLALANINE 67 MG PER PACKET.
Maximum Strength TYLENOL® FLU NightTime Liquid:
Do not take for pain for more than 7 days or for fever for more than 3 days unless directed by a doctor. If pain or fever persists, or gets worse, if new symptoms occur, or if redness or swelling is present, consult a doctor because these could be signs of a serious condition. If sore throat is severe, persists for more than 2 days, is accompanied or followed by fever, headache, rash, nausea, or vomiting, consult a doctor promptly. A persistent cough may be a sign of a serious condi-

tion. If cough persists for more than 1 week, tends to recur or is accompanied by fever, rash or persistent headache, consult a doctor. Do not take this product for persistent or chronic cough such as occurs with smoking, asthma, or emphysema or if cough is accompanied by excessive phlegm (mucus) unless directed by a doctor.

Do not exceed recommended dosage. If nervousness, dizziness or sleeplessness occur, discontinue use and consult a doctor. May cause excitability especially in children.

Do not take this product, unless directed by a doctor, if you have a breathing problem such as emphysema or chronic bronchitis, or if you have glaucoma or difficulty in urination due to enlargement of the prostate gland. Do not take this product if you have heart disease, high blood pressure, thyroid disease or diabetes unless directed by a doctor.

May cause marked drowsiness; alcohol, sedatives and tranquilizers may increase the drowsiness effect. Avoid alcoholic beverages while taking this product. Do not take this product if you are taking sedatives or tranquilizers, without first consulting your doctor. Use caution when driving a motor vehicle or operating machinery.

Keep this and all drugs out of the reach of children. In case of accidental overdose, contact a doctor or poison control center immediately. Prompt medical attention is critical for adults as well as for children even if you do not notice any signs or symptoms. As with any drug, if you are pregnant or nursing a baby, seek the advice of a health professional before using this product. Do not use with other products containing acetaminophen.

DO NOT USE IF CARTON IS OPENED OR IF BOTTLE WRAP OR FOIL INNER SEAL IMPRINTED "SAFETY SEAL®" IS BROKEN OR MISSING.

Alcohol Warning: *Maximum Strength TYLENOL® FLU Medication No Drowsiness Formula, Maximum Strength TYLENOL® FLU NightTime Medication, Maximum Strength TYLENOL® FLU NightTime Hot Medication and Maximum Strength TYLENOL® FLU NightTime Liquid:* If you consume 3 or more alcoholic drinks every day, ask your doctor whether you should take acetaminophen or other pain relievers/fever reducers. Acetaminophen may cause liver damage.

Drug Interaction Precaution: *Maximum Strength TYLENOL® FLU Medication No Drowsiness Formula, Maximum Strength TYLENOL® FLU NightTime Medication, Maximum Strength TYLENOL® FLU NightTime Hot Medication and Maximum Strength TYLENOL® FLU NightTime Liquid:* Do not use this product if you are now taking a prescription monoamine oxidase inhibitor (MAOI) (certain drugs for depression, psychiatric or emotional conditions, or Parkinson's disease), or for 2 weeks after stopping the MAOI drug. If you are un-

certain whether your prescription drug contains an MAOI, consult a health professional before taking this product.

PROFESSIONAL INFORMATION

Overdosage Information: *Maximum Strength TYLENOL® FLU Medication No Drowsiness Formula, Maximum Strength TYLENOL® FLU NightTime Medication, Maximum Strength TYLENOL® FLU NightTime Hot Medication and Maximum Strength TYLENOL® FLU NightTime Liquid:* Acetaminophen in massive overdosage may cause hepatic toxicity in some patients. In adults and adolescents, hepatic toxicity has rarely been reported following ingestion of acute overdoses of less than 7.5 to 10 grams. Fatalities are infrequent (less than 3–4% of untreated cases) and have rarely been reported with overdosage of less than 15 grams. In children, an acute overdosage of less than 150 mg/kg has not been associated with hepatic toxicity.

Early symptoms following a potentially hepatotoxic overdose may include: nausea, vomiting, diaphoresis and general malaise. Clinical and laboratory evidence of hepatic toxicity may not be apparent until 48 to 72 hours postingestion. In adults and adolescents, regardless of the quantity of acetaminophen reported to have been ingested, administer acetylcysteine immediately if 24 hours or less have elapsed from the reported time of ingestion. For full prescribing information, refer to the acetylcysteine package insert. Do not await results of assays for plasma acetaminophen levels before initiating treatment with acetylcysteine. The following additional procedures are recommended: Promptly initiate gastric decontamination of the stomach. A plasma acetaminophen assay should be obtained as early as possible, but not sooner than four hours following ingestion. If plasma level falls above the lower treatment line on the acetaminophen overdose nomogram, acetylcysteine therapy should be continued. Liver function studies should be obtained initially and repeated at 24-hour intervals.

Serious toxicity or fatalities are extremely infrequent in children, possibly due to differences in the way they metabolize acetaminophen. In children, the maximum potential amount ingested can be more easily estimated. If more than 150 mg/kg or an unknown amount was ingested, obtain an plasma acetaminophen level. The plasma acetaminophen level should be obtained as soon as possible, but no sooner than 4 hours following ingestion. If plasma level falls above the lower treatment line on the acetaminophen overdose nomogram, the acetylcysteine therapy should be initiated and continued for a full course of therapy. If plasma acetaminophen assay capability is not available, and the estimated acetaminophen ingestion exceeds 150 mg/kg, acetylcysteine therapy should be initiated and continued for a full course of therapy.

For additional emergency information, call your regional poison center or call the Rocky Mountain Poison Center toll-free, (1-800-525-6115).

Symptoms from pseudoephedrine overdose consist most often of mild anxiety, tachycardia and/or mild hypertension. Symptoms usually appear within 4 to 8 hours of ingestion and are transient, usually requiring no treatment.

Acute dextromethorphan overdose usually does not result in serious signs and symptoms unless massive amounts have been ingested. Signs and symptoms of a substantial overdose may include nausea and vomiting, visual disturbances, CNS disturbances, and urinary retention.

Diphenhydramine and doxylamine toxicity should be treated as you would an antihistamine/anticholinergic overdose and is likely to be present within a few hours after acute ingestion.

Alcohol Information: *Maximum Strength TYLENOL® FLU Medication No Drowsiness Formula, Maximum Strength TYLENOL® FLU NightTime Medication, Maximum Strength TYLENOL® FLU NightTime Hot Medication, and Maximum Strength TYLENOL® FLU NightTime Liquid:* Chronic heavy alcohol abusers may be at increased risk of liver toxicity from excessive acetaminophen use, although reports of this event are rare. Reports usually involve cases of severe chronic alcoholics and the dosages of acetaminophen most often exceed recommended doses and often involve substantial overdose. Professionals should alert their patients who regularly consume large amounts of alcohol not to exceed recommended doses of acetaminophen.

Inactive Ingredients: *Maximum Strength TYLENOL® FLU Medication No Drowsiness Gelcaps:* Benzyl Alcohol, Butylparaben, Castor Oil, Cellulose, Corn Starch Edetate Calcium Disodium, Gelatin, Hydroxypropyl Methylcellulose, Iron Oxide Black, Magnesium Stearate, Methylparaben, Propylparaben, Sodium Lauryl Sulfate, Sodium Propionate, Sodium Starch Glycolate, Titanium Dioxide, Red #40 and Blue #1.

Maximum Strength TYLENOL® FLU NightTime Medication Gelcaps: Benzyl Alcohol, Butylparaben, Castor Oil, Cellulose, Corn Starch, Edetate Calcium Disodium, Gelatin, Hydroxypropyl Methylcellulose, Iron Oxide Black, Magnesium Stearate, Methylparaben, Propylparaben, Sodium Citrate, Sodium Lauryl Sulfate, Sodium Propionate, Sodium Starch Glycolate, Titanium Dioxide, D&C Red #28 and FD&C Blue #1.

Maximum Strength TYLENOL® FLU Hot Medication Packets: Ascorbic Acid (Vitamin C), Aspartame, Citric Acid, Flavors, Sodium Citrate, Sucrose, Yellow #10, Blue #1, Red #40, and Yellow #6. May Also Contain: Silicon Dioxide.

Maximum Strength TYLENOL® FLU NightTime Liquid: Citric Acid, Corn

Continued on next page

Tylenol Flu—Cont.

Syrup, D&C Red #33, FD&C Red #40, Flavors, High Fructose Corn Syrup, Polyethylene Glycol, Propylene Glycol, Purified Water, Saccharin Sodium, Sodium Benzoate, Sorbitol.

How Supplied: *Maximum Strength TYLENOL® FLU Medication No Drowsiness Formula:* **Gelcaps** (colored burgundy and white, imprinted "TYLENOL FLU") in blister packs of 10 and 20.
Maximum Strength TYLENOL® FLU NightTime Medication: **Gelcaps** (colored blue and white, imprinted "TYLENOL FLU NT") in blister packs of 10 and 20.
Maximum Strength TYLENOL® FLU Hot Medication Packets: **Packets of powder** (yellow colored) in cartons of 6 tamper-evident foil packets.
Maximum Strength TYLENOL® FLU NightTime Liquid: red-colored liquid in 8 oz bottle with child resistant safety cap and tamper evident packaging.

Shown in Product Identification Guide, page 512

**Extra Strength
TYLENOL® PM
Pain Reliever/Sleep Aid Caplets, Geltabs and Gelcaps**

Description: Each *Extra Strength TYLENOL® PM Caplet, Geltab* or *Gelcap* contains acetaminophen 500 mg and diphenhydramine HCl 25 mg.

Actions: *Extra Strength TYLENOL® PM Caplets, Geltabs* and *Gelcaps* contain a clinically proven analgesic-antipyretic and an antihistamine. Maximum allowable non-prescription levels of acetaminophen and diphenhydramine provide temporary relief of occasional headaches and minor aches and pains accompanying sleeplessness. Acetaminophen is equal to aspirin in analgesic and antipyretic effectiveness and it is unlikely to produce many of the side effects associated with aspirin containing products. Acetaminophen produces analgesia by elevation of the pain threshold. Diphenhydramine HCl is an antihistamine with sedative properties.

Uses: *Extra Strength TYLENOL® PM Caplets, Geltabs* and *Gelcaps* provide temporary relief of occasional headaches and minor aches and pains with accompanying sleeplessness.

Precautions: If a rare sensitivity reaction occurs, the drug should be discontinued.

Directions: Adults and children 12 years of age and older: Take 2 caplets, geltabs or gelcaps at bedtime or as directed by a doctor. **Children under 12 years of age:** Do not use this adult product in children under 12 years of age. This will provide more than the recommended dose (overdose) and could cause serious health problems.

Warnings: Do not use if carton is opened or neck wrap or foil inner seal imprinted with "Safety Seal®" is broken. If sleeplessness persists continuously for more than 2 weeks, consult your doctor. Insomnia may be a symptom of serious underlying medical illness. Do not take for pain for more than 10 days or for fever for more than 3 days unless directed by a doctor. If pain or fever persists, or gets worse, if new symptoms occur, or if redness or swelling is present, consult a doctor because these could be signs of a serious condition. Do not take this product, unless directed by a doctor, if you have a breathing problem such as emphysema or chronic bronchitis, or if you have glaucoma or difficulty in urination due to enlargement of the prostate gland. Avoid alcoholic beverages while taking this product. Do not take this product if you are taking sedatives or tranquilizers without first consulting your doctor. **Do not exceed recommended dose.** Keep this and all drugs out of the reach of children. In case of accidental overdose, contact a doctor or poison control center immediately. Prompt medical attention is critical for adults as well as for children even if you do not notice any signs or symptoms. As with any drug, if you are pregnant or nursing a baby, seek the advice of a health professional before using this product. Do not use with other products containing acetaminophen.

CAUTION: This product will cause drowsiness. **Do not drive a motor vehicle or operate machinery after use.**

Alcohol Warning: If you consume 3 or more alcoholic drinks every day, ask your doctor whether you should take acetaminophen or other pain relievers/fever reducers. Acetaminophen may cause liver damage.

PROFESSIONAL INFORMATION

Overdosage Information: Acetaminophen in massive overdosage may cause hepatic toxicity in some patients. In adults and adolescents, hepatic toxicity has rarely been reported following ingestion of acute overdoses of less than 7.5 to 10 grams. Fatalities are infrequent (less than 3–4% of untreated cases) and have rarely been reported with overdoses of less than 15 grams. In children, an acute overdosage of less than 150 mg/kg has not been associated with hepatic toxicity. Early symptoms following a potentially hepatotoxic overdose may include: nausea, vomiting, diaphoresis and general malaise. Clinical and laboratory evidence of hepatic toxicity may not be apparent until 48 to 72 hours postingestion.
In adults and adolescents, regardless of the quantity of acetaminophen reported to have been ingested, administer acetylcysteine immediately if 24 hours or less have elapsed from the reported time of ingestion. For full prescribing information, refer to the acetylcysteine package insert. Do not await results of assays for plasma acetaminophen levels before initiating treatment with acetylcysteine. The following additional procedures are recommended: Promptly initiate gastric decontamination of the stomach. A plasma acetaminophen assay should be obtained as early as possible, but no sooner than four hours following ingestion. If plasma level falls above the lower treatment line on the acetaminophen overdose nomogram, acetylcysteine therapy should be continued. Liver function studies should be obtained initially and repeated at 24-hour intervals.

Serious toxicity or fatalities are extremely infrequent in children, possibly due to differences in the way they metabolize acetaminophen. In children, the maximum potential amount ingested can be more easily estimated. If more than 150 mg/kg or an unknown amount was ingested, obtain a plasma acetaminophen level. The plasma acetaminophen level should be obtained as soon as possible, but no sooner than 4 hours following ingestion. If the plasma level falls above the lower treatment line on the acetaminophen overdose nomogram, the acetylcysteine therapy should be initiated and continued for a full course of therapy. If plasma acetaminophen assay capability is not available, and the estimated acetaminophen ingestion exceeds 150 mg/kg, acetylcysteine therapy should be initiated and continued for a full course of therapy.

For additional emergency information, call your regional poison center or call the Rocky Mountain Poison Center toll-free, (1-800-525-6115).

Diphenhydramine toxicity should be treated as you would an antihistamine/anticholinergic overdose and is likely to be present within a few hours after acute ingestion.

Alcohol Information: Chronic heavy alcohol abusers may be at increased risk of liver toxicity from excessive acetaminophen use, although reports of this event are rare. Reports usually involve cases of severe chronic alcoholics and the dosages of acetaminophen most often exceed recommended doses and often involve substantial overdose. Professionals should alert their patients who regularly consume large amounts of alcohol not to exceed recommended doses of acetaminophen.

Inactive Ingredients: Caplets: Cellulose, Cornstarch, FD&C Blue #1, FD&C Blue #2, Hydroxypropyl Methylcellulose, Magnesium Stearate, Polyethylene Glycol, Polysorbate 80, Sodium Citrate, Sodium Starch Glycolate, Titanium Dioxide.

Geltabs/Gelcaps: Benzyl Alcohol, Butylparaben, Castor Oil, Cellulose, Corn Starch, D&C Red #28, Edetate Calcium Disodium, FD&C Blue #1, Gelatin, Hydroxypropyl Methylcellulose, Magnesium Stearate, Methylparaben, Propylparaben, Sodium Citrate, Sodium Lauryl Sulfate, Sodium Propionate, Sodium Starch Glycolate, Titanium Dioxide.

How Supplied: Caplets (colored light blue imprinted "Tylenol PM") vials of 10 and tamper-evident bottles of 24, 50, 100, and 150.
Gelcaps (colored blue and white imprinted "TYLENOL PM") tamper-evident bottles of 24 and 50.
Geltabs (colored blue and white imprinted "TYLENOL PM") tamper-evident bottles of 24, 50, and 100.

Shown in Product Identification Guide, page 512

TYLENOL® SEVERE ALLERGY
Medication Caplets

Maximum Strength
TYLENOL® ALLERGY SINUS NIGHTTIME
Caplets

Maximum Strength
TYLENOL® ALLERGY SINUS
Caplets, Gelcaps and Geltabs

Product information for all dosage forms of TYLENOL ALLERGY have been combined under this heading.

Description: Each *TYLENOL® SEVERE ALLERGY Caplet* contains acetaminophen 500 mg, and diphenhydramine HCl 12.5 mg. Each *Maximum Strength TYLENOL® ALLERGY SINUS NightTime Caplet* contains acetaminophen 500 mg, pseudoephedrine HCl 30 mg, and diphenhydramine HCl 25 mg. Each *Maximum Strength TYLENOL® ALLERGY SINUS Caplet Gelcap and Geltab* contains acetaminophen 500 mg, chlorpheniramine maleate 2 mg, and pseudoephedrine HCl 30 mg.

Actions: *TYLENOL® SEVERE ALLERGY Caplets* contain a clinically proven analgesic-antipyretic and antihistamine. Acetaminophen produces analgesia by elevation of the pain threshold and antipyresis through action on the hypothalamic heat-regulating center. Acetaminophen is equal to aspirin in analgesic and antipyretic effectiveness, and it is unlikely to produce many of the side effects associated with aspirin and aspirin-containing products.
Diphenhydramine is an antihistamine which helps provide temporary relief of itchy, watery eyes, runny nose, sneezing, itching of the nose or throat due to hay fever or other respiratory allergies.
Maximum Strength TYLENOL® ALLERGY SINUS NightTime Caplets contain, in addition to the above ingredients, a decongestant, pseudoephedrine. Pseudoephedrine is a sympathomimetic amine which provides temporary relief of nasal and sinus congestion.
Maximum Strength TYLENOL® ALLERGY SINUS Caplets, Gelcaps and Geltabs contain acetaminophen, pseudoephedrine and the antihistamine, chlorpheniramine. Chlorpheniramine is an antihistamine which helps provide temporary relief of runny nose, sneezing and watery and itchy eyes.

Indications: *TYLENOL® SEVERE ALLERGY* provides effective temporary relief of itchy, watery eyes, runny nose, sneezing, sore or scratchy throat and itching of the nose or throat due to hay fever or other upper respiratory allergies.
TYLENOL® ALLERGY SINUS Night-Time and TYLENOL® ALLERGY SINUS provide effective temporary relief of runny nose, sneezing, itching of the nose or throat, and itchy, watery eyes due to hay fever or other upper respiratory allergies, nasal and sinus congestion, and sinus pain and headaches.

Precautions: *TYLENOL® SEVERE ALLERGY:* If a rare sensitivity reaction occurs, the drug should be stopped.
TYLENOL® ALLERGY SINUS Night-Time and *TYLENOL® ALLERGY SINUS:* If a rare sensitivity reaction occurs, the drug should be stopped. Although pseudoephedrine is virtually without pressor effect in normotensive patients, it should be used with caution in hypertensives.

Directions: *TYLENOL® SEVERE ALLERGY:* **Adults and children 12 years of age and older:** Take 2 caplets every 4–6 hours. Do not take more than 8 caplets in 24 hours, or as directed by a doctor. **Children under 12 years:** Do not use this adult product in children under 12 years of age. This will provide more than the recommended dose (overdose) and could cause serious health problems.
TYLENOL® ALLERGY SINUS Night-Time: **Adults and children 12 years of age and older:** Take 2 caplets at bedtime. May repeat every 4–6 hours. Do not take more than 8 caplets in 24 hours, or as directed by a doctor. **Children under 12 years:** Do not use this adult product in children under 12 years of age. This will provide more than the recommended dose (overdose) and could cause serious health problems.
TYLENOL® ALLERGY SINUS: **Adults and children 12 years of age and older:** Take two every 4–6 hours. Do not take more than 8 in 24 hours, or as directed by a doctor. **Children under 12 years:** Do not use this adult product in children under 12 years of age. This will provide more than the recommended dose (overdose) and could cause serious health problems.

Warnings: *TYLENOL® SEVERE ALLERGY:* **DO NOT USE IF CARTON IS OPEN OR IF A BLISTER UNIT IS BROKEN.** Do not take for pain for more than 10 days or for fever for more than 3 days unless directed by a doctor. If pain or fever persists, or gets worse, if new symptoms occur, or if redness or swelling is present, consult a doctor because these could be signs of a serious condition. If sore throat is severe, persists for more than 2 days, is accompanied or followed by fever, headache, rash, nausea or vomiting, consult a doctor promptly. May cause excitability especially in children. Do not take this product, unless directed

by a doctor, if you have a breathing problem such as emphysema or chronic bronchitis, or if you have glaucoma or difficulty in urination due to enlargement of the prostate gland. May cause marked drowsiness; alcohol, sedatives and tranquilizers may increase the drowsiness effect.
Avoid alcoholic beverages while taking this product. Do not take this product if you are taking sedatives or tranquilizers without first consulting your doctor. Use caution while driving a motor vehicle or operating machinery. As with any drug, if you are pregnant or nursing a baby, seek the advice of a health professional before using this product. Keep this and all drugs out of the reach of children. In case of accidental overdose, contact a doctor or poison control center immediately. Prompt medical attention is critical for adults as well as for children even if you do not notice any signs or symptoms. Do not use with other products containing acetaminophen.
TYLENOL® ALLERGY SINUS Night-Time and TYLENOL® ALLERGY SINUS: **Do not use if carton is open or if a blister unit is broken.** Do not take for pain for more than 7 days or for fever for more than 3 days unless directed by a doctor. If pain or fever persists, or gets worse, if new symptoms occur, or if redness or swelling is present, consult a doctor because these could be signs of a serious condition. **Do not exceed recommended dosage.** If nervousness, dizziness or sleeplessness occur, discontinue use and consult a doctor.
May cause excitability, especially in children. Do not take this product unless directed by a doctor, if you have a breathing problem such as emphysema or chronic bronchitis, or if you have glaucoma or difficulty in urination due to enlargement of the prostate gland. Do not take this product if you have heart disease, high blood pressure, thyroid disease or diabetes unless directed by a doctor. May cause marked drowsiness; alcohol, sedatives and tranquilizers may increase the drowsiness effect. Avoid alcoholic beverages while taking this product. Do not take this product if you are taking sedatives or tranquilizers without first consulting your doctor. Use caution when driving a motor vehicle or operating machinery.
As with any drug, if you are pregnant or nursing a baby, seek the advice of a health professional before using this product. Keep this and all drugs out of the reach of children. In case of accidental overdose, contact a doctor or poison control center immediately. Prompt medical attention is critical for adults as well as for children even if you do not notice any signs or symptoms. Do not use with other products containing acetaminophen.

Alcohol Warning: If you consume 3 or more alcoholic drinks every day, ask your doctor whether your should take aceta-

Continued on next page

Tylenol Allergy—Cont.

minophen or other pain relievers/fever reducers. Acetaminophen may cause liver damage.

Drug Interaction Precaution: *TY-LENOL® ALLERGY SINUS NightTime and TYLENOL® ALLERGY SINUS:* Do not use this product if you are now taking a prescription monamine oxidase inhibitor (MAOI) (certain drugs for depression, psychiatric or emotional condition, or Parkinson's disease), or for 2 weeks after stopping the MAOI drug. If you are uncertain whether your prescription drug contains an MAOI, consult a health professional before taking this product.

PROFESSIONAL INFORMATION

Overdosage Information: Acetaminophen in massive overdosage may cause hepatic toxicity in some patients. In adults and adolescents, hepatic toxicity has rarely been reported following ingestion of acute overdoses of less than 7.5 to 10 grams. Fatalities are infrequent (less than 3–4% of untreated cases) and have rarely been reported with overdoses of less than 15 grams. In children, an acute overdosage of less than 150 mg/kg has not been associated with hepatic toxicity. Early symptoms following a potentially hepatotoxic overdose may include: nausea, vomiting, diaphoresis and general malaise. Clinical and laboratory evidence of hepatic toxicity may not be apparent until 48 to 72 hours postingestion. In adults and adolescents, regardless of the quantity of acetaminophen reported to have been ingested, administer acetylcysteine immediately if 24 hours or less have elapsed from the reported time of ingestion. For full prescribing information, refer to the acetylcysteine package insert. Do not await results of assays for plasma acetaminophen levels before initiating treatment with acetylcysteine. The following additional procedures are recommended: Promptly initiate gastric decontamination of the stomach. A plasma acetaminophen assay should be obtained as early as possible, but no sooner than four hours following ingestion. If plasma level falls above the lower treatment line on the acetaminophen overdose nomogram, acetylcysteine therapy should be continued. Liver function studies should be obtained initially and repeated at 24-hour intervals.

Serious toxicity or fatalities are extremely infrequent in children, possibly due to differences in the way they metabolize acetaminophen. In children, the maximum potential amount ingested can be more easily estimated. If more than 150 mg/kg or an unknown amount was ingested, obtain a plasma acetaminophen level. The plasma acetaminophen level should be obtained as soon as possible, but no sooner than 4 hours following ingestion. If plasma level falls above the lower treatment line on the acetaminophen overdose nomogram, the acetylcysteine therapy should be initiated and continued for a full course of

therapy. If plasma acetaminophen assay capability is not available, and the estimated acetaminophen ingestion exceeds 150 mg/kg, acetylcysteine therapy should be initiated and continued for a full course of therapy.

For additional emergency information, call your regional poison center or call the Rocky Mountain Poison Center toll-free (1–800–525–6115).

Symptoms for pseudoephedrine overdose consist most often of mild anxiety, tachycardia and/or hypertension. Symptoms usually appear within 4 to 8 hours of ingestion and are transient, usually requiring no treatment.

Diphenhydramine and chlorpheniramine toxicity should be treated as you would an antihistamine/anticholinergic overdose and is likely to be present within a few hours after acute ingestion.

Alcohol Information: Chronic heavy alcohol abusers may be at increased risk of liver toxicity from excessive acetaminophen use, although reports of this event are rare. Reports usually involve cases of severe chronic alcoholics and the dosages of acetaminophen most often exceed recommended doses and often involve substantial overdose. Professionals should alert their patients who regularly consume large amounts of alcohol not to exceed recommended doses of acetaminophen.

Inactive Ingredients: *TYLENOL® SEVERE ALLERGY Caplets:* Cellulose, Corn Starch, Hydroxpropyl Cellulose, Hydroxypropyl Methylcellulose, Iron Oxide Black, Magnesium Stearate, Polyethylene Glycol, Sodium Citrate, Sodium Starch Glycolate, Titanium Dioxide, Yellow #6 and Yellow #10.

TYLENOL® ALLERGY SINUS Night-Time Caplets: Cellulose, Corn Starch, Hydroxypropyl Methylcellulose, Iron Oxide Black, Magnesium Stearate, Polyethylene Glycol, Polysorbate 80, Sodium Citrate, Sodium Starch Glycolate, Titanium Dioxide, Blue #1, and Yellow #10.

TYLENOL® ALLERGY SINUS: Caplets: Carnauba Wax, Cellulose, Cornstarch, Hydroxypropyl Cellulose, Hydroxypropyl Methylcellulose, Iron Oxide Black, Magnesium Stearate, Polyethylene Glycol, Sodium Starch Glycolate, Titanium Dioxide, Blue #1, Yellow #6, and Yellow #10. **Gelcaps and Geltabs:** Benzyl Alcohol, Butylparaben, Castor Oil, Cellulose, Corn Starch, D&C Yellow No. 10, Edetate Calcium Disodium, FD&C Blue No. 1, FD&C Blue No. 2, Gelatin, Hydroxypropyl Methylcellulose, Magnesium Stearate, Methylparaben, Propylparaben, Sodium Lauryl Sulfate, Sodium Propionate, Sodium Starch Glycolate, Titanium Dioxide.

How Supplied: *TYLENOL® SEVERE ALLERGY:* **Caplets** (dark yellow, imprinted "TYLENOL Severe Allergy") blister packs of 12 and 24.

TYLENOL® ALLERGY SINUS Night-Time: **Caplets** (light blue, imprinted "TYLENOL A/S NightTime") child-resistant blister packs of 24.

TYLENOL® ALLERGY SINUS: **Caplets:** (dark yellow, imprinted "TYLENOL Allergy Sinus") Blister packs of 24 and 48. **Gelcaps and Geltabs:** (dark green and dark yellow, imprinted "TYLENOL A/S") Blister packs of 24 and 48.

Shown in Product Identification Guide, page 511 and 512

**Maximum Strength
TYLENOL® SINUS
Geltabs, Gelcaps, Caplets and Tablets**

**Maximum Strength
TYLENOL® SINUS
NightTime Caplets**

Description: Each *Maximum Strength TYLENOL® SINUS Geltab, Gelcap, Caplet or Tablet* contains acetaminophen 500 mg and pseudoephedrine hydrochloride 30 mg. Each *Maximum Strength TYLENOL® SINUS NightTime Caplet* contains acetaminophen 500 mg, doxylamine succinate 6.25 mg and pseudoephedrine HCl 30 mg.

Actions: *Maximum Strength TYLENOL® SINUS* contains a clinically proven analgesic-antipyretic and a decongestant. Maximum allowable nonprescription levels of acetaminophen and pseudoephedrine provide temporary relief of sinus headache and congestion. Acetaminophen is equal to aspirin in analgesic and antipyretic effectiveness and it is unlikely to produce many of the side effects associated with aspirin and aspirin-containing products.

Acetaminophen produces analgesia by elevation of the pain threshold and antipyresis through action on the hypothalamic heat-regulating center. Pseudoephedrine hydrochloride is a sympathomimetic amine which promotes sinus cavity drainage by reducing nasopharyngeal mucosal congestion.

Maximum Strength TYLENOL® SINUS NightTime Caplets contain, in addition to the above ingredients, an antihistamine which provides temporary relief of runny nose and itching of the nose or throat.

Indications: *Maximum Strength TYLENOL® SINUS* provides for the temporary relief of nasal and sinus congestion and sinus pain and headaches. *Maximum Strength TYLENOL® SINUS* is particularly well-suited in patients with aspirin allergy, hemostatic disturbances (including anticoagulant therapy), and bleeding diatheses (e.g., hemophilia) and upper gastrointestinal disease (e.g., ulcer, gastritis, hiatus hernia).

Maximum Strength TYLENOL® SINUS NightTime provides for the temporary relief of nasal congestion, sinus congestion and pressure, sinus pain, headache, runny nose, and itching of the nose or throat.

Precautions: If a rare sensitivity occurs, the drug should be discontinued. Although pseudoephedrine is virtually without pressor effect in normotensive patients, it should be used with caution in hypertensives.

Directions:
Maximum Strength TYLENOL® SINUS:
Adults and children 12 years of age and older: Take two every 4–6 hours. Do not take more than 8 in 24 hours, or as directed by a doctor. **Children under 12 years:** Do not use this adult product in children under 12 years of age. This will provide more than the recommended dose (overdose) and could cause serious health problems.
Maximum Strength TYLENOL® SINUS NightTime: **Adults and children 12 years of age and older:** Take 2 caplets at bedtime. May repeat every 4 to 6 hours. Do not take more than 8 caplets in 24 hours, or as directed by a doctor.
Children under 12 years: Do not use this adult product in children under 12 years of age. This will provide more than the recommended dose (overdose) and could cause serious health problems.

Warnings: *Maximum Strength TYLENOL® SINUS* Do not use if carton is opened or if blister unit is broken. Do not take for pain for more than 7 days or for fever for more than 3 days unless directed by a doctor. If pain or fever persists, or gets worse, if new symptoms occur, or if redness or swelling is present, consult a doctor because these could be signs of a serious condition. **Do not exceed recommended dosage.** If nervousness, dizziness or sleeplessness occur, discontinue use and consult a doctor. Do not take this product if you have heart disease, high blood pressure, thyroid disease, diabetes, or difficulty in urination due to enlargement of the prostate gland unless directed by a doctor. As with any drug, if you are pregnant or nursing a baby, seek the advice of a health professional before using this product. Keep this and all drugs out of the reach of children. In case of accidental overdose, contact a doctor or poison control center immediately. Prompt medical attention is critical for adults as well as for children even if you do not notice any signs or symptoms. Do not use with other products containing acetaminophen.
Maximum Strength TYLENOL® SINUS NightTime Caplets: Do not take for pain for more than 7 days or for fever for more than 3 days unless directed by a doctor. If pain or fever persists, or gets worse, if new symptoms occur, or if redness or swelling is present, consult a doctor because these could be signs of a serious condition. May cause excitability especially in children. If nervousness, dizziness or sleeplessness occur, discontinue use and consult a doctor. May cause marked drowsiness; alcohol, sedatives and tranquilizers may increase the drowsiness effect. Avoid alcoholic beverages while taking this product. Do not take this product if you are taking sedatives or tranquilizers, without first consulting your doctor. Use caution when driving a motor vehicle or operating ma-

chinery. Do not take this product, unless directed by a doctor, if you have a breathing problem such as emphysema or chronic bronchitis, or if you have glaucoma, or difficulty in urination due to enlargement of the prostate gland. Do not take this product if you have heart disease, high blood pressure, thyroid disease or diabetes unless directed by a doctor.
Do not exceed recommended dosage. Keep this and all drugs out of the reach of children. In case of accidental overdose, contact a doctor or poison control center immediately. Prompt medical attention is critical for adults as well as for children even if you do not notice any signs or symptoms. As with any drug. If you are pregnant or nursing a baby, seek the advice of a health care professional before using this product. Do not use with other products containing acetaminophen.

Alcohol Warning: If you consume 3 or more alcoholic drinks every day, ask your doctor whether you should take acetaminophen or other pain relievers/fever reducers. Acetaminophen may cause liver damage.

Drug Interactions Precaution: Do not use this product if you are now taking a prescription monoamine oxidase inhibitor (MAOI) (certain drugs for depression, psychiatric or emotional conditions, or Parkinson's disease), or for 2 weeks after stopping the MAOI drug. If you are uncertain whether your prescription drug contains an MAOI, consult a health professional before taking this product.

PROFESSIONAL INFORMATION
Overdosage Information: Acetaminophen in massive overdosage may cause hepatic toxicity in some patients. In adults and adolescents, hepatic toxicity has rarely been reported following ingestion of acute overdoses of less than 7.5 to 10 grams. Fatalities are infrequent (less than 3–4% of untreated cases) and have rarely been reported with overdoses of less than 15 grams. In children, an acute overdosage of less than 150 mg/kg has not been associated with hepatic toxicity. Early symptoms following a potentially hepatotoxic overdose may include: nausea, vomiting, diaphoresis and general malaise. Clinical and laboratory evidence of hepatic toxicity may not be apparent until 48 to 72 hours postingestion.
In adults and adolescents, regardless of the quantity of acetaminophen reported to have been ingested, administer acetylcysteine immediately if 24 hours or less have elapsed from the reported time of ingestion. For full prescribing information, refer to the acetylcysteine package insert. Do not await results of assays for plasma acetaminophen levels before initiating treatment with acetylcysteine. The following additional procedures are recommended: Promptly initiate gastric decontamination of the stomach. A plasma acetaminophen assay should be obtained as early as possible, but no

sooner than four hours following ingestion. If plasma level falls above the lower treatment line on the acetaminophen overdose nomogram, acetylcysteine therapy should be continued. Liver function studies should be obtained initially and repeated at 24-hour intervals.
Serious toxicity or fatalities are extremely infrequent in children, possibly due to differences in the way they metabolize acetaminophen. In children, the maximum potential amount ingested can be more easily estimated. If more than 150 mg/kg or an unknown amount was ingested, obtain a plasma acetaminophen level. The plasma acetaminophen level should be obtained as soon as possible, but no sooner than 4 hours following ingestion. If plasma level falls above the lower treatment line on the acetaminophen overdose nomogram, the acetylcysteine therapy should be initiated and continued for a full course of therapy. If plasma acetaminophen assay capability is not available, and the estimated acetaminophen ingestion exceeds 150 mg/kg, acetylcysteine therapy should be initiated and continued for a full course of therapy.
For additional emergency information, call your regional poison center or call the Rocky Mountain Poison Center toll-free (1-800-525-6115).
Symptoms from pseudoephedrine overdose consist most often of mild anxiety, tachycardia and/or mild hypertension. Symptoms usually appear within 4 to 8 hours after ingestion and are transient, usually requiring no treatment.
Doxylamine toxicity should be treated as you would an antihistamine/anticholinergic overdose and is likely to be present within a few hours after acute ingestion.
Alcohol Information: Chronic heavy alcohol abusers may be at increased risk of liver toxicity from excessive acetaminophen use, although reports of this event are rare. Reports usually involve cases of severe chronic alcoholics and the dosages of acetaminophen most often exceed recommended doses and often involve substantial overdose. Professionals should alert their patients who regularly consume large amounts of alcohol not to exceed recommended doses of acetaminophen.

Inactive Ingredients: *Maximum Strength TYLENOL® SINUS:* **Caplets:** Carnauba Wax, Cellulose, Corn Starch, Hydroxypropyl Methylcellulose, Magnesium Stearate, Polyethylene Glycol, Polysorbate 80, Sodium Starch Glycolate, Titanium Dioxide, Blue #1, Red #40, Yellow #10.
Tablets: Cellulose, Corn Starch, Magnesium Stearate, Sodium Starch Glycolate,. Blue #1, Yellow #6, and Yellow #10.
Gelcaps: Benzyl Alcohol, Butylparaben, Castor Oil, Cellulose, Corn Starch, Edetate Calcium Disodium, Gelatin, Hydroxypropyl Methylcellulose, Iron Oxide Black, Magnesium Stearate, Methylparaben, Propylparaben, Sodium Lauryl

Continued on next page

Tylenol Sinus—Cont.

Sulfate, Sodium Propionate, Sodium Starch Glycolate, Titanium Dioxide, Blue #1 and Yellow #10.

Geltabs: Benzyl Alcohol, Butylparaben, Castor Oil, Cellulose, Corn Starch, Edetate Calcium Disodium, Gelatin, Hydroxypropyl Methylcellulose, Iron Oxide Black, Magnesium Stearate, Methylparaben, Propylparaben, Sodium Lauryl Sulfate, Sodium Propionate, Sodium Starch Glycolate, Titanium Dioxide, D&C Yellow #10, FD&C Blue #1

Maximum Strength TYLENOL® SINUS NightTime Caplets: Cellulose, Cornstarch, FD&C Blue #1, FD&C Blue #2, Hydroxypropyl Methylcellulose, Iron Oxide, Silicon Dioxide, Sodium Starch Glycolate, Stearic Acid, Titanium Dioxide, Triacetin.

How Supplied: *Maximum Strength TYLENOL® SINUS:* **Tablets:** (colored light green, imprinted "Maximum Strength TYLENOL SINUS")—in blister packs of 24.
Caplets: (light green coating, printed "TYLENOL SINUS" in dark green) in blister packs of 24 and 48.
Gelcaps: (colored green and white), printed "TYLENOL SINUS" in blister packs of 24 and 48.
Geltabs: (colored green and white), printed "TYLENOL SINUS" in blister packs of 24 and 48.
Maximum Strength TYLENOL® SINUS NightTime Caplets: (teal green coating), printed "TYLENOL SINUS NT" in blister packs of 24.

Shown in Product Identification Guide, page 513

Medeva
Pharmaceuticals, Inc.
PO BOX 1710
ROCHESTER, NY 14603

Direct Inquiries to:
Customer Service Department
P.O. Box 1766
Rochester, NY 14603
(716) 274-5300
(888) 9–MEDEVA

DELSYM® Cough Formula
[del 'sĭm]
(dextromethorphan polistirex)
Extended-Release Suspension
12-Hour Cough Relief

Active Ingredient: Each teaspoonful (5 mL) contains dextromethorphan polistirex equivalent to 30 mg dextromethorphan hydrobromide.

Inactive Ingredients: Citric acid, ethylcellulose, FD&C Yellow No. 6, flavor, high fructose corn syrup, methylparaben, polyethylene glycol 3350, polysor-

bate 80, propylene glycol, propylparaben, purified water, sucrose, tragacanth, vegetable oil, xanthan gum.

Indications: Temporarily relieves cough due to minor throat and bronchial irritation as may occur with the common cold or inhaled irritants.

Warnings: Do not take this product for persistent or chronic cough such as occurs with smoking, asthma, or emphysema, or if cough is accompanied by excessive phlegm (mucus) unless directed by a physician. A persistent cough may be a sign of a serious condition. If cough persists for more than 1 week, tends to recur, or is accompanied by fever, rash, or persistent headache, consult a physician. As with any drug, if you are pregnant or nursing a baby, seek the advice of a health professional before using this product. **Keep this and all drugs out of the reach of children.** In case of accidental overdose, seek professional assistance or contact a Poison Control Center immediately.

Drug Interaction Precaution: Do not use this product if you are now taking a prescription monoamine oxidase inhibitor (MAOI) (certain drugs for depression, psychiatric or emotional conditions, or Parkinson's disease), or for 2 weeks after stopping the MAOI drug. If you are uncertain whether your prescription drug contains an MAOI, consult a health professional before taking this product.

Directions: Shake Bottle Well Before Using. Dose as follows or as directed by a physician.
Adults and Adolescents 12 years of age and over: 2 teaspoonfuls every 12 hours, not to exceed 4 teaspoonfuls in 24 hours.
Children 6 to under 12 years of age: 1 teaspoonful every 12 hours, not to exceed 2 teaspoonfuls in 24 hours.
Children 2 to under 6 years of age: $1/2$ teaspoonful every 12 hours, not to exceed 1 teaspoonful in 24 hours.
Pediatric Patients under 2 years of age: Consult a physician.

How Supplied: 89 mL (3 fl oz) bottles NDC 53014-842-61
Store at 15°–30°C (59°–86°F).
MEDEVA Pharmaceuticals
Medeva Pharmaceuticals, Inc.
Rochester, NY 14623 USA

UNKNOWN DRUG?
Consult the
Product Identification Guide
(Gray Pages)
for full-color photos of
leading over-the-counter
medications

Mission Pharmacal
Company
10999 IH 10 WEST
SUITE 1000
SAN ANTONIO, TX 78230-1355

Direct Inquiries to:
PO Box 786099
San Antonio, TX 78278-6099
TOLL FREE: (800) 292-7364
(210) 696-8400
FAX: (210) 696-6010
For Medical Information Contact:
In Emergencies:
George Alexandrides
(830) 249-9822
FAX: (830) 816-2545

THERA-GESIC®
[thĕr'ə-jē-zik]
(Methyl Salicylate 15%, Menthol 1%)
TOPICAL THERAPEUTIC ANALGESIC CREME

Description: THERA-GESIC® contains methyl salicylate and menthol in a rapidly absorbed greaseless base containing carbomer 934, dimethicone, glycerine, methylparaben, propylparaben, sodium lauryl sulfate, trolamine, and water.

Indications: For the temporary relief of minor aches and pains of muscles and joints associated with arthritis, simple backache, strains, sprains and sports injuries.

Warnings: FOR EXTERNAL USE ONLY. Use only as directed. Keep away from children to avoid accidental poisoning. Keep away from eyes, mucous membranes, broken or irritated skin. Do not use THERA-GESIC® if you have skin sensitive to oil of wintergreen (methyl salicylate). If skin irritation develops, if pain lasts 7 days or more, or if redness is present, discontinue use and consult a physician immediately. DO NOT SWALLOW. If swallowed induce vomiting, call a physician. Contact a physician before applying this medicine to children, including teenagers with chicken pox or flu.

Directions: ADULTS AND CHILDREN 12 OR MORE YEARS OF AGE: An application of THERA-GESIC® is the gentle massaging of several thin layers of creme into and around the sore or painful area. The number of thin layers controls the intensity of the action. One thin layer provides a mild effect, two thin layers provide a strong effect and three thin layers provide a very strong effect. Do not apply more than 3 to 4 times daily. Once THERA-GESIC® has penetrated the skin, the area may be washed, leaving it dry, clean and fragrance-free without decreasing the effectiveness of the products. IF YOU INTEND TO WRAP, BANDAGE OR COVER THE AREA WHERE YOU HAVE APPLIED THERA-GESIC®,

IT MUST BE WASHED THOROUGHLY TO AVOID EXCESSIVE IRRITATION. DO NOT USE A HEATING PAD AFTER APPLICATION OF THERA-GESIC®.

How Supplied:
NDC 0178-0320-03   3 oz. tube
NDC 0178-0320-05   5 oz. tube
Store at room temperature.

Novartis Consumer Health, Inc.
**560 MORRIS AVE.
SUMMIT, NJ 07901-1312**

Direct Product Inquiries to:
Consumer & Professional Affairs
(800) 452-0051
Fax: (800) 635-2801

Or write to above address.

ASCRIPTIN®
[ă "skrĭp 'tin]
**Regular Strength
Maximum Strength
Arthritis Pain**

**Analgesic
Aspirin buffered with Maalox®**

Active Ingredients: Regular Strength and Arthritis Pain Ascriptin®:
Each tablet/caplet contains Aspirin (325 mg), buffered with Maalox® (Alumina-Magnesia) and Calcium Carbonate.
Maximum Strength Ascriptin®:
Each caplet contains Aspirin (500 mg), buffered with Maalox® (Alumina-Magnesia) and Calcium Carbonate.

Inactive Ingredients: Regular Strength—carnauba wax, corn starch, croscarmellose sodium, FD&C Red No. 40 Aluminum Lake, granular sugar, hydroxypropyl methylcellulose, magnesium stearate, mannitol, microcrystalline cellulose, propylene glycol, sodium saccharin, sorbitol, talc, titanium dioxide.

Inactive Ingredients: Arthritis Pain—ammonium hydroxide, carnuba wax, corn starch, croscarmellose sodium, granular sugar, hydroxypropyl methylcellulose, iron oxide, magnesium stearate, mannitol, microcrystalline cellulose, propylene glycol, sodium saccharin, sorbitol, talc, titanium dioxide.

Inactive Ingredients: Maximum Strength—carnauba wax, corn starch, croscarmellose sodium, FD&C Blue No. 1 Aluminum Lake, granular sugar, hydroxypropyl methylcellulose, magnesium stearate, mannitol, microcrystalline cellulose, propylene glycol, sodium saccharin, sorbitol, talc, titanium dioxide.

Description: Ascriptin is an excellent analgesic, antipyretic agent for general use, and is buffered with Maalox®. Coated tablets/caplets make swallowing easy.

Indications: Regular Strength/Maximum Strength Ascriptin®: For the temporary relief of minor aches and pains associated with headaches, muscle aches, toothaches, menstrual cramps, and discomfort of the common cold. Also provides relief from the minor aches and pains of arthritis.
Arthritis Pain Ascriptin®: For effective temporary relief of minor aches and pains associated with arthritis. Also provides relief from the minor aches and pains associated with headaches, muscle aches, toothaches, menstrual cramps and discomfort of the common cold.

Directions: Regular Strength and Arthritis Pain Ascriptin®:
Adults: Two tablets/caplets with water every 4 hours while symptoms persist, not to exceed 12 tablets/caplets in 24 hours, or as directed by a doctor. Drink a full glass of water with each dose. **Children under 12 years of age:** Consult a doctor.
Maximum Strength Ascriptin®:
Adults: Two caplets with water every 6 hours while symptoms persist, not to exceed 8 caplets in 24 hours, or as directed by a doctor. Drink a full glass of water with each dose. **Children under 12 years of age:** Consult a doctor.

Warnings: Children and teenagers should not use this medicine for chicken pox or flu symptoms before a doctor is consulted about Reye's syndrome, a rare but serious illness reported to be associated with aspirin. Keep this and all drugs out of the reach of children. Do not take this product for pain for more than 10 days or for fever for more than 3 days unless directed by a doctor. If pain or fever persists or gets worse, if new symptoms occur, or if redness or swelling is present, consult a doctor because these could be signs of a serious condition. Do not take this product if you are allergic to aspirin or if you have asthma unless directed by a doctor. Do not take this product if you have stomach problems (such as heartburn, upset stomach, or stomach pain) that persist or recur, or if you have ulcers or bleeding problems, unless directed by a doctor. As with any drug, if you are pregnant or nursing a baby, seek the advice of a health professional before using this product. **IT IS ESPECIALLY IMPORTANT NOT TO USE ASPIRIN DURING THE LAST 3 MONTHS OF PREGNANCY UNLESS SPECIFICALLY DIRECTED TO DO SO BY A DOCTOR BECAUSE IT MAY CAUSE PROBLEMS IN THE UNBORN CHILD OR COMPLICATIONS DURING DELIVERY.** If ringing in the ears or loss of hearing occurs, consult a doctor before taking any more of this product. **In case of accidental overdose, seek professional assistance or contact a poison control center immediately.**

Drug Interaction Precaution: Do not use if taking a prescription drug for anticoagulation (blood thinning), diabetes, gout or arthritis unless directed by a doctor. Antacids may interact with certain prescription drugs. If you are presently taking a prescription drug, do not take this product without checking with your doctor or other health professional.

Alcohol Warning: If you consume 3 or more alcoholic drinks every day, ask your doctor whether you should take aspirin or other pain relievers/fever reducers. Aspirin may cause stomach bleeding.

Professional Labeling
For professional uses of this product, see Professional Labeling at the end of the product information for Ascriptin® enteric.

How Supplied: Regular Strength: Bottles of 100 tablets, 160 tablets, and 225 tablets. Bottles of 500 tablets without child-resistant closures.
Maximum Strength: Bottles of 50 caplets and 85 caplets.
Arthritis Pain: Bottles of 60 caplets, 100 caplets, and 225 caplets. Bottles of 500 caplets without child-resistant closures.
Shown in Product Identification Guide, page 513

ASCRIPTIN® enteric
**Pain Reliever
For Aspirin Therapy Users**

Ascriptin® enteric is enteric safety coated to help prevent the stomach upset caused by aspirin.

Active Ingredient: Regular Strength Ascriptin® enteric: Aspirin 325 mg. **Adult Low Strength Ascriptin® enteric:** Aspirin 81 mg.

Inactive Ingredients: Hydroxypropyl Methylcellulose, Methacrylic Acid Copolymer, Microcrystalline Cellulose, Polyethylene Glycol, Polysorbate 80, Pregelatinized Starch, Sodium Lauryl Sulfate, Talc, Titanium Dioxide, Triacetin. May also contain Carnauba Wax.

Indications: For the temporary relief of minor aches and pains associated with headaches, muscle aches, toothaches, and menstrual cramps. Ascriptin® enteric also provides relief from the minor aches and pains of arthritis.

Regular Strength Ascriptin® enteric

Directions: Adults: Two tablets every four hours while symptoms persist, not to exceed 12 tablets in 24 hours, or as directed by a doctor. **Children under 12 years of age:** Consult a doctor. Drink a full glass of water with each dose.

Adult Low Strength Ascriptin® enteric

Directions: Adults: 4–8 tablets every four hours while symptoms persist, not

Continued on next page

Information on Novartis Consumer Health, Inc., products appearing on these pages is effective as of November 1998.

Ascriptin Enteric—Cont.

to exceed 48 tablets in 24 hours, or as directed by a doctor. **Children under 12 years of age:** Consult a doctor. Drink a full glass of water with each dose.

Warnings: Children and teenagers should not use this medicine for chicken pox or flu symptoms before a doctor is consulted about Reye's syndrome, a rare but serious illness reported to be associated with aspirin. Keep this and all drugs out of the reach of children. Do not take this product for pain for more than 10 days or for fever for more than 3 days unless directed by a doctor. If pain or fever persists or gets worse, if new symptoms occur, or if redness or swelling is present, consult a doctor because these could be signs of a serious condition. Do not take this product if you are allergic to aspirin or if you have asthma unless directed by a doctor. Do not take this product if you have stomach problems (such as heartburn, upset stomach, or stomach pain) that persist or recur, or if you have ulcers or bleeding problems, unless directed by a doctor. As with any drug, if you are pregnant or nursing a baby, seek the advice of a health professional before using this product. **IT IS ESPECIALLY IMPORTANT NOT TO USE ASPIRIN DURING THE LAST 3 MONTHS OF PREGNANCY UNLESS SPECIFICALLY DIRECTED TO DO SO BY A DOCTOR BECAUSE IT MAY CAUSE PROBLEMS IN THE UNBORN CHILD OR COMPLICATIONS DURING DELIVERY.** If ringing in the ears or loss of hearing occurs, consult a doctor before taking any more of this product. **In case of accidental overdose, seek professional assistance or contact a poison control center immediately.**

Drug Interaction Precaution: Do not use if taking a prescription drug for anticoagulation (blood thinning), diabetes, gout, or arthritis unless directed by a doctor.

Alcoholic Warning: If you consume 3 or more alcoholic drinks every day, ask your doctor whether you should take aspirin or other pain relievers/fever reducers. Aspirin may cause stomach bleeding.

IMPORTANT: See your doctor before taking this product for your heart or for other new uses of aspirin, because serious side effects could occur with self treatment.

COMPREHENSIVE PRESCRIBING INFORMATION

Description: Regular Strength and Arthritis Pain Ascriptin®: Each tablet/ caplet contains the active ingredient aspirin (325 mg), buffered with Maalox® (alumina-magnesia) and calcium carbonate. Maximum Strength Ascriptin®: Each caplet contains the active ingredient, aspirin (500 mg), buffered with Maalox® (alumina-magnesia) and calcium carbonate. The inactive ingredients in these Ascriptin® products are: car-

nauba wax, hydroxypropyl methylcellulose, magnesium stearate, microcrystalline cellulose, propylene glycol, starch, talc, titanium dioxide, Regular Strength Ascriptin® enteric: Each table contains the active ingredient aspirin (325 mg). Adult Low Strength Ascriptin® enteric: Each tablet contains the active ingredient, aspirin (81 mg). The inactive ingredients in Ascriptin® enteric are: hydroxypropyl methylcellulose, methacrylic acid copolymer, microcrystalline cellulose, polyethylene glycol, polysorbate 80, pregelatinized starch, sodium lauryl sulfate, talc, titanium dioxide, triacetin. May also contain carnauba wax. All Ascriptin® products contain aspirin, a nonsteroidal anti-inflammatory analgesic, and are for oral administration for analgesic, antipyretic and anti-inflammatory use. Aspirin is an odorless white, needle-like crystalline or powdery substance. When exposed to moisture, aspirin hydrolyzes into salicylic and acetic acids, and gives off a vinegary-odor. It is highly lipid soluble and slightly soluble in water.

aspirin

Clinical Pharmacology: *Mechanism of Action:* Apririn is a more potent inhibitor of both prostaglandin synthesis and platelet aggregation than other salicylic acid derivatives. The differences in activity between aspirin and salicylic acid are thought to be due to the acetyl group on the aspirin molecule. This acetyl group is responsible for the inactivation of cyclooxygenase via acetylation.

Pharmacokinetics: *Absorption:* In general, immediate release aspirin is well and completely absorbed from the gastrointestinal (GI) tract. Following absorption, aspirin is hydrolyzed to salicylic acid with peak plasma levels of salicylic acid occurring within 1–2 hours of dosing (see **Pharmacokinetics**—*Metabolism*). The rate of absorption from the GI tract is dependent upon the dosage form, the presence or absence of food, gastric pH (the presence or absence of GI antacids or buffering agents), and other physiologic factors. Enteric coated aspirin products are erratically absorbed from the GI tract.

Distribution: Salicylic acid is widely distributed to all tissues and fluids in the body including the central nervous system (CNS), breast milk, and fetal tissues. The highest concentrations are found in the plasma, liver, renal cortex, heart, and lungs. The protein binding of salicylate is concentration-dependent, i.e., non-linear. At low concentrations (< 100 micrograms/milliliter (μg/mL)), approximately 90 percent of plasma salicylate is bound to albumin while at higher concentrations ($> 400\mu$g/mL), only about 75 percent is bound. The early signs of salicylic overdose (salicylism), including tinnitus (ringing in the

ears), occur at plasma concentrations approximating 200 μg/mL. Severe toxic effects are associated with levels $> 400\mu$g/mL. (See **Adverse Reactions** and **Overdosage**.)

Metabolism: Aspirin is rapidly hydrolyzed in the plasma to salicylic acid such that plasma levels of aspirin are essentially undetectable 1–2 hours after dosing. Salicylic acid is primarily conjugated in the liver to form salicyluric acid, a phenolic glucuronide, an acyl glucuronide, and a number of minor metabolites. Salicylic acid has a plasma half-life of approximately 6 hours. Salicylate metabolism is saturable and total body clearance decreases at higher serum concentrations due to the limited ability of the liver to form both salicyluric acid and phenolic glucuronide. Following toxic doses (10–20 grams (g)), the plasma half-life may be increased to over 20 hours.

Elimination: The elimination of salicylic acid follows zero order pharmacokinetics; (i.e., the rate of drug elimination is constant in relation to plasma concentration). Renal excretion of unchanged drug depends upon urine pH. As urinary pH rises above 6.5, the renal clearance of free salicylate increases from < 5 percent to > 80 percent.

Alkalinization of the urine is a key concept in the management of salicylate overdose. (See **Overdosage**.) Following therapeutic doses, approximately 10 percent is found excreted in the urine as salicylic acid, 75 percent as salicyluric acid, as the phenolic and acyl glucuronides, respectively.

Pharmacodynamics: Aspirin affects platelet aggregation by irreversibly inhibiting prostglandin cyclo-oxygenase. This effect lasts for the life of the platelet and prevents the formation of the platelet aggregating factor thromboxane A2. Non-acetylated salicylates do not inhibit this enzyme and have no effect on platelet aggregation. At somewhat higher doses, aspirin reversibly inhibits the formation of prostaglandin I_2 (prostacyclin), which is an arterial vasodilator and inhibits platelet aggregation.

At higher doses aspirin is an effective anti-inflammatory agent, partially due to inhibition of inflammatory mediators via cyclo-oxygenase inhibition in peripheral tissues. In vitro studies suggest that other mediators of inflammation may also be suppressed by aspirin administration, although the precise mechanism of action has not been elucidated. It is this non-specific suppression of cyclo-oxygenase activity in peripheral tissues following large doses that leads to its primary side effect of gastric irritation. (See **Adverse Reactions**.)

Clinical Studies: *Ischemic Stroke and Transient Ischemic Attack (TIA):* In clinical trials of subjects with TIA's due to fibrin platelet emboli or ischemic stroke, aspirin has been shown to significantly reduce the risk of the combined endpoint of stroke or death and the combined endpoint of TIA, stroke, or death by about 13–18 percent.

Suspected Acute Myocardial Infarction (MI): In a large, multi-center study of aspirin, streptokinase, and the combination of aspirin and streptokinase in 17,187 patients with suspected acute MI, aspirin treatment produced a 23-percent reduction in the risk of vascular mortality. Aspirin was also shown to have an additional benefit in patients given a thrombolytic agent.

Prevention of Recurrent MI and Unstable Angina Pectoris: These indications are supported by the results of six large, randomized, multi-center, placebo-controlled trials of predominantly male-post-MI subjects and one randomized placebo-controlled study of men with unstable angina pectoris. Aspirin therapy in MI subjects was associated with a significant reduction (about 20 percent) in the risk of the combined endpoint of subsequent death and/or nonfatal reinfarction in these patients. In aspirin-treated unstable angina patients the event rate was reduced to 5 percent from the 10 percent rate in the placebo group.

Chronic Stable Angina Pectoris: In a randomized, multi-center, double-blind trial designed to assess the roll of aspirin for prevention of MI in patients with chronic stable angina pectoris, aspirin significantly reduced the primary combined endpoint of nonfatal MI, fatal MI, and sudden death by 34 percent. The secondary endpoint for vascular events (first occurrence of MI, stroke, or vascular death) was also significantly reduced (32 percent).

Revascularization Procedures: Most patients who undergo coronary artery revascularization procedures have already had symptomatic coronary artery disease for which aspirin is indicated. Similarly, patients with lesions of the carotid bifurcation sufficient to require carotid endarterectomy are likely to have had a precedent event. Aspirin is recommended for patients who undergo revascularization procedures if there is a pre-existing condition for which aspirin is already indicated.

Rheumatologic Diseases: In clinical studies in patients with rheumatoid arthritis, juvenile rheumatoid arthritis, ankylosing spondylitis and osteoarthritis, aspirin has been shown to be effective in controlling various indices of clinical disease activity.

Animal Toxicology: The acute oral 50 percent lethal dose in rats is about 1.5 g/kilogram (kg) and in mice 1.1 g/kg. Renal papilary necrosis and decreased urinary concentrating ability occur in rodents chronically administered high doses. Dose-dependent gastric mucosal injury occurs in rats and humans. Mammals may develop aspirin toxicosis associated with GI symptoms, circulatory effects, and central nervous system depressioin. (See **Overdosage**.)

Indications And Usage: *Vascular Indications (Ischemic Stroke, TIA, Acute MI, Prevention of Recurrent MI, Unstable Angina Pectoris, and Chronic Stable Angina Pectoris):* Aspirin is indicated to:

(1) Reduce the combined risk of death and nonfatal stroke in patients who have had ischemic stroke or transient ischemia of the brain due to fibrin platelet emboli, (2) reduce the risk of vascular mortality in patients with a suspected acute MI, (3) reduce the combined risk of death and nonfatal MI in patients with a previous MI or unstable angina pectoris, and (4) reduce the combined risk of MI and sudden death in patients with chronic stable angina pectoris.

Revascularization Procedures (Coronary Artery Bypass Graft (CABG), Percutaneous Transluminal Coronary Angioplasty (PTCA), and Carotid Endarterectomy): Aspirin is indicated in patients who have undergone revascularization procedures (i.e., CABG, PTCA, or carotid endarterectomy) when there is a preexisting condition for which aspirin is already indicated.

Rheumatologic Disease Indications (Rheumatoid Arthritis, Juvenile Rheumatoid Arthritis, Spondyloarthropathies, Osteoarthritis, and the Arthritis and Pleurisy of Systemic Lupus Erythematosus (SLE)): Aspirin is indicated for the relief of the signs and symptoms of rheumatoid arthritis, juvenile rheumatoid arthritis, osteoarthritis, spondyloarthropathies, and arthritis and pleurisy associated with SLE.

Contraindications: *Allergy:* Aspirin is contraindicated in patients with known allergy to nonsteroidal anti-inflammatory drug products and in patients with the syndrome of asthma, rhinitis, and nasal polyps. Aspirin may cause severe urticaria, angioedema, or bronchospasm (asthma).

Reye's Syndrome: Aspirin should not be used in children or teenagers for viral infections, with or without fever, because of the risk of Reye's syndrome with concomitant use of aspirin in certain viral illnesses.

Warnings: *Alcohol Warning:* Patients who consume three or more alcoholic drinks every day should be counseled about the bleeding risks involved with chronic, heavy alcohol use while taking aspirin.

Coagulation Abnormalities: Even low doses of aspirin can inhibit platelet function leading to an increase in bleeding time. This can adversely affect patients with inherited (hemophilia) or acquired (liver disease or vitamin K deficiency) bleeding disorders.

GI Side Effects: GI side effects include stomach pain, heartburn, nausea, vomiting, and gross GI bleeding. Although minor upper GI symptoms, such as dyspepsia, are common and can occur anytime during therapy, physicians should remain alert for signs of ulceration and bleeding, even in the absence of previous GI symptoms. Physicians should inform patients about the signs and symptoms of GI side effects and what steps to take if they occur.

Peptic Ulcer Disease: Patients with a history of active peptic ulcer disease should

avoid using aspirin, which can cause gastric mucosal irritation and bleeding.

Precautions: General—*Renal Failure:* Avoid aspirin in patients with severe renal failure (glomerular filtration rate less than 10 mL/minute).

Hepatic Insufficiency: Avoid aspirin in patients with severe hepatic insufficiency.

Sodium Restricted Diets: Patients with sodium-retaining states, such as congestive heart failure or renal failure, should avoid sodium-containing buffered aspirin preparations because of their high sodium content.

Laboratory Tests: Aspirin has been associated with elevated hepatic enzymes, blood urea nitrogen and serum creatinine, hyperkalemia, proteinuria, and prolonged bleeding time.

Drug Interactions

Angiotensin Converting Enzyme (ACE) Inhibitors: The hyponatremic and hypotensive effects of ACE inhibitors may be diminished by the concomitant administration of aspirin due to its indirect effect on the renin-angiotensin conversion pathway.

Acetazolamide: Concurrent use of aspirin and acetazolamide can lead to high serum concentrations of acetazolamide (and toxicity) due to competition at the renal tubule for secretion.

Anticoagulant Therapy (Heparin and Warfarin): Patients on anticoagulation therapy are at increased risk for bleeding because of drug-drug interactions and the effect on platelets. Aspirin can displace warfarin from protein binding sites, leading to prolongation of both the prothrombin time and the bleeding time. Aspirin can increase the anticoagulant activity of heparin, increasing bleeding risk.

Anticonvulsants: Salicylate can displace protein-bound phenytoin and valproic acid, leading to a decrease in the total concentration of phenytoin and an increase in serum valproic acid levels.

Beta Blockers: The hypotensive effects of beta blockers may be diminished by the concomitant administration of aspirin due to inhibition of renal prostaglandins, leading to decreased renal blood flow, and salt and fluid retention.

Diuretics: The effectiveness of diuretics in patients with underlying renal or cardiovascular disease may be diminished by the concomitant administration of aspirin due to inhibition of renal prostaglandins, leading to decreased renal blood flow and salt and fluid retention.

Methotrexate: Salicylate can inhibit renal clearance of methotrexate, leading to bone marrow toxicity, especially in the elderly or renal impaired.

Continued on next page

Information on Novartis Consumer Health, Inc., products appearing on these pages is effective as of November 1998.

Ascriptin Enteric—Cont.

Nonsteroidal Anti-inflammatory Drugs (NSAID's): The concurrent use of aspirin with other NSAID's should be avoided because this may increase bleeding or lead to decreased renal function.

Oral Hypoglycemics: Moderate doses of aspirin may increase the effectiveness of oral hypoglycemic drugs, leading to hypoglycemia.

Uricosuric Agents (Probenecid and Sulfinpyrazone): Salicylates antagonize the uricosuric action of uricosuric agents.

Carcinogenesis, Mutagenesis, Impairment of Fertility: Administration of aspirin for 68 weeks at 0.5 percent in the feed of rats was not carcinogenic. In the Ames Salmonella assay, aspirin was not mutagenic; however, aspirin did induce chromosome aberrations in cultured human fibroblasts. Aspirin inhibits ovulation in rats. (See *Pregnancy.*)

Pregnancy: Pregnant women should only take aspirin if clearly needed. Because of the known effects of NSAID's on the fetal cardiovascular system (closure of the ductus arteriosus), use during the third trimester of pregnancy should be avoided. Salicylate products have also been associated with alterations in maternal and neonatal hemostasis mechanisms, decreased birth weight, and with perinatal mortality.

Labor and Delivery: Aspirin should be avoided 1 week prior to and during labor and delivery because it can result in excessive blood loss at delivery. Prolonged gestation and prolonged labor due to prostaglandin inhibition have been reported.

Nursing Mothers: Nursing mothers should avoid using aspirin because salicylate is excreted in breast milk. Use of high doses may lead to rashes, platelet abnormalities, and bleeding in nursing infants.

Pediatric Use: Pediatric dosing recommendations for juvenile rheumatoid arthritis are based on well-controlled clinical studies. An initial dose of 90–130 mg/kg/day in divided doses, with an increase as needed for anti-inflammatory efficacy (target plasma salicylate levels of 150–300 µg/mL) are effective. At high doses (i.e., plasma levels of greater than 200 mg/mL), the incidence of toxicity increases.

Adverse Reactions: Many adverse reactions due to aspirin ingestion are dose-related. The following is a list of adverse reactions that have been reported in the literature. (See **Warnings.**)

Body as a Whole: Fever, hypothermia, thirst.

Cardiovascular: Dysrhythmias, hypotension, tachycardia.

Central Nervous System: Agitation, cerebral edema, coma, confusion, dizziness, headache, subdural or intracranial hemorrhage, lethargy, seizures.

Fluid and Electrolyte: Dehydration, hyperkalemia, metabolic acidosis, respiratory alkalosis.

Gastrointestinal: Dyspepsia, GI bleeding, ulceration and perforation, nausea, vomiting, transient elevations of hepatic enzymes, hepatitis, Reye's Syndrome, pancreatitis.

Hematologic: Prolongation of the prothrombin time, disseminated intravascular coagulation, coagulopathy, thrombocytopenia.

Hypersensitivity: Acute anaphylaxis, angioedema, asthma, bronchospasm, laryngeal edema, urticaria.

Musculoskeletal: Rhabdomyolysis.

Metabolism: Hypoglycemia (in children), hyperglycemia.

Reproductive: Prolonged pregnancy and labor, stillbirths, lower birth weight infants, antepartum and postpartum bleeding.

Respiratory: Hyperpnea, pulmonary edema, tachypnea.

Special Senses: Hearing loss, tinnitus. Patients with high frequency hearing loss may have difficulty perceiving tinnitus. In these patients, tinnitus cannot be used as a clinical indicator of salicylism.

Urogenital: Interstitial nephritis, papillary necrosis, proteinuria, renal insufficiency and failure.

Drug Abuse and Dependence: Aspirin is non-narcotic. There is no known potential for addiction associated with the use of aspirin.

Overdosage: Salicylate toxicity may result from acute ingestion (overdose) or chronic intoxication. The early signs of salicylic overdose (salicylism), including tinnitus (ringing in the ears), occur at plasma concentrations approaching 200 µg/mL. Plasma concentrations of aspirin above 300 µg/mL are clearly toxic. Severe toxic effects are associated with levels above 400 µg/mL. (See **Clinical Pharmacology.**) A single lethal dose of aspirin in adults is not known with certainty but death may be expected at 30 g. For real or suspected overdose, a Poison Control Center should be contacted immediately. Careful medical management is essential.

Signs and Symptoms: In acute overdose, severe acid-base and electrolyte disturbances may occur and are complicated by hyperthermia and dehydration. Respiratory alkalosis occurs early while hyperventilation is present, but is quickly followed by metabolic acidosis.

Treatment: Treatment consists primarily of supporting vital functions, increasing salicylate elimination, and correcting the acid-base disturbance. Gastric emptying and/or lavage is recommended as soon as possible after ingestion, even if the patient has vomited spontaneously. After lavage and/or emesis, administration of activated charcoal, as a slurry, is beneficial, if less than 3 hours have passed since ingestion. Charcoal adsorption should not be employed prior to emesis and lavage.

Severity of aspirin intoxication is determined by measuring the blood salicylate level. Acid-base status should be closely followed with serial blood gas and serum pH measurements. Fluid and electrolyte balance should also be maintained.

In severe cases, hyperthermia and hypovolemia are the major immediate threats to life. Children should be sponged with tepid water. Replacement fluid should be administered intravenously and augmented with correction of acidosis. Plasma electrolytes and pH should be monitored to promote alkaline diuresis of salicylate if renal function is normal. Infusion of glucose may be required to control hypoglycemia.

Hemodialysis and peritoneal dialysis can be performed to reduce the body drug content. In patients with renal insufficiency or in cases of life-threatening intoxication, dialysis is usually required. Exchange transfusion may be indicated in infants and young children.

Dosage And Administration: Each dose of aspirin should be taken with a full glass of water unless patient is fluid restricted. Anti-inflammatory and analgesic dosages should be individualized. When apsirin is used in high doses, the development of tinnitus may be used as a clinical sign of elevated plasma salicylate levels except in patients with high frequency hearing loss.

Ischemic Stroke and TIA: 50–325 mg once a day. Continue therapy indefinitely.

Suspected Acute MI: The initial dose of 160–162.5 mg is administered as soon as an MI is suspected. The maintenance dose of 160–162.5 mg a day is continued for 30 days post-infarction. After 30 days, consider further therapy based on dosage and administration for prevention of recurrent MI.

Prevention of Recurrent MI: 75–325 mg once a day. Continue therapy indefinitely.

Unstable Angina Pectoris: 75–325 mg once a day. Continue therapy indefinitely.

Chronic Stable Angina Pectoris: 75–325 mg once a day. Continue therapy indefinitely.

CABG: 325 mg daily starting 6 hours post-procedure. Continue therapy for 1 year post-procedure.

PTCA: The initial dose of 325 mg should be given 2 hours pre-surgery. Maintenance dose is 160–325 mg daily. Continue therapy indefinitely.

Carotid Endarterectomy: Doses of 80 mg once daily to 650 mg twice daily, started presurgery, are recommended. Continue therapy indefinitely.

Rheumatoid Arthritis: The initial dose is 3 g a day in divided doses. Increase as needed for anti-inflammatory efficacy with target plasma salicylate levels of 150–300 µg/mL. At high doses (i.e., plasma levels of greater than 200 mg/mL), the incidence of toxicity increases.

Juvenile Rheumatoid Arthritis: Initial dose is 90–130 mg/kg/day in divided doses. Increase as needed for anti-inflammatory efficacy with target plasma salicylate levels of 150–200 µg/mL. At high doses (i.e., plasma levels of greater than 200 mg/mL), the incidence of toxicity increases.

Spondyloarthropathies: Up to 4 g per day in divided doses.

Osteoarthritis: Up to 3 g per day in divided doses.

Arthritis and Pleurisy of SLE: The initial dose is 3 g a day in divided doses. Increase as needed for anti-inflammatory efficacy with target plasma salicylate levels of 150–300 µg/mL. At high doses (i.e., plasma levels of greater than 200 mg/mL), the incidence of toxicity increases.

How Supplied: Refer to specific Ascriptin® products listed above.

Keep tightly closed in a dry place. Do not expose to excessive heat.

Store in a tight container at 25°C (77°F); excursions permitted to 15–30°C (59–86°F).

Do not use if the imprinted foil seal under the cap is broken or missing.

Questions? Call 1-800-548-3708, weekdays 9 am – 5 pm ET.

October 23, 1998

Shown in Product Identification Guide, page 513

CRUEX® ANTIFUNGALS
[kru 'ex]

Available in Prescription Strength varieties (see below)

Active Ingredients: *Spray Powder —* Miconazole nitrate 2%. *Cream*—Clotrimazole 1%.

Inactive Ingredients: *Spray Powder —*Aloe vera gel, aluminum starch octenylsuccinate, isopropyl myristate, propylene carbonate, SD alcohol 40-B (10% w/w), sorbitan monooleate, stearalkonium hectorite. Propellant: Isobutane/propane. *Cream —*Benzyl alcohol (1%), cetostearyl alcohol, cetyl esters wax, 2-octyldodecanol, polysorbate-60, sorbitan monostearate, purified water.

Indications: Cures jock itch (tinea cruris). Relieves itching and burning. Cruex powder also absorbs perspiration.

Warnings: Do not use on children under 2 years of age unless directed by a doctor. For external use only. Avoid contact with the eyes. If irritation occurs, or if there is no improvement within 2 weeks, discontinue use and consult a doctor. **Keep this and all drugs out of the reach of children.** In case of accidental ingestion, seek professional assistance or contact a poison control center immediately. Use only as directed. *For Spray only—*Avoid inhaling. Avoid contact with the eyes or other mucous membranes. Contents under pressure. Do not puncture or incinerate. Flammable mixture, do not use near fire or flame. Do not expose to heat or temperatures above 49°C (120°F). Use only as directed. Intentional misuse by deliberately concentrating and inhaling the contents can be harmful or fatal.

Directions: Clean the affected area and dry thoroughly. Apply a thin layer of the product over affected area twice daily (morning and night) or as directed by a doctor. (For Sprays: **Shake spray can well,** and hold 4″ to 6″ from skin when applying.) Supervise children in the use of these products. For jock itch, use daily for 2 weeks. If condition persists longer, consult a doctor. This product is not effective on the scalp or nails.

Important *(Cream)*: UNSCREW THE CAP. THE TUBE OPENING IS SEALED. DO NOT USE IF SEAL IS PUNCTURED OR NOT VISIBLE AND RETURN PRODUCT TO PLACE OF PURCHASE. TO PUNCTURE THE SEAL, REVERSE THE CAP AND PLACE THE PUNCTURE-TOP ONTO THE TUBE. PUSH DOWN FIRMLY UNTIL SEAL IS OPEN. TO CLOSE, SCREW THE CAP BACK ONTO THE TUBE.

How Supplied: *Spray Powder —*3 oz. aerosol container. *Cream —*0.5 oz. tube.' Store **spray powder** at room temperature, 15°–30°C (59°–86°F). See container bottom for lot number and expiration date. Spray powders: Tamper-resistant aerosol can for your protection. If clogging occurs, remove button and clean nozzle with pin.

Store **Cream** between 2° and 30° (36°–86°F). See box or tube crimp for lot number and expiration date.

CRUEX is a registered trademark of Novartis.

Shown in Product Identification Guide, page 513

DESENEX® ANTIFUNGALS
[dess 'i-nex]

Available in Prescription Strength (see below)

Active Ingredients: *Shake Powder, Spray Powder and Spray Liquid —*Miconazole nitrate 2%. *Cream —*Clotrimazole 1%.

Inactive Ingredients: *CREAM—*Benzyl alcohol (1%) as a preservative, cetostearyl alcohol, cetyl esters wax, 2-octyldodecanol, polysorbate-60, purified water, sorbitan monostearate.

*SHAKE POWDER—*Corn starch, corn starch/acrylamide/sodium acrylate polymer, fragrance, talc.

*LIQUID SPRAY—*Polyethylene glycol 300, polysorbate 20, SD alcohol 40-B (15% w/w).

PROPELLANT: Dimethyl ether.

*SPRAY POWDER—*Aloe vera gel, aluminum starch octenylsuccinate, isopropyl myristate, propylene carbonate, SD alcohol 40-B (10% w/w), sorbitan monooleate, stearalkonium hectorite.

PROPELLANT: Isobutane/propane.

*JOCK ITCH SPRAY POWDER—*Aloe vera gel, aluminum starch octenylsuccinate, isopropyl myristate, propylene carbonate, SD alcohol 40-B (10% w/w), sorbitan monooleate, stearalkonium hectorite.

PROPELLANT: Isobutane/propane.

Indications: Cures athlete's foot (tinea pedis), jock itch (tinea cruris) and ringworm (tinea corporis). For effective relief of the itching, cracking, and burning which can accompany these conditions. Desenex powders also help keep feet dry.

Warnings: Do not use on children under 2 years of age unless directed by a doctor. For external use only. Avoid contact with the eyes. If irritation occurs, or if there is no improvement in 4 weeks (for athlete's foot or ringworm), or within 2 weeks for jock itch, discontinue use and consult a doctor. **Keep this and all drugs out of the reach of children.** In case of accidental ingestion, seek professional assistance or contact a poison control center immediately. Use only as directed. *For Spray Powders and Spray Liquid —*Avoid inhaling. Avoid contact with the eyes or other mucous membranes. Contents under pressure. Do not puncture or incinerate. Flammable mixture, do not use near fire or flame. Do not expose to heat or temperatures above 49°C (120°F). Use only as directed. Intentional misuse by deliberately concentrating and inhaling the contents can be harmful or fatal.

Directions: Clean the affected area and dry thoroughly. Apply a thin layer of the product over affected area twice daily (morning and night) or as directed by a doctor. (For Sprays: **Shake Spray can well,** and hold 4″ to 6″ from skin when applying.) For athlete's foot, pay special attention to the spaces between the toes. Wear well-fitting, ventilated shoes and change shoes and socks at least once daily. For athlete's foot or ringworm, use daily for 4 weeks. For jock itch, use daily for 2 weeks. If condition persists longer, consult a doctor. Supervise children in the use of this product. This product is not effective on the scalp or nails.

Important *(For Cream)*: UNSCREW THE CAP. THE TUBE OPENING IS SEALED. DO NOT USE IF SEAL IS PUNCTURED OR NOT VISIBLE AND RETURN PRODUCT TO PLACE OF PURCHASE. TO PUNCTURE THE SEAL, REVERSE THE CAP AND PLACE THE PUNCTURE-TOP ONTO THE TUBE. PUSH DOWN FIRMLY UNTIL SEAL IS OPEN. TO CLOSE, SCREW THE CAP BACK ONTO THE TUBE.

How Supplied:
*Cream—*¹/₂ oz, .66 oz, 1 oz, 1.33 oz.
*Shake Powder—*1.5 oz, 3 oz, 4 oz.
*Spray Powder—*3 oz, 4 oz.
*Liquid Spray—*3.5 oz, 4.6 oz.
Store **powders/spray powders** and **Liquid sprays** at room temperature, 15°–

Continued on next page

Information on Novartis Consumer Health, Inc., products appearing on these pages is effective as of November 1998.

PROPELLANT: Isobutane/propane.

Desenex—Cont.

30°C (59°–86°F). For powders, see container bottom for lot number and expiration date. Spray powders: Tamper-resistant aerosol can for your protection. If clogging occurs, remove button and clean nozzle with pin.

Store **Cream** between 2° and 30° (36°–86°F). See box or tube crimp for lot number and expiration date.
DESENEX is a registered trademark of Novartis.

Shown in Product Identification Guide, page 513

REGULAR STRENGTH DOAN'S®
Analgesic Caplets

EXTRA STRENGTH DOAN'S®
Analgesic Caplets

Active Ingredient: Regular Strength Doan's: Each caplet contains Magnesium Salicylate Tetrahydrate 377 mg (equivalent to 303.7 mg of anhydrous Magnesium Salicylate). **Extra Strength Doan's:** Each caplet contains Magnesium Salicylate Tetrahydrate 580 mg (equivalent to 467.2 mg of anhydrous Magnesium Salicylate).

Also contains: Regular Strength Doan's: FD&C Blue #1 Aluminum Lake, FD&C Yellow #6 Aluminum Lake, FD&C Yellow #10 Aluminum Lake, Hydroxypropyl Methylcellulose, Magnesium Stearate, Microcrystalline Cellulose, Polyethylene Glycol, Polysorbate 80, Stearic Acid, Titanium Dioxide. **Extra Strength Doan's:** Hydroxypropyl Methylcellulose, Magnesium Stearate, Microcrystalline Cellulose, Polyethylene Glycol, Polysorbate 80, Stearic Acid, Titanium Dioxide.

Indications: For temporary relief of minor backache pain.

Directions: Regular Strength Doan's: Adults—Two caplets every 4 hours while symptoms persist, not to exceed 12 caplets during a 24-hour period or as directed by a doctor. Drink a full glass of water with each dose. Children under 12: consult a doctor. **Extra Strength Doan's:** Adults—Two caplets every 6 hours while symptoms persist, not to exceed 8 caplets during a 24-hour period or as directed by a doctor. Drink a full glass of water with each dose. Children under 12: consult a doctor.

Warnings: Children and teenagers should not use this medicine for chicken pox or flu symptoms before a doctor is consulted about Reye's Syndrome, a rare but serious illness. As with any drug, if you are pregnant or nursing a baby, seek the advice of a health professional before using this product. Do not take this product for pain for more than 10 days or for fever for more than 3 days unless directed by a doctor. If pain or fever persists or gets worse, if new symptoms occur, or if redness or swelling is present, consult a doctor because these could be signs of a serious condition. Do not take this product if you are allergic to salicylates (including aspirin), have stomach problems (such as heartburn, upset stomach, or stomach pain) that persist or recur, or if you have ulcers or bleeding problems, unless directed by a doctor. If ringing in the ears or a loss of hearing occurs, consult a doctor before taking any more of this product.
Keep this and all drugs out of the reach of children. In case of accidental overdose, seek professional assistance or contact a poison control center immediately.

Drug Interaction Precaution: Do not take this product if you are taking a prescription drug for anticoagulation (thinning of the blood), diabetes, gout, or arthritis unless directed by a doctor.

Alcohol Warning: If you consume 3 or more alcoholic drinks every day, ask your doctor whether you should take magnesium salicylate or other pain relievers/fever reducers. Magnesium salicylate may cause stomach bleeding.

How Supplied: Blister packages of 24 and 48 caplets.
Store at 15°–30°C (59°–86°F). Protect from moisture.

Extra Strength DOAN'S® P.M.
Magnesium Salicylate/Diphenhydramine
Analgesic/Nighttime Sleep Aid Caplets

Active Ingredients: Each caplet contains Magnesium Salicylate Tetrahydrate 580mg. (equivalent to 467.2mg. of anhydrous Magnesium Salicylate) and Diphenydramine HCl 25mg.

Also Contains: Carnauba Wax, Colloidal Silicon Dioxide, Croscarmellose Sodium, FD&C Blue #2 Aluminum Lake, Hydroxypropyl Methylcellulose, Magnesium Stearate, Microcrystalline Cellulose, Polyethylene Glycol, Polysorbate 80, Stearic Acid, Talc, Titanium Dioxide.

Indications: For temporary relief of minor back pain accompanied by sleeplessness.

Directions: Adults and children 12 years of age or older: Take 2 caplets at bedtime if needed, or as directed by a doctor. Drink a full glass of water with each dose.

Warnings: Children and teenagers should not use this medicine for chicken pox or flu symptoms before a doctor is consulted about Reye's syndrome, a rare but serious illness. **Keep this and all drugs out of the reach of children.** In case of accidental overdose, seek professional assistance or contact a poison control center immediately. Do not give this product to children under 12 years of age. As with any drug, if you are pregnant or nursing a baby, seek the advice of a health professional before using this product. Do not take this product for pain for more than 10 days or for fever for more than 3 days unless directed by a doctor. If pain or fever persists or gets worse, if new symptoms occur, or if redness or swelling is present, consult a doctor because these could be signs of a serious condition. If sleeplessness persists continuously for more than 2 weeks, consult your doctor. Insomnia may be a symptom of serious underlying medical illness. Do not take this product, unless directed by a doctor, if you have a breathing problem such as emphysema or chronic bronchitis, or if you have glaucoma, difficulty in urination due to enlargement of the prostate gland, stomach problems (such as heartburn, upset stomach, or stomach pain) that persist or recur, ulcers or bleeding problems, or if you are allergic to aspirin or salicylates. If ringing in the ears or a loss of hearing occurs, consult a doctor before taking any more of this product. Avoid alcoholic beverages while taking this product. Do not take this product if you are taking sedatives or tranquilizers without first consulting your doctor. **DO NOT USE with any other product containing diphenhydramine, including one applied topically.**

Drug Interaction Precaution: Do not take this product if you are taking a prescription drug for anticoagulation (thinning of the blood), diabetes, gout, or arthritis unless directed by a doctor.

Alcohol Warning: If you consume 3 or more alcoholic drinks every day, ask your doctor whether you should take magnesium salicylate or other pain relievers/fever reducers. Magnesium salicylate may cause stomach bleeding.

How Supplied: Blister packages of 20 caplets supplied in child-resistant packaging.
Store at 15°–30°C (59°–86°F). Protect from moisture.

DULCOLAX®
[dul 'co-lax]
**brand of bisacodyl USP
Tablets of 5 mg
Suppositories of 10 mg
Laxative**

Active Ingredients: Dulcolax Tablets-Bisacodyl USP 5 mg.
Dulcolax Suppositories-Bisacodyl USP 10 mg.

Inactive Ingredients: Dulcolax Tablets-acacia, acetylated monoglyceride, carnauba wax, cellulose acetate phthalate, corn starch, D&C Red No. 30 aluminum lake, D&C Yellow No. 10 aluminum lake, dibutyl phthalate, docusate sodium, gelatin, glycerin, iron oxides, kaolin, lactose, magnesium stearate, methylparaben, pharmaceutical glaze, polyethylene glycol, povidone, propylparaben, sodium benzoate, sorbitan monooleate, sucrose, talc, titanium dioxide, white wax. **Dulcolax Suppositories**-Hydrogenated vegetable oil.

Sodium Content: Tablets and suppositories contain less than 0.2 mg per dosage unit and are thus dietetically sodium free.

Indications: For the relief of occasional constipation and irregularity. Physicians should refer to the "Professional Labeling" section for additional indications and information.

Directions:
Tablets
Adults and children 12 years of age and over: Take 2 or 3 tablets (usually 2) in a single dose once daily.
Children 6 to under 12 years of age: Take 1 tablet once daily.
Children under 6 years of age: Consult a physician.
Expect results in 8–12 hours if taken at bedtime or within 6 hours if taken before breakfast.
Suppositories
Adults and children 12 years of age and over: 1 suppository once daily. Remove foil wrapper. Lie on your side and, with pointed end first, push suppository high into the rectum so it will not slip out. Retain it for 15 to 20 minutes. If you feel the suppository must come out immediately, it was not inserted high enough and should be pushed higher.
Children 6 to under 12 years of age: $^{1}/_{2}$ suppository once daily.
Children under 6 years of age: Consult a physician.
If the suppository seems soft, hold in foil wrapper under cold water for one or two minutes before use. In the presence of anal fissures or hemorrhoids, suppository may be coated at the tip with petroleum jelly before insertion.

Warnings: Do not use laxative products when abdominal pain, nausea, or vomiting are present unless directed by a physician. If you have noticed a sudden change in bowel habits that persists over a period of 2 weeks, consult a physician before using a laxative. Restoration of normal bowel function by using this product may cause abdominal discomfort including cramps. Laxative products should not be used for a period longer than 1 week unless directed by a physician. Rectal bleeding or failure to have a bowel movement after use of a laxative may indicate a serious condition. If this occurs, discontinue use and consult your physician. As with any drug, if you are pregnant or nursing a baby, seek the advice of a health care professional before using this product. **Keep this and all drugs out of the reach of children.** In case of accidental overdose or ingestion, seek professional assistance or contact a poison control center immediately. For tablets: Do not chew or crush. Do not give to children under 6 years of age unless directed by a physician. Do not take this product within 1 hour after taking an antacid or milk.

How Supplied: Dulcolax, brand of bisacodyl: Yellow, enteric-coated tablets of 5 mg in boxes of 10, 25, 50 and 100; suppositories of 10 mg in boxes of 4, 8, 16 and 50.

Store Dulcolax suppositories and tablets at temperatures below 77°F (25°C). Avoid excessive humidity.

Also Available: Dulcolax® Bowel Prep Kit. Each kit contains:
1 Dulcolax suppository of 10 mg bisacodyl;
4 Dulcolax tablets of 5 mg bisacodyl;
Complete patient instructions.

Professional Labeling

Description and Clinical Pharmacology: Dulcolax is a contact stimulant laxative, administered either orally or rectally, which acts directly on the colonic mucosa to produce normal peristalsis throughout the large intestine. The active ingredient in Dulcolax, bisacodyl, is a colorless, tasteless compound that is practically insoluble in water or alkaline solution. Its chemical name is: bis(p-acetoxyphenyl)-2-pyridylmethane. Bisacodyl is very poorly absorbed, if at all, in the small intestine following oral administration, nor in the large intestine following rectal administration. On contact with the mucosa or submucosal plexi of the large intestine, bisacodyl stimulates sensory nerve endings to produce parasympathetic reflexes resulting in increased peristaltic contractions of the colon. It has also been shown to promote fluid and ion accumulation in the colon, which increases the laxative effect. A bowel movement is usually produced approximately 6 hours after oral administration (8–12 hours if taken at bedtime), and approximately 15 minutes to 1 hour after rectal administration, providing satisfactory cleansing of the bowel which may, under certain circumstances, obviate the need for colonic irrigation.

Indications and Usage: For use as part of a bowel cleansing regimen in preparing the patient for surgery or for preparing the colon for x-ray endoscopic examination. Dulcolax will not replace the colonic irrigations usually given patients before intracolonic surgery, but is useful in the preliminary emptying of the colon prior to these procedures.
Also for use as a laxative in postoperative care (i.e., restoration of normal bowel hygiene), antepartum care, postpartum care, and in preparation for delivery.

Contraindications: Stimulant laxatives, such as Dulcolax, are contraindicated for patients with acute surgical abdomen, appendicitis, rectal bleeding, gastroenteritis, or intestinal obstruction.

Precautions: Long-term administration of Dulcolax is not recommended in the treatment of chronic constipation.

Dosage and Administration:
Preparation for x-ray endoscopy: For barium enemas, no food should be given following oral administration to prevent

reaccumulation of material in the cecum, and a suppository should be administered one to two hours prior to examination.
Children under 6 years of age: Oral administration is not recommended due to the requirement to swallow tablets whole. For rectal administration, the suppository dosage is 5 mg ($^{1}/_{2}$ of 10 mg suppository) in a single daily dose.

Shown in Product Identification Guide, page 513

EX–LAX® Chocolated Laxative Pieces

Active Ingredient: Sennosides, USP, 15mg

Use: For Relief of
• OCCASIONAL CONSTIPATION (IRREGULARITY). This product generally produces bowel movement in 6 to 12 hours.

Directions: Adults and children 12 years of age and over: chew 2 chocolated pieces once or twice daily. Children 6 to under 12 years of age: chew 1 chocolated piece once or twice daily. Children under 6 years of age: consult a doctor.

Warnings:
• as with any drug, if you are pregnant or nursing a baby, seek the advice of a health professional before using the product.
Unless directed by a doctor, do not use
• laxative products when abdominal pain, nausea, or vomiting is present.
• laxative products for a period longer than 1 week.
Consult a doctor before using a laxative if
• you have noticed a sudden change in bowel habits that persists over a period of 2 weeks.
Consult a doctor and stop using a laxative if
• rectal bleeding occurs or you fail to have a bowel movement after use because this may indicate a serious condition.
Keep this and all drugs out of the reach of children
In case of accidental overdose, seek professional assistance or contact a poison control center immediately.

Inactive Ingredients: cocoa, confectioners sugar, hydrogenated palm kernel oil, lecithin, non-fat dry milk, vanillin.

How Supplied: Available in boxes of 6, 18, 48, chewable chocolated pieces.

Shown in Product Identification Guide, page 513

Continued on next page

Information on Novartis Consumer Health, Inc., products appearing on these pages is effective as of November 1998.

EX–LAX® Laxative Pills
Regular Strength Ex-Lax®
Laxative Pills
Maximum Strength Ex-Lax®
Laxative Pills

Active Ingredients: Regular Strength Ex-Lax Laxative Pills—Sennosides, USP, 15 mg. **Maximum Relief Formula Ex-Lax Laxative Pills**—Sennosides, USP, 25 mg.

USE: For Relief of
- OCCASIONAL CONSTIPATION (IRREGULARITY). This product generally produces bowel movement in 6 to 12 hours.

WARNINGS:
- as with any drug, if you are pregnant or nursing a baby, seek the advice of a health professional before using this product.

Unless directed by a doctor, do not use
- laxative products when abdominal pain, nausea, or vomiting is present.
- laxative products for a period longer than 1 week.

Consult a doctor before using a laxative if
- you have noticed a sudden change in bowel habits that persists over a period of 2 weeks.

Consult a doctor and stop using a laxative if
- rectal bleeding occurs or you fail to have a bowel movement after use because this may indicate a serious condition.

Keep this and all drugs out of the reach of children. In case of accidental overdose, seek professional assistance or contact a poison control center immediately.

Dosage and Administration: Regular Strength Ex-Lax Laxative Pills, and Maximum Strength Ex-Lax Laxative Pills—Adults and children 12 years of age and over: take 2 pills once or twice daily with a glass of water. Children 6 to under 12 years of age: take 1 pill once or twice daily with a glass of water. Children under 6 years of age: consult a doctor.

Inactive Ingredients: Regular Strength Ex-Lax Laxative Pills—acacia, alginic acid, carnauba wax, colloidal silicon dioxide, dibasic calcium phosphate, iron oxides, magnesium stearate, microcrystalline cellulose, sodium benzoate, sodium lauryl sulfate, starch, stearic acid, sucrose, talc, titanium dioxide. Sodium-free. **Maximum Strength Ex-Lax Laxative Pills**—acacia, alginic acid, FD&C Blue No. 1 aluminum lake, carnauba wax, colloidal silicon dioxide, dibasic calcium phosphate, magnesium stearate, microcrystalline cellulose, povidone, sodium benzoate, sodium lauryl sulfate, starch, stearic acid, sucrose, talc, titanium dioxide. Sodium-free.

How Supplied: Regular Strength Ex-Lax Laxative Pills—Available in boxes of 8, 30, and 60 pills. **Maximum Strength Ex-Lax Laxative Pills**—Available in boxes of 24 and 48 pills.
Shown in Product Identification Guide, page 513

EX-LAX® STOOL SOFTENER CAPLETS
docusate sodium 100mg
stimulant-free
mild, natural-feeling relief
for sensitive systems

Active Ingredient: Docusate Sodium, 100 mg per caplet.

Indications: Relief of occasional constipation (irregularity), especially for sensitive systems. This gentle, stimulant-free formula generally works within 12–72 hours after the first dose.

Directions: Take Ex-Lax stool softener caplets with a glass of water at any time. Adults and children 12 years of age and over: 1 to 3 caplets daily as needed. Children 2 to under 12 years of age: 1 caplet daily. This dose may be taken as a single daily dose or in divided doses. Children under 2 years of age: consult a doctor.

Warnings: Keep this and all drugs out of the reach of children. In case of accidental overdose, seek professional assistance or contact a poison control center immediately. Do not use laxative products when abdominal pain, nausea, or vomiting are present unless directed by a doctor. If you have noticed a sudden change in bowel habits that persists over a period of 2 weeks, consult a doctor before using a laxative. Laxative products should not be used for a period longer than 1 week unless directed by a doctor. Rectal bleeding or failure to have a bowel movement after use of a laxative may indicate a serious condition. Discontinue use and consult your doctor. As with any drug, if you are pregnant or nursing a baby, seek the advice of a health care professional before using this product.

Inactive Ingredients: alginic acid, Blue 1, colloidal silicon dioxide, croscarmellose sodium, dibasic calcium phosphate, hydroxypropyl methylcellulose, magnesium stearate, methylparaben, microcrystalline cellulose, polydextrose, polyethylene glycol, silicon dioxide, sodium benzoate, stearic acid, talc, titanium dioxide, triacetin, Yellow 10. Sodium content: 8.4 mg per caplet.

Drug Interaction Precaution: Do not take this product if you are presently taking mineral oil, unless directed by a doctor.

Store in a dry place at controlled room temperature 15°–30°C (59°–86°F).

How Supplied: Available in boxes of 40 caplets.
Shown in Product Identification Guide, page 513

GAS–X®
EXTRA STRENGTH GAS-X®
Antiflatulent, Anti-Gas Chewable Tablets
Extra Strength Softgels
Extra Strength Liquids

Active Ingredients: GAS-X®—Each chewable tablet contains simethicone 80 mg.

EXTRA STRENGTH GAS-X®—Each chewable tablet contains simethicone, 125 mg, each swallowable softgel contains simethicone, USP, 125 mg and each teaspoon of liquid contains simethicone, 50 mg.

Inactive Ingredients
Extra Strength Peppermint Creme: calcium phosphate tribasic, colloidal silicon dioxide, dextrose, flavors, maltodextrin, D&C Red 30, D&C Yellow 10.
Extra Strength Cherry Creme: calcium phosphate tribasic, colloidal silicon dioxide, dextrose, flavors, maltodextrin, D&C Red 30.
GAS-X Peppermint Creme: calcium carbonate, dextrose, flavors, maltodextrin. Sodium-free.
GAS-X Cherry Creme: calcium carbonate, dextrose, flavors, maltodextrin, D&C Red 30.
Sodium-free.
Extra Strength Softgels: FD&C Blue 1, gelatin, glycerin, peppermint oil, FD&C Red 40, sorbitol, titanium dioxide water, D&C Yellow 10.
Sodium-free.
Liquids: benzoic acid, carboxymethylcellulose sodium, flavors, hydrochloric acid, microcrystalline cellulose, propylene glycol, propylparaben, purified water, sucrose, titanium dioxide, (cherry creme contains FD&C Red 40).

Indications: Relieves the symptoms referred to as gas.

Actions: GAS-X relieves the bloating, pressure and fullness commonly referred to as gas.

Warning: Keep this and all drugs out of the reach of children.

Drug Interaction Precautions: No known drug interaction.

Dosage and Administration: For Chewable Tablets: Adults: Chew thoroughly and swallow one or two tablets as needed after meals or at bedtime. Do not exceed six GAS-X chewable tablets or four EXTRA STRENGTH GAS-X chewable tablets in 24 hours. Do not increase dosage unless recommended by your physician.
For Extra Strength GAS-X Softgels: Adults: Swallow with water 1 or 2 softgels as needed after meals or at bedtime. Do not exceed 4 softgels in 24 hours unless recommended by your physician.
For Extra Strength GAS-X Liquids: Adults: 2–4 teaspoons as needed after meals or at bedtime. Do not exceed 10 teaspoons in a 24 hour period. Children (2–12 years): 1 teaspoon as needed after meals or at bedtime. Do not exceed 4 teaspoons in 24 hours. Consult a physician before increasing dosage.

Professional Labeling: GAS-X may be used in the alleviation of postoperative bloating/pressure, and for use in endoscopic examination.

How Supplied: GAS-X Chewable tablets are available in peppermint creme and cherry creme flavored, chewable, scored tablets in boxes of 12 tablets and 36 tablets.

EXTRA STRENGTH GAS-X Chewable tablets are available in peppermint creme and cherry creme flavored, chewable, scored tablets in boxes of 18 tablets and 48 tablets.
Easy-to-swallow, tasteless Extra Strength Gas-X Softgels are available in boxes of 10 pills, 30 pills and 50 pills.
Extra Strength GAS-X Liquids are available in peppermint creme and cherry creme in 10 oz. bottles.
Shown in Product Identification Guide, page 513 and 514

MAXIMUM STRENGTH MAALOX® ANTACID/ANTI-GAS Liquid
(formerly called Extra Strength Maalox® Antacid Anti-Gas)
Oral Suspension Antacid/Anti-Gas

Liquids
☐ **Refreshing Lemon**
  Smooth Cherry
  Cooling Mint
☐ **Physician-proven Maalox® formula for antacid effectiveness.**
☐ **Simethicone, at a recognized clinical dose, for antiflatulent action.**

Description: Maximum Strength Maalox® Antacid/Anti-Gas, a balanced combination of magnesium and aluminum hydroxides plus simethicone, is a nonconstipating antacid/anti-gas product to provide symptomatic relief of acid indigestion, heartburn, sour stomach, upset stomach associated with these symptoms and relief of pressure and bloating commonly referred to as gas.

Composition: To provide symptomatic relief of hyperacidity plus alleviation of gas symptoms, each teaspoonful contains:

Active Ingredients	Maximum Strength Maalox® Antacid/Anti-Gas Per Tsp. (5 mL)
Magnesium Hydroxide	450 mg
Aluminum Hydroxide (equivalent to dried gel, USP)	500 mg
Simethicone	40 mg

Inactive Ingredients: calcium saccharin, FD&C Red. No. 40, flavors, guar gum, methylparaben, propylparaben, purified water, sorbitol.

Directions for Use: 2 to 4 teaspoonfuls, 4 times per day, or as directed by a physician.

Patient Warnings: Do not take more than 12 teaspoonfuls in a 24-hour period or use the maximum dosage for more than 2 weeks or use if you have kidney disease except under the advice and supervision of a physician. **Keep this and all drugs out of the reach of children.**

Drug Interaction Precaution: Antacids may interact with certain prescription drugs. If you are presently taking a prescription drug, do not take this product without checking with your physician or other health professional.
To aid in establishing proper dosage schedules, the following information is provided:

	Maximum Strength Maalox® Antacid/Anti-Gas Per 2 Tsp. (10 mL) (Minimum Recommended Dosage)
Acid neutralizing capacity	59.6 mEq
Sodium content*	<2 mg

*Dietetically insignificant.

Professional Labeling
Indications: As an antacid for symptomatic relief of hyperacidity associated with the diagnosis of peptic ulcer, gastritis, peptic esophagitis, gastric hyperacidity, heartburn, or hiatal hernia. As an antiflatulent to alleviate the symptoms of gas, including postoperative gas pain.

Warnings: Prolonged use of aluminum-containing antacids in patients with renal failure may result in or worsen dialysis osteomalacia. Elevated tissue aluminum levels contribute to the development of the dialysis encephalopathy and osteomalacia syndromes. Small amounts of aluminum are absorbed from the gastrointestinal tract and renal excretion of aluminum is impaired in renal failure. Aluminum is not well removed by dialysis because it is bound to albumin and transferrin, which do not cross dialysis membranes. As a result, aluminum is deposited in bone, and dialysis osteomalacia may develop when large amounts of aluminum are ingested orally by patients with impaired renal function. Aluminum forms insoluble complexes with phosphate in the gastrointestinal tract, thus decreasing phosphate absorption. Prolonged use of aluminum-containing antacids by normophosphatemic patients may result in hypophosphatemia if phosphate intake is not adequate. In its more severe forms, hypophosphatemia can lead to anorexia, malaise, muscle weakness, and osteomalacia.

Advantages: Among antacids, Maximum Strength Maalox® Antacid/Anti-Gas Suspension is uniquely palatable—an important feature which encourages patients to follow your dosage directions. Maximum Strength Maalox® Antacid/Anti-Gas Suspension has the time-proven, nonconstipating, sodium-free* Maalox® formula—useful for those patients suffering from the problems associated with hyperacidity. Additionally, Maximum Strength Maalox® Antacid/Anti-Gas Suspension contains simethicone to alleviate discomfort associated with entrapped gas.
*Dietetically insignificant.

How Supplied:
Maximum Strength Maalox® Antacid/Anti-Gas Suspension
Refreshing Lemon is available in plastic bottles of 5 fl. oz. (148 mL), 12 fl. oz. (355 mL), and 26 fl. oz. (769 mL).
Smooth Cherry is available in plastic bottles of 12 fl. oz. (355 mL) and 26 fl. oz. (769 mL).
Cooling Mint is available in plastic bottles of 12 fl. oz. (355 mL) and 26 fl. oz. (769 mL).
Shown in Product Identification Guide, page 514

MAALOX® ANTI-GAS
(Simethicone)
Tablets (Regular Strength)
Peppermint and Sweet Lemon Flavors

Description: Maalox Anti-Gas relieves the symptoms of bloating, pressure, and fullness, commonly referred to as gas.

Active Ingredient: Simethicone (80 mg per tablet).

Inactive Ingredients: Corn starch, flavor, gelatin, mannitol, sucrose, and tribasic calcium phosphate. Peppermint: D&C red no. 27 aluminum lake. Sweet Lemon: D&C red no. 30 aluminum lake, D&C yellow no. 10 aluminum lake.

Indications: Relieves the symptoms of gas, in the digestive tract.
Gas symptoms may be caused by excessive swallowing of air or by eating foods that disagree.

Directions for Use: Chew 1 to 2 tablets thoroughly. Use after meals or at bedtime, or as directed by a physician. May also be taken as needed, up to 6 tablets daily. If symptoms persist, contact your physician. **DO NOT EXCEED 6 TABLETS A DAY UNLESS DIRECTED BY A PHYSICIAN.**

Warnings: Keep this and all drugs out of the reach of children.

How Supplied: Peppermint: Cartons of 12 tablets. Sweet Lemon: Cartons of 12 tablets.
Shown in Product Identification Guide, page 514

Continued on next page

Information on Novartis Consumer Health, Inc., products appearing on these pages is effective as of November 1998.

EXTRA STRENGTH MAALOX® ANTI-GAS
(Simethicone) Tablets
Peppermint and Sweet Lemon Flavors

Description: Extra Strength Maalox Anti-Gas relieves bloating, pressure, and fullness, commonly referred to as gas. It is formulated with an additional amount of the active ingredient.

Active Ingredient: Simethicone (150 mg per tablet).

Inactive Ingredients: Corn starch, flavor, gelatin, mannitol, sucrose, and tribasic calcium phosphate. Peppermint: D&C red no. 27 aluminum lake. Sweet Lemon: D&C red no. 30 aluminum lake, D&C yellow no. 10 aluminum lake.

Indications: Relieves the symptoms of gas in the digestive tract.
Gas symptoms may be caused by excessive swallowing of air or by eating foods that disagree.

Directions for Use: Chew 1 to 2 tablets thoroughly. Use after meals or at bedtime, or as directed by a physician. May also be taken as needed, up to 3 tablets daily. If symptoms persist, contact your physician. **DO NOT EXCEED 3 TABLETS A DAY UNLESS DIRECTED BY A PHYSICIAN.**

Warnings: Keep this and all drugs out of the reach of children.

How Supplied: Peppermint: Cartons of 10 tablets. Sweet Lemon: Cartons of 10 tablets.
Shown in Product Identification Guide, page 514

MAALOX®
Magnesia and Alumina
Oral Suspension
Antacid

Liquids
Cooling Mint
Smooth Cherry
Refreshing Lemon

Description: Maalox® Antacid, a balanced combination of magnesium and aluminum hydroxides, is a nonconstipating product to provide symptomatic relief of acid indigestion, heartburn, sour stomach and upset stomach associated with these symptoms.

Active Ingredients	Maalox Suspension 5 mL teaspoon
Magnesium Hydroxide	200 mg
Aluminum Hydroxide (equivalent to dried gel, USP)	225 mg

Inactive Ingredients: Calcium saccharin, flavors, methylparaben, propyl-

paraben, purified water, sorbitol, xanthan gum (Smooth Cherry & Refreshing Lemon only), guar gum (Cooling Mint) and other ingredients.

Maalox Suspension Per 2 Tsp. (10 mL) (Minimum Recommended Dosage)	
Acid neutralizing capacity	26.6 mEq
Sodium content	<3 mg

Directions for Use: Two to four teaspoonfuls, four times a day or as directed by a physician.

Patient Warnings: Do not take more than 16 teaspoonfuls in a 24-hour period or use the maximum dosage for more than 2 weeks or use if you have kidney disease except under the advice and supervision of a physician. **Keep this and all drugs out of the reach of children.**

Drug Interaction Precaution: Antacids may interact with certain prescription drugs. If you are presently taking a prescription drug, do not take this product without checking with your physician or other health professional.

Professional Labeling

Indications: As an antacid for symptomatic relief of hyperacidity associated with the diagnosis of peptic ulcer, gastritis, peptic esophagitis, gastric hyperacidity, heartburn, or hiatal hernia.

Warnings: Prolonged use of aluminum-containing antacids in patients with renal failure may result in or worsen dialysis osteomalacia. Elevated tissue aluminum levels contribute to the development of the dialysis encephalopathy and osteomalacia syndromes. Small amounts of aluminum are absorbed from the gastrointestinal tract and renal excretion of aluminum is impaired in renal failure. Aluminum is not well removed by dialysis because it is bound to albumin and transferrin, which do not cross dialysis membranes. As a result, aluminum is deposited in bone, and dialysis osteomalacia may develop when large amounts of aluminum are ingested orally by patients with impaired renal function. Aluminum forms insoluble complexes with phosphate in the gastrointestinal tract, thus decreasing phosphate absorption. Prolonged use of aluminum-containing antacids by normophosphatemic patients may result in hypophosphatemia if phosphate intake is not adequate. In its more severe forms, hypophosphatemia can lead to anorexia, malaise, muscle weakness, and osteomalacia.

Advantages: Among antacids, Maalox® Suspension is uniquely palatable—an important feature which encourages patients to follow your dosage directions. Maalox® has the time-proven, nonconstipating Maalox® formula—useful for those patients suffering from the problems associated with hyperacidity.

How Supplied:
Maalox® Cooling Mint Suspension is available in plastic bottles of 5 oz. (148 mL), 12 oz. (355 mL) and 26 oz. (769 mL)
Maalox® Smooth Cherry Suspension is available in plastic bottles of 12 oz. (355 mL) and 26 oz. (769 mL)
Maalox® Refreshing Lemon Suspension is available in plastic bottles of 12 oz. (355 mL) and 26 oz. (769 mL)
Shown in Product Identification Guide, page 514

Quick Dissolve
MAALOX® Antacid
Calcium Carbonate Chewable Antacid Tablets
Regular Strength and Maximum Strength
Lemon, Wild Berry, and Wintergreen Flavors
Fast Dissolving Tablets

Description: Quick Dissolve Maalox® Antacid Calcium Carbonate Chewable Tablets have a unique form that dissolves quickly to relieve heartburn, acid indigestion, and sour stomach fast.

Composition: To provide symptomatic relief of hyperacidity, each Quick Dissolve Maalox® Antacid Calcium Carbonate Tablets contains:

Active Ingredients:
Regular Strength—600 mg Calcium Carbonate
Maximum Strength—1000 mg Calcium Carbonate
The acid neutralizing capacity (per minimum recommended dosage) for Regular Strength is 21.6 mEq; for Maximum Strength, 18 mEq.

Inactive Ingredients: Aspartame, colloidal silicon dioxide, croscarmellose sodium, dextrose, flavors, magnesium stearate, maltodextrin, mannitol, pregelatinized starch. Depending on the flavor, may also contain Blue #1 lake, Red #30 lake and or Yellow #10 lake.
Sodium Content: 1 mg per tablet for Regular Strength; 2 mg per tablet for Maximum Strength.

Directions for Use: Regular Strength—Chew 2 to 4 tablets as symptoms occur or as directed by a physician. Maximum Strength—Chew 1 to 2 tablets as symptoms occur or as directed by a physician.

Patient Warnings: Do not take more than 12 (8 for Maximum Strength) tablets in a 24-hour period or use the maximum dosage for more than 2 weeks except under the advice and supervision of a physician.
Keep out of reach of children.
Phenylketonurics: Contains Phenylalanine .5 mg Per Tablet (.9 mg per Tablet for Maximum Strength)

Drug Interaction Precaution: Ask a doctor before use if you are presently taking a prescription drug.

Advantages: Quick Dissolve Maalox® Calcium Carbonate Antacid Tablets have a unique form that dissolves quickly to relieve heartburn fast.

How Supplied: Quick Dissolve Maalox® Antacid Calcium Carbonate Tablets are available in plastic bottles of 45 and 85 tablets (Regular Strength) and 35 and 65 tablets (Maximum Strength).

Wild Berry flavored tablets are not available in the larger sizes. Wintergreen flavored tablets are not available in the smaller sizes. Plastic bottles of Assorted Flavored and Lemon Flavor tablets are available in 45 and 85 tablet sizes (Regular Strength) and 35 and 65 tablet sizes (Maximum Strength). Regular Strength 3-roll packs of 30 tablets are also available in Lemon and Assorted flavors.

Shown in Product Identification Guide, page 514

MYOFLEX® PAIN RELIEVING CREAM
[mī 'ō-flex]

Description: Odorless, greaseless and non-burning topical pain reliever.

Active Ingredient: Trolamine salicylate 10%.

Other Ingredients: Cetyl alcohol, disodium EDTA, fragrance, propylene glycol, purified water, sodium lauryl sulfate, stearyl alcohol, white wax.

Indications: For the temporary relief of minor aches and pains of muscles and joints associated with arthritis, strains and sprains, and simple backache.

Warning: FOR EXTERNAL USE ONLY. Do not apply to irritated skin or if excessive irritation develops. Avoid contact with eyes. If condition worsens, or if symptoms persist for more than 7 days or clear up and occur again within a few days, discontinue use of this product and consult a physician. **Keep this and all drugs out of the reach of children.** In case of accidental ingestion, seek professional assistance or contact a poison control center immediately. As with any drug, if you are pregnant or nursing a baby, seek the advice of a health professional before using this product.

Directions: Use only as directed. **Adults and children 2 years of age and older:** Apply to affected area not more than three to four times daily. Affected areas may be wrapped loosely with two- or three-inch elastic bandage. **Children under 2 years of age:** Consult a physician.

How Supplied: Myoflex is supplied in 2 oz. and 4 oz. easy-squeeze tubes, and 8 oz. and 16 oz. jars. Store at room temperature 15°–30°C (59°–86°F).
MYOFLEX is a registered trademark of Novartis.
Shown in Product Identification Guide, page 514

NUPERCAINAL®
Dibucaine
Hemorrhoidal and Anesthetic Ointment

Ingredient: 1% dibucaine USP. Also contains: acetone sodium bisulfite, lanolin, light mineral oil, purified water, and white petrolatum.

Indications: For prompt, temporary relief of pain, itching and burning due to hemorrhoids or other anorectal disorders. May also be used topically for temporary relief of pain and itching associated with sunburn, minor burns, cuts, scrapes, insect bites, or minor skin irritation.

Directions: Adults: When practical, cleanse the affected area with mild soap and warm water and rinse thoroughly. Gently dry by patting or blotting with toilet tissue or a soft cloth before application of this product. Puncture tube seal with cap or sharp object. Apply externally to the affected area up to 3 or 4 times daily. Children 2–12: Do not use except under the advice and supervision of a physician. DO NOT USE ON INFANTS UNDER 2 YEARS OF AGE OR LESS THAN 35 LBS. WEIGHT.

Warnings: FOR EXTERNAL USE ONLY. IF SWALLOWED, CONSULT A PHYSICIAN OR POISON CONTROL CENTER IMMEDIATELY. **Do not use in or near the eyes.** If condition worsens or does not improve within 7 days, consult a physician. Do not put this product into the rectum by using fingers or any mechanical device. Do not exceed recommended daily dosage unless directed by a physician. Certain persons can develop allergic reactions to ingredients in this product. If the symptom being treated does not subside or if redness, irritation, swelling, pain, bleeding or other symptoms develop or increase, discontinue use and consult a physician promptly. As with any drug, if you are pregnant or nursing a baby, seek the advice of a health care professional before using this product. **Keep this and all medication out of reach of children.**

How Supplied: Nupercainal Hemorrhoidal and Anesthetic Ointment is available in tubes of 1 and 2 ounces. See crimp of tube for lot number and expiration date.
Store between 15°–30°C (59°–86°F).
Nupercainal is a registered trademark of Novartis.
Made in Canada
Distributed by Novartis Consumer Health, Inc., Summit NJ 07901-1312
Shown in Product Identification Guide, page 514

NUPERCAINAL®
HYDROCORTISONE 1% CREAM
Anti-Itch Cream

Active Ingredient: Hydrocortisone Acetate USP (equivalent to Hydrocortisone Free Base 1%).

Inactive Ingredients: Cetostearyl Alcohol, Sodium Lauryl Sulfate, White Petrolatum, Propylene Glycol, Purified Water.

Indications: For the temporary relief of external anal itching. May also be used for the temporary relief of itching associated with minor skin irritations and rashes due to eczema, insect bites, poison ivy, poison oak, poison sumac, soaps, detergents, cosmetics, jewelry, seborrheic dermatitis, or psoriasis. Other uses of this product should be only under the advice and supervision of a physician.

Directions: Adults: When practical, cleanse the affected area with mild soap and warm water and rinse thoroughly. Gently dry by patting or blotting with toilet tissue or a soft cloth before application of this product. Apply to affected area not more than 3 to 4 times daily. **Children under 12 years of age:** Consult a physician.

Warnings: For external use only. Avoid contact with the eyes. If condition worsens, or if symptoms persist for more than 7 days or clear up and occur again within a few days, stop use of this product and do not begin use of any other hydrocortisone product unless you have consulted a physician. Do not use for the treatment of diaper rash; consult a physician. Do not exceed the recommended daily dosage unless directed by a physician. In case of bleeding, consult a physician promptly. Do not put this product into the rectum by using fingers or any mechanical device or applicator. **Keep this and all medication out of reach of children.** In case of accidental ingestion, seek professional assistance or contact a poison control center immediately.

How Supplied: Nupercainal Hydrocortisone Cream is available in a 1 ounce tube. See crimp of tube for lot number and expiration date.
Store at controlled room temperature 15–30°C (59°–86°F).
Nupercainal is a registered trademark of Novartis.
Made in Canada
Distributed by Novartis Consumer Health, Inc., Summit, NJ 07901-1312

NUPERCAINAL®
Suppositories

Ingredients: 2.1 grams cocoa butter, NF and .25 gram zinc oxide. Also contains acetone sodium bisulfite and bismuth subgallate.

Indications: For temporary relief of itching, burning, and discomfort associated with hemorrhoids or other anorectal disorders.

Continued on next page

Information on Novartis Consumer Health, Inc., products appearing on these pages is effective as of November 1998.

Nupercainal Supp.—Cont.

Directions: ADULTS—When practical, cleanse the affected area. Tear one suppository at the "V" cut, peel foil downward and remove foil wrapper before inserting into the rectum. Gently insert the suppository rectally, rounded end first. Use one suppository up to 6 times daily or after each bowel movement. CHILDREN UNDER 12 YEARS OF AGE—Consult a physician.

WARNING: IF ACCIDENTALLY SWALLOWED, CONSULT A PHYSICIAN OR POISON CONTROL CENTER IMMEDIATELY.

If condition worsens or does not improve within 7 days, consult a physician. Do not exceed the recommended daily dosage unless directed by a physician. In case of bleeding consult a physician promptly. As with any drug, if you are pregnant or nursing a baby, seek the advice of a health professional before using this product.

Keep this and all medications out of reach of children.

How Supplied: Nupercainal Suppositories are available in tamper-evident packages of 12 or 24.

Do not store above 30°C (86°F).

Nupercainal is a registered trademark of Novartis.

OTRIVIN®
Nasal Decongestant

Active Ingredient: xylometazoline hydrochloride USP (Nasal Spray and Nasal Drops 0.1%, Pediatric Nasal Drops 0.05%).

Inactive Ingredients: Otrivin Nasal Spray/Nasal Drops—benzalkonium chloride, dibasic sodium phosphate, disodium edetate, monobasic sodium phosphate, purified water and sodium chloride.

Otrivin Pediatric Nasal Drops—benzalkonium chloride, dibasic sodium phosphate, disodium edetate, monobasic sodium phosphate, purified water and sodium chloride.

Indications: For the temporary relief of nasal congestion due to the common cold, hay fever or other upper respiratory allergies, or associated with sinusitis.

Otrivin has been provide support apt for many years. Here is how you use it:

Directions: Nasal Spray 0.1%—for adults and children 12 years and over: Spray 2 or 3 times into each nostril not more often than every 8 to 10 hours. **Do not give Nasal Spray 0.1% to children under 12 years of age unless directed by a doctor.**

Nasal Drops 0.1%—for adults and children 12 years and over: 2 or 3 drops in each nostril not more often than every 8 to 10 hours. **Do not give Nasal Drops 0.1% to children under 12 years except under the advice and supervision of a physician.**

Pediatric Nasal Drops 0.05%—children 6 to 12 years of age (with adult supervision): 2 or 3 drops in each nostril not more often than every 8 to 10 hours. Children 2 to 6 years of age (with adult supervision): 2 to 3 drops in each nostril not more often than every 8 to 10 hours. Use dropper provided. Use only recommended amount. Do not exceed 3 doses in any 24 hour period. Children under 2 years of age: consult a doctor.

Warning: Do not exceed recommended dosage. This product may cause temporary discomfort such as burning, stinging, sneezing, or an increase in nasal discharge. Do not use this product for more than 3 days. Use only as directed. Frequent or prolonged use may cause nasal congestion to recur or worsen. If symptoms persist, consult a doctor. Do not use this product if you have heart disease, high blood pressure, thyroid disease, diabetes, or difficulty in urination due to enlargement of the prostate gland unless directed by a doctor. The use of this container by more than one person may spread infection.

Keep this and all drugs out of the reach of children. In case of accidental ingestion, seek professional assistance or contact a Poison Control Center immediately.

Overdosage in young children may cause marked sedation.

Caution: Do not use if the clear overwrap with the name Otrivin® or the printed band on the bottle is missing or damaged.

How Supplied: Nasal Spray—unbreakable plastic spray bottle of 0.66 fl. oz. (20 ml).

Nasal Drops—plastic dropper bottle of 0.83 fl. oz. (25 ml).

Pediatric Nasal Drops—Plastic dropper bottle of 0.83 fl. oz. (25 ml).

Store at 15°–30°C (59°–86°F).

Shown in Product Identification Guide, page 514

Overnight Relief
PERDIEM®
[pĕr "dē 'ŭm]
Natural Bulk Fiber Plus Vegetable Laxative

Description: Overnight Relief Perdiem® is a 100% Natural Fiber *plus* Vegetable Laxative. Perdiem's unique combination of natural ingredients provides gentle, predictable overnight relief of constipation without chemical additives. Perdiem's unique form is easy to swallow and requires no mixing. Overnight Relief Perdiem generally takes effect within 12 hours.

Indications: For relief of occasional constipation. This product generally produces bowel movement within 12 hours.

Active Ingredients: 82% psyllium (Plantago Hydrocolloid), a natural grain substance and 18% senna (Cassia Pod Concentrate), a natural vegetable derivative.

Each rounded (6 gram) teaspoonful contains:

3.25 grams psyllium   35.5 mg potassium
0.74 gram senna   1.8 mg sodium
only 4 calories

Inactive Ingredients: acacia, iron oxides, natural flavors, paraffin, sucrose, talc. Perdiem is "Dye-Free" and contains no artificial sweeteners.

Directions For Use: TAKE THIS PRODUCT (CHILD OR ADULT DOSE) WITH AT LEAST 8 OUNCES (A FULL GLASS) OF COOL WATER OR OTHER FLUID. TAKING THIS PRODUCT WITHOUT ENOUGH LIQUID MAY CAUSE CHOKING. SEE WARNINGS.
Four easy steps for using Perdiem

1. Moisten your mouth with a drink of water or any cool beverage.

2. Place a teaspoonful of granules on your tongue. If you prefer take only a partial teaspoonful at a time.

3. Without chewing, wash granules down with water or any cool beverage.

4. Repeat steps 1–3 until the recommended dose has been swallowed. Be sure to drink at least 8 ounces of cool liquid.

Adults and Children 12 years and older: In the evening and/or before breakfast, 1 to 2 rounded teaspoonfuls one to two times daily should be placed in the mouth and swallowed with at least 8 ounces of cool liquid.

Children 7 to 11 years: One (1) rounded teaspoonful one to two times daily with at least 8 ounces of cool liquid.

For severe Cases of Constipation: Perdiem may be taken more frequently, up to 2 rounded teaspoonfuls every 6 hours not to exceed 5 teaspoonfuls in a 24-hour period.

PERDIEM SHOULD NOT BE CHEWED.

WARNINGS: TAKING THIS PRODUCT WITHOUT ADEQUATE FLUID MAY CAUSE IT TO SWELL AND BLOCK YOUR THROAT OR ESOPHAGUS AND MAY CAUSE CHOKING. DO NOT TAKE THIS PRODUCT IF YOU HAVE DIFFICULTY IN SWALLOWING. IF YOU EXPERIENCE CHEST PAIN, VOMITING OR DIFFICULTY IN SWALLOWING OR BREATHING AFTER TAKING THIS PRODUCT, SEEK IMMEDIATE MEDICAL ATTENTION.

People with esophageal narrowing should not use bulk-forming agents.

If you have noticed a sudden change in bowel habits that persists over a two-week period, consult a doctor before using any laxative product.

If use of this product for one week has produced no effect or if rectal bleeding occurs after use of any bulk fiber or laxative, discontinue use and consult a doctor.

Do not use if you have a history of psyllium allergy or experience abdominal pain, nausea or vomiting unless directed by a doctor.

In case of accidental overdose, seek professional assistance or contact a poison control center immediately.

If you are pregnant or nursing a baby, seek the advice of a health professional before using this product.

Keep this and all drugs out of the reach of children.

How Supplied: Granules: 400–gram (14 oz) canisters, and 250-gram (8.8 oz) canisters.

Store at room temperature 15–30°C (59–86°F). Avoid exposure to moisture.

Shown in Product Identification Guide, page 514

FIBER THERAPY PERDIEM®
[pĕr "dē 'ŭm]
Bulk Fiber Laxative

Description: Fiber Therapy Perdiem® is a 100% Natural Bulk-Forming Fiber that helps maintain regularity and prevent constipation (irregularity) without chemical stimulants and may be used daily by those who lack sufficient dietary fiber. Perdiem's unique form is easy to swallow and requires no mixing. Fiber Therapy Perdiem generally takes effect after 12 hours; 48 to 72 hours may be required for optimal relief.

Indications: For relief of occasional constipation. This product generally takes effect after 12 hours; 48 to 72 hours may be required for optimal relief.

Active Ingredients: 100% psyllium (Plantago Hydrocolloid), a natural grain substance with no chemical stimulants.

Each rounded (6 gram) teaspoonful contains:
4.03 grams psyllium, 36.1 mg potassium, 1.80 mg sodium.
only 4 calories

Inactive Ingredients: acacia, iron oxides, natural flavors, paraffin, sucrose, talc, titanium dioxide. Fiber Therapy Perdiem is "Dye-Free" and contains no artificial sweeteners.

Directions For Use: TAKE THIS PRODUCT (CHILD OR ADULT DOSE) WITH AT LEAST 8 OUNCES (A FULL GLASS) OF COOL WATER OR OTHER FLUID. TAKING THIS PRODUCT WITHOUT ENOUGH LIQUID MAY CAUSE CHOKING. SEE WARNINGS.

Four easy steps for using Perdiem

1. Moisten your mouth with a drink of water or any cool beverage.

2. Place a teaspoonful of granules on your tongue. If you prefer, take only a partial teaspoonful at a time.

3. Without chewing, wash granules down with water or any cool beverage.

4. Repeat steps 1–3 until the recommended dose has been swallowed. Be sure to drink at least 8 ounces of cool liquid.

Adults and Children 12 years and older: In the evening and/or before breakfast, 1 to 2 rounded teaspoonfuls one to two times daily should be placed in the mouth and swallowed with at least 8 ounces of cool liquid.

Children 7 to 11 years: One (1) rounded teaspoonful one to two times daily with at least 8 ounces of cool liquid.

For Severe Cases of Constipation: Perdiem may be taken more frequently, up to 2 rounded teaspoonfuls every 6 hours not to exceed 5 teaspoonfuls in a 24-hour period.

PERDIEM SHOULD NOT BE CHEWED.

WARNINGS: TAKING THIS PRODUCT WITHOUT ADEQUATE FLUID MAY CAUSE IT TO SWELL AND BLOCK YOUR THROAT OR ESOPHAGUS AND MAY CAUSE CHOKING. DO NOT TAKE THIS PRODUCT IF YOU HAVE DIFFICULTY IN SWALLOWING. IF YOU EXPERIENCE CHEST PAIN, VOMITING OR DIFFICULTY IN SWALLOWING OR BREATHING AFTER TAKING THIS PRODUCT, SEEK IMMEDIATE MEDICAL ATTENTION.

People with esophageal narrowing should not use bulk-forming agents.

If you have noticed a sudden change in bowel habits that persists over a two-week period, consult a doctor before using any laxative product.

If use of this product for constipation has produced no effect within one week or if rectal bleeding occurs after use of any bulk fiber or laxative, discontinue use and consult a doctor.

Do not use if you have a history of psyllium allergy or experience abdominal pain, nausea or vomiting unless directed by a doctor.

In case of accidental overdose, seek professional assistance or contact a poison control center immediately.

Keep this and all drugs out of the reach of children.

How Supplied: Granules: 250-gram (8.8 oz) plastic container.

Store at room temperature. 15°–30°C (59°–86°F). Avoid exposure to moisture.

Shown in Product Identification Guide, page 514

TAVIST® Allergy Tablets (formerly TAVIST-1®)

Description: Active Ingredients: clemastine fumarate, USP 1.34 mg (equivalent to 1 mg clemastine). **Inactive Ingredients:** lactose, povidone, starch, stearic acid, and talc.

Sodium Free.

Indications: Temporarily reduces runny nose and sneezing due to hay fever or other respiratory allergies due to the common cold. Temporarily reduces itching of the nose or throat and itchy, watery eyes due to hay fever or other upper respiratory allergies.

Warnings: Keep this and all drugs out of the reach of children. In case of accidental overdose, seek professional assistance or contact a poison control center immediately. May cause drowsiness; alcohol, sedatives, and tranquilizers may increase the drowsiness effect. Avoid alcoholic beverages while taking this product. Do not take this product if you are taking sedatives or tranquilizers without first consulting your doctor. Use caution when driving a motor vehicle or operating machinery. May cause excitability especially in children. Do not take this product, unless directed by a doctor, if you have a breathing problem such as emphysema or chronic bronchitis, or if you have glaucoma or difficulty in urination due to enlargement of the prostate gland. As with any drug, if you are pregnant or nursing a baby, seek the advice of a health professional before using this product.

Directions: Adults and children 12 years of age and older: Swallow 1 tablet every 12 hours, not to exceed 2 tablets in 24 hours unless directed by a doctor. Children under 12 years of age: Consult a doctor.

How Supplied: Tavist Allergy tablets (white) imprinted Tavist on one side and Allergy on the other side in blister packs of 8, 16, and 32.
Formerly Tavist-1®
Shown in Product Identification Guide, page 514

TAVIST•D® Caplets
Antihistamine/Nasal Decongestant

Description: Active Ingredients: clemastine fumarate, USP, 1.34 mg

Continued on next page

Information on Novartis Consumer Health, Inc., products appearing on these pages is effective as of November 1998.

Tavist-D Caplets—Cont.

(equivalent to 1 mg clemastine) immediate release and phenylpropanolamine hydrochloride, USP, 75 mg extended release. **Inactive Ingredients:** Carnauba wax, hydroxypropyl methylcellulose, lactose monohydrate, methylparaben, polydextrose, polyethylene glycol, silicon dioxide (colloidal), starch (pregelatinized), stearic acid, titanium dioxide, triacetin. Sodium free.

Indications: Temporarily relieves the following symptoms associated with the common cold and hay fever or other upper respiratory allergies: nasal congestion, runny nose, sneezing. Temporarily relieves the following symptoms associated with hay fever or other upper respiratory allergies: itching of the nose or throat, itchy watery eyes. Temporarily relieves nasal congestion associated with sinusitis.

Warnings: Keep this and all drugs out of the reach of children. In case of accidental overdose, seek professional assistance or contact a poison control center immediately. May cause drowsiness; alcohol, sedatives, and tranquilizers may increase the drowsiness effect. Avoid alcoholic beverages while taking this product. Do not take this product if you are taking sedatives or tranquilizers without first consulting your doctor. Use caution when driving a motor vehicle or operating machinery. May cause excitability especially in children.

Do not exceed recommended dosage. If nervousness, dizziness, or sleeplessness occur, discontinue use and consult a doctor. If symptoms do not improve within 7 days, or are accompanied by fever, consult a doctor. Do not take this product if you have heart disease, high blood pressure, thyroid disease, diabetes, glaucoma, a breathing problem such as emphysema or chronic bronchitis, or difficulty in urination due to enlargement of the prostate gland unless directed by a doctor. As with any drug, if you are pregnant or nursing a baby, seek the advice of a health professional before using this product.

Drug Interaction Precaution: Do not take this product if you are presently taking another product containing phenylpropanolamine. Do not use this product if you are now taking a prescription monoamine oxidase inhibitor [MAOI] (certain drugs for depression, psychiatric or emotional conditions, or Parkinson's disease), or for 2 weeks after stopping the MAOI drug. If you are uncertain whether your prescription drug contains an MAOI, consult a health professional before taking this product.

Directions: Adults and children 12 years of age and older: Swallow 1 caplet whole every 12 hours, not to exceed 2 caplets in 24 hours or as directed by a doctor. Children under 12 years of age: Consult a doctor.

How Supplied: Tavist•D caplets (white) imprinted "Tavist•D" on one side, in blister packs of 8 and 16.

TAVIST•D® TABLETS

Description: Active Ingredients: clemastine fumarate, USP, 1.34 mg (equivalent to 1 mg clemastine) immediate release and 75 mg phenylpropanolamine hydrochloride, USP, extended release. **Inactive Ingredients:** Colloidal silicon dioxide, dibasic calcium phosphate, lactose, magnesium stearate, methylcellulose, polyethylene glycol, Sodium Free povidone, starch, synthetic polymers, titanium dioxide and D&C Yellow 10.

Sodium Free

Indications: Temporarily relieves the following symptoms associated with the common cold and hay fever or other upper respiratory allergies: nasal congestion, runny nose, sneezing. Temporarily relieves the following symptoms associated with hay fever or other upper respiratory allergies: itching of the nose or throat, itchy watery eyes. Temporarily relieves nasal congestion associated with sinusitis.

Warnings: Keep this and all drugs out of the reach of children. In case of accidental overdose, seek professional assistance or contact a poison control center immediately. May cause drowsiness; alcohol, sedatives, and tranquilizers may increase the drowsiness effect. Avoid alcoholic beverages while taking this product. Do not take this product if you are taking sedatives or tranquilizers without first consulting your doctor. Use caution when driving a motor vehicle or operating machinery. May cause excitability especially in children.

Do not exceed recommended dosage. If nervousness, dizziness or sleeplessness occur, discontinue use and consult a doctor. If symptoms do not improve within 7 days or are accompanied by fever consult a doctor. Do not take this product if you have heart disease, high blood pressure, thyroid disease, diabetes, glaucoma, a breathing problem such as emphysema or chronic bronchitis, or difficulty in urination due to enlargement of the prostate glan unless directed by a doctor. As with any drug, if you are pregnant or nursing a baby, seek the advice of a health professional before using this product.

Drug Interaction Precaution: Do not take this product if you are presently taking another product containing phenylpropanolamine. Do not use this product if you are now taking a prescription monoamine oxidase inhibitor [MAOI] (certain drugs for depression, psychiatric or emotional conditions, or Parkinson's disease), or for 2 weeks after stopping the MAOI drug. If you are uncertain whether your prescription drug contains an MAOI, consult a health professional before taking this product.

Directions: Adults and children 12 years of age and older: Swallow 1 tablet whole every 12 hours, not to exceed 2 tablets in 24 hours unless directed by a doctor. Children under 12 years of age: Consult a doctor.

How Supplied: Tavist•D tablets (white) imprinted "Tavist•D" on both sides, in blister packs of 8, 16, 32, and 48.

Shown in Product Identification Guide, page 515

TAVIST® SINUS

Description: Active Ingredients: acetaminophen, 500 mg and pseudoephedrine HCl, 30 mg. **Inactive Ingredients:** Colloidal silicon dioxide, croscarmellose sodium, hydroxypropyl cellulose, hydroxypropyl methylcellulose, lactose monohydrate, magnesium stearate, methylparaben, polydextrose powder, polyethylene glycol, pregelatinized starch, titanium dioxide, triacetin.

Sodium content: 3 mg per caplet.

Indications: Temporarily relieves nasal and sinus congestion and pressure. For temporary relief of minor aches and pains associated with common cold, and sinus pain and headache.

Warnings: Keep this and all drugs out of the reach of children. In case of accidental overdose, seek professional assistance or contact a poison control center immediately. Prompt medical attention is critical for adults as well as children even if you do not notice any signs or symptoms. As with any drug, if you are pregnant or nursing a baby, seek the advice of a health professional before using this product. **Do not exceed recommended dosage.**

Unless directed by a doctor, do not use if you have: heart disease, high blood pressure, thyroid disease, diabetes or difficulty in urination due to enlargement of the prostate gland or pain for more than 10 days or fever for more than 3 days.

Consult a doctor if: pain or fever persists or gets worse, if new symptoms occur or if redness or swelling is present, because these could be signs of a serious condition or if symptoms do not improve within 7 days or are accompanied by fever.

Consult a doctor and stop using this drug if: nervousness, dizziness, or sleeplessness occur.

Drug Interaction Precaution: Do not use this product if you are now taking a prescription monoamine oxidase inhibitor [MAOI] (certain drugs for depression, psychiatric or emotional conditions, or Parkinson's disease), or for 2 weeks after stopping the MAOI drug. If you are uncertain whether your prescription drug contains an MAOI, consult a health professional before taking this product.

Directions: Adults and children 12 years of age and older: Take 2 caplets and gelcaps every 6 hours, not to exceed 8 caplets and gelcaps in 24 hours, or as directed by a doctor. Children under 12 years of age: Consult a doctor.

How Supplied: Tavist Sinus coated caplets (white) imprinted "Tavist" on one side and "Sinus" on the other, in blister packs of 24.
Tavist Sinus coated gelcaps (red and white) imprinted with "Tavist" on one side in blister packs of 24.
Shown in Product Identification Guide, page 515

THERAFLU®
Flu and Cold Medicine
Flu, Cold & Cough Medicine

Description: Each packet of TheraFlu Flu and Cold Medicine contains: acetaminophen 650 mg, pseudoephedrine hydrochloride 60 mg, and chlorpheniramine maleate 4 mg. Each packet of TheraFlu Flu, Cold & Cough Medicine also contains dextromethorphan hydrobromide 20 mg. **Inactive ingredients:** ascorbic acid (vitamin C), citric acid, D&C Yellow 10, natural lemon flavors, pregelatinized starch, silicon dioxide, sodium citrate, sucrose, titanium dioxide and tribasic calcium phosphate.

Sodium content: 25 mg per packet.

Indications: Provides temporary relief of the symptoms associated with flu, common cold and other upper respiratory allergies including: headache, body aches, fever, minor sore throat pain, nasal and sinus congestion, runny nose and sneezing. TheraFlu Flu, Cold & Cough Medicine also suppresses coughs due to minor throat and bronchial irritation.

Warnings: Keep this and all drugs out of the reach of children. In case of accidental overdose, seek professional assistance or contact a poison control center immediately. Prompt medical attention is critical for adults as well as children even if you do not notice any signs or symptoms.
Do not exceed recommended dosage. If nervousness, dizziness, or sleeplessness occur, discontinue use and consult a doctor. If symptoms do not improve within 7 days or are accompanied by fever, consult a doctor. May cause excitability especially in children. Do not take this product if you have heart disease, high blood pressure, thyroid disease, diabetes, glaucoma, a breathing problem such as emphysema or chronic bronchitis, or difficulty in urination due to enlargement of the prostate gland, unless directed by a doctor.
Do not take this product for pain for more than 10 days or for fever for more than 3 days unless directed by a doctor. If pain or fever persists or gets worse, if new symptoms occur, or if redness or swelling is present, consult a doctor because these could be signs of a serious

condition. If sore throat is severe, persists for more than 2 days, is accompanied or followed by fever, headache, rash, nausea, or vomiting, consult a doctor promptly.
May cause marked drowsiness; alcohol, sedatives, and tranquilizers may increase the drowsiness effect. Avoid alcoholic beverages while taking this product. Do not take this product if you are taking sedatives or tranquilizers, without first consulting your doctor. Use caution when driving a motor vehicle or operating machinery.
A persistent cough may be a sign of a serious condition. If cough persists for more than 1 week, tends to recur, or is accompanied by a fever, rash, or persistent headache, consult a doctor. Do not take the Flu, Cold & Cough formula for persistent or chronic cough such as occurs with smoking, asthma, or emphysema, or if cough is accompanied by excessive phlegm (mucus) unless directed by a doctor.
As with any drug, if you are pregnant or nursing a baby, seek the advice of a health professional before using this product.

Drug Interaction Precaution: Do not take this product if you are now taking a prescription monoamine oxidase inhibitor [MAOI] (certain drugs for depression, psychiatric or emotional conditions, or Parkinson's disease), or for 2 weeks after stopping the MAOI drug. If you are uncertain whether your prescription drug contains an MAOI, consult a health professional before taking this product.

Alcohol Warning: If you consume 3 or more alcoholic drinks everyday ask your doctor whether you should take acetaminophen or other pain relievers/fever reducers. Acetaminophen may cause liver damage.

Directions: Adults and children 12 years of age and over—dissolve one packet in 6 oz. hot water; sip while hot. One packet of Flu and Cold formula every 4 to 6 hours; one packet of Flu, Cold and Cough formula every six hours. Not to exceed 4 packets in 24 hours, or as directed by a doctor. Children under 12 years of age: consult a doctor. **Microwave heating instructions:** Add contents of packet and 6 oz. of cool water to a microwave-safe cup and stir briskly. Microwave on high $1^{1}/_{2}$ minutes or until hot. Do not boil water or overheat, and remember to stir liquid between reheatings. Sweeten to taste if desired.

How Supplied: TheraFlu Flu and Cold Medicine powder in foil packets, 6 or 12 packets per carton. TheraFlu Flu, Cold & Cough Medicine powder in foil packets, 6 or 12 packets per carton.
Shown in Product Identification Guide, page 515

THERAFLU® MAXIMUM STRENGTH
Flu and Cold Medicine
For Sore Throat

Each packet of Theraflu Maximum Strength Sore Throat formula contains:

acetaminophen 1000 mg, pseudoephedrine HCl 60 mg, chlorpheniramine maleate 4 mg. **Inactive Ingredients:** Acesulfame K, ascorbic acid, aspartame, citric acid, D&C Yellow 10, FD&C Blue 1, FD&C Red 40, maltodextrin, natural apple and cinnamon flavors, silicon dioxide, sodium citrate, sucrose and tribasic calcium phosphate.

Sodium content: 30 mg per packet.

Indications: Provides temporary relief of minor sore throat pain, body aches, pains, and headaches and reduces fever. Temporarily relieves runny nose, sneezing and nasal congestion due to flu, the common cold, hay fever or other upper respiratory allergies.

Warnings: Keep this and all drugs out of the reach of children. In case of accidental overdose, seek professional assistance or contact a poison control center immediately. Prompt medical attention is critical for adults as well as children even if you do not notice any signs or symptoms.
Do not exceed recommended dosage. If nervousness, dizziness, or sleeplessness occur, discontinue use and consult a doctor. If symptoms do not improve within 7 days or are accompanied by fever, consult a doctor. May cause excitability, especially in children. Do not take this product if you have heart disease, high blood pressure, thyroid disease, diabetes, glaucoma, a breathing problem such as emphysema or chronic bronchitis, or difficulty in urination due to enlargement of the prostate gland, unless directed by a doctor.
Do not take this product for pain for more than 10 days or for fever for more than 3 days unless directed by a doctor. If pain or fever persists or gets worse, if new symptoms occur, or if redness or swelling is present, consult a doctor because these could be signs of a serious condition. If sore throat is severe, persists for more than 2 days, is accompanied or followed by fever, headache, rash, nausea, or vomiting, consult a doctor promptly.
May cause marked drowsiness; alcohol, sedatives and tranquilizers may increase the drowsiness effect. Avoid alcoholic beverages while taking this product. Do not take this product if you are taking sedatives or tranquilizers without first consulting your doctor. Use caution when driving a motor vehicle or operating machinery.
As with any drug, if you are pregnant or nursing a baby, seek the advice of a health professional before using this product.

Drug Interaction Precaution: Do not use this product if you are now tak-

Continued on next page

Information on Novartis Consumer Health, Inc., products appearing on these pages is effective as of November 1998.

Theraflu/Sore Throat—Cont.

ing a prescription monoamine oxidase inhibitor [MAOI] (certain drugs for depression, psychiatric or emotional conditions, or Parkinson's Disease), or for 2 weeks after stopping the MAOI drug. If you are uncertain whether your prescription drug contains an MAOI, consult a health professional before taking this product.

Phenylketonurics: Contains Phenylalanine 25 mg per adult dose.

Alcohol Warning: If you consume 3 or more alcoholic drinks everyday ask your doctor whether you should take acetaminophen or other pain relievers/fever reducers. Acetaminophen may cause liver damage.

Directions: Adults and children 12 years of age and over: dissolve one packet in 6 oz. of hot water; sip while hot. One packet every 6 hours, not to exceed 4 packets in 24 hours, or as directed by a doctor. Children under 12 years of age: consult a doctor. **Microwave Heating Instructions:** Add contents of packet and 6 oz. of cool water to a microwave-safe cup and stir briskly. Microwave on high 1 1/2 minutes or until hot. Do not boil water or overheat, and remember to stir liquid between reheatings.
Sweeten to taste if desired. May repeat every 6 hours, but not to exceed 4 doses in 24 hours.

How Supplied: Theraflu Maximum Strength flu and Cold Medicine for Sore Throat powder in foil packets, 6 packets per carton.

Shown in Product Identification Guide, page 515

Maximum Strength
THERAFLU® Flu, Cold and Cough Medicine
Sore Throat and Cough

Description: Maximum Strength TheraFlu Sore Throat and Cough formula combines effective medicines with the hot liquids recommended by most doctors to provide maximum relief of your flu and cold symptoms, so you can get the sleep you need. And TheraFlu is alcohol-free.
[See table below]

Inactive Ingredients: acesulfame K, ascorbic acid (Vitamin C), aspartame,

FD&C Blue 1, calcium phosphate tribasic, cherry flavor, citric acid, maltodextrin, FD&C Red 40 silicon dioxide sodium citrate, and sucrose.
Sodium content 26 mg per packet.

Directions: Adults and children 12 years of age and over: dissolve contents of one packet in 6 oz. hot water; sip while hot. One packet every 6 hours, not to exceed 4 packets in 24 hours, or as directed by a doctor. Children under 12 years of age: consult a doctor.
Microwave heating instructions: Add contents of one packet and 6 oz. of cool water to a microwave-safe cup and stir briskly. Microwave on high 1½ minutes or until hot. Do not boil water or overheat, and remember to stir liquid between reheatings.
Sweeten to taste if desired.
DO NOT USE IF SEALED THERAFLU PACKET IS TORN OR BROKEN.

Warning: Keep this and all drugs out of the reach of children. In case of accidental overdose, seek professional assistance or contact a poison control center immediately. Prompt medical attention is critical for adults as well as for children even if you do not notice any signs or symptoms.
Do not exceed recommended dosage. If nervousness, dizziness, or sleeplessness occur, discontinue use and consult a doctor. If symptoms do not improve within 7 days or are accompanied by fever, consult a doctor. May cause excitability, especially in children. Do not take this product if you have heart disease, high blood pressure, thyroid disease, diabetes, glaucoma, a breathing problem such as emphysema or chronic bronchitis, or difficulty in urination due to enlargement of the prostate gland, unless directed by a doctor.
A persistent cough may be a sign of a serious condition. If cough persists for more than 1 week, tends to recur, or is accompanied by fever, rash, or persistent headache, consult a doctor. Do not take this product for persistent or chronic cough such as occurs with smoking, asthma, emphysema, or if cough is accompanied by excessive phlegm (mucus) unless directed by a doctor.
Do not take this product for pain for more than 10 days or for fever for more than 3 days unless directed by a doctor. If pain or fever persists or gets worse, if new symptoms occur, or if redness or

swelling is present, consult a doctor because these could be signs of a serious condition. If sore throat is severe, persists for more than 2 days, is accompanied or followed by fever, headache, rash, nausea, or vomiting, consult a doctor promptly.
May cause marked drowsiness; alcohol, sedatives, and tranquilizers may increase the drowsiness effect. Avoid alcoholic beverages while taking this product. Do not take this product if you are taking sedatives or tranquilizers, without first consulting your doctor. Use caution when driving a motor vehicle or operating machinery.
As with any drug, if you are pregnant or nursing a baby, seek the advice of a health professional before using this product.

Drug interaction precaution: Do not use this product if you are now taking a prescription monoamine oxide inhibitor [MAOI] (certain drugs for depression, psychiatric or emotional conditions, or Parkinson's disease), or for 2 weeks after stopping the MAOI drug. If you are uncertain whether your prescription drug contains an MAOI, consult a health professional before taking this product.

Alcohol Warning: If you consume 3 or more alcoholic drinks every day ask your doctor whether you should take acetaminophen or other pain relievers/fever reducers. Acetaminophen may cause liver damage.
Phenylketonurics: CONTAINS PHENYLALANINE 26 mg per adult dose.

How Supplied: Available in 6 packet carton.
Shown in Product Identification Guide, page 515

THERAFLU®
MAXIMUM STRENGTH NIGHTTIME
Hot Liquid and Caplet
Flu, Cold & Cough Medicine

Description: Each packet of TheraFlu Maximum Strength NightTime Flu, Cold & Cough Hot Liquid Medicine contains: acetaminophen 1000 mg, dextromethorphan HBr 30 mg, pseudoephedrine HCl 60 mg, and chlorpheniramine maleate 4 mg. **Inactive Ingredients:** ascorbic acid (Vitamin C), citric acid, D&C Yellow 10, natural lemon flavors, maltol, pregelatinized starch, silicon dioxide, sodium citrate, sucrose, titanium dioxide and tribasic calcium phosphate.

Sodium content: 25 mg per packet.

TheraFlu NIGHTTIME Caplets: each caplet contains acetaminophen 500 mg, pseudo-ephedrine HCl 30 mg. dextromethorphan HBr 15 mg. and chlorpheniramine maleate 2 mg. **Inactive Ingredients:** colloidal silicon dioxide, croscarmellose sodium gelatin, D&C Yellow 10, FD&C Blue 1, FD&C Yellow 6, hydroxypropyl cellulose, hydroxypropyl methylcellulose, lactose, magnesium stearate, methylparaben, polydextrose, polyethylene glycol, pregelatinized starch, titanium dioxide and triacetin.

EACH PACKET CONTAINS THESE ACTIVE INGREDIENTS	INDICATIONS FOR THESE FLU AND COLD SYMPTOMS:
PAIN RELIEVER-FEVER REDUCER (Acetaminophen 1000mg)	*Relieves headache, body aches, pain, reduces fever and soothes minor sore throat pain.*
COUGH SUPPRESSANT (Dextromethrophan HBr 30mg)	*Provides up to 8 hours of cough relief so you get the sleep you need.*
NASAL DECONGESTANT (Pseudoephedrine HCl 60mg)	*Helps clear nasal and sinus congestion.*
ANTIHISTAMINE (Chlorpheniramine Maleate 4mg)	*Relieves runny nose and sneezing.*

Sodium content: 3 mg per caplet.

Indications: TheraFlu Hot Liquid and caplets provide temporary relief of the symptoms associated with flu, common cold and other upper respiratory allergies including: headache, body aches, fever, minor sore throat pain, nasal and sinus congestion, runny nose and sneezing. TheraFlu Maximum Strength Flu, Cold, & Cough Medicine also suppresses coughs due to minor throat and bronchial irritation.

Warnings: Keep this and all drugs out of the reach of children. In case of accidental overdose, seek professional assistance or contact a poison control center immediately. Prompt medical attention is critical for adults as well as children even if you do not notice any signs or symptoms.
Do not exceed recommended dosage. If nervousness, dizziness, or sleeplessness occur, discontinue use and consult a doctor. If symptoms do not improve within 7 days or are accompanied by fever, consult a doctor. May cause excitability, especially in children. Do not take this product if you have heart disease, high blood pressure, thyroid disease, diabetes, glaucoma, a breathing problem such as emphysema or chronic bronchitis, or difficulty in urination due to enlargement of the prostate gland, unless directed by a doctor. A persistent cough may be a sign of a serious condition. If cough persists for more than 1 week, tends to recur, or is accompanied by a fever, rash, or persistent headache, consult a doctor. Do not take this product for persistent or chronic cough such as occurs with smoking, asthma, or emphysema, or if cough is accompanied by excessive phlegm (mucus) unless directed by a doctor.
Do not take this product for pain for more than 10 days or for fever for more than 3 days unless directed by a doctor. If pain or fever persists or gets worse, if new symptoms occur, or if redness or swelling is present, consult a doctor because these could be signs of a serious condition. If sore throat is severe, persists for more than 2 days, is accompanied or followed by fever, headache, rash, nausea, or vomiting, consult a doctor promptly.
May cause marked drowsiness; alcohol, sedatives, and tranquilizers may increase the drowsiness effect. Avoid alcoholic beverages while taking this product. Do not take this product if you are taking sedatives or tranquilizers, without first consulting your doctor. Use caution when driving a motor vehicle or operating machinery.
As with any drug, if you are pregnant or nursing a baby, seek the advice of a health professional before using this product.

Drug Interaction Precaution: Do not use this product if you are now taking a prescription monoamine oxidase inhibitor [MAOI] (certain drugs for depression, psychiatric or emotional conditions, or

Parkinson's disease), or for 2 weeks after stopping the MAOI drug. If you are uncertain whether your prescription drug contains an MAOI, consult a health professional before taking this product.

Alcohol Warning: If you consume 3 or more alcoholic drinks everyday ask your doctor whether you should take acetaminophen or other pain relievers/fever reducers. Acetaminophen may cause liver damage.

Directions: Adults and children 12 years of age and over: dissolve contents of one packet in 6 oz. cup of hot water; sip while hot. One packet every 6 hours, not to exceed 4 packets in 24 hours, or as directed by a doctor. Children under 12 years of age: consult a doctor. **Microwave Heating Instructions:** Add contents of packet and 6 oz. of cool water to a microwave-safe cup and stir briskly. Microwave on high $1^1/_2$ minutes or until water is hot. Do not boil water or overheat, and remember to stir liquid between reheatings. Sweeten to taste if desired.
TheraFlu NIGHTTIME Caplets: Adults and children 12 years of age and over: two caplets every 6 hours, not to exceed 8 caplets in 24 hours or as directed by a doctor. Children under 12 years of age: consult a doctor.

How Supplied: TheraFlu Maximum Strength NightTime Flu, Cold, & Cough Medicine powder in foil packets, 6, or 12, packets per carton. TheraFlu maximum strength NIGHTTIME Formula Caplets in blister packs of 12's.
Shown in Product Identification Guide, page 515

**THERAFLU®
MAXIMUM STRENGTH
NO-DROWSINESS FORMULA
THERAFLU® MAXIMUM
STRENGTH NON-DROWSY
FORMULA CAPLETS
Flu, Cold & Cough Medicine**

Description: Each packet of TheraFlu Maximum Strength Non-Drowsy Hot Liquid Formula contains: acetaminophen 1000 mg, pseudoephedrine HCl 60 mg, dextromethorphan 30 mg. **Inactive Ingredients:** Ascorbic acid (Vitamin C), citric acid, D&C Yellow 10, natural lemon flavors, maltol, pregelatinized starch, silicon dioxide, sodium citrate, sucrose, titanium dioxide and tribasic calcium phosphate.

Sodium content: 25 mg per packet.

Each TheraFlu Maximum Strength Non-Drowsy caplet contains: Dextromethorphan HBr, 15 mg, pseudoephedrine HCl 30 mg, and acetaminophen 500 mg. **Inactive ingredients:** colloidal silicon dioxide, croscarmellose sodium, D&C Yellow 10, FD&C Red 40, FD&C Yellow 6, gelatin, hydroxypropyl cellulose, hydroxypropyl methylcellulose, lactose, magnesium stearate, methylparaben, polydextrose, polyethylene glycol, pregelatinized starch, titanium dioxide and triacetin.

Sodium content: 3 mg per caplet.

Indications: Provides temporary relief of the symptoms associated with flu, common cold and other upper respiratory allergies including: headache, body aches, fever, minor sore throat pain, nasal and sinus congestion. TheraFlu Maximum Strength Non-Drowsy Formula also suppresses coughs due to minor throat and bronchial irritation.

Warnings: Keep this and all drugs out of the reach of children. In case of accidental overdose, seek professional assistance or contact a poison control center immediately. Prompt medical attention is critical for adults as well as children even if you do not notice any signs or symptoms.
Do not exceed recommended dosage. If nervousness, dizziness, or sleeplessness occur, discontinue use and consult a doctor. If symptoms do not improve within 7 days or are accompanied by fever, consult a doctor. Do not take this product if you have heart disease, high blood pressure, thyroid disease, diabetes, or difficulty in urination due to enlargement of the prostate gland unless directed by a physician.
A persistent cough may be a sign of a serious condition. If cough persists for more than 1 week, tends to recur, or is accompanied by a fever, rash, or persistent headache, consult a doctor. Do not take this product for persistent or chronic cough such as occurs with smoking, asthma, or emphysema, or if cough is accompanied by excessive phlegm (mucus) unless directed by a doctor.
Do not take this product for pain for more than 10 days or for fever for more than 3 days unless directed by a doctor. If pain or fever persists or gets worse, if new symptoms occur, or if redness or swelling is present, consult a doctor, because these could be signs of a serious condition. If sore throat is severe, persists for more than 2 days, is accompanied or followed by fever, headache, rash, nausea, or vomiting, consult a doctor promptly.
As with any drug, if you are pregnant or nursing a baby, seek the advice of a health professional before using this product.

Drug Interaction Precaution: Do not take this product if you are now taking a prescription monoamine oxidase inhibitor [MAOI] (certain drugs for depression, psychiatric or emotional conditions, or Parkinson's disease), or for 2 weeks after stopping the MAOI drug. If you are uncertain whether your prescription drug contains an MAOI, consult a health professional before taking this product.

Continued on next page

Information on Novartis Consumer Health, Inc., products appearing on these pages is effective as of November 1998.

Theraflu Non-Drowsy—Cont.

Alcohol Warning: If you consume 3 or more alcoholic drinks everyday ask your doctor whether you should take acetaminophen or other pain relievers/fever reducers. Acetaminophen may cause liver damage.

Directions: Adults and children 12 years of age and over: dissolve one packet in 6 oz. cup of hot water; sip while hot. One packet every 6 hours, not to exceed 4 packets in 24 hours, or as directed by a doctor. Children under 12 years of age: consult a doctor. Microwave Heating Instructions: Add contents of packet and 6 oz. of cool water to a microwave-safe cup and stir briskly. Microwave on high 1 1/2 minutes or until hot. Do not boil or overheat, and remember to stir liquid between reheatings. Sweeten to taste if desired.

TheraFlu Maximum Strength Non-Drowsy Caplet: Adults and Children 12 years of age and over: two caplets every 6 hours, not to exceed eight caplets in 24 hours or as directed by a doctor. Children under 12 years of age—Consult a doctor.

How Supplied: TheraFlu Maximum Strength No-Drowsiness Flu, Cold, & Cough Medicine powder in foil packets, 6 or 12 packets per carton. TheraFlu Maximum Strength Non-Drowsy Formula gelatin coated caplets (yellow) in blister packs of 12 and 24.

Shown in Product Identification Guide, page 515

TRIAMINIC® AM COUGH AND DECONGESTANT FORMULA

Description: Each teaspoon (5 mL) of TRIAMINIC® AM COUGH AND DECONGESTANT FORMULA contains: pseudoephedrine hydrochloride, USP 15 mg and dextromethorphan hydrobromide, USP 7.5 mg in a palatable, orange/stawberry flavored, dye-free, non-drowsy, alcohol-free liquid. **Inactive Ingredients:** benzoic acid, citric acid, dibasic sodium phosphate, edetate disodium, flavors, propylene glycol, purified water, sorbitol, sucrose.

Sodium content: 7 mg per teaspoon.

Indications: Temporarily quiets coughs due to minor throat and bronchial irritations and relieves stuffy noses.

Warnings: Keep this and all drugs out of the reach of children. In case of accidental overdose, seek professional assistance or contact a Poison Control Center immediately.

Do not exceed recommended dosage. If nervousness, dizziness, or sleeplessness occur, discontinue use and consult a doctor. If symptoms do not improve within 7 days or are accompanied by fever, consult a doctor. Do not take this product if you have heart disease, high blood pressure, thyroid disease, diabe-

tes, or difficulty in urination due to enlargement of the prostate gland, unless directed by a doctor.

A persistent cough may be a sign of a serious condition. If cough persists for more than 1 week, tends to recur, or is accompanied by fever, rash or persistent headache, consult a doctor. Do not take this product for persistent or chronic cough such as occurs with smoking, asthma, or emphysema or if cough is accompanied by excessive phlegm (mucus) unless directed by doctor.

As with any drug, if you are pregnant or nursing a baby, seek the advice of a health professional before using this product.

Drug Interaction Precaution: Do not use this product if you are now taking a prescription monoamine oxidase inhibitor [MAOI] (certain drugs for depression, psychiatric or emotional conditions, or Parkinson's disease), or for 2 weeks after stopping the MAOI drug. If you are uncertain whether your prescription drug contains an MAOI, consult a health professional before taking this product.

Dosage and Administration: Adults and children 12 and over (96+ lbs)—4 teaspoons every 6 hours. Children 6 to under 12 years (48–95 lbs)—2 teaspoons every 6 hours. Children 2 to under 6 years (24–47 lbs)—1 teaspoon every 6 hours. Do not exceed 4 doses in 24 hours, or as directed by a doctor. Dosing to children under 2 years of age is to be under the direction of a physician. For convenience, a True-Dose® dosage cup is provided with each 4 fl. oz. bottle.

Professional Labeling: The suggested dosage for pediatric patients is:

4–12 months	1.25 ml ($^1/_4$ tsp)
(12–17 lbs)	every 6 hours
12–24 months	2.5 ml ($^1/_2$ tsp)
(18–23 lbs)	every 6 hours

Do not exceed 4 doses in 24 hours.

How Supplied: TRIAMINIC AM COUGH AND DECONGESTANT FORMULA (clear liquid) in 4 fl. oz. plastic bottles with tamper-evident band around child-resistant cap. Dosage cup included. Orange/strawberry flavored. Alcohol-free. Dye-free. Non-drowsy.

Shown in Product Identification Guide, page 515

TRIAMINIC® AM DECONGESTANT FORMULA

Description: Each teaspoon (5 mL) of TRIAMINIC® AM DECONGESTANT FORMULA contains: pseudoephedrine hydrochloride, USP 15 mg in a palatable, orange/strawberry flavored, dye-free, non-drowsy, alcohol-free liquid. **Inactive ingredients:** benzoic acid, edetate disodium, flavors, purified water, sodium hydroxide, sorbitol, sucrose.

Sodium content: 1 mg per teaspoon.

Indications: For temporary relief of nasal congestion due to the common cold,

hay fever or other upper respiratory allergies, or associated with sinusitis. Reduces swelling of nasal passages; shrinks swollen membranes.

Warnings: Keep this and all drugs out of the reach of children. In case of accidental overdose, seek professional assistance or contact a poison control center immediately.

Do not exceed recommended dosage. If nervousness, dizziness, or sleeplessness occur, discontinue use and consult a doctor. If symptoms do not improve within 7 days or are accompanied by fever, consult a doctor. Do not take this product if you have heart disease, high blood pressure, thyroid disease, diabetes, or difficulty in urination due to enlargement of the prostate gland, unless directed by a doctor.

As with any drug, if you are pregnant or nursing a baby, seek the advice of a health professional before using this product.

Drug Interaction Precaution: Do not use this product if you are now taking a prescription monoamine oxidase inhibitor [MAOI] (certain drugs for depression, psychiatric or emotional conditions, or Parkinson's disease) or for 2 weeks after stopping the MAOI drug. If you are uncertain whether your prescription drug contains an MAOI, consult a health professional before taking this product.

Dosage and Administration: Adults and children 12 and over (96+ lbs)—4 teaspoons every 4–6 hours. Children 6 to under 12 years (48–95 lbs)—2 teaspoons every 4–6 hours. Children 2 to under 6 years (24–47 lbs)—1 teaspoon every 4–6 hours. Do not exceed 4 doses in 24 hours, or as directed by a doctor. Dosing to children under 2 years of age is to be under the direction of a physician. For convenience, a True-Dose® dosage cup is provided with each 4 fl. oz. bottle.

Professional Labeling: The suggested dosage for pediatric patients is:

4–12 months	1.25 ml ($^1/_4$ tsp)
(12–17 lbs)	every 4 to 6 hours
12–24 months	2.5 ml ($^1/_2$ tsp)
(18–23 lbs)	every 4 to 6 hours

Do not exceed 4 doses in 24 hours.

How Supplied: TRIAMINIC AM DECONGESTANT FORMULA (clear liquid) in 4 fl oz plastic bottles with tamper-evident band around child-resistant cap. Dosage cup included. Orange/strawberry flavored. Alcohol-free. Dye-free. Non-drowsy.

Shown in Product Identification Guide, page 515

TRIAMINIC® EXPECTORANT

Description: Each teaspoon (5 mL) of TRIAMINIC® Expectorant contains: guaifenesin, USP 50 mg, and phenylpropanolamine hydrochloride, USP 6.25 mg in a palatable, citrus-flavored alcohol-free liquid. **Inactive ingredients:** benzoic acid, D&C Yellow 10, edetate disodium, FD&C Yellow 6, flavors, glycerin, polyethylene glycol, propylene glycol, purified water, sorbitol and sucrose.

Sodium-free.

Indications: Relieves chest congestion by loosening phlegm to help clear bronchial passageways. Temporarily relieves stuffy nose.

Warnings: Keep this and all drugs out of the reach of children. In case of accidental overdose, seek professional assistance or contact a poison control center immediately.

Do not exceed recommended dosage. If nervousness, dizziness, or sleeplessness occur, discontinue use and consult a doctor. If symptoms do not improve within 7 days or are accompanied by fever, consult a doctor. A persistent cough may be a sign of a serious condition. If cough persists for more than 1 week, tends to recur, or is accompanied by fever, rash, or persistent headache, consult a doctor. Do not take this product: 1) if cough is accompanied by excessive phlegm (mucus), 2) for persistent or chronic cough such as occurs with smoking, asthma, chronic bronchitis or emphysema. 3) if you have heart disease, high blood pressure, thyroid disease, diabetes, difficulty in urination due to enlargement of the prostate gland, or 4) if you are presently taking another product containing phenylpropanolamine, unless directed by a doctor.

As with any drug, if you are pregnant or nursing a baby, seek the advice of a health professional before using this product.

Drug Interaction Precaution: Do not use this product if you are now taking a prescription monoamine oxidase inhibitor [MAOI] (certain drugs for depression, psychiatric or emotional conditions, or Parkinson's disease), or for 2 weeks after stopping the MAOI drug. If you are uncertain whether your prescription drug contains an MAOI, consult a health professional before taking this product.

Dosage and Administration: Adults and children 12 and over (96+ lbs)—4 teaspoons every 4 hours. Children 6 to under 12 years (48–95 lbs)—2 teaspoons every 4 hours. Children 2 to under 6 years (24–47 lbs)—1 teaspoon every 4 hours. Do not exceed 6 doses in 24 hours, or as directed by a doctor. Dosing to children under 2 years of age is to be under the direction of a physician. For convenience, a True-Dose® dosage cup is provided with each 4 fl. oz. and 8 fl. oz. bottle.

Professional Labeling: The suggested dosage for pediatric patients is:

4–12 months	1.25 ml ($^1/_4$ tsp)
(12–17 lbs)	every 4 hours
12–24 months	2.5 ml ($^1/_2$ tsp)
(18–23 lbs)	every 4 hours

Do not exceed 6 doses in 24 hours.

How Supplied: TRIAMINIC Expectorant (yellow), in 4 fl oz and 8 fl oz plastic bottles with tamper-evident band around child-resistant cap. Dosage cup included. Citrus flavored, Alcohol free.

Shown in Product Identification Guide, page 515

TRIAMINIC® INFANT
Oral Decongestant Drops

Description: Each dropperful (0.8mL) of Triaminic Infant Oral Decongestant Drops contains: pseudoephedrine hydrochloride, USP 7.5 mg in a palatable, grape-flavored alcohol-free, dye-free liquid. **Inactive ingredients:** benzoic acid, edetate disodium, flavors, purified water, sodium chloride, sorbitol solution, sucrose.

Sodium-free.

Indications: For temporary relief of nasal congestion due to the common cold, hay fever or other upper respiratory allergies, or nasal congestion associated with sinusitis. The decongestant is provided in an alcohol-free and antihistamine-free formula.

Warnings: Keep this and all drugs out of the reach of children. In case of accidental overdose, seek professional assistance or contact a poison control center immediately.

Do not exceed recommended dosage. If nervousness, dizziness, or sleeplessness occur, discontinue use and consult a doctor. If symptoms do not improve within 7 days or are accompanied by fever, consult a doctor. Do not give this product to a child who has heart disease, high blood pressure, thyroid disease, or diabetes unless directed by a doctor.

Drug Interaction Precaution: Do not give this product to a child who is taking a prescription monoamine oxidase inhibitor [MAOI] (certain drugs for depression, psychiatric or emotional conditions) or for 2 weeks after stopping the MAOI drug. If you are uncertain whether your child's prescription drug contains an MAOI, consult a health professional before giving this product.

Dosage and Administration: Children 2 to 3 years of age (24–35 lbs.): Two dropperfuls (1.6mL) every 4–6 hours (or as directed by a doctor). Children under 2 years of age: consult a doctor. **Do not exceed 4 doses in a 24-hour period. Give by mouth only.** Not for use in the nose. For convenience, a True-Dose® dosing child-resistant dropper is provided.
Professional Labeling: The suggested dosage for pediatric patients is:

Age	Weight	Amount
4–11 months	12–17 lbs.	1 dropperful (0.8mL)
12–23 months	18–23 lbs.	1½ dropperfuls (1.2mL)
2–3 years	24–35 lbs.	2 dropperfuls (1.6mL)

The dose may be repeated every 4 to 6 hours, not to exceed 4 doses in 24 hours or as directed by a doctor.

How Supplied: Triaminic Infant Oral Decongestant Drops (clear), in a $^1/_2$ fl. oz. (15mL) glass bottle with tamper evident band around cap. True-Dose® dosing child-resistant dropper is also provided. Grape flavored, alcohol-free, antihistamine-free, crystal clear, non-staining formula.

TRIAMINIC® Night Time
Maximum Strength
Nighttime Cough and Cold Medicine

Description: Each teaspoon (5 mL) of Triaminic® Night Time contains: pseudoephedrine hydrochloride USP 15 mg, dextromethorphan hydrobromide, USP 7.5 mg, chlorpheniramine maleate, USP 1 mg, in a palatable, grape-flavored, alcohol-free liquid.

Inactive ingredients: benzoic acid, citric acid, D&C Red 33, dibasic sodium phosphate, FD&C Blue 1, flavors, propylene glycol, purified water, sorbitol, sucrose.

Sodium content: 23 mg per teaspoon.

Indications: Temporarily relieves cold and allergy symptoms, including coughs due to minor throat and bronchial irritation, runny nose; stuffy nose; sneezing; itching of the nose or throat; and itchy, watery eyes.

Warnings: Keep this and all drugs out of the reach of children. In case of accidental overdose, seek professional assistance or contact a poison control center immediately.

Do not exceed recommended dosage. If nervousness, dizziness, or sleeplessness occur, discontinue use and consult a doctor. If symptoms do not improve within 7 days or are accompanied by fever, consult a doctor. A persistent cough may be a sign of a serious condition. If cough persists for more than 1 week, tends to recur, or is accompanied by fever, rash, or persistent headache, consult a doctor. Do not take this product: 1) if cough is accompanied by excessive phlegm (mucus), 2) for persistent or chronic cough such as occurs with smoking, asthma or emphysema, 3) if you have heart disease, high blood pressure, thyroid disease, diabetes, glaucoma, a breathing problem such as emphysema or chronic bronchitis, or difficulty in urination due to enlargement of the prostate gland, or 4) if you are taking sedatives or tranquilizers, unless directed by a doctor. May cause excitability especially in children. May cause drowsiness; alcohol, sedatives or tranquilizers may increase the drowsiness effect. Avoid al-

Continued on next page

Information on Novartis Consumer Health, Inc., products appearing on these pages is effective as of November 1998.

Triaminic Night Time—Cont.

coholic beverages while taking this product. Use caution when driving a motor vehicle or operating machinery. Do not use this product if you are on a sodium restricted diet unless directed by a doctor. As with any drug, if you are pregnant or nursing a baby, seek the advice of a health professional before using this product.

Drug Interaction Precaution: Do not use this product if you are now taking a prescription monoamine oxidase inhibitor (MAOI) (certain drugs for depression, psychiatric or emotional conditions, or Parkinson's disease) or for 2 weeks after stopping the MAOI drug. If you are uncertain whether your prescription drug contains an MAOI, consult a health professional before taking this product.

Dosage and Administration: Adults and children 12 and over (96+ lbs.)—4 teaspoons every 6 hours. Children 6 to under 12 years (48–95 lbs.)—2 teaspoons every 6 hours. Do not exceed 4 doses in 24 hours, or as directed by a doctor. Dosing to children under 6 years of age is to be under the direction of a physician. For convenience, a True-Dose® dosage cup is provided with each 4 fl. oz. and 8 fl. oz. bottle.

Professional Labeling: The suggested dosage for pediatric patients is:

4 to under 12 months (12–17 lbs.)	$1/4$ teaspoon or 1.25 ml every 6 hours
12 months to under 2 years (18–23 lbs.)	$1/2$ teaspoon or 2.5 ml every 6 hours
2 to under 6 years	1 teaspoon or 5 ml every 6 hours

Not to exceed 4 doses in 24 hours

How Supplied: Triaminic® Night Time Cough and Cold Medicine for Children (purple), in 4 fl. oz. and 8 fl. oz. plastic bottles packaged in cartons with tamper-evident band around child-resistant cap. Grape flavored. Alcohol free.

Shown in Product Identification Guide, page 515

TRIAMINIC
Severe Cold & Fever

Directions: Children 6 to under 12 years of age: 2 teaspoons every 6 hours. Children 12 years of age and over and adults: 4 teaspoons every 6 hours. Do not exceed 4 doses in 24 hours, or as directed by a doctor. Children under 6 years of age: consult a doctor.

AGE	WEIGHT	DOSAGE
Under 6 yrs.	Under 48 lbs.	Consult a Doctor
6 to Under 12 yrs.	48-95 lbs.	2 Teaspoons

The dose may be repeated every 6 hours—not to exceed 4 doses in 24 hours, or as directed by a doctor.

Indications: Temporarily relieves fever, minor aches and pains, headaches and sore throat, quiets coughs, relieves stuffy nose; sneezing; itching of the nose or throat; and itchy, watery eyes.

Each Teaspoon (5ML) Contains: acetaminophen, USP, 160 mg, pseudoephedrine hydrochloride, USP, 15 mg, dextromethorphan hydrobromide, USP, 7.5 mg, and chlorpheniramine maleate, USP, 1 mg. **Inactive Ingredients:** Acesulfame K, benzoic acid, citric acid, dibasic potassium phosphate, disodium edetate, flavors, glycerin, polyethylene glycol, potassium chloride, propylene glycol, purified water, D&C Red No. 33, FD&C Red No. 40, sucrose and other ingredients.

Warnings: Keep this and all drugs out of the reach of children. In case of accidental overdose, seek professional assistance or contact a poison control center immediately. Prompt medical attention is critical for adults as well as children even if you do not notice any signs or symptoms. **Do not exceed recommended dosage.** If nervousness, dizziness, or sleeplessness occur, discontinue use and consult a doctor. Do not take for pain for more than 5 days or for fever for more than 3 days unless directed by a doctor. If pain or fever persists, or gets worse, if new symptoms occur, or if redness or swelling is present, consult a doctor promptly because these could be signs of a serious condition. If sore throat is severe, persists for more than 2 days, is accompanied or followed by fever, headache, rash, nausea or vomiting, consult a doctor promptly. If symptoms do not improve within 7 days or are accompanied by fever, consult a doctor. A persistent cough may be a sign of a serious condition. If cough persists for more than 1 week, tends to recur or is accompanied by a rash, persistent headache, fever that lasts for more than 3 days, or if new symptoms occur, consult a doctor. Do not give this product: 1) if cough is accompanied by excessive phlegm (mucus). 2) for persistent or chronic cough such as occurs with smoking, asthma, chronic bronchitis or emphysema, or 3) if you have heart disease, high blood pressure, thyroid disease, diabetes, glaucoma, or difficulty in urination due to enlargement of the prostate gland, unless directed by a doctor. May cause excitability especially in children. May cause drowsiness; alcohol, sedatives and tranquilizers may increase the drowsiness effect. Avoid alcoholic beverages while taking this product. Use caution when driving a motor vehicle or operating machinery. As with any drug, if you are pregnant or nursing a baby, seek the advice of a health professional before using this product.

Drug Interaction Precaution: Do not use this product if you are now taking a prescription monamine oxidase inhibitor [MAOI] (certain drugs for depression,

psychiatric or emotional conditions, or Parkinson's disease), or for 2 weeks after stopping the MAOI drug. If you are uncertain whether your prescription drug contains an MAOI, consult a health professional before taking this product.

> **Triaminic Severe Cold and Fever contains acetaminophen. It should not be taken in combination with other products containing acetaminophen, such as Children's Tylenol*, except as directed by your doctor.**

*Children's Tylenol is a registered trademark of McNeil Consumer.

How Supplied: 4 fl. oz. (118 mL)
STORE AT ROOM TEMPERATURE. PROTECT FROM LIGHT. CONTAINS NO ASPIRIN.
NOVARTIS
©1998 Novartis Consumer Health, Inc. Summit, NJ 07901-1312

Shown in Product Identification Guide, page 515

TRIAMINIC® SOFTCHEWS®
Cold & Allergy
Nasal Decongestant, Antihistamine

Clears Stuffy Noses
Relieves Runny Noses
Relieves Sneezing & Itchy, Watery Eyes

Directions: Let *Softchews®* tablet dissolve in mouth or chew *Softchews®* tablet before swallowing, whichever is preferred. Children 6 to under 12 years of age: 2 tablets every 4 to 6 hours. Children 12 years of age and over and adults: 4 tablets every 4 to 6 hours. Do not exceed 4 doses in 24 hours, or as directed by a doctor. Children under 6 years of age, consult a doctor.

AGE	WEIGHT	DOSAGE
UNDER 6 YEARS	UNDER 48 lbs.	CONSULT A DOCTOR
6 TO UNDER 12 YEARS	48–95 lbs.	TWO (2) SOFTCHEWS® TABLETS
12 YEARS TO ADULT	96+ lbs.	FOUR (4) SOFTCHEWS® TABLETS

The dose may be repeated every 4–6 hours, not to exceed 4 doses in 24 hours, or as directed by a doctor.

Indications: Temporarily relieves cold and allergy symptoms, including runny nose; stuffy nose; sneezing; itching of the nose or throat; and itchy, watery eyes.

Each SOFTCHEWS® Tablet Contains: pseudoephedrine hydrochloride, USP, 15mg, chlorpheniramine maleate, USP, 1 mg. **Inactive ingredients:** aspartame, citric acid, crospovidone D&C Red No. 27 aluminum lake, D&C Yellow No. 10 aluminum lake, distilled acetylated monoglycerides, ethylcellulose, flavors, mannitol, magnesium stearate, silicon dioxide and sodium bicarbonate.

Sodium content: 5.1mg per *Softchews®* Tablet.

Warnings: Keep this and all drugs out of the reach of children. In case of accidental overdose, seek professional assistance or contact a poison control center immediately. Prompt medical attention is critical for adults, as well as for children, even if you do not notice any signs or symptoms.

Do not exceed recommended dosage. If nervousness, dizziness, or sleeplessness occur, discontinue use and consult a doctor. If symptoms do not improve within 7 days or are accompanied by fever, consult a doctor. Do not take this product: 1) if you have heart disease, high blood pressure, thyroid disease, diabetes, glaucoma, a breathing problem such as emphysema or chronic bronchitis, or difficulty in urination due to enlargement of the prostate gland: 2) if you are taking sedatives or tranquilizers, unless directed by a doctor. May cause excitability, especially in children. May cause drowsiness; alcohol, sedatives, and tranquilizers may increase the drowsiness effect. Avoid alcoholic beverages while taking this product. Use caution when driving a motor vehicle or operating machinery. As with any drug, if you are pregnant or nursing a baby, seek the advice of a health professional before using this product.

Drug Interaction Precaution: Do not use this product if you are now taking a prescription monoamine oxidase inhibitor [MAOI] (certain drugs for depression, psychiatric or emotional conditions, or Parkinson's disease), or for 2 weeks after stopping the MAOI drug. If you are uncertain whether your prescription drug contains an MAOI, consult a health professional before taking this product.
STORE AT ROOM TEMPERATURE. CONTAINS NO ASPIRIN.
Phenylketonurics: Contains phenylalanine, 17.4mg per *Softchews®* Tablet.

How Supplied: 18 Softchews® Tablets.
Distributed by:
NOVARTIS
©1998 Novartis Consumer Health, Inc.
Summit, NJ 07901–1312
U.S. Pat. No. 5,178,878
Shown in Product Identification Guide, page 516

TRIAMINIC® SOFTCHEWS®
Cold & Cough
Nasal Decongestant, Cough Suppressant, Antihistamine

Quiets Coughs
Clears Stuffy Noses
Relieves Runny Noses
Relieves Sneezing & Itchy, Watery Eyes

Directions: Let *Softchews®* tablet dissolve in mouth or chew *Softchews®* tablet before swallowing, whichever is preferred. Children 6 to under 12 years of age: 2 tablets every 4 to 6 hours. Children 12 years of age and over and adults: 4 tablets every 4 to 6 hours. Do not exceed 4 doses in 24 hours, or as directed by a doctor. Children under 6 years of age, consult a doctor.

AGE	WEIGHT	DOSAGE
UNDER 6 YEARS	UNDER 48 lbs.	CONSULT A DOCTOR
6 TO UNDER 12 YEARS	48–95 lbs.	TWO (2) *SOFTCHEWS®* TABLETS
12 YEARS TO ADULT	96+ lbs.	FOUR (4) *SOFTCHEWS®* TABLETS

The dose may be repeated every 4–6 hours, not to exceed 4 doses in 24 hours, or as directed by a doctor.

Indications: Temporarily relieves cold and allergy symptoms, including coughs due to minor throat and bronchial irritation; runny nose; stuffy nose; sneezing; itching of the nose or throat; and itchy, water eyes.

Each *SOFTCHEWS®* Tablet Contains: pseudoephedrine hydrochloride, USP, 15mg, dextromethorphan hydrobromide, USP, 5mg, and chlorpheniramine maleate, USP, 1mg.

Inactive ingredients: aspartame, citric acid, crospovidone, D&C Red No. 27 aluminum lake, distilled acetylated monoglycerides, ethylcellulose, flavors, mannitol, magnesium stearate, silicon dioxide and sodium bicarbonate.

Sodium content: 5.1mg per *Softchews®* Tablet.

Warnings: Keep this and all drugs out of the reach of children. In case of accidental overdose, seek professional assistance or contact a poison control center immediately. Prompt medical attention is critical for adults, as well as for children, even if you do not notice any signs or symptoms.
Do not exceed recommended dosage. If nervousness, dizziness, or sleeplessness occur, discontinue use and consult a doctor. If symptoms do not improve within 7 days or are accompanied by fever, consult a doctor. A persistent cough may be a sign of a serious condition. If cough persists for more than 7 days, tends to recur, or is accompanied by fever, rash, or persistent headache, or if new symptoms occur, consult a doctor. Do not take this product: 1) if cough is accompanied by excessive phlegm (mucus); 2) for persistent or chronic cough such as occurs with smoking, asthma, or emphysema; 3) if you have heart disease, high blood pressure, thyroid disease, diabetes, glaucoma, a breathing problem

such as emphysema or chronic bronchitis, or difficulty in urination due to enlargement of the prostate gland; or 4) if you are taking sedatives or tranquilizers, unless directed by a doctor. May cause excitability, especially in children. May cause drowsiness; alcohol, sedatives, and tranquilizers may increase the drowsiness effect. Avoid alcoholic beverages while taking this product. Use caution when driving a motor vehicle or operating machinery. As with any drug, if you are pregnant or nursing a baby, seek the advice of a health professional before using this product.

Drug Interaction Precaution: Do not use this product if you are now taking a prescription monoamine oxidase inhibitor [MAOI] (certain drugs for depression, psychiatric or emotional conditions, or Parkinson's disease), or for 2 weeks after stopping the MAOI drug. If you are uncertain whether your prescription drug contains an MAOI, consult a health professional before taking this product.
STORE AT ROOM TEMPERATURE. CONTAINS NO ASPIRIN.
Phenylketonurics: Contains phenylalanine, 17.4mg per *Softchews®* Tablet.

How Supplied: 18 Softchews® Tablets
Distributed by:
NOVARTIS
©1998 Novartis Consumer Health, Inc.
Summit, NJ 07901-1312
U.S. Pat. No. 5,178,878
Shown in Product Identification Guide, page 516

TRIAMINIC® SOFTCHEWS®
Throat Pain & Cough
Pain Reliever-Fever Reducer, Nasal Decongestant, Cough Suppressant

Eases Sore Throat Pain
Quiets Coughs
Clears Stuffy Noses
Reduces Fever

Directions: Let *Softchews®* tablet dissolve in mouth or chew *Softchews®* tablet before swallowing, whichever is preferred. Children 2 to under 6 years of age: 1 tablet every 4 to 6 hours. Children 6 to under 12 years of age: 2 tablets every 4 to 6 hours. Children 12 years of age and over and adults: 4 tablets every 4 to 6 hours. Do not exceed 4 doses in 24 hours, or as directed by a doctor. Children under 2 years of age, consult a doctor.

AGE	WEIGHT	DOSAGE
UNDER 2 YEARS	UNDER 24 lbs.	CONSULT A DOCTOR

Continued on next page

Information on Novartis Consumer Health, Inc., products appearing on these pages is effective as of November 1998.

Triaminic Softchews—Cont.

2 TO UNDER 6 YEARS	24–47 lbs.	ONE (1) *SOFTCHEWS®* TABLET
6 TO UNDER 12 YEARS	48–95 lbs.	TWO (2) *SOFTCHEWS®* TABLETS
12 YEARS TO ADULT	96+ lbs.	FOUR (4) *SOFTCHEWS®* TABLETS

The dose may be repeated every 4–6 hours, not to exceed 4 doses in 24 hours, or as directed by a doctor.

Indications: Temporarily relieves sore throat pain and other minor aches and pains, quiets coughs due to minor throat and bronchial irritation, relieves stuffy nose, and reduces fever.

Each *SOFTCHEWS®* Tablet Contains: acetaminophen, USP, 160mg, pseudoephedrine hydrochloride, USP, 15mg, dextromethorphan hydrobromide, USP, 5mg. **Inactive Ingredients:** aspartame, citric acid, crospovidone, FD&C Blue No. 1 aluminum lake, D&C Red No. 27 aluminum lake, distilled acetylated monoglycerides, ethylcellulose, flavors, mannitol, magnesium stearate, silicon dioxide and sodium bicarbonate.

Sodium content: 8.2mg per *Softchews®* Tablet.

Warnings: Keep this and all drugs out of the reach of children. In case of accidental overdose, seek professional assistance or contact a poison control center immediately. Prompt medical attention is critical for adults, as well as for children, even if you do not notice any signs or symptoms.

Do not exceed recommended dosage. If nervousness, dizziness, or sleeplessness occur, discontinue use and consult a doctor. Do not take this product for more than 7 days (for adults) or 5 days (for children). Do not take for sore throat pain for more than 2 days, or for fever for more than 3 days. If pain or fever persists or gets worse. If new symptoms occur, or if redness or swelling is present, consult a doctor because these could be signs of a serious condition. If sore throat is severe, persists for more than 2 days, is accompanied or followed by fever, headache, rash, nausea or vomiting, consult a doctor promptly. If symptoms do not improve within 7 days or are accompanied by fever, consult a doctor. A persistent cough may be a sign of a serious condition. If cough persists for more than 7 days, tends to recur, or is accompanied by rash, persistent headache, fever that lasts for more than 3 days or if new symptoms occur, consult a doctor. Do not take this product: 1) if cough is accompanied by excessive phlegm (mucus); 2) for persistent or chronic cough such as occurs with smoking, asthma or emphysema; or 3) if you have heart disease, high blood pressure, thyroid disease, diabetes, or difficulty in urination due to enlargement of the prostate gland unless directed by a doctor. As with any drug, if you are pregnant or nursing a baby, seek the advice of a health professional before using this product. **Triaminic®** *Softchews®* **Throat Pain & Cough formula contains acetaminophen. It should not be taken in combination with other products containing acetaminophen such as Children's Tylenol*, except as directed by your doctor.**

Alcohol Warning: If you consume 3 or more alcoholic drinks everyday ask your doctor whether you should take acetaminophen or other pain relievers/fever reducers. Acetaminophen may cause liver damage.

Drug Interaction Precaution: Do not use this product if you are now taking a prescription monoamine oxidase inhibitor [MAOI] (certain drugs for depression, psychiatric or emotional conditions, or Parkinson's disease), or for 2 weeks after stopping the MAOI drug. If you are uncertain whether your prescription drug contains an MAOI, consult a health professional before taking this product.

STORE AT ROOM TEMPERATURE. CONTAINS NO ASPIRIN.

Phenylketonurics: Contains phenylalanine, 28.1mg per *Softchews®* Tablet.

*Children's Tylenol is a registered trademark of McNeil Consumer.

How Supplied: 18 Softchews Tablets
Distributed by:
NOVARTIS
©1998 Novartis Consumer Health, Inc.
Summit, NJ 07901-1312
U.S. Pat. No. 5,178,878

Shown in Product Identification Guide, page 516

TRIAMINIC®
Sore Throat Formula

Description: Each teaspoon (5 mL) of Triaminic® Sore Throat Formula contains: acetaminophen, USP 160 mg, pseudoephedrine hydrochloride, USP 15 mg and dextromethorphan hydrobromide, USP 7.5 mg, in a palatable, grape-flavored, alcohol-free liquid. **Inactive ingredients:** benzoic acid, D&C Red 33, dibasic sodium phosphate, edetate disodium, FD&C Blue 1, FD&C Red 40, flavors, glycerin, polyethylene glycol, propylene glycol, purified water, sucrose and tartaric acid.

Sodium content: 12 mg per teaspoon.

Indications: Temporarily relieves sore throat pain and other minor aches and pains, quiets coughs due to minor throat and bronchial irritations, relieves stuffy nose, and reduces fever.

Warnings: Keep this and all drugs out of the reach of children. In case of accidental overdose, seek professional assistance or contact a poison control center immediately. Prompt medical attention is critical for adults as well as for children even if you do not notice any signs or symptoms.

Do not exceed recommended dosage. If nervousness, dizziness, or sleeplessness occur, discontinue use and consult a doctor. Do not take this product for more than 7 days (for adults) or 5 days (for children). Do not take for sore throat pain for more than 2 days, and for fever for more than 3 days. If pain or fever persists or gets worse, if new symptoms occur, or if redness or swelling is present, consult a doctor because these could be signs of a serious condition. If sore throat is severe, persists for more than 2 days, is accompanied or followed by fever, headache, rash, nausea, or vomiting, consult a doctor promptly. If symptoms do not improve within 7 days or are accompanied by fever, consult a doctor. A persistent cough may be a sign of a serious condition. If cough persists for more than 1 week, tends to recur, or is accompanied by rash, persistent headache, fever that lasts for more than 3 days, or if new symptoms occur, consult a doctor. Do not take this product: 1) if cough is accompanied by excessive phlegm (mucus), 2) for persistent or chronic cough such as occurs with smoking, asthma or emphysema, or 3) if you have heart disease, high blood pressure, thyroid disease, diabetes, difficulty in urination due to enlargement of the prostate gland, unless directed by a doctor. As with any drug, if you are pregnant or nursing a baby, seek advice from a health professional before using this product. Do not use this product if you are on a sodium restricted diet unless directed by a doctor.

Alcohol Warning: If you consume 3 or more alcoholic drinks every day, ask your doctor whether you should take acetaminophen or other pain relievers/fever reducers. Acetaminophen may cause liver damage.

Drug Interaction Precaution: Do not use this product if you are now taking a prescription monoamine oxidase inhibitor [MAOI] (certain drugs for depression, psychiatric or emotional conditions, or Parkinson's disease) or for 2 weeks after stopping the MAOI drug. If you are uncertain whether your prescription drug contains an MAOI, consult a health professional before taking this product. Triaminic Sore Throat Formula contains acetaminophen. It should not be taken in combination with other products containing acetaminophen, such as Children's Tylenol®*, except as directed by your doctor. (*Children's Tylenol is a registered trademark of McNeil Consumer)

Dosage and Administration: Adults and children 12 and over (96+lbs)—4 teaspoons every 6 hours. Children 6 to under 12 years (48–95 lbs)—2 teaspoons every 6 hours. Children 2 to under 6 years (24–47 lbs)—1 teaspoon every 6 hours. Do not exceed 4 doses in 24 hours, or as directed by a doctor. Dosing to children under 2 years of age is to be under the direction of a physician. For convenience, a True-Dose® dosage cup is provided with each 4 fl. oz and 8 fl. oz. bottle.

Professional Labeling: The suggested dosage for pediatric patients is:

4–12 months　　　1.25 ml ($^1/_4$ tsp)
(12–17 lbs)　　　　every 6 hours
12–24 months　　　2.5 ml ($^1/_2$ tsp)
(18–23 lbs)　　　　every 6 hours
2–6 years　　　　　5 ml (1 tsp)
(24–47 lbs)　　　　every 6 hours
Do not exceed 4 doses in 24 hours.

How Supplied: Triaminic Sore Throat Formula (purple), in 4 fl. oz. and 8 fl. oz. plastic bottles with tamper-evident band around child resistant cap. Grape flavored, alcohol-free.

Shown in Product Identification Guide, page 516

TRIAMINIC® SYRUP

Description: Each teaspoon (5 mL) of TRIAMINIC® Syrup contains: phenylpropanolamine hydrochloride, USP 6.25 mg and chlorpheniramine maleate USP 1 mg in a palatable, orange-flavored, alcohol-free liquid. **Inactive ingredients:** benzoic acid, edetate disodium, FD&C Yellow 6, flavors, purified water, sodium hydroxide, sorbitol, and sucrose.

Sodium content: 1 mg per teaspoon.

Indications: Temporarily relieves cold and allergy symptoms, including runny nose; stuffy nose; itching of the nose or throat; and itchy, watery eyes.

Warnings: Keep this and all drugs out of the reach of children. In case of accidental overdose, seek professional assistance or contact a poison control center immediately.

Do not exceed recommended dosage. If nervousness, dizziness or sleeplessness occur, discontinue use and consult a doctor. If symptoms do not improve within 7 days or are accompanied by fever, consult a doctor. Do not take this product: 1) if you have heart disease, high blood pressure, thyroid disease, diabetes, glaucoma, a breathing problem such as emphysema or chronic bronchitis, or difficulty in urination due to enlargement of the prostate gland, 2) if you are taking sedatives or tranquilizers, or 3) if you are presently taking another product containing phenylpropanolamine, unless directed by a doctor. May cause excitability, especially in children. May cause drowsiness; alcohol, sedatives or tranquilizers may increase the drowsiness effect. Avoid alcoholic beverages while taking this product. Use caution when driving a motor vehicle or operating machinery.
As with any drug, if you are pregnant or nursing a baby, seek the advice of a health professional before using this product.

Drug Interaction Precaution: Do not use this product if you are now taking a prescription monoamine oxidase inhibitor [MAOI] (certain drugs for depression, psychiatric or emotional conditions, or Parkinson's disease) or for 2 weeks after stopping the MAOI drug. If you are uncertain whether your prescription

drug contains an MAOI, consult a health professional before taking this product.

Dosage and Administration: Adults and children 12 and over (96+ lbs)—4 teaspoons every 4 to 6 hours. Children 6 to under 12 years (48–95 lbs)—2 teaspoons every 4 to 6 hours. Do not exceed 6 doses in 24 hours, or as directed by a doctor. Dosing to children under 6 years of age is to be under the direction of a physician. For convenience, a True-Dose® dosage cup is provided with each 4 fl. oz. and 8 fl. oz. bottle.

Professional Labeling: The suggested dosage for pediatric patients is:

4–12 months　　　1.25 ml ($^1/_4$ tsp)
(12–17 lbs)　　　　every 4 to 6 hours
12–24 months　　　2.5 ml ($^1/_2$ tsp)
(18–23 lbs)　　　　every 4 to 6 hours
2–6 years　　　　　5 ml (1 tsp)
(24–47 lbs)　　　　every 4 to 6 hours
Do not exceed 6 doses in 24 hours.

How Supplied: TRIAMINIC Syrup (orange), in 4 fl oz and 8 fl oz plastic bottles with tamper-evident band around child-resistant cap. Dosage cup included. Orange flavored. Alcohol-free.

Shown in Product Identification Guide, page 516

TRIAMINIC®
TRIAMINICOL® Cold & Cough

Description: Each teaspoon (5 mL) of TRIAMINIC® Cold & Cough contains: phenylpropanolamine hydrochloride, USP 6.25 mg, dextromethorphan hydrobromide, USP 5 mg, chlorpheniramine maleate, USP 1 mg in a palatable, cherry flavored alcohol-free liquid. **Inactive ingredients:** benzoic acid, FD&C Red 40, flavor, propylene glycol, purified water, sodium chloride, sorbitol, sucrose.

Sodium content: 5 mg per teaspoon.

Indications: Temporarily relieves cold and allergy symptoms, including coughs due to minor throat and bronchial irritation, runny nose, stuffy nose, sneezing, itching of the nose or throat and itchy, watery eyes.

Warnings: Keep this and all drugs out of the reach of children. In case of accidental overdose, seek professional assistance or contact a poison control center immediately.

Do not exceed recommended dosage. If nervousness, dizziness, or sleeplessness occur, discontinue use and consult a doctor. If symptoms do not improve within 7 days or are accompanied by fever, consult a doctor. A persistent cough may be a sign of a serious condition. If cough persists for more than 1 week, tends to recur, or is accompanied by fever, rash, or persistent headache, consult a doctor. Do not take this product: 1) if cough is accompanied by excessive phlegm (mucus), 2) for persistent or chronic cough such as occurs with smoking, asthma or emphysema, 3) if you have heart disease, high blood pressure, thyroid disease, diabetes, glaucoma, a

breathing problem such as emphysema or chronic bronchitis, or difficulty in urination due to enlargement of the prostate gland, 4) if you are presently taking another product containing phenylpropanolamine, or 5) if you are taking sedatives or tranquilizers, unless directed by a doctor. May cause excitability, especially in children. May cause drowsiness; alcohol, sedatives and tranquilizers may increase the drowsiness effect. Avoid alcoholic beverages while taking this product. Use caution when driving a motor vehicle or operating machinery.
As with any drug, if you are pregnant or nursing a baby, seek the advice of a health professional before using this product.

Drug Interaction Precaution: Do not use this product if you are now taking a prescription monoamine oxidase inhibitor [MAOI] (certain drugs for depression, psychiatric or emotional conditions, or Parkinson's disease) or for 2 weeks after stopping the MAOI drug. If you are uncertain whether your prescription drug contains an MAOI, consult a health professional before taking this product.

Dosage and Administration: Adults and children 12 and over (96+ lbs)—4 teaspoons every 4 to 6 hours. Children 6 to under 12 years (48–95 lbs)—2 teaspoons every 4 to 6 hours. Unless directed by physician, do not exceed 6 doses in 24 hours or give to children under 6 years of age. For convenience, a True-Dose® Dosage cup is provided with each 4 fl. oz. and 8 fl. oz. bottle.

Professional Labeling: The suggested dosage for pediatric patients is:

4–12 months　　　1.25 ml ($^1/_4$ tsp)
(12–17 lbs)　　　　every 4 to 6 hours
12–24 months　　　2.5 ml ($^1/_2$ tsp)
(18–23 lbs)　　　　every 4 to 6 hours
2–6 years　　　　　5 ml (1 tsp)
(24–47 lbs)　　　　every 4 to 6 hours
Do not exceed 4 doses in 24 hours

How Supplied: TRIAMINICOL (red), in 4 fl oz and 8 fl oz plastic bottles with tamper-evident band around child-resistant cap. Dosage cup included. Cherry flavored. Alcohol-free.

Shown in Product Identification Guide, page 516

TRIAMINIC® DM SYRUP

Description: Each teaspoon (5 mL) of TRIAMINIC® DM Syrup contains: phenylpropanolamine hydrochloride, USP 6.25 mg and dextromethorphan hydrobromide, USP 5 mg in a palatable, berry-flavored alcohol-free liquid. **Inactive in-**

Continued on next page

Information on Novartis Consumer Health, Inc., products appearing on these pages is effective as of November 1998.

Triaminic DM—Cont.

gredients: benzoic acid, FD&C Blue 1, FD&C Red 40, flavors, propylene glycol, purified water, sodium chloride, sorbitol, sucrose.

Sodium content: 10 mg per teaspoon.

Indications: Temporarily quiets coughs due to minor throat and bronchial irritation, and relieves stuffy nose.

Warnings: Keep this and all drugs out of the reach of children. In case of accidental overdose, seek professional assistance or contact a poison control center immediately.

Do not exceed recommended dosage. If nervousness, dizziness, or sleeplessness occur, discontinue use and consult a doctor. If symptoms do not improve within 7 days or are accompanied by fever, consult a doctor. A persistent cough may be a sign of a serious condition. If cough persists for more than 1 week, tends to recur, or is accompanied by fever, rash, or persistent headache, consult a doctor. Do not take this product: 1) if cough is accompanied by excessive phlegm (mucus), 2) for persistent or chronic cough such as occurs with smoking, asthma or emphysema, 3) if you have heart disease, high blood pressure, thyroid disease, diabetes, difficulty in urination due to enlargement of the prostate gland, or 4) if you are presently taking another product containing phenylpropanolamine, unless directed by a doctor. Do not use this product if you are on a sodium restricted diet unless directed by a doctor.
As with any drug, if you are pregnant or nursing a baby, seek the advice of a health professional before using this product.

Drug Interaction Precaution: Do not use this product if you are now taking a prescription monoamine oxidase inhibitor [MAOI] (certain drugs for depression, psychiatric or emotional conditions, or Parkinson's disease), or for 2 weeks after stopping the MAOI drug. If you are uncertain whether your prescription drug contains an MAOI, consult a health professional before taking this product.

Dosage and Administration: Adults and children 12 and over (96+ lbs)—4 teaspoons every 4 hours. Children 6 to under 12 years (48–95 lbs)—2 teaspoons every 4 hours. Children 2 to under 6 years (24–47 lbs) 1 teaspoon every 4 hours. Do not exceed 6 doses in 24 hours, or as directed by a doctor. Dosing to children under 2 years of age is to be under the direction of a physician. For convenience, a True-Dose® dosage cup is provided with each 4 fl. oz. and 8 fl. oz. bottle.

Professional Labeling: The suggested dosage for pediatric patients is:

4–12 months   1.25 ml ($^1/_4$ tsp)
(12–17 lbs)   every 4 hours
12–24 months   2.5 ml ($^1/_2$ tsp)

(18–23 lbs)   every 4 hours
Do not exceed 6 doses in 24 hours.

How Supplied: TRIAMINIC DM Syrup (dark red), in 4 fl oz and 8 fl oz plastic bottles with tamper-evident band around child-resistant cap. Dosage cup included. Berry flavored. Alcohol-free.
Shown in Product Identification Guide, page 515

TRIAMINICIN® TABLETS

Description: Each tablet contains: acetaminophen 650 mg, phenylpropanolamine hydrochloride 25 mg, and chlorpheniramine maleate 4 mg. **Inactive Ingredients:** colloidal silicon dioxide, croscarmellose sodium, D&C Yellow 10, FD&C Red 40, hydroxypropyl cellulose, lactose, magnesium stearate, methylcellulose, methylparaben, polyethylene glycol, povidone, pregelatinized starch, titanium dioxide.

Sodium-free.

Indications: Temporarily relieves minor aches, pains, headache, muscular aches, and fever associated with the common cold, nasal congestion associated with sinusitis, or nasal congestion, runny nose, sneezing, itching of the nose or throat and itchy, watery eyes due to hay fever (allergic rhinitis) or other upper respiratory allergies.

Warnings: Keep this and all drugs out of the reach of children. In case of accidental overdose, seek professional assistance or contact a poison control center immediately. Prompt medical attention is critical for adults as well as children even if you do not notice any signs or symptoms.

Do not exceed recommended dosage. If nervousness, dizziness, or sleeplessness occur, discontinue use and consult a doctor. Do not take this product for pain for more than 10 days or for fever for more than 3 days unless directed by a doctor. If pain or fever persists or gets worse, if new symptoms occur, or if redness or swelling is present, consult a doctor because these could be signs of a serious condition. May cause excitability especially in children. Do not take this product if you have heart disease, high blood pressure, thyroid disease, diabetes, glaucoma, a breathing problem such as emphysema or chronic bronchitis, difficulty in urination due to enlargement of the prostate gland, or you are now taking another product containing phenylpropanolamine, unless directed by a doctor.
May cause drowsiness; alcohol, sedatives and tranquilizers may increase the drowsiness effect. Avoid alcoholic beverages while taking this product. Do not take this product if you are taking sedatives or tranquilizers, without first consulting your doctor. Use caution when driving a motor vehicle or operating machinery.

As with any drug, if you are pregnant or nursing a baby, seek the advice of a health professional before using this product.

Alcohol Warning: If you consume 3 or more alcoholic drinks every day, ask your doctor whether you should take acetaminophen or other pain relievers/fever reducers. Acetaminophen may cause liver damage.

Drug Interaction Precaution: Do not use this product if you are now taking a prescription monoamine oxidase inhibitor [MAOI] (certain drugs for depression, psychiatric or emotional conditions, or Parkinson's disease), or for 2 weeks after stopping the MAOI drug. If you are uncertain whether your prescription drug contains an MAOI, consult a health professional before taking this product.

Directions: Adults and children 12 years of age and over: 1 tablet every 4 to 6 hours, not to exceed 6 tablets in 24 hours, or as directed by a doctor. Children under 12 years of age: consult a doctor.

How Supplied: TRIAMINICIN Tablets (yellow) imprinted "TRIAMINICIN" on one side, in blister packs of 12, 24 and 48.
Shown in Product Identification Guide, page 516

P & S Laboratories

See Standard Homeopathic Company

The Parthenon Co., Inc.
**3311 W. 2400 SOUTH
SALT LAKE CITY, UTAH 84119**

Direct Inquiries to:
(801) 972-5184
FAX: (801) 972-4734

For Medical Emergency Contact:
Nick G. Mihalopoulos
(801) 972-5184

DEVROM® CHEWABLE TABLETS

Description: DEVROM® is a safe and effective internal (oral) deodorant. Each tablet contains 200 mg of Bismuth Subgallate powder.

Indications: DEVROM® is indicated for the control of odors from ileostomies, colostomies and fecal incontinence.

Dosage: Take one or two tablets of DEVROM® three times a day with meals or as directed by physician. Chew or swallow whole if desired.

Note: The beneficial ingredient in DEVROM® may coat the tongue which may also darken in color. This condition is harmless and temporary. Darkening of the stool is also possible and equally harmless.

Warning: This product cannot be expected to be effective in the reduction of odor due to faulty personal hygiene. **KEEP THIS BOTTLE AND ALL MEDICATION OUT OF THE REACH OF CHILDREN.**

Inactive Ingredients: Mannitol, Lactose, Corn Starch, Confectioner's Sugar, Acacia Powder, Magnesium Stearate, Natural Banana Flavor.
NO PHYSICIAN'S PRESCRIPTION IS NECESSARY

How Supplied: DEVROM® is supplied in bottles of 100 tablets.
   DO NOT USE IF PRINTED OUTER SAFETY SEAL OR PRINTED INNER SAFETY SEAL IS BROKEN.
THE PARTHENON CO., INC./
3311 W. 2400 So./
Salt Lake City, Utah 84119

Pfizer
Consumer Health Care Group

Address Questions & Comments to:
Consumer Relations
(800) 723-7529

For Medical Emergencies/Information Contact:
(800) 723-7529

BENGAY® External Analgesic Products

Description: BENGAY products contain menthol in an alcohol base gel, combinations of methyl salicylate and menthol in cream and ointment bases, as well as a combination of methyl salicylate, menthol and camphor in a non-greasy cream base; all suitable for topical application.
In addition to the Original Formula Pain Relieving Ointment (methyl salicylate, 18.3%; menthol, 16%), BENGAY is offered as BENGAY Greaseless Pain Relieving Cream (methyl salicylate, 15%; menthol, 10%), an Arthritis Formula NonGreasy Pain Relieving Cream (methyl salicylate, 30%; menthol, 8%), an Ultra Strength NonGreasy Pain Relieving Cream (methyl salicylate 30%; menthol 10%; camphor 4%), Vanishing Scent NonGreasy Pain Relieving Gel (2.5% menthol), and S.P.A. (Site Penetrating Action) Pain Relieving Cream (10% menthol) with a fresh scent.

Action and Uses: Methyl salicylate, menthol and camphor are external analgesics which stimulate sensory receptors of warmth and/or cold. This produces a counter-irritant response which provides temporary relief of minor aches and pains of muscles and joints associated with simple backache, arthritis, strains and sprains.

Several double-blind clinical studies of BENGAY products containing menthol-methyl salicylate have shown the effectiveness of this combination in counteracting minor pain of skeletal muscle stress and arthritis.
Three studies involving a total of 102 normal subjects in which muscle soreness was experimentally induced showed statistically significant beneficial results from use of the active product vs. placebo for lowered Muscle Action Potential (spasms), greater rise in threshold of muscular pain and greater reduction in perceived muscular pain.
Six clinical studies of a total of 207 subjects suffering from minor pain due to osteoarthritis and rheumatoid arthritis showed the active product to give statistically significant beneficial results vs. placebo for greater relief of perceived pain, increased range of motion of the affected joints and increased digital dexterity. In two studies designed to measure the effect of topically applied BENGAY vs. placebo on muscular endurance, discomfort, onset of exercise pain and fatigue, 30 subjects performed a submaximal three-hour run and another 30 subjects performed a maximal treadmill run. BENGAY was found to significantly decrease the discomfort during the submaximal and maximal runs, and increase the time before onset of fatigue during the maximal run.
Applied before workouts, BENGAY relaxes tight muscles and increases circulation to make exercising more comfortable, longer.
To help reduce muscle ache and soreness after exercise, BENGAY can be applied and allowed to work before taking a shower.

Directions: Apply generously and gently massage into painful area until BENGAY disappears. Repeat 3 to 4 times daily.

Warnings: For external use only. Do not use with a heating pad. Keep away from children to avoid accidental poisoning. Do not bandage tightly. Do not swallow. If swallowed, induce vomiting and call a physician. Keep away from eyes, mucous membranes, broken or irritated skin. If skin redness or irritation develops, pain lasts for more than 10 days, or with arthritis—like conditions in children under 12, do not use and call a physician.

Shown in Product Identification Guide, page 516

BONINE®
(Meclizine hydrochloride)
Chewable Tablets

Action: BONINE (meclizine) is an H_1 histamine receptor blocker of the piperazine side chain group. It exhibits its action by an effect on the Central Nervous System (CNS), possibly by its ability to block muscarinic receptors in the brain.

Indications: BONINE is effective in the management of nausea, vomiting and dizziness associated with motion sickness.

Contraindications: Do not take this product, unless directed by a doctor, if you have a breathing problem such as emphysema or chronic bronchitis, or if you have glaucoma or difficulty in urination due to enlargement of the prostate gland.

Warnings: May cause drowsiness; alcohol, sedatives and tranquilizers may increase the drowsiness effect. Avoid alcoholic beverages while taking this product. Do not take this product if you are taking sedatives or tranquilizers without first consulting your doctor. Do not drive or operate dangerous machinery while taking this medication.

Usage in Children: Clinical studies establishing safety and effectiveness in children have not been done; therefore, usage is not recommended in children under 12 years of age.

Usage in Pregnancy: As with any drug, if you are pregnant or nursing a baby, seek advice of a health care professional before taking this product.

Adverse Reactions: Drowsiness, dry mouth, and on rare occasions, blurred vision have been reported.

Dosage and Administration: For motion sickness, take one or two tablets of Bonine once daily, one hour before travel starts, for up to 24 hours of protection against motion sickness. The tablet can be chewed with or without water or swallowed whole with water. Thereafter, the dose may be repeated every 24 hours for the duration of the travel.

How Supplied: BONINE (meclizine HCl) is available in convenient packets of 8 chewable tablets of 25 mg. meclizine HCl.

Inactive Ingredients: FD&C Red #40, Lactose, Magnesium Stearate, Purified Siliceous Earth, Raspberry Flavor, Saccharin Sodium, Starch, Talc.

CORTIZONE•5®
Creme and Ointment
CORTIZONE FOR KIDS™
Creme Anti-itch
(0.5% hydrocortisone)

Description: CORTIZONE•5® creme (with aloe) and ointment are topical anti-itch preparations.

Active Ingredient: Hydrocortisone 0.5%.

Inactive Ingredients: Creme: Aloe Barbadensis Gel, Aluminum Sulfate, Calcium Acetate, Cetearyl Alcohol, Glycerin, Light Mineral Oil, Maltodextrin, Methylparaben, Potato Dextrin, Propylparaben, Purified Water, Sodium Cetearyl Sulfate,

Continued on next page

Cortizone 5/For Kids—Cont.

Sodium Lauryl Sulfate, White Petrolatum, White Wax.
Ointment: Aloe Barbadensis Extract, White Petrolatum.

Indications: CORTIZONE•5® is recommended for the temporary relief of itching associated with minor skin irritations, inflammation and rashes due to: eczema, insect bites, poison ivy, oak, sumac, soaps, detergents, cosmetics, jewelry, seborrheic dermatitis, psoriasis, external anal and genital itching. Other uses of this product should be only under the advice and supervision of a doctor.

Warnings: For external use only. Avoid contact with the eyes. If condition worsens, or if symptoms persist for more than 7 days or clear up and occur again within a few days, stop use of this product and do not begin use of any other hydrocortisone product unless you have consulted a doctor. Do not use in genital area if you have a vaginal discharge, consult a doctor. Do not use for the treatment of diaper rash or for the treatment of chicken pox, consult a doctor.
Warnings For External Anal Itching Users: Do not exceed the recommended daily dosage unless directed by a doctor. In case of bleeding, consult a doctor promptly. Do not put this product into the rectum by using fingers or any mechanical device or applicator.
Keep this and all drugs out of the reach of children. In case of accidental ingestion, seek professional assistance or contact a poison control center immediately.

Dosage and Administration: Adults and children 2 years of age and older: Apply to affected area not more than 3 to 4 times daily. Children under 2 years of age: Do not use, consult a doctor.
Directions For External Anal Itching Users: Adults: When practical, cleanse the affected area with mild soap and warm water and rinse thoroughly. Gently dry by patting or blotting with toilet tissue or a soft cloth before application of this product. Children under 12 years of age: Consult a doctor.

How to Store: Store at controlled room temperature 15°–30°C (59°–86°F).

How Supplied: CORTIZONE•5® creme: 1 oz. and 2 oz. tubes. CORTIZONE•5® ointment: 1 oz. tube. CORTIZONE for KIDS™ creme: $1/_2$ oz. and 1 oz. tubes.

Shown in Product Identification Guide, page 516

CORTIZONE•10®
Creme and Ointment
CORTIZONE•10®
Quick Shot Spray

Description: CORTIZONE•10® creme (with aloe), ointment and Quick Shot Spray are topical anti-itch preparations and are the maximum strength available without a prescription.

Active Ingredient: Hydrocortisone 1%.

Inactive Ingredients: Creme: Aloe Barbadensis Gel, Aluminum Sulfate, Calcium Acetate, Cetearyl Alcohol, Glycerin, Light Mineral Oil, Maltodextrin, Methylparaben, Potato Dextrin, Propylparaben, Purified Water, Sodium Cetearyl Sulfate, Sodium Lauryl Sulfate, White Petrolatum, White Wax.
Ointment: White Petrolatum.
Quick Shot Spray: Benzyl Alcohol, Propylene Glycol, Purified Water, SD Alcohol 40-2 (60% v/v).

Indications: Cortizone•10® is recommended for the temporary relief of itching associated with minor skin irritations, inflammation and rashes due to: eczema, insect bites, poison ivy, oak, sumac, soaps, detergents, cosmetics, jewelry, seborrheic dermatitis, psoriasis, external anal and genital itching. Other uses of this product should be only under the advice and supervision of a doctor.

Warnings: For external use only. Avoid contact with the eyes. If condition worsens, or if symptoms persist for more than 7 days or clear up and occur again within a few days, stop use of this product and do not begin use of any other hydrocortisone product unless you have consulted a doctor. Do not use in genital area if you have a vaginal discharge, consult a doctor. Do not use for the treatment of diaper rash, consult a doctor. CORTIZONE•10® Creme and Ointment only:
Warnings For External Anal Itching Users: Do not exceed the recommended daily dosage unless directed by a doctor. In case of bleeding, consult a doctor promptly. Do not put this product into the rectum by using fingers or any mechanical device or applicator.
Keep this and all drugs out of the reach of children. In case of accidental ingestion, seek professional assistance or contact a poison control center immediately.

Dosage and Administration: Adults and children 2 years of age and older: Apply to affected area not more than 3 to 4 times daily. Children under 2 years of age: Do not use, consult a doctor.
CORTIZONE•10® Creme and Ointment Only:

Directions For External Anal Itching Users: Adults: When practical, cleanse the affected area with mild soap and warm water. Rinse thoroughly. Gently dry by patting or blotting with toilet tissue or a soft cloth before application of this product. Children under 12 years of age: Consult a doctor.

How to Store: Store at controlled room temperature 15°–30°C (59°–86°F).
Quick Shot Spray only:
Flammable—Keep away from fire or flame.

How Supplied: CORTIZONE•10® creme: .5 oz, 1 oz. and 2 oz. tubes. CORTIZONE•10® ointment: 1 oz. and 2 oz. tubes.

CORTIZONE•10® Quick Shot Spray: 1.5 oz. pump bottle.
Shown in Product Identification Guide, page 516

CORTIZONE•10® Plus
Creme

Description: CORTIZONE•10® Plus creme is a topical anti-itch preparation containing 10 moisturizers.

Active Ingredient: Hydrocortisone 1%.

Inactive Ingredients: Aloe Barbadensis Gel, Aluminum Sulfate, Calcium Acetate, Cetearyl Alcohol, Cetyl Alcohol, Corn Oil, Glycerin, Isopropyl Palmitate, Light Mineral Oil, Maltodextrin, Methylparaben, Potato Dextrin, Propylene Glycol, Propylparaben, Purified Water, Sodium Cetearyl Sulfate, Sodium Lauryl Sulfate, Vitamin A Palmitate, Vitamin D, Vitamin E, White Petrolatum, White Wax.

Indications: CORTIZONE•10® Plus is recommended for the temporary relief of itching associated with minor skin irritations, inflammation and rashes due to: eczema, insect bites, poison ivy, oak, sumac, soaps, detergents, cosmetics, jewelry, seborrheic dermatitis, psoriasis, external anal and genital itching. Other uses of this product should be only under the advice and supervision of a doctor.

Warnings: For external use only. Avoid contact with the eyes. If condition worsens, or if symptoms persist for more than 7 days or clear up and occur again within a few days, stop use of this product and do not begin use of any other hydrocortisone product unless you have consulted a doctor. Do not use in genital area if you have a vaginal discharge, consult a doctor. Do not use for the treatment of diaper rash consult a doctor.
Warnings For External Anal Itching Users: Do not exceed the recommended daily dosage unless directed by a doctor. In case of bleeding, consult a doctor promptly. Do not put this product into the rectum by using fingers or any mechanical device or applicator.
Keep this and all drugs out of the reach of children. In case of accidental ingestion, seek professional assistance or contact a poison control center immediately.

Dosage and Administration: Adults and children 2 years of age and older: Apply to affected area not more than 3 to 4 times daily. Children under 2 years of age: Do not use, consult a doctor.
Directions For External Anal Itching Users: Adults: When practical, cleanse the affected area with mild soap and warm water and rinse thoroughly. Gently dry by patting or blotting with toilet tissue or a soft cloth before application of this product. Children under 12 years of age: Consult a doctor.

How to Store: Store at controlled room temperature 15°–30°C (59°–86°F).

How Supplied: CORTIZONE•10® Plus creme: 1 oz and 2 oz. tubes.

Shown in Product Identification Guide, page 516

DESITIN® CORNSTARCH BABY POWDER
(with Zinc Oxide)

Description: Desitin Cornstarch Baby Powder combines zinc oxide (10%) with topical starch (cornstarch) for topical application. Also contains: fragrance and tribasic calcium phosphate.

Actions and Uses: Desitin Cornstarch Baby Powder with zinc oxide and topical starch (cornstarch) is designed to protect from wetness, help prevent and treat diaper rash, and other minor skin irritations. It offers all the benefits of a talc-free, absorbent cornstarch powder, but with the addition of zinc oxide, the same protective ingredient found in Desitin Ointment. Cornstarch also prevents friction. Zinc oxide provides an additional physical barrier by forming a protective coating over the skin or mucous membranes which serves to reduce further effects of irritants on affected areas.

Directions: Change wet and soiled diapers promptly, cleanse the diaper area, and allow to dry.
Apply powder close to the body away from child's face. Carefully shake the powder into the diaper or into the hand and apply to diaper area. Apply liberally as often as necessary with each diaper change, especially at bedtime, or anytime when exposure to wet diapers may be prolonged. Use liberally in all body creases, and whenever chafing, prickly heat or other minor skin irritations occur.

Warning: For external use only. Do not use on broken skin. Avoid contact with eyes. Keep powder away from child's face to avoid inhalation. If diaper rash worsens or does not improve within 7 days, consult a doctor.

How Supplied: Desitin Cornstarch Baby Powder with Zinc Oxide is available in 14 ounce (397g) containers with sifter-top caps.

Shown in Product Identification Guide, page 516

DESITIN® CREAMY
Diaper Rash Ointment
(10% Zinc Oxide)

Description: Desitin Creamy contains Zinc Oxide (10%) in a white petrolatum base suitable for topical application. Also contains: cyclomethicone, dimethicone, fragrance, methylparaben, microcrystalline wax, mineral oil, propylparaben, purified water, sodium borate, sorbitan sesquioleate, white petrolatum and white wax.

Actions and Uses: Desitin Creamy treats diaper rash and soothes irritated skin. It also prevents diaper rash by forming a protective barrier that helps seal out wetness and irritants that can cause diaper rash. Desitin Creamy has a pleasant hypoallergenic formula that is easy to apply, easy to clean off, and has a fresh scent.

Directions: 1) Change wet and soiled diapers promptly. 2) Cleanse the diaper area. 3) Allow to dry. 4) Apply ointment liberally as often as necessary, with each diaper change, especially at bedtime or anytime when exposure to wet diapers may be prolonged.

Warnings: For external use only. Avoid contact with eyes. If condition worsens or does not improve within 7 days, consult your doctor. Keep this and all drugs out of the reach of children. In case of accidental ingestion, seek professional assistance or contact a poison control center immediately. Store between 15° and 30°C (59° and 86°F).

How Supplied: Desitin Creamy is available in 2 oz. (57g) and 4 oz. (113g) tubes.

Shown in Product Identification Guide, page 516

DESITIN® OINTMENT

Description: Desitin Ointment combines Zinc Oxide (40%) with Cod Liver Oil in a petrolatum-lanolin base suitable for topical application. Also contains: BHA, fragrances, methylparaben, talc and water.

Actions and Uses: Desitin Ointment helps treat and prevent diaper rash. Desitin also protects chafed skin due to diaper rash and helps seal out wetness. In addition to healing diaper rash, Desitin is excellent first aid to treat and protect minor burns, cuts, scrapes, sunburn, and skin irritations. Use for superficial non-infected wounds and burns only.
Relief and protection is afforded by Zinc Oxide in a unique hypoallergenic formula. This ingredient together with cod liver oil and the petrolatum-lanolin base provide a physical barrier by forming a protective coating over skin or mucous membranes which serves to reduce further effects of irritants on the affected area and relieves burning, pain or itch produced by them.
Several studies have shown the effectiveness of Desitin Ointment in the relief and prevention of diaper rash.
Two clinical studies involving 90 infants demonstrated the effectiveness of Desitin Ointment in curing diaper rash. The diaper rash area was treated with Desitin Ointment at each diaper change for a period of 24 hours, while the untreated site served as controls. A significant reduction was noted in the severity and area of diaper dermatitis on the treated area.
Ninety-seven (97) babies participated in a 12-week study to show that Desitin Ointment helps prevent diaper rash. Approximately half of the infants (49) were treated with Desitin Ointment on a regular daily basis. The other half (48) received the ointment as necessary to treat any diaper rash which occurred. The incidence as well as the severity of diaper rash was significantly less among the babies using the ointment on a regular daily basis.

In a comparative study of the efficacy of Desitin Ointment vs. a baby powder, forty-five (45) babies were observed for a total of eight (8) weeks. Results support the conclusion that Desitin Ointment is a better prophylactic against diaper rash than the baby powder.
In another study, Desitin was found to be dramatically more effective in reducing the severity of medically diagnosed diaper rash than a commercially available diaper rash product in which only anhydrous lanolin and petrolatum were listed as ingredients. Fifty (50) infants participated in the study, half of whom were treated with Desitin and half with the other product. In the group (25) treated with Desitin, seventeen (17) infants showed significant improvement within 10 hours which increased to twenty-three improved infants within 24 hours. Of the group (25) treated with the other product, only three showed improvement at ten hours with a total of four improved within twenty-four hours. These results are statistically valid to conclude that Desitin Ointment reduces severity of diaper rash within ten hours.
Several other studies show that Desitin Ointment helps relieve other skin disorders, such as contact dermatitis.

Directions: To treat and prevent diaper rash, change wet and soiled diapers promptly, cleanse the diaper area and allow to dry. Apply Desitin Ointment liberally as often as necessary, with each diaper change, especially at bedtime or anytime when exposure to wet diapers may be prolonged.
Treatment: If diaper rash is present, or at the first sign of redness, minor skin irritation or chafing, simply apply Desitin Ointment three or four times daily as needed. In superficial noninfected surface wounds and minor burns, apply a thin layer of Desitin Ointment, using a gauze dressing, if necessary. For external use only.

Warnings: For external use only. Avoid contact with eyes. If condition worsens or does not improve within 7 days, consult your doctor. Keep this and all drugs out of the reach of children. In case of accidental ingestion, seek professional assistance or contact a poison control center immediately. Store between 15° and 30°C (59° and 86° F).

How Supplied: Desitin Ointment is available in 1 ounce (28g), 2 ounce (57g), and 4 ounce (114g) tubes, and 9 ounce (255g) and 1 lb. (454g) jars.

Shown in Product Identification Guide, page 516

Continued on next page

OCUHIST®
Eye Allergy Relief
Itching & Redness Reliever
Eye Drops
ANTIHISTAMINE & DECONGESTANT

OcuHist is an antihistamine/decongestant eye drop, clinically proven to temporarily relieve itching and redness of the eye.

Indications: For the temporary relief of itching and redness of the eye due to pollen, ragweed, grass, animal hair and dander.

Directions: Adults and children 6 years of age or older: Place 1 or 2 drops in the affected eye(s) up to four times a day. Some users may experience a brief tingling sensation.

Active Ingredients: pheniramine maleate 0.3%, naphazoline hydrochloride 0.025%.

Inactive Ingredients: boric acid and sodium borate buffer system preserved with benzalkonium chloride (0.01%) and edetate disodium (0.1%), sodium hydroxide and/or hydrochloric acid (to adjust pH) and purified water. The solution has a pH of 5.5–6.5 and a tonicity of 245–305 mOsm/Kg.

Warnings: If you experience eye pain, changes in vision, continued redness or irritation of the eye, or if the condition worsens or persists for more than 72 hours, discontinue use and consult a physician.

Do not use this product if you have heart disease, high blood pressure, difficulty in urination due to enlargement of the prostate gland or narrow angle glaucoma unless directed by a physician. Accidental oral ingestion in infants and children may lead to coma and marked reduction in body temperature.

To avoid contamination, do not touch tip of container to any surface. Replace cap after using. Do not use if solution changes color or becomes cloudy.

Remove contact lenses before using.

Overuse of this product may produce increased redness of the eye.

Use before the expiration date marked on the carton or bottle.

Keep this and all drugs out of the reach of children.

Store between 15° and 25°C (59° and 77°F).

Parents Note: Before using with children under 6 years of age, consult your physician. Keep this and all drugs out of the reach of children. In case of accidental ingestion, seek professional assistance or contact a Poison Control Center immediately.

Caution: Do not use if Pfizer imprinted neckband on bottle is broken or missing.

Distributed By:
CONSUMER HEALTH CARE GROUP, PFIZER INC, NEW YORK, NEW YORK 10017

Shown in Product Identification Guide, page 517

MAXIMUM STRENGTH
RID®
LICE KILLING SHAMPOO
Pediculicide (Lice Treatment)

Product Description: Kills lice and their eggs (head lice, crab lice and body lice).

Indications: For the treatment of head, pubic (crab) and body lice.

Head lice: Head lice live on the scalp and lay small white eggs (nits) on the hair shaft close to the scalp. The nits are most easily found on the nape of the neck or behind the ears. All personal headgear, scarfs, coats, and bed linen should be disinfected by machine washing in hot water and drying, using the hot cycle of a dryer for at least 20 minutes. Personal articles of clothing or bedding that cannot be washed may be dry-cleaned, sealed in a plastic bag for a period of about 2 weeks, or sprayed with a product specifically designed for this purpose. Personal combs and brushes may be disinfected by soaking in hot water (above 130°F, 54°C) for 5 to 10 minutes. Thorough vacuuming of rooms inhabited by infected patients is recommended.

Pubic (Crab) lice: Pubic lice may be transmitted by sexual contact; therefore, sexual partners should be treated simultaneously to avoid reinfestation. The lice are very small and look almost like brown or grey dots on the skin. Pubic lice usually cause intense itching and lay small white eggs (nits) on the hair shaft generally close to the skin surface. In hairy individuals, pubic lice may be present on the short hairs of the thighs and trunk, underarms, and occasionally on the beard and mustache. Underwear should be disinfected by machine washing in hot water; then drying, using the hot cycle for at least 20 minutes.

Body lice: Body lice and their eggs are generally found in the seams of clothing, particularly in the waistline and armpit area. They move to the skin to feed, then return to the seams of the clothing where they lay their eggs. Clothing worn and not laundered before treatment should be disinfected by the same procedure as described for head lice, except that sealing clothing in a plastic bag is not recommended for body lice because the nits (eggs) from these lice can remain dormant for a period of up to 30 days.

Actions: RID® kills head lice (Pediculus humanus capitis), body lice (Pediculus humanus humanus), and pubic (crab) lice (Phthirus pubis), and their eggs. The pyrethrum extract affects the parasite's nervous system, resulting in paralysis and death. The efficacy of the pyrethrum extract is enhanced by a synergist, piperonyl butoxide. RID® rinses out completely after treatment and leaves no active residue. Pyrethrum extract is poorly absorbed through the skin. Of the relatively minor amounts that are absorbed, they are rapidly metabolized to water-soluble compounds and eliminated from the body without ill effects.

Sizes Available: 2 FL OZ (59mL), 4 FL OZ (118mL), 8 FL OZ (236mL), and Lice Elimination Kit containing 4 FL OZ (118mL) Lice Killing Shampoo and 5 OZ (141.8g) Lice Control Spray For Bedding & Furniture.

Application:

A. Helpful hints
1. Use RID® on dry hair. Hair should not be wet prior to applying RID® because it may dilute the active ingredients and reduce its effectiveness.
2. You must thoroughly comb out the lice eggs in order to prevent reinfestation. This will take time, but is very important. Using your favorite shampoo and conditioner after treatment with RID® will help make combing easier. Comb out tangles with your regular comb before using the RID® Egg Removal Comb. Then, follow combing instructions on the package insert.
3. For more helpful hints call 1-800-RID-LICE (1-800-743-5423) or visit us at www.licerid.com.

B. Directions
IMPORTANT: READ WARNINGS BEFORE USING.
1. Apply to affected area until all the hair is thoroughly wet with product.
2. Allow product to remain on area for 10 minutes but no longer.
3. Add sufficient warm water to form a lather and shampoo as usual. Rinse thoroughly.
4. A fine-toothed comb or special lice/nit removing comb may be used to help remove dead lice or their eggs (nits) from hair.
5. A second treatment must be done in 7 to 10 days to kill any newly hatched lice.

Warnings:
☐ Use with caution on persons allergic to ragweed.
☐ For external use only. Do not use near the eyes or permit contact with mucous membranes, such as inside the nose, mouth, or vagina, as irritation may occur. Keep out of eyes when rinsing hair. Adults and children: Close eyes tightly and do not open eyes until product is rinsed out. Also, protect children's eyes with washcloth, towel or other suitable material, or by a similar method. If product gets into the eyes, immediately flush with water.
☐ If skin irritation or infection is present or develops, discontinue use and consult a doctor. Consult a doctor if infestation of eyebrows or eyelashes occurs.
☐ In case of accidental ingestion, seek professional assistance or contact a Poison Control Center immediately.
☐ Keep this and all drugs out of the reach of children.

Prevent Reinfestation:
Since there is no immunity from lice, personal cleanliness and the avoidance of infested persons and their bedding and clothes will aid in preventing infestation. These additional steps are important in order to minimize the chance of possible reinfestation.
☐ Inspect all family members daily for at least two weeks, and if they become infested, treat with RID®.

☐ Wash all personal clothing, nightwear and bedding of any infested person in hot water, at least 130°F (54°C) or by dry cleaning.

☐ Soak all personal articles such as combs, brushes, etc. in RID® solution or hot soapy water, at least 130°F (54°C), for ten minutes.

☐ Tell children not to use any borrowed combs or brushes, nor to wear anyone else's clothes.

Active Ingredients: Piperonyl Butoxide 4%, Pyrethrum Extract equivalent to 0.33% Pyrethrins.

Inactive Ingredients: C_{13}–C_{14} Isoparaffin, Fragrance, Isopropyl Alcohol, PEG-25 Hydrogenated Castor Oil, Water, Xanthan Gum.

Storage and disposal:

☐ Store at room temperature 59°–86°F (15°–30°C).

☐ Do not reuse original container.

☐ Securely wrap original container in several layers of newspaper and discard in trash.

Additional Information:
Call 1-800-RID-LICE (1-800-743-5423) or visit www.licerid.com for further information. Comprehensive patient education materials are available free of charge through 1-800-RID-LICE.

Shown in Product Identification Guide, page 517

RID® LICE CONTROL SPRAY
For Bedding & Furniture.

NOT FOR USE ON HUMANS

Product description: Contains the synthetic pyrethroid permethrin. Kills lice and their eggs. For use on bedding, furniture, and other inanimate objects infested with lice.

Actions: A highly active synthetic pyrethroid for the control of lice and louse eggs on bedding, furniture and other inanimate objects.

Sizes available: 5 OZ (141.8g) and in a Lice Elimination Kit containing 4 FL OZ (118mL) Lice Killing Shampoo and 5 OZ (141.8g) Lice Control Spray for Bedding & Furniture.

Directions for use: It is a violation of Federal Law to use this product in a manner inconsistent with its labeling. Shake well before using.

To kill lice and louse eggs: Spray in an inconspicuous area to test for possible staining or discoloration. Inspect again after drying, then proceed to spray entire area to be treated. Hold container upright with nozzle away from you. Depress valve and spray from a distance of 8 to 10 inches. Spray each square foot for 3 seconds. Spray only those garments

and parts of bedding, including mattresses and furniture, that cannot be either laundered or dry cleaned. Allow all sprayed articles to dry thoroughly before use. Buyer assumes all risks of use, storage or handling of this material not in strict accordance with directions given herewith.

Precautionary statements:
HAZARDS TO HUMANS AND DOMESTIC ANIMALS
Caution: KEEP OUT OF REACH OF CHILDREN
Harmful if swallowed. May be absorbed through skin. Avoid inhalation of spray mist. Avoid contact with skin, eyes or clothing. Wash thoroughly after handling and before smoking or eating. Avoid contamination of feed and foodstuffs. Remove pets and birds and cover fish aquaria before space spraying or surface applications. *This product is not for use on humans.* If lice infestation should occur on humans, use a product labeled for use on humans. Vacate room after treatment and ventilate before reoccupying. Do not allow children or pets to contact treated areas until surfaces are dry.

Animals: Do not spray directly in/on eyes, mouth or genitalia of pets. Do not treat or cause exposure to kittens or puppies less than four weeks old.

Environmental hazards: This product is toxic to fish. Do not apply directly to any body of water. Do not contaminate water when disposing of equipment washwaters.

Statement of practical treatment:
IF INHALED: Remove affected person to fresh air. Apply artificial respiration if indicated.
IF IN EYES: Flush with plenty of water. Contact a physician if irritation persists.
IF ON SKIN: Wash affected areas immediately with soap and water. Get medical attention if irritation persists.

Physical or chemical hazards: Contents under pressure. Do not use or store near heat or open flame. Do not puncture or incinerate container. Exposure to temperatures above 130° F (54° C) may cause bursting.

Ingredients:
[See table below]

Storage and disposal:
☐ Store in cool, dry area.
☐ Do not transport or store below 32° F (0° C).
☐ Wrap container in several layers of newspaper and dispose of in trash.
☐ Do not incinerate or puncture.

Additional information:
Call 1-800-RID-LICE (1-800-743-5423) or visit www.licerid.com for further in-

formation. Comprehensive patient education materials are available free of charge through 1-800-RID-LICE.

EPA Reg. No. 4816-690-25354
EPA Est. No. 54487-GA-1

MAXIMUM STRENGTH UNISOM SLEEPGELS
Nighttime Sleep Aid

Description: Maximum Strength Unisom SleepGels are liquid-filled, blue soft gelatin capsules.
Active Ingredient: Diphenhydramine Hydrochloride 50 mg.
Inactive Ingredients: FD&C Blue No. 1, Gelatin, Glycerin, Pharmaceutical Glaze, Polyethylene Glycol, Propylene Glycol, Purified Water, Sorbitol, Titanium Dioxide.

Indications: Helps to reduce difficulty falling asleep.

Action: Diphenhydramine Hydrochloride is an ethanolamine antihistamine with anticholinergic and sedative effects.

Administration and Dosage: Adults and children 12 years of age and over: Oral dosage is one softgel (50 mg) at bedtime if needed, or as directed by a doctor.

Warnings: Do not take this product, unless directed by a doctor, if you have a breathing problem such as emphysema or chronic bronchitis, or if you have glaucoma or difficulty in urination due to enlargement of the prostate gland. Do not take this product if pregnant or nursing a baby.

• Do not give to children under 12 years of age.
• If sleeplessness persists continuously for more than two weeks, consult your doctor. Insomnia may be a symptom of serious underlying medical illness.
• Avoid alcoholic beverages while taking this product. Do not take this product if you are taking sedatives or tranquilizers, without first consulting your doctor.
• **Do Not Use:** with any other product containing diphenhydramine, including one applied topically.
• Keep this and all drugs out of the reach of children.
• In case of accidental overdose, seek professional assistance or contact a poison control center immediately.

Drug Interaction: Monoamine oxidase (MAO) inhibitors prolong and intensify the anticholinergic effects of antihistamines. The CNS depressant effect is heightened by alcohol and other CNS depressant drugs.

Symptoms of Oral Overdosage: Antihistamine overdosage reactions may vary from central nervous system depression to stimulation.
Stimulation is particularly likely in children. Atropine-like signs and symptoms, such as dry mouth, fixed and dilated pupils, flushing, and gastrointestinal symptoms, may also occur.

ACTIVE INGREDIENT:	Permethrin*	0.50%
INERT INGREDIENTS:		99.50%
		100.00%

*(3-phenoxyphenyl) methyl (±) cis/trans 3-(2,2-dichloroethenyl) 2,2-dimethylcyclopropanecarboxylate. Cis/trans ratio: min. 35% (±) cis and max. 65% (±) trans.

Continued on next page

Unisom Max. Str.—Cont.

Attention: Use only if softgel blister seals are unbroken.

How Supplied: Boxes of 16 liquid filled softgels in child resistant blisters and boxes of 8 with non-child resistant packaging. Also in a 32 count easy to open child resistant bottle.
Store between 15° and 30°C (59° and 86°F)

UNISOM®
[yu 'na-som]
Nighttime Sleep Aid
(doxylamine succinate)

PRODUCT OVERVIEW

Key Facts: Unisom is an ethanol-amine antihistamine (doxylamine) which characteristically shows a high incidence of sedation. It produces a reduced latency to end of wakefulness and early onset of sleep.

Major Uses: Unisom has been shown to be clinically effective as a sleep aid when 1 tablet is given 30 minutes before retiring.

Safety Information: Unisom is contraindicated in pregnancy and nursing mothers. It is also contraindicated in patients with asthma, glaucoma, and enlargement of the prostate. Caution should be used if taken when alcohol is being consumed. Caution is also indicated when taken concurrently with other medications due to the anticholinergic properties of antihistamines.

PRESCRIBING INFORMATION
UNISOM®
[yu 'na-som]
Nighttime Sleep Aid
(doxylamine succinate)

Description: Pale blue oval scored tablets containing 25 mg. of doxylamine succinate, 2-[α-(2-dimethylaminoethoxy)α-methylbenzyl]pyridine succinate.

Inactive Ingredients: Dibasic Calcium Phosphate, FD&C Blue #1 Aluminum Lake, Magnesium Stearate, Microcrystalline Cellulose, Sodium Starch Glycolate.

Administration and Dosage: One tablet 30 minutes before going to bed. Take once daily or as directed by a doctor. Not for children under 12 years of age.

Warnings: Do not take this product, unless directed by a doctor, if you have a breathing problem such as emphysema or chronic bronchitis, or if you have glaucoma or difficulty in urination due to enlargement of the prostate gland. Do not take this product if pregnant or nursing a baby.
- If sleeplessness persists continuously for more than two weeks, consult your doctor. Insomnia may be a symptom of a serious underlying medical illness.
- Do not take this product if presently taking any other drug, without consulting your doctor or pharmacist.

- Take this product with caution if alcohol is being consumed.
- For adults only. Do not give to children under 12 years of age.
- Keep this and all medications out of the reach of children. This product contains an antihistamine and will cause drowsiness. It should be used only at bedtime.

Side Effects: Occasional anticholinergic effects may be seen.

Attention: Use only if tablet blister seals are unbroken.

How Supplied: Boxes of 8, 16, 32 or 48 tablets.

UNISOM® WITH PAIN RELIEF®
[yu 'na-som]
Nighttime Sleep Aid and Pain Reliever

PRODUCT OVERVIEW

Key Facts: Unisom With Pain Relief (diphenhydramine sleep aid/acetaminophen pain relief formula) is a product with a dual antihistamine sleep aid/analgesic action to utilize the sedative effects of an antihistamine and relieve mild to moderate pain that may disturb normal sleep patterns. If patients have difficulty in falling asleep but are not experiencing pain at the same time, regular Unisom Sleep Aid which contains doxylamine succinate or Maximum Strength Unisom SleepGels which contains diphenhydramine is indicated.

Major Uses: One Unisom With Pain Relief is indicated 30 minutes before retiring to help reduce difficulty in falling asleep while relieving accompanying minor aches and pains, such as headache, muscle aches or menstrual discomfort.

Safety Information: Do not take this product, unless directed by a doctor, if you have a breathing problem such as emphysema or chronic bronchitis, or if you have glaucoma or difficulty in urination due to enlargement of the prostate gland. Unisom With Pain Relief is contraindicated in pregnancy or in nursing mothers. Excessive dosing may lead to liver damage. Product is intended for patients 12 years and older. Alcoholic beverages should be avoided while taking this product. This product should not be taken without first consulting a physician if sedatives or tranquilizers are being taken.

PRESCRIBING INFORMATION
UNISOM WITH PAIN RELIEF®
[yu 'na-som]
Nighttime Sleep Aid and Pain Reliever

Description: Unisom With Pain Relief® is a pale blue, capsule-shaped, coated tablet.

Active Ingredients: 650 mg acetaminophen and 50 mg diphenhydramine HCl per tablet.

Inactive Ingredients: Crospovidone, FD&C Blue #1 Aluminum Lake, FD&C Blue #2 Aluminum Lake, Hydroxypropyl Methylcellulose, Magnesium Stearate, Polyethylene Glycol, Polysorbate 80, Povidone, Pregelantinized Starch, Stearic Acid, Titanium Dioxide.

Indications: Unisom With Pain Relief (diphenhydramine sleep aid formula) is indicated to help reduce difficulty in falling asleep while relieving accompanying minor aches and pain such as headache, muscle ache or menstrual discomfort. If there is difficulty in falling asleep, but pain is not being experienced at the same time, use regular Unisom sleep aid which contains doxylamine succinate as its active ingredient.

Administration and Dosage: One tablet at bedtime if needed, or as directed by a physician.

Warnings: Do not take this product, unless directed by a doctor, if you have a breathing problem such as emphysema or chronic bronchitis, or if you have glaucoma or difficulty in urination due to enlargement of the prostate gland. Do not take this product if pregnant or nursing a baby.
Do not take this product for treatment of arthritis except under the advice and supervision of a physican.
Do not exceed recommended dosage because severe liver damage may occur. If symptoms persist continuously for more than ten days, consult your physician. Insomnia may be a symptom of serious underlying medical illness. Avoid alcoholic beverages while taking this product. Do not take this product if you are taking sedatives or tranquilizers, without first consulting your doctor. For adults only. Do not give to children under 12 years of age. Keep this and all medications out of reach of children. In case of accidental overdose seek professional advice or contact a poison control center immediately.

Caution: This product contains an antihistamine and will cause drowsiness. It should be used only at bedtime.

Drug Interaction: Monoamine oxidase (MAO) inhibitors prolong and intensify the anticholinergic effects of antihistamines. The CNS depressant effect is heightened by alcohol and other CNS depressant drugs.

Attention: Use only if tablet blister seals are unbroken. Child resistant packaging.

How Supplied: Boxes of 8 and 16 tablets in child resistant blisters.

ADVANCED RELIEF VISINE®
Lubricant/Redness Reliever Eye Drops

Description: Advanced Relief Visine is a sterile, isotonic, buffered ophthalmic solution containing polyethylene glycol 400 1%, povidone 1%, dextran 70 0.1%, tetrahydrozoline hydrochloride 0.05%.

Advanced Relief Visine is an ophthalmic solution combining the effects of the decongestant, tetrahydrozoline hydrochloride, with the demulcent effects of polyethylene glycol, povidone and dextran 70. It provides symptomatic relief of conjunctival edema and hyperemia secondary to minor irritations. Tetrahydrozoline hydrochloride is a sympathomimetic agent, which brings about decongestion by vasoconstriction. Reddened eyes are rapidly whitened by this effective vasoconstrictor, which limits the local vascular response by constricting the small blood vessels. The onset of vasoconstriction becomes apparent within minutes. Additional effects include amelioration of burning, irritation and excessive lacrimation. Relief is afforded by three moisturizers: polyethylene glycol 400, povidone and dextran 70.

Polyethylene glycol 400, povidone and dextran 70 are ophthalmic demulcents which have been shown to be effective for the temporary relief of discomfort of minor irritations of the eye due to exposure to wind or sun. They are effective as protectants and lubricants against further irritation or to relieve dryness of the eye. The effectiveness of tetrahydrozoline hydrochloride in relieving conjunctival hyperemia and associated symptoms has been demonstrated by numerous clinicals, including several double-blind studies, involving more than 2,000 subjects suffering from acute or chronic hyperemia induced by a variety of conditions. Advanced Relief Visine is a unique eye drop formulation that combines the redness-relieving effects of a vasoconstrictor and the soothing, moisturizing and protective effects of three demulcents.

Indications: Relieves redness of the eye due to minor eye irritations. For use as a protectant against further irritation or to relieve dryness.

Directions: Instill 1 to 2 drops in the affected eye(s) up to 4 times daily.

Active Ingredients: Polyethylene glycol 400 1%; povidone 1%; dextran 70 0.1%; tetrahydrozoline hydrochloride 0.05%.

Inactive Ingredients: Benzalkonium chloride; boric acid; edetate disodium; purified water; sodium borate; sodium chloride.

Warnings: If you experience eye pain, changes in vision, continued redness or irritation of the eye, or if the condition worsens or persists for more than 72 hours, discontinue use and consult a physician. If you have glaucoma, do not use this product except under the advice and supervision of a physician. As with any drug, if you are pregnant or nursing a baby, seek the advice of a health professional before using this product. Overuse of this product may produce increased redness of the eye. If solution changes color or becomes cloudy, do not use. To avoid contamination, do not touch tip of container to any surface. Replace cap after using. Remove contact lenses before using this product.

Parents Note: Before using with children under 6 years of age, consult your physician. Keep this and all drugs out of the reach of children. In case of accidental ingestion, seek professional assistance or contact a Poison Control Center immediately.

Caution: Should not be used if Visine-imprinted neckband on bottle is broken or missing.

Storage: Store between 15° and 30°C (59° and 86°F).

How Supplied: In 0.5 fl. oz. and 1.0 fl. oz. plastic dispenser bottle.
Shown in Product Identification Guide, page 517

VISINE L.R.® Long Lasting Oxymetazoline Hydrochloride/ Redness Reliever Eye Drops

Description: Visine L.R. is a sterile, isotonic, buffered ophthalmic solution containing the vasoconstrictor, oxymetazoline hydrochloride. Visine L.R. is specially formulated to relieve redness of the eye in minutes with effective relief that lasts up to 6 hours.

Indications: Visine L.R. is a decongestant ophthalmic solution designed for the relief of redness of the eye due to minor eye irritations.

Directions: Adults and children 6 years of age or older: Place 1 or 2 drops in the affected eye(s). This may be repeated as needed every 6 hours or as directed by a physician.

Active Ingredients: Oxymetazoline hydrochloride 0.025%.

Inactive Ingredients: Sodium chloride; boric acid; sodium borate; with benzalkonium chloride 0.01% and edetate disodium 0.1% added as preservatives; purified water.

Warnings: If you experience eye pain, changes in vision, continued redness or irritation of the eye, or if the condition worsens or persists for more than 72 hours, discontinue use and consult a physician. If you have glaucoma, do not use this product except under the advice and supervision of a physician. As with any drug, if you are pregnant or nursing a baby, seek the advice of a health professional before using this product. Overuse of this product may produce increased redness of the eye. If solution changes color or becomes cloudy, do not use. To avoid contamination, do not touch tip of container to any surface. Replace cap after using. Remove contact lenses before using this product.
Parents: Before using with children under 6 years of age, consult your physician. Keep this and all drugs out of the reach of children. In case of accidental ingestion, seek professional assistance or contact a Poison Control Center immediately.
Caution: Should not be used if Visine-imprinted neckband on bottle is broken or missing.

Storage: Store between 2° and 30°C (36° and 86°F).

How Supplied: In 0.5 fl. oz. and 1 fl. oz. plastic dispenser bottle.
Shown in Product Identification Guide, page 517

VISINE A.C.® Seasonal Relief From Pollen & Dust Astringent/Redness Reliever Eye Drops

Description: Visine A.C. is a sterile, isotonic, buffered ophthalmic solution containing tetrahydrozoline hydrochloride 0.05% and zinc sulfate 0.25%. Visine A.C. is a fast-acting, dual-action ophthalmic solution combining the effects of the vasoconstrictor, tetrahydrozoline hydrochloride, with the astringent effects of zinc sulfate. The vasoconstrictor provides temporary relief of conjunctival edema, hyperemia and discomfort due to airborne irritants such as pollen, dust and ragweed, while zinc sulfate relieves itching and burning eye discomfort.

Tetrahydrozoline hydrochloride is a sympathomimetic agent, which brings about decongestion by vasoconstriction. Reddened eyes are rapidly whitened by this effective vasoconstrictor which limits the local vascular response by constricting the small blood vessels. The onset of vasoconstriction becomes apparent within minutes. Zinc sulfate is an ocular astringent which, by precipitating protein, helps to clear mucus from the outer surface of the eye. The effectiveness of Visine A.C. in temporarily relieving conjunctival hyperemia and eye discomfort due to pollen, dust and ragweed has been clinically demonstrated. In one double-blind study of subjects who experienced acute episodes of minor eye irritation, Visine A.C. produced statistically significant beneficial results versus a placebo of normal saline solution in relieving irritation of bulbar conjunctivae, irritation of palpebral conjunctivae and mucus buildup. Treatment with Visine A.C. also significantly relieved eye discomfort.

Indications: For temporary relief of discomfort and redness due to minor eye irritations.

Directions: Instill 1 to 2 drops in the affected eye(s) up to 4 times daily.
Note: As drops go to work, some users may notice a brief tingling sensation which will quickly pass.

Active Ingredients: Zinc sulfate 0.25%; tetrahydrozoline hydrochloride 0.05%.

Inactive Ingredients: Benzalkonium chloride; boric acid; edetate disodium; purified water; sodium chloride; sodium citrate.

Warnings: If you experience eye pain, changes in vision, continued redness or

Continued on next page

Visine A.C.—Cont.

irritation of the eye, or if the condition worsens or persists for more than 72 hours, discontinue use and consult a physician. If you have glaucoma, do not use this product except under the advice and supervision of a physician. As with any drug, if you are pregnant or nursing a baby, seek the advice of a health professional before using this product. Overuse of this product may produce increased redness of the eye. If solution changes color or becomes cloudy, do not use. To avoid contamination, do not touch tip of container to any surface. Replace cap after using. Remove contact lenses before using this product.

Parents Note: Before using with children under 6 years of age, consult your physician. Keep this and all drugs out of the reach of children. In case of accidental ingestion, seek professional assistance or contact a Poison Control Center immediately.

Caution: Should not be used if Visine-imprinted neckband on bottle is broken or missing.

Storage: Store between 15° and 30°C (59° and 86°F).

How Supplied: In 0.5 fl. oz. and 1.0 fl. oz. plastic dispenser bottle.

Shown in Product Identification Guide, page 517

VISINE® ORIGINAL
Tetrahydrozoline Hydrochloride/ Redness Reliever Eye Drops

Description: Visine is a sterile, isotonic, buffered ophthalmic solution containing tetrahydrozoline hydrochloride 0.05%. Visine is a decongestant ophthalmic solution designed to provide symptomatic relief of conjunctival edema and hyperemia secondary to minor irritations, due to conditions such as smoke, dust, other airborne pollutants and swimming. Relief is afforded by tetrahydrozoline hydrochloride, a sympathomimetic agent, which brings about decongestion by vasoconstriction. Reddened eyes are rapidly whitened by this effective vasoconstrictor, which limits the local vascular response by constricting the small blood vessels. The onset of vasoconstriction becomes apparent within minutes.

The effectiveness of Visine in relieving conjunctival hyperemia has been demonstrated by numerous clinicals, including several double-blind studies, involving more than 2,000 subjects suffering from acute or chronic hyperemia induced by a variety of conditions.

Indications: Relieves redness of the eye due to minor eye irritations.

Directions: Instill 1 to 2 drops in the affected eye(s) up to four times daily.

Active Ingredient: Tetrahydrozoline hydrochloride 0.05%.

Inactive Ingredients: Benzalkonium chloride 0.01%; boric acid; edetate disodium 0.1%; sodium borate; sodium chloride; purified water.

Warnings: If you experience eye pain, changes in vision, continued redness or irritation of the eye, or if the condition worsens or persists for more than 72 hours, discontinue use and consult a physician. If you have glaucoma, do not use this product except under the advice and supervision of a physician. As with any drug, if you are pregnant or nursing a baby, seek the advice of a health professional before using this product. Overuse of this product may produce increased redness of the eye. If solution changes color or becomes cloudy, do not use. To avoid contamination, do not touch tip of container to any surface. Replace cap after using. Remove contact lenses before using this product.

Parents Note: Before using with children under 6 years of age, consult your physician. Keep this and all drugs out of the reach of children. In case of accidental ingestion, seek professional assistance or contact a Poison Control Center immediately.

Caution: Should not be used if Visine-imprinted neckband on bottle is broken or missing.

Storage: Store between 2° and 30°C (36° and 86°F).

How Supplied: In 0.5 fl. oz., 0.75 fl. oz. and 1.0 fl. oz. plastic dispenser bottle and 0.5 fl. oz. plastic bottle with dropper.

Shown in Product Identification Guide, page 517

VISINE® TEARS™
Lubricant Eye Drops

Description:
Visine Tears is specially formulated to cool and comfort dry, irritated eyes. It relieves the dryness caused by computer use, reading, wind, heat and air conditioning, while it protects your eyes from further irritation. Visine Tears is safe to use as often as needed.

Indications: For the temporary relief of burning and irritation due to dryness of the eye and for use as a protectant against further irritation.

Directions: Instill 1 to 2 drops in the affected eye(s) as needed.

Active Ingredients: Polyethylene glycol 400 1%; glycerin 0.2%; hydroxypropyl methylcellulose 0.2%.

Inactive Ingredients: Ascorbic acid; benzalkonium chloride; boric acid; dextrose; disodium phosphate; glycine; magnesium chloride; potassium chloride; purified water; sodium borate; sodium chloride; sodium citrate; sodium lactate.

Warnings: If you experience eye pain, changes in vision, continued redness or irritation of the eye, or if the condition

worsens or persists for more than 72 hours, discontinue use and consult a physician.

As with any drug, if you are pregnant or nursing a baby, seek the advice of a health professional before using this product.

If solution changes color or becomes cloudy, do not use.

To avoid contamination, do not touch tip of container to any surface.

Replace cap after using.

Remove contact lenses before using this product.

Parents note: Before using with children under 6 years of age, consult your physician.

Keep this and all drugs out of the reach of children.

In case of accidental ingestion, seek professional assistance or contact a Poison Control Center immediately.

Caution: Should not be used if Visine-imprinted neckband on bottle is broken or missing.

Storage: Store between 15° and 30°C (59° and 86°F).

How Supplied: In 0.5 FL. OZ. and 1 FL. OZ. plastic dispenser bottles.

Shown in Product Identification Guide, page 517

WART–OFF®
Liquid

Active Ingredient: Salicylic Acid 17% w/w.

Inactive Ingredients: Alcohol, 26.35% w/w, Flexible Collodion, Propylene Glycol Dipelargonate.

Indications: For the removal of common warts and plantar warts on the bottom of the foot. The common wart is easily recognized by the rough "cauliflower-like" appearance of the surface. The plantar wart is recognized by its location only on the bottom of the foot, its tenderness, and the interruption of the footprint pattern.

Warnings: For external use only. Keep this and all medications out of the reach of children to avoid accidental poisoning. In case of accidental ingestion, contact a physician or a Poison Control Center immediately. Do not use this product on irritated skin, on any area that is infected or reddened, if you are a diabetic, or if you have poor blood circulation. Do not use on moles, birthmarks, warts with hair growing from them, genital warts, or warts on the face or mucous membranes. If product gets into the eye, flush with water for 15 minutes. Avoid inhaling vapors. If discomfort persists, see your doctor.

Extremely Flammable—Keep away from fire or flame. Cap bottle tightly and store at room temperature away from heat (59°–86°F) (15°–30°C).

Instructions For Use: Read warnings and enclosed instructional brochure.

Wash affected area. Dry area thoroughly. Using the special pinpoint applicator, apply one drop at a time to sufficiently cover each wart. Apply Wart-Off to warts only—not to surrounding skin. Let dry. Repeat this procedure once or twice daily as needed (until wart is removed) for up to 12 weeks. Replace cap tightly to prevent evaporation.

How Supplied: 0.45 fluid ounce (13.3mL) bottle with special pinpoint plastic applicator and instructional brochure.

EDUCATIONAL MATERIAL

All materials available to physicians, pharmacists, nurses and consumers free of charge by calling 1-800-RID-LICE (1-800-743-5423)
- Parent's Guide to Head Lice & Their Eggs (English and Spanish)
- "Back to Normal" Video (English and Spanish)
- ABCs of Lice Poster
- Lice Outbreak Notification Letters
- "From Eradication to Resistance: Five Continuing Concerns About Pediculosis", Reprinted from Journal of School Health, April 1988.
- "Pediculicides: Is Resistance Emerging?", Reprinted from US Pharmacist, August 1997
- "Lice: Resistance and Treatment," Reprinted from Contemporary Pediatrics, November 1998

Pharmacia & Upjohn
KALAMAZOO, MI 49001

For Medical and Pharmaceutical Information, Including Emergencies:
(616) 833-4000
(800) 253-8600

CORTAID®
Maximum Strength, Sensitive Skin Formula, Intensive Therapy, and FastStick®.
Cream, Ointment, and Roll-on Stick (hydrocortisone 1% and ¹/₂%)
Anti-itch products

Indications: Use CORTAID for the temporary relief of itching associated with minor skin irritations, inflammation, and rashes due to eczema, psoriasis, seborrheic dermatitis, poison ivy, poison oak, or poison sumac, insect bites, soaps, detergents, cosmetics, jewelry, and for external feminine and anal itching. Other uses of this product should be only under the advice and supervision of a physician.

Description: CORTAID provides safe, effective relief of many different types of itches and rashes and no brand is recommended by more physicians and pharmacists. Maximum Strength CORTAID 1%

hydrocortisone is the same strength and form of hydrocortisone relief formerly available only with a prescription. CORTAID Sensitive Skin Formula has been specially formulated with aloe and ¹/₂% hydrocortisone. CORTAID Intensive Therapy Cream's special formula of 1% hydrocortisone is specific for eczema & psoriasis sufferers. CORTAID FastStick provides the relief of Maximum Strength CORTAID in a convenient roll-on-stick—Great for insect bites. CORTAID is available in 1) a greaseless, odorless vanishing cream that leaves no residue; 2) a soothing, lubricating ointment; 3) a quick-drying non-staining, roll-on stick (Maximum Strength only).

Active Ingredients: Cortaid Maximum Strength Cream: Hydrocortisone 1%
Cortaid Maximum Strength Ointment: Hydrocortisone acetate 1%
Cortraid Intensive Therapy Cream: Hydrocortisone 1%
Cortaid Sensitive Skin Cream: Hydrocortisone acetate ¹/₂%
Cortaid FastStick: Hydrocortisone 1%

Other Ingredients:
Maximum Strength Products: *Maximum Strength Cream:* Aloe vera gel, ceteareth-20, ceteareth alcohol, cetyl palmitate, glycerin, isopropyl myristate, isostearyl neopentanoate, methylparaben, and purified water.
Maximum Strength Ointment: butylparaben, cholesterol, methylparaben, microcrystalline wax, mineral oil, and white petrolatum.
FastStick: alcohol (55%), butylated hydroxytoluene, glycerin, methylparaben, and purified water.
Sensitive Skin Products:
Sensitive Skin Formula Cream: aloe vera, butylparaben, cetyl palmitate, glyceryl stearate, methylparaben, polyethylene glycol, stearamidoethyl diethylamine, and purified water.
Intensive Therapy Products:
Intensive Therapy Cream: cetyl alcohol, citric acid, glyceryl stearate, isopropyl myristate, methylparaben, polyoxyl 40 stearate, polysorbate 60, propylene glycol, propylparaben, purified water, sodium citrate, sorbic acid, sorbitan monostearate, stearyl alcohol and white wax.

Uses: The vanishing action of CORTAID Cream makes it cosmetically acceptable when the skin itch or rash treated is on exposed parts of the body such as the hands or arms. CORTAID Ointment is best used where protection lubrication and soothing of dry and scaly lesions is required. The ointment is also recommended for treating itchy genital and anal areas. CORTAID FastStick delivers quick-drying, non-staining medicine via a convenient and highly portable roll-on stick.

Warnings: For external use only. Avoid contact with the eyes. If condition worsens, or if symptoms persist for more than 7 days or clear up and occur again within a few days, stop use of this product and do not begin use of any other hydrocortisone product unless you have consulted a

physician. Do not use for the treatment of diaper rash. Consult a physician. For external feminine itching, do not use if you have a vaginal discharge. Consult a physician. For external anal itching, do not exceed the recommended daily dosage unless directed by a physician. In case of bleeding, consult a physician promptly. Do not put this product into the rectum by using fingers or any mechanical device or applicator.
Keep this and all drugs out of the reach of children. In case of accidental ingestion, seek professional assistance or contact a poison control center immediately.

Dosage and Administration: *Adults and children 2 years of age and older:* Apply to affected area not more than 3 to 4 times daily. *Children under 2 years of age:* Do not use, consult a physician. *Adults:* For external anal itching, when practical, cleanse the affected area with mild soap and warm water and rinse thoroughly by patting or blotting with an appropriate cleansing pad. Gently dry by patting or blotting with toilet tissue or a soft cloth before application of this product. *Children under 12 years of age:* For external anal itching, consult a physician.

How Supplied: Maximum Strength Cream: ¹/₂ oz. and 1 oz. tubes
Maximum Strength Ointment: ¹/₂ oz. and 1 oz. tubes
Sensitive Skin Cream: ¹/₂ oz. tube
Intensive Therapy Cream: 2 oz. tube
FastStick: .23 fl. oz. vial
Shown in Product Identification Guide, page 517

DOXIDAN® LIQUI-GELS®
Stimulant/Stool Softener Laxative

Indications: DOXIDAN is a safe reliable laxative for the relief of occasional constipation. The combination of a stimulant/stool softener laxative allows positive laxative action on a softened stool for gentle evacuation without straining. DOXIDAN generally produces a bowel movement in 6 to 12 hours.

Active Ingredients: Each soft gelatin Liqui-gel contains 30 mg casanthranol and 100 mg docusate sodium.

Inactive Ingredients: Also contains FD&C Blue #1 and Red #40, gelatin, glycerin, polyethylene glycol, sorbitol, titanium dioxide.

Dosage and Administration: Adults and children 12 years of age and over: one to three Liqui-Gels by mouth in a single daily dose. Children 2 to under 12 years of age: one Liqui-Gel daily. Children under 2 years of age: consult a doctor.

Warnings: Do not use laxative products when abdominal pain, nausea, or vomiting are present unless directed by a doctor. If you have noticed a sudden

Continued on next page

Doxidan—Cont.

change in bowel habits that persists over a period of 2 weeks, consult a doctor before using a laxative. Laxative products should not be used for a period longer than 1 week unless directed by a doctor. Rectal bleeding or failure to have a bowel movement after use of a laxative may indicate a serious condition. Discontinue use and consult your doctor. Keep this and all drugs out of the reach of children. In case of accidental overdose, seek professional assistance or contact a poison control center immediately. As with any drug, if you are pregnant or nursing a baby, seek the advice of a health professional before using this product.

Drug Interaction Precaution: Do not take this product if you are presently taking mineral oil, unless directed by a doctor.

How Supplied: Packages of 10, 30, 100, and Unit Dose 100s (10 × 10 strips). LIQUI-GELS® Reg TM R P Scherer Corp

Shown in Product Identification Guide, page 517

DRAMAMINE® Tablets
(dimenhydrinate USP)
DRAMAMINE® Chewable Tablets
(dimenhydrinate USP)
DRAMAMINE® Children's Liquid
(dimenhydrinate syrup USP)

Indications: For the prevention and treatment of the nausea, vomiting, or dizziness associated with motion sickness.

Description: Dimenhydrinate is the chlorotheophylline salt of the antihistaminic agent diphenhydramine. Dimenhydrinate contains not less than 53% and not more than 56% of diphenhydramine, and not less than 44% and not more than 47% of 8-chlorotheophylline, calculated on the dried basis.

Active Ingredients: DRAMAMINE Tablets and Chewable Tablets: Dimenhydrinate 50 mg.
DRAMAMINE Children's: Dimenhydrinate 12.5 mg. per 5 ml.

Inactive Ingredients: DRAMAMINE Tablets: Colloidal Silicon Dioxide, Croscarmellose Sodium, Lactose, Magnesium Stearate, Microcrystalline Cellulose.
DRAMAMINE Children's: FD&C Red No. 40, Flavor, Glycerin, Methylparaben, Sucrose, and Water.
DRAMAMINE Chewable Tablets: Aspartame, Citric Acid, FD&C Yellow No. 5 (Tartrazine) and FD&C Yellow No. 6 as color additives, Flavor, Magnesium Stearate, Methacrylic Acid Copolymer, Sorbitol.
Phenylketonurics: Contains Phenylalanine 1.5 mg per tablet.

Actions: While the precise mode of action of dimenhydrinate is not known, it is thought to have a depressant action on hyperstimulated labyrinthine function.

Directions:
DRAMAMINE Tablets and Chewable Tablets: To prevent motion sickness, the first dose should be taken one half to one hour before starting activity. ADULTS: 1 to 2 tablets every 4 to 6 hours, not to exceed 8 tablets in 24 hours or as directed by a doctor.
CHILDREN 6 TO UNDER 12 years: $1/2$ to 1 tablet every 6 to 8 hours, not to exceed 3 tablets in 24 hours or as directed by a doctor.
CHILDREN 2 to UNDER 6 years: $1/4$ to $1/2$ tablet every 6 to 8 hours not to exceed $1^1/2$ tablets in 24 hours or as directed by a doctor.
Children may also be given DRAMAMINE Cherry Flavored Liquid in accordance with directions for use.
DRAMAMINE Children's: To prevent motion sickness, the first dose should be taken one half to one hour before starting activity. CHILDREN 2 TO UNDER 6 years: 1 to 2 teaspoonfuls (5 ml per teaspoonful) every 6 to 8 hours, not to exceed 6 teaspoonfuls in 24 hours or as directed by a doctor. CHILDREN 6 TO UNDER 12 years: 2 to 4 teaspoonfuls every 6 to 8 hours, not to exceed 12 teaspoonfuls in 24 hours or as directed by a doctor. CHILDREN 12 YEARS OR OLDER (and adults): 4 to 8 teaspoonfuls every 4 to 6 hours, not to exceed 32 teaspoonfuls in 24 hours or as directed by a doctor. Use of a measuring device is recommended for all liquid medication.

Warnings: Do not take this product, unless directed by a doctor, if you have a breathing problem such as emphysema or chronic bronchitis, or if you have glaucoma or difficulty in urination due to enlargement of the prostate gland. Do not give to children under 2 years of age unless directed by a doctor. May cause marked drowsiness; alcohol, sedatives, and tranquilizers may increase the drowsiness effect. Avoid alcoholic beverages while taking this product. Do not take this product if you are taking sedatives or tranquilizers, without first consulting your doctor. Use caution when driving a motor vehicle or operating machinery. Not for frequent or prolonged use except on advice of a doctor. Do not exceed recommended dosage. Keep this and all drugs out of the reach of children. In case of accidental overdose, seek professional assistance or contact a poison control center immediately. As with any drug, if you are pregnant or nursing a baby, seek the advice of a health professional before using this product.

How Supplied: *Tablets*—scored, white tablets available in 12 ct. vials, 36 ct. and 100 ct. packages; *Chewables*—scored, orange tablets available in packages of 8 ct. and 24 ct; *Liquid*—Available in bottles of 4 fl oz.

Shown in Product Identification Guide, page 517

DRAMAMINE Less Drowsy Formula
(Meclizine hydrochloride)

Indications: For the prevention and treatment of the nausea, vomiting, or dizziness associated with motion sickness.

Description: Meclizine hydrochloride is an antihistamine of the piperazine class with antiemetic action.

Actions: While the precise mode of action of meclizine hydrochloride is not known, it is thought to have a depressant action on hyperstimulated labyrinthine function.

Active Ingredients: Each tablet contains 25 mg. meclizine hydrochloride.

Inactive Ingredients: Colloidal silicon dioxide, Corn starch, Lactose, D&C Yellow No. 10 (Aluminum Lake), Microcrystalline Cellulose, Magnesium Stearate.

Directions: To prevent motion sickness, the first dose should be taken one hour before starting your activity. **Adults (12 years and older):** Take 1 to 2 tablets daily or as directed by a doctor. Do not exceed 2 tablets in 24 hours.

Warnings: Do not take this product, unless directed by a doctor, if you have a breathing problem such as emphysema or chronic bronchitis, or if you have glaucoma or difficulty in urination due to enlargement of the prostate gland. Do not give to children under 12 years of age unless directed by a doctor. May cause drowsiness; alcohol, sedatives, and tranquilizers may increase the drowsiness effect. Avoid alcoholic beverages while taking this product. Do not take this product if you are taking sedatives or tranquilizers, without first consulting your doctor. Use caution when driving a motor vehicle or operating machinery. Not for frequent or prolonged use except on the advice of a doctor. Do not exceed recommended dosage. Keep this and all drugs out of reach of children. In case of accidental overdose, seek professional assistance or contact a poison control center immediately. As with any drug, if you are pregnant or nursing a baby, seek the advice of a health professional before using this product.

How Supplied: Dramamine Less Drowsy Formula is supplied as a yellow tablet in 8 ct. vials.
Shown in Product Identification Guide, page 517

EMETROL®
(Phosphorated Carbohydrate Solution)
For the relief of nausea associated with upset stomach

Description: EMETROL is an oral solution containing balanced amounts of dextrose (glucose) and levulose (fructose) and phosphoric acid with controlled hydrogen ion concentration. Available in original lemon-mint or cherry flavor.

Ingredients: Each 5 mL teaspoonful contains dextrose (glucose), 1.87 g; levulose (fructose), 1.87 g; phosphoric acid, 21.5 mg; and the following inactive ingredients: glycerin, methylparaben, purified water; D&C yellow No. 10 and natural lemon-mint flavor in lemon-mint Emetrol; FD&C red No. 40 and artificial cherry flavor in cherry Emetrol.

Action: EMETROL quickly relieves nausea by local action on the wall of the hyperactive G.I. tract. No delay in therapeutic action such as that associated with systemic drugs.

Indications: For the relief of nausea due to upset stomach from intestinal flu and food or drink indiscretions. For other conditions, take only as directed by your physician.

Advantages:
1. **Fast Action**—works quickly through local action on contact with the hyperactive G.I. tract.
2. **Effectiveness**—clinically proven to stop nausea.
3. **Safety**—all natural active ingredients won't mask symptoms of organic pathology. No known drug interactions.
4. **Convenience**—no Rx required.
5. **Patient Acceptance**—pleasant tasting lemon-mint or cherry flavor.

Usual Adult Dose: One or two tablespoonfuls. Repeat every 15 minutes until distress subsides.

Usual Children's Dose (2 to 12 years): One or two teaspoonfuls. Repeat dose every 15 minutes until distress subsides.

Important: For maximum effectiveness never dilute EMETROL or drink fluids of any kind immediately before or after taking a dose.

Caution: Not to be taken for more than one hour (5 doses) without consulting a physician. If upset stomach continues or recurs frequently, consult a physician promptly as it may be a sign of a serious condition.

WARNING: This product contains fructose and should not be taken by persons with hereditary fructose intolerance (HFI).
As with any drug, if you are pregnant or nursing a baby, seek the advice of a health professional before using this product.

> **This product contains sugar and should not be taken by diabetics except under the advice and supervision of a physician.**

In case of accidental overdose, contact a poison control center, emergency medical facility, or physician immediately for advice.
KEEP THIS AND ALL MEDICATIONS OUT OF THE REACH OF CHILDREN.

How Supplied: Each 5 mL teaspoonful of EMETROL contains dextrose (glucose), 1.87 g; levulose (fructose), 1.87 g;

and phosphoric acid, 21.5 mg in a yellow, lemon-mint or red, cherry-flavored syrup.
Yellow, Lemon-Mint
NDC 0009-7573-01—Bottle of 4 fluid ounces (118 mL)
NDC 0009-7573-02—Bottle of 8 fluid ounces (236 mL)
Red, Cherry
NDC 0009-7574-01—Bottle of 4 fluid ounces (118 mL)
NDC 0009-7574-02—Bottle of 8 fluid ounces (236 mL)
NDC 0009-7574-03—Bottle of 1 pint (473 mL)
STORE AT ROOM TEMPERATURE
NOTICE: Each bottle is protected by a printed band around the cap. Do not use if band is damaged or missing.
Shown in Product Identification Guide, page 517

KAOPECTATE®
Anti-Diarrheal,
Regular Flavor, Peppermint Flavor and Children's Cherry Flavored Liquids. Maximum Strength Caplets.

Indications: For the fast relief of diarrhea and cramping.

Active Ingredients: Each tablespoon of Kaopectate Regular and Peppermint Flavored Liquids and each Maximum Strength Caplet contains 750 mg attapulgite. Each tablespoon of Children's Cherry Flavored Liquid contains 600 mg attapulgite.

Inactive Ingredients: Liquids: flavors, glucono-delta-lactone, magnesium aluminum silicate, methylparaben, sorbic acid, sucrose, titanium dioxide, xanthan gum and purified water; Peppermint flavor and Children's Cherry flavor contain FD&C Red #40. Maximum Strength Caplets: Carnauba Wax, Croscarmellose Sodium, Hydroxypropyl Cellulose, Hydroxypropyl Methylcellulose, Methylparaben, Pectin, Propylene Glycol, Propylparaben, Sucrose, Titanium Dioxide, Zinc Stearate. May also contain Talc.

Dosage and Administration: Liquids: For best results, take full recommended dose at first sign of diarrhea and after each subsequent bowel movement. (Maximum 6 times in 24 hours.) Adults and children 12 years of age and over: 2 tablespoons. Children 6 to under 12 years of age: 1 tablespoon. Children 3 to 6 years of age: $\frac{1}{2}$ tablespoon. Maximum Strength Tablets: Swallow whole caplets with water; do not chew. For best results, take full recommended dose. Adults: Take 2 caplets after the initial bowel movement and 2 caplets after each subsequent bowel movement, not to exceed 12 caplets in 24 hours. Children 6 to 12 years of age: Take 1 caplet after the initial bowel movement and 1 caplet after each subsequent movement, not to exceed 6 caplets in 24 hours. Children 3 to

under 6 years of age can use Children's Cherry Flavored Liquid or Advanced Formula KAOPECTATE Liquid.

Warnings: **DO NOT USE FOR MORE THAN TWO DAYS UNLESS DIRECTED BY A DOCTOR.** Do not use if diarrhea is accompanied by fever or if blood or mucus is present in stool. Do not use in infants or children under 3 years of age unless directed by a doctor. If you are taking a prescription medicine, consult your doctor before taking this product. In case of accidental overdose, seek professional assistance or contact a poison control center immediately.

How Supplied: Regular flavor available in 8 oz., 12 oz. and 16 oz. bottles. Peppermint flavor available in 8 oz. and 12 oz. bottles. Children's Cherry flavor available in 6 oz. bottle. Maximum Strength Caplets available in blister packs of 12 and 20 caplets.
Shown in Product Identification Guide, page 517

MICATIN®
Antifungal for Athlete's Foot and Ringworm

MICATIN®
Antifungal for Jock Itch

Description: An antifungal containing the active ingredient miconazole nitrate 2%, clinically proven to cure athlete's foot, ringworm, and jock itch.

Indications: Proven clinically effective in the treatment of athlete's foot (tinea pedis), jock itch (tinea cruris), and ringworm (tinea corporis). For effective relief of the itching, cracking, scaling, burning and discomfort that can accompany these conditions.

Professional Labeling: For the treatment of superficial skin infections caused by yeast (*Candida albicans*)

Directions: Clean the affected area and dry thoroughly. Apply or spray a thin layer of MICATIN over affected area twice daily (morning and night) or as directed by a doctor. Supervise children in the use of the product. For athlete's foot, pay special attention to the spaces between the toes; wear well-fitting, ventilated shoes and change shoes and socks at least once daily. For athlete's foot and ringworm, use daily 4 weeks; for jock itch, use daily for 2 weeks. If condition persist longer, consult a doctor. This product is not effective on the scalp or nails.

Warnings: Do not use on children under 2 years of age unless directed by a doctor. For external use only. Avoid contact with the eyes. If irritation occurs or if there is no improvement within 4 weeks (for athlete's foot and ringworm) or within 2 weeks (for jock itch), discontinue use and consult a doctor. Keep this and all drugs out of the reach of children.

Continued on next page

Micatin—Cont.

In case of accidental ingestion, seek professional assistance or contact a Poison Control Center immediately.

How Supplied:
MICATIN® Antifungal Cream is available in a 0.5 oz. tube and 1.0 oz. tube.
MICATIN Antifungal Spray Powder is available in a 3.0 oz. aerosol can.
MICATIN Antifungal Odor Control Spray Powder is available in a 3.0 oz. aerosol can.
MICATIN Antifungal Powder is available in a 3.0 oz. plastic bottle.
MICATIN Antifungal Spray Liquid is available in a 3.5 oz. aerosol can.
MICATIN Antifungal Cooling Action Spray Liquid is available in a 3 oz. bottle.
MICATIN Jock Itch Cream is available in a 1/2 oz. and 1 oz. tube.
MICATIN Jock Itch Spray Powder is available in a 3.0 oz. aerosol can.

Inactive Ingredients:
MICATIN Antifungal Cream: Benzoic Acid, BHA, Mineral Oil, Peglicol 5 Oleate, Pegoxol 7 Stearate, Purified Water.
MICATIN Antifungal Spray Powder: Alcohol SD 40 (10%), Sorbitan Sesquioleate, Stearalkonium Hectorite, Talc. Propellant: Isobutane, Propane.
MICATIN Antifungal Odor Control Spray Powder: Alcohol SD 40 (10%), Fragrance, Sorbitan Sesquioleate, Stearalkonium Hectorite, Talc. Propellant: Isobutane, Propane.
MICATIN Antifungal Powder: Talc.
MICATIN Antifungal Spray Liquid: Alcohol SD 40 (16.8%), Benzyl Alcohol, Cocamide DEA, Sorbitan Sesquioleate, Tocopherol. Propellant: Isobutane, Propane.
MICATIN Antifungal Cooling Action Spray Liquid: Dimethyl Ether, Lactic Acid, Menthol, Polysorbate 60, Polysorbate 65, SD Alcohol 40-B, Sodium Hydroxide, Sorbitan Stearate, Water.
MICATIN Jock Itch Cream: Benzoic Acid, BHA, Mineral Oil, Peglicol 5 Oleate, Pegoxol 7 Stearate, Purified Water.
MICATIN Jock Itch Spray Powder: Alcohol SD 40 (10%), Sorbitan Sesquioleate, Stearalkonium Hectorite, Talc. Propellant: Isobutane, Propane.

Storage: Store at room temperature.

Shown in Product Identification Guide, page 517

NASALCROM™ Nasal Spray
CHILDREN'S NASALCROM™
Nasal Spray
Nasal Allergy Symptom Controller

Description: NASALCROM Nasal Spray and CHILDREN'S NASALCROM Nasal Spray contain a unique formulation of cromolyn sodium that stabilizes mast cells that contain and release histamine. By taking NASALCROM Nasal Spray or CHILDREN'S NASALCROM Nasal Spray prior to exposure to irritating allergens, a layer of protection is built up on the mast cells preventing degranulation and the release of histamine.

Indications: NASALCROM Nasal Spray and CHILDREN'S NASALCROM Nasal Spray are indicated for the prevention and treatment of the symptoms of seasonal and perennial allergic rhinitis such as runny/itchy nose, sneezing, and allergic stuffy nose.

Ingredients: Each mL of NASALCROM Nasal Spray and CHILDREN'S NASALCROM Nasal Spray contains 40 mg. of cromolyn sodium in purified water with 0.01% benzalkonium chloride to preserve and 0.01% EDTA (edetate disodium) to stabilize the solution. Each metered spray releases the same amount of medicine, 5.2 mg. cromolyn sodium. CHILDREN'S NASALCROM Nasal Spray comes with a special child friendly applicator, designed for easier use by children.

What Makes NasalCrom Unique?
• **Prevention and relief.**
NasalCrom relieves nasal allergy symptoms and, if used as directed, prevents symptoms from occurring.
• **Non-drowsy.**
Many allergy medications contain antihistamines, which may cause drowsiness. NasalCrom's unique formula works only in the nose without drowsiness.
• **Builds protection.**
NasalCrom works by building protection against nasal allergy symptoms. To maintain protection, continue to use NasalCrom daily.
• **Can be used every day protection is needed.**
NasalCrom is a gentle nasal spray that works differently from decongestant sprays. Unlike those products, it continues to be safe and effective when used every day.
• **Can be used with other medications.**
NasalCrom can be used safely with other medications, including other allergy medications.

Directions:
Adults and children 6 years of age and older:
• Spray once into each nostril. Repeat 3–4 times a day (every 4–6 hours). If needed, may be used up to 6 times a day. Directions on how to use pump spray are detailed on carton and package insert.
• Use every day while in contact with the cause of the allergies (pollens, molds, pets, and dust).
• To **prevent** nasal allergy symptoms, use before contact with the cause of the allergies. For best results, start using up to one week before contact.
• If desired, NASALCROM Nasal Spray and CHILDREN'S NASALCROM Nasal Spray can be used with other allergy medications.

Children under 6 years of age: Do not use unless directed by a doctor.

Warnings:
Ask a doctor before use if you have:
• Fever
• Discolored nasal discharge
• Sinus pain
• Wheezing

When using this product:
• It may take several days of use to notice an effect. The best effect may not be seen for 1 to 2 weeks.
• Brief stinging or sneezing may occur right after use.
• Do not use this product to treat sinus infection, asthma, or cold symptoms.
• Do not share this bottle with anyone else as this may spread germs.

Stop using this product if:
• Symptoms worsen.
• New symptoms occur.
• Symptoms do not begin to improve within two weeks.

See your doctor because these could be signs of a serious illness.
As with any drug, if you are pregnant or nursing a baby, seek the advice of a healthcare professional before using this product. Keep this and all drugs out of the reach of children. In case of accidental ingestion/overdose, seek professional assistance or contact a poison control center immediately.

Do not use if printed plastic bottle wrap imprinted with "Safety Seal®" is broken or missing.

How Supplied: NASALCROM Nasal Spray and CHILDREN'S NASALCROM Nasal Spray are available in 13mL (100 metered sprays) and 26mL (200 metered sprays) sizes. CHILDREN'S NASALCROM comes with a special child friendly applicator, designed for easier use by children.

Shown in Product Identification Guide, page 517

NASALCROM™ A
NASALCROM™ CA
Allergy Prevention Packs

Desciption: NASALCROM A and CA are unique combination packs containing NASALCROM Nasal Spray and allergy relief tablets or caplets. The tablets or caplets are used for quick, short-term allergy relief while NASALCROM Nasal Spray builds to full strength. Both prevention packs contain NASALCROM Nasal Spray, a unique formulation of cromolyn sodium that stabilizes mast cells that contain and release histamine. By taking NASALCROM Nasal Spray prior to exposure to irritating allergens, a layer of protection is built up on the mast cells preventing degranulation and the release of histamine.

Indications: NASALCROM Nasal Spray is indicated for the prevention and treatment of the symptoms of seasonal and perennial allergic rhinitis. NASALCROM Nasal Spray contains 4% cromolyn sodium solution. Each metered spray releases the same amount of medicine, 5.2 mg. cromolyn sodium. NASALCROM A antihistamine tablets contain 4 mg. of chlorpheniramine maleate for the temporary relief of runny nose, sneezing, itching of the nose or throat, and itchy, watery eyes due to hay fever or allergic rhinitis. NASALCROM CA decongestant caplets contain 30 mg. of pseudoephedrine HCl and 500 mg. of acetaminophen for relief of nasal congestion, sinus congestion and pressure, and sinus headache pain due to hay fever or respiratory allergies (allergic rhinitis).

Active Ingredients: Each mL of NASALCROM Nasal Spray contains 40 mg. cromolyn sodium in purified water. Each metered spray releases the same amount of medicine, 5.2 mg. cromolyn sodium. Each tablet of NASALCROM A tablets contains 4 mg. of chlorpheniramine maleate. Each caplet of NASALCROM CA caplets contains 30 mg. of Pseudoephedrine HCl and 500 mg. of acetaminophen.

Inactive Ingredients: NASALCROM Nasal Spray contains 0.01% benzalkonium chloride to preserve and 0.01% EDTA (edetate disodium) to stabilize the solution. NASALCROM A tablets contain D&C Yellow No. 10 Aluminum Lake, Lactose, Microcrystalline Cellulose, Starch. May Also Contain: Crospovidone, Magnesium Stearate, Silicon Dioxide, Stearic Acid. NASALCROM CA caplets contain Croscarmellose Sodium, D&C Yellow No. 10, FD&C Blue No. 1, FD&C Red No. 40, FD&C Yellow No. 6, Hydroxypropyl Methylcellulose, Magnesium Stearate, Microcrystalline Cellulose, Polyethylene Glycol, Polysorbate 80, Propylene Glycol, Silicon Dioxide, Titanium Dioxide.

Directions for NASALCROM Nasal Spray:
Adults and children 6 years of age and older: Spray once into each nostril. Repeat 3–4 times a day (every 4–6 hours). If needed, may be used up to 6 times a day. See side panel on how to use pump. Use every day while in contact with the cause of your allergies (pollens, molds, pets, and dust). To **prevent** nasal allergy symptoms, use before contact with the cause of the allergies. For best results, start using up to one week before contact. If desired, NASALCROM can be used with other medicines, including other allergy medicines.
Children 6–12 years: Use spray only.
Children under 6 years: Do not use unless directed by a doctor.

Directions for NASALCROM A Allergy Relief Tablets:
Adults and children over 12 years: Take 1 tablet every 4 to 6 hours as needed. Do not take more than 6 tablets in 24 hours, unless directed by a doctor.
Children 6 to under 12 years: Take ½ tablet every 4 to 6 hours as needed. Do not take more than 3 tablets in 24 hours, unless directed by a doctor.
Children under 6 years: Do not use unless directed by a doctor.

Directions for NASALCROM CA Congested Allergy Relief Caplets:
Adults and children over 12 years: Take 2 caplets every 4 to 6 hours. Do not take more than 8 caplets in 24 hours, unless directed by a doctor.
Children under 12 years: Do not use unless directed by a doctor.

Warnings for NASALCROM Nasal Spray:
Ask a doctor before use if you have:
• Fever

• Discolored nasal discharge
• Sinus pain
• Wheezing
When using this product:
• It may take several days of use to notice an effect. Your best effect may not be seen for 1 to 2 weeks.
• Brief stinging or sneezing may occur right after use.
• Do not use this product to treat sinus infection, asthma, or cold symptoms.
• Do not share this bottle with anyone else as this may spread germs.
Stop using this product if:
• Symptoms worsen.
• New symptoms occur.
• Symptoms do not begin to improve within two weeks.
See your doctor because these could be signs of a serious illness.
As with any drug, if you are pregnant or nursing a baby, seek the advice of a healthcare professional before using this product. Keep this and all drugs out of the reach of children. In case of accidental ingestion/overdose, seek professional assistance or contact a poison control center immediately.
Do not use if printed plastic bottle wrap imprinted with "Safety Seal®" is broken or missing.

Warnings for NASALCROM A Allergy Relief Tablets:
May cause excitability, especially in children. Do not take this product, unless directed by a doctor, if you have a breathing problem such as emphysema or chronic bronchitis, or if you have glaucoma or difficulty in urination due to enlargement of the prostate gland. May cause drowsiness; alcohol, sedatives and tranquilizers may increase the drowsiness effect. Avoid alcoholic beverages while taking this product. Do not take this product if you are taking sedatives or tranquilizers, without first consulting your doctor. Use caution when driving a motor vehicle or operating machinery. As with any drug, if you are pregnant or nursing a baby, seek the advice of a health professional before using this product. Keep this and all drugs out of the reach of children. In case of accidental overdose, seek professional assistance or contact a poison control center immediately.

Warnings for NASALCROM CA Congested Allergy Relief Caplets:
Sealed in blister unit for your protection. Do not take for pain for more than 7 days or for fever for more than 3 days unless directed by a doctor. If pain or fever persists, or gets worse, or if new symptoms occur, or if redness or swelling is present, consult a doctor because these could be signs of a serious condition. Do not exceed recommended dosage. If nervousness, dizziness or sleeplessness occur, discontinue use and consult a doctor. Do not take this product if you have heart disease, high blood pressure, thyroid disease, diabetes or difficulty in urination due to enlargement of the prostate gland unless directed by a doctor. As with any drug, if you are pregnant or nursing a baby, seek the advice

of a health professional before using this product. Keep this and all drugs out of the reach of children. In case of accidental overdose, contact a doctor or poison control center immediately. Prompt medical attention is critical for adults as well as for children even if you do not notice any signs or symptoms. Do not use with other products containing acetaminophen.

Alcohol Warning: If you consume three or more alcoholic drinks every day, ask your doctor whether you should take acetaminophen or other pain relievers/fever reducers. Acetaminophen may cause liver damage.

DRUG INTERACTION PRECAUTION: Do not use this product if you are now taking a prescription monoamine oxidase inhibitor (MAOI) (certain drugs for depression, psychiatric or emotional conditions or Parkinson's disease), or for 2 weeks after stopping the MAOI drug. If you are uncertain whether your prescription drug contains MAOI, consult a health professional before taking this product.

How Supplied: NASALCROM A Prevention Pack has 1–13mL NASALCROM Nasal Spray and 12 Allergy Relief Tablets and NASALCROM CA Prevention Pack has 1–13mL NASALCROM Nasal Spray and 12 Congested Allergy Relief Caplets.

Shown in Product Identification Guide, page 517

PEDIACARE® Cough-Cold Liquid and Chewable Tablets
PEDIACARE® NightRest Cough-Cold Liquid
PEDIACARE® Infants' Drops Decongestant
PEDIACARE® Infants' Drops Decongestant Plus Cough

Description: Each 5 ml of *PEDIACARE® Cough-Cold Liquid* contains pseudoephedrine hydrochloride 15 mg, chlorpheniramine maleate 1 mg and dextromethorphan hydrobromide 5 mg. Each *PEDIACARE® Cough-Cold Chewable Tablet* contains pseudoephedrine hydrochloride 15 mg, chlorpheniramine maleate 1 mg and dextromethorphan hydrobromide 5 mg. Each 0.8 ml oral dropper of *PEDIACARE® Infants' Drops Decongestant* contains pseudoephedrine hydrochloride 7.5 mg. Each 0.8 oral dropper of *PEDIACARE® Infants' Drops Decongestant Plus Cough* contains pseudoephedrine hydrochloride 7.5 mg and dextromethorphan hydrobromide 2.5 mg. *PEDIACARE® NightRest Cough-Cold Liquid* contains pseudoephedrine hydrochloride 15 mg, chlorpheniramine maleate 1 mg and dextromethorphan hydrobromide 7.5 mg per 5 ml. *PEDIACARE® Cough-Cold Liquid* and *NightRest Cough-Cold Liquid* are stable, cherry flavored and red in color. *PEDIACARE® In-*

Continued on next page

Pediacare—Cont.

fants' Drops are fruit flavored alcohol free and red in color. PEDIACARE® Infants' Drops Decongestant Plus Cough are cherry flavored, alcohol free and clear, non-staining in color. PEDIACARE® Cough-Cold Chewable Tablets are fruit flavored and pink in color.

Actions: PEDIACARE Products are available in four different formulas, allowing you to select the ideal product to temporarily relieve the patient's symptoms. PEDIACARE® Cough-Cold Liquid and Chewable Tablets contain an antihistamine, chlorpheniramine maleate, a nasal decongestant, pseudoephedrine HCl, and a cough suppressant, dextromethorphan hydrobromide, to provide temporary relief of nasal congestion, runny nose, sneezing and coughing due to the common cold, hay fever or other upper respiratory allergies. PEDIACARE® NightRest Cough-Cold Liquid contains a decongestant, pseudoephedrine hydrochloride, an antihistamine, chlorpheniramine maleate, and a cough suppressant, dextromethorphan hydrobromide, to provide temporary relief of coughs, nasal congestion, runny nose and sneezing due to the common cold hayfever or other upper respiratory allergies. PEDIACARE® NightRest may be used day or night to relieve cough and cold symptoms. PEDIACARE® Infants' Drops Decongestant contain a decongestant, pseudoephedrine hydrochloride, to provide temporary relief of nasal congestion due to the common cold, hay fever or other upper respiratory allergies. PEDIACARE® Infants' Drops Decongestant Plus Cough contain a decongestant, pseudoephedrine hydrochloride, and a cough suppressant, dextromethorphan hydrobromide to provide temporary relief of nasal congestion and coughing due to common cold, hay fever or other upper respiratory allergies.

Professional Dosage: A calibrated dosage cup is provided for accurate dosing of the PEDIACARE Liquid formulas. A calibrated oral dropper is provided for accurate dosing of PEDIACARE® Infants'

Drops. All doses of PEDIACARE® Cough-Cold Liquid and Chewable Tablets, as well as PEDIACARE® Infants' Drops may be repeated every 4–6 hours, not to exceed 4 doses in 24 hours. PEDIACARE® NightRest Liquid may be repeated every 6–8 hrs, not to exceed 4 doses in 24 hours.
[See table below]

Warnings: DO NOT USE IF CARTON IS OPENED, OR IF PRINTED PLASTIC BOTTLE WRAP OR FOIL INNER SEAL IS BROKEN. KEEP THIS AND ALL MEDICATION OUT OF THE REACH OF CHILDREN. IN CASE OF ACCIDENTAL OVERDOSAGE, CONTACT A PHYSICIAN OR POISON CONTROL CENTER IMMEDIATELY.
The following information appears on the appropriate package labels:
PEDIACARE® Cough-Cold Chewable Tablets:
PHENYLKETONURICS: CONTAINS PHENYLALANINE 6MG PER TABLET.
PEDIACARE® Cough-Cold Liquid and Chewable Tablets, Night Rest Cough-Cold Liquid: Do not exceed recommended dosage. If nervousness, dizziness or sleeplessness occur, discontinue use and consult a doctor. If symptoms do not improve within 7 days or are accompanied by fever, consult a doctor. A persistent cough may be a sign of a serious condition. If cough persists for more than one week, tends to recur or is accompanied by fever, rash, or persistent headache, consult a doctor. Do not give this product for persistent or chronic cough such as occurs with asthma or if cough is accompanied by excessive phlegm (mucus) unless directed by a doctor. May cause excitability especially in children. May cause drowsiness. Sedatives and tranquilizers may increase the drowsiness effect. Do not give this product to children who are taking sedatives or tranquilizers without first consulting the child's doctor. Do not give this product to children who have a breathing problem such as chronic bronchitis, or who have glaucoma, heart disease, high blood pressure, thyroid disease or diabetes, without first consulting the child's doctor.

PEDIACARE® Infants' Drops Decongestant: Do not exceed the recommended dosage. If nervousness, dizziness or sleeplessness occur discontinue use and consult a doctor. If symptoms do not improve within 7 days or are accompanied by fever, consult a physician. Do not give this product to a child who has heart disease, high blood pressure, thyroid disease or diabetes unless directed by a doctor. Take by mouth only. Not for nasal use.
**PEDIACARE® Infants' Drops Decongestant Plus
Cough:** Do not exceed recommended dosage. If nervousness, dizziness, or sleeplessness occur, discontinue use and consult a doctor. If symptoms do not improve within 7 days or are accompanied by fever, consult a doctor. A persistent cough may be a sign of a serious condition. If cough persists for more than one week, tends to recur or is accompanied by fever, rash, or persistent headache, consult a doctor. Do not give this product for persistent or chronic cough such as occurs with asthma or if cough is accompanied by excessive phlegm (mucus) unless directed by a doctor. Do not give this product to a child who has heart disease, high blood pressure, thyroid disease or diabetes unless directed by a doctor. Take by mouth only. Not for nasal use.
Drug Interaction Precaution: Do not give this product to a child who is taking a prescription monoamine oxidase inhibitor (MAOI) (certain drugs for depression, psychiatric or emotional conditions), or for 2 weeks after stopping the MAOI drug. If you are uncertain whether your child's prescription drug contains an MAOI, consult a health professional before giving this product.

Inactive Ingredients: PEDIACARE® Cough-Cold Liquid: Citric acid, corn syrup, flavors, glycerin, propylene glycol, sodium benzoate, sodium carboxymethylcellulose, sorbitol, purified water and Red #40.
PEDIACARE® NightRest Cough-Cold Liquid: Citric acid, corn syrup, flavors, glycerin, propylene glycol, sodium benzoate, sodium carboxymethylcellulose, sorbitol, purified water and Red #40.

Age Group	0–3 mos	4–11 mos	12–23 mos	2–3 yrs	4–5 yrs	6–8 yrs	9–10 yrs	11 yrs	Dosage
Weight (lbs)	6–11 lb	12–17 lb	18–23 lb	24–35 lb	36–47 lb	48–59 lb	60–71 lb	72–95 lb	
PEDIACARE® Infants' Drops Decongestant*	$^{1}/_{2}$ dropper (0.4 ml)	1 dropper (0.8 ml)	$1^{1}/_{2}$ droppers (1.2 ml)	2 droppers (1.6 ml)					q4–6h
PEDIACARE® Infants' Drops Decongestant Plus Cough*	$^{1}/_{2}$ dropper (0.4 ml)	1 dropper (0.8 ml)	$1^{1}/_{2}$ droppers (1.2 ml)	2 droppers (1.6 ml)					q4–6h
PEDIACARE® Cough-Cold Liquid**				1 tsp	$1^{1}/_{2}$ tsp	2 tsp	$2^{1}/_{2}$ tsp	3 tsp	q4–6h
and Chewable Tablets**				1 tab	$1^{1}/_{2}$ tabs	2 tabs	$2^{1}/_{2}$ tabs	3 tabs	q4–6h
PEDIACARE® NightRest Liquid**				1 tsp	$1^{1}/_{2}$ tsp	2 tsp	$2^{1}/_{2}$ tsp	3 tsp	q6–8h

*Administer to children under 2 years only on the advice of a physician.
**Administer to children under 6 years only on the advice of a physician.

PEDIACARE® Cough-Cold Chewable Tablets: Aspartame, cellulose, citric acid, flavors, magnesium stearate, magnesium trisilicate, mannitol, corn starch and Red #7.

PEDIACARE® Infants' Drops Decongestant: Benzoic acid, citric acid, flavors, glycerin, polyethylene glycol, propylene glycol, purified water, sodium benzoate, sorbitol, sucrose and Red #40.

PEDIACARE® Infants' Drops Decongestant Plus Cough: Citric acid, flavors, glycerin, purified water, sodium benzoate, and sorbitol.

Overdosage: Acute dextromethorphan overdose usually does not result in serious signs and symptoms unless massive amounts have been ingested. Signs and symptoms of a substantial overdose may include nausea and vomiting, visual disturbances, CNS disturbances, and urinary retention. Symptoms from pseudoephedrine overdose consist most often of mild anxiety, tachycardia and/or mild hypertension. Symptoms usually appear within 4 to 8 hours of ingestion and are transient, usually requiring no treatment. Chlorpheniramine toxicity should be treated as you would an antihistamine/anticholinergic overdose and is likely to be present within a few hours after acute ingestion. Symptoms from pseudoephedrine overdose consist often of mild anxiety, tachycardia and/or mild hypertension. Symptoms usually appear within 4 to 8 hours of ingestion and are transient, usually requiring no treatment.

How Supplied: *PEDIACARE® Cough-Cold Liquid and NightRest Cough-Cold Liquid* (colored red)—bottles of 4 fl. oz. (120 ml) with child-resistant safety cap and calibrated dosage cup. *PEDIACARE® Cough-Cold Chewable Tablets* (pink, scored)—blister packs of 16. *PEDIACARE® Infants' Drops Decongestant* (colored red) and *PEDIACARE® Infants' Drops Decongestant Plus Cough* (clear)—bottles of ½ fl. oz (15 ml) with calibrated dropper.

Shown in Product Identification Guide, page 518

PEDIACARE Fever Liquid
Ibuprofen Oral Suspension Liquid
PEDIACARE Fever Drops
Ibuprofen Oral Suspension Drops

Description: PEDIACARE Fever Liquid and PEDIACARE Fever Drops are alcohol-free, berry-flavored liquids especially developed for children. Each 5 mL (teaspoon) of PEDIACARE Fever Liquid contains 100 mg. of ibuprofen. Each 1.25 mL (dropperful) of PEDIACARE Fever Drops contains 50 mg. of ibuprofen.

Active Ingredient: Ibuprofen

Inactive Ingredients for PEDIACARE Fever Liquid:
Citric acid, cornstarch, D&C Yellow #10, FD&C Red #40, Artificial flavors, glycerin, polysorbate 80, purified water, sodium benzoate, sucrose, xanthan gum.

Age	Weight	Fever Drops Every 6–8 hours* <102.5°F Fever	Fever Drops Every 6–8 hours* ≥102.5°F† Fever	Fever Liquid Every 6–8 hours* <102.5°F Fever	Fever Liquid Every 6–8 hours* ≥102.5°F† Fever
6–11 months	12–17 lbs.	1/2 dropper‡	1 dropper‡	1/4 teaspoon	1/2 teaspoon
12–23 months	18–23 lbs.	1 dropper‡	2 droppers‡	1/2 teaspoon	1 teaspoon
2–3 years	24–35 lbs.	2 droppers‡		1 teaspoon	
4–5 years	36–47 lbs.			1 1/2 teaspoons	
6–8 years	48–59 lbs.			2 teaspoons	
9–10 years	60–71 lbs.			2 1/2 teaspoons	
11 years	72–95 lbs.			3 teaspoons	

☐ Professional Dosing

*Do not exceed 4 doses in 24 hours.
†For persistent high fever, contact your Healthcare Professional.
‡dropper fever drops = 1.25 mL dropperful every 6–8 hours.   lbs = pounds
Recommended maximum daily dose is 40 mg/kg.

Inactive Ingredients for PEDIACARE Fever Drops:
Citric acid, cornstarch, artificial flavors, glycerin, polysorbate 80, purified water, sodium benzoate, sorbitol, sucrose, xanthan gum, FD&C #40.

Indications:
- **Reduces fever**
- **Relieves minor aches and pains** due to the common cold, flu, sore throat, headaches and toothaches

Directions for PEDIACARE Fever Liquid:
1. Do not take more than directed.
2. Shake well before using.
3. Find right dose on chart below. If possible, use weight to dose; otherwise use age.
4. Only use enclosed measuring cup.
5. Replace bottle cap tightly to maintain child resistance.
6. If needed, repeat dose every **6–8 hours.**
7. Do not use more than **4 times** a day.
8. If stomach upset occurs while taking this product, give with food or milk.

Directions for PEDIACARE Fever Drops: This product is intended for use in children ages 2–3 years.
1. Do not take more than directed.
2. Shake well before using.
3. Find right dose on chart below. If possible, use weight to dose; otherwise use age.
4. Only use enclosed dropper; fill to prescribed level and dispense liquid slowly into child's mouth, toward inner cheek.
5. Replace bottle cap tightly to maintain child resistance.
6. If needed, repeat dose every **6–8 hours.**
7. Do not use more than **4 times a day.**
8. If stomach upset occurs while taking this product, give with food or milk.

[See table above]

Warnings:
Allergy Alert: Ibuprofen may cause a severe allergic reaction which may include:
- Hives
- Facial swelling

- Asthma (wheezing)
- Shock

Do not use if you have ever had an allergic reaction to any other pain reliever/fever reducer.

Stop use and ask a doctor if an allergic reaction occurs. Seek medical help right away.

Call Your Doctor If:
- Your child is under a doctor's care for any serious condition or is taking any other drug.
- Your child has problems or serious side effects from taking fever reducers or pain relievers.
- Your child does not get any relief within first day (24 hours) of treatment, or pain or fever gets worse.
- Stomach upset gets worse or lasts.
- Redness or swelling is present in the painful area.
- Sore throat is severe, lasts for more than 2 days or occurs with fever, headache, rash, nausea or vomiting.
- Any new symptoms appear.

Do Not Use:
- With any other product that contains ibuprofen, or any other pain reliever/fever reducer, unless directed by a doctor.
- For more than **3 days** for fever or pain unless directed by a doctor.
- For stomach pain unless directed by a doctor.
- If your child is dehydrated (significant fluid loss) due to continued vomiting, diarrhea or lack of fluid intake.
- **If plastic bottle wrap on PEDIACARE Fever Drops imprinted "Safety Seal®" and "Use With Enclosed Dropper Only" is broken or missing or if plastic bottle wrap on PEDIACARE Fever Liquid is broken or missing.**

Important:
Keep this and all drugs out of the reach of children. In case of accidental overdose, seek professional assistance or contact a poison control center immediately.

Continued on next page

Pediacare Fever Drops—Cont.

Warnings for PediaCare Fever Liquid:
ALLERGIC REACTIONS: PediaCare Fever Liquid may cause a severe allergic reaction which may include:
- wheezing (asthma)
- hives
- fast, irregular pulse or heartbeat
- shortness of breath
- swelling of the face
- changing color of the skin (shock)

ASPIRIN SENSITIVE PATIENTS: Although PediaCare Fever Liquid does not contain aspirin, it may cause a severe reaction similar to that listed above, in people allergic to aspirin or other pain relievers/fever reducers. **Any of these reactions could be serious. Stop using this product and get emergency medical help immediately. These reactions can occur after taking a single dose or any subsequent dose in persons both with, and without, prior reaction to PediaCare Fever Liquid or other pain relievers/fever reducers.**

How Supplied: PEDIACARE Fever Liquid is available in 4 fl. Oz. Bottles and PEDIACARE Fever Drops is available in ½ fl. Oz. Bottles.

Shown in Product Identification Guide, page 517 and 518

ROGAINE EXTRA STRENGTH FOR MEN
Hair Regrowth Treatment
5% Minoxidil Topical Solution

Description: ROGAINE Extra Strength For Men is a colorless liquid medication for use only on the scalp to help regrow hair in men. It contains the highest concentration available in a specially formulated ROGAINE to provide more hair regrowth. Also, results may occur in as early as 2 months, compared to 4 months or more for regular strength products.

Active Ingredients: Minoxidil 5% w/v

Inactive Ingredients: Alcohol, 30% v/v, propylene glycol, 50% v/v, and purified water.

How Supplied: ROGAINE Extra Strength For Men is available in single, twin or triple packs.

Indication: ROGAINE Extra Strength For Men is medically proven to regrow hair.

Directions: FOR EXTERNAL USE ONLY. Apply one mL 2 times a day, every day, directly onto the scalp in the hair loss area. Using more or using more often will not improve results. Each bottle should last about 25–30 days, if used as directed. It is not necessary to use fingertips when applying ROGAINE Extra Strength For Men. However, if you use your hands, wash them afterwards. If you miss one or two daily doses of ROGAINE Extra Strength For Men continue with your next dose. You should not make up for missed doses. Allow 2 to 4 hours for ROGAINE Extra Strength For Men to completely dry. Do not apply to other parts of the body. Do not take ROGAINE Extra Strength For Men by mouth. **Keep this and all drugs out of the reach of children. In case of accidental ingestion, seek professional assistance or contact a Poison Control Center immediately.**

Use a mild shampoo if you wash your scalp before applying ROGAINE Extra Strength For Men. There is no need to change your usual hair care routine when using ROGAINE Extra Strength For Men. However, you should apply ROGAINE Extra Strength For Men first and wait for it to dry before applying your styling aids.

Instructions for use of Applicators:

How to use the applicators.

Applicator options
Two applicators are included in the carton which have been designed especially for men.

A. Dropper
The child-resistant dropper can be useful for a broad range of hair styles or hair loss because it allows for easy application through the hair and directly onto the scalp.

B. Sprayer
The sprayer may be more useful for larger areas of hair loss. When using the sprayer it is important to make sure that the medicine gets to the scalp. Also, one dose with the sprayer is 6 pumps.

Using the applicators
Important: When applying Rogaine Extra Strength For Men, make sure the medicine comes in direct contact with the scalp. The medicine will not work if it is sprayed only on your hair and does not reach your scalp.

A. Dropper
1. Squeeze the rubber bulb and put the dropper into the bottle. Release the bulb, allowing the dropper to fill to the 1 mL line. If the level of medicine is above the 1 mL line, squeeze the extra amount back into the bottle.
2. Next, place the tip of the dropper near the part of the scalp you want to treat and gently squeeze the bulb to gradually release the solution. To prevent the solution from running off the scalp, apply a small amount at a time.

B. B. Sprayer
The spray applicator is NOT child-resistant. If you have small children, keep the original child-resistant cap and place it back on the bottle after each use.
1. Put the spray applicator into the bottle and twist it on firmly.
2. Next, holding the bottle upright, pump the spray attachment 6 times to get one full dose (1ml). Be careful not to inhale the mist.

WARNINGS:
Do not use Rogaine Extra Strength if you are:
- a woman
- not sure of the reason for your hair loss
- under 18 years of age. Not for babies and children.
- using other medicines on the scalp

Not For Use By Women:
May grow facial hair. May be harmful if used during pregnancy or breast-feeding.

Do not use if you have:
- no family history of hair loss
- sudden and/or patchy hair loss
- a red, inflamed, infected, irritated or painful scalp

Stop use and see a doctor if you get:
- chest pain, a rapid heartbeat faintness, or dizziness
- sudden unexplained weight gain
- swollen hands or feet
- scalp irritation that continues or worsens

For external use only.
Avoid contact with eyes in case of accidental contact rinse with large amounts of cool tap water.
Keep this and all drugs out of the reach of children. Do not use on babies or children. In case of accidental ingestion, seek professional assistance or contact a Poison Control Center immediately.

Side Effects:
The most common side effects are itching and skin irritation of the treated area of the scalp. If scalp irritation continues, stop use and see a doctor. Rogaine Extra Strength For Men contains alcohol, which will cause burning or irritation of the eyes. If Rogaine Extra Strength For Men accidentally gets into eyes, rinse with large amounts of cool tap water.

Additional Information:
Who should NOT use Rogaine Extra Strength For Men?
Women should not use Rogaine Extra Strength For Men because studies have shown it works no better in women than Rogaine For Women. Some women may also grow facial hair. In addition, Rogaine Extra Strength For Men may be harmful if used during pregnancy or breast-feeding.
Rogaine Extra Strength For Men should not be used on babies or for children under 18 years old.
Rogaine Extra Strength For Men will not prevent or improve hair loss which may occur with the use of some prescription and non-prescription medications, certain severe nutritional problems (very low body iron; too much vitamin A intake), low thyroid states (hypothyroidism), chemotherapy, or diseases which cause scarring of the scalp. Also, Rogaine Extra Strength For Men will not improve hair loss due to: damage from the use of hair care products which cause scarring or deep burns of the scalp; hair grooming methods such as cornrowing or ponytails which require pulling the hair tightly back from the scalp.
Do not use if you are not sure of the reason for your hair loss.
Rogaine Extra Strength For Men differs from Regular Strength For Men products in the following ways:
- Contains 5% minoxidil (Rogaine Regular Strength contains 2%).
- Regrows more hair.
- With Rogaine Extra Strength For Men, results may occur at 2 months with twice daily use. For some men, it may take at least 4 months for results to be seen.

• Is more likely to cause scalp irritation. If scalp irritation continues or worsens, stop use and see a doctor. See Warnings on carton or bottle label.

Will Rogaine Extra Strength For Men work for me?

The amount of hair regrowth is different for each person. Not everyone will respond to Rogaine Extra Strength For Men. The response to Rogaine Extra Strength For Men cannot be predicted. It is unlikely anyone will be able to grow back all their hair.

However, to see your best results with Rogaine Extra Strength For Men, make sure you get the medicine directly to the scalp and apply it twice a day, everyday. You may get better results if you have been losing your hair for a short period of time or have little hair loss. However, for some men Rogaine Extra Strength For Men may not work.

How soon can I expect results from using Rogaine Extra Strength For Men?

Since normal hair usually grows only 1/2 to 1 inch per month, hair regrowth with Rogaine Extra Strength For Men also takes time.

Results may be seen as early as 2 months with twice daily use. For some men, it may take at least 4 months for results to be seen. If you do not see any results after 4 months, stop using Rogaine Extra Strength For Men.

When you first begin to use Rogaine Extra Strength For Men, your hair loss may increase temporarily for up to 2 weeks. This is likely a sign that you are getting rid of old hairs in order to regrow more new hairs. This temporary increase in hair loss is expected and is a part of the process for how Rogaine Extra Strength For Men regrows hair. Remember, this increased hair loss is temporary. However, if it continues after two weeks, see your doctor.

If Rogaine Extra Strength For Men is working, what will the hair look like?

At first, hair growth is usually soft, downy, colorless hairs (like peach fuzz). After further use, the new hairs should be the same color and thickness as the other hairs on your scalp.

How long do I need to use Rogaine Extra Strength For Men?

If you experience hair regrowth, continued use of Rogaine Extra For Men is necessary or the hair loss will begin again. In studies with Rogaine Extra Strength For Men, hair regrowth has not been shown to last longer than 48 weeks of continuous treatment in large clinical trials.

What happens if I completely stop using Rogaine Extra Strength For Men? Will I keep the new hair?

Continuous use of Rogaine Extra Strength For Men is needed to maintain hair regrowth.

If you stop using Rogaine Extra Strength For Men, you will lose your newly regrown hair in 3 to 4 months.

When do I use Rogaine Extra Strength For Men?

Apply Rogaine Extra Strength For Men once in the morning and once at night.

The nighttime application should occur 2 to 4 hours before going to bed to allow for drying. Each bottle should last about 25–30 days, if used as directed.

What if I miss a dose or forget to use Rogaine Extra Strength For Men?

If you miss one or two daily doses of Rogaine Extra Strength For Men, just continue with your next dose. You should not make up for missed doses.

Can I use Rogaine Extra Strength For Men more than twice a day? Will it work faster, better?

No. Rogaine Extra Strength For Men will not work faster or better if used more than two times a day. Studies have been carefully conducted to determine the correct amount of Rogaine Extra Strength For Men needed to get the best results. More frequent use or larger doses have not been shown to speed up hair growth and may increase your chance of side effects.

What kind of shampoo should I use with Rogaine Extra Strength For Men?

If you wash your scalp before applying Rogaine Extra Strength For Men, use a mild shampoo.

Can I use hair sprays, mousses, conditioners, gels, etc.?

Hair sprays, spritz, or styling aids may be used on your hair while using Rogaine Extra Strength For Men. For best results, Rogaine Extra Strength For Men should be allowed to soak into the scalp before using any styling products. Try to develop a good routine of applying Rogaine Extra Strength For Men first, and then applying styling products and style as usual. Keep in mind that your best results will be seen with proper application.

Can I have my hair colored or permed or use hair relaxers while using Rogaine Extra Strength For Men?

We have no evidence that coloring or perming your hair or that the use of relaxers change the effect of Rogaine Extra Strength For Men. However, because the use of a permanent wave and hair color can cause scalp irritation on certain people, we recommend the following precautions:

1) To avoid possible scalp irritation, you should make sure all of the Rogaine Extra Strength For Men has been washed off the hair and scalp before using color or perm chemicals.
2) For best results, do not apply Rogaine Extra Strength For Men on the same day that you use a chemical treatment on your hair.
3) Do not use Rogaine Extra Strength For Men for 24 hours after using any chemicals to make sure your scalp has not been irritated by the perm or color treatment. If no irritation occurs, continue use of Rogaine Extra Strength For Men as usual.
4) Simply restart your normal Rogaine Extra Strength For Men routine. There is no need to use more Rogaine Extra Strength For Men to make up for missed applications. Missing one day of Rogaine Extra Strength For Men will not affect your hair regrowth results.

Can I apply Rogaine Extra Strength For Men and wash my hair an hour later?

No. For Rogaine Extra Strength For Men to work best, you should allow it to stay on the scalp for about 4 hours before washing.

Can Rogaine Extra Strength For Men produce unwanted hair growth?

Unwanted hair growth on the face and other parts of the body has been reported in women. But it is rare and reversible. If you develop unwanted hair, stop using Rogaine Extra Strength For Men. Over time, the unwanted hair, if caused by Rogaine Extra Strength For Men, will go away. You can take the following steps to decrease the chances of unwanted hair growth: 1) limit the application of Rogaine Extra Strength For Men only to the scalp; 2) if you use your hands to apply Rogaine Extra Strength For Men, wash your hands well immediately afterwards; and 3) after your nighttime application of Rogaine Extra Strength For Men, allow enough drying time before going to bed (usually 2 to 4 hours).

Can I use Rogaine Extra Strength For Men for baldness or hair loss in babies or children?

No. Rogaine Extra Strength For Men must not be used to treat baldness or hair loss in babies and children.

Store at controlled room temperature 20° to 25°C (68° to 77°F)

Shown in Product Identification Guide, page 518

ROGAINE® Regular Strength For Men
Hair Regrowth Treatment
2% Minoxidil Topical Solution

Description: ROGAINE Regular Strength For Men is a colorless liquid medication for use only on the scalp to help regrow hair.

Active Ingredients: Minoxidil 2% w/v
Inactive Ingredients: Alcohol, 60% v/v, propylene glycol, and purified water.

How Supplied: ROGAINE Regular Strength For Men is available in single, twin or triple packs.

Indication: ROGAINE is medically proven to regrow hair. ROGAINE is the only product ever prescribed by doctors for men and women.

Directions: FOR EXTERNAL USE ONLY. Apply one mL 2 times a day, every day, directly onto the scalp in the hair loss area. Each applicator contains one dose of medicine. Using more or using more often will not improve results. Each bottle should last about 25–30 days, if used as directed. It is not necessary to use fingertips when applying ROGAINE Regular Strength For Men. However, if you use your hands, wash them afterwards. If you miss one or two daily doses of ROGAINE Regular Strength For Men, continue with your next dose. You should not make up for missed doses. Do not apply to other parts of the body. Do not take

Continued on next page

Rogaine For Men—Cont.

ROGAINE Regular Strength For Men by mouth. **Keep this and all drugs out of the reach of children. In case of accidental ingestion, seek professional assistance or contact a Poison Control Center immediately.**

Use a mild shampoo if you wash your scalp before applying ROGAINE Regular Strength For Men. There is no need to change your usual hair care routine when using ROGAINE Regular Strength For Men. However, you should apply ROGAINE Regular Strength For Men first and wait for it to dry before applying your styling aids.

Instructions for use of Applicators:
APPLICATOR OPTIONS

Dropper: The child-resistant dropper can be useful for a broad range of hair styles or hair loss because it allows for easy application through the hair and directly onto the scalp.

Sprayer: This may be more useful for broader areas of hair loss.

When using the sprayer, it is important to make sure that ROGAINE Regular Strength For Men gets to the scalp. Also, one dose with the sprayer is 6 pumps.

Using the Applicators
DROPPER

Squeeze the rubber bulb and insert the dropper into the bottle. Release the bulb, allowing the dropper to fill to the 1 mL line. If the level of the solution is above the 1 mL line, squeeze the extra amount back into the bottle. Next, place the tip near the part of the scalp you want to treat and gently squeeze the bulb to gradually release the solution. To prevent the solution from running off the scalp, apply a small amount at a time.

SPRAYER

The sprayer applicator is NOT child-resistant. If you have small children, keep the original child-resistant cap and place it back on the bottle after each use. Insert the spray applicator into the bottle and twist on firmly. Next, holding the bottle upright, pump the spray attachment six (6) times to get one full dose (1 mL). Be careful not to inhale the mist.

Warnings: Do not use if
- you have no family history of hair loss.
- hair loss is sudden and/or patchy.
- scalp is red, inflamed, infected, irritated or painful.
- you do not know the reason for your hair loss.
- you are under 18 years of age. Do not use on babies and children.
- you use other topical prescription products on the scalp.

Stop use of ROGAINE Regular Strength For Men and see your doctor if you get:
- chest pain, rapid heatbeat, faintness, or dizziness;
- sudden unexplained weight gain,
- swollen hands or feet,
- redness or irritation on your scalp.

Side Effects:
The most common side effects are itching and other skin irritations of the treated area of the scalp. ROGAINE Regular Strength For Men contains alcohol, which would cause burning or irritation of the eyes or sensitive skin areas. If ROGAINE Regular Strength For Men accidentally gets into these areas, rinse with large amounts of cold tap water. Contact your doctor if irritation persists.

Additional Information:
Who may use ROGAINE Regular Strength For Men?
ROGAINE Regular Strength For Men may be appropriate for you if you are an adult who is at least 18 years old and experiencing gradually thinning hair or gradual hair loss on the top of the head. The common hereditary thinning or hair loss process begins slowly and may become noticeable only after years of gradual loss. Many of those experiencing hair loss have other family members with gradual thinning hair or hair loss. **If there is no family history of gradual thinning hair or gradual hair loss, or hair loss is patchy, talk to your doctor.**
Who should NOT use ROGAINE Regular Strength For Men?
ROGAINE Regular Strength For Men will not prevent or improve hair loss which may occur with the use of some prescription and non-prescription medications, certain severe nutritional problems (very low body iron; excessive vitamin A intake), low thyroid states (hypothyroidism), chemotherapy, or diseases which cause scarring of the scalp. Also, ROGAINE Regular Strength For Men will not improve hair loss due to damage from the use of hair care products which cause scarring or deep burns of the scalp or hair grooming methods such as cornrowing or ponytails which require pulling the hair tightly back from the scalp. **You should ask your doctor if you are unsure of the cause of your hair loss.**
Will ROGAINE Regular Strength For Men work for me?
The amount of hair regrowth is different for each person. Not everyone will respond to ROGAINE Regular Strength For Men. The response to ROGAINE Regular Strength For Men cannot be predicted. No one will be able to grow back all their hair. You may respond better if you have been losing your hair for a short period of time or have little initial hair loss.
Will ROGAINE Regular Strength For Men help prevent hair loss?
Yes. ROGAINE Regular Strength For Men is the only brand clinically shown to help stop hair loss.
How soon can I expect results from using ROGAINE Regular Strength For Men?
Since normal hair usually grows only $\frac{1}{2}$ to 1 inch per month, hair regrowth with ROGAINE Regular Strength For Men also takes time. Generally new hair growth is slow for a ROGAINE Regular Strength For Men user. Continued use 2 times a day, everyday, for at least 4 months is usually needed before you notice hair regrowth. Up to 12 months of use may be needed to see your best results from ROGAINE Regular Strength For Men. However, if you do not see hair regrowth in 12 months, stop using ROGAINE Regular Strength For Men and see your doctor. When you first begin to use ROGAINE Regular Strength For Men, your hair loss may continue for up to 2 weeks. This hair loss is temporary. If you continue to lose hair after two weeks, see your doctor.
If ROGAINE Regular Strength For Men is working, what will the hair look like?
At first, hair growth may be soft, downy, colorless hairs. After further use, the new hair should be the same color and thickness as the other hairs on your scalp.
How long do I need to use ROGAINE Regular Strength For Men?
If you respond to ROGAINE Regular Strength For Men, you will need to use it 2 times a day, every day, to keep and continue the hair regrowth. Up to 12 months of use may be needed to see your best results with ROGAINE Regular Strength For Men.
What happens if I completely stop using ROGAINE Regular Strength For Men? Will I keep the new hair?
Continuous use of ROGAINE Regular Strength For Men is needed to maintain hair regrowth. If you stop using ROGAINE Regular Strength For Men, the normal hair loss process will start again. You will probably lose your newly regrown hair in three to four months.
Can I have my hair colored or permed or use hair relaxers while using ROGAINE Regular Strength For Men?
We have no evidence that coloring or perming your hair or that the use of relaxers interferes in any way with the effectiveness of ROGAINE Regular Strength For Men. However, because the use of a permanent wave and hair color can cause scalp irritation on certain people, we recommend the following precautions:
1. To avoid possible scalp irritation, you should make sure all of the ROGAINE Regular Strength For Men has been washed off the hair and scalp before using color or perm chemicals.
2. Refrain form using ROGAINE Regular Strength For Men for 24 hours after using any chemicals to ensure your scalp has not been irritated by the perm or color treatment. If no irritation occurs, continue use of ROGAINE Regular Strength For Men as usual. Simply resume your normal ROGAINE Regular Strength For Men routine. There is no need to use additional quantities to make up for missed applications. One day of not using ROGAINE Regular Strength For Men will not affect your hair regrowth chances.
Can I apply ROGAINE Regular Strength For Men and wash my hair an hour later?
No. For ROGAINE Regular Strength For Men to work best, you should allow ROGAINE Regular Strength For Men to remain on the scalp for about 4 hours before washing.

Can I go swimming or out in the rain?

Yes, as long as you use good judgment. Avoid washing off ROGAINE Regular Strength For Men. If possible, apply ROGAINE Regular Strength For Men to a dry scalp after swimming, or wait about 4 hours after application before going swimming. Do not let your scalp get wet from the rain after applying ROGAINE Regular Strength For Men.

Can ROGAINE Regular Strength For Men produce unwanted hair growth?

Although unwanted hair growth has been reported, on the face, and on other parts of the body, it is rare. To prevent unwanted hair growth, limit the application of ROGAINE Regular Strength For Men only to the scalp. If you experience unwanted hair, discontinue using ROGAINE Regular Strength For Men. After stopping use of ROGAINE Regular Strength For Men, over time the unwanted hair, if caused by the use of ROGAINE Regular Strength For Men, will go away. You can take steps to decrease the chances for unwanted hair growth:
1) limit the application of ROGAINE Regular Strength For Men only to the scalp, 2) if you use your hands to apply ROGAINE Regular Strength For Men, wash your hands thoroughly afterwards, and 3) allow sufficient drying time (usually 2 to 4 hours) before going to bed after your nighttime application of ROGAINE Regular Strength For Men.

Shown in Product Identification Guide, page 518

ROGAINE® For Women
Hair Regrowth Treatment
2% Minoxidil Topical Solution

Description: ROGAINE For Women is a colorless liquid medication for use only on the scalp to help regrow hair.
Active Ingredients: Minoxidil 2% w/v
Inactive Ingredients: Alcohol, 60% v/v, propylene glycol, and purified water.

How Supplied: ROGAINE For Women is available in single, twin, and triple packs.

Indication: ROGAINE For Women is medically proven to regrow hair. ROGAINE For Women is the only product ever prescribed by doctors for men and women. And, ROGAINE For Women is now available without a prescription in its original, full prescription strength.

Directions: FOR EXTERNAL USE ONLY. Apply one mL 2 times a day, every day, directly onto the scalp in the hair loss area. Each applicator contains one dose of medicine. Using more or using more often will not improve results. Each bottle should last about 25–30 days, if used as directed. It is not necessary to use fingertips when applying ROGAINE For Women. However, if you use your hands, wash them afterwards. If you miss one or two daily doses of ROGAINE

For Women, continue with your next dose. You should not make up for missed doses. Do not apply to other parts of the body. Do not take ROGAINE For Women by mouth. **Keep this and all drugs out of the reach of children. In case of accidental ingestion, seek professional assistance or contact a Poison Control Center Immediately.**
Use a mild shampoo if you wash your scalp before applying ROGAINE For Women. There is no need to change your usual hair care routine when using ROGAINE For Women. However, you should apply ROGAINE For Women first and wait for it to dry before applying your styling aids.

Instructions for use of Applicators:
APPLICATOR OPTIONS
Dropper: The child-resistant dropper can be useful for a broad range of hair styles or hair loss because it allows for easy application through the hair and directly onto the scalp.
Extender Sprayer: The extender sprayer is designed to help you spray through the hair directly onto the scalp. This applicator should not be used for broad spraying on the scalp. ROGAINE For Women must get to the scalp for maximum effectiveness.

How to use the applicators
DROPPER
Squeeze the rubber bulb and insert the dropper into the bottle. Release the bulb, allowing the dropper to fill to the 1 mL line. If the level of the solution is above the 1 mL line, squeeze the extra amount back into the bottle. Next, place the tip near the part of the scalp you want to treat and gently squeeze the bulb to gradually release the solution. To prevent the solution from running off the scalp, apply a small amount at a time.
EXTENDER SPRAYER
The sprayer applicator is NOT child-resistant. If you have small children, keep the original child-resistant cap and place it back on the bottle after each use. Insert the spray applicator into the bottle and twist on firmly. Pull off the small spray head from the plastic tube. Fit the extender spray onto the plastic tub and push down firmly. Remove the cap from the end of the extended spray. Pump the extender spray six (6) times to get one full dose (1 mL). With each pump, make sure ROGAINE For Women is applied directly onto the scalp. Be careful not to inhale the mist. Note: With the sprayer applicator, one dose = 6 pumps.

Warnings: Do not use if
• you have no family history of hair loss.
• hair loss is sudden and/or patchy.
• scalp is red, inflamed, infected, irritated or painful.
• you do not know the reason for your hair loss.
• you are under 18 years of age. Do not use on babies and children.
• you use other topical prescription products on the scalp.
• you have ever had an allergic reaction to ROGAINE For Women.
• you have normal hair loss associated with childbirth.

Stop use of ROGAINE For Women and see your doctor if you get:
• chest pain, rapid heartbeat, faintness, or dizziness,
• sudden unexplained weight gain,
• swollen hands or feet,
• redness or irritation.
As with any drug, if you are pregnant or nursing a baby, seek the advice of a health professional before using this product.
Side Effects:
The most common side effects are itching and other skin irritations of the treated area of scalp. ROGAINE For Women contains alcohol, which would cause burning or irritation of the eyes or sensitive skin areas. If ROGAINE For Women accidentally gets into these areas, rinse with large amounts of cold tap water. Contact your doctor if irritation persists.

Additional Information:
Who may use ROGAINE For Women?
ROGAINE For Women may be appropriate for you if you are an adult who is at least 18 years old and experiencing gradually thinning hair or gradual hair loss on the top of the head. The common hereditary thinning or hair loss process begins slowly and may become noticeable only after years of gradual loss. Many of those experiencing hair loss have other family members with gradual thinning hair or hair loss. **If there is no family history of gradual thinning hair or gradual hair loss, or hair loss is patchy, talk to your doctor.**
Who should NOT use ROGAINE For Women?
ROGAINE For Women will not prevent or improve hair loss which may occur with the use of some prescription and non-prescription medications, certain severe nutritional problems (very low body iron; excessive vitamin A intake), low thyroid states (hypothyroidism), chemotherapy, or diseases which cause scarring of the scalp. Also, ROGAINE For Women will not improve hair loss due to damage from the use of hair care products which cause scarring or deep burns of the scalp or hair grooming methods such as cornrowing or ponytails which require pulling the hair tightly back from the scalp. **You should ask your doctor if you are unsure of the cause of your hair loss.**
What can I expect from ROGAINE For Women use?
The amount of hair regrowth is different for each person. Not everyone will respond to ROGAINE For Women. The response to ROGAINE For Women cannot be predicted. No one will be able to grow back all their hair. You may respond better if you have been losing your hair for a short period of time or have little initial hair loss.
Will ROGAINE For Women help prevent hair loss?
Yes. ROGAINE For Women is the only brand clinically shown to help stop hair loss.

Continued on next page

Rogaine For Women—Cont.

How soon can I expect results from using ROGAINE For Women?

Since normal hair usually grows only $1/2$ to 1 inch per month, hair regrowth with ROGAINE For Women also takes time. Generally new hair growth is slow for a ROGAINE For Women user. Continued use 2 times a day for at least 4 months is usually needed before you notice hair regrowth. Up to 8 months of use may be needed to see your best results from ROGAINE For Women. However, if you do not see hair regrowth in 8 months, stop using ROGAINE For Women and see your doctor. When you first begin to use ROGAINE For Women, your hair loss may continue for up to 2 weeks. This hair loss is temporary. If you continue to lose hair after two weeks, see your doctor.

If ROGAINE For Women is working, what will the hair look like?

At first, hair growth may be soft, downy, colorless hairs. After further use, the new hair should be the same color and thickness as the other hairs on your scalp.

How long do I need to use ROGAINE For Women?

If you respond to ROGAINE For Women, you will need to use it 2 times a day to keep and continue the hair regrowth. Up to 8 months of use may be needed to see your best results with ROGAINE For Women.

What happens if I completely stop using ROGAINE For Women? Will I keep the new hair?

Continuous use of ROGAINE For Women is needed to maintain hair regrowth. If you stop using ROGAINE For Women, the normal hair loss process will start again. You will probably lose your newly regrown hair in three to four months.

Can I have my hair colored or permed or use hair relaxers while using ROGAINE For Women?

We have no evidence that coloring or perming your hair or that the use of relaxers interferes in any way with the effectiveness of ROGAINE For Women.

However, because the use of a permanent wave and hair color can cause scalp irritation on certain people, we recommend the following precautions:
1. To avoid possible scalp irritation, you should make sure all of the ROGAINE For Women has been washed off the hair and scalp before using color or perm chemicals.
2. Refrain from using ROGAINE For Women for 24 hours after using any chemicals to ensure your scalp has not been irritated by the perm or color treatment. If no irritation occurs, continue use of ROGAINE For Women as usual. Simply resume your normal ROGAINE For Women routine. There is no need to use additional quantities to make up for missed applications. One day of not using ROGAINE For Women will not affect your hair regrowth chances.

Can I apply ROGAINE For Women and wash my hair an hour later?

No. For ROGAINE For Women to work best, you should allow ROGAINE For Women to remain on the scalp for about 4 hours before washing.

Can I go swimming or out in the rain?

Yes, as long as you use good judgment. Avoid washing off ROGAINE For Women. If possible, apply ROGAINE For Women to a dry scalp after swimming, or wait about 4 hours after application before going swimming. Do not let your scalp get wet from the rain after applying ROGAINE For Women.

Can ROGAINE For Women produce unwanted hair growth?

Although unwanted hair growth has been reported on the face and other parts of the body, it is rare. This may be due to the frequent application of ROGAINE For Women on the areas of the skin other than the scalp. To prevent unwanted hair growth, limit the application of ROGAINE For Women only to the scalp. If you experience unwanted hair, discontinue using ROGAINE For Women. After stopping use of ROGAINE For Women, over time the unwanted hair, if caused by the use of ROGAINE For Women, will go away.

You can take steps to decrease the chances for unwanted hair growth:
1) limit the application of ROGAINE For Women only to the scalp, 2) if you use your hands to apply ROGAINE For Women, wash your hands thoroughly afterwards, and 3) allow sufficient drying time (usually 2 to 4 hours) before going to bed after your nighttime application of ROGAINE For Women.

Shown in Product Identification Guide, page 518

SURFAK® LIQUI-GELS®
Stool Softener Laxative

Indications: Surfak®, a stool softener, is indicated for the relief of occasional constipation. Unlike some other types of laxatives, Surfak contains no harsh stimulants that can upset your stomach or cause cramps. Instead, Surfak works gently by drawing water into the stool, making it softer and easier to pass. Regularity can be expected to return in 12 to 72 hours.

Active Ingredients: Each soft gelatin Liqui-gel contains 240 mg docusate calcium.

Inactive Ingredients: Also contains corn oil, FD&C Blue #1 and Red #40, gelatin, glycerin, parabens, sorbitol, and other ingredients.

Dosage and Administration: Adults and children 12 years of age and over: one capsule by mouth daily for several days or until bowel movements are normal. For use in children under 12, consult a physician.

Warnings: Do not use laxative products when abdominal pain, nausea, or vomiting are present unless directed by a doctor. If you have noticed a sudden change in bowel habits that persists over a period of 2 weeks, consult a doctor before using a laxative. Laxative products should not be used for a period longer than 1 week unless directed by a doctor. Rectal bleeding or failure to have a bowel movement after use of a laxative may indicate a serious condition. Discontinue use and consult your doctor. Keep this and all drugs out of the reach of children. In case of accidental overdose, seek professional assistance or contact a poison control center immediately. As with any drug, if you are pregnant or nursing a baby, seek the advice of a health professional before using this product.

Drug Interaction Precaution: Do not take this product if you are presently taking mineral oil, unless directed by a doctor.

How Supplied: Packages of 10, 30, 100 and 500 red soft gelatin capsules and Unit Dose 100s (10×10 strips). LIQUI-GELS® Reg TM R P Scherer Corp

Shown in Product Identification Guide, page 518

Procter & Gamble
P. O. BOX 5516
CINCINNATI, OH 45201

Direct Inquiries to:
Charles Lambert
(800) 358-8707

For Medical Emergencies:
Call Collect: (513) 558-4422

CREST® Sensitivity Protection Toothpaste for sensitive teeth and cavity prevention

Active Ingredients: Potassium Nitrate (5%), Sodium Fluoride (0.15% w/v fluoride ion).

Actions: Builds protection against sensitive tooth pain. Contains **Fluoride** for cavity prevention. Gentle on tooth enamel, leaves teeth feeling clean.

WHAT ARE SENSITIVE TEETH?

If you experience flashes of tooth pain or discomfort from cold or hot foods and drinks, or even when you touch your teeth with your toothbrush, you may suffer from **Dentinal Hypersensitivity** (or "sensitive teeth.") **Hypersensitivity** can occur when dentin, which surrounds the pulp cavity and tooth nerve, is not protected. Dentin can become exposed when gums recede and the protective layer covering the root surface is worn away, leaving dentin exposed. Crest Sensitivity Protection helps relieve the pain of sensitive teeth by soothing the nerves in your teeth when the dentin is exposed. This product has the Seal of Acceptance from the Council on Scientific Affairs–ADA.

Fiber Laxative/Dietary Fiber Supplement

Versions/Flavors	Ingredients (alphabetical order)	Sodium mg dose	Calcium mg/ dose	Potassi- um mg/ dose	Calories kcal/ dose	Total Carbo- hydrate g/dose	Dietary Fiber/ (Soluble) g/dose	Dosage (Weight in gms)	How Supplied
Smooth Texture Orange Flavor Metamucil Powder	Citric Acid, FD&C Yellow #6, Natural and Artificial Flavor, Psyllium Husk, Sucrose	5	7	30	45	12	3 (2.3)	1 rounded tablespoon ~12g	Canisters: Doses: 48, 72, 114; Cartons: 30 single-dose packets.
Smooth Texture Sugar-Free Orange Flavor Metamucil Powder	Aspartame, Citric Acid, FD&C Yellow #6, Maltodextrin, Natural and Artificial Flavor, Psyllium Husk	5	7	30	20	5	3 (2.3)	1 rounded teaspoon ~5.8g	Canisters: Doses: 48, 72 114, 180; Cartons: 30 single-dose packets.
Smooth Texture Sugar-Free Regular Flavor Metamucil Powder	Citric Acid, Maltodextrin, Psyllium Husk	4	7	30	20	5	3 (2.3)	1 rounded teaspoon ~5.4g	Canisters: Doses: 48, 72 114; Cartons: 30 single-dose packets.
Original Texture Regular Flavor Metamucil Powder	Psyllium Husk, Sucrose	3	6	30	20	6	3 (2.3)	1 rounded teaspoon ~7g	Canisters: Doses: 48, 72 114.
Original Texture Orange Flavor Metamucil Powder	Citric Acid, FD&C Yellow #6, Natural and Artificial Flavor, Psyllium Husk, Sucrose	5	6	30	40	10	3 (2.3)	1 rounded tablespoon ~11g	Canisters: Doses: 48,72 114).
Fiber Laxative									
Wafers									
Apple Crisp Metamucil Wafers	(1)	20	14	60	120	17	6	2 wafers 25 g	Cartons: 12 doses
Cinnamon Spice Metamucil Wafers	(2)	20	14	60	120	17	6	2 wafers 25 g	Cartons: 12 doses

(1) Ascorbic Acid, Brown Sugar, Cinnamon, Corn Oil, Flavoring, Fructose, Lecithin, Modified Food Starch, Molasses, Oat Hull Fiber, Sodium Bicarbonate, Sucrose, Water, Wheat Flour
(2) Ascorbic Acid, Cinnamon, Corn Oil, Flavoring, Fructose, Lecithin, Modified Food Starch, Molasses, Nutmeg, Oat Hull Fiber, Oats, Sodium Bicarbonate, Sucrose, Water, Wheat Flour

Uses: When used regularly, builds increasing protection against painful sensitivity of the teeth to cold, heat, acids, sweets, or contact, and aids in the prevention of cavities.

Directions: Adults and children 12 years of age and older: Apply at least a 1-inch strip of the product onto a soft bristle toothbrush. Brush teeth thoroughly for at least 1 minute twice a day (morning and evening) or as recommended by a dentist or physician. Make sure to brush all sensitive areas of the teeth. Do not swallow. Children under 12 years of age: ask a dentist or physician.

Warnings: Sensitive teeth may indicate a serious problem that may need prompt care by a dentist. See your dentist if the problem persists or worsens. Do not use this product longer than four weeks unless recommended by a dentist or physician. **Keep this and all drugs out of the reach of children.** If you accidentally swallow more than used for brushing, seek professional help or contact a poison control center immediately.

Inactive Ingredients: Water, Hydrated Silica, Glycerin, Sorbitol, Trisodium Phosphate, Sodium Lauryl Sulfate, Cellulose Gum, Flavor, Xanthan Gum, Sodium Saccharin, Titanium Dioxide.

How Supplied: 6.2 OZ (175g), 2.5 OZ (70g) and 1.0 OZ (28g) tubes in cartons.

METAMUCIL® Fiber Laxative
[*met uh-mū sil*]
(psyllium husk)
Also see Metamucil Dietary Fiber Supplement in Dietary Supplement Section

Description: Metamucil contains psyllium husk (from the plant *Plantago ovata*), a bulk forming, natural therapeutic fiber for restoring and maintaining regularity when recommended by a physician. Metamucil contains no chemical stimulants and does not disrupt normal bowel function. Each dose contains approximately 3.4 grams of psyllium husk (or 2.3 grams of soluble fiber). Inactive ingredients, sodium, calcium, potassium, calories, carbohydrate, dietary fiber, and phenylalanine content are shown in the following table for all versions and flavors. Metamucil Smooth Texture Sugar-Free Regular flavor contains no sugar and no artificial sweeteners; Metamucil Smooth Texture Sugar-Free Orange Flavor contains aspartame (phenylalanine content per dose is 25 mg). Metamucil powdered products are gluten-free. Metamucil Fiber Wafers contain gluten: Apple Crisp contains 0.7g/dose, Cinnamon Spice contains 0.5g/dose. Each two-wafer dose contains 5 grams of fat.

Actions: The active ingredient in Metamucil is psyllium husk, a natural fiber which promotes elimination due to its bulking effect in the colon. This bulking effect is due to both the water-holding capacity of undigested fiber and the increased bacterial mass following partial fiber digestion. These actions result in enlargement of the lumen of the colon, and softer stool, thereby decreasing in-

Continued on next page

Metamucil—Cont.

traluminal pressure and straining, and speeding colonic transit in constipated patients.

Indications: Metamucil is indicated for the treatment of occasional constipation, and when recommended by a physician, for chronic constipation and constipation associated with irritable bowel syndrome, diverticulosis, hemorrhoids, convalescence, senility and pregnancy. Pregnancy: Category B. If considering use of Metamucil as part of a cholesterol-lowering program, see **Metamucil Dietary Fiber Supplement** in Dietary Supplement Section.

Contraindications: Intestinal obstruction, fecal impaction, allergy to any component.

Warnings: Patients are advised they should consult a doctor before using this product if they have abdominal pain, nausea, vomiting or rectal bleeding, if they have noticed a sudden change in bowel habits that persists over a period of two weeks, or if they are considering use of this product as part of a cholesterol-lowering program. Patients are advised to consult a physician if constipation persists for longer than one week, as this may be a sign of a serious medical condition. **Patients are cautioned that taking this product without adequate fluid may cause it to swell and block the throat or esophagus and may cause choking. They should not take the product if they have difficulty in swallowing. If they experience chest pain, vomiting, or difficulty in swallowing or breathing after taking this product, they are advised to seek immediate medical attention.** Psyllium products may cause allergic reaction in people sensitive to inhaled or ingested psyllium. Keep out of the reach of children. In case of accidental overdose, seek professional assistance or contact a poison control center immediately.

Precaution: Notice to Health Care Professionals: To minimize the potential for allergic reaction, health care professionals who frequently dispense powdered psyllium products should avoid inhaling airborne dust while dispensing these products. Handling and Dispensing: To minimize generating airborne dust, spoon product from the canister into a glass according to label directions.

Dosage and Administration: The usual adult dosage is one rounded teaspoon, or tablespoon, depending on the product version. Some versions are available in single-dose packets. For children (6 to 12 years old) use ½ the adult dose; for children under 6, consult a doctor. The appropriate dose should be mixed with 8 oz. of liquid (e.g., cool water, fruit juice, milk) following the label instructions. Metamucil Fiber Wafers should be consumed with 8 oz. of liquid. **The product (child or adult dose) should be** taken with at least 8 oz. (a full glass) of water or other fluid. Taking this product without enough liquid may cause choking (see warnings). Metamucil can be take one to three times per day, depending on the need and response. It may require continued use for 2 to 3 days to provide optimal benefit. Generally produces effect in 12–72 hours.

Laxatives, including bulk fibers, may affect how well other medicines work. If you are taking a prescription medicine by mouth, take this product at least 2 hours before or 2 hours after the prescribed medicine. As your body adjusts to increased fiber intake, you may experience changes in bowel habits or minor bloating.

How Supplied: Powder: canisters and cartons of single-dose packets. Wafers: cartons of single dose packets. (See Table 1)

[See table at top of previous page]

Shown in Product Identification Guide, page 519

OIL OF OLAY®—Complete UV Protective Moisturizer (Lotion/ Cream)
SPF 15—Original & Fragrance Free Versions
(Olay Co., Inc.)

Oil of Olay Complete UV Protective Moisturizer is a light, greaseless Lotion/ Cream that is specially formulated to provide effective moisturization and broad-spectrum UV protection against UVA and UVB (SPF 15) rays. It has minimal migration thus reduce the likelihood of eye sting. It is PABA free, non-comedogenic, and is suitable for daily use under facial make-up.

Active Ingredients: Octyl Methoxycinnamate, Zinc Oxide

Inactive Ingredients: Water, Isohexadecane, Glycerin, Polyacrylamide, C13-14 Isoparaffin, Laureth-7, Cyclomethicone, Dimethicone Copolyol, Steareth-21, Stearyl Alcohol, Sucrose Polycottonseedate, Behenyl Alcohol, Cetyl Alcohol, DMDM Hydantoin, Iodopropynyl Butylcarbamate, Fragrance, Tocopheryl Acetate, Disodium Edta, Steareth-2, Dea Oleth-3 Phosphate.

Available in both lightly scented original version and a 100% color free and fragrance free version.

Indications: Filters out the sun's harmful rays to help prevent skin damage. Provides broad-spectrum UV protection against UVA and UVB (SPF 15) rays in a light, greaseless moisturizer. Regular use over the years may reduce the chance of skin damage, some types of skin cancer, and other harmful effects due to the sun.

Directions: Adults and children 6 months of age and over: Apply liberally as often as necessary. Children under 6 months of age: Consult a doctor.

WARNINGS: For external use only, not to be swallowed. Avoid contact with the eyes. If contact occurs, rinse eyes thoroughly with water. Discontinue use if signs of irritation or rash appear. If irritation or rash persists, consult a doctor. **KEEP OUT OF REACH OF CHILDREN.**

How Supplied: Available in 4.0 fl. oz. and 6.0 fl. oz. plastic bottles.

PEPTO-BISMOL®
ORIGINAL LIQUID,
ORIGINAL AND CHERRY TABLETS
AND EASY-TO-SWALLOW CAPLETS
For upset stomach, indigestion, diarrhea, heartburn and nausea.

Multi-symptom Pepto-Bismol contains bismuth subsalicylate and is the only leading OTC stomach remedy clinically proven effective for both upper and lower GI symptoms. Pepto-Bismol is in more households than any other stomach remedy, making it a convenient recommendation with a name your patients will know. It has been clinically proven in double-blind placebo-controlled trials for relief of upset stomach symptoms and diarrhea.

Description: Each tablespoon (15 ml) of Pepto-Bismol Liquid contains 262 mg bismuth subsalicylate. Each tablespoonful of liquid contains a total of 130 mg non-aspirin salicylate. Pepto-Bismol liquid contains no sugar. Inactive ingredients: benzoic acid, D&C Red No. 22, D&C Red No. 28, flavor, magnesium aluminum silicate, methylcellulose, saccharin sodium, salicylic acid, sodium salicylate, sorbic acid and water.

Each Pepto-Bismol Tablet contains 262 mg bismuth subsalicylate. Each tablet contains a total of 102 mg non-aspirin salicylate (99 mg non-aspirin salicylate for Cherry). Pepto-Bismol tablets contain no sugar. Inactive ingredients include: adipic acid (in Cherry only), calcium carbonate, D&C Red No. 27 aluminum lake, FD&C Red No. 40 aluminum lake (in Cherry only), flavor, magnesium stearate, mannitol, povidone, saccharin sodium and talc.

Each Pepto-Bismol Caplet contains 262 mg bismuth subsalicylate. Each caplet contains a total of 99 mg non-aspirin salicylate. Caplets contain no sugar. Inactive ingredients include: calcium carbonate, D&C Red No. 27 aluminum lake, magnesium stearate, mannitol, microcrystalline cellulose, povidone, polysorbate 80, silicon dioxide, and sodium starch glycolate.

Indications: Pepto-Bismol controls diarrhea within 24 hours, relieving associated abdominal cramps; soothes heartburn and indigestion without constipating; and relieves nausea and upset stomach.

Actions: For upset stomach symptoms (i.e., indigestion, heartburn, nausea and fullness caused by over-indulgence), the active ingredient is believed to work via a topical effect on the stomach mucosa. For diarrhea, it is believed to work by several mechanisms in the gastrointestinal tract, including: 1) normalizing fluid movement via an antisecretory mechanism, 2) binding bacterial toxins and 3) antimicrobial activity.

Warnings: Children and teenagers who have or are recovering from chicken pox or flu should not use this medicine to treat nausea or vomiting. If nausea or vomiting is present, patients are advised to consult a doctor because this could be an early sign of Reye syndrome, a rare but serious illness.

This product contains non-aspirin salicylates. If taken with aspirin and ringing in the ears occurs, discontinue use. This product does not contain aspirin, but should not be administered to those patients who have a known allergy to aspirin or other non-aspirin salicylates as an adverse reaction may occur. Caution is advised in the administration to patients taking medication for anticoagulation, diabetes and gout.

If diarrhea is accompanied by a high fever or continues more than 2 days, patients are advised to consult a physician. As with any drug, caution is advised in the administration to pregnant or nursing women.

Keep all medicines out of the reach of children.

Note: This medication may cause a temporary and harmless darkening of the tongue and/or stool. Stool darkening should not be confused with melena.

Overdosage: In case of overdose, patients are advised to contact a physician or Poison Control Center. Emesis induced by ipecac syrup is indicated in large ingestions provided ipecac can be administered within one hour of ingestion. Activated charcoal should be administered after gastric emptying. Patients should be evaluated for signs and symptoms of salicylate toxicity.

Dosage and Administration: Liquid: Shake well before using.

Adults— 2 tablespoonsful
    (1 dose cup, 30 ml)
Children (according to age)—
  9–12 yrs. 1 tablespoonful
    ($^1/_2$ dose cup, 15 ml)
  6–9 yrs. 2 teaspoonsful
    ($^1/_3$ dose cup, 10 ml)
  3–6 yrs. 1 teaspoonful
    ($^1/_6$ dose cup, 5 ml)

Repeat dosage every $^1/_2$ to 1 hour, if needed, to a maximum of 8 doses in a 24-hour period. Drink plenty of clear fluids to help prevent dehydration which may accompany diarrhea.

For children under 3 years of age, consult a physician.

Tablets:
  Adults—Two tablets
  Children (according to age)—
    9–12 yrs. 1 tablet
    6–9 yrs. $^2/_3$ tablet
    3–6 yrs. $^1/_3$ tablet

Chew or dissolve in mouth. Repeat every $^1/_2$ to 1 hour as needed, to a maxi-

mum of 8 doses in a 24-hour period. Drink plenty of clear fluids to help prevent dehydration, which may accompany diarrhea. For children under 3 years of age, consult a physician.

Caplets:
  Adults—Two caplets
  Children (according to age)—
    9–12 yrs. 1 caplet
    6–9 yrs. $^2/_3$ caplet
    3–6 yrs. $^1/_3$ caplet

Swallow caplet(s) with water, do not chew. Repeat every $^1/_2$ to 1 hour as needed, to a maximum of 8 doses in a 24-hour period. Drink plenty of clear fluids to help prevent dehydration, which may accompany diarrhea. For children under 3 years of age, consult a physician.

How Supplied: Pepto-Bismol Liquid is available in: 4, 8, 12, 16 and FL OZ bottles. Pepto-Bismol Tablets are pink, round, chewable tablets imprinted with a debossed triangle and "Pepto-Bismol" on one side. Tablets are available in: boxes of 30 and 48. Caplets are available in bottles of 24 and 40. Caplets are imprinted with "Pepto-Bismol" on one side.

Shown in Product Identification Guide, page 519

PEPTO-BISMOL®
MAXIMUM STRENGTH LIQUID
For upset stomach, indigestion, diarrhea, heartburn and nausea.

Multi-symptom Pepto-Bismol contains bismuth subsalicylate and is the only leading OTC stomach remedy clinically proven effective for both upper and lower GI symptoms. Pepto-Bismol is in more households than any other stomach remedy, making it a convenient recommendation with a name your patients will know. It has been clinically-proven in double-blind placebo-controlled trials for relief of upset stomach symptoms and diarrhea.

Description: Each tablespoonful (15 ml) of Maximum Strength Pepto-Bismol Liquid contains 525 mg bismuth subsalicylate (236 mg non-aspirin salicylate). Maximum Strength Pepto-Bismol Liquid contains no sugar. Inactive ingredients include: benzoic acid, D&C Red No. 22, D&C Red No. 28, flavor, magnesium aluminum silicate, methylcellulose, saccharin sodium, salicylic acid, sodium salicylate, sorbic acid and water.

Indications: Maximum Strength Pepto-Bismol soothes upset stomach and indigestion without constipating; controls diarrhea within 24 hours, relieving associated abdominal cramps; and relieves heartburn and nausea.

Actions: For upset stomach symptoms (i.e. indigestion, heartburn, nausea and fullness caused by over-indulgence), the active ingredient is believed to work via a topical effect on the stomach mucosa. For diarrhea, it is believed to work by several mechanisms in the gastrointestinal tract, including: 1) normalizing fluid

movement via an antisecretory mechanism, 2) binding bacterial toxins, and 3) antimicrobial activity.

Warnings: Children and teenagers who have or are recovering from chicken pox or flu should not use this medicine to treat nausea or vomiting. If nausea or vomiting is present, patients are advised to consult a doctor because this could be an early sign of Reye syndrome, a rare but serious illness.

This product contains non-aspirin salicylates. If taken with aspirin and ringing in the ears occurs, discontinue use. This product does not contain aspirin, but should not be administered to those patients who have a known allergy to aspirin or other non-aspirin salicylates as an adverse reaction may occur. Caution is advised in the administration to patients taking medication for anticoagulation, diabetes and gout.

If diarrhea is accompanied by a high fever or continues more than 2 days, patients are advised to consult a physician. As with any drug, caution is advised in the administration to pregnant or nursing women.

Keep all medicines out of the reach of children.

Note: This medication may cause a temporary and harmless darkening of the tongue and/or stool. Stool darkening should not be confused with melena.

Overdosage: In case of overdose, patients are advised to contact a physician or Poison Control Center. Emesis induced by ipecac syrup is indicated in large ingestions provided ipecac can be administered within one hour of ingestion. Activated charcoal should be administered after gastric emptying. Patients should be evaluated for signs and symptoms of salicylate toxicity.

Dosage and Administration: Shake well before using.

Adults— 2 tablespoonsful
    (1 dose cup, 30 ml)
Children (according to age)—
  9–12 yrs. 1 tablespoonful
    ($^1/_2$ dose cup, 15 ml)
  6–9 yrs. 2 teaspoonsful
    ($^1/_3$ dose cup, 10 ml)
  3–6 yrs. 1 teaspoonful
    ($^1/_6$ dose cup, 5 ml)

Repeat dosage every hour, if needed, to a maximum of 4 doses in a 24-hour period. Drink plenty of clear fluids to help prevent dehydration, which may accompany diarrhea.

How Supplied: Maximum Strength Pepto-Bismol is available in: 4, 8, and 12 FL OZ bottles.

VICKS® 44 COUGH
RELIEF
Dextromethorphan HBr/
Cough Suppressant
Alcohol 5%

Active Ingredient
per 3 tsp. (15 ml):
Dextromethorphan Hydrobromide 30 mg

Continued on next page

Vicks 44—Cont.

Inactive Ingredients: Alcohol, Blue 1, Carboxymethylcellulose Sodium, Citric Acid, Flavor, High Fructose Corn Syrup, Polyethylene Oxide, Polyoxyl 40 Stearate, Propylene Glycol, Purified Water, Red 40, Saccharin Sodium, Sodium Benzoate, Sodium Citrate.

SODIUM CONTENT: 31 mg per 15 mL dose.

Use: Temporary relieves coughs due to minor throat and bronchial irritation associated with a cold.

Directions: Use teaspoon (tsp) or dose cup.

Under 6 yrs.: Ask a doctor.

6–11 yrs.	1½ tsp or 7½ ml
12 yrs. & older	3 tsp or 15 ml

Repeat every 6–8 hours, not to exceed 4 doses per day or use as directed by a doctor.

Warnings: A persistent cough may be a sign of a serious condition. If cough persists for more than 1 week, tends to recur, or is accompanied by fever, rash, or persistent headache, ask a doctor. Do not take this product for persistent or chronic cough such as occurs with smoking, asthma, emphysema, or if cough is accompanied by excessive phlegm (mucus) unless directed by a doctor.

Keep this and all drugs out of the reach of children.

In case if accidental overdose, seek professional advice or contact a poison control center immediately. As with any drug, if you are pregnant or nursing a baby, seek the advice of a health professional before using this product.

Drug Interaction Precaution: Do not use this product without first asking a doctor if you take a prescription monoamine oxidase inhibitor (MAOI) (certain drugs for depression, psychiatric or emotional conditions, or Parkinson's disease), or for 2 weeks after stopping the MAOI drug or if you are uncertain whether your prescription drug contains an MAOI.

How Supplied: Available in 4 FL OZ (118 ml) plastic bottle. A calibrated dose cup accompanies each bottle.

VICKS® 44D
COUGH & HEAD CONGESTION RELIEF
Cough Suppressant/
Nasal Decongestant
Alcohol 5%

Active Ingredients per 3 tsp. (15 ml): Dextromethorphan Hydrobromide 30 mg, Pseudoephedrine Hydrochloride 60 mg.

Inactive Ingredients: Alcohol, Blue 1, Carboxymethylcellulose Sodium, Citric Acid, Flavor, High Fructose Corn Syrup, Polyethylene Oxide, Polyoxyl 40 Stearate, Propylene Glycol, Purified Water, Red 40, Saccharin Sodium, Sodium Benzoate, Sodium Citrate.

Sodium Content: 31 mg per 15 mL dose.

Uses: Temporary relieves coughs and nasal congestion due to a common cold.

Directions: Use teaspoon (tsp) or dose cup.

Under 6 yrs.: Ask a doctor.

6–11 yrs.	1½ tsp or 7½ ml
12 yrs. & older	3 tsp or 15 ml

Repeat every 6 hours, not to exceed 4 doses per day or use as directed by a doctor.

Warnings: Do not exceed recommended dosage.
If nervousness, dizziness, or sleeplessness occur, discontinue use and ask a doctor.
Do not take unless directed by a doctor if you have:
• heart disease
• asthma
• emphysema
• thyroid disease
• diabetes
• high blood pressure
• excessive phlegm (mucus)
• persistent or chronic cough
• cough associated with smoking
• difficulty in urination due to enlarged prostate gland

Keep this and all drugs out of the reach of children. In the case of accidental overdose, seek professional advice or contact a poison control center immediately. As with any drug, if you are pregnant or nursing a baby, seek the advice of a health professional before using this product.

Drug Interaction Precaution: Do not use this product without first asking a doctor if you take a prescription monoamine oxidase inhibitor (MAOI) (certain drugs for depression, psychiatric or emotional conditions, or Parkinson's disease), or for 2 weeks after stopping the MAOI drug or if you are uncertain whether your prescription drug contains an MAOI.

Dosing Duration and When to Ask a Doctor:
• If symptoms do not improve within 7 days or are accompanied by fever.
• If a cough persists for more than 7 days, recurs, or is accompanied by fever, rash or persistent headache. A persistent cough may be the sign of a serious condition.

How Supplied: Available in 4 FL OZ (118 ml) and 8 FL OZ (236 ml) plastic bottles. A calibrated dose cup accompanies each bottle.

VICKS® 44E
Cough & Chest Congestion Relief
Cough Suppressant/Expectorant
Alcohol 5%

Active Ingredients: per 3 teaspoons (15 ml): Dextromethorphan Hydrobromide 20 mg, Guaifenesin 200 mg

Inactive Ingredients: Alcohol, Blue 1, Carboxymethylcellulose Sodium, Citric Acid, Flavor, High Frutose Corn Syrup, Polyethylene Oxide, Polyoxyl 40 Stearate, Propylene Glycol, Purified Water, Red 40, Saacharin Sodium, Sodium Benzoate, Sodium Citrate.

Sodium Content: 31 mg per 15 mL dose.

Uses: Temporarily relieves coughs due to a common cold. Helps loosen phlegm to rid the bronchial passageways of bothersome mucus.

Directions: Use teaspoon (tsp) or dose cup.

Under 6 yrs.: Ask a doctor.

6–11 yrs.	1½ tsp or 7½ ml
12 yrs. & older	3 tsp or 15 ml

Repeat every 4 hours, not to exceed 6 doses per day or use as directed by a doctor.

Warnings: *Do not take unless directed by a doctor if you have:*
• asthma
• emphysema
• excessive phlegm (mucus)
• persistent or chronic cough
• chronic bronchitis
• cough associated with smoking

Keep this and all drugs out of the reach of children.
In the case of accidental overdose, seek professional advice or contact a poison control center immediately. As with any drug, if you are pregnant or nursing a baby, seek the advice of a health professional before using this product. Do not use this product if you are on a sodium-restricted diet unless directed by a doctor.

Drug Interaction Precaution: Do not use this product without first asking a doctor if you take a prescription monoamine oxidase inhibitor (MAOI) (certain drugs for depression, psychiatric or emotional conditions, or Parkinson's disease), or for 2 weeks after stopping the MAOI drug or if you are uncertain whether your prescription drug contains an MAOI.

Dosing Duration & When to Ask a Doctor:
• If a cough persists for more than 7 days, recurs, or is accompanied by fever, rash or persistent headache. A persistent cough may be the sign of a serious condition.

How Supplied: Available in 4 FL OZ (118 ml) and 8 FL OZ (236 ml) plastic bottles. A calibrated dose cup accompanies each bottle.

VICKS® 44M
COUGH, COLD & FLU RELIEF
Cough Suppressant/Nasal Decongestant/Antihistamine/ Pain Reliever–Fever Reducer Alcohol 10%

Actives: per 4 tsp. (20 ml): Dextromethorphan Hydrobromide 30 mg, Pseudoephedrine Hydrochloride 60 mg, Chlorpheniramine Maleate 4 mg, Acetaminophen 650 mg

Inactives: Alcohol, Blue 1, Carboxymethylcellulose Sodium, Citric Acid, Flavor, High Fructose Corn Syrup, Polyethylene Glycol, Polyethylene Oxide, Propylene Glycol, Purified Water, Red 40, Saccharin Sodium, Sodium Citrate.

Sodium Content: 32 mg per 20 mL dose.

Uses: Temporarily relieves cough/cold/ flu symptoms:
• cough
• nasal congestion
• runny nose
• sneezing
• headache
• fever
• muscular aches
• sore throat pain

Directions: **Use teaspoon (tsp) or dose cup.**

12 yrs. & older	4 tsp or 20 ml

Under 12 yrs.: Ask a doctor.
Repeat every 6 hours, not to exceed 4 doses per day, or use as directed by a doctor.
Failure to follow these warnings could result in serious consequences.

Warnings: Do not exceed recommended dosage. Do not use with other products containing Acetaminophen.
If nervousness, dizziness, or sleeplessness occur, discontinue use and ask a doctor. May cause drowsiness. May cause excitability especially in children.
Do not take unless directed by a doctor if you have:
• heart disease
• asthma
• emphysema
• thyroid disease
• diabetes
• glaucoma
• high blood pressure
• excessive phlegm (mucus)
• breathing problems
• chronic bronchitis
• difficulty in breathing
• persistent or chronic cough
• cough associated with smoking
• difficulty in urination due to enlarged prostate gland

Alcohol Warning: If you consume 3 or more alcoholic drinks every day, ask your doctor whether you should take acetaminophen or other pain relievers/fever reducers. Acetaminophen may cause liver damage.
Keep this and all drugs out of the reach of children. In the case of accidental overdose, seek professional advice or contact a poison control center immedi-

ately. Prompt medical attention is critical for adults as well as for children even if you do not notice any signs or symptoms. As with any drug, if you are pregnant or nursing a baby, seek the advice of a health professional before using this product.
Alcohol, sedatives, and tranquilizers may increase the drowsiness effect. Avoid alcoholic beverages while taking this product. Use caution when driving a motor vehicle or operating machinery.
Drug Interaction Precaution: Do not use this product without first asking a doctor if you take:
• sedatives
• tranquilizers
• a prescription monoamine oxidase inhibitor (MAOI) (certain drugs for depression, psychiatric or emotional conditions, or Parkinson's disease), or for 2 weeks after stopping the MAOI drug or if you are uncertain whether your prescription drug contains an MAOI.
Dosing Duration: Do not use over 7 days. *Ask a Doctor:*
• If sore throat is severe, persists for more than 2 days, is accompanied or followed by fever, headache, rash, nausea, or vomiting.
• If symptoms do not improve or are accompanied by a fever that lasts more than 3 days, or if new symptoms occur.
• If a cough presists for more than 7 days, recurs, or is accompanied by a rash or persistent headache. A persistent cough may be the sign of a serious condition.

How Supplied: Available in 4 FL OZ (118 ml) and 8 FL OZ (236 ml) plastic bottles. A calibrated dose cup accompanies each bottle.

CHILDREN'S VICKS® NYQUIL® COLD/COUGH RELIEF
Antihistamine/Nasal Decongestant/ Cough Suppressant

Children's NyQuil was specially formulated with three effective ingredients to relieve nighttime cough, nasal congestion, and runny nose so children can rest. Children's NyQuil® is alcohol free and analgesic free and has a pleasant cherry flavor.

Active Ingredients: Per 1 TBSP.: Chlorpheniramine Maleate 2 mg, Pseudoephedrine HCl 30 mg, Dextromethorphan Hydrobromide 15 mg.

Inactive Ingredients: Citric Acid, Flavor, Potassium Sorbate, Propylene Glycol, Purified Water, Red 40, Sodium Citrate, Sucrose.

Sodium Content: 141 mg per 30 ml dose.

Uses: Temporarily relieves cold symptoms:
• nasal congestion
• runny nose
• sneezing
• cough

Directions: Use Tablespoon (TBSP) or dose cup.

Under 6 yrs.	Ask a doctor.
6–11 yrs.	1 TBSP or 15 ml
12 yrs. & older	2 TBSP or 30 ml

Repeat every 6 hours, not to exceed 4 doses per day or use as directed by a doctor.
Warnings: Do not exceed recommended dosage.
If nervousness, dizziness, or sleeplessness occur, discontinue use and ask a doctor. May cause marked drowsiness. May cause excitability, especially in children.
Do not take unless directed by a doctor if you have:
• heart disease
• asthma
• emphysema
• thyroid disease
• diabetes
• glaucoma
• high blood pressure
• excessive phelgm (mucus)
• breathing problems
• chronic bronchitis
• difficulty in breathing
• persistent or chronic cough
• cough associated with smoking
• difficulty in urination due to enlarged prostate gland
Keep this and all drugs out of the reach of children. In the case of accidental overdose, seek professional advice or contact a poison control center immediately. As with any drug, if you are pregnant or nursing a baby, seek the advice of a health professional before using this product.
Alcohol, sedatives, and tranquilizers may increase the drowsiness effect. Avoid alcoholic beverages while taking this product. Use caution when driving a motor vehicle or operating machinery.
Do not use this product if you are on a sodium-restricted diet unless directed by a doctor.

Drug Interaction Precaution: Do not take this product without first asking a doctor if you take:
• sedatives
• tranquilizers
• a prescription monoamine oxidase inhibitor (MAOI) (certain drugs for depression, psychiatric or emotional conditions, or Parkinson's disease), or for 2 weeks after stopping the MAOI drug or if you are uncertain whether your prescription drug contains an MAOI.

Dosing Duration: Do not use over 7 days. *Ask a Doctor:*
• If symptoms do not improve within 7 days or are accompanied by a fever.
• If a cough persists for more than 7 days, recurs, or is accompanied by a fever, rash or persistent headache. A persistent cough may be the sign of a serious condition.

How Supplied: Available in 4 FL OZ (115 ml) plastic bottles with child-resistant, tamper-evident cap and a calibrated medicine cup.

Continued on next page

VICKS® CHLORASEPTIC®
SORE THROAT LOZENGES
Menthol/Benzocaine
Oral Anesthetic
Menthol and Cherry Flavors

Active Ingredients: Benzocaine 6 mg, Menthol 10 mg (per lozenge).

Inactive Ingredients: Menthol Lozenges: Blue 1, Corn Syrup, Flavor, Sucrose, Yellow 6, Yellow 10. Cherry Lozenges: Blue 1, Corn Syrup, Flavor, Red 40, Sucrose.

Uses: Temporary relieves:
• sore mouth
• sore throat
• occasional minor mouth irritation and pain
• pain associated with canker sores

Directions: 5 yrs. & older:
Allow 1 lozenge to dissolve slowly in mouth. May be repeated every 2 hours as needed or as directed by a physician or dentist.
Under 5 yrs: ask a physician or dentist.

Warnings: *Do not use this product if you have a history of allergy to local anesthetics like:*
• procaine
• butacaine
• benzocaine
• other 'caine' anesthetics
Keep this and all drugs out of the reach of children.
In case of accidental overdose, seek professional advice or contact a poison control center immediately. As with any drug if you are pregnant or nursing a baby, seek the advice of a health professional before using this product.
Dosing Duration and When to Ask a Doctor:
• If sore throat is severe, persists for more than 2 days, or is accompanied by difficulty in breathing.
• If sore throat is accompanied or followed by fever, headache, rash, swelling, nausea, or vomiting.
• If sore mouth symptoms do not improve in 7 days, or if irritation, pain, or redness persists or worsens.

How Supplied: Available in Menthol and Cherry, lozenges in packages of 18. Each green or red lozenge is debossed with "VC".

VICKS® CHLORASEPTIC®
SORE THROAT SPRAY
Phenol/oral anesthetic/antiseptic
Menthol and Cherry Flavors

Active: Spray—Phenol 1.4%.

Inactives: Menthol Liquid: Green 3, Green 5, flavor, glycerin, purified water, saccharin sodium, Yellow 10. Cherry Liquid: flavor, glycerin, purified water, Red 40, saccharin sodium.

Uses: Temporarily relieves:
• sore mouth
• sore throat pain
• minor irritation or injury of the mouth and gums

• pain due to minor dental procedures, dentures or orthodontic appliances
• pain associated with canker sores

Directions: Chloraseptic may be used every 2 hours or use as directed by a physician or dentist.
12 yrs. & older: For each application, spray 5 times onto throat or affected area.
2–11 yrs. (with adult supervision): For each application, spray 3 times onto throat or affected area.
Under 2 yrs.: Ask a doctor or dentist.

Warnings: Keep this and all drugs out of the reach of children. In case of accidental overdose, seek professional advice or contact a poison control center immediately. As with any drug, if you are pregnant or nursing a baby, seek the advice of a health professional before using this product.
Dosing Duration and When to Ask a Doctor:
• If sore throat is severe, persists for more than 2 days, or is accompanied by difficulty in breathing.
• If sore throat is accompanied or followed by fever, headache, rash, swelling, nausea, or vomiting.
• If sore mouth symptoms do not improve in 7 days, or if irritation, pain, or redness persists or worsens.

How Supplied: Available in Menthol and Cherry flavors in 6 FL OZ (175 mL) plastic bottles with sprayer.

VICKS® Cough Drops
Menthol Cough Suppressant/
Oral Anesthetic
Menthol and Cherry Flavors

Uses: Temporarily relieves sore throat and coughs due to colds or inhaled irritants.

Active Ingredient: Menthol 3.3mg (Menthol), 1.7mg (Cherry)

Inactive Ingredients: [Menthol] Ascorbic Acid, Blue 1, Caramel, Corn Syrup, Eucalyptus Oil, Flavor, Sucrose. [Cherry] Ascorbic Acid, Citric Acid, Corn Syrup, Ecualyptus Oil, Red 40, Sucrose.

Directions: 5 yrs. & older:
Menthol: Allow 2 drops to dissolve slowly in mouth.
Cherry: Allow 3 drops to dissolve slowly in mouth.
COUGH: May be repeated every hour as needed or as directed by a doctor.
SORE THROAT: May be repeated every 2 hours as needed or as directed by a doctor.
Under 5 yrs.: Ask a doctor.

Warnings: A persistent cough may be a sign of a serious condition. If cough persists for more than 1 week, tends to recur, or is accompanied by fever, rash, or persistent headache, ask a doctor. Do not take this product for persistent or chronic cough such as occurs with smoking, asthma, emphysema, or if cough is accompanied by excessive phlegm (mucus) unless directed by a doctor. If sore

throat is severe, is accompanied by difficulty in breathing, or persists for more than 2 days, do not use, and ask a doctor promptly. If sore throat is accompanied or followed by fever, headache, rash, swelling, nausea, or vomiting, ask a doctor promptly. **Keep this and all drugs out of the reach of children.** As with any drug, if you are pregnant or nursing a baby, seek the advice of a health professional before using this product.

How Supplied: Vicks® Cough Drops are available in boxes of 20 triangular drops. Each red or green drop is debossed with "V."

VICKS® COUGH
DROPS
Menthol Cough Suppressant/
Oral Anesthetic

Active Ingredient: Menthol 6.6 mg (menthol), 3.1 mg (cherry)

Menthol and Cherry Flavors.

Inactive Ingredients: Menthol Flavor: Benzyl Alcohol, Camphor, Caramel, Corn Syrup, Eucalyptus Oil, Flavor, Sucrose, Tolu Balsam, Thymol.

Cherry Flavor: Citric Acid, Corn Syrup, Blue 1, Red 40, Flavor, Sucrose.

Uses: Temporarily relieves sore throat and coughs due to colds or inhaled irritants.

Directions: Adults and children 5 to 12 years: [Menthol] Allow drop to dissolve slowly in mouth. [Cherry] Allow 2 drops to dissolve slowly in mouth.

Cough: may be repeated every hour as needed or as directed by a doctor. **Sore Throat:** may be repeated every 2 hours—as needed or as directed by a doctor. **Children under 5 years of age:** ask a doctor.

Warnings: A persistent cough may be a sign of a serious condition. If cough persists for more than 1 week, tends to recur, or is accompanied by fever, rash, or persistent headache, ask a doctor. Do not take this product for persistent or chronic cough such as occurs with smoking, asthma, emphysema, or if cough is accompanied by excessive phlegm (mucus), unless directed by a doctor. If sore throat is severe, or is accompanied by difficulty in breathing, or persists for more than 2 days, do not use, and ask a doctor promptly. If sore throat is accompanied or followed by fever, headache, rash, swelling, nausea, or vomiting, ask a doctor promptly. **Keep this and all drugs out of the reach of children.** As with any drug, if you are pregnant or nursing a baby, seek the advice of a health professional before using this product.

How Supplied: Vicks® Cough Drops are available in boxes of 20 drops.

VICKS® DAYQUIL® LIQUID
VICKS® DAYQUIL® LIQUICAPS®
Multi-Symptom Cold/Flu Relief
Nasal Decongestant/
Pain Reliever/Cough
Suppressant/Fever Reducer

Active Ingredients: LIQUID—per 2 TBSP or LIQUICAPS—per two softgels, contains: Pseudoephedrine Hydrochloride 60 mg, Acetaminophen 650 mg (Liquid) or 500 mg (softgels), Dextromethorphan Hydrobromide 20 mg.

Inactive Ingredients: Liquid: Citric Acid, Flavor, Glycerin, Polyethylene Glycol, Propylene Glycol, Purified Water, Saccharin Sodium, Sodium Citrate, Sucrose, Yellow 6. Softgels: Gelatin, Glycerin, Polyethylene Glycol, Povidone, Propylene Glycol, Purified Water, Red 40, Sorbitol Special, Yellow 6.
Sodium Content: Liquid, 141 mg per 30 ml dose.

Uses: Temporarily relieves common cold/flu symptoms:
• minor aches
• pains
• headache
• muscular aches
• sore throat pain
• fever
• nasal congestion
• cough

Liquid

Directions: **Use measuring spoon or dose cup.**

Under 6 years	Ask a doctor.
6–11 years	1 Tablespoon (TBSP) or 15 ml
12 yrs. and older	2 Tablespoons (TBSP) or 30 ml

Repeat every 4 hours, not to exceed 4 doses per day or use as directed by a doctor. If taking NyQuil® and DayQuil®, limit total to 4 doses per day.

LiquiCaps

Directions: Under 6 years—Ask a doctor.

6–11 years	Swallow 1 softgel with water.
12 yrs. and older	Swallow 2 softgels with water.

Repeat every 4 hours, not to exceed 4 doses per day or use as directed by a doctor. If taking DayQuil and NyQuil® limit total to 4 doses per day.

Failure to follow these warnings could result in serious consequences.

Warnings: Do not exceed recommended dosage. Do not use with other products containing acetaminophen. If nervousness, dizziness or sleeplessness occur, discontinue use and ask a doctor.
Do not take unless directed by a doctor if you have:
• heart disease
• asthma
• emphysema
• thyroid disease
• diabetes
• high blood pressure
• persistent or chronic cough
• cough associated with smoking
• excessive phlegm (mucus)
• breathing problems
• difficulty in urination due to enlargement of the prostate gland

Alcohol Warning: If you consume 3 or more alcoholic drinks every day, ask your doctor whether you should take acetaminophen or other pain relievers/fever reducers. Acetaminophen may cause liver damage.
Keep this and all drugs out of the reach of children. In case of accidental overdose, seek professional advice or contact a poison control center immediately. Prompt medical attention is critical for adults as well as for children even if you do not notice any signs or symptoms. As with any drug, if you are pregnant or nursing a baby, seek the advice of a health professional before using this product. Liquid only: Do not use this product if you are on a sodium-restricted diet unless directed by a doctor.
Drug Interaction Precaution: Do not use this product without first asking a doctor if you take:
• a prescription monoamine oxidase inhibitor (MAOI) (certain drugs for depression, psychiatric or emotional conditions, or Parkinson's disease), for 2 weeks after stopping the MAOI drug or if you are uncertain whether your prescription drug contains an MAOI.
Dosing Duration: Do not use over 7 days (for adults) or 5 days (for children).
Ask A Doctor:
• If sore throat is severe, persists for more than 2 days, is accompanied or followed by fever, headache, rash, nausea or vomiting.
• If symptoms do not improve, are accompanied by a fever that lasts more than 3 days or if new symptoms occur.
• If a cough persists for more than 7 days (adults) or 5 days (children), recurs or is accompanied by a rash or persistent headache. A persistent cough may be the sign of a serious condition.

How Supplied: Available in: **LIQUID** 6 FL OZ (175 ml) plastic bottles with child-resistant, tamper-evident cap and a calibrated medicine cup.
LIQUICAP: in 12-count child-resistant packages and 20- and 36-count nonchild-resistant packages. Each softgel is imprinted: "DayQuil."

VICKS® DAYQUIL® SINUS
Pressure & PAIN Relief
WITH IBUPROFEN
IBUPROFEN/PSEUDOEPHEDRINE HCL
Pain Reliever/Fever Reducer/
Nasal Decongestant

Warning: **ASPIRIN SENSITIVE PATIENTS.** Do not take this product if you have had a severe allergic reaction to aspirin e.g., asthma, swelling, shock or hives, because even though this product contains no aspirin or salicylates, cross-reactions may occur in patients allergic to aspirin.

Uses: For temporary relief of symptoms associated with the common cold, sinusitis or flu including nasal congestion, headache, fever, body aches, and pains.

Directions: 12 yrs. and older: Take 1 caplet every 4 to 6 hours while symptoms persist. If symptoms do not respond to 1 caplet, 2 caplets may be used but do not exceed 6 caplets in 24 hours, unless directed by a doctor. The smallest effective dose should be used. Take with food or milk if occasional and mild heartburn, upset stomach, or stomach pain occurs with use. Ask a doctor if these symptoms are more than mild or they persist.
Under 12 yrs.: Do not give this product to children under 12 years of age except under the advice and supervision of a doctor.

Warnings: Do not take for colds for more than 7 days or for fever for more than 3 days unless directed by a doctor. If the cold or fever persists or gets worse or if new symptoms occur, ask a doctor. These could be signs of serious illness. As with aspirin and acetaminophen, if you have any condition which requires you to take prescription drugs or if you have had problems or serious side effects from taking any non-prescription pain reliever, do not take this product without first discussing it with your doctor. IF YOU EXPERIENCE ANY SYMPTOMS WHICH ARE UNUSUAL OR SEEM UNRELATED TO THE CONDITION FOR WHICH YOU TOOK THIS PRODUCT, CONSULT A DOCTOR BEFORE TAKING ANY MORE OF IT. If you are under a doctor's care for any serious condition, ask a doctor before taking this product. **Do not exceed recommended dosage.** If nervousness, dizziness or sleeplessness occur, discontinue use and ask a doctor. Do not take this product if you have high blood pressure, heart disease, diabetes, thyroid disease or difficulty in urination due to enlargement of the prostate gland, unless directed by a doctor. Do not combine this product with other non-prescription pain relievers. Do not combine this product with any other ibuprofen-containing product. As with any drug, if you are pregnant or nursing a baby, seek the advice of a health professional before using this product. IT IS ESPECIALLY IMPORTANT NOT TO USE THIS PRODUCT DURING THE LAST 3 MONTHS OF PREGNANCY UNLESS SPECIFICALLY DIRECTED TO DO SO BY A DOCTOR BECAUSE IT MAY CAUSE PROBLEMS IN THE UNBORN CHILD OR COMPLICATIONS DURING DELIVERY. Keep this and all drugs out of reach of children. In case of accidental overdose, seek professional as-

Continued on next page

Vicks Dayquil Sinus—Cont.

sistance or contact a poison control center immediately. DRUG INTERACTION PRECAUTION: Do not take this product if you are taking a prescription monoamine oxidase inhibitor (MAOI) (certain drugs for depression, psychiatric or emotional conditions, or Parkinson's disease), or for 2 weeks after stopping the MAOI drug. If you are uncertain whether your prescription drug contains an MAOI, ask a health professional before taking this product.

Alcohol Warning: If you consume 3 or more alcoholic drinks every day, ask your doctor whether you should take ibuprofen or other pain relievers/fever reducers. Ibuprofen may cause stomach bleeding.

Active Ingredients: each caplet contains Ibuprofen 200 mg, Pseudoephedrine Hydrochloride 30 mg.

Inactive Ingredients: Carnuba or Equivalent Wax, Croscarmellose Sodium, Iron Oxide, Methylparaben, Microcrystalline Cellulose, Propylparaben, Silicon Dioxide, Sodium Benzoate, Sodium Lauryl Sulfate, Starch, Stearic Acid, Sucrose, Titanium Dioxide.

How Supplied: Available in 20 count blister package.

VICKS® NYQUIL® LIQUICAPS®
VICKS® NYQUIL® LIQUID
(Original and Cherry)
Multi-Symptom Cold/Flu Relief
Antihistamine/Cough
Suppressant/Pain Reliever/
Nasal Decongestant/
Fever Reducer

Active Ingredients (per softgel): Doxylamine Succinate 6.25 mg, Dextromethorphan HBr 10 mg, Acetaminophen 250 mg, Pseudoephedrine HCl 30 mg. **(per 2 TBSP):** Doxylamine succinate 12.5 mg, Dextromethorphan HBr 30 mg, Acetaminophen 1000 mg, Pseudoephedrine HCl 60 mg.

Inactive Ingredients: (per softgel): Blue 1, Gelatin, Glycerin, Polyethylene Glycol, Povidone, Propylene Glycol and Purified Water, Sorbitol Special, Yellow 10. **(Liquid):** Alcohol 10%, Citric Acid, Flavor, High Fructose Corn Syrup, Polyethylene Glycol, Propylene Glycol, Purified Water, Saccharin Sodium, Sodium Citrate.
Original flavor also has Green 3, Yellow 6, Yellow 10.
Cherry flavor also has Blue 1, Red 40.
Sodium Content: Original flavor, 35 mg per 30 ml dose. Cherry flavor, 35 mg per 30 ml dose.

Uses: Temporarily relieves common cold/flu symptoms:
- minor aches
- pains
- headache
- muscular aches
- sore throat pain

- fever
- runny nose and sneezing
- nasal congestion
- cough due to minor throat and bronchial irritation

Liquid

Directions: Adults Dose (12 yrs. and older):
Take 2 Tablespoons (TBSP) or 30 ml in dose cup provided. Repeat every 6 hours. Do not take more than 4 doses a day or use as directed by a doctor. If taking NyQuil and DayQuil®, limit total to 4 doses per day.
Ask a doctor for use in children under 12 yrs. of age.

LiquiCaps

Directions: Adults 12 yrs. and older: Swallow two softgels with water. A total of 4 doses may be taken per day, each 4 hours apart or as directed by a doctor. If taking both NyQuil and DayQuil, limit total to 4 doses per day. **NOT RECOMMENDED FOR CHILDREN.**

Failure to follow these warnings could result in serious consequences.

Warnings: Do not exceed recommended dosage. Do not use with other products containing acetaminophen.
If nervousness, dizziness or sleeplessness occur, discontinue use and ask a doctor. May cause marked drowsiness. May cause excitability especially in children.
Do not take unless directed by a doctor if you have:
- heart disease
- asthma
- emphysema
- thyroid disease
- diabetes
- glaucoma
- high blood pressure
- excessive phlegm (mucus)
- breathing problems
- chronic bronchitis
- persistent or chronic cough
- cough associated with smoking
- difficulty in urination due to enlargement of the prostate gland

Alcohol Warning: If you consume 3 or more alcoholic drinks every day, ask your doctor whether you should take acetaminophen or other pain relievers/fever reducers. Acetaminophen may cause liver damage. **Keep this and all drugs out of the reach of children.** In case of accidental overdose, seek professional assistance or contact a poison control center immediately. Prompt medical attention is critical for adults as well as children even if you do not notice any signs or symptoms. As with any drug, if you are pregnant or nursing a baby, seek the advice of a health professional before using this product. Alcohol, sedatives and tranquilizers may increase the drowsiness effect. Avoid alcoholic beverages while taking this product. Use caution when driving a motor vehicle or operating heavy machinery.

Drug Interaction Precaution: Do not use this product without first asking a doctor if you take:
- sedatives
- tranquilizers
- a prescription monoamine oxidase inhibitor (MAOI) (certain drugs for depression, psychiatric or emotional conditions, or Parkinson's disease), for 2 weeks after stopping the MAOI drug or if you are uncertain whether your prescription drug contains an MAOI.
DOSING DURATION: Do not use over 7 days. *ASK A DOCTOR:*
- If sore throat is severe, persists for more than 2 days, is accompanied or followed by fever, headache, rash, nausea or vomiting.
- If symptoms do not improve or are accompanied by a fever that lasts more than 3 days or if new symptoms occur.
- If a cough persists for more than 7 days, recurs or is accompanied by a rash or persistent headache.
A persistent cough may be the sign of a serious condition.

How Supplied: (LiquiCaps®) Available in 12-count child-resistant blister packages and 20- and 36-count non-child resistant blister packages. Each softgel is imprinted: "NyQuil".
(Liquid) Available in 6 and 10 FL OZ (175 and 295 ml, respectively) plastic bottles with child-resistant, tamper-evident cap and calibrated medicine cup.

PEDIATRIC VICKS® 44®e
Cough & Chest Congestion Relief

Active Ingredients
per 1 tablespoon (TBSP.) (15 ml):
Dextromethorphan Hydrobromide 10 mg, Guaifenesin 100 mg.

CONTAINS NO ALCOHOL

Inactive Ingredients: Carboxymethylcellulose Sodium, Citric Acid, Flavor, High Fructose Corn Syrup, Polyethylene Oxide, Polyoxyl 40 Stearate, Propylene Glycol, Purified Water, Red 40, Saccharin Sodium, Sodium Benzoate, Sodium Citrate.
Sodium Content: 60 mg per 30 mL dose.

Uses: Temporary relieves cough due to a common cold. Helps loosen phlegm to rid the bronchial passageways of bothersome mucus.
Directions: Use Tablespoon (TBSP) or dose cup.

Under 2 yrs.	Ask a doctor.
2–5 yrs.	$1/2$ TBSP or $7^1/2$ ml
6–11 yrs.	1 TBSP or 15 ml
12 yrs. & older	2 TBSP or 30 ml

Repeat every 4 hours. Not to exceed 6 doses per day or use as directed by a doctor.

*Professional Dosage:

Physicians: Suggested doses for children under 2 years of age.

Age	Dose
* 6–11 mo.	1 teaspoon (tsp.) (5 ml)
*12–23 mo.	1¼ teaspoon (tsp.) (6.25 ml)

Repeat every 4 hours. Not to exceed 6 doses per day or use as directed by doctor.

*Based on extrapolation from studies on the safety and efficacy of active ingredients conducted among older children and adults. Use caution in treating children under 2 years who were born prematurely.

Warnings:

Do not take unless directed by a doctor if you have:
• asthma
• emphysema
• excessive phlegm (mucus)
• persistent or chronic cough
• chronic bronchitis
• cough associated with smoking

Keep this and all drugs out of the reach of children.
In the case of accidental overdose, seek professional advice or contact a poison control center immediately. As with any drug, if you are pregnant or nursing a baby, seek the advice of a health professional before using this product. Do not use this product if you are on a sodium-restricted diet unless directed by a doctor.

Drug Interaction Precaution: Do not use this product without first asking a doctor if you are take a prescription monoamine oxidase inhibitor (MAOI) (certain drugs for depression, psychiatric or emotional conditions, or Parkinson's disease), or for 2 weeks after stopping the MAOI drug or if you are uncertain whether your prescription drug contains an MAOI.

Dosing Duration & When to Ask a Doctor:
• If a cough persists for more than 7 days, recurs, or is accompanied by fever, rash or persistent headache. A persistent cough may be the sign of a serious condition.

How Supplied: 4 FL OZ (118 ml) plastic bottles. A calibrated dose cup accompanies each bottle.

PEDIATRIC VICKS® 44®m
Cough & Cold Relief
Cough Suppressant/Nasal
Decongestant/Antihistamine

Active Ingredients Per 1 tablespoon (TBSP) (15 ml): Dextromethorphan Hydrobromide 15 mg, Pseudoephedrine Hydrochloride 30 mg, Chlorpheniramine Maleate 2 mg

CONTAINS NO ALCOHOL

Inactive Ingredients: Carboxymethylcellulose Sodium, Citric Acid, Flavor, High Fructose Corn Syrup, Polyethylene Oxide, Polyoxyl 40 Stearate, Propylene Glycol, Purified Water, Red 40, Saccharin Sodium, Sodium Benzoate, Sodium Citrate.

Sodium Content: 60 mg per 30 mL dose.

Uses: Temporary relieves cough/cold symptoms:
• cough
• nasal congestion
• runny nose
• sneezing

Directions: Use Tablespoon (TBSP) or dose cup.

Under 6 yrs.	Ask a doctor.
6–11 yrs.	1 TBSP or 15 ml
12 yrs. & older	2 TBSP or 30 ml

Repeat every 6 hours, not to exceed 4 doses per day or use as directed by a doctor.

Professional Dosage:

*Physicians: Suggested doses for children under 6 years of age.

Age	Dose
* 6–11 mo.	1 teaspoon (tsp.) (5 ml)
*12–23 mo.	1¼ teaspoon (tsp.) (6.25 ml)
2–5 yrs.	½ TABLESPOON (TBSP.) (7.5 ml)

Repeat every 6 hours, no more than 4 doses in 24 hours, or as directed by doctor.

*Based on extrapolation from studies on the safety and efficacy of active ingredients conducted among older children and adults. Use caution in treating children under 2 years of age who were born prematurely.

Warnings: Do not exceed recommended dosage.
If nervousness, dizziness, or sleeplessness occur, discontinue use and ask a doctor. May cause drowsiness. May cause excitability especially in children.

Do not take unless directed by a doctor if you have:
• heart disease
• asthma
• emphysema
• thyroid disease
• diabetes
• glaucoma
• high blood pressure
• excessive phlegm (mucus)
• breathing problems
• chronic bronchitis
• difficulty in breathing
• persistent or chronic cough
• cough associated with smoking
• difficulty in urination due to enlarged prostate gland

Keep this and all drugs out of the reach of children. In case of accidental overdose, seek professional advice or contact a poison control center immediately. As with any drug, if you are pregnant or nursing a baby, seek the advice of a health professional before using this product.

Alcohol, sedatives, and tranquilizers may increase the drowsiness effect. Avoid alcoholic beverages while taking this product. Use caution when driving a motor vehicle or operating machinery. Do not use this product if you are on a sodium-restricted diet unless directed by a doctor.

Drug Interaction Precaution: Do not take this product without first asking a doctor if you take:
• sedatives
• tranquilizers
• a prescription monoamine oxidase inhibitor (MAOI) (certain drugs for depression, psychiatric or emotional conditions, or Parkinson's disease), or for 2 weeks after stopping the MAOI drug or if you are uncertain whether your prescription drug contains an MAOI.

Dosing Duration: Do not use over 7 days. *Ask a Doctor:*
• If symptoms do not improve within 7 days or are accompanied by a fever.
• If a cough persists for more than 7 days, recurs, or is accompanied by fever, rash or persistent headache. A persistent cough may be a sign of a serious condition.

How Supplied: 4 FL OZ (118 ml) plastic bottles. A calibrated dose cup accompanies each bottle.

VICKS® SINEX® [NASAL SPRAY]
[Ultra Fine Mist] for Sinus Relief
[sī 'nĕx]
Nasal Decongestant

Active Ingredient: Phenylephrine Hydrochloride 0.5%.

Inactives: Benzalkonium Chloride, Camphor, Chlorhexidine Gluconate, Citric Acid, Disodium EDTA, Eucalyptol, Menthol, Purified Water, Tyloxapol.

Use: For temporary relief of sinus/nasal congestion due to colds, hay fever, upper respiratory allergies or sinusitis.

Dosage: Ultra Fine Mist: Remove protective cap. Before using for the first time, prime the pump by firmly depressing its rim several times. Hold container with thumb at base and nozzle between first and second fingers. Without tilting your head, insert nozzle into nostril. Fully depress rim with a firm even stroke and inhale deeply.
12 yrs. & over: 2 or 3 sprays in each nostril not more often than every 4 hours. Under 12 yrs. ask a doctor.
Nasal Spray: 12 yrs & over: 2 or 3 sprays in each nostril without tilting your head, not more often than every 4 hours. Under 12 yrs. ask a doctor.

Warnings: Do not exceed recommended dosage. This product may cause temporary discomfort such as burning, stinging, sneezing, or an increase of nasal discharge. The use of this container by more than one person may

Continued on next page

Vicks Sinex—Cont.

spread infection. Do not use this product for more than 3 days. Use only as directed. Frequent or prolonged use may cause nasal congestion to recur or worsen. If symptoms persist, ask a doctor. Do not use this product if you have heart disease, high blood pressure, thyroid disease, diabetes, or difficulty in urination due to enlargement of the prostate gland unless directed by a doctor. **Keep this and all drugs out of the reach of children.** In case of accidental ingestion, seek professional assistance or contact a poison control center immediately.

How Supplied: Available in $1/2$ FL OZ (15 ml) plastic squeeze bottle and $1/2$ FL OZ (15 ml) measured dose Ultra Fine mist pump.

VICKS® SINEX®

[sī 'něx]
12-HOUR [Nasal Spray]
[Ultra Fine Mist] for Sinus Relief

Active Ingredient: Oxymetazoline Hydrochloride 0.05%.

Inactives: Benzalkonium Chloride, Camphor, Chlorhexidine Gluconate, Disodium EDTA, Eucalyptol, Menthol, Potassium Phosphate, Purified Water, Sodium Chloride, Sodium Phosphate, Tyloxapol.

Use: For temporary relief of nasal congestion due to colds, hay fever, upper respiratory allergies or sinusitis.

Dosage and Administration:

Ultra Fine Mist: Remove protective cap. Before using for the first time, prime the pump by firmly depressing its rim several times. Hold container with thumb at base and nozzle between first and second fingers. Without tilting head, insert nozzle into nostril. Fully depress rim with a firm even stroke and inhale deeply.
6 yrs. & older (with adult supervision): 2 or 3 sprays in each nostril not more often than every 10 to 12 hours. Do not exceed 2 applications in any 24-hour period. Under 6 yrs. ask a doctor.
Squeeze Bottle: 6 yrs. & older: (with adult supervision): 2 or 3 sprays in each nostril without tilting your head, not more often than every 10 to 12 hours. Do not exceed 2 applications in any 24-hour period. Under 6 yrs. ask a doctor.

Warnings: Do not exceed recommended dosage. This product may cause temporary discomfort such as burning, stinging, sneezing or an increase of nasal discharge. The use of this container by more than one person may spread infection. Do not use this product for more than 3 days. Use only as directed. Frequent or prolonged use may cause nasal congestion to recur or worsen. If symptoms persist, ask a doctor. Do not use this product if you have heart disease, high blood pressure, thy-

roid disease, diabetes, or difficulty in urination due to enlargement of the prostate gland unless directed by a doctor.
Keep this and all drugs out of the reach of children. In case of accidental ingestion, seek professional assistance or contact a poison control center immediately.

How Supplied: Available in $1/2$ FL OZ (15 ml) plastic squeeze bottle and $1/2$ FL OZ (15 ml) measured-dose Ultra Fine mist pump.

VICKS® VAPOR INHALER
Leumetamfetamine/Nasal Decongestant

Active Ingredient per inhaler: Leumetamfetamine 50 mg.

Inactive Ingredients: Bornyl acetate, camphor, lavender oil, menthol.

Indications: For the temporary relief of nasal congestion due to the common cold, hay fever, upper respiratory allergies or sinusitis.

Directions: 12 yrs. & older: 2 inhalations in each nostril not more often than every 2 hours. 6–11 yrs. (with adult supervision): 1 inhalation in each nostril not more often than every 2 hours. Under 6 yrs.: ask a doctor.

Warnings: Do not exceed recommended dosage. This product may cause temporary discomfort such as burning, stinging, sneezing, or an increase of nasal discharge. The use of this container by more than one person may spread infection. Do not use this product for more than 3 days. Frequent or prolonged use may cause nasal congestion to recur or worsen. If symptoms persist, ask a doctor. Do not use this product if you have heart disease, high blood pressure, thyroid disease, diabetes or difficulty in urination due to enlargement of the prostate gland unless directed by a doctor.
Keep this and all drugs out of the reach of children. In case of accidental ingestion, seek professional assistance or contact a poison control center immediately.

VICKS® VAPOR INHALER is effective for a minimum of 3 months after first use. Keep tightly closed.

How Supplied: Available as a cylindrical plastic nasal inhaler.
Net weight: 0.007 OZ (200 mg).

VICKS® VAPORUB®
VICKS® VAPORUB® CREAM
[vā 'pō-rub]
Nasal Decongestant/Cough Suppressant/Topical Analgesic

Active Ingredients: Camphor (5.2% cream) (4.8% oint.), Menthol (2.8% cream) (2.6% oint.), Eucalyptus Oil 1.2%.

USE on Chest & Throat: For temporary relief of nasal congestion and coughs associated with a cold.

Active Ingredients: Camphor (5.2% cream) (4.8% oint.), Menthol (2.8% cream) (2.6% oint.).

USE: For temporary relief of minor aches and pains of muscles.

Inactive Ingredients: (ointment) Cedarleaf Oil, Nutmeg Oil, Special Petrolatum, Thymol, Turpentine Oil. **(cream)** Carbomer 954, Cedarleaf Oil, Cetyl Alcohol, Cetyl Palmitate, Cyclomethicone, Dimethicone Copolyol, Dimethicone, EDTA, Glycerin, Imidazolidinyl Urea, Isopropyl Palmitate, Methylparaben, Nutmeg Oil, PEG-100, Stearate, Propylparaben, Purified Water, Sodium Hydroxide, Stearic Acid, Stearyl Alcohol, Thymol, Titanium Dioxide, Turpentine Oil.

Directions: 2 yrs. & older:
Chest & Throat: Rub on a thick layer. Keep clothing loose to let vapors rise to the nose and mouth.
Rub on sore area.
Repeat up to three times daily or as directed by a doctor.
Under 2 yrs.: ask a doctor.
Do not heat. Never expose VapoRub to flame, microwave, or place in any container in which you are heating water. Such improper use may cause the mixture to splatter.

Warnings: For external use only. Avoid contact with eyes.
Do not use unless directed by a doctor if you have cough associated with:
- smoking
- excessive phlegm (mucus)
- asthma
- emphysema
- a persistent or chronic cough
Do not:
- take by mouth
- place in nostrils
- bandage tightly
- apply to wounds or damaged skin
Ask a doctor:
- If a cough persists for more than 7 days, recurs or is accompanied by a fever, rash or persistent headache. A persistent cough may be the sign of a serious condition.
- If muscle aches/pains persist for more than 7 days or recur.
Keep this and all drugs out of the reach of children. In case of accidental overdose, seek professional assistance or contact a poison control center immediately.

How Supplied: (ointment) Available in 1.5 OZ (40 g), 3.0 OZ (90 g) and 6.0 OZ (170 g) plastic jars. **(cream)** 2.0 OZ (60 g) tube.

VICKS® VAPOSTEAM®
[vā 'pō "stēm]
Liquid Medication for Hot Steam Vaporizers.
Camphor/Cough Suppressant

Active Ingredients: Camphor 6.2%.

Inactive Ingredients: Alcohol 78%, Cedarleaf Oil, Eucalyptus Oil, Laureth .

7, Menthol, Nutmeg Oil, Poloxamer 124, Silicone.

Indications: Temporarily relieves cough due to minor throat and bronchial irritation associated with a cold.

Directions:
2 yrs. & older: For each quart of water add one tablespoon of solution directly to the water in a hot steam vaporizer. Breathe in medicated vapors. May be repeated up to 3 times daily or as directed by a doctor.
Under 2 yrs.: ask a doctor.
In Hot/Warm Steam Vaporizers: VAPOSTEAM is formulated to be added directly to the water in your hot/warm steam vaporizer. Do not direct steam from vaporizer too close to face. For best performance, vaporizer should be thoroughly cleaned after each use according to manufacturer's instructions. To promote steaming, follow directions of vaporizer manufacturer.
Never expose VAPOSTEAM to flame, microwave, or place in any container in which you are heating water except for a hot-warm steam vaporizer. Never use VAPOSTEAM in any bowl or washbasin with hot water. Improper use may cause the mixture to splatter and cause burns.
Caution not for Internal Use: For steam inhalation only. Do not take by mouth.

Warnings: A persistent cough may be a sign of a serious condition. If cough persists for more than one week, tends to recur or is accompanied by fever, rash, or persistent headache, consult a doctor. Do not use this product for persistent or chronic cough such as occurs with smoking, asthma, emphysema, or if cough is accompanied by excessive phlegm (mucus) unless directed by a doctor. **Keep this and all drugs out of the reach of children.**
Flammable

Accidental Ingestion: In case of accidental ingestion, seek professional assistance or contact a poison control center immediately.

Eye Exposure: In case of eye contact, flush with water. Seek professional assistance or contact a poison control center immediately.

How Supplied: Available in 4 FL OZ (118 mL) and 8 FL OZ (236 mL) bottles.

EDUCATIONAL MATERIAL

Procter & Gamble offers to health care professionals a variety of journal reprints and patient education materials on:
- fiber therapy and related bowel disorders (Metamucil),
- H. pylori research and healthy traveling advice (Pepto-Bismol),
- caffeine reduction (Folgers), and
- pharmacy practice issues (Pharmacy Digest newsletter).

Additionally, selected professional samples of Procter & Gamble Health Care and Skin Care products are available to targeted health care specialists. For these materials, please call 1-800/358-8707, or write:
Charles Lambert
Manager, Scientific Communications
The Procter & Gamble Company
Two Procter & Gamble Plaza
Cincinnati, OH 45201

The Purdue Frederick Company
100 CONNECTICUT AVENUE
NORWALK, CT 06850-3590

For Medical Information Contact:
Medical Department
(203) 853-0123

BETADINE® BRAND First Aid Antibiotics + Moisturizer Ointment

Actions: Topical broad-spectrum antibiotics polymyxin B sulfate and bacitracin zinc in a cholesterolized ointment* (moisturizer) base to help prevent infection. Formulated with a special blend of waxes and oils to help retain vital moisture needed to aid in healing.

Indications: First aid to help prevent infection in minor cuts, scrapes and burns.

Administration: Clean affected area. Apply small amount of this product (an amount equal to the surface area of the tip of the finger) on the area 1 to 3 times daily. May be covered with a sterile bandage.

Warnings: For External Use Only. Do not use in the eyes or apply over large areas of the body. In case of deep or puncture wounds, animal bites, or serious burns, consult a physician. Stop use and consult a physician if the condition persists or gets worse. Do not use longer than 1 week unless directed by a physician. Keep this and all medications out of the reach of children. In case of accidental ingestion, seek professional assistance or contact a Poison Control Center immediately.

Active Ingredients: Per gram: Polymyxin B sulfate (10,000 IU) and bacitracin zinc (500 IU).

How Supplied: 1/2 oz. plastic tube with applicator tip.
• Formulated with Aquaphor®—a registered trademark of Beiersdorf AG.

Copyright 1998, The Purdue Frederick Company
Shown in Product Identification Guide, page 519

BETADINE® BRAND PLUS
First Aid Antibiotics + Pain Reliever Ointment
[bā 'tăh-dīn"]

Actions: Topical broad-spectrum antibiotics polymyxin B sulfate and bacitracin zinc plus topical anesthetic in a cholesterolized ointment* (moisturizer) base to help prevent infection and relieve pain.

Indications: Helps prevent infection in minor cuts, scrapes and burns.

Administration: Clean affected area. Apply small amount of this product (an amount equal to the surface area of the tip of the finger) on the area 1 to 3 times daily. May be covered with a sterile bandage.

Warnings: For External Use Only. Do not use in the eyes or apply over large areas of the body. In case of deep or puncture wounds, animal bites, or serious burns, consult a physician. Stop use and consult a physician if the condition persists or gets worse. Do not use longer than 1 week unless directed by a physician. Keep this and all medications out of the reach of children. In case of accidental ingestion, seek professional assistance or contact a Poison Control Center immediately.

Active Ingredients: Per gram: Polymyxin B sulfate (10,000 IU), bacitracin zinc (500 IU), and pramoxine HCl 10 mg.

How Supplied: 1/2 oz. plastic tube with an applicator tip.
*Formulated with Aquaphor® — a registered trademark of Beiersdorf AG.
Copyright 1998, The Purdue Frederick Company.
Shown in Product Identification Guide, page 519

BETADINE® OINTMENT
(povidone-iodine, 10%)
BETADINE® SOLUTION
(povidone-iodine, 10%)
BETADINE® SKIN CLEANSER
(povidone-iodine, 7.5%)
Topical Antiseptic
Bactericide/Virucide

Action: Topical microbicides active against organisms commonly encountered in minor skin wounds and burns.

Indications: **Ointment**—For the prevention of infection in minor burns, cuts and abrasions. Kills microorganisms promptly. **Solution**—Kills microorganisms in minor burns, cuts and scrapes. First aid to help prevent infection in minor cuts, scrapes and burns. **Skin Cleanser**—Helps prevent infection in minor cuts, scrapes and burns. Use routinely for general hygiene.

Administration: **Ointment**—For the prevention of infection in minor burns, cuts and abrasions, apply directly to af-

Continued on next page

Betadine Antiseptic—Cont.

fected areas as needed. Nonocclusive: allows air to reach the wound. May be bandaged. **Solution**—For minor cuts, scrapes and burns, apply directly to affected area as needed. May be covered with gauze or adhesive bandage. **Skin Cleanser**—Wet skin and apply a sufficient amount to work up a rich, golden lather. Allow lather to remain about 3 minutes and rinse off. Repeat 2–3 times a day or as directed by physician.

Warnings: For External Use Only. In case of deep or puncture wounds or serious burns, consult physician. If redness, irritation, swelling or pain persists or increases, or if infection occurs, discontinue use and consult physician. Keep out of reach of children.

How Supplied:
Ointment: 1/32 and 1/8 oz. packettes; 1 oz. tubes
Solution: 1/2 oz., 4 oz., 8 oz., 16 oz. (1 pt.), 32 oz. (1 qt.), and 1 gal. plastic bottles.
Skin Cleanser: 4 fl. oz. plastic bottles
Copyright 1991, 1998, The Purdue Frederick Company
Shown in Product Identification Guide, page 519

SENOKOT® Tablets/Granules
SenokotXTRA® Tablets
(standardized senna concentrate)

SENOKOT® Syrup
SENOKOT® Children's Syrup
(extract of senna concentrate)

SENOKOT-S® Tablets
(standardized senna concentrate and docusate sodium)

Natural Vegetable Laxative

Actions: Senna provides a virtually colon-specific action which is gentle, effective, and predictable, generally producing bowel movement in 6 to 12 hours. Senokot-S tablets also contain a stool softener for smoother, easier evacuation.

Indications: Senokot products generally produce bowel movement in 6 to 12 hours.

Dosage and Administration: Take according to product-package instructions or as directed by a doctor. Take preferably at bedtime. For older, debilitated patients, a doctor may consider prescribing $1/2$ the initial dose recommended on the package. For use of Senokot Laxatives in children under 2 years of age, consult a doctor.

Warnings: Do not use a laxative product when abdominal pain, nausea or vomiting are present unless directed by a doctor. If you have noticed a sudden change in bowel movements that persists over a period of 2 weeks, consult a doctor before using a laxative. Laxative products should not be used for a period longer than 1 week unless directed by a doctor. Rectal bleeding or failure to have a bowel movement after the use of a laxative may indicate a serious condition. Discontinue use and consult your doctor. As with any drug, if you are pregnant or nursing a baby, seek the advice of a health professional before using this product. In case of accidental overdose, seek professional assistance or contact a Poison Control Center immediately. Keep out of children's reach.

How Supplied: Senokot Tablets: Boxes of 10 and 20; bottles of 50, 100, and 1000; Unit Strip Packs in boxes of 100 individually sealed tablets. Each Senokot Tablet contains 8.6 mg sennosides.
SenokotXTRA Tablets: Boxes of 12 and 36. Each SenokotXTRA Tablet contains 17 mg sennosides.
Senokot-S Tablets: Packages of 10; bottles of 30, 60 and 1000; Unit Strip boxes of 100. Each Senokot-S Tablet contains 8.6 mg sennosides and 50 mg docusate sodium.
Senokot Granules: 2, 6, and 12 oz. plastic containers. Each teaspoon of Senokot Granules contains 15 mg sennosides.
Senokot Syrup: 2 and 8 fl. oz. bottles.
Senokot Children's Syrup: Chocolate-flavored, alcohol-free syrup in 2.5 fl. oz. plastic bottle packaged with measuring cup. Each teaspoon of Senokot Syrup or Senokot Children's Syrup contains 8.8 mg sennosides.
Copyright 1991, 1998 The Purdue Frederick Company.
Shown in Product Identification Guide, page 519

EDUCATIONAL MATERIAL

Samples Available:
1) Senokot-S® Tablets Samples– 1 display of 12 (4 tablets per packette)
2) Betadine® Antibiotic Ointment Samples– 1 display of 48 packettes

---

Richardson-Vicks Inc.
(See Procter & Gamble.)

**FACED WITH AN
Rx SIDE EFFECT?**
Turn to the
Companion Drug Index
(Green Pages)
for products that
provide symptomatic
relief.

Roberts Pharmaceutical Corporation
4 INDUSTRIAL WAY WEST
EATONTOWN, NJ 07724-2274

Direct Inquiries to:
Customer Service Department:
(732) 389-1182
(800) 828-2088
FAX: (908) 389-1014

For Medical Emergencies Contact:
Medical Services Department
(800) 992-9306

COLACE®
[kōlās]
docusate sodium,
capsules • syrup • liquid (drops)

Description: Colace® (docusate sodium) is a stool softener.
Colace® Capsules, 50 mg, contain the following inactive ingredients: D&C Red No. 33, FD&C Red No. 40, polyethylene glycol, propylene glycol, sorbitol, gelatin, and glycerin.
Colace® Capsules, 100 mg, contain the following inactive ingredients: D&C Red No. 33, FD&C Red No. 40, FD&C Yellow No. 6, polyethylene glycol, propylene glycol, sorbitol, gelatin, titanium dioxide, methylparaben, propylparaben, and glycerin.
Colace® Liquid, 1%, (10 mg/mL), contains the following inactive ingredients: citric acid, D&C Red No. 33, methylparaben, poloxamer, polyethylene glycol, propylene glycol, propylparaben, sodium citrate, vanillin, and purified water.
Colace® Syrup, 20 mg/5 mL, contains the following inactive ingredients: alcohol (not more than 1%), citric acid, D&C Red No. 33, FD&C Red No. 40, flavor (natural), menthol, methylparaben, peppermint oil, poloxamer, polyethylene glycol, propylparaben, sodium citrate, sucrose, and purified water.

Actions and Uses: Colace®, a surface-active agent, helps to keep stools soft for easy, natural passage and is not a laxative, thus, not habit forming. Useful in constipation due to hard stools, in painful anorectal conditions, in cardiac and other conditions in which maximum ease of passage is desirable to avoid difficult or painful defecation, and when peristaltic stimulants are contraindicated.

Note: When peristaltic stimulation is needed due to inadequate bowel motility, see Peri-Colace® (laxative and stool softener).

Contraindications: There are no known contraindications to Colace®.

Warning: As with any drug, pregnant or nursing women should seek the advice of a health professional before using this product. Keep this and all medication out of the reach of children.

Side Effects: The incidence of side effects—none of a serious nature—is exceedingly small. Bitter taste, throat irritation, and nausea (primarily associated with the use of the syrup and liquid) are the main side effects reported. Rash has occurred.

Administration and Dosage: *Orally*—Suggested daily Dosage: *Adults and older children:* 50 to 200 mg *Children 6 to 12:* 40 to 120 mg *Children 3 to 6:* 20 to 60 mg. *Infants and children under 3:* 10 to 40 mg. The higher doses are recommended for initial therapy. Dosage should be adjusted to individual response. The effect on stools is usually apparent 1 to 3 days after the first dose. Colace® liquid or syrup must be given in a 6 oz. to 8 oz. glass of milk or fruit juice or in infant's formula to prevent throat irritation. In *enemas*—Add 50 to 100 mg Colace® (5 to 10 mL Colace® liquid) to a retention or flushing enema.

How Supplied: Colace® capsules, 50 mg
    NDC 54092-052-30 Bottles of 30
    NDC 54092-052-60 Bottles of 60
    NDC 54092-052-52 Cartons of 100
        single unit packs
Colace® capsules, 100 mg
    NDC 54092-053-30 Bottles of 30
    NDC 54092-053-60 Bottle of 60
    NDC 54092-053-02 Bottles of 250
    NDC 54092-053-10 Bottles of 1000
    NDC 54092-053-52 Cartons of 100
        single unit packs
Note: Colace® capsules should be stored at controlled room temperature (59°–86°F or 15°–30°C)
Colace® liquid, 1% solution; 10 mg/mL (with calibrated dropper)
    NDC 54092-414-16 Bottles of 16 fl oz
    NDC 54092-414-30 Bottles of 30 mL
Colace® syrup, 20 mg/5 mL teaspoon; contains not more than 1% alcohol
    NDC 54092-415-08 Bottles of 8 fl oz
    NDC 54092-415-16 Bottles of 16 fl oz
Manufactured for
Roberts Laboratories Inc.,
a subsidiary of
ROBERTS PHARMACEUTICAL CORPORATION
Eatontown, NJ 07724 USA

COLACE MICROENEMA
[kō lās]
(docusate sodium)
(for rectal use only)

Description: Active ingredient: Each 5 mL contains 200 mg of docusate sodium.
Inactive ingredients: Citric acid, sodium benzoate, hydroxypropyl methylcellulose, apricot kernel oil PEG-8 esters. PEG-6 and PEG-32 and glycol stearate, glycerin 96%, and purified water.
Indications: For relief of occasional constipation (irregularity).
Directions for use: Adults and children 3 years of age and older: Express a drop of the mixture to lubricate the tip if necessary. Slowly insert the full length

(half length for children 3 to 12 years old) of the nozzle into the rectum. Squeeze out the entire contents of the tube. Remove the nozzle completely before releasing grip on the tube, otherwise the contents may flow back into the tube. Do not use in children under 3 years of age, except under the advise of a physician.
This product generally produces bowel movement in 2 to 15 minutes.

Warnings: Do not use laxative products when abdominal pain, nausea, or vomiting are present, unless directed by a doctor. If you have noticed a sudden change in bowel habits that persists over a period of 2 weeks, consult a doctor before using a laxative. Laxative products should not be used for a period longer than 1 week unless directed by a doctor. Rectal bleeding or failure to have a bowel movement after use of a laxative may indicate a serious condition. Discontinue use and consult your doctor.
Keep this and all medication out of the reach of children.
Store from 15°C to 30°C.

How Supplied: 200 mg
3 × 5 mL Microenemas
NDC 54092-491-70
Manufactured for
Roberts Laboratories Inc., a subsidiary of
ROBERTS PHARMACEUTICAL CORP.
Eatontown, NJ 07724, USA
Copyright ©1995 Roberts Laboratories Inc.
491 7004 001   10/95

PERI-COLACE® capsules • syrup
(casanthranol and docusate sodium)

Description: Peri-Colace® is a combination of the mild stimulant laxative casanthranol, and the stool-softener Colace® (docusate sodium). Each capsule contains 30 mg of casanthranol and 100 mg of Colace®; the syrup contains 30 mg of casanthranol and 60 mg of Colace® per 15-mL tablespoon (10 mg of casanthranol and 20 mg of Colace® per 5-mL teaspoon) and 10% alcohol.
Peri-Colace® Capsules contain the following inactive ingredients: FD&C Red No. 40, FD&C Blue No. 1, polyethylene glycol, propylene glycol, sorbitol, titanium dioxide, methylparaben, propylparaben, glycerin, and gelatin.
Peri-Colace® Syrup contains the following inactive ingredients: alcohol (10% v/v), citric acid, flavors, methyl salicylate, methylparaben, poloxamer, polyethylene glycol, propylparaben, sodium citrate, sorbitol solution, sucrose, and purified water.

Action and Uses: Peri-Colace® provides gentle peristaltic stimulation and helps to keep stools soft for easier passage. Bowel movement is induced gently—usually overnight or in 8 to 12 hours. Nausea, griping, abnormally loose stools,

and constipation rebound are minimized. Useful in management of chronic or temporary constipation.
Note: To prevent hard stools when laxative stimulation is not needed or undesirable, see Colace® (stool softener).

Warnings: Do not use when abdominal pain, nausea, or vomiting is present. Frequent or prolonged use of this preparation may result in dependence on laxatives.
As with any drug, pregnant or nursing women should seek the advice of a health professional before using this product.
Keep this and all medication out of the reach of children.

Side Effects: The incidence of side effects—none of a serious nature—is exceedingly small. Nausea, abdominal cramping or discomfort, diarrhea, and rash are the main side effects reported.

Administration and Dosage: *Adults*—1 or 2 capsules, or 1 or 2 tablespoons syrup at bedtime, or as indicated. In severe cases, dosage may be increased to 2 capsules or 2 tablespoons twice daily, or 3 capsules at bedtime. *Children*—1 to 3 teaspoons of syrup at bedtime, or as indicated. Peri-Colace® syrup must be given in a 6 oz. to 8 oz. glass of milk or fruit juice or in infant's formula to prevent throat irritation.

Overdosage: In addition to symptomatic treatment, gastric lavage, if timely, is recommended in cases of large overdosage.

How Supplied: Peri-Colace® Capsules
    NDC 54092-054-30 Bottles of 30
    NDC 54092-054-60 Bottles of 60
    NDC 54092-054-02 Bottles of 250
    NDC 54092-054-10 Bottles of 1000
    NDC 54092-054-52 Cartons of 100 single unit packs
Note: Peri-Colace® capsules should be stored at controlled room temperatures (59°–86°F or 15°–30°C).
Peri-Colace® Syrup
    NDC 54092-418-08 Bottles of 8 fl oz
    NDC 54092-418-16 Bottles of 16 fl oz
Manufactured for
Roberts Laboratories Inc.,
a subsidiary of
ROBERTS PHARMACEUTICAL CORPORATION
Eatontown, NJ 07724 USA

UNKNOWN DRUG?
Consult the
Product Identification Guide
(Gray Pages)
for full-color photos of
leading over-the-counter
medications

Schering-Plough HealthCare Products
LIBERTY CORNER, NJ 07938

Direct Product Requests to:
(908) 604-1983 Telephone Number
(908) 604-1776 Fax Number

For Medical Emergencies Contact:
Clinical Department
(908) 604-1805

A + D® Ointment with Zinc Oxide

Active Ingredients: Dimethicone 1%, Zinc Oxide 10%.

Inactive Ingredients: Aloe Extract, Benzyl Alcohol, Cod Liver Oil (contains Vitamin A and Vitamin D), Fragrance, Glyceryl Oleate, Light Mineral Oil, Ozokerite, Paraffin, Propylene Glycol, Sorbitol, Synthetic Beeswax, Water.

Indications: Helps treat and prevent diaper rash. Protects chafed skin or minor skin irritation associated with diaper rash and helps seal out wetness.

Directions: Change wet and soiled diapers promptly, cleanse the diaper area and allow to dry. Apply ointment liberally as often as necessary with each diaper change especially at bedtime or anytime when exposure to wet diapers may be prolonged.

Warning: For external use only. Avoid contact with eyes. If condition worsens or does not improve within 7 days, consult a doctor. Not to be applied over deep or puncture wounds, infections, or lacerations. Consult a doctor. Keep this and all drugs out of the reach of children. In case of accidental ingestion, seek professional assistance or contact a Poison Control Center immediately.

How Supplied: A and D® Ointment with Zinc Oxide is available in 1 1/2-ounce (42.5g) 3 ounce (81g) and 4-ounce (113g) tubes.

Store between 15° and 30°C (59° and 86°F).

Shown in Product Identification Guide, page 520

A + D ® Original Ointment

Active Ingredients: Petrolatum 53.4%, Lanolin 15.5%.

Inactive Ingredients: Cod Liver Oil (Contains Vitamin A and Vitamin D), Fragrance, Light Mineral Oil, Microcrystalline Wax, Paraffin.

A+D Original Ointment for Diaper Rash:

Indications: Helps treat and prevent diaper rash. Protects chafed skin or minor skin irritation associated with diaper rash and helps seal out wetness.

Directions: Change wet and soiled diapers promptly, cleanse the diaper area, and allow to dry. Apply **A+D Original Ointment** liberally as often as necessary with each diaper change especially at bedtime or anytime when exposure to wet diapers may be prolonged.

A+D Original Ointment for Skin Irritations:

Indications: Helps prevent and temporarily protects chafed, chapped, cracked or windburn skin and lips. Provides temporary protection of minor cuts, scrapes, burns and sunburn.

Directions: Apply **A+D Original Ointment** liberally as often as necessary.

Warnings: For external use only. Avoid contact with eyes. If condition worsens or does not improve within 7 days, consult a doctor. Not to be applied over deep or puncture wounds, infections or lacerations. Consult a doctor. Keep this and all drugs out of the reach of children. In case of acidental ingestion, seek professional assistance or contact a Poison Control Center immediately.

How Supplied: A and D Ointment is available in 1¹/₂-ounce (42.5g) 3 ounce (81g) and 4-ounce (113g) tubes and 1-pound (454g) jars.

Store between 15° and 30°C (59° and 86°F)

Shown in Product Identification Guide, page 520

AFRIN® 12 Hour
[á frin]
Original Nasal Spray 0.05%
Pump Mist 0.05%
Sinus Nasal Spray 0.05%
Severe Congestion Nasal Spray 0.05%
Extra Moisturizing Nasal Spray 0.05%
Nose Drops 0.05%

Description: AFRIN 12 Hour products contain oxymetazoline hydrochloride, the longest acting topical nasal decongestant available.
Each mL of **AFRIN Original Nasal Spray, Pump Mist, and Nose Drops** contains Oxymetazoline Hydrochloride, 0.05%. **Also contains:** Benzalkonium Chloride, Edetate Disodium, Polyethlene Glycol 1450, Povidone, Propylene Glycol, Sodium Phosphate Dibasic, Sodium Phosphate Monobasic, Water.
Each mL of **AFRIN Sinus Nasal Spray** contains Oxymetazoline Hydrochloride 0.05%. **Also contains:** Benzalkonium Chloride, Benzyl Alcohol, Edetate Disodium, Polysorbate 80, Propylene Glycol, Sodium Phosphate Dibasic, Sodium Phosphate Monobasic, Vapornase™ (Camphor, Eucalyptol, Menthol), Water.
Each mL of **AFRIN Extra Moisturizing Nasal Spray** contains Oxymetazoline Hydrochloride, 0.05%. **Also contains:** Benzalkonium Chloride, Edetate Disodium, Povidone, Sodium Phosphate Dibasic, Sodium Phosphate Monobasic, Soothate™ (Glycerin, Polyethlene Glycol 1450, Propylene Glycol), Water.
AFRIN Extra Moisturizing Nasal Spray with Soothate™ ingredients is specially formulated to soothe dry, irritated nasal passages.
Each mL of **AFRIN Severe Congestion Nasal Spray** contains Oxymetazoline Hydrochloride 0.05%. **Also contains:** Benzalkonium Chloride, Benzyl Alcohol, Camphor, Edetate Disodium, Eucalyptol, Menthol, Polysorbate 80, Propylene Glycol, Sodium Phosphate Dibasic, Sodium Phosphate Monobasic, Water.

Indications: For the temporary relief of nasal congestion due to a cold, due to hay fever or other upper respiratory allergies, or associated with sinusitis. Skrinks swollen nasal membranes so you can breathe more freely.

Actions: The sympathomimetic action of AFRIN products constricts the smaller arterioles of the nasal passages, producing a prolonged, gentle and predictable decongesting effect. In just a few minutes a single dose, as directed, provides prompt, temporary relief of nasal congestion that lasts up to 12 hours. AFRIN products last up to 3 or 4 times longer than most ordinary nasal sprays.

Warnings: Do not exceed recommended dosage. This product may cause temporary discomfort such as burning, stinging, sneezing, or an increase in nasal discharge. Do not use this product for more than 3 days. Use only as directed. Frequent or prolonged use may cause nasal congestion to recur or worsen. If symptoms persist, consult a doctor. The use of this container by more than one person may spread infection. Do not use this product if you have heart disease, high blood pressure, thyroid disease, diabetes, or difficulty in urination due to enlargement of the prostate gland unless directed by a doctor. As with any drug, if you are pregnant or nursing a baby, seek the advice of a health professional before using this product. Keep this and all medicines out of the reach of children. In case of accidental ingestion, seek professional assistance or contact a Poison Control Center immediately.

Directions for Afrin Original Nasal Spray Pump Mist, Sinus Nasal Spray, Severe Congestion Nasal Spray and Extra Moisturizing Nasal Spray: Adults and children 6 to under 12 years of age (with adult supervision): 2 or 3 sprays in each nostril not more often than every 10 to 12 hours. Do not exceed 2 doses in any 24-hour period. **Children under 6 years of age:** consult a doctor. To spray, squeeze bottle quickly and firmly. Do not tilt head backward while spraying. Wipe nozzle clean after use.

Directions for Afrin Original Nose Drops: Adults and children 6 to under 12 years of age (with adult supervision): 2 or 3 drops in each nostril not more often than every 10 to 12 hours.

Do not exceed 2 doses in any 24-hour period. **Children under 6 years of age:** consult a doctor. Wipe dropper clean after use.

How Supplied: AFRIN Nasal Spray 0.05%-15 ml and 30 ml plastic squeeze bottles.
AFRIN Pump Mist 0.05% (1:2000)-15 ml pump bottle.
AFRIN Sinus Nasal Spray 0.05%-15 ml and 30 ml plastic squeeze bottles.
AFRIN Extra Moisturizing Nasal Spray 0.05%-15 ml and 30 ml plastic squeeze bottles.
AFRIN Severe Congestion Nasal Spray 0.05% (1:2000)-15 ml plastic squeeze bottle.
AFRIN Nose Drops 0.05% (1:2000)-20 ml dropper bottle.
Store all nasal sprays and nose drops between 2° and 30°C (36° and 86°F)

Shown in Product Identification Guide, page 519 and 520

AFRIN® Allergy Nasal Spray
[*á frin*]

Each ml of **AFRIN Allergy Nasal Spray** contains Phenylephrine Hydrochloride 0.5%. **Also contains:** Benzalkonium Chloride, Edetate Disodium, Glycerin, Polyethylene Glycol 1450, Povidone, Propylene Glycol, Sodium Phosphate Dibasic, Sodium Phosphate Monobasic, Water.

Indications: For the temporary relief of nasal congestion due to hay fever or other upper respiratory allergies. Shrinks swollen nasal membranes so you can breathe more freely.

Warning: Do not exceed recommended dosage. This product may cause temporary discomfort such as burning, stinging, sneezing, or an increase in nasal discharge. Do not use this product for more than 3 days. Use only as directed. Frequent or prolonged use may cause nasal congestion to recur or worsen. If symptoms persist, consult a doctor. The use of this container by more than one person may spread infection. Do not use this product if you have heart disease, high blood pressure, thyroid disease, diabetes, or difficulty in urination due to enlargement of the prostate gland unless directed by a doctor. As with any drug, if you are pregnant or nursing a baby, seek the advice of a health professional before using this product. Keep this and all drugs out of the reach of children. In case of accidental ingestion seek professional assistance or contact a Poison Control Center immediately.

Directions: Adults and children 12 years of age and over: 2 or 3 sprays in each nostril not more often than every 4 hours. Do not give to children under 12 years of age unless directed by a doctor. To spray, squeeze bottle quickly and firmly. Do not tilt head backward while spraying. Wipe nozzle clean after use.

How Supplied: 15 mL plastic squeeze bottle.
Store between 2° and 30°C (36° and 86°F).

Shown in Product Identification Guide, page 519

AFRIN® Saline Mist w/Eucalyptol and Menthol
[*á frin*]

Ingredients: Water, PEG-32, Propylene Glycol, Sodium Chloride, PVP, Disodium Phosphate, Sodium Phosphate, Benzyl Alcohol, Polysorbate 80, Benzalkonium Chloride, Menthol, Camphor, Eucalyptol, Disodium EDTA.

Indications: Provides gentle, soothing moisture to irritated dry, nasal passages due to colds, allergies, air pollution, smoke, dry air (low humidity) and air travel. AFRIN Saline Mist loosens and thins mucous secretions to clear stuffy, blocked nasal passages. And since it is non-medicated, AFRIN Saline Mist is safe to use with cold, allergy and sinus medications; it is also safe enough for infants.

Directions: For infants, children and adults: 2 to 6 sprays in each nostril as often as needed or as directed by a doctor. For a fine mist, keep bottle upright; for a stream, keep bottle horizontal. Wipe nozzle clean after use.
Keep out of the reach of children. The use of this dispenser by more than one person may spread infection.

How Supplied: Afrin Saline Mist with Eucalyptol and Menthol—45 mL plastic squeeze bottle.

Shown in Product Identification Guide, page 520

AFRIN® Moisturizing Saline Mist
[*á frin*]

Ingredients: Water, PEG-32, Sodium Chloride, PVP, Disodium Phosphate, Sodium Phosphate, Benzalkonium Chloride, Disodium EDTA.

CONTAINS NO ALCOHOL

Indications: Provides soothing moisture to dry, irritated nasal passages caused by colds, allergies, low humidity, and other minor nasal irritations. Afrin Moisturizing Saline Mist loosens and thins mucus secretions to aid removal of mucus from nose and sinuses. Afrin Moisturizing Saline Mist can be used as often as needed, and is safe to use with cold, allergy, and sinus medications. It is also safe enough for infants.

Directions: For infants, children, and adults, 2 to 6 sprays in each nostril as often as needed or as directed by a doctor. For a fine mist, keep bottle upright; for a stream, keep bottle horizontal. Wipe nozzle clean after use.

Keep out of the reach of children.

The use of this dispenser by more than one person may spread infection.

How Supplied: Afrin Moisturizing Saline Mist—45 mL plastic squeeze bottle.

AFRIN® NASAL DECONGESTANT CHILDREN'S Pump Mist
Phenylephrine Hydrochloride

• Safe for kids 6–12 years old
• Clears stuffy noses fast
• Specially formulated to be mild and moisturizing
• Easy action pump delivers a precise, measured dose each time

Active Ingredient: Phenylephrine Hydrochloride 0.25%.

Inactive Ingredients: Benzalkonium Chloride, Edetate Disodium, Glycerin, Polyethylene Glycol 1450, Propylene Glycol, Sodium Phosphate Dibasic, Sodium Phosphate Monobasic, Water.

Indications: For temporary relief of nasal congestion due to colds, hay fever or other upper respiratory allergies, or associated with sinusitis. Shrinks swollen nasal membranes so you can breathe more freely.

Warnings: Do not exceed recommended dosage. This product may cause temporary discomfort such as burning, stinging, sneezing, or an increase in nasal discharge. Do not use this product for more than 3 days. Use only as directed. Frequent or prolonged use may cause nasal congestion to recur or worsen. If symptoms persist, consult a doctor. The use of this container by more than one person may spread infection. Do not use this product if you have heart disease, high blood pressure, thyroid disease, diabetes, or difficulty in urination due to enlargement of the prostate gland unless directed by a doctor. As with any drug, if you are pregnant or nursing a baby, seek the advice of a health professional before using this product. Keep this and all drugs out of the reach of children. In case of accidental ingestion, seek professional assistance or contact a Poison Control Center immediately.

Important: RETAIN CARTON FOR FUTURE REFERENCE ON FULL LABELING AND WARNINGS.

Directions: Adults and children 6 to under 12 years of age (with adult supervision): 2 or 3 sprays in each nostril not more often than every 4 hours. Do not give to children under 6 years of age unless directed by a doctor.
To spray, remove protective cap. Hold bottle with thumb at base and nozzle between first and second fingers. Without tilting head, insert nozzle into nostril.

Continued on next page

Information on Schering-Plough HealthCare Products appearing on these pages is effective as of November 1998.

Afrin Children's Pump—Cont.

Fully depress rim with a firm, even stroke and sniff deeply. Wipe nozzle clean after use. Before using the first time, remove the protective cap from the tip and prime metered pump by depressing pump firmly several times.

How Supplied: Afrin Nasal Decongestant
Children's Pump Mist—1/2 FL OZ (15 mL)
Store between 2° and 30°C (36° and 86°F).
21029700/05591-00
©1994, 1997 Distributed by Schering-Plough HealthCare Products, Inc., Memphis, TN 38151 USA. All rights reserved. Patent Pending. Made in USA.

CHLOR–TRIMETON®
[klor-tri 'mě-ton]
4 Hour Allergy Tablets
8 Hour Allergy Tablets
12 Hour Allergy Tablets

Active Ingredients: Each 4 Hour Allergy Tablet contains: 4 mg chlorpheniramine maleate, also contains: Corn Starch, D&C Yellow No. 10 Aluminum Lake, Lactose, Magnesium Stearate. **Each 8 Hour Allergy Tablet contains:** 8 mg chlorpheniramine maleate; also contains: Acacia, Butylparaben, Calcium Phosphate, Calcium Sulfate, Carnauba Wax, Corn Starch, D&C Yellow No. 10 Aluminum Lake, FD&C Yellow No. 6 Aluminum Lake, FD&C Yellow No. 6, Lactose, Magnesium Stearate, Neutral Soap, Oleic Acid, Potato Starch, Rosin, Sugar, Talc, White Wax, Zein. **Each 12 Hour Allergy Tablet contains:** 12 mg chlorpheniramine maleate; also contains: Acacia, Butylparaben, Calcium Phosphate, Calcium Sulfate, Carnauba Wax, Corn Starch, D&C Yellow No. 10 Aluminum Lake, FD&C Blue No. 2 Aluminum Lake, FD&C Yellow No. 6, FD&C Yellow No. 6 Aluminum Lake, Lactose, Magnesium Stearate, Neutral Soap, Oleic Acid, Potato Starch, Rosin, Sugar, Talc, White Wax, Zein.

Indications: For effective temporary relief of sneezing, itchy, watery eyes, itchy throat, and runny nose due to hay fever and other upper respiratory allergies.

Warnings: May cause excitability especially in children. Do not give the 8 Hour or 12 Hour Allergy Tablets to children under 12 years, or 4 Hour Allergy Tablets to children under 6 years except under the advice and supervision of a doctor. Do not take this product, unless directed by a doctor, if you have a breathing problem such as emphysema or chronic bronchitis, or if you have glaucoma, difficulty in urination due to enlargement of the prostate gland. May cause drowsiness; alcohol, sedatives and tranquilizers may increase the drowsiness effect. Avoid alcoholic beverages while taking this product. Do not take this product if you are taking sedatives or tranquilizers, without first consulting your doctor. Use caution when driving a motor vehicle or operating machinery. As with any drug, if you are pregnant or nursing a baby, seek the advice of a health professional before using this product. Keep this and all drugs out of the reach of children. In case of accidental overdose, seek professional assistance or contact a Poison Control Center immediately.

Dosage and Administration: 4 Hour Allergy Tablets—Adults and Children 12 years of age and over: Oral dosage is one tablet (4 mg) every 4 to 6 hours, not to exceed 6 tablets (24 mg) in 24 hours or as directed by a doctor. Children 6 to under 12 years of age: Oral dosage is one half the adult dose (2 mg) (break tablet in half) every 4 to 6 hours, not to exceed 3 whole tablets (12 mg) in 24 hours, or as directed by a doctor. Children under 6 years of age: consult a doctor.
8 Hour Allergy Tablets—Adults and Children 12 years and over—One tablet every 8 to 12 hours. Do not take more than one tablet every 8 hours or 3 tablets in 24 hours. Children under 12 years of age: Consult a doctor.
12 Hour Allergy Tablets—Adults and children 12 years and over—One tablet every 12 hours. Do not exceed 2 tablets in 24 hours. Children under 12 years of age: Consult a doctor.

How Supplied: CHLOR-TRIMETON 4 Hour Allergy Tablets, box of 24, bottles of 100.
CHLOR-TRIMETON 8 Hour Allergy Tablets, boxes of 15, bottles of 100.
CHLOR-TRIMETON 12 Hour Allergy Tablets, boxes of 10 and 24, bottles of 100.
Store between 2° and 30°C (36° and 86°F). Protect from excessive moisture.
Shown in Product Identification Guide, page 520

CHLOR–TRIMETON®
[klortri 'mě-ton]
4 Hour Allergy/Decongestant Tablets
12 Hour Allergy/Decongestant Tablets

Active Ingredients: Each 4 Hour Allergy/Decongestant Tablet contains: 4 mg chlorpheniramine maleate, and 60 mg pseudoephedrine sulfate; also contains: Corn Starch, FD&C Blue No. 1, Lactose, Magnesium Stearate, Povidone.
Each 12 Hour Allergy/Decongestant Tablet contains: 8 mg chlorpheniramine maleate and 120 mg pseudoephedrine sulfate; also contains: Acacia, Butylparaben, Calcium Sulfate, Carnauba Wax, Corn Starch, D&C Yellow No. 10 Aluminum Lake, FD&C Blue No. 1 Aluminum Lake, FD&C Yellow No. 6 Aluminum Lake, Gelatin, Lactose, Magnesium Stearate, Neutral Soap, Oleic Acid, Povidone, Rosin, Sugar, Talc, White Wax, Zein.

Indications: For the temporary relief of runny nose, sneezing, itching of the nose or throat, itchy, watery eyes and nasal congestion due to hay fever or other upper respiratory allergies. Helps decongest sinus openings and passages. Reduces swelling of nasal passages, shrinks swollen membranes, and temporarily restores freer breathing through the nose.
Warnings: CHLOR-TRIMETON 4 HOUR ALLERGY/DECONGESTANT: Do not exceed recommended dosage. If nervousness, dizziness, or sleeplessness occur, discontinue use and consult a doctor. If symptoms do not improve within 7 days or are accompanied by fever, consult a doctor. Do not take this product unless directed by a doctor, if you have a breathing problem such as emphysema, chronic bronchitis, or if you have glaucoma, heart disease, high blood pressure, thyroid disease, diabetes, or difficulty in urination due to enlargement of the prostate gland. May cause excitability, especially in children. May cause drowsiness; alcohol, sedatives, and tranquilizers may increase the drowsiness effect. Avoid alcoholic beverages while taking this product. Do not take this product if you are taking sedatives or tranquilizers, without first consulting your doctor. Use caution when driving a motor vehicle or operating machinery. As with any drug, if you are pregnant or nursing a baby, seek the advice of a health professional before using this product. Keep this and all drugs out of the reach of children. In case of accidental overdose, seek professional assistance or contact a Poison Control Center immediately.

Drug Interaction Precaution: Do not use this product if you are taking a prescription monoamine oxidase inhibitor (MAOI) (certain drugs for depression, psychiatric or emotional conditions, or Parkinson's disease), or for 2 weeks after stopping the MAOI drug. If you are uncertain whether your prescription drug contains an MAOI, consult a health professional before taking this product.
CHLOR-TRIMETON 12 HOUR ALLERGY/DECONGESTANT: Do not exceed recommended dosage. If nervousness, dizziness, or sleeplessness occur, discontinue use and consult a doctor. If symptoms do not improve within 7 days or are accompanied by fever, consult a doctor. Do not take this product unless directed by a doctor if you have a breathing problem such as emphysema, chronic bronchitis, or if you have glaucoma, heart disease, high blood pressure, thyroid disease, diabetes, or difficulty in urination due to enlargement of the prostate gland, or give this product children under 12 years of age. May cause excitability especially in children. May cause drowsiness; alcohol, sedatives, and tranquilizers may increase the drowsiness effect. Avoid alcoholic beverages while taking this product. Do not take this product if you are taking sedatives or tranquilizers without first consulting a doctor. Use caution when driving a motor vehicle or

operating machinery. As with any drug, if you are pregnant or nursing a baby, seek the advice of a health professional before using this product. Keep this and all drugs out of the reach of children. In case of accidental overdose, seek professional assistance or contact a Poison Control Center immediately.

Drug Interaction Precaution: Do not use this product if you are taking a prescription monoamine oxidase inhibitor (MAOI) (certain drugs for depression, psychiatric or emotional conditions, or Parkinson's disease), or for 2 weeks after stopping the MAOI drug. If you are uncertain whether your prescription drug contains an MAOI, consult a health professional before taking this product.

Dosage and Administration: 4 Hour Allergy/Decongestant Tablets— ADULTS AND CHILDREN 12 YEARS OF AGE AND OVER: Oral dosage is one tablet every 4 to 6 hours, not to exceed 4 tablets in 24 hours, or as directed by a doctor. CHILDREN 6 TO UNDER 12 YEARS OF AGE: Oral dosage is one half the adult dose (break tablet in half) every 4 to 6 hours, not to exceed 2 whole tablets in 24 hours, or as directed by a doctor. CHILDREN UNDER 6 YEARS OF AGE: Consult a doctor. **12 Hour Allergy/Decongestant Tablets**—ADULTS AND CHILDREN 12 YEARS AND OVER: one tablet every 12 hours. Do not exceed 2 tablets in 24 hours. CHILDREN UNDER 12 YEARS OF AGE: Consult a doctor.

How Supplied: CHLOR-TRIMETON 4 Hour Allergy/Decongestant Tablets— boxes of 24. CHLOR-TRIMETON 12 Hour Allergy/Decongestant Tablets boxes of 10 and 24.
Store these CHLOR-TRIMETON Products between 2° and 30°C (36°and 86°F); and protect from excessive moisture.
Shown in Product Identification Guide, page 520

**CLEAR AWAY®
ONE STEP FOR KIDS
Medicated Wart Removal Strips**

Active Ingredient: Medicated strips contain Salicylic Acid 40% in a rubber-based vehicle.

Indications: For removal of common warts on hands, recognized by the rough, cauliflower-like appearance of the surface.

Warning: For external use only. Do not use this product on irritated skin, on any area that is infected or reddened, if you are a diabetic, or if you have poor blood circulation. If discomfort persists, see your doctor. Do not use on moles, birthmarks, warts with hair growing from them, genital warts or warts on the face or mucous membranes. Keep this and all drugs out of the reach of children. In case of accidental ingestion, seek professional assistance or contact a Poison Control Center immediately. Not recommended for children under the age of 2 except at the advice of a doctor.

Directions:
Parents should supervise use by children.
1. Wash affected area. Dry area thoroughly.
2. Apply medicated pad. Repeat procedure every 48 hours as needed (until wart is removed) up to 12 weeks.
NOTE: When applying medicated pad to wart, secure adhesive strips firmly to skin.

How Supplied: Clear Away One Step For Kids includes 14 medicated strips in a variety of fun, multi-colored designs that help to protect and conceal while treatment is ongoing.

Store between 15° and 30°C (59° and 86°F).

Shown in Product Identification Guide, page 520

**CLEAR AWAY®
ONE STEP WART REMOVAL
SYSTEM**

Active Ingredient: Medicated strips contain Salicylic Acid 40% in a rubber-based vehicle.

Indications: For removal of common warts on hands, recognized by the rough, cauliflower-like appearance of the surface.

Warning: For external use only. Do not use this product on irritated skin, on any area that is infected or reddened, if you are a diabetic, or if you have poor blood circulation. If discomfort persists, see your doctor. Do not use on moles, birthmarks, warts with hair growing from them, genital warts or warts on the face or mucous membranes. Keep this and all drugs out of the reach of children. In case of accidental ingestion, seek professional assistance or contact a Poison Control Center immediately.

Directions:
1. Wash affected area. Dry area thoroughly.
2. Apply medicated pad. Repeat procedure every 48 hours as needed (until wart is removed) up to 12 weeks.
NOTE: When applying medicated pad to wart, secure adhesive strips firmly to skin.

How Supplied: Clear Away One Step includes 14 all-in-one medicated strips that protect and conceal while treatment is ongoing. Conceals as it Heals™.

Store between 15°C and 30°C (59° and 86°F).

Shown in Product Identification Guide, page 520

CORICIDIN® HBP™ Cold & Flu Tablets
[*kor-a-see 'din*]

CORICIDIN® HBP™ Cough & Cold Tablets

CORICIDIN HBP™ NightTime Cold & Cough Liquid

CORICIDIN D® Decongestant Tablets

Active Ingredients: CORICIDIN HBP Cold & Flu Tablets—325 mg acetaminophen, 2 mg chlorpheniramine maleate. **CORICIDIN® HBP Cough & Cold Tablets**—4 mg chlorpheniramine maleate, 30 mg dextromethorphan hydrobromide. **CORICIDIN HBP NightTime Cold & Cough Liquid**—per tablespoon ($^1/_2$ fl. oz.)—325 mg Acetaminophen, 12.5 mg Diphenhydramine Hydrochloride. **CORICIDIN D Decongestant Tablets**— 325 mg acetaminophen, 2 mg chlorpheniramine maleate, 12.5 mg phenylpropanolamine hydrochloride.

Inactive Ingredients: CORICIDIN HBP Cold & Flu Tablets—Acacia, Butylparaben, Calcium Sulfate, Carnauba Wax, Cellulose, Corn Starch, FD&C Red No. 40 Aluminum Lake, FD&C Yellow No. 6 Aluminum Lake, Lactose, Magnesium Stearate, Povidone, Sugar, Talc, Titanium Dioxide, White Wax. **CORICIDIN® HBP Cough & Cold Tablets**—Acacia, Calcium Sulfate, Carnauba Wax, Croscarmellose Sodium, D&C Red No. 27 Aluminum Lake, FD&C Yellow No. 6 Aluminum Lake, Lactose, Magnesium Stearate, Microcrystalline Cellulose, Povidone, Sodium Benzoate, Sugar, Talc, Titanium Dioxide, White Wax. **CORICIDIN® HBP NightTime Cold & Cough Liquid**—Citric Acid, FD&C Blue No. 1, FD&C Red No. 40, Flavor, Glycerin, Polyethylene Glycol, Propylene Glycol, Sodium Citrate, Sodium Saccharin, Sugar, Water. **CORICIDIN D Decongestant Tablets**— Acacia, Butylparaben, Calcium Sulfate, Carnauba Wax, Cellulose, Corn Starch, Magnesium Stearate, Povidone, Sugar, Talc, Titanium Dioxide, White Wax.

Indications: CORICIDIN HBP Cold & Flu Tablets temporarily relieve minor aches, pains and headache, and reduce the fever associated with colds or flu; temporarily relieve sneezing, runny nose and itchy watery eyes due to hay fever, other upper respiratory allergies or the common cold. **Unlike most cold remedies, CORICIDIN HBP Cold & Flu Tablets do not contain a decongestant and therefore are suitable for hypertensive patients.**

Continued on next page

Information on Schering-Plough HealthCare Products appearing on these pages is effective as of November 1998.

Coricidin HBP/D—Cont.

CORICIDIN HBP Cough & Cold Tablets temporarily relieve coughs due to minor throat irritations as may occur with a cold; temporarily relieve sneezing, runny nose and itchy, watery eyes due to the common cold, hayfever or other respiratory allergies. **Unlike most cold remedies, CORICIDIN HBP Cough & Cold Tablets do not contain a decongestant and therefore are suitable for hypertensive patients.**

CORICIDIN® HBP NightTime Cold & Cough Liquid Temporarily relieves common cold/flu symptoms: minor aches, pain, headache, sore throat, fever, runny nose, sneezing, cough due to minor throat and bronchial irritation. **Unlike most cold remedies, CORICIDIN HBP NightTime Cold & Cough Liquid does not contain a decongestant and therefore is suitable for hypertensive patients.**

CORICIDIN D Tablets temporarily relieve minor aches and pains, and reduces the fever associated with a cold or flu. Provides temporary relief of: sneezing and runny nose; nasal congestion due to the common cold and associated with sinusitis; stuffy nose; sinus congestion and pressure. Helps decongest sinus openings and passages.

Warnings: CORICIDIN HBP Cold & Flu Tablets—Do not take this product for pain for more than 10 days (adults) or 5 days (children 6 to under 12 years of age) and do not take for fever for more than 3 days unless directed by a doctor. If pain or fever persists or gets worse, if new symptoms occur, or if redness or swelling is present, consult a doctor because these could be signs of a serious condition. May cause excitability especially in children. Do not take this product, unless directed by a doctor, if you have a breathing problem such as emphysema or chronic bronchitis, or if you have glaucoma or difficulty in urination due to enlargement of the prostate gland. May cause drowsiness; alcohol, sedatives, and tranquilizers may increase the drowsiness effect. Avoid alcoholic beverages while taking this product. Do not take this product if you are taking sedatives or tranquilizers without first consulting your doctor. Use caution when driving a motor vehicle or operating machinery. As with any drug if you are pregnant or nursing a baby, seek the advice of a health professional before using this product. Keep this and all drugs out of the reach of children. In case of accidental overdose, seek professional assistance or contact a Poison Control Center immediately. Prompt medical attention is critical for adults as well as for children even if you do not notice any signs or symptoms.

Alcohol Warning: If you generally consume 3 or more alcohol containing drinks per day, you should consult your doctor on when and how you should take this product and other pain relievers.

CORICIDIN HBP Cough & Cold Tablets—A persistent cough may be a sign of a serious condition. If cough persists for more than 1 week, tends to recur, or is accompanied by fever, rash or persistent headache, consult a doctor. Do not take this product for persistent or chronic cough such as occurs with smoking, asthma, emphysema, or if cough is accompanied by excessive phlegm (mucus) unless directed by a doctor. May cause excitability, especially in children. Do not take this product, unless directed by a doctor, if you have a breathing problem such as emphysema or chronic bronchitis, or if you have glaucoma or difficulty in urination due to enlargement of the prostate gland. May cause marked drowsiness; alcohol, sedatives, and tranquilizers may increase the drowsiness effect. Avoid alcoholic beverages while taking this product. Do not take this product if you are taking sedatives or tranquilizers, without first consulting your doctor. Use caution when driving a motor vehicle or operating machinery. As with any drug, if you are pregnant or nursing a baby, seek the advice of a health professional before using this product. Keep this and all drugs out of the reach of children. In case of accidental overdose, seek professional assistance or contact a Poison Control Center immediately.

DRUG INTERACTION PRECAUTION: Do not use this product if you are now taking a prescription monoamine oxidase inhibitor (MAOI) (certain drugs for depression, psychiatric or emotional conditions, or Parkinson's disease), or for 2 weeks after stopping the MAOI drug. If you are uncertain whether your prescription drug contains an MAOI, consult a health professional before taking this product.

CORICIDIN® HBP NightTime Cold & Cough Liquid—Do not take this product for pain for more than 10 days (adults) or 5 days (children) or for fever for more than 3 days unless directed by a doctor. If pain or fever persists or gets worse, if new symptoms occur, if redness or swelling is present, or if cough persists, consult a doctor because these could be signs of a serious condition. If cough persists for more than 1 week, tends to recur is accompanied by fever, rash, or persistent headache, consult a doctor. If sore throat is severe, persists for more than 2 days, is accompanied or followed by fever, headache, rash, nausea or vomiting, consult a doctor promptly. Do not take this product for persistent or chronic cough such as occurs with smoking, asthma, or emphysema, or if cough is accompanied by excessive phlegm (mucus) unless directed by a doctor. May cause excitability especially in children. Do not take this product, unless directed by a doctor, if you have a breathing problem, such as emphysema or chronic bronchitis, or if you have glaucoma or difficulty in urination due to enlargement of the prostate gland. May cause marked drowsiness; alcohol, sedatives, and tranquilizers may increase the drowsiness effect. Avoid alcoholic bever-

ages while taking this product. Use caution when driving a motor vehicle or operating machinery. As with any drug, if you are pregnant or nursing a baby, seek the advice of a health professional before using this product. Keep this and all drugs out of the reach of children. In case of accidental overdose, seek the advice assistance or contact a Poison Control Center immediately. Prompt medical attention is critical for adults as well as for children even if you do not notice any signs or symptoms.

Do not use with any other product containing diphenhydramine, including one applied topically.

Alcohol Warning: If you generally consume 3 or more alcohol-containing drinks per day, you should consult your doctor on when and how you should take this product and other pain relievers.

CORICIDIN D Decongestant Tablets—Do not exceed recommended dosage. If nervousness, dizziness, or sleeplessness occur, discontinue use and consult a doctor. If congestion does not improve within 7 days, consult a doctor. Do not take this product for pain for more than 10 days (adults) or 5 days (children 6 to under 12 years) or for fever for more than 3 days unless directed by a doctor. If pain or fever persists or gets worse, if new symptoms occur, or if redness or swelling is present, consult a doctor because these could be signs of a serious condition. May cause excitability, especially in children. Do not take this product, unless directed by a doctor if you have a breathing problem such as emphysema or chronic bronchitis, or if you have glaucoma, heart disease, high blood pressure, thyroid disease, diabetes, or difficulty in urination due to enlargement of the prostate gland. May cause drowsiness; alcohol, sedatives, and tranquilizers may increase the drowsiness effect. Avoid alcoholic beverages while taking this product. Do not take this product if you are taking sedatives or tranquilizers without first consulting your doctor. Use caution when driving a motor vehicle or operating machinery. As with any drug, if you are pregnant or nursing a baby, seek the advice of a health professional before using this product. Keep this and all drugs out of the reach of children. In case of accidental overdose, seek professional assistance or contact a Poison Control Center immediately. Prompt medical attention is critical for adults as well as for children even if you do not notice any signs or symptoms.

Alcohol Warning: If you generally consume 3 or more alcohol-containing drinks per day, you should consult your doctor on when and how you should take this product and other pain relievers.

Drug Interaction Precaution: Do not use this product if you are now taking a prescription monoamine oxidase inhibitor (MAOI) (certain drugs for depression, psychiatric or emotional conditions, or Parkinson's disease), or for 2 weeks after stopping the MAOI drug. If you are uncertain whether your prescription drug contains an MAOI, consult a health professional before taking this product. Do not use this product if you are now taking an appetite-controlling medication containing phenylpropanolamine.

Dosage and Administration: CORICIDIN HBP Cold & Flu Tablets— Adults and children 12 years of age and over: oral dosage is 2 tablets every 4 to 6 hours, not to exceed 12 tablets in 24 hours, or as directed by a doctor. **Children 6 to under 12 years of age:** oral dosage is 1 tablet every 4 to 6 hours, not to exceed 5 tablets in 24 hours, or as directed by a doctor. **Children under 6 years of age:** consult a doctor.
CORICIDIN HBP Cough & Cold Tablets— Adults and Children 12 years of age and over: one tablet every 6 hours, not to exceed 4 tablets in 24 hours. This product is not for children under 12 years of age.
CORICIDIN HBP NightTime Cold & Cough Liquid—Adults and children 12 years of age and over: Oral dosage is two tablespoons (1 fl oz) every 4 hours, not to exceed 6 doses in 24 hours, or as directed by a doctor. **Children 6 to under 12 years of age:** Oral dosage is one tablespoon ($^{1}/_{2}$ fl oz) every 4 hours, not to exceed 5 doses in 24 hours, or as directed by a doctor. **Children under 6 years of age:** Consult a doctor.
CORICIDIN D Decongestant Tablets — Adults and children 12 years of age and over: oral dosage is 2 tablets every 4 hours not to exceed 12 tablets in 24 hours, or as directed by a doctor. **Children 6 to under 12 years of age:** oral dosage is 1 tablet every 4 hours not to exceed 5 tablets in 24 hours, or as directed by a doctor. **Children under 6 years of age:** consult a doctor.

How Supplied: CORICIDIN HBP Cold & Flu Tablets— Bottles of 48, and 100 tablets, blisters of 12 and 24.
CORICIDIN HBP Cough & Cold Tablets— blisters of 16.
CORICIDIN HBP NightTime Cold & Cough Liquid—6 oz. bottles.
CORICIDIN D Decongestant Tablets— blisters of 12, 24, and 48.
Store between 2° and 30°C (36° and 86°F).

Shown in Product Identification Guide, page 520

CORRECTOL®
Laxative Tablets and Caplets

Active Ingredient: Bisacodyl, 5 mg.

Inactive Ingredients: Acetylated monoglycerides, calcium sulfate, carnauba wax, D&C Red no. 7 calcium lake, gelatin, hydroxypropyl methylcellulose phthalate, lactose, magnesium stearate, sugar, talc, titanium dioxide, white wax.

Indications: For gentle, overnight relief of occasional constipation and irregularity. Correctol Laxative generally produces a bowel movement in 6 to 12 hours.

Warnings: Do not chew tablets or caplets. Do not give to children under 6 years of age, or to persons who cannot swallow without chewing, unless directed by a doctor. Do not take this product within 1 hour after taking an antacid or milk. Do not use laxative products when abdominal pain, nausea, or vomiting are present unless directed by a doctor. If you have noticed a sudden change in bowel habits that persists over a period of 2 weeks, consult a doctor before using a laxative. Laxative products should not be used for a period longer than 1 week unless directed by a doctor. Rectal bleeding or failure to have a bowel movement after use of a laxative may indicate a serious condition. Discontinue use and consult a doctor. All stimulant laxatives may cause abdominal discomfort, faintness, and cramps. As with any drug, if you are pregnant or nursing a baby, seek the advice of a health professional before using this product. Keep this and all drugs out of the reach of children. In case of accidental overdose, seek professional assistance or contact a Poison Control Center immediately. Store at temperatures not above 86°F (30°C). Protect from excessive moisture.

Directions: Adults and children 12 years of age and older: Take 1 to 3 tablets or caplets in a single dose once daily. **Children 6 to under 12 years of age:** Take 1 tablet or caplet once daily. **Children under 6 years of age:** consult a doctor. **Do not chew or crush tablets or caplets.**

Each laxative works differently. Adults and children over 12 may need fewer tablets or caplets of Correctol to get the same effect as more tablets or caplets of another brand. **We recommend you start with one Correctol tablet or caplet and take with water.** If one tablet or caplet does not produce desired results, then try two or three Correctol tablets or caplets daily. Do not take more than 3 tablets or caplets of Correctol daily.

How Supplied: Tablets: Individual foil-backed safety sealed blister packaging in boxes of 10, 30, 60, & 90 tablets. Caplets: Individual foil-backed safety sealed blister packaging in boxes of 30 caplets.

Shown in Product Identification Guide, page 520

CORRECTOL® STOOL SOFTENER
Laxative

Active Ingredient: Docusate sodium 100 mg. per soft gel.
Also Contains—D&C Red No. 33, FD&C Red No. 40, FD&C Yellow No. 6, gelatin, glycerin, polyethylene glycol 400, propylene glycol, sorbitol.

Indications: For relief of occasional constipation. Correctol Stool Softener generally produces a bowel movement in 12 to 72 hours.

Warning: Do not use laxative products when abdominal pain, nausea, or vomiting are present unless directed by a doctor. If you have noticed a sudden change in bowel habits that persists over two weeks, consult a doctor before using a laxative. Laxative products should not be used for longer than 1 week unless directed by a doctor. Rectal bleeding or failure to have a bowel movement after use of a laxative may indicated a serious condition. Discontinue use and consult your doctor. As with any drug, if you are pregnant or nursing a baby, seek the advice of a health professional before using this product. Keep this and all drugs out of the reach of children. In case of accidental overdose, seek professional assistance or contact a Poison Control Center immediately.

Drug Interaction Precaution: Do not take this product if you are presently taking mineral oil, unless directed by a doctor.

Directions: Adults and Children 12 years of age and older: Take 1 to 3 soft gels daily. **Children 2 to under 12 years of age:** Take 1 soft gel daily. **Children under 2 years of age:** Consult a doctor.

How Supplied: Tablets—individual foil-backed safety sealed blister packaging in boxes of 30 tablets.
Store below 86°F. Protect from freezing.

Shown in Product Identification Guide, page 520

DI–GEL®
Antacid · Anti-Gas
Tablets

DI-GEL Tablets: Active Ingredients: (Per Tablet)—Simethicone 20 mg., Calcium Carbonate 280 mg., Magnesium Hydroxide 128 mg. **Inactive Ingredients:** D & C yellow No. 10 aluminum lake, dextrin, FD&C yellow No. 6 aluminum lake, flavor, magnesium stearate, mannitol, povidone, stearic acid, sucrose, talc.
Dietetically sodium free, calcium rich.

Indications: For fast, temporary relief of acid indigestion, heartburn, sour stomach and accompanying symptoms of gas.

Actions: When excess acid and bubbles of gas are trapped in the stomach, they can cause heartburn and acid indigestion.
The white layer of Di-Gel goes to work fast to neutralize excess acid. And unlike plain antacids, the Simethicone in the yellow layer breaks up gas bubbles rapidly.

Continued on next page

Information on Schering-Plough HealthCare Products appearing on these pages is effective as of November 1998.

Di-Gel—Cont.

Warnings: Do not take more than 24 tablets in a 24 hour period, or use the maximum dosage of this product for more than 2 weeks, except under the advice and supervision of a physician. If you have kidney disease do not use this product except under the advice and supervision of a physician. Tablets may cause constipation or have a laxative effect. Keep this and all drugs out of the reach of children.

Drug Interaction: Antacids may interact with certain prescription drugs. If you are presently taking a prescription drug, do not take this product without checking with your doctor or other health professional.

Directions: TABLETS: Chew 2 to 4 tablets every 2 hours, after or between meals and at bedtime, or as directed by a doctor.

How Supplied:
DI-GEL Tablets in Mint and Lemon/Orange Flavor - In boxes of 30 and 90 in handy portable safety sealed blister packaging.
Shown in Product Identification Guide, page 521

DRIXORAL® COLD & ALLERGY
[*dricks-or 'al*]
Sustained-Action Tablets

Description: EACH DRIXORAL® COLD & ALLERGY SUSTAINED-ACTION TABLET CONTAINS: 120 mg of pseudoephedrine sulfate and 6 mg of dexbrompheniramine maleate. Half of the medication is released after the tablet is swallowed and the remaining amount of medication is released hours later providing continuous long-lasting relief for 12 hours. Inactive Ingredients: Acacia, Butylparaben, Calcium Sulfate, Carnauba Wax, Corn Starch, D&C Yellow No. 10 Aluminum Lake, FD&C Blue No. 1 Aluminum Lake, FD&C Yellow No. 6 Aluminum Lake, Gelatin, Lactose, Magnesium Stearate, Neutral Soap, Oleic Acid, Povidone, Rosin, Sugar, Talc, White Wax, Zein.

Indications: The decongestant (pseudoephedrine sulfate) temporarily relieves nasal congestion due to the common cold, hay fever or other upper respiratory allergies, and associated with sinusitis. Helps decongest sinus openings and sinus passages. Reduces swelling of nasal passages; shrinks swollen membranes; and temporarily restores freer breathing through the nose. The antihistamine (dexbrompheniramine maleate) alleviates runny nose, sneezing, itching of the nose or throat and itchy and watery eyes as may occur in allergic rhinitis (such as hay fever).

Warnings: Do not exceed recommended dosage. If nervousness, dizziness, or sleeplessness occur, discontinue use and consult a doctor. If symptoms do not improve within 7 days, or are accompanied by fever, consult a doctor. May cause excitability especially in children. Do not take this product if you have a breathing problem such as emphysema or chronic bronchitis, or if you have glaucoma, heart disease, high blood pressure, thyroid disease, diabetes, or difficulty in urination due to enlargement of the prostate gland, or give this product to children under 12 years of age, unless directed by a doctor. May cause drowsiness; alcohol, sedatives, and tranquilizers may increase the drowsiness effect. Avoid alcoholic beverages while taking this product. Do not take this product if you are taking sedatives or tranquilizers without first consulting your doctor. Use caution when driving a motor vehicle or operating machinery. As with any drug, if you are pregnant or nursing a baby, seek the advice of a health professional before using this product. Keep this and all drugs out of the reach of children. In case of accidental overdose, seek professional assistance or contact a Poison Control Center immediately.

Drug Interaction Precaution: Do not use this product if you are now taking a prescription monoamine oxidase inhibitor (MAOI) (certain drugs for depression, psychiatric or emotional conditions, or Parkinson's disease),or for 2 weeks after stopping the MAOI drug. If you are uncertain whether your prescription drug contains an MAOI, consult a health professional before taking this product.

Dosage and Administration: ADULTS AND CHILDREN 12 YEARS AND OVER—one tablet every 12 hours. Do not exceed two tablets in 24 hours.
Children under 12 years of age: Consult a doctor.

How Supplied: DRIXORAL® Cold & Allergy Sustained-Action Tablets, green, sugar-coated tablets branded in black with the product name, boxes of 10, 20, and 30, bottle of 100 (for institutional sale only).
Store between 2° and 25°C (36° and 77°F).
Protect from excessive moisture.
Shown in Product Identification Guide, page 521

DRIXORAL® Nasal Decongestant
[*dricks-or 'al*]
Long-Acting Nasal Decongestant

DRIXORAL® Nasal Decongestant Long-Acting Nasal Decongestant Tablets contain 120 mg pseudoephedrine sulfate, a nasal decongestant, in an extended-release tablet providing up to 12 hours of continuous relief ...without drowsiness. Inactive Ingredients: Acacia, Butylparaben, Calcium Sulfate, Carnauba Wax, Corn Starch, FD&C Blue No. 1 Aluminum Lake, Gelatin, Lactose, Magnesium Stearate, Neutral Soap, Oleic Acid, Povidone, Rosin, Sugar, Talc, White Wax, Zein.

Indications: For temporary relief of nasal congestion due to the common cold, hay fever or other upper respiratory allergies, and associated with sinusitis. Helps decongest sinus openings and sinus passages.

Directions: Adults and Children 12 Years and Over—One tablet every 12 hours. Do not exceed two tablets in 24 hours. **Children under 12 years of age:** Consult a doctor.

Warnings: Do not exceed recommended dosage. If nervousness, dizziness, or sleeplessness occur, discontinue use and consult a doctor. If symptoms do not improve within 7 days or are accompanied by fever, consult a doctor. Do not take this product if you have heart disease, high blood pressure, thyroid disease, diabetes, or difficulty in urination due to enlargement of the prostate gland, or give this product to children under 12 years of age, unless directed by a doctor. As with any drug, if you are pregnant or nursing a baby, seek the advice of a health professional before using this product. Keep this and all drugs out of the reach of children. In case of accidental overdose, seek professional assistance or contact a Poison Control Center immediately.

Drug Interaction Precaution: Do not use this product if you are now taking a prescription monoamine oxidase inhibitor (MAOI) (certain drugs for depression, psychiatric or emotional conditions, or Parkinson's disease), or for 2 weeks after stopping the MAOI drug. If you are uncertain whether your prescription drug contains an MAOI, consult a health professional before taking this product.

How Supplied: DRIXORAL® Nasal Decongestant Long-Acting Non-Drowsy Tablets are available in boxes of 10's and 20's.
Store between 2° and 25°C (36° and 77°F).
Protect from excessive moisture.
Shown in Product Identification Guide, page 521

DRIXORAL® COLD & FLU
[*dricks-or 'al*]
Extended-Release Tablets

Active Ingredients: 500 mg Acetaminophen, 3 mg Dexbrompheniramine Maleate, 60 mg Pseudoephedrine Sulfate.

Inactive Ingredients: Calcium Phosphate, Carnauba Wax, D&C Yellow No. 10 Aluminum Lake, FD&C Blue No. 1 Aluminum Lake, FD&C Yellow No. 6 Aluminum Lake, Hydroxypropyl Methylcellulose, Magnesium Stearate, Methylparaben, PEG, Propylparaben, Stearic Acid.
DRIXORAL® COLD & FLU Extended-Release Tablets combine a nasal decongestant and an antihistamine with a pain reliever-fever reducer in a special 12-hour continuous-acting timed-release tablet.

Indications: The *decongestant* temporarily relieves nasal congestion due to the common cold, hay fever or other upper respiratory allergies, and associated with sinusitis. Reduces swelling of nasal passages; shrinks swollen membranes; and temporarily restores freer breathing through the nose. Also helps decongest sinus openings, sinus passages. The pain reliever-fever reducer temporarily relieves minor aches, pains, and headache and reduces fever due to the common cold. The *antihistamine* temporarily relieves runny nose and sneezing associated with the common cold.

Directions: ADULTS AND CHILDREN 12 YEARS AND OVER—two tablets every 12 hours. Do not exceed four tablets in 24 hours. **CHILDREN UNDER 12 YEARS OF AGE:** Consult a doctor.

Warnings: Do not exceed recommended dosage. If nervousness, dizziness, or sleeplessness occur, discontinue use and consult a doctor. If symptoms do not improve within 7 days , or are accompanied by fever that lasts for more than 3 days or recurs, consult a doctor before continuing use. If pain or fever persists or gets worse, if new symptoms occur, or if redness or swelling is present, consult a doctor because these could be signs of a serious condition. May cause excitability especially in children. Do not take this product if you have a breathing problem such as emphysema or chronic bronchitis, or if you have glaucoma, heart disease, high blood pressure, thyroid disease, diabetes, or difficulty in urination due to enlargement of the prostate gland, or give this product to children under 12 years of age, unless directed by a doctor. May cause drowsiness; alcohol, sedatives, and tranquilizers may increase the drowsiness effect. Avoid alcoholic beverages while taking this product. Do not take this product if you are taking sedatives or tranquilizers without first consulting your doctor. Use caution when driving a motor vehicle or operating machinery. As with any drug, if you are pregnant or nursing a baby, seek the advice of a health professional before using this product. Keep this and all drugs out of the reach of children. In case of accidental overdose, seek professional assistance or contact a Poison Control Center immediately. Prompt medical attention is critical for adults as well as for children even if you do not notice any signs or symptoms.

Alcohol Warning: If you generally consume 3 or more alcohol containing drinks per day, you should consult your doctor on when and how you should take this product and other pain relievers.

Drug Interaction Precaution: Do not use this product if you are now taking a prescription monoamine oxidase inhibitor (MAOI) (certain drugs for depression, psychiatric or emotional conditions, or Parkinson's disease), or for 2 weeks after stopping the MAOI drug. If you are uncertain whether your prescription drug contains an MAOI, consult a health professional before taking this product.

How Supplied: DRIXORAL® COLD & FLU Extended-Release Tablets are available in boxes of 12's and 24's.
Store between 2° and 25°C (36° and 77°F).
Protect from excessive moisture.
Shown in Product Identification Guide, page 521

DRIXORAL® ALLERGY/SINUS
[*dricks-or 'al*]
Nasal decongestant/Pain reliever/ Antihistamine

DRIXORAL® ALLERGY/SINUS Extended-Release Tablets combine a nasal decongestant, a non-aspirin pain-reliever, and an antihistamine in a 12-hour timed-release tablet.

Indications: The *decongestant* temporarily relieves nasal congestion due to sinusitis, the common cold, and hay fever or other upper respiratory allergies. Helps decongest sinus openings, sinus passages; relieves sinus pressure. Reduces swelling of nasal passages; shrinks swollen membranes; and temporarily restores freer breathing through the nose. The pain reliever temporarily relieves headaches, and minor aches and pains. The *antihistamine* alleviates runny nose, sneezing, itching of the nose or throat, and itchy and watery eyes as may occur in allergic rhinitis (such as hay fever).

Each DRIXORAL® ALLERGY/SINUS Extended-Release Tablet Contains: 60 mg of pseudoephedrine sulfate, 3 mg of dexbrompheniramine maleate, and 500 mg of acetaminophen. These ingredients are released continuously, providing long-lasting relief for 12 hours. Inactive Ingredients: Calcium Phosphate, Carnauba Wax, D&C Yellow No. 10 Aluminum Lake, FD&C Yellow No. 6 Aluminum Lake, Hydroxypropyl Methylcellulose, Magnesium Stearate, Methylparaben, PEG, Propylparaben, Stearic Acid.

Directions: ADULTS AND CHILDREN 12 YEARS AND OVER—two tablets every 12 hours. Do not exceed four tablets in 24 hours. **CHILDREN UNDER 12 YEARS OF AGE:** consult a physician. **Store between 2° and 25°C (36° and 77°F).** Protect from excessive moisture.

Warnings: Do not exceed recommended dosage. If nervousness, dizziness, or sleeplessness occur, discontinue use and consult a doctor. If symptoms do not improve within 7 days, or are accompanied by fever that lasts for more than 3 days or recurs, consult a doctor before continuing use. If pain or fever persists or gets worse, if new symptoms occur, or if redness or swelling is present, consult a doctor because these could be signs of a serious condition. May cause excitability especially in children. Do not take this product if you have a breathing problem such as emphysema or chronic bronchi-

tis, or if you have glaucoma, heart disease, high blood pressure, thryoid disease, diabetes, or difficulty in urination due to enlargement of the prostate gland, or give this product to children under 12 years of age, unless directed by a doctor. May cause drowsiness; alcohol, sedatives, and tranquilizers may increase the drowsiness effect. Avoid alcoholic beverages while taking this product. Do not take this product if you are taking sedatives or tranquilizers without first consulting your doctor. Use caution when driving a motor vehicle or operating machinery. As with any drug, if you are pregnant or nursing a baby, seek the advice of a health professional before using this product. Keep this and all drugs out of the reach of children. In case of accidental overdose, seek professional assistance or contact a Poison Control Center immediately. Prompt medical attention is critical for adults as well as for children even if you do not notice any signs or symptoms.

Alcohol Warning: If you generally consume 3 or more alcohol containing drinks per day, you should consult your doctor on when and how you should take this product and other pain relievers.

Drug Interaction Precaution: Do not use this product if you are now taking a prescription monoamine oxidase inhibitor (MAOI) (certain drugs for depression, psychiatric or emotional conditions, or Parkinson's disease), or for 2 weeks after stopping the MAOI drug. If you are uncertain whether your prescription drug contains an MAOI, consult a health professional before taking this product.

How Supplied: DRIXORAL® ALLERGY/SINUS Extended-Release Tablets are available in boxes of 12's and 24's.
Shown in Product Identification Guide, page 521

DUOFILM® LIQUID
Wart Remover

Active Ingredient: Salicylic Acid 17% (w/w).

Inactive Ingredients: Alcohol 15.8% w/w, castor oil, ether 42.6% w/w, ethyl lactate, and polybutene in flexible collodion.

Indications: For the removal of common and plantar warts. Common warts can be easily recognized by the rough, cauliflower-like appearance of the surface. Plantar warts are found on the bottom of the foot.

Warnings: For external use only. Do not use this product on irritated skin, on

Continued on next page

Information on Schering-Plough HealthCare Products appearing on these pages is effective as of November 1998.

DuoFilm—Cont.

any area that is infected or reddened, if you are a diabetic, or if you have poor blood circulation. If discomfort persists, see your doctor. Do not use on moles, birthmarks, warts with hair growing from them, genital warts, or warts on the face or mucous membranes. Keep this and all drugs out of the reach of children. In case of accidental ingestion, seek professional assistance or contact a Poison Control Center immediately. If product gets in eyes, flush with water for 15 minutes. Avoid inhaling vapors. HIGHLY FLAMMABLE. Keep away from fire or flame. Cap bottle tightly when not in use. Store at room temperature away from heat.

Directions: Wash affected area. May soak wart in warm water for 5 minutes. Dry area thoroughly. Apply one thin layer (with brush applicator) at a time to sufficiently cover each wart. Let dry. Repeat this procedure once or twice daily as needed (until wart is removed) for up to 12 weeks.

Note: Adhesive bandage may be used to cover treated area.

How Supplied: DuoFilm Liquid is available in $1/2$ fluid oz. spill-resistant bottles with brush applicator and cover-up discs for pinpoint application.

Shown in Product Identification Guide, page 521

DUOFILM® PATCH FOR KIDS
Wart Remover

Active Ingredient: Salicylic Acid 40% in a rubber-based vehicle.

Indications: For the concealment and removal of common warts. Common warts can be easily recognized by the rough, cauliflower-like appearance of the surface.

Warnings: For external use only. Do not use this product on irritated skin, on any area that is infected or reddened, if you are a diabetic, or if you have poor blood circulation. If discomfort persists, see your doctor. Do not use on moles, birthmarks, warts with hair growing from them, genital warts, or warts on the face or mucous membranes. Keep this and all drugs out of the reach of children. In case of accidental ingestion, seek professional assistance or contact a Poison Control Center immediately. Not recommended for children under two, except at the advice of a physician.

Directions: Parents should supervise use by children. Wash affected area. May soak wart in warm water for five minutes. Dry area thoroughly. Apply Medicated Patch (packet A). If necessary, cut patch to fit wart. Repeat procedure every 48 hours as needed (until wart is removed) for up to 12 weeks.

Note: Self-adhesive cover-up patches (packet B) may be used to conceal Medicated Patch and wart.

How Supplied: DuoFilm Patch includes 18 Medicated Patches and 20 self-adhesive Cover-Up patches for concealment while treatment is ongoing.

Store between 15° and 30°C (59° and 86°F).

Shown in Product Identification Guide, page 521

DUOPLANT® GEL
Plantar Wart Remover

Active Ingredient: Salicylic Acid 17% (w/w).

Inactive Ingredients: Alcohol 57.6% w/w, ether 16.42% w/w, ethyl lactate, hydroxypropyl cellulose, and polybutene in flexible collodion, USP.

Indications: For the removal of plantar and common warts. Plantar warts are found on the bottom of the foot. Common warts can be easily recognized by the rough, cauliflower-like appearance of the surface.

Warnings: For external use only. Do not use this product on irritated skin, on any area that is infected or reddened, if you are a diabetic, or if you have poor blood circulation. If discomfort persists, see your doctor. Do not use on moles, birthmarks, warts with hair growing from them, genital warts, or warts on the face or mucous membranes. If product gets in eyes, flush with water for 15 minutes. Avoid inhaling vapors. Highly Flammable. Keep away from fire or flame. Cap tube tightly and store at room temperature away from heat. Keep out of the reach of children. In case of accidental ingestion, seek professional assistance or contact a Poison Control Center immediately.

Directions: Wash affected area. May soak wart in warm water for five minutes. Dry area thoroughly. Apply a thin layer to sufficiently cover each wart. Let dry. Repeat this procedure once or twice daily as needed (until wart is removed) for up to 12 weeks.

Note: Adhesive bandage may be used to cover treated area.

How Supplied: DuoPlant Gel is available in $1/2$ oz. tubes with applicator tip for pinpoint application.

Shown in Product Identification Guide, page 521

GYNE-LOTRIMIN 3®-DAY
COMBINATION PACK
[gī-něh-lōtrimin]
Clotrimazole
Vaginal Inserts and External Vulvar Cream Antifungal

Active Ingredients: Inserts: Clotrimazole 200 mg per insert. Cream: Clotrimazole 1%.

Inactive Ingredients: Inserts: Corn starch, crospovidone, lactose, magnesium stearate, povidone. Cream: Benzyl alcohol, cetearyl alcohol, cetyl esters wax, octyldodecanol, polysorbate 60, purified water, sorbitan monostearate.

Gyne-Lotrimin3 antifungal vaginal inserts and external vulvar cream can kill the yeast that may cause vaginal infection. They do not stain clothes.

Indications: For the treatment of vaginal yeast (*Candida*) infection and the relief of external vulvar itching and irritation associated with a yeast infection. Starts to relieve itching and other symptoms within 1-2 days.

IF THIS IS THE FIRST TIME YOU HAVE HAD VAGINAL OR VULVAR ITCH AND DISCOMFORT, CONSULT YOUR DOCTOR. IF YOU HAVE HAD A DOCTOR DIAGNOSE A VAGINAL YEAST INFECTION BEFORE AND HAVE THE SAME SYMPTOMS NOW, USE THESE INSERTS AND CREAM AS DIRECTED FOR 3 CONSECUTIVE DAYS.

Warnings: DO NOT USE IF YOU HAVE ABDOMINAL PAIN, FEVER, OR FOUL-SMELLING DISCHARGE. CONTACT YOUR DOCTOR IMMEDIATELY. IF YOUR SYMPTOMS DO NOT IMPROVE IN 3 DAYS, YOU MAY HAVE A CONDITION OTHER THAN A YEAST INFECTION. CONSULT YOUR DOCTOR. If your symptoms return within 2 months or if you have infections that do not clear up easily with proper treatment, consult your doctor. You could be pregnant or there could be a serious underlying medical cause for your infections, including diabetes, or a damaged immune system (including damage from infection with HIV - the virus that causes AIDS). (PLEASE READ ENCLOSED EDUCATIONAL PAMPHLET). Do not use during pregnancy except under the advice and supervision of a doctor. Do not use tampons while using this medication. Keep these and all drugs out of the reach of children. In case of accidental ingestion, seek professional assistance or contact a Poison Control Center immediately. NOT FOR USE IN CHILDREN LESS THAN 12 YEARS OF AGE.

Dosage and Administration: Before using, read the enclosed pamphlet.

Directions: (Inserts): Unwrap one insert, place it in the applicator, and use the applicator to place the insert into the vagina, preferably at bedtime. Repeat this procedure daily for 3 consecutive days to treat vaginal yeast (*Candida*) infection.

(Cream): Squeeze a small amount of cream onto your finger and gently spread the cream into the irritated area of the vulva. Use once or twice a day for up to 7 days as needed to relieve external vulvar itching. **THE CREAM SHOULD NOT BE USED FOR VULVAR ITCHING DUE TO CAUSES OTHER THAN A YEAST INFECTION.**

How Supplied: 3 vaginal inserts with applicator (3-day therapy) and a 7g tube of external vulvar cream.

Store at room temperature between 2° and 30°C (36° and 86°F).

See end pane of carton, tube crimp, and foil wrappers for lot numbers and expiration date.

Shown in Product Identification Guide, page 521

LOTRIMIN® AF ANTIFUNGAL

[*lo-tre-min*]
Clotrimazole
Cream 1%
Solution 1%
Lotion 1%
Jock Itch Cream 1%

Description: Lotrimin® AF Cream 1% is a white fully vanishing homogeneous cream containing 1% clotrimazole. The cream contains no sensitizing parabens and is totally grease free and nonstaining.

Lotrimin® AF Solution 1% is a non-aqueous liquid, containing 1% clotrimazole. Also contains polyethylene glycol.

Lotrimin® AF Lotion 1% is a light penetrating buffered emulsion containing 1% clotrimazole. Does not contain common sensitizing agents. Also is greaseless and nonstaining.

Indications: Lotrimin AF Cream, Solution and Lotion cure athlete's foot (tinea pedis), jock itch (tinea cruris) and ringworm (tinea corporis). For effective relief of the itching, cracking, burning, scaling and discomfort which can accompany these conditions.

Directions: Cleanse skin with soap and water and dry thoroughly. Apply a thin layer over affected area morning and evening or as directed by a doctor. For athlete's foot, pay special attention to the spaces between the toes. It is also helpful to wear well-fitting, ventilated shoes and to change shoes and socks at least once daily. Best results in athlete's foot and ringworm are usually obtained with 4 weeks use of this product, and in jock itch with 2 weeks use. If satisfactory results have not occurred within these times, consult a doctor or pharmacist. Children under 12 years of age should be supervised in the use of this product. This product is not effective on the scalp or nails.

Warnings: For external use only. Avoid contact with the eyes. Do not use on children under 2 years of age except under the advice and supervision of a doctor. If irritation occurs or if there is no improvement within 4 weeks (for athlete's foot or ringworm) or within 2 weeks (for jock itch), discontinue use and consult a doctor or pharmacist. Keep this and all drugs out of the reach of children. In case of accidental ingestion, seek professional assistance or contact a Poison Control Center immediately.

How Supplied: Lotrimin® AF Antifungal Cream is available in a 0.42 oz.

tube (12 grams) and a 0.84 oz. tube (24 grams). Lotrimin® AF Jock Itch Cream is available in a 0.42 oz tube (12 grams). Inactive ingredients include: cetearyl alcohol, cetyl esters wax, octyldodecanol, polysorbate, sorbitan monostearate and water and as a preservative, benzyl alcohol (1%).

Lotrimin® AF Antifungal Solution is available in a 0.33 fl. oz. (10 milliliters) bottle. Inactive ingredient is PEG.

Lotrimin® AF Antifungal Lotion is available in a 0.66 fl. oz. (20 milliliters) bottle. Inactive ingredients include cetearyl alcohol, cetyl esters wax, octyldodecanol, polysorbate, sodium biphosphate, sodium phosphate dibasic, sorbitan monostearate and water and as a preservative, benzyl alcohol (1%).

Storage: Keep Lotrimin® AF Cream and Solution products between 2° and 30°C (36° and 86°F), and Lotrimin® AF Lotion product between 2° and 25°C (36° and 77°F).

Shown in Product Identification Guide, page 521

LOTRIMIN® AF ANTIFUNGAL
Miconazole Nitrate 2%
Athlete's Foot Spray Liquid
Athlete's Foot Spray Powder
Athlete's Foot Spray Deodorant Powder
Athlete's Foot Powder
Jock Itch Spray Powder

Active Ingredients: SPRAY LIQUID contains Miconazole Nitrate 2%. Also contains: Alcohol SD-40 (17% w/w), Cocamide DEA, Isobutane, Propylene Glycol, Tocopherol (vitamin E).

SPRAY POWDER (Athlete's Foot) contains Miconazole Nitrate 2%. Also contains: Alcohol SD-40 (10% w/w), Isobutane, Starch/Acrylates/Acrylamide Copolymer, Stearalkonium Hectorite, Talc.

SPRAY POWDER (Jock Itch) contains Miconazole Nitrate 2%. Also contains Alcohol SD-40 (10% w/w), Isobutane, Stearalkonium Hectorite, Talc.

SPRAY DEODORANT POWDER contains Miconazole Nitrate 2%. Also contains: Isobutane, Alcohol SD-40 (10% w/w), Talc, Starch/Acrylates/Acrylamide Copolymer, Stearalkonium Hectorite, Fragrance.

POWDER contains Miconazole Nitrate 2%. Also contains: Benzethonium Chloride, Corn Starch, Kaolin, Sodium Bicarbonate, Starch/Acrylates/Acrylamide Copolymer, Zinc Oxide.

Indications: LOTRIMIN® AF Athlete's Foot Spray Liquid, Spray Powder, Spray Deodorant Powder and Powder are proven clinically effective in the treatment of athlete's foot (tinea pedis), jock itch (tinea cruris) and ringworm (tinea corporis). For effective relief of the itching, cracking, burning, scaling and discomfort that can accompany these conditions.

LOTRIMIN AF Powder also aids in the drying of naturally moist areas.

LOTRIMIN® AF Jock Itch Spray Powder cures jock itch (tinea cruris). For effective relief of the itching, burning, scaling and discomfort associated with jock itch.

Warnings: For Athlete's Foot Spray Powder, Spray Liquid, Spray Deodorant Powder and Jock Itch Spray Powder: Do not use on children under 2 years of age unless directed by a doctor. For external use only. Avoid contact with the eyes. If irritation occurs or if there is no improvement within 4 weeks (for athlete's foot and ringworm) or 2 weeks (for jock itch), discontinue use and consult a doctor. Flammable. Do not use while smoking or near heat or flame. Avoid spraying in eyes. Contents under pressure. Do not puncture or incinerate. Do not store at temperature above 120°F. Use only as directed. Intentional misuse by deliberately concentrating and inhaling contents can be harmful or fatal. Keep this and all drugs out of the reach of children. In case of accidental ingestion, seek professional assistance or contact a Poison Control Center immediately.

Lotrimin® AF Powder: Do not use on children under 2 years of age unless directed by a doctor. For external use only. Avoid contact with the eyes. If irritation occurs, or if there is no improvement within 4 weeks (for athlete's foot or ringworm) or within 2 weeks (for jock itch), discontinue use and consult a doctor. Keep this and all drugs out of the reach of children. In case of accidental ingestion, seek professional assistance or contact a Poison Control Center immediately.

Directions: For Athlete's Foot Spray Liquid, Spray Powder, Spray Deodorant Powder and Jock Itch Spray Powder: Wash affected area and dry thoroughly. Shake can well. Spray a thin layer of product over affected area twice daily (morning and night) or as directed by a doctor. Supervise children in the use of this product. For athlete's foot, pay special attention to the spaces between the toes; wear well-fitting, ventilated shoes and change shoes and socks at least once daily. For athlete's foot and ringworm use daily for 4 weeks; for jock itch use daily for 2 weeks. If condition persists longer, consult a doctor. This product is not effective on the scalp or nails.

Powder: Wash affected area and dry thoroughly. Sprinkle a thin layer of product over affected area twice daily (morning and night) or as directed by a doctor. Supervise children in the use of this product. For athlete's foot, pay special attention to the spaces between the toes; wear well-fitting, ventilated shoes and change shoes and socks at least once

---

Continued on next page

Information on Schering-Plough HealthCare Products appearing on these pages is effective as of November 1998.

Lotrimin AF Spray—Cont.

daily. For athlete's foot and ringworm use daily for 4 weeks; for jock itch use daily for 2 weeks. If condition persists longer, consult a doctor. This product is not effective on the scalp or nails.

Store between 2° and 30° C (36° and 86°F).

How Supplied: LOTRIMIN® AF Athlete's Foot Spray Powder, Spray Deodorant Powder and Jock Itch Spray Powder—3.5 oz. cans. LOTRIMIN® AF Spray Liquid—4 oz. can. LOTRIMIN® AF Powder—3 oz. plastic bottle.

Shown in Product Identification Guide, page 521

SmithKline Beecham Consumer Healthcare, L.P.

POST OFFICE BOX 1467 PITTSBURGH, PA 15230

For Medical Information Contact:
(800) 245-1040 (Consumer Inquiries)
(800) 378-4055 (Healthcare Professional Inquiries)

Direct Healthcare Professional Sample Requests to:
(800) BEECHAM

Orange Flavor CITRUCEL®

[sĭt 'rə-sĕl]
(Methylcellulose)
Bulk-forming Fiber Laxative

Description: Each 19 g adult dose (approximately one heaping measuring tablespoonful) contains Methylcellulose 2 g. Each 9.5 g child's dose (one-half the adult dose) contains Methylcellulose 1 g. Methylcellulose is a nonallergenic fiber. Also contains: Citric Acid, FD&C Yellow No. 6, Orange Flavors (natural and artificial), Potassium Citrate, Riboflavin, Sucrose, and other ingredients. Each adult dose contains approximately 3 mg of sodium, 105 mg of potassium, and contributes 60 calories from Sucrose.

Actions: Promotes elimination by providing additional fiber (bulk) to the diet. This product generally produces bowel movement in 12 to 72 hours.

Indications: For relief of constipation (irregularity). May also be used for relief of constipation associated with other bowel disorders such as irritable bowel syndrome, diverticular disease, and hemorrhoids as well as for bowel management during postpartum, postsurgical, and convalescent periods when recommended by a physician.

Contraindications: Intestinal obstruction, fecal impaction, known hypersensitivity to formula ingredients.

Warnings: Patients should be instructed to consult their physician before using any laxative if they have noticed a sudden change in bowel habits which persists for two weeks. Unless directed by a physician, patients should be advised not to use laxative products when abdominal pain, nausea, or vomiting is present. Patients should also be advised to discontinue use and consult a physician if rectal bleeding or failure to have a bowel movement occurs after use of any laxative product. Unless recommended by a physician, patients should not exceed the recommended maximum daily dose. Patients should not use laxative products for a period longer than one week unless directed by a physician. **TAKING THIS PRODUCT WITHOUT ADEQUATE FLUID MAY CAUSE IT TO SWELL AND BLOCK YOUR THROAT OR ESOPHAGUS AND MAY CAUSE CHOKING. DO NOT TAKE THIS PRODUCT IF YOU HAVE DIFFICULTY IN SWALLOWING. IF YOU EXPERIENCE CHEST PAIN, VOMITING, OR DIFFICULTY IN SWALLOWING OR BREATHING AFTER TAKING THIS PRODUCT, SEEK IMMEDIATE MEDICAL ATTENTION. KEEP THIS AND ALL DRUGS OUT OF THE REACH OF CHILDREN.**

Dosage and Administration: Adult Dose: dissolve one leveled scoop (one heaping tablespoon – 19g) in 8 ounces of cold water up to three times daily at the first sign of constipation. Children age 6 to 12 years of age: *one-half the adult dose* stirred briskly in 8 ounces of cold water, once daily at the first sign of constipation. The mixture should be administered promptly and drinking another glass of water is highly recommended (see warnings). Children under 6 years of age: *Use only as directed by a physician.* Continued use for 12 to 72 hours may be necessary for full benefit. **TAKE THIS PRODUCT (CHILD OR ADULT DOSE) WITH AT LEAST 8 OZ. (A FULL GLASS) OF WATER OR OTHER FLUID. TAKING THIS PRODUCT WITHOUT ENOUGH LIQUID MAY CAUSE CHOKING. SEE WARNINGS.**

How Supplied: 16 oz. and 30 oz. containers.
Boxes of 20-single-dose packets.
Store below 86°F (30°C). Protect contents from humidity; keep tightly closed.

Shown in Product Identification Guide, page 521

Sugar Free Orange Flavor CITRUCEL®

[sĭt 'rə-sĕl]
(Methylcellulose)
Bulk-forming Fiber Laxative

Description: Each 10.2 g adult dose (approximately one rounded measuring tablespoonful) contains Methylcellulose 2 g. Each 5.1 g child's dose (one-half the adult dose) contains Methylcellulose 1 g. Methylcellulose is a nonallergenic fiber.

Also contains: Aspartame, Dibasic Calcium Phosphate, FD&C Yellow No. 6, Malic Acid, Maltodextrin, Orange Flavors (natural and artificial), Potassium Citrate and Riboflavin. Each 10.2 g dose contributes 24 calories from Maltodextrin.

Actions: Promotes elimination by providing additional fiber (bulk) to the diet. This product generally produces bowel movement in 12 to 72 hours.

Indications: For relief of constipation (irregularity). May also be used for relief of constipation associated with other bowel disorders such as irritable bowel syndrome, diverticular disease, and hemorrhoids as well as for bowel management during postpartum, postsurgical, and convalescent periods when recommended by a physician.

Contraindications and Warnings: See entry for "Orange Flavor Citrucel".

Phenylketonurics: CONTAINS PHENYLALANINE 52 mg per adult dose. Individuals with phenylketonuria and other individuals who must restrict their intake of phenylalanine should be warned that each 10.2 g adult dose contains aspartame which provides 52 mg of phenylalanine.

Dosage and Administration: Adult Dose: dissolve one leveled scoop (one rounded measuring tablespoon – 10.2g) in 8 ounces of cold water up to three times daily at the first sign of constipation. Children age 6 to 12 years of age: *one-half the adult dose* stirred briskly into at least 8 ounces of cold water, once daily at the first sign of constipation. The mixture should be administered promptly and drinking another glass of water is highly recommended (see warnings). Children under 6 years of age: *Use only as directed by a physician.* Continued use for 12 to 72 hours may be necessary for full benefit. **TAKE THIS PRODUCT (CHILD OR ADULT DOSE) WITH AT LEAST 8 OZ. (A FULL GLASS) OF WATER OR OTHER FLUID. TAKING THIS PRODUCT WITHOUT ENOUGH LIQUID MAY CAUSE CHOKING. SEE WARNINGS.**

How Supplied:
8.6 oz and 16.9 oz containers.
Boxes of 20 single-dose packets.
Store below 86°F (30°C). Protect contents from humidity; keep tightly closed.

Shown in Product Identification Guide, page 521

CONTAC®
Continuous Action Nasal Decongestant/Antihistamine 12 Hour Capsules & Caplets

Product Information: Each CONTAC timed release capsule or caplet has a portion of its medicines that work right away while the balance are dissolved slowly to provide 12-Hours of relief.

Indications: Temporarily relieves nasal congestion due to the common cold, hay fever or other upper respiratory allergies and associated with sinusitis. Temporarily relieves runny nose and reduces sneezing, itching of the nose or throat and itchy, watery eyes due to hay fever or other upper respiratory allergies. Helps clear nasal passages; shrinks swollen membranes. Helps decongest sinus openings and passages; temporarily relieves sinus congestion and pressure.

Directions: Adults and children over 12 years of age: One capsule or caplet every 12 hours, not to exceed 2 capsules or caplets in 24 hours, or as directed by a doctor. Children under 12 years of age: consult a doctor.

TAMPER-EVIDENT PACKAGING FEATURES FOR YOUR PROTECTION:

Each capsule or caplet is encased in a plastic cell with a foil back; do not use if cell or foil is broken. The carton is protected by a clear overwrap printed with "safety-sealed"; do not use if overwrap is missing or broken.

In addition, each CONTAC capsule is protected by a red Perma-Seal™ band which bonds the two capsule halves together; do not use if capsule or band is broken.

Warnings: Do not exceed the recommended dosage. If nervousness, dizziness, or sleeplessness occur, discontinue use and consult a doctor. If symptoms do not improve within 7 days or are accompanied by high fever, consult a doctor. Do not take this product, unless directed by a doctor, if you have a breathing problem such as emphysema or chronic bronchitis, or if you have heart disease, high blood pressure, thyroid disease, diabetes, glaucoma or difficulty in urination due to enlargement of the prostate gland. Do not take this product if you are taking another medication containing phenylpropanolamine. Use caution when driving a motor vehicle or operating machinery. May cause drowsiness; alcohol, sedatives and tranquilizers may increase the drowsiness effect. Avoid alcoholic beverages while taking this product. Do not take this product if you are taking sedatives or tranquilizers, without first consulting your doctor. May cause excitability especially in children. KEEP THIS AND ALL DRUGS OUT OF REACH OF CHILDREN. IN CASE OF ACCIDENTAL OVERDOSE, SEEK PROFESSIONAL ASSISTANCE OR CONTACT A POISON CONTROL CENTER IMMEDIATELY. As with any drug, if you are pregnant or nursing a baby, seek the advice of a health professional before using this product. Store in a dry place at controlled room temperature 15°–30°C (59°–86°F).

Drug Interaction Precaution: Do not use this product if you are now taking a prescription monoamine oxidase inhibitor (MAOI) (certain drugs for depression, psychiatric or emotional conditions, or Parkinson's disease), or for 2 weeks after stopping the MAOI drug. If you are uncertain whether your prescription drug contains an MAOI, consult a health professional before taking this product.

Capsule Active Ingredients: Phenylpropanolamine Hydrochloride 75 mg. and Chlorpheniramine Maleate 8 mg.

Caplet Active Ingredients: Phenylpropanolamine Hydrochloride 75 mg. and Chlorpheniramine Maleate 12 mg.

Each Capsule Also Contains: Benzyl Alcohol, Butylparaben, D&C Red No. 33, D&C Yellow No. 10, Edetate Calcium Disodium, FD&C Red No. 3, FD&C Yellow No. 6, Gelatin, Methylparaben, Pharmaceutical Glaze, Propylparaben, Sodium Lauryl Sulfate, Sodium Propionate, Starch, Sucrose and other ingredients, may also contain: Polysorbate 80.

Each Caplet Also Contains: Acetylated Monoglycerides, Carnuba Wax, Colloidal Silicon Dioxide, Ethylcellulose Hydroxypropyl Methylcellulose, Lactose, Stearic Acid, Titanium Dioxide.

How Supplied: Consumer packages of 10 and 20 capsules or caplets.
Note: There are other CONTAC products. Make sure this is the one you are interested in. See the table below for all of the products in the CONTAC line.
Shown in Product Identification Guide, page 521

CONTAC®
Severe Cold and Flu
Caplets Maximum Strength
Analgesic• Decongestant
Antihistamine• Cough Suppressant

Composition: Phenylpropanolamine HCl, 25 mg, Chlorpheniramine Maleate 4 mg, Acetaminophen 1000 mg, Dextromethorphan Hydrobromide 30 mg.

Product Information: Two caplets every 6 hours to help relieve the discomforts of severe colds with flu-like symptoms.

Product Benefits: CONTAC Severe Cold and Flu contains a Non-Aspirin Analgesic, a Decongestant, an Antihistamine and a Cough Suppressant.

Indications: Temporarily relieves nasal congestion, runny nose, sneezing, itchy, watery eyes and coughing due to the common cold. Provides temporary relief of fever, sore throat, headache and minor aches associated with the flu.

Directions: Adults (12 years and older): Two caplets every 6 hours, not to exceed 8 caplets in any 24-hour period, or as directed by a doctor. Children under 12 years of age: consult a doctor.

TAMPER-EVIDENT PACKAGING FEATURES FOR YOUR PROTECTION:

Caplets are encased in a plastic cell with a foil back; do not use if cell or foil is broken. The letters SCF appear on each caplet; do not use this product if these letters are missing.

Warnings: Do not take this product for more than 10 days. If symptoms do not improve or are accompanied by fever that lasts for more than 3 days, or if new symptoms occur, consult a doctor. If sore throat is severe, persists for more than 2 days, is accompanied or followed by fever, headache, rash, nausea, or vomiting, consult a doctor promptly. A persistent cough may be a sign of a serious condition. If cough persists for more than 7 days, tends to recur, or is accompanied by rash, persistent headache, fever that lasts for more than 3 days, or if new symptoms occur, consult a doctor. Do not take this product for persistent or chronic cough such as occurs with smoking, asthma, emphysema, or if cough is accompanied by excessive phlegm (mucus) unless directed by a doctor. May cause excitability especially in children. Do not take this product, unless directed by a doctor, if you have a breathing problem such as emphysema or chronic bronchitis, or if you have heart disease, high blood pressure, thyroid disease, diabetes, glaucoma or difficulty in urination due to enlargement of the prostate gland. May cause marked drowsiness: alcohol, sedatives, and tranquilizers may increase the drowsiness effect. Avoid taking alcoholic beverages while taking this product. Do not take this product if you are taking sedatives or tranquilizers, without first consulting your doctor. Use caution when driving a motor vehicle or operating machinery. **Do not exceed recommended dosage.** If nervousness, dizziness, or sleeplessness occur, discontinue use and consult a doctor. **KEEP THIS AND ALL DRUGS OUT OF THE REACH OF CHILDREN.** Prompt medical attention is critical for adults as well as for children even if you do not notice any signs or symptoms. In case of accidental overdose, seek professional assistance or contact a Poison Control Center immediately. As with any drug, if you are pregnant or nursing a baby, seek the advice of a health professional before using this product.

Drug Interaction Precaution: Do not use this product if you are now taking a prescription monoamine oxidase inhibitor (MAOI) (certain drugs for depression, psychiatric or emotional conditions, or Parkinson's disease), or for 2 weeks after stopping the MAOI drug. If you are uncertain whether your prescription drug contains an MAOI, consult a health professional before taking this product.

Formula: Active Ingredients: Each caplet contains Acetaminophen, 500 mg., Dextromethorphan Hydrobromide, 15 mg.; Phenylpropanolamine Hydrochloride, 12.5 mg.; Chlorpheniramine Maleate, 2 mg. **Inactive Ingredients:** FD&C Blue 1, Hydroxypropyl Methylcellulose, Microcrystalline Cellulose, Polyethylene Glycol, Polysorbate 80, Povidone, Sodium Starch Glycolate, Starch, Stearic Acid, Titanium Dioxide.

Continued on next page

Contac Sev. Cold/Flu—Cont.

Avoid storing at high temperature (greater than 100°F).

How Supplied: Consumer packages of 16 and 30 caplets.

Shown in Product Identification Guide, page 521

Product Change: During middle of 1999, Phenylpropanolamine Hydrochloride 12.5 mg will be replaced by Pseudoephedrine Hydrochloride 30 mg.

Note: There are other CONTAC products. Make sure this is the one you are interested in. See the table below for all of the products in the CONTAC line.
[See table below]

DEBROX® Drops
Ear Wax Removal Aid

Description: Carbamide peroxide 6.5%. Also contains citric acid, glycerin, propylene glycol, sodium stannate, water, and other ingredients.

Actions: DEBROX®, used as directed, cleanses the ear with sustained microfoam. DEBROX Drops foam on contact with earwax due to the release of oxygen (there may be an associated crackling sound). DEBROX Drops provide a safe, nonirritating method of softening and removing ear wax.

Indications: For occasional use as an aid to soften, loosen, and remove excessive earwax.

Directions: FOR USE IN THE EAR ONLY. Adults and children over 12 years of age: tilt head sideways and place 5 to 10 drops into ear. Tip of applicator should not enter ear canal. Keep drops in ear for several minutes by keeping head tilted or placing cotton in the ear. Use twice daily for up to four days if needed, or as directed by a doctor. Any wax remaining after treatment may be removed by gently flushing the ear with warm water, using a soft rubber bulb ear syringe. Children under 12 years of age: consult a doctor.

Warnings: Do not use if you have ear drainage or discharge, ear pain, irritation or rash in the ear, or are dizzy; consult a doctor. Do not use if you have an injury or perforation (hole) of the eardrum or after ear surgery unless directed by a doctor. Do not use for more than four days. If excessive earwax remains after use of this product, consult a doctor. Avoid contact with the eyes.

Cautions: Avoid exposing bottle to excessive heat and direct sunlight. Keep tip on bottle when not in use. Keep this and all drugs out of the reach of children. In case of accidental ingestion, seek professional assistance or contact a poison control center immediately.

How Supplied: DEBROX Drops are available in $^1/_2$- or 1-fl-oz (15 or 30 ml) plastic squeeze bottles with applicator spouts.

Shown in Product Identification Guide, page 521

ECOTRIN®
Enteric-Coated Aspirin
Antiarthritic, Antiplatelet

Description: 'Ecotrin' is enteric-coated aspirin (acetylsalicylic acid, ASA) available in tablet form in 81 mg, 325 mg and 500 mg dosage units.

The enteric coating covers a core of aspirin and is designed to resist disintegration in the stomach, dissolving in the more neutral-to-alkaline environment of the duodenum. Such action helps to protect the stomach from injury that may result from ingestion of plain, buffered or highly buffered aspirin (see SAFETY).

Indications: 'Ecotrin' is indicated for:
• conditions requiring chronic or long-term aspirin therapy for pain and/or inflammation, e.g., rheumatoid arthritis, juvenile rheumatoid arthritis, systemic lupus erythematosus, osteoarthritis (degenerative joint disease), ankylosing spondylitis, psoriatic arthritis, Reiter's syndrome and fibrositis,
• antiplatelet indications of aspirin (see the ANTIPLATELET EFFECT section) and
• situations in which compliance with aspirin therapy may be affected because of the gastrointestinal side effects of plain, i.e., non-enteric-coated, or buffered aspirin.

Dosage: For analgesic or anti-inflammatory indications, the OTC maximum dosage for aspirin is 4000 mg per day in divided doses, i.e., up to 650 mg every 4 hours or 1000 mg every 6 hours.

For antiplatelet effect dosage: see the ANTIPLATELET EFFECT section.

Under a physician's direction, the dosage can be increased or otherwise modified as appropriate to the clinical situation. When 'Ecotrin' is used for anti-inflammatory effect, the physician should be attentive to plasma salicylate levels, and may also caution the patient to be alert to the development of tinnitus as an indicator of elevated salicylate levels. It should be noted that patients with a high frequency hearing loss (such as may occur in older individuals) may have difficulty perceiving the tinnitus. Tinnitus would then not be a reliable indicator in such individuals.

Inactive Ingredients: 81 mg: Carnauba Wax, D&C Yellow 10, FD&C Yellow 6, Hydroxypropyl Methylcellulose, Methacrylic Acid Copolymer, Microcrystalline Cellulose, Polyethylene Glycol, Polysorbate 80, Propylene Glycol, Silicon Dioxide, Starch, Stearic Acid, Talc, Titanium Dioxide, Triethyl Citrate.

325 mg and 500 mg: Carnauba wax, Colloidal Silicon Dioxide, FD&C Yellow #6, Hydroxypropyl Methylcellulose, Maltodextrin, Methacrylic Acid Copolymer, Microcrystalline Cellulose, Pregelatinized Starch, Propylene Glycol, Simethicone, Sodium Hydroxide, Sodium Starch Glycolate, Stearic Acid, Talc, Titanium Dioxide, Triethyl Citrate.

Bioavailability: The bioavailability of aspirin from 'Ecotrin' has been demonstrated in a number of salicylate excretion studies. The studies show levels of salicylate (and metabolites) in urine excreted over 48 hours for 'Ecotrin' do not differ statistically from plain, i.e., non-enteric-coated, aspirin.

Plasma studies, in which 'Ecotrin' has been compared with plain aspirin in steady-state studies over eight days, also demonstrate that 'Ecotrin' provides plasma salicylate levels not statistically different from plain aspirin.

Information regarding salicylate levels over a range of doses was generated in a

---

PDR For Nonprescription Drugs

	CONTAC 12 Hour Cold Caplets Maximum Strength	CONTAC 12 Hour Cold Capsules	CONTAC Severe Cold and Flu Caplets (each 2 caplet dose)	CONTAC Severe Cold and Flu Non-Drowsy Caplet (each 2 caplet dose)	CONTAC Day & Night Cold & Flu Day Caplets	CONTAC Day & Night Cold & Flu Night Caplets
Phenylpropanolamine HCl	75.0 mg	75.0 mg	25.0 mg	—	—	—
Chlorpheniramine Maleate	12.0 mg	8.0 mg	4.0 mg	—	—	—
Pseudoephedrine HCl	—	—	—	60.0 mg	60.0 mg	60.0 mg
Acetaminophen	—	—	1000.0 mg	650.0 mg	650.0 mg	650.0 mg
Dextromethorphan Hydrobromide	—	—	30.0 mg	30.0 mg	30.0 mg	—
Diphenhydramine HCl	—	—	—	—	—	50.0 mg

study in which 24 healthy volunteers (12 male and 12 female) took daily (divided) doses of either 2600 mg, 3900 mg, or 5200 mg of 'Ecotrin'. Plasma salicylate levels generally acknowledged to be anti-inflammatory (15 mg/dL) were attained at daily doses of 5200 mg, on Day 2 by females and Day 3 by males. At 3900 mg, anti-inflammatory levels were attained at Day 3 by females and Day 4 by males. Dissolution of the enteric coating occurs at a neutral-to-basic pH and is therefore dependent on gastric emptying into the duodenum. With continued dosing, appropriate plasma levels are maintained.

Safety: The safety of 'Ecotrin' has been demonstrated in a number of endoscopic studies comparing 'Ecotrin', plain aspirin, buffered aspirin, and highly buffered aspirin preparations. In these studies, all forms of aspirin was dosed to the OTC maximum (3900–4000 mg per day) for up to 14 days. The normal healthy volunteers participating in these studies were gastroscoped before and after the courses of treatment and 14-day drug-free periods followed active drug. Compared to all the other preparations, there was less gastric damage at a statistically significant level during the 'Ecotrin' courses. There was also statistically less duodenal damage when compared with the plain i.e., non-enteric-coated aspirin.

Details of studies demonstrating the safety and bioavailability of 'Ecotrin' are available to health care professionals. Write: Professional Services Department, SmithKline Beecham Consumer Healthcare, P.O. Box 1467, Pittsburgh, Pa. 15230.

Warnings: Children and teenagers should not use this product for chicken pox or flu symptoms before a doctor is consulted about Reye Syndrome, a rare but serious illness reported to be associated with aspirin. Do not take this product for pain for more than 10 days or for fever for more than 3 days, or in conditions affecting children under 12 years of age, unless directed by a doctor. If pain or fever persists or gets worse, if new symptoms occur, or if redness or swelling is present, consult a doctor because these could be signs of a serious condition. Do not take this product if you are allergic to aspirin, have asthma, have stomach problems that persist or recur, or if you have ulcers or bleeding problems unless directed by a doctor. If ringing in the ears or a loss of hearing occurs, consult a doctor before taking any more of this product. **Keep this and all drugs out of the reach of children**. In case of accidental overdose, seek professional assistance or contact a poison control center immediately. As with any medicine, if you are pregnant or nursing a baby, seek the advice of a health professional before using this product. **IT IS ESPECIALLY IMPORTANT NOT TO USE ASPIRIN DURING THE LAST 3 MONTHS OF PREGNANCY UNLESS SPECIFICALLY DIRECTED TO DO SO BY A DOCTOR BECAUSE IT MAY CAUSE PROBLEMS IN THE UNBORN CHILD OR COMPLICATIONS DURING DELIVERY.**

Alcohol Warning: If you consume three or more alcoholic drinks every day, ask your doctor whether you should take aspirin or other pain relievers/fever reducers. Aspirin may cause stomach bleeding.

Drug Interaction Precaution:
Do not take this product if you are taking a prescription drug for anticoagulation (thinning of the blood), diabetes, gout, or arthritis unless directed by a doctor.

Professional Warning: There have been occasional reports in the literature concerning individuals with impaired gastric emptying in whom there may be retention of one or more enteric coated aspirin tablets over time. This unusual phenomenon may occur as a result of outlet obstruction from ulcer disease alone or combined with hypotonic gastric peristalsis. Because of the integrity of the enteric coating in an acidic environment, these tablets may accumulate and form a bezoar in the stomach. Individuals with this condition may present with complaints of early satiety or of vague upper abdominal distress. Diagnosis may be made by endoscopy or by abdominal films which show opacities suggestive of a mass of small tablets (*Ref.: Bogacz, K. and Caldron, P.: Enteric-coated Aspirin Bezoar: Elevation of Serum Salicylate Level by Barium Study. Amer. J. Med. 1987:83, 783-6.*). Management may vary according to the condition of the patient. Options include: gastrotomy and alternating slightly basic and neutral lavage (*Ref.: Baum, J.: Enteric-Coated Aspirin and the Problem of Gastric Retention. J. Rheum., 1984:11, 250-1.*). While there have been no clinical reports, it has been suggested that such individuals may also be treated with parenteral cimetidine (to reduce acid secretion) and then given sips of slightly basic liquids to effect gradual dissolution of the enteric coating. Progress may be followed with plasma salicylate levels or via recognition of tinnitus by the patient. It should be kept in mind that individuals with a history of partial or complete gastrectomy may produce reduced amounts of acid and therefore have less acidic gastric pH. Under these circumstances, the benefits offered by the acid-resistant enteric coating may not exist.

Antiarthritic and Anti-inflammatory Indications: For rheumatoid arthritis, juvenile rheumatoid arthritis, systemic lupus erythematosus, osteoarthritis (degenerative joint disease), ankylosing spondylitis, psoriatic arthritis, Reiter's syndrome, and fibrositis.

Antiplatelet Effect: Aspirin may be recommended to reduce the risk of death and/or nonfatal myocardial infarction (MI) in patients with a previous infarction or unstable angina pectoris and its use in reducing the risk of transient ischemic attacks in men.

Aspirin is also indicated to reduce the risk of vascular mortality in patients with suspected acute MI. Indications for these conditions follow:

Aspirin for Myocardial Infarction Indications: Recurrent Myocardial Infarction (MI) (Reinfarction) or Unstable Angina Pectoris: Aspirin is indicated to reduce the risk of death and/or nonfatal MI in patients with a previous MI or unstable angina pectoris.

Suspected Acute MI: Aspirin is indicated to reduce the risk of vascular mortality in patients with a suspected acute MI.

Clinical Trials: Recurrent MI (Reinfarction) and Unstable Angina Pectoris: The indication is supported by the results of six large, randomized multicenter, placebo-controlled studies involving 10,816, predominantly male, post-myocardial infarction (MI) patients and one randomized placebo-controlled study of 1,266 men with unstable angina (1–7). Therapy with aspirin was begun at intervals after the onset of acute MI varying from less than 3 days to more than 5 years and continued for periods of from less than 1 year to 4 years. In the unstable angina study, treatment was started within 1 month after the onset of unstable angina and continued for 12 weeks, and congestive heart failure were not included in the study.

Aspirin therapy in MI patients was associated with about a 20-percent reduction in the risk of subsequent death and/or non-fatal reinfarction, a median absolute decrease of 3 percent from the 12- to 22-percent event rates in the placebo groups. In aspirin-treated unstable angina patients the reduction in risk was about 50 percent, a reduction in event rate of 5 percent from the 10-percent rate in the placebo group over the 12-weeks of the study.

Daily dosage of aspirin in the post-myocardial infarction studies was 300 milligrams in one study and 900 to 1,500 milligrams in 5 studies. A dose of 325 milligrams was used in the study of unstable angina.

Suspected Acute MI: The use of aspirin in patients with a suspected acute MI is supported by the results of a large, multicenter 2×2 factorial study of 17,187 subjects with suspected acute MI (8). Subjects were randomized within 24 hours of the onset of symptoms so that 8,587 subjects received oral aspirin (162.5 milligrams, enteric-coated) daily for 1 month (the first dose crushed, sucked, or chewed) and 8,600 received oral placebo. Of the subjects, 8,592 were also randomized to receive a single dose of streptokinase (1.5 million units) infused intravenously for about 1 hour, and 8,595 received a placebo infusion. Thus, 4,295 subjects received aspirin plus placebo, 4,300 received streptokinase plus placebo, 4,292 received aspirin plus streptokinase, and 4,300 received double placebo.

Continued on next page

Ecotrin—Cont.

Vascular mortality (attributed to cardiac, cerebral, hemorrhagic, other vascular, or unknown causes) occurred in 9.4 percent of the subjects in the aspirin group and in 11.8 percent of the subjects in the oral placebo group in the 35-day followup. This represents an absolute reduction of 2.4 percent in the mean 35-day vascular mortality attributable to aspirin and a 23 percent reduction in the odds of vascular death ($2p < 0.0001$).

Significant absolute reductions in mortality and corresponding reductions in specific clinical events favoring aspirin were found for reinfarction (1.5 percent absolute reduction, 45 percent odds reduction, $2p < 0.0001$), cardiac arrest (1.2 percent absolute reduction, 14.2 percent odds reduction, $2p < 0.01$), and total stroke (0.4 percent absolute reduction, 41.5 percent odds reduction, $2p < 0.01$). The effect of aspirin over and above its effect on mortality was evidenced by small, but significant, reductions in vascular morbidity in those subjects who were discharged.

The beneficial effects of aspirin on mortality were present with or without streptokinase infusion. Aspirin reduced vascular mortality from 10.4 to 8.0 percent for days 0 to 35 in subjects given streptokinase and reduced vascular mortality from 13.2 to 10.7 percent in subjects given no streptokinase.

The effects of aspirin and thrombolytic therapy with streptokinase in this study were approximately additive. subjects who received the combination of streptokinase infusion and daily aspirin had significantly lower vascular mortality at 35 days than those who received either active treatment alone (combination 8.0 percent, aspirin 10.7 percent, streptokinase 10.4 percent, and no treatment 13.2 percent). While this study demonstrated that aspirin has an additive benefit in patients given streptokinase, there is no reason to restrict its use to that specific thrombolytic.

Adverse Reactions: Gastrointestinal Reactions: Doses of 1,000 milligrams per day of aspirin caused gastrointestinal symptoms and bleeding that in some cases were clinically significant. In the largest post-infarction study (the Aspirin Myocardial Infarction Study (AMIS) with 4,500 people), the percentage incidences of gastrointestinal symptoms for the aspirin (1,000 milligrams of a standard, solid-tablet formulation) and placebo-treated subjects, respectively, were: stomach pain (14.5 percent; 4.4 percent); heartburn (11.9 percent; 4.8 percent); nausea and/or vomiting (7.6 percent; 2.1 percent); hospitalization for gastrointestinal disorder (4.8 percent; 3.5 percent). Symptoms and signs of gastrointestinal irritation were not significantly increased in subjects treated for unstable angina with 325 milligrams buffered aspirin in solution.

Bleeding: In the AMIS and other trials, aspirin-treated subjects had increased rates of gross gastrointestinal bleeding. In the ISIS-2 study (8), there was no significant difference in the incidence of major bleeding (bleeds requiring transfusion) between 8,587 subjects taking 162.5 milligrams aspirin daily and 8,600 subjects taking placebo (31 versus 33 subjects). There were five confirmed cerebral hemorrhages in the aspirin group compared with two in the placebo group, but the incidence of stroke of all causes was significantly reduced from 81 to 47 for the placebo versus aspirin group (0.4 percent absolute change). There was a small and statistically significant excess (0.6 percent) of minor bleeding in people taking aspirin (2.5 percent for aspirin, 1.9 percent for placebo). No other significant adverse effects were reported.

Cardiovascular and Biochemical: In the AMIS trial, the dosage of 1,000 milligrams per day of aspirin was associated with small increases in systolic blood pressure (BP) (average 1.5 to 2.1 millimeters), depending upon whether maximal or last available readings were used. Blood urea nitrogen and uric acid levels were also increased, but by less than 1.0 milligram percent.

Subjects with marked hypertension or renal insufficiency had been excluded from the trial so that the clinical importance of these observations for such subjects or for any subjects treated over more prolonged periods is not known. It is recommended that patients placed on long-term aspirin treatment, even at doses of 300 milligrams per day, be seen at regular intervals to assess changes in these measurements.

Sodium in Buffered Aspirin for Solution Formulations: One tablet daily of buffered aspirin in solutions adds 553 milligrams of sodium to that in the diet and may not be tolerated by patients with active sodium-retaining states such as congestive heart or renal failure. This amount of sodium adds about 30 percent to the 70- to 90-millieqivalents intake suggested as appropriate for dietary treatment of essential hypertension in the "1984 Report of the Joint National Committee on Detection, Evaluation, and Treatment of High Blood Pressure" (9).

Dosage and Administration: Recurrent MI (Reinfarction) and Unstable Angina Pectoris: Although most of the studies used dosages exceeding 300 milligrams, 2 trials used only 300 millgrams and pharmacologic data indicate that this dose inhibits platelet function fully. Therefore, 300 milligrams or a conventional 325 milligram aspirin dose is a reasonable, routine dose that would minimize gastrointestinal adverse reactions. This use of aspirin applies to both solid, oral dosage forms (buffered and plain aspirin) and buffered aspirin in solution.

Suspected Acute MI: The recommended dose of aspirin to treat suspected acute MI is 160 to 162.5 milligrams taken as soon as the infarct is suspected and then daily for at least 30 days. (One-half of a conventional 325-milligram aspirin tablet or two 80- or 81-milligram aspirin tablets may be taken.) This use of aspirin applies to both solid, oral dosage forms buffered, plain, and enteric-coated aspirin) and buffered aspirin in solution. If using a solid dosage form, the first dose should be crushed, sucked, or chewed. After the 30-day treatment, physicians should consider further therapy based on the labeling for dosage and administration of aspirin for prevention of recurrent MI (reinfarction).

References: (1) Elwood, P.C. et al., "A Randomized Controlled Trial of Acetylsalicylic Acid in the Secondary Prevention of Mortality from Myocardial Infarction," British Medical Journal, 1:436–440, 1974.
(2) The Coronary Drug Project Research Group, "Aspirin in Coronary Heart Disease," Journal of Chronic Diseases, 29:625–642, 1976.
(3) Breddin, K. et al., "Secondary Prevention of Myocardial Infarction: A Comparison of Acetylsalicylic Acid, Phenprocoumon or Placebo," Homeostasis, 470:263–268, 1979.
(4) Aspirin Myocardial Infarction Study Research Group, "A Randomized, Controlled Trial of Aspirin in Persons Recovered from Myocardial Infarction," Journal of the American Medical Aassociation, 243:661–669, 1980.
(5) Elwood, P.C., and P.M. Sweetnam, "Aspirin and Secondary Mortality After Myocardial Infarction," Lancet, II:1313–1315, December 22–29, 1979.
(6) The Persantine-Aspirin Reinfarction Study Research Group, "Persantine and Aspirin in Coronary Heart Disease," Circulation, 62:449–461, 1980.
(7) Lewis, H.D. et al., "Protective Effects of Aspirin Against Acute Myocardial Infarction and Death in Men with Unstable Angina, Results of a Veterans Administration Cooperative Study," New England Journal of Medicine, 309:396–403, 1983.
(8) ISIS-2 (Second International Study of Infarct Survival) Collaborative Group, "Randomized Trial of Intravenous Streptokinase, Oral Aspirin, Both, or Neither Among 17,187 Cases of Suspected Acute Myocardial Infarction: ISIS-2," Lancet, 2:349-360, August 13, 1988.
(8) "1984 Report of the Joint National Committee on Detection, Evaluation, and Treatment of High Blood Pressure," United States Department of Health and Human Services and United States Public Health Service, National Institutes of Health, Publication No. NIH 84-1088, 1984.

"ASPIRIN FOR TRANSIENT ISCHEMIC ATTACKS"

Indication: For reducing the risk of recurrent Transient Ischemic Attacks (TIA's) or stroke in men who have had transient ischemia of the brain due to fibrin platelet emboli. There is inadequate evidence that aspirin or buffered aspirin is effective in reducing TIA's in women at the recommended dosage. There is no evidence that aspirin or buffered aspirin is of benefit in the treatment of completed strokes in men or women.

Clinical Trials: The indication is supported by the results of a Canadian study (1) in which 585 patients with threatened stroke were followed in a randomized clinical trial for an average of 26 months to determine whether aspirin or sulfinpyrazone, singly or in combination, was superior to placebo in preventing transient ischemic attacks, stroke or death. The study showed that, although sulfinpyrazone had no statistically significant effect, aspirin reduced the risk of continuing transient ischemic attacks, stroke or death by 19 percent and reduced the risk of stroke or death by 31 percent. Another aspirin study carried out in the United States with 178 patients, showed a statistically significant number of "favorable outcomes," including reduced transient ischemic attacks, stroke and death (2).

Precautions: Patients presenting with signs and/or symptoms of TIA's should have a complete medical and neurologic evaluation. Consideration should be given to other disorders that resemble TIA's. Attention should be given to risk factors: it is important to evaluate and treat, if appropriate, other diseases associated with TIA's and stroke, such as hypertension and diabetes.

Concurrent administration of absorbable antacids at therapeutic doses may increase the clearance of salicylates in some individuals. The concurrent administration of nonabsorbable antacids may alter the rate of absorption of aspirin, thereby resulting in a decreased acetylsalicylic acid/salicylate ratio in plasma. The clinical significance of these decreases in available aspirin is unknown.

Aspirin at dosages of 1,000 milligrams per day has been associated with small increases in blood pressure, blood urea nitrogen, and serum uric acid levels. It is recommended that patients placed on long-term aspirin treatment be seen at regular intervals to assess changes in these measurements.

Adverse Reactions: At dosages of 1,000 milligrams or higher of aspirin per day, gastrointestinal side effects include stomach pain, heartburn, nausea and/or vomiting, as well as increased rates of gross gastrointestinal bleeding.

Dosage and Administration: Adult dosage for men is 1,300 mg a day, in divided doses of 650 mg twice a day or 325 mg four times a day.

References: (1) The Canadian Cooperative Study Group, "Randomized Trial of Aspirin and Sulfinpyrazone in Threatened Stroke," *New England Journal of Medicine,* 299:53–59, 1978.
(2) Fields, W. S., et al., "Controlled Trial of Aspirin in Cerebral Ischemia," *Stroke* 8:301–316, 1977."

How Supplied: 'Ecotrin' Tablets
81 mg in bottle of 36
325 mg in bottles of 100* and 250
500 mg in bottles of 60* and 150
*Without child-resistant caps.

TAMPER-RESISTANT PACKAGE FEATURES FOR YOUR PROTECTION:
• Bottle has imprinted seal under cap.
• The words ECOTRIN LOW or ECOTRIN REG or ECOTRIN MAX appear on each tablet.
• **DO NOT USE THIS PRODUCT IF ANY OF THESE TAMPER-RESISTANT FEATURES ARE MISSING OR BROKEN.**

Comments or Questions? Call Toll-Free 800-245-1040 weekdays.

Shown in Product Identification Guide, page 521 and 522

FEOSOL® Caplets
Hematinic
Iron Supplement

Description: FEOSOL Caplets contain pure iron micro particles called carbonyl iron. Replacing FEOSOL Capsules, this advanced formula is specially designed to be well absorbed, gentle on the stomach and offers enhanced safety in the event of an accidental overdose. Each FEOSOL carbonyl iron caplet delivers 50 mg of pure elemental iron, the same amount of elemental iron contained in the 250 mg ferrous sulfate capsule. At equivalent doses, carbonyl iron and ferrous sulfate were shown to be equally efficacious in correcting hemoglobin, hematocrit and serum iron levels in iron-deficient patients[1].

Safety: According to the American Association of Poison Control Centers, iron containing supplements are the leading cause of pediatric poisoning deaths for children under six in the United States[2]. Widely used as a food additive, carbonyl iron must be gastrically solubilized before it can be absorbed, giving it lower toxicity and enhancing its safety versus any of the ferrous salts[3]. As a result, carbonyl iron presents less chance of harm from accidental overdose. In addition, at equivalent doses, carbonyl iron side effects are no greater than those experienced with ferrous sulfate[4].

Warnings: Do not exceed recommended dosage. The treatment of any anemic condition should be under the advice and supervision of a physician. Since oral iron products interfere with absorption of oral tetracycline antibiotics, these products should not be taken within two hours of each other. Occasional gastrointestinal discomfort (such as nausea) may be minimized by taking with meals. Iron containing medication may occasionally cause constipation or diarrhea.
WARNING: Accidental overdose of iron-containing products is a leading cause of fatal poisoning in children under 6. Keep this product out of reach of children. In case of accidental overdose, call a doctor or poison control center immediately.

NUTRITION FACTS
Serving Size: 1 Caplet

Amount per Caplet	% Daily Value
Iron 50 mg	280%

Formula Ingredients: Lactose, Sorbitol, Carbonyl Iron, Crospovidone, Magnesium Stearate, Polyethylene Glycol, Stearic Acid, Hydroxypropyl Methylcellulose, Polydextrose, Carnauba Wax, Titanium Dioxide, Triacetin, Blue #2 A1 Lake, Red #40 A1 Lake, Yellow #6 A1 Lake.

Directions: Adults—one caplet daily or as directed by a physician. Children under 12 years: Consult a physician.

Tamper-Evident Feature: Each caplet is encased in a plastic cell with a foil back; do not use if cell or foil is broken.

References: [1]Devasthali SD, Gordeuk VR, Brittenham GM, et al, "Bioavailability of Carbonyl Iron: A randomized, double-blind study." Eur J Haematology, 1991; 46:272–278.
[2]FDA Consumer; March 1996:7
[3]Heubers, JA, Brittenham GM, Csiba E and Finch CA. "Absorption of carbonyl iron." J Lab Clin Med 1986; 108:473–78.
[4]Devasthali SD, Gordeuk VR, Brittenham GM, et al, "Bioavailability of a Carbonyl Iron: A randomized, double-blind study." Eur J Haematology, 1991; 46:272–278.
Store at room temperature, avoid excessive heat (greater than 100°F) or humidity.

How Supplied: Boxes of 30 and 60 caplets in blisters. Also available in single unit packages of 100 caplets intended for institutional use
Also available: Feosol Tablets, and Feosol Elixir
Comments or Questions? Call Toll-Free 1-800-245-1040 Weekdays.
SmithKline Beecham Consumer Healthcare, L.P.
Pittsburgh, PA 15230   Made in USA
Shown in Product Identification Guide, page 522

FEOSOL® ELIXIR
Iron Supplement

Description: 'Feosol' Elixir, an unusually palatable iron elixir, provides the body with ferrous sulfate—the standard elixir for simple iron deficiency and iron-deficiency anemia when the need for such therapy has been determined by a physician.

NUTRITION FACTS
Serving Size: 1 teaspoonful
Servings per Container: 94

Amount per teaspoonful	% Daily Value
Iron 44 mg	240%

Continued on next page

Feosol Elixir—Cont.

Formula:
INGREDIENTS
Purified Water, Sucrose, Glucose, Ferrous Sulfate, Alcohol 5%, Citric Acid, Saccharin Sodium, FD&C Yellow #6, Flavors.

Directions: Adults—1 teaspoonful daily or as directed by a doctor. Children under 12 years—Consult a physician. Mix with water or fruit juice to avoid temporary staining of teeth; do not mix with milk or wine-based vehicles.

TAMPER-RESISTANT PACKAGE FEATURE:
IMPRINTED SEAL AROUND BOTTLE CAP: DO NOT USE IF BROKEN.

Warnings: Do not exceed recommended dosage. The treatment of any anemic condition should be under the advice and supervision of a physician. Since oral iron products interfere with absorption of oral tetracycline antibiotics, these products should not be taken within two hours of each other. Occasional gastrointestinal discomfort (such as nausea) may be minimized by taking with meals. Iron containing medication may occasionally cause constipation or diarrhea and liquids may cause temporary staining of the teeth (this is less likely when diluted).
WARNING: Accidental overdose of iron-containing products is a leading cause of fatal poisoning in children under 6. Keep this product out of reach of children. In case of accidental overdose, call a doctor or poison control center immediately.
If you are pregnant or nursing a baby, seek the advice of a health professional before using this product.
STORE AT ROOM TEMPERATURE (59–86 F), PROTECT FROM FREEZING.

How Supplied: A clear orange liquid in 16 fl. oz. child-resistant bottles.

Also Available: 'Feosol' Tablets, 'Feosol' Caplets.
Comments or Questions? Call Toll-Free 1-800-245-1040 Weekdays.
SmithKline Beecham Consumer Healthcare, L.P.
Pittsburgh, PA 15230
Made in USA
Shown in Product Identification Guide, page 522

FEOSOL® TABLETS
Iron Supplement

Description: Feosol tablets provide the body with ferrous sulfate—an iron supplement for iron deficiency and iron deficiency anemia when the need for such therapy has been determined by a physician.

NUTRITION FACTS
Serving Size: 1 Tablet

Amount per Tablet	% Daily Value
Iron 65 mg	360%

Formula:
INGREDIENTS
Dried ferrous sulfate 200 mg (65 mg of elemental iron) equivalent to 325 mg of ferrous sulfate USP per tablet. Calcium Sulfate, Starch, Glucose, Hydroxypropyl Methylcellulose, Talc, Stearic Acid, Polyethylene Glycol, Sodium Lauryl Sulfate, Mineral Oil, Titanium Dioxide, D&C Yellow 10, FD&C Blue 2.

Directions: Adults and children 12 years and over—One tablet daily or as directed by a physician. Children under 12 years—Consult a physician.
Tamper-Evident Feature: Each tablet is encased in a plastic cell with a foil back; do not use if cell or foil is broken.

Warnings: Do not exceed recommended dosage. The treatment of any anemic condition should be under the advice and supervision of a physician. Since oral iron products interfere with absorption of oral tetracycline antibiotics, these products should not be taken within two hours of each other. Occasional gastrointestinal discomfort (such as nausea) may be minimized by taking with meals. Iron containing medication may occassionally cause constipation or diarrhea.
WARNING: Accidental overdose of iron-contraining products is a leading cause of fatal poisoning in children under 6. Keep this product out of reach of children. In case of accidental overdose, call a doctor, or poison control center immediately. If you are pregnant or nursing a baby, seek the advice of a health professional before using this product.
Store at room temperature (59–86°F). Not USP for dissolution.

How Supplied: Cartons of 100 tablets in child-resistant blisters.
Previously packaged in bottles.
Also available: Feosol caplets and Feosol elixir.

Comments or Questions?
Call toll-free 800-245-1040 weekdays.
SmithKline Beecham Consumer Healthcare, L.P.
Pittsburgh, PA 15230   Made in USA
Shown in Product Identification Guide, page 522

GAVISCON® Regular Strength
Antacid Tablets
[găv 'ĭs-kŏn]

Composition: Each chewable tablet contains the following active ingredients:
Aluminum hydroxide dried gel... 80 mg
Magnesium trisilicate .... 20 mg
and the following inactive ingredients: alginic acid, calcium stearate, flavor, sodium bicarbonate, starch (may contain cornstarch), and sucrose.

Actions: Unique formulation produces soothing foam which floats on stomach contents. Foam containing antacid precedes stomach contents into the esophagus when reflux occurs to help protect the sensitive mucosa from further irritation. GAVISCON® acts locally without neutralizing entire stomach contents to help maintain integrity of the digestive process. Endoscopic studies indicate that GAVISCON Antacid Tablets are equally as effective in the erect or supine patient.

Indications: GAVISCON is specifically formulated for the temporary relief of heartburn (acid indigestion) due to acid reflux. GAVISCON is not indicated for the treatment of peptic ulcers.

Directions: Chew 2 to 4 tablets four times a day or as directed by a physician. Tablets should be taken after meals and at bedtime or as needed. For best results follow by a half glass of water or other liquid. DO NOT SWALLOW WHOLE.

Warnings: Do not take more than 16 tablets in a 24-hour period or 16 tablets daily for more than 2 weeks, except under the advice and supervision of a physician. Do not use this product except under the advice and supervision of a physician if you are on a sodium-restricted diet. Each GAVISCON Tablet contains approximately 0.8 mEq sodium.

Drug Interaction Precaution: Antacids may interact with certain prescription drugs. If you are presently taking a prescription drug, do not take this product without checking with your physician or other health professional.
Store at a controlled room temperature in a dry place.

Keep this and all drugs out of the reach of children. In case of accidental overdose, seek professional assistance or contact a poison control center immediately.

How Supplied: Bottles of 100 tablets and in foil-wrapped 2s in boxes of 30 tablets.
Shown in Product Identification Guide, page 522

GAVISCON® EXTRA STRENGTH
Antacid Tablets
[găv 'ĭs-kŏn]

Composition: Each chewable tablet contains the following active ingredients:
Aluminum hydroxide .... 160 mg
Magnesium carbonate .... 105 mg
and the following inactive ingredients: alginic acid, calcium stearate, flavor, sodium bicarbonate, and sucrose. May contain stearic acid. Contains sorbitol or mannitol. May contain starch.

Actions: Gavison's unique antacid foam barrier neutralizes stomach acid.

Indications: For the relief of heartburn, sour stomach, acid indigestion and upset stomach associated with these conditions.

Directions: Chew 2 to 4 tablets four times a day or as directed by a physician. Tablets should be taken after meals and at bedtime or as needed. For best results follow by a half glass of water or other liquid. DO NOT SWALLOW WHOLE.

Warnings: Do not take more than 16 tablets in a 24-hour period or 16 tablets daily for more than 2 weeks, except under the advice and supervision of a physician. Do not use this product except under the advice and supervision of a physician if you are on a sodium-restricted diet. Each tablet contains approximately 1.3 mEq sodium.

Drug Interaction Precaution: Antacids may interact with certain prescription drugs. If you are presently taking a prescription drug, do not take this product without checking with your physician or other health professional.

Store at a controlled room temperature in a dry place.

Keep this and all drugs out of the reach of children. In case of accidental overdose, seek professional assistance or contact a poison control center immediately.

How Supplied: Bottles of 100 tablets and in foil-wrapped 2s in boxes of 6 and 30 tablets.

Shown in Product Identification Guide, page 522

GAVISCON® EXTRA STRENGTH
Liquid Antacid

[găv ʹĭs-kŏn]

Composition: Each 2 teaspoonfuls (10 mL) contains the following active ingredients:
Aluminum hydroxide .... 508 mg
Magnesium carbonate .... 475 mg
and the following inactive ingredients: benzyl alcohol, edetate disodium, flavor, glycerin, saccharin sodium, simethicone emulsion, sodium alginate, sorbitol solution, water, and xanthan gum.

Actions: Gaviscon's unique antacid foam barrier neutralizes stomach acid.

Indications: For the relief of heartburn, sour stomach, acid indigestion & upset stomach associated with these conditions.

Directions: SHAKE WELL BEFORE USING. Take 2 to 4 teaspoonfuls four times a day or as directed by a physician. GAVISCON Extra Strength Liquid should be taken after meals and at bedtime, followed by half a glass of water. Dispense product only by spoon or other measuring device.

Warnings: Except under the advice and supervision of a physician, do not take more than 16 teaspoonfuls in a 24-hour period or 16 teaspoonfuls daily for more than 2 weeks. May have laxative effect. Do not use this product if you have a kidney disease. Do not use this product if you are on a sodium-restricted diet. Each teaspoonful contains approximately 0.9 mEq sodium.

Drug Interaction Precaution: Antacids may interact with certain prescription drugs. If you are presently taking a prescription drug, do not take this prod-

uct without checking with your physician or other health professional.

Keep tightly closed. Avoid freezing. Store at a controlled room temperature.

Keep this and all drugs out of the reach of children. In case of accidental overdose, seek professional assistance or contact a poison control center immediately.

How Supplied: 12 fl oz (355 mL) bottles.

Shown in Product Identification Guide, page 522

GAVISCON® Regular Strength
Liquid Antacid

[găv ʹĭs-kŏn]

Composition: Each tablespoonful (15 ml) contains the following active ingredients:
Aluminum hydroxide .... 95 mg
Magnesium carbonate .... 358 mg
and the following inactive ingredients: benzyl alcohol, D&C Yellow #10, edetate disodium, FD&C Blue #1, flavor, glycerin, saccharin sodium, sodium alginate, sorbitol solution, water, and xanthan gum.

Actions: Gaviscon's unique antacid foam barrier neutralizes stomach acid.

Indications: For the relief of heartburn, sour stomach, acid indigestion & upset stomach associated with these conditions.

Directions: SHAKE WELL BEFORE USING. Take 1 or 2 tablespoonfuls four times a day or as directed by a physician. GAVISCON Regular Strength Liquid should be taken after meals and at bedtime, followed by half a glass of water. Dispense product only by spoon or other measuring device.

Warnings: Except under the advice and supervision of a physician, do not take more than 8 tablespoonfuls in a 24-hour period or 8 tablespoonfuls daily for more than 2 weeks. May have laxative effect. Do not use this product if you have a kidney disease. Do not use this product if you are on a sodium-restricted diet. Each tablespoonful of GAVISCON Liquid contains approximately 1.7 mEq sodium.

Drug Interaction Precaution: Antacids may interact with certain prescription drugs. If you are presently taking a prescription drug, do not take this product without checking with your physician or other health professional.

Keep tightly closed. Avoid freezing. Store at a controlled room temperature.

Keep this and all drugs out of the reach of children. In case of accidental overdose, seek professional assistance or contact a poison control center immediately.

How Supplied: 12 fluid oz (355 ml) bottles.

Shown in Product Identification Guide, page 522

GLY–OXIDE® Liquid

Description/Active Ingredient: GLY-OXIDE® Liquid contains carbamide peroxide 10%.

Actions: GLY-OXIDE® Liquid has an oxygen-rich formula that works to relieve the pain of canker sores by cleaning and debriding damaged tissue so natural healing can occur. GLY-OXIDE Liquid's dense oxygenating microfoam helps destroy odor-forming germs and flushes out food particles that ordinary brushing can miss.

Indications For Temporary Use: Gly-Oxide liquid is for temporary use in cleansing canker sores and minor wound or gum inflammation resulting from minor dental procedures, dentures, orthodontic appliances, accidental injury, or other irritations of the mouth and gums. Gly-Oxide can also be used to guard against the risk of infections in the mouth and gums.

Everyday Uses: Gly-Oxide may be used routinely to improve oral hygiene as an aid to regular brushing or when regular brushing is inadequate or impossible such as total care geriatrics, etc. Gly-Oxide kills germs to reduce mouth odors and/or odors on dental appliances. Gly-Oxide penetrates between teeth and other areas of the mouth to flush out food particles ordinary brushing can miss. This can be especially useful when brushing is made more difficult by the presence of orthodontics or other dental appliances. Plus, Gly-Oxide helps remove stains on dental appliances to improve appearance.

Directions For Temporary Use: Do not dilute. Replace tip on bottle when not in use. **Adults and children 2 years of age and older:** Apply several drops directly from bottle onto affected area; spit out after 2 to 3 minutes. Use up to four times daily after meals and at bedtime or as directed by dentist or doctor. OR place 10 drops on tongue, mix with saliva, swish for several minutes, and then spit out. Use by children under 12 years of age should be supervised. **Children under 2 years of age:** Consult a dentist or doctor.

Directions For Everyday Use: The product may be used following the temporary use directions above. OR apply Gly-Oxide to the toothbrush (it will sink into the brush), cover with toothpaste, brush normally, and spit out.

Warnings: Severe or persistent oral inflammation, denture irritation, or gingivitis may be serious. If sore mouth symptoms do not improve in 7 days, or if irritation, pain, or redness persists or worsens, or if swelling, rash, or fever develops, discontinue use of product and see your dentist or doctor promptly. Avoid contact with eyes. **KEEP THIS AND ALL DRUGS OUT OF THE REACH OF CHILDREN.** In case of accidental overdose, seek professional assistance or contact a poison control center immediately.

Continued on next page

Gly-Oxide—Cont.

Inactive Ingredients: Citric Acid, Flavor, Glycerin, Propylene Glycol, Sodium Stannate, Water, and Other Ingredients.

Protect from excessive heat and direct sunlight.

How Supplied: GLY-OXIDE® Liquid is available in $^1/_2$-fl-oz and 2-fl-oz plastic squeeze bottles with applicator spouts. Comments or Questions? Call Toll-free 1-800-245-1040 Weekdays SmithKline Beecham Consumer Healthcare, L.P.
Pittsburgh, PA 15230   Made in U.S.A.
Shown in Product Identification Guide, page 522

MASSENGILL® Douches, Towelettes and Cleansing Wash
[*mas 'sen-gil*]

PRODUCT OVERVIEW

Key Facts: Massengill is the brand name for a line of feminine hygiene products which are recommended for routine cleansing and for temporary relief of vaginal itching and irritation. Massengill disposable douches are available in two Vinegar & Water formulas (Extra Mild and Extra Cleansing), and four other cosmetic solutions (Country Flowers, Fresh Baby Powder Scent, Fresh Mountain Breeze, and Spring Rain Freshness), and a Medicated formula (with povidone-iodine). Massengill also has products specially designed to safely and gently cleanse the external vaginal area: Baby Powder Soft Cloth Towelettes, Medicated Soft Cloth Towelettes and Feminine Cleansing Wash.

Major Uses: Massengill's Vinegar & Water, and other cosmetic douches are recommended for routine douching, or for cleansing following menstruation, prescribed use of vaginal medication or use of contraceptives. Massengill Medicated is recommended in a seven day regimen for the symptomatic relief of minor itching and irritation associated with vaginitis due to Candida albicans, Trichomonas vaginalis, and Gardnerella vaginalis. Massengill Feminine Cleansing Wash is a gentle soapfree way to clean the external vaginal area. Massengill Non-medicated Soft Cloth Towelettes are a convenient and portable way to cleanse the external vaginal area and wash odor away. Massengill Medicated Soft Cloth Towelettes provide temporary relief of minor external itching associated with irritation or skin rashes.

Safety Information: Do not douche during pregnancy unless directed by a physician. Douching does not prevent pregnancy. Do not use this product and consult your physician if you are experiencing any of the following symptoms: unusual vaginal discharge, vaginal bleeding, painful and/or frequent urina-

tion, lower abdominal/pelvis pain, or you or your sex partner have genital sores or ulcers.
Massengill Vinegar & Water, and other Cosmetic Douches—If vaginal dryness or irritation occurs, discontinue use.
Massengill Medicated — Women with iodine-sensitivity should not use this product. If symptoms persist after seven days, or if redness, swelling or pain develop, consult a physician. Do not use while nursing unless directed by a physician.

PRODUCT INFORMATION
MASSENGILL®
[*mas 'sen-gil*]
Disposable Douches

Ingredients: DISPOSABLES: Extra Mild Vinegar and Water—Purified Water, Sodium Citrate, Citric Acid, and Vinegar.
Extra Cleansing Vinegar and Water—Purified Water, Sodium Citrate, Citric Acid, Vinegar, Diazolidinyl Urea, Octoxynol-9, Cetylpyridinium Chloride, Edetate Disodium.
Fresh Baby Powder Scent—Purified Water, Sodium Citrate, Citric Acid, SD Alcohol 40, Diazolidinyl Urea, Octoxynol-9, Fragrance, Cetylpyridinium Chloride, Edetate Disodium, FD&C Blue #1.
Country Flowers—Purified Water, Sodium Citrate, Citric Acid, SD Alcohol 40, Diazolidinyl Urea, Octoxynol-9, Fragrance, Cetylpyridinium Chloride, Edetate Disodium, D&C Red #28, FD&C Blue #1.
Fresh Mountain Breeze—Purified Water, SD Alcohol 40, Diazolindinyl Urea, Citric Acid, Sodium Citrate, Octoxynol-9, Fragrance, Cetylpyridinium Chloride, Edetate Disodium, FD&C Blue #1, D&C Yellow #10.
Spring Rain Freshness—Purified Water, SD Alcohol 40, Diazolidinyl Urea, Citric Acid, Sodium Citrate, Octoxynol-9, Fragrance, Cetylpyridinium Chloride, Edetate Disodium.

Indications: Recommended for routine cleansing at the end of menstruation, after use of contraceptive creams or jellies (check the contraceptive package instructions first) or to rinse out the residue of prescribed vaginal medication (as directed by physician).

Actions: The buffered acid solutions of Massengill Douches are valuable adjuncts to specific vaginal therapy following the prescribed use of vaginal medication or contraceptives and in feminine hygiene.

Directions: DISPOSABLES: Twist off flat, wing-shaped tab from bottle containing premixed solution, attach nozzle supplied and use. The unit is completely disposable.

Warning: Douching does not prevent pregnancy. Do not use during pregnancy except under the advice and supervision of your physician. If vaginal dryness or irritation occurs, discontinue use. Use this product only as directed for routine

cleansing. You should douche no more than twice a week except on the advice of your doctor.
An association has been reported between douching and pelvic inflammatory disease (PID), a serious infection of your reproductive system which can lead to sterility and/or ectopic (tubal) pregnancy. PID requires immediate medical attention.
PID's most common symptoms are pain and/or tenderness in the lower part of the abdomen and pelvis. You may also experience a vaginal discharge, vaginal bleeding, nausea or fever. Other sexually transmitted diseases (STDs) have similar symptoms and/or frequent urination, genital sores, or ulcers. Douches should not be used for the self treatment of any STDs or PID. If you suspect you have one of these infections or PID, stop using this product and see your doctor immediately.
See the enclosed insert for important health information concerning sexually transmitted diseases and PID.

How Supplied: Disposable—6 oz. disposable plastic bottle.

MASSENGILL®
[*mas 'sen-gil*]
Baby Powder Scent Soft Cloth Towelette

Ingredients: Water, Lactic Acid, Sodium Lactate, Potassium Sorbate, Octoxynol-9, Disodium EDTA, Cetylpyridinium Chloride, and Fragrance.

Indications: For cleansing and refreshing the external vaginal area.

Actions: Massengill Baby Powder Scent Soft Cloth Towelette safely cleanse the external vaginal area. The towelette delivery system makes the application soft and gentle.

Directions: Remove towelette from foil packet, unfold, and gently wipe. Throw away towelette after it has been used once.

How Supplied: Sixteen individually wrapped, disposable towelettes per carton.

MASSENGILL Feminine Cleansing Wash
[*mas 'sen-gil*]

Ingredients: Water, sodium laureth sulfate, magnesium laureth sulfate, sodium laureth-8 sulfate, magnesium laureth-8 sulfate, sodium oleth sulfate, magnesium oleth sulfate, lauramidopropyl betaine, myristamine oxide, lactic acid, PEG-120 methyl glucose dioleate, fragrance, sodium methylparaben, sodium ethylparaben, sodium propylparaben, methylchloroisothiazolinone, methylisothiazolinone, D&C Red #33.

Indications: For cleansing and refreshing of external vaginal area.

Actions: Massengill feminine cleansing wash safely and gently cleanses the external vaginal area.

Directions: Pour small amount into palm of hand or wash cloth and lather into wet skin. Rinse clean. Safe to use daily. For external use only.

How Supplied: 8 fl. oz plastic flip-top bottle.

MASSENGILL® Medicated
[mas 'sen-gil]
Disposable Douche

Active Ingredient: Povidone-iodine: When mixed as directed a 0.30% solution is formed (Cepticin™).

Indications: For symptomatic relief of minor vaginal irritation or itching associated with vaginitis due to Candida albicans, Trichomonas vaginalis, and Gardnerella vaginalis.

Action: Povidone-iodine is widely recognized as an effective broad spectrum microbicide against both gram negative and gram positive bacteria, fungi, yeasts and protozoa. While remaining active in the presence of blood, serum or bodily secretions, it possesses virtually none of the irritating properties of iodine.

Warning: Douching does not prevent pregnancy. Do not use during pregnancy or while nursing except under the advice and supervision of your physician. If vaginal dryness or irritation occurs discontinue use. Use this product only as directed. Do not use this product for routine cleansing.
An association has been reported between douching and pelvic inflammatory disease (PID), a serious infection of your reproductive system, which can lead to sterility and/or ectopic (tubal) pregnancy. PID requires immediate medical attention.
PID's most common symptoms are pain and/or tenderness in the lower part of the abdomen and pelvis. You may also experience a vaginal discharge, vaginal bleeding, nausea or fever. Other sexually transmitted diseases (STDs) have similar symptoms and/or frequent urination, genital sores, or ulcers. Douches should not be used for self-treatment of any STDs or PID. If you suspect you have one of these infections or PID, stop using this product and see your doctor immediately.
See the enclosed insert for important health information concerning sexually transmitted diseases and PID.
Women with iodine sensitivity should not use this product.
Keep out of the reach of children.
Avoid storing at high temperature (greater than 100°F).
Protect from freezing.

Dosage and Administration: Dosage is provided as a single unit concentrate to be added to 6 oz. of sanitized water supplied in a disposable bottle. A specially designed nozzle is provided. After use, the unit is discarded. Use one bottle a day for seven days. Although symptoms may be relieved earlier, for maximum relief, treatment should be continued for the full seven days.

How Supplied: 6 oz. bottle of sanitized water with 0.17 oz. vial of povidone-iodine and nozzle.
Shown in Product Identification Guide, page 522

MASSENGILL® Medicated
[mas 'sen-gil]
Soft Cloth Towelette

Active Ingredient: Hydrocortisone (0.5%).

Inactive Ingredients: Diazolidinyl Urea, DMDM Hydantoin, Isopropyl Myristate, Methylparaben, Polysorbate 60, Propylene Glycol, Propylparaben, Sorbitan Stearate, Steareth-2, Steareth-21, Water.
Also available in non-medicated (Baby Powder Scent) to freshen and cleanse the external vaginal area.

Indications: For soothing relief of minor external feminine itching or other itching associated with minor skin irritations, and rashes. Other uses of this product should be only under the advice and supervision of a physician.

Action: Massengill Medicated Soft Cloth Towelettes contain hydrocortisone, a proven anti-inflammatory, anti-pruritic ingredient. The towelette delivery system makes the application soothing, soft, and gentle.

Warnings: For external use only. Avoid contact with eyes. If condition worsens, symptoms persist for more than seven days, or symptoms recur within a few days, do not use this or any other hydrocortisone product unless you have consulted a physician. If experiencing a vaginal discharge, see a physician. Do not use this product for the treatment of diaper rash.
Keep this and all drugs out of the reach of children. As with any drug, if pregnant or nursing a baby, seek the advice of a health professional before using this product. In case of accidental ingestion, seek professional assistance or contact a Poison Control Center immediately.

Directions: Adults and Children two years of age and older—apply to the affected area not more than three to four times daily. Remove towelette from foil packet, gently wipe, and discard. Throw away towelette after it has been used once. Children under 2 years of age: DO NOT USE.

How Supplied: Ten individually wrapped, disposable towelettes per carton.

"The facts about Vaginal Infections and STDs"
A guide for women on vaginal infections and sexually transmitted diseases (STDs).
Free to physicians, pharmacists and patients in limited quantities by writing SmithKline Beecham Consumer Healthcare, L.P. PO Box 1469, Pittsburgh, PA 15230 or calling 1-800-233-2426.

NICODERM® CQ®
Nicotine Transdermal System/Stop Smoking Aid

Available as:
　　　　Step 1 - 21 mg/24 hours
　　　　Step 2 - 14 mg/24 hours
　　　　Step 3 - 7 mg/24 hours

If you smoke: Over 10 cigarettes a Day: Start with Step 1
10 Cigarettes a Day or Less: Start with Step 2

WHAT IS THE NICODERM CQ PATCH AND HOW IS IT USED?
NicoDerm CQ is a small, nicotine containing patch. When you put on a NicoDerm CQ patch, nicotine passes through the skin and into your body. NicoDerm CQ is very thin and uses special material to control how fast nicotine passes through the skin. Unlike the sudden jolts of nicotine delivered by cigarettes, the amount of nicotine you receive remains relatively smooth throughout the 24 or 16 hours period you wear the NicoDerm CQ patch. This helps to reduce cravings you may have for nicotine.

Active Ingredient: Nicotine

Purpose: Stop Smoking Aid

Use: To reduce withdrawal symptoms, including nicotine craving, associated with quitting smoking.

Directions:
• Stop smoking completely when you begin using NicoDerm CQ.

NicoDerm CQ Program

STEP 1 (21 mg)	STEP 2 (14 mg)	STEP 3 (7 mg)
Initial Treatment Period	Step Down Treatment Period	
Weeks 1–6	Weeks 7–8	Weeks 9–10

• Light Smokers (10 cigarettes a day or less): Do not use STEP 1 (21 mg). Use STEP 2 (14 mg) for six weeks and STEP 3 (7 mg) for two weeks and then stop.
• STEPS 2 and 3 allow you to gradually reduce your level of nicotine. Completing the full program will increase your chances of quitting successfully.
• A the end of 10 weeks (8 weeks for light smokers), stop using NicoDerm CQ. If you still feel the need for NicoDerm CQ, talk with your doctor.

Continued on next page

Nicoderm CQ—Cont.

- Each day apply a new patch to a different place on skin that is dry, clean and hairless.
- You may wear the patch for 16 or 24 hours.
- If you crave cigarettes when you wake up, wear the patch for 24 hours.
- If you begin to have vivid dreams or other disruptions of your sleep while wearing the patch for 24 hours, try taking the patch off at bedtime (after about 16 hours) and putting on a new one when you get up the next day.
- Remove the used patch and put on a new patch at the same time every day. Do not leave patch on for more than 24 hours because it may irritate your skin and loses strength after 24 hours.
- Wash your hands after applying or removing NicoDerm QC.

WARNINGS:
- Keep this and all medication away from children and pets. Used patches have enough nicotine to poison children and pets. Fold sticky ends together and insert in the disposal tray in the box. For accidental overdose, seek professional assistance or contact a poison control center immediately.
- Nicotine can increase your baby's heart rate. First try to stop smoking without the nicotine patch. As with any drug, if you are pregnant or nursing a baby, seek the advice of a health professional before using this product.
- Do not smoke even when not wearing the patch. The nicotine in your skin will still be entering your bloodstream for several hours after you take off the patch.

DO NOT USE IF YOU
- Continue to smoke, chew tobacco, use snuff, or use nicotine or other nicotine containing products.

ASK YOUR DOCTOR BEFORE USE IF YOU
- Are under 18 years of age.
- Have heart disease, recent heart attack, or irregular heartbeat. Nicotine can increase your heart rate.
- Have high blood pressure not controlled with medication. Nicotine can increase blood pressure.
- Take prescription medicine for depression or asthma. Your prescription dose may need to be adjusted.
- Are allergic to adhesive tape or have skin problems, because you are more likely to get rashes.

STOP USE AND SEE YOUR DOCTOR IF YOU HAVE
- Skin redness caused by the patch that does not go away after four days, or if your skin swells or you get a rash.
- Irregular heartbeat or palpitations.
- Symptoms of nicotine overdose such as nausea, vomiting, dizziness, weakness and rapid heartbeat.

READ THE LABEL
Read the carton and the User's Guide before using this product. Keep the carton and User's Guide. They contain important information.

Inactive Ingredients: Ethylene vinyl acetate-copolymer, polyisobutylene and high density polyethylene between pigmented and clear polyester backings.
Do not store above 30°C (86°F).

TO INCREASE YOUR SUCCESS IN QUITTING:
1. You must be motivated to quit.
2. Complete the full treatment program, applying a new patch every day.
3. Use with a support program as described in the enclosed Users Guide.

USER'S GUIDE:
HOW TO USE NICODERM CQ TO HELP YOU QUIT SMOKING
KEYS TO SUCCESS
1) You must really want to quit smoking for NicoDerm CQ to help you.
2) Apply a new patch every day.
3) NicoDerm CQ works best when used together with a support program.
4) If you have trouble using NicoDerm CQ, ask your doctor or pharmacist or call SmithKline Beecham at 1-800-834-5895 weekdays (10:00am - 4:30 pm EST).

SO YOU'VE DECIDED TO QUIT
Congratulations. Your decision to stop smoking is one of the most important things you can do to improve your health. Quitting smoking is a two-part process that involves:
1) overcoming your physical need for nicotine, and 2) breaking your smoking habit. Nico-Derm CQ helps smokers quit by reducing nicotine withdrawal symptoms. Many NicoDerm CQ users will be able to stop smoking for a few days but often will start smoking again. Most smokers try to quit several times before they completely stop. Your own chances of quitting smoking depend how strongly you are addicted to nicotine, how much you want to quit, and how closely you follow a quitting plan like the one that comes with NicoDerm CQ.

QUITTING SMOKING IS HARD!
If you find you cannot stop or if you start smoking again after using NicoDerm CQ please talk to a health care professional who can help you find a program that may work better for you. Breaking this addiction doesn't happen overnight. Because NicoDerm CQ provides some nicotine, the NicoDerm CQ patch will help you stop smoking by reducing nicotine withdrawal symptoms such as nicotine craving, nervousness and irritability. This User's Guide will give you support as you become a non-smoker. It will answer common questions about NicoDerm CQ and give tips to help you stop smoking, and should be referred to often.

WHERE TO GET HELP
You are more likely to stop smoking by using NicoDerm CQ with a support program that helps you break your smoking habit. There may be support groups in your area for people trying to quit. Call your local chapter of the American Lung Association (1-800-586-4872), American Cancer Society (1-800-227-2345) or American Heart Association (1-800-242-8721) for further information. If you find you cannot stop smoking or if you start smoking again after using NicoDerm CQ, remember breaking this addiction doesn't happen overnight. You may want to talk to a health care professional who can help you improve your chances of quitting the next time you try NicoDerm CQ or another method.

LET'S GET ORGANIZED
Your reason for quitting may be a combination of concerns about health, the effect of smoking on your appearance, and pressure from your family and friends to stop smoking. Or maybe you're concerned about the dangerous effect of second-hand smoke on the people you care about. All of these are good reasons. You probably have others. Decide your most important reasons, and write them down on the wallet card inside the back cover of the User's Guide. Carry this card with you. In difficult moments, when you want to smoke, the card will remind you why you are quitting.

WHAT YOU'RE UP AGAINST
Smoking is addictive in two ways. Your need for nicotine has become both physical and mental. You must overcome both addictions to stop smoking. So while NicoDerm CQ will lessen your body's physical addiction to nicotine, you've got to want to quit smoking to overcome the mental dependence on cigarettes. Once you've decided that you're going to quit, it's time to get started. But first, there are some important cautions you should consider.

SOME IMPORTANT CAUTIONS
This product is only for those who want to stop smoking. If you smoke, chew tobacco, use snuff or use nicotine gum or other nicotine containing products while using NicoDerm CQ, you may get a nicotine overdose. Ask your doctor before using NicoDerm CQ if you have heart disease, had a recent heart attack, irregular heartbeat. Nicotine can increase your blood pressure. If you take a prescription medication for asthma or depression, be sure your doctor knows you are quitting smoking. Your prescription medication dose may need to be adjusted. You should ask your doctor before using NicoDerm CQ if you are allergic to adhesive tape or have skin problems, because you are more likely to get rashes. Nicotine can increase your baby's heart rate. First try to stop smoking without the nicotine patch. As with any drug, if you are pregnant or nursing a baby, seek the advice of a health professional before using this product. Ask your doctor before using NicoDerm CQ if you are under 18 years of age.

You should stop use and see your doctor if you have skin redness caused by the patch that does not go away after four days, or if your skin swells or you get a rash, or if you have irregular heartbeat or palpitations.

Also, stop use if you have symptoms of nicotine overdose. These may include nausea, vomiting, diarrhea, dizziness, weakness and rapid heartbeat. Also, seizures have been seen in children who swallowed cigarettes. They may have a similar reaction to nicotine patches.

Keep this and all drugs out of the reach of children and pets. Even used patches have enough nicotine to poison children and pets. Be sure to fold the sticky ends together and insert in the disposal tray provided in the box. In case of accidental overdose, seek professional assistance or contact a poison control center immediately.

LET'S GET STARTED

Becoming a non-smoker starts today. Your first step is to read through the entire User's Guide carefully.

First, check that you bought the right starting dose. If you smoke more than 10 cigarettes a day, begin with Step 1 (21 mg). As the carton indicates, light smokers should not use Step 1 (21 mg). They should start with Step 2 (14 mg). Light smokers are people who smoke 10 cigarettes or less a day. Throughout this User's Guide we will give specific instructions for light smokers.

Next set your personalized quitting schedule.

Take out a calendar that you can use to track your progress. Pick a quit date, and mark this on your calendar using the stickers in the middle of the User's Guide.

For people who smoke over 10 cigarettes a day:

STEP 1. Initial Treatment Period (weeks 1–6): 21 mg patches. Choose your quit date (it should be soon). This is the day you will quit smoking cigarettes entirely and begin using NicoDerm CQ to reduce your cravings for nicotine. Place the Step 1 sticker on this date. For the first six weeks you'll use the highest-strength (21 mg) NicoDerm CQ patches. Be sure to follow the directions on page 10 of the User's Guide.

Completing the full program will increase your chances of quitting successfully. This is done by changing over to the Step 2 (14 mg) patch for 2 weeks followed by a final 2 weeks with the Step 3 (7mg) patch. The four week step down treatment period allows you to gradually reduce the amount of nicotine you get, rather than stopping suddenly, and will increase your chances of quitting.

STEP 2. First step down treatment period (Weeks 7–8): 14 mg patches. Switching to Step 2 (14 mg) patches after 6 weeks begins to gradually reduce your nicotine usage. Place the Step 2 sticker on this date (the first day of week seven). Use the 14 mg patches for two weeks.

STEP 3. Final step down treatment period (Weeks 9–10): 7 mg patches. After eight weeks, nicotine intake is further reduced by moving down to Step 3 (7 mg) patches. Place the Step 3 sticker on this date (the first day of week nine). Use the 7 mg patches for two weeks.

See the chart in the "DIRECTIONS" section above for the recommended usage schedule for NicoDerm CQ. **Stop using NicoDerm CQ at the end of week 10.** If you still feel the need to use NicoDerm CQ after Week 10, talk with your doctor or health professional.

LIGHT SMOKER DIRECTIONS

Do not use Step 1 (21 mg). You should start with Step 2 (14 mg).

For LIGHT SMOKERS–People who smoke 10 cigarettes or less a day: Begin with STEP 2–Initial Treatment Period (Weeks 1–6): 14 mg patches.

Choose your quit date (it should be soon). This is the day you will quit smoking cigarettes entirely and begin using NicoDerm CQ to reduce your cravings for nicotine. Place the Step 2 sticker on this date. For the first six weeks, you'll use the Step 2 (14 mg) NicoDerm CQ patches. Be sure to follow the directions on page 10.

Continue with STEP 3–Step Down Treatment Period (Weeks 7–8): 7 mg patches.

Completing the full program will increase your chances of quitting successfully. This is done by changing over to the Step 3 (7mg) patches for 2 weeks. The two week step down treatment period allows you to gradually reduce the amount of nicotine you get, rather than stopping suddenly, and will increase your chances of quitting. Place the Step 3 sticker on the first day of week seven. Use the 7 mg patches for two weeks.

Light smokers should not use NicoDerm CQ for longer than 8 weeks. If you still feel the need to use NicoDerm CQ after 8 weeks, talk with your doctor.

PLAN AHEAD

Because smoking is an addiction, it is not easy to stop. After you've given up nicotine, you may still have a strong urge to smoke. Plan ahead NOW for these times, so you're not tempted to start smoking again in a moment of weakness. The following tips may help:

- Keep the phone numbers of supportive friends and family members handy.
- Keep a record of your quitting process. Track when you have a craving for nicotine if it occurs. If you smoke at all, write down what you think caused the slip.
- Put together an Emergency Kit that includes items that will help take your mind off occasional urges to smoke. You might include cinnamon gum or lemon drops to suck on, a relaxing cassette tape and something for your hands to play with, like a smooth rock, rubber band or small metal balls.
- Set aside some small rewards, like a new magazine or a gift certificate from your favorite store, which you'll 'give' yourself after passing difficult hurdles.
- Think now about the times when you most often want a cigarette, and then plan what else you might do instead of smoking. For instance, you might plan to take your coffee break in a new location, or take a walk right after dinner, so you won't be tempted to smoke.

HOW NICODERM CQ WORKS

NicoDerm CQ patches provide nicotine to your system—they work as a temporary aid to help you quit smoking by reducing nicotine withdrawal symptoms, including nicotine craving. NicoDerm CQ provides a lower level of nicotine to your blood than cigarettes, and allows you to gradually do away with your body's need for nicotine. Because Nico-

Derm CQ does not contain the tar or carbon monoxide of cigarette smoke, it does not have the same health dangers as tobacco. However, it still delivers nicotine, the addictive part of cigarette smoke. Nicotine can cause side effects such as headache, nausea, upset stomach and dizziness.

HOW TO USE NICODERM CQ PATCHES

Read all the following instructions, and the instructions on the outer carton, before using NicoDerm CQ. Refer to them often to make sure your're using NicoDerm CQ correctly. Please refer to the audio tape for additional help.

1. Stop smoking completely before you start using NicoDerm CQ.
2. To reduce craving and other withdrawal symptoms, use NicoDerm CQ according to the dosage schedule in the "directions" section above.

Insert used NicoDerm CQ patches in the child resistant disposal tray provided in the box—safely away from children and pets.

When to apply and remove NicoDerm CQ patches.

Each day apply a new patch to a different place on skin that is dry, clean and hairless. **You can wear a NicoDerm CQ patch for either 16 or 24 hours.** If you crave cigarettes when you wake up, wear the patch for 24 hours. If you begin to have vivid dreams or other disruptions of your sleep while wearing the patch 24 hours, try taking the patch off at bedtime (after about 16 hours) and putting on a new one when you get up the next day. **Do not smoke even when you are not wearing the patch.**

Remove the used patch and put on a new patch at the same time every day. Applying the patch at about the same time each day (first thing in the morning, for instance) will help you remember when to put on a new patch. Do not leave the same NicoDerm CQ patch on for more than 24 hours because it may irritate your skin and because it loses strength after 24 hours. Do not use NicoDerm CQ continuously for more than 10 weeks (8 weeks for light smokers).

How to apply a NicoDerm CQ patch.

1. Do not remove the NicoDerm CQ patch from its sealed protective pouch until you are ready to use it. NicoDerm CQ patches will lose nicotine to the air if you store them out of the pouch.
2. Choose a non-hairy, clean, dry area of skin. Do not put a NicoDerm CQ patch on skin that is burned, broken out, cut or irritated in any way. Make sure your skin is free of lotion and soap before applying a patch.
3. A clear, protective liner covers the sticky silver side of the NicoDerm CQ patch—the side that will be put on your skin. The liner has a slit down the middle to help you remove it from the patch. With the silver side facing you, put half the liner away from the NicoDerm CQ patch starting at the middle slit, as shown in the illustration above. Hold the NicoDerm CQ patch at one of the outside edges

Continued on next page

Nicoderm CQ—Cont.

(touch the silver side as little as possible), and pull off the other half of the protective liner. Place this liner in the slot in the disposable tray provided in the NicoDerm CQ package where it will be out of reach of children and pets.

4. Immediately apply the sticky side of the NicoDerm CQ patch to your skin. **Press the patch firmly on your skin with the heel of your hand for at least 10 seconds.** Make sure it sticks well to your skin, especially around the edges.

5. Wash your hands when you have finished applying the NicoDerm CQ patch. Nicotine on your hands could get into your eyes and nose, and cause stinging, redness, or more serious problems.

6. After 24 or 16 hours, remove the patch you have been wearing. Fold the used NicoDerm CQ patch in half with the silver side together. Careful dispose of the used patch in the slot of the disposal tray provided in the NicoDerm CQ package where it will be out of the reach of children and pets. Even used patches have enough nicotine to poison children and pets. Wash your hands.

7. Chose a different place on your skin to apply the next NicoDerm CQ patch and repeat Steps 1 to 6. Do not apply a new patch to a previously used skin site for at least one week.

If your NicoDerm CQ patch gets wet during wearing. Water will not harm the NicoDerm CQ patch you are wearing if applied properly. You can bathe, swim or shower for short periods while you are wearing the NicoDerm CQ patch.

If your NicoDerm CQ patch comes off while wearing. NicoDerm CQ patches generally stick well to most people's skin, However, a patch may occasionally come off. If your NicoDerm CQ patch falls off during the day, put on a new patch, making sure you select a non-hairy, non-irritated area of the skin that is clean and dry. If the soap you use has lanolin or moisturizers, the patch may not stick well. Using a different soap may help. Body creams, lotions and sunscreens can also cause problems with keeping your patch on. Do not apply creams or lotions to the place on your skin where you will put the patch. If you have followed the directions and the patch still does not stick to you, try using medical adhesive tape over the patch.

Disposing of NicoDerm CQ patches. Fold the used patch in half with the silver side together. Carefully dispose of the patch in the disposal slot of the tray provided in the NicoDerm CQ package where it will be out of the reach of children and pets. Small amounts of nicotine, even from a used patch can poison children and pets. **Keep all nicotine patches away from children and pets.** Wash. YOUR HANDS AFTER DISPOSING OF THE PATCH.

If your skin reacts to the NicoDerm CQ patch. When you first put on a Nico-Derm CQ patch, mild itching, burning or tingling is normal and should go away within an hour. After you remove a Nico-Derm CQ patch, the skin under the patch might be somewhat red. Your skin should not stay red for more than a day after removing the patch. **If you get a skin rash after using a NicoDerm CQ patch, or if the skin under the patch becomes swollen or very red, call your doctor. Do not put on a new patch.**

Storage Instructions

Keep each NicoDerm CQ patch in its protective pouch, unopened, until you are ready to use it, because the patch will lose nicotine to the air if it's outside the pouch. Do not store NicoDerm CQ patches above 86°F (30°C) because they are sensitive to heat. Remember, the inside of your car can reach temperatures much higher than this. A slight yellowing of the silver side of the patch is normal. Do not use NicoDerm CQ patches stored in pouches that are damaged or open.

TIPS TO MAKE QUITTING EASIER

Within the first few weeks of giving up smoking, you may be tempted to smoke for pleasure, particularly after completing a difficult task, or at a party or bar. Here are some tips to help get you through the important first stages of becoming a non-smoker:

On Your Quit Date:

• Ask your family, friends and co-workers to support you in your efforts to stop smoking.
• Throw away all your cigarettes, matches, lighters, ashtrays, etc.
• Keep busy on your quit day. Exercise. Go to a movie. Take a walk. Get together with friends.
• Figure out how much money you'll save by not smoking. Most ex-smokers can save more than $1,000 a year on the price of cigarettes alone.
• Write down what you will do with the money you save.
• Know your high risk situations and plan ahead how you will deal with them.
• Visit your dentist and have your teeth cleaned to get rid of the tobacco stains.
• Use a whitening toothpaste to keep your new smile.

Right after Quitting:

• During the first few days after you've stopped smoking, spend as much time as possible at places where smoking is not allowed.
• Drink large quantities of water and fruit juices.
• Try to avoid alcohol, coffee and other beverages you associate with smoking.
• Remember that temporary urges to smoke will pass, even if you don't smoke a cigarette.
• Keep your hands busy with something like a pencil or a paper clip.
• Find other activities which help you relax without cigarettes. Swim, jog, take a walk, play basketball.
• Don't worry too much about gaining weight. Watch what you eat, take time for daily exercise, and change your eating habits if you need to.
• Laughter helps. Watch or read something funny.

WHAT TO EXPECT

Your body is now coming back into balance. During the first few days after you stop smoking, you might feel edgy and nervous and have trouble concentrating.

You might get headaches, feel dizzy and a little out of sorts, feel sweaty or have stomach upsets. You might even have trouble sleeping at first. These are typical withdrawal symptoms that will go away with time. Your smoker's cough will get worse before it gets better. But don't worry, that's a good sign. Coughing helps clear the tar deposits out of your lungs.

After a week or two

By now you should be feeling more confident that you can handle those smoking urges. Many of your nicotine withdrawal symptoms have left by now, and you should be noticing some positive signs: less coughing, better breathing and an improved sense of taste and smell, to name a few.

After a month

You probably have the urge to smoke much less often now. But urges may still occur, and when they do, they are likely to be powerful ones that come out of nowhere. Don't let them catch you off guard. Plan ahead for these difficult times. Concentrate on the ways non-smokers are more attractive than smokers. Their skin is less likely to wrinkle. Their teeth are whiter, cleaner. Their breath is fresher. Their hair and clothes smell better. That cough that seems to make even a laugh sound more like a rattle is a thing of the past. Their children and others around them are healthier, too.

What To Do About Relapse.

What should you do if you slip and start smoking again? The answer is simple.

A lapse of one or two or even a few cigarettes should not spoil your efforts! Throw away your cigarettes forgive yourself and continue with the program. Listen to the Audio Tape again and re-read the User's Guide to ensure that you're using NicoDerm CQ correctly and following the other important tips for dealing with the mental and social dependence on nicotine. Your doctor, pharmacist or other health professional can also provide useful counseling on the importance of stopping smoking. You should consider them partners in your quit attempt.

What To Do About Relapse After a Successful Quit Attempt. If you have taken up regular smoking again, don't be discouraged. Research shows that the best thing you can do is to try again, since several quitting attempts may be needed before your're successful. And your chances of quitting successfully increase with each quit attempt. The important thing is to learn from your last attempt.

• Admit that you've slipped, but don't treat yourself as a failure.
• Try to identify the 'trigger' that caused you to slip, and prepare a better plan for dealing with this problem next time.
• Talk positively to yourself—tell yourself that you have learned something from this experience.
• Make sure you used NicoDerm CQ patches correctly.
• Remember that it takes practice to do anything and quitting smoking is no exception.

WHEN THE STRUGGLE IS OVER

Once you've stopped smoking, take a second and pat yourself on the back. Now do it again. You deserve it. Remember now why you decided to stop smoking in the first place. Look at your list of reasons. Read them again. And smile. Now think about all the money you are saving and what you'll do with it. All the non-smoking places you can go, and what you might do there. All those years you may have added to your life, and what you'll do with them. Remember that temptation may not be gone forever. However, the hard part is behind you, so look forward with a positive attitude and enjoy your new life as a non-smoker.

QUESTIONS & ANSWERS

1. How will I feel when I stop smoking and start using NicoDerm CQ?
You'll need to prepare yourself for some nicotine withdrawal symptoms. These begin almost immediately after you stop smoking, and are usually at their worst during the first three or four days. Understand that any of the following is possible
- craving for nicotine
- anxiety, irritability, restlessness, mood changes, nervousness
- disruptions of your sleep
- drowsiness
- trouble concentrating
- increased appetite and weight gain
- headaches, muscular pain, constipation, fatigue.

NicoDerm CQ reduces nicotine withdrawal symptoms such as irritability and nervousness, as well as the craving for nicotine you used to satisfy by having a cigarette.

2. Is NicoDerm CQ just substituting one form of nicotine for another? NicoDerm CQ does contain nicotine. The purpose of NicoDerm CQ is to provide you with enough nicotine to reduce the physical withdrawal symptoms so you can deal with the mental aspects of quitting.

3. Can I be hurt by using NicoDerm CQ? For most adults, the amount of nicotine in the gum is less than from smoking. If you believe you may be sensitive to even this amount of nicotine, you should not use this product without advice from your doctor (see p. 4 of the User's Guide). There are also some important cautions in the User's Guide (See p. 4).

4. Will I gain weight? Many people do tend to gain a few pounds the first 8–10 weeks after they stop smoking. This is a very small price to pay for the enormous gains that you will make in your overall health and attractiveness. If you continue to gain weight after the first two months, try to analyze what you're doing differently. Reduce your fat intake, choose healthy snacks, and increase your physical activity to burn off the extra calories. Drink lots of water. This is good for your body and skin, and also helps to reduce the amount you eat.

5. Is NicoDerm CQ more expensive than smoking? The total cost of NicoDerm CQ for the twelve week program is similar to what a person who smokes one and a half packs of cigarettes a day would spend on cigarettes for the same period of time. Also use of NicoDerm CQ is only a short-term cost, while the cost of smoking is a long-term cost, because of the health problems smoking causes.

6. What if I slip up? Discard your cigarettes, forgive yourself and then get back on track. Don't consider yourself a failure or punish yourself. In fact, people who have already tried to quit are more likely to be successful the next time. **GOOD LUCK!**

Copyright © 1997 Smithkline Beecham

For your family's protection, NicoDerm CQ patches are supplied in child resistant pouches. Do not use if individual pouch is damaged or open.

Manufactured by ALZA Corporation, Palo Alto, CA 94304 for SmithKline Beecham Consumer Healthcare, L.P. Comments or Questions? Call 1–800–834–5895 Weekdays. (10 a.m.–4:30 p.m. EST).

- **Not for sale to those under 18 years of age.**
- **Proof of age required.**
- **Not for sale in vending machines or from any source where proof of age cannot be verified.**

Available as

NicoDerm CQ Step 1 (21 mg/24 hours)–7 Patches*
NicoDerm CQ Step 1 (21 mg/24 hours)–14 Patches*
NicoDerm CQ Step 2 (14 mg/24 hours)–7 Patches*
NicoDerm CQ Step 2 (14 mg/24 hours)–14 patches*
NicoDerm CQ Step 3 (7 mg/24 hours)–7 Patches**
NicoDerm CQ Step 3 (7 mg/24 hours)–14 patches**

*   User's Guide, Audio Tape & Child Resistant Disposal Tray
** User's Guide, & Child Resistant Disposal Tray

Shown in Product Identification Guide, page 522

NICORETTE®
Nicotine Polacrilex Gum/Stop Smoking Aid
Available in 2mg and 4mg Strength

If you smoke:
UNDER 25 CIGARETTES A DAY: Use 2 mg
OVER 24 CIGARETTES A DAY: Use 4 mg

Action: Stop Smoking Aid

Use:
- To reduce withdrawal symptoms, including nicotine craving, associated with quitting smoking.

Directions:
- Stop smoking completely when you begin using Nicorette.
- Read the enclosed User's Guide before using Nicorette.
- Use properly as directed in the User's Guide.
- Don't eat or drink for 15 minutes before using Nicorette or while chewing a piece.
- Use according to the following 12 week schedule:

Weeks 1 to 6	Weeks 7 to 9	Weeks 10 to 12
1 piece every 1 to 2 hours	1 piece every 2 to 4 hours	1 piece every 4 to 8 hours

- Do not exceed 24 pieces a day.
- Stop using Nicorette at the end of week 12. If you still feel the need for Nicorette, talk with your doctor.

Warnings:
- Keep this and all drugs out of the reach of children and pets. In case of accidental overdose, seek professional assistance or contact a poison control center immediately.
- Nicorette can increase your baby's heart rate; if you are pregnant or nursing a bay, seek the advice of a health professional before using this product.

DO NOT USE IF YOU
- Continue to smoke, chew tobacco, use snuff, or use a nicotine patch or other nicotine containing products.

ASK YOUR DOCTOR BEFORE USE IF YOU
- Are under 18 years of age.
- Have heart disease, recent heart attack, or irregular heartbeat. Nicotine can increase your heart rate.
- Have high blood pressure not controlled with medication. Nicotine can increase blood pressure.
- Have stomach ulcer or take insulin for diabetes.
- Take prescription medicine for depression or asthma. Your prescription dose may need to be adjusted.

STOP USE AND SEE YOUR DOCTOR IF YOU HAVE
- Mouth, teeth or jaw problems.
- Irregular heartbeat, palpitations.
- Symptoms of nicotine overdose such as nausea, vomiting, dizziness, weakness and rapid heartbeat.

READ THE LABEL
Read the carton and the User's Guide before taking this product. Do not discard carton or User's Guide. They contain important information.

[2 mg] Inactive Ingredients: Flavors, glycerin, gum base, sodium carbonate, sorbitol, sodium bicarbonate.
[4 mg] Inactive Ingredients: Flavors, glycerin, gum base, sodium carbonate, sorbitol, D&C Yellow 10.
Do not store above 86°F (30°C). Protect from light.

TO INCREASE YOUR SUCCESS IN QUITTING:
1. **You must be motivated to quit.**
2. **Use Enough** —Chew **at least 9 pieces** of Nicorette per day during the first six weeks.
3. **Use long enough** —Use Nicorette for the full 12 weeks.
4. **Use with a support program** as described in the enclosed User's Guide.

USER'S GUIDE:
HOW TO USE NICORETTE TO HELP YOU QUIT SMOKING
KEYS TO SUCCESS
1) You must really want to quit smoking for Nicorette to help you.
2) You can greatly increase your chances for success by using at least 9 to 12

Continued on next page

Nicorette—Cont.

pieces every day when you start using Nicorette.

3) You should continue to use Nicorette as explained in the User's Guide for 12 full weeks.

4) Nicorette works best when used together with a support program.

5) If you have trouble using Nicorette, ask your doctor or pharmacist or call SmithKline Beecham at 1-800-419-4766 weekdays (10:00am–4:30pm EST).

SO YOU DECIDED TO QUIT

Congratulations. Your decision to stop smoking is an important one. That's why you've made the right choice in choosing Nicorette gum. Your own chances of quitting smoking depend on how much you want to quit, how strongly you are addicted to tobacco, and how closely you follow a quitting program like the one that comes with Nicorette.

QUITTING SMOKING IS HARD!

If you've tried to quit before and haven't succeeded, don't be discouraged! Quitting isn't easy. It takes time, and most people try a few times before they are successful. The important thing is to try again until you succeed. This User's Guide will give you support as you become a non-smoker. It will answer common questions about Nicorette and give tips to help you stop smoking, and should be referred to often.

WHERE TO GET HELP

You are more likely to stop smoking by using Nicorette with a support program that helps you break your smoking habit. There may be support groups in your area for people trying to quit. Call your local chapter of the American Lung Association (1-800-586-4872), American Cancer Society (1-800-227-2345) or American Heart Association (1-800-242-8721) for further information. If you find you cannot stop smoking or if you start smoking again after using Nicorette, remember breaking this addiction doesn't happen overnight. You may want to talk to a health care professional who can help you improve your chances of quitting the next time you try Nicorette or another method.

LET'S GET ORGANIZED

Your reason for quitting may be a combination of concerns about health, the effect of smoking on your appearance, and pressure from your family and friends to stop smoking. Or maybe you're concerned about the dangerous effect of second-hand smoke on the people you care about. All of these are good reasons. You probably have others. Decide your most important reasons, and write them down on the wallet card inside the back cover of the User's Guide. Carry this card with you. In difficult moments, when you want to smoke, the card will remind you why you are quitting.

WHAT YOU'RE UP AGAINST

Smoking is addictive in two ways. Your need for nicotine has become both physical and mental. You must overcome both addictions to stop smoking. So while Nicorette will lessen your body's physical addition to nicotine, you've got to want to quit smoking to overcome the mental dependence on cigarettes. Once you've decided that you're going to quit, it's time to get started. But first, there are some important cautions you should consider.

SOME IMPORTANT CAUTIONS

This product is only for those who want to stop smoking. Do not smoke, chew tobacco, use snuff or nicotine patches while using Nicorette. If you have heart disease, a recent heart attack, irregular heartbeats, palpitations, high blood pressure not controlled with medication, stomach ulcer, or take insulin for diabetes, ask your doctor whether you should use Nicorette. As with any drug, if you are pregnant or nursing a baby, seek the advice of a health professional before using this product. If you take a prescription medication for asthma or depression, be sure your doctor knows you are quitting smoking. Your prescription medication dose may need to be adjusted. Those under 18 should use this product under a doctor's care. Symptoms of nicotine overdose may include vomiting and diarrhea. Young children are more likely to have additional symptoms, including weakness. Also, seizures have been seen in children who swallowed cigarettes. Keep this and all drugs out of the reach of children. In case of accidental overdose, seek professional assistance or contact a poison control center immediately.

LET'S GET STARTED

Becoming a non-smoker starts today. Your first step is to read through the entire User's Guide carefully. **Next, set your personalized quitting schedule.** Take out a calendar that you can use to track your progress, and identify four dates, using the stickers in the User's Guide.

STEP 1: Your quit date (and the day you'll start using Nicorette gum). Choose your quit date (it should be soon). This is the day you will quit smoking cigarettes entirely and begin using Nicorette to satisfy your craving for nicotine. For the first six weeks, you'll use a piece of Nicorette every hour or two. Be sure to follow the directions on pages 8 and 11 of the User's Guide. Place the Step 1 sticker on this date.

STEP 2: The day you'll start reducing your use of Nicorette. After six weeks, you'll begin gradually reducing your Nicorette usage to one piece every two to four hours. Place the Step 2 sticker on this date (the first day of week seven).

STEP 3: The day you'll further reduce your use of Nicorette. Nine weeks after you begin using Nicorette, you will further reduce your nicotine intake by using one piece every four to eight hours. Place the Step 3 sticker on this date (the first day of week ten). For the next three weeks, you'll use a piece of Nicorette every four to eight hours. **End of treatment: The day you'll complete Nicorette therapy.** Nicorette should not be used for longer than twelve weeks. Identify the date thirteen weeks after the date you chose in Step 1 and place the "EX-Smoker" sticker on your calendar.

PLAN AHEAD

Because smoking is an addiction, it is not easy to stop. After you've given up cigarettes, you will still have a strong urge to smoke. Plan ahead NOW for these times, so you're not defeated in a moment of weakness. The following tips may help:

• Keep the phone numbers of supportive friends and family members handy.

• Keep a record of your quitting process. Track the number of Nicorette pieces you use each day, and whether you feel a craving for cigarettes. If you smoke at all, write down what you think caused the slip.

• Put together an Emergency Kit that includes items that will help take your mind off occasional urges to smoke. Include cinnamon gum or lemon drops to suck on, a relaxing cassette tape and something for your hands to play with, like a smooth rock, rubber band or small metal balls.

• Set aside some small rewards, like a new magazine or a gift certificate from your favorite store, which you'll 'give' yourself after passing difficult hurdles.

• Think now about the times when you most often want a cigarette, and then plan what else you might do instead of smoking. For instance, you might plan to take your coffee break in a new location, or take a walk right after dinner, so you won't be tempted to smoke.

HOW NICORETTE GUM WORKS

Nicorette's sugar-free chewing pieces provide nicotine to your system—they work as a temporary aid to help you quit smoking by reducing nicotine withdrawal symptoms. Nicorette provides a lower level of nicotine to your blood than cigarettes, and allows you to gradually do away with your body's need for nicotine. Because Nicorette does not contain the tar or carbon monoxide of cigarette smoke, it does not have the same health dangers as tobacco. However, it still delivers nicotine, the addictive part of cigarette smoke. Nicotine can cause side effects such as headache, nausea, upset stomach and dizziness.

HOW TO USE NICORETTE GUM

Before you can use Nicorette correctly, you have to practice! That sounds silly, but it isn't.

Nicorette isn't like ordinary chewing gum. It's a medicine, and must be chewed a certain way to work right. Chewed like ordinary gum, Nicorette won't work well and can cause side effects. An overdose can occur if you chew more than one piece of Nicorette at the same time, or if you chew many pieces one after another. Read all the following instructions before using Nicorette. Refer to them often to make sure you're using Nicorette gum correctly. If you chew too fast, or do not chew correctly, you may get hiccups, heartburn, or other stomach problems.

1. Stop smoking completely before you start using Nicorette.

2. To reduce craving and other withdrawal symptoms, use Nicorette according to the dosage schedule on page 11 of the User's Guide.

3. Chew each Nicorette piece <u>very slowly several times.</u>
4. Stop chewing when you notice a peppery taste, or a slight tingling in your mouth. (This usually happens after about 15 chews, but may vary from person to person.)
5. "PARK" the Nicorette piece between your cheek and gum and leave it there.
6. When the peppery taste or tingle is almost gone (in about a minute), start to chew a few times slowly again. When the taste or tingle returns, stop again.
7. Park the Nicorette piece again (in a different place in your mouth).
8. Repeat steps 3 to 7 (chew, chew, park) until most of the nicotine is gone from the Nicorette piece (usually happens in about half an hour; the peppery taste or tingle won't return).

Throw away the used Nicorette piece, safely away from children and pets.

See the chart in the **"DIRECTIONS"** section above for the recommended usage schedule for Nicorette.

To improve your chances of quitting, use at least 9 pieces of Nicorette a day. Heavier smokers may need more pieces to reduce their cravings. Don't eat or drink for 15 minutes before using Nicorette or while chewing a piece. The effectiveness of Nicorette may be reduced by some foods and drinks, such as coffee, juices, wine or soft drinks.

HOW TO REDUCE YOUR NICORETTE USAGE

The goal of using Nicorette is to slowly reduce your dependence on nicotine. The schedule for using Nicorette will help you reduce your nicotine craving gradually. Here are some tips to help you cut back during each step:

- After a while, start chewing each Nicorette piece for only 10 to 15 minutes, instead of half an hour. Then gradually begin to reduce the number of pieces used.
- Or, try chewing each piece for longer than half an hour, but reduce the number of pieces you use each day.
- Substitute ordinary chewing gum for some of the Nicorette pieces you would normally use. Increase the number of pieces of ordinary gum as you cut back on the Nicorette pieces.

STOP USING NICORETTE AT THE END OF WEEK 12. If you still feel the need to use Nicorette after Week 12, talk with your doctor.

TIPS TO MAKE QUITTING EASIER

Within the first few weeks of giving up smoking, you may be tempted to smoke for pleasure, particularly after completing a difficult task, or at a party or bar. Here are some tips to help get you through the important first stages of becoming a non-smoker:

On your Quit Date:

- Ask your family, friends, and co-workers to support you in your efforts to stop smoking.
- Throw away all your cigarettes, matches, lighters, ashtrays, etc.
- Keep busy on your quit day. Exercise. Go to a movie. Take a walk. Get together with friends.
- Figure out how much money you'll save by not smoking. Most ex-smokers can save more than $1,000 a year.

- Write down what you will do with the money you save.
- Know your high risk situations and plan ahead how you will deal with them.
- Keep Nicorette gum near your bed, so you'll be prepared for any nicotine cravings when you wake up in the morning.
- Visit your dentist and have your teeth cleaned to get rid of the tobacco stains.

Right after Quitting:

- During the first few days after you've stopped smoking, spend as much time as possible at places where smoking is not allowed.
- Drink large quantities of water and fruit juices.
- Try to avoid alcohol, coffee and other beverages you associate with smoking.
- Remember that temporary urges to smoke will pass, even if you don't smoke a cigarette.
- Keep your hands busy with something like a pencil or a paper clip.
- Find other activities which help you relax without cigarettes. Swim, jog, take a walk, play basketball.
- Don't worry too much about gaining weight. Watch what you eat, take time for daily exercise, and change your eating habits if you need to.
- Laughter helps. Watch or read something funny.

WHAT TO EXPECT

Your body is now coming back into balance. During the first few days after you stop smoking, you might feel edgy and nervous and have trouble concentrating. You might get headaches, feel dizzy and a little out of sorts, feel sweaty or have stomach upsets. You might even have trouble sleeping at first. These are typical withdrawal symptoms that will go away with time. Your smoker's cough will get worse before it gets better. But don't worry, that's a good sign. Coughing helps clear the tar deposits out of your lungs.

After a Week or Two.

By now you should be feeling more confident that you can handle those smoking urges. Many of your withdrawal symptoms have left by now, and you should be noticing some positive signs: less coughing, better breathing and an improved sense of taste and smell, to name a few.

After a Month.

You probably have the urge to smoke much less often now. But urges may still occur, and when they do, they are likely to be powerful ones that come out of nowhere. Don't let them catch you off guard. Plan ahead for these difficult times. Concentrate on the ways non-smokers are more attractive than smokers. Their skin is less likely to wrinkle. Their teeth are whiter, cleaner. Their breath is fresher. Their hair and clothes smell better. That cough seems to make even a laugh sound more like a rattle is a thing of the past. Their children and others around them are healthier, too.

What To Do About Relapse.

What should you do if you slip and start smoking again? The answer is simple. A lapse of one or two or even a few cigarettes has not spoiled your efforts! Dis-

card your cigarettes, forgive yourself and try again. If you start smoking again, keep your box of Nicorette for your next quit attempt. If you have taken up regular smoking again, don't be discouraged. Research shows that the best thing you can do is to try again. The important thing is to learn from your last attempt.

- Admit that you've slipped, but don't treat yourself as a failure.
- Try to identify the 'trigger' that caused you to slip, and prepare a better plan for dealing with this problem next time.
- Talk positively to yourself—tell yourself that you have learned something from this experience.
- Make sure you used Nicorette gum correctly over the full 12 weeks to reduce your craving for nicotine.
- Remember that it takes practice to do anything, and quitting smoking is no exception.

WHEN THE STRUGGLE IS OVER

Once you've stopped smoking, take a second and pat yourself on the back. Now do it again. You deserve it. Remember now why you decided to stop smoking in the first place. Look at your list of reasons. Read them again. And smile. Now think about all the money you are saving and what you'll do with it. All the non-smoking places you can go, and what you might do there. All those years you may have added to your life, and what you'll do with them. Remember that temptation may not be gone forever. However, the hard part is behind you, so look forward with a positive attitude and enjoy your new life as a non-smoker.

QUESTIONS & ANSWERS

1. How will I feel when I stop smoking and start using Nicorette? You'll need to prepare yourself for some nicotine withdrawal symptoms. These begin almost immediately after you stop smoking, and are usually at their worst during the first three to four days. Understand that any of the following is possible

- craving for cigarettes
- anxiety, irritability, restlessness, mood changes, nervousness
- drowsiness
- trouble concentrating
- increased appetite and weight gain
- headaches, muscular pain, constipation, fatigue.

Nicorette can help provide relief from withdrawal symptoms such as irritability and nervousness, as well as the craving for nicotine you used to satisfy by having a cigarette.

2. Is Nicorette just substuting one form of nicotine for another? Nicorette does contain nicotine. The purpose of Nicorette is to provide you with enough nicotine to help control the physical withdrawal symptoms so you can deal with the mental aspects of quitting. During the 12 week program, you will gradually reduce your nicotine intake by switching to fewer pieces each day. Remember, don't use Nicorette together with nicotine patches or other nicotine containing products.

3. Can I be hurt by using Nicorette? For most adults, the amount of nicotine in the gum is less than from smoking. Some people will be sensitive to even this

Continued on next page

Nicorette—Cont.

amount of nicotine and should not use this product without advice from their doctor. Because Nicorette is a gum-based product, chewing it can cause dental fillings to loosen and aggravate other mouth, tooth and jaw problems. Nicorette can also cause hiccups, heartburn and other stomach problems especially if chewed too quickly or not chewed correctly.

4. Will I gain weight? Many people do tend to gain a few pounds in the first 8–10 weeks after they stop smoking. This is a very small price to pay for the enormous gains that you will make in your overall health and attractiveness. If you continue to gain weight after the first two months, try to analyze what you're doing differently. Reduce your fat intake, choose healthy snacks, and increase your physical activity to burn off the extra calories.

5. Is Nicorette more expensive than smoking? The total cost of Nicorette for the twelve week program is about equal to what a person who smokes one and a half packs of cigarettes a day would spend one cigarettes for the same period of time. Also use of Nicorette is only a short-term cost, while the cost of smoking is a long-term cost, because of the health problems smoking causes.

6. What if I slip up? Discard your cigarettes, forgive yourself and then get back on track. Don't consider yourself a failure or punish yourself. In fact, people who have already tried to quit are more likely to be successful the next time.

GOOD LUCK!

[End User's Guide]

Copyright © 1997 Smithkline Beecham

To remove the gum, tear off a single unit.

Peel off backing starting at corner with loose edge.

Push gum through foil.

Blister Packaged for your protection. Do not use if individual seals are broken.

Manufactured by Pharmacia & Upjohn AB, Stockholm, Sweden for SmithKline Beecham Consumer Healthcare, LP Pittsburgh, PA 15230

Comments or Questions? Call 1-800-419-4766 weekdays.

(10 a.m.–4:30 p.m. EST).

- **Not for sale to those under 18 years of age.**
- **Proof of age required.**
- **Not for sale in vending machines or from any source where proof of age cannot be verified.**

Available as:

Nicorette 2 mg Gum—108 Pieces*

Nicorette 2 mg Gum—48 pieces (refill)

Nicorette 4 mg Gum—108 Pieces*

Nicorette 4 mg Gum—48 pieces (refill)

***User's Guide and Audio Tape included in Kit**

Shown in Product Identification Guide, page 522

SINGLET® For Adults
Nasal Decongestant/Antihistamine/Analgesic (pain reliever)/Antipyretic (fever reducer)

Indications: For temporary relief of nasal congestion and sinus and headache pain associated with sinusitis or due to a cold, hay fever or other upper respiratory allergies. Also temporarily relieves nasal congestion, sinus headache, runny nose, sneezing, itching of the nose or throat, and itchy, watery eyes due to hay fever or other upper respiratory allergies. Also temporarily relieves fever due to the common cold.

Directions: Adults (12 years and older): 1 caplet every 4 to 6 hours, **not to exceed 4 caplets in any 24-hour period,** or as directed by a doctor. Children under 12 years of age: Consult a doctor.

Warnings: Do not take this product for more than 10 days. If symptoms do not improve or are accompanied by fever that lasts for more than 3 days, or if new symptoms occur, consult a doctor. Do not take this product, unless directed by a doctor, if you have a breathing problem such as emphysema or chronic bronchitis, or if you have heart disease, high blood pressure, thyroid disease, diabetes, glaucoma or difficulty in urination due to enlargement of the prostate gland. May cause excitability especially in children. May cause drowsiness; alcohol, sedatives, and tranquilizers may increase the drowsiness effect. Avoid alcoholic beverages while taking this product. Do not take this product if you are taking sedatives or tranquilizers, without first consulting your doctor. Use caution when driving a motor vehicle or operating machinery. **Do not exceed recommended dosage.** If nervousness, dizziness, or sleeplessness occur, discontinue use and consult a doctor. **KEEP THIS AND ALL DRUGS OUT OF THE REACH OF CHILDREN.** Prompt medical attention is critical for adults as well as for children even if you do not notice any signs or symptoms. In case of accidental overdose, seek professional assistance or contact a Poison Control Center immediately. As with any drug, if you are pregnant or nursing a baby, seek the advice of a health professional before using this product.

Drug Interaction Precaution: Do not use this product if you are now taking a prescription monoamine oxidase inhibitor (MAOI) (certain drugs for depression, psychiatric or emotional conditions, or Parkinson's disease), or for 2 weeks after stopping the MAOI drug. If you are uncertain whether your prescription drug contains an MAOI, consult a health professional before taking this product.

Active Ingredients: Each caplet contains: Pseudoephedrine Hydrochloride 60 mg, Chlorpheniramine Maleate 4 mg, Acetaminophen 650 mg.

Inactive Ingredients: D&C Red 27, D&C Yellow 10, FD&C Blue 1, Hydroxy-propyl Cellulose, Hydroxypropyl Methylcellulose, Magnesium Stearate, Microcrystalline Cellulose, Polyethylene Glycol, Pregelatinized Corn Starch, Sodium Starch Glycolate, Sucrose and Titanium Dioxide.

Store at room temperature (59°–86°F). Avoid excessive heat and humidity.

Comments or Questions? Call toll-free 1-800-245-1040 weekdays

Distributed by: SmithKline Beecham Consumer Healthcare, L.P.

Pittsburgh, PA 15230. Made in U.S.A.

SOMINEX Original Formula
Nighttime Sleep Aid
Doctor-preferred sleep ingredient

Indications: Helps to reduce difficulty falling asleep.

Directions: Adults and children 12 years and over: Take 2 tablets at bedtime if needed, or as directed by a doctor. For best results, take recommended dose. This will provide approximately six to eight hours of restful sleep.

Warnings: Do not give to children under 12 years of age. If sleeplessness persists continually for more than 2 weeks, consult your doctor. Insomnia may be a symptom of serious underlying medical illness. Do not take this product, unless directed by a doctor, if you have a breathing problem such as emphysema or chronic bronchitis, or if you have glaucoma or difficulty in urination due to enlargement of the prostate gland. Avoid alcoholic beverages while taking this product. Do not take this product if you are taking sedatives or tranquilizers, without first consulting your doctor. As with any drug, if you are pregnant or nursing a baby, seek the advice of a health professional before using this product. **Keep this and all drugs out of the reach of children.** In case of accidental overdose, seek professional assistance or contact a poison control center immediately.

Active Ingredients: Each tablet contains 25 mg Diphenhydramine HCl.

Inactive Ingredients: Dibasic Calcium Phosphate, FD&C Blue #1, Magnesium Stearate, Microcrystalline Cellulose, Silicon Dioxide, Starch.

Tamper Evident Feature: Individually sealed in foil for your protection. Do not use if foil or plastic bubble is torn or punctured.

Store at room temperature, avoid excessive heat (greater than 100°F) or humidity.

How Supplied: Consumer Packages of 16, 32 and 72 tablets

Also Available in Maximum Strength and Pain Relief Formulas.

Comments or Questions? Call Toll-Free 1-800-245-1040 Weekdays.

SmithKline Beecham Consumer Healthcare, L.P.

Pittsburgh, PA 15230. Made in U.S.A.

SUCRETS® Maximum Strength
[su 'krets]
Wintergreen
**SUCRETS® Wild Cherry Regular
Strength**
**SUCRETS® Children's Cherry
Flavored
Sore Throat Lozenges**
**SUCRETS® Regular Strength
Original Mint**
**SUCRETS® Regular Strength
Vapor Lemon**
**SUCRETS® Maximum Strength
Vapor Black Cherry**
SUCRETS® Assorted

Active Ingredient: Maximum Strength
Wintergreen: Dyclonine Hydrochloride
3.0 mg. per lozenge. Wild Cherry, Regular Strength: Dyclonine Hydrochloride
2.0 mg. per lozenge. Children's Cherry:
Dyclonine Hydrochloride 1.2 mg. per lozenge. Regular Strength–Original Mint:
Hexylresorcinol 2.4 mg. per lozenge. Regular Strength–Vapor Lemon: Dyclonine
Hydrochloride 2.0 mg. per lozenge. Maximum Strength–Vapor Black Cherry: Dyclonine Hydrochloride 3.0 mg. per lozenge.

Inactive Ingredients: Maximum
Strength Wintergreen: Citric Acid, Corn
Syrup, D&C Yellow #10, Flavors, Mineral
Oil, Silicon Dioxide, Sucrose. Wild
Cherry Regular Strength: Corn Syrup,
FD&C Blue #1, FD&C Red #40, Flavor,
Mineral Oil, Silicon Dioxide, Sucrose,
Tartaric Acid. Children's Cherry: Citric
Acid, Corn Syrup, FD&C Blue #1, FD&C
Red #40, Flavor, Mineral Oil, Silicon Di-
oxide, Sucrose. Regular Strength–Origi-
nal Mint: Corn Syrup, D&C Yellow #10,
FD&C Blue #1, Flavors, Mineral Oil, Sil-
icon Dioxide, Sucrose. Regular Strength–
Vapor Lemon: Citric Acid, Corn Syrup,
D&C Yellow #10, Flavors, Mineral Oil,
Silicon Dioxide, Sucrose. Maximum
Strength–Vapor Black Cherry: Corn
Syrup, FD&C Blue #1, FD&C Red #40,
Flavors, Menthol, Mineral Oil, Silicon
Dioxide, Sucrose, Tartaric Acid.

Indications: For temporary relief of
occasional minor irritation, pain, sore
mouth and sore throat.

Actions: Dyclonine Hydrochloride's
soothing anesthetic action relieves minor
throat irritations.

Warnings: If sore throat is severe, persists for more than 2 days, is accompanied or followed by fever, headache, rash,
swelling, nausea, or vomiting, do not use
and consult a doctor promptly. If sore
mouth symptoms do not improve in 7
days or if irritation, pain, or redness persists or worsens, see your dentist or doctor promptly. Do not exceed recommended dosage. KEEP THIS AND ALL
MEDICINES OUT OF THE REACH OF
CHILDREN. In case of accidental overdose, seek professional assistance or contact a poison control center immediately.

Drug Interaction: No known drug interaction.

**Symptoms and Treatment of Oral
Overdosage:** Reactions due to large
overdosage are systemic and involve the
central nervous system and cardiovascular system. Central nervous system reactions are characterized by excitation
and/or depression. Nervousness, dizziness, blurred vision or tremors may occur. Reactions involving the cardiovascular system include depression of the myo-
cardium, hypotension or bradycardia.
Should a large overdose be suspected
seek professional assistance. Call your
physician, local poison control center or
the Rocky Mountain Poison Control Center at 303-592-1710 (Collect), 24 hours a
day.

**Dosage and Administration: Adults
and children 2 years of age or older:**
Allow one lozenge to dissolve slowly in
the mouth. May be repeated every two
hours as needed or as directed by a dentist or doctor. **Children under 2 years
of age:** Consult a dentist or doctor.

Professional Labeling: For the temporary relief of pain associated with ton-
sillitis, pharyngitis, throat infections or
stomatitis.

How Supplied: Available in plastic
packages of 18 lozenges.
*Shown in Product Identification
Guide, page 523*

TAGAMET HB® 200
**Acid Reducer/Cimetidine Tablets
200 mg**

**Tagamet HB® 200 relieves and pre-
vents heartburn, acid indigestion and
sour stomach when used as directed. It
contains the same ingredient found in
prescription strength Tagamet. Tagamet HB 200 reduces the production of
stomach acid.**
ACTIVE INGREDIENT Cimetidine Tablets, 200 mg. Acid Reducer.
INACTIVE INGREDIENTS Cellulose,
cornstarch, hydroxypropyl methylcellulose, magnesium stearate, polyethylene glycol, polysorbate 80, povidone, sodium lauryl sulfate, sodium starch glycolate, titanium dioxide.
USES For **relief** of heartburn associated with acid indigestion and sour
stomach. For **prevention** of heartburn
associated with acid indigestion and
sour stomach brought on by certain food
and beverages.

Directions: For relief of symptoms,
swallow 1 tablet with a glass of water.
For prevention of symptoms, swallow 1
tablet with a glass of water **right before
or anytime up to 30 minutes before**
eating a meal you expect to cause symptoms.
Tagamet HB 200 can be used up to twice
daily (up to 2 tablets in 24 hours). This
product should not be given to children
under 12 years old unless directed by a
doctor.

Warnings:
Allergy Warning: Do not use if you
are allergic to Tagamet HB 200 (cimetidine) or other acid reducers.
**Ask a Doctor Before Use If You are Tak-
ing:**
• theophylline (oral asthma medicine)
• warfarin (blood thinning medicine)
• phenytoin (seizure medicine)
If you are not sure whether your medication contains one of these drugs or
have any other questions about medicines you are taking, call our consumer
affairs specialist at 1-800-482-4394.
• Do not take the maximum daily dosage for more than 2 weeks continuously except under the advice and supervision of a doctor.
• If you have trouble swallowing, or persistent abdominal pain, see your doctor promptly. You may have a serious
condition that may need a different
treatment.
• As with any drug, if you are pregnant
or nursing a baby, seek the advice of a
health professional before using this
product.
• Keep this and all medications out of
the reach of children.
• In case of accidental overdose, seek
professional assistance or contact a
poison control center immediately.
READ THE LABEL
**Read the directions and warnings be-
fore taking this medication.**
Store at 15°–30°C (59–86°F).
Comments or questions? Call Toll-Free
1-800-482-4394 weekdays.
PHARMACOKINETIC INTERACTIONS
Cimetidine at prescription doses is
known to inhibit various P450 metabolizing isoenzymes, which could affect metabolism of other drugs and increase
their blood concentration. Investigation
of pharmacokinetic interactions at the
recommended OTC doses of cimetidine
have thus far shown only small effects.
A pharmacokinetic study conducted in
26 normal male subjects (mean age, 38
years) at steady state using the maximum recommended OTC dose level (200
mg twice a day), showed that Tagamet
HB 200, on average, increased the 24
hour AUC of theophylline by 14% and increased peak theophylline levels by 15%.
This interaction should be borne in mind
in advising patients on the use of Tagamet HB 200. At the prescription doses of
cimetidine, clinically significant pharmacokinetic interactions between cimetidine and warfarin, phenytoin, and theophylline have been reported. At prescription doses, pharmacokinetic
interactions have been reported for a
number of other drugs as well, such as
with dihydropyridine calcium channel
blockers or some short acting benzodiazepines. At the maximum recommended
OTC dose level (200 mg twice a day), a
pharmacokinetic study conducted in 21
normal male subjects (mean age, 38
years) showed that Tagamet HB 200, on
average, increased the total AUC of triazolam by 26–28% and increased peak
triazolam levels by 11–23%. Tagamet HB
200 did not alter the apparent terminal
elimination half-life of triazolam.

Continued on next page

Tagamet HB 200—Cont.

This labeling information is current as of Oct. 30, 1998.

How Supplied: Tagamet HB 200 (cimetidine Tablets 200 mg) is available in boxes of blister strips in 6, 12, 18, 30, 50, 70 & 80 tablet sizes.

Shown in Product Identification Guide, page 523

TUMS® Regular Antacid/Calcium Supplement Tablets
TUMS E–X® and TUMS E–X® Sugar Free Antacid/Calcium Supplement Tablets
TUMS ULTRA® Antacid/Calcium Supplement Tablets

Indications: For fast relief of acid indigestion, heartburn, sour stomach, and upset stomach associated with these symptoms.

Professional Labeling: Indicated for the symptomatic relief of hyperacidity associated with the diagnosis of peptic ulcer, gastritis, peptic esophagitis, gastric hyperacidity, and hiatal hernia.

Active Ingredient:
Tums, Calcium Carbonate 500 mg
Tums E-X, Calcium Carbonate 750 mg
Tums ULTRA, Calcium Carbonate 1000 mg

Actions: Tums provides rapid neutralization of stomach acid. Each Tums tablet has an acid-neutralizing capacity (ANC) of 10 mEq. Each Tums E-X tablet has an ANC of 15 mEq and each Tums ULTRA tablet, an ANC of 20 mEq. This high neutralization capacity makes Tums tablets an ideal antacid for management of conditions associated with hyperacidity. It effectively neutralizes free acid yet does not cause systemic alkalosis in the presence of normal renal function. A double-blind placebo-controlled clinical study demonstrated that calcium carbonate taken at a dosage of 16 Tums tablets daily for a two-week period was non-constipating/non-laxative.

Warnings: Tums: Do not take more than 16 tablets in a 24-hour period or use the maximum dosage of this product for more than 2 weeks, except under the advice and supervision of a physician. If symptoms persist for 2 weeks, stop using this product and see a physician. Keep this and all drugs out of the reach of children.
Tums E-X: Do not take more than 10 tablets in a 24-hour period or use the maximum dosage of this product for more than two weeks, except under the advice and supervision of a physician. If symptoms persist for two weeks, stop using this product and see a physician. Keep this and all drugs out of the reach of children.
Additionally, for Tums Ex Sugar Free: Phenylketonurics: Contains phenylalanine, less than 1 mg per tablet.

Supplement Facts

	Tums 2 Tablets	Tums E-X 2 Tablets	Tums E-X Sugar Free 2 Tablets	Tums Ultra 2 Tablets
Serving Size				
Amount Per Serving				
Calories	5	10	5	10
Sorbitol (g)	—	—	1	—
Sugars (g)	1	2	—	3
Calcium (mg)	400	600	600	800
% Daily Value	40	60	60	80
Sodium (mg)		5		10
% Daily Value	—	<1%	—	<1%

Tums ULTRA: Do not take more than 8 tablets in 24-hour period or use the maximum dosage of this product for more than two weeks, except under the advice and supervision of a physician. If symptoms persist for two weeks, stop using and see a physician. Keep this and all drugs out of the reach of children.

Drug Interaction Precaution: Antacids may interact with certain prescription drugs. If you are presently taking a prescription drug, do not take this product without checking with your physician or other health professional.

Dosage and Administration:
Tums: Chew 2-4 tablets as symptoms occur. Repeat hourly if symptoms return, or as directed by physician.
Tums E-X: Chew 2-4 tablets as symptoms occur. Repeat hourly if symptoms return, or as directed by a physician.
Tums ULTRA: Chew 2-3 tablets as symptoms occur. Repeat hourly if symptoms return, or as directed by a physician.

AS A DIETARY SUPPLEMENT:
Calcium Supplement Directions
Tums, Tums E-X, & Tums ULTRA:
USES: As a daily source of extra calcium. Tums is recommended by the National Osteoporosis Foundation.

IMPORTANT INFORMATION ON OSTEOPOROSIS: Regular exercise and a healthy diet with enough calcium helps teen and young adult white and Asian women maintain good bone health and may reduce their risk of osteoporosis later in life. Adequate calcium intake is important, but daily intakes above 2,000 mg are not likely to provide any additional benefit.

DIRECTIONS: Chew 2 tablets twice daily.
[See table above]

Ingredients (all variants except sugar free): Sucrose, Corn Starch, Talc, Mineral Oil, Flavors (natural and/or artificial), Sodium Polyphosphate. May also contain 1% or less of Adipic Acid, Blue 1 Lake, Yellow 6 Lake, Yellow 10 Lake, Red 27 Lake, Red 30 Lake, Red 40 Lake.

Ingredients (Sugar Free): Sorbitol, Acacia, Natural and Artificial Flavors, Calcium Stearate, Adipic Acid, Yellow 6 Lake, Aspartame.

How Supplied:
Tums: Peppermint flavor is available in 12-tablet rolls, 3-roll wraps, and bottles of 75 and 150. **Assorted Flavors**

(Cherry, Lemon, Orange, and Lime), are available in 12-tablet rolls, 3-roll wraps, and bottles of 75, 150, and 400.
Tums E-X: Wintergreen, Assorted Fruit Assorted Tropical Fruit Flavors, and **Assorted Berries** 8-tablet rolls, 3-roll wraps and bottles of 48 and 96 tablets. Tropical fruit is also available in bottles of 250 tablets.
Tums EX Sugar Free: Orange Cream; bottles of 48 and 96 tablets.
Tums Ultra: Assorted Fruit, Assorted Tropical Fruit and **Assorted Mint Flavors;** bottles of 36 and 72 tablets. Assorted Tropical Fruit & Assorted Fruit also available in bottles of 250 tablets.

Shown in Product Identification Guide, page 523

TUMS 500™ Calcium Supplement

Each Tablet Contains: 1,250 mg calcium carbonate, which provides 500 mg elemental calcium (50% of the U.S. RDI, or Daily Value). Each tablet contains less than 4 mg sodium.

Supplement Facts
Serving size: 1 tablet

Amount per Tablet
Calories: 10
Sugars 2g
Calcium 500mg
% Daily Value 50%

Ingredients: Sucrose, Calcium Carbonate, Corn Starch, Natural and/or Artificial Flavors, Talc, Mineral Oil and Sodium Polyphosphate. May also contain Adipic Acid, Blue 1 Lake, Yellow 6 Lake, Yellow 10 Lake, Red 27 Lake, Red 30 Lake.

Directions: Chew one tablet with meals, two to three times a day or as recommended by a physician.

IMPORTANT INFORMATION ON OSTEOPOROSIS
Osteoporosis affects older persons, especially middle-aged, white and Asian women and those whose families tend to have fragile bones in later years. A lifetime of regular exercise and eating a healthful diet that includes enough calcium, especially during teen and early adult years, builds and maintains good bone health and may reduce the risk of osteoporosis later in life. Adequate calcium intake is important, but intakes above 2,000 mg elemental calcium are not likely to provide any additional benefit.

How Supplied: Tums 500™ is available in **Assorted Fruit and Peppermint,** Flavors, in bottles of 60 tablets.

VIVARIN Tablets & Caplets
Alertness Aid with Caffeine
Maximum Strength

Each Tablet or Caplet Contains 200 mg. Caffeine, Equal to About Two Cups of Coffee

Take Vivarin for a safe, fast pick up anytime you feel drowsy and need to be alert. The caffeine in Vivarin is less irritating to your stomach than coffee, according to a government appointed panel of experts.

FDA APPROVED USES: Helps restore mental alertness or wakefulness when experiencing fatigue or drowsiness.

Active Ingredients: Caffeine 200 mg.

Inactive Ingredients: Tablet: Colloidal Silicon Dioxide, D&C Yellow #10 Al. Lake, Dextrose, FD&C Yellow #6 Al. Lake, Magnesium Stearate, Microcrystalline Cellulose, Starch.
Caplet: Carnauba Wax, Colloidal Silicon Dioxide, D&C Yellow #10 Al Lake, Dextrose, FD&C Yellow #6 Al Lake, Hydroxypropyl Methylcellulose, Magnesium Stearate, Microcrystalline Cellulose, Polyethylene Glycol, Polysorbate 80, Starch, Titanium Dioxide.

Directions: Adults and children 12 years and over: Take 1 tablet (200 mg) not more often than every 3 to 4 hours.

Warnings: The recommended dose of this product contains about as much caffeine as two cups of coffee. Limit the use of caffeine containing medications, foods, or beverages while taking this product because too much caffeine may cause nervousness, irritability, sleeplessness, and occasionally, rapid heartbeat. For occasional use only. Not intended for use as a substitute for sleep. If fatigue or drowsiness persists or continues to recur, consult a doctor. Do not give to children under 12 years of age. As with any drug, if you are pregnant or nursing a baby, seek the advice of a health professional before using this product. In case of accidental overdose, seek professional assistance or contact a poison control center immediately. Keep this and all drugs out of the reach of children.

Tamper Evident Feature: Individually sealed in foil for your protection. Do not use if foil or plastic bubble is torn or punctured.

Store at room temperature, avoid excessive heat (greater than 100°F) or humidity.

How Supplied:
Tablets: Consumer packages of 16, 40 and 80 tablets
Caplets: Consumer packages of 24 and 48 caplets
Comments or Questions? Call Toll-Free 1-800-245-1040 Weekdays.
SmithKline Beecham Consumer Healthcare, L.P.
Pittsburgh, PA 15230. Made in U.S.A.
©1996 SmithKline Beecham
Shown in Product Identification Guide, page 523

Standard Homeopathic Company
210 WEST 131st STREET
BOX 61067
LOS ANGELES, CA 90061

Direct Inquiries to:
Jay Borneman
(800) 624-9659 x20

HYLAND'S BLADDER IRRITATION

Active Ingredients: Rhus Aromatica 3X, HPUS; Benzoicum Acidum 3X, HPUS; Equisetum Hyemale 3X, HPUS; Argentum Nitricum 6X, HPUS; Cantharis 12X, HPUS.

Inactive Ingredients: Lactose NF

Indications: Relief of symptoms of burning and painful urination associated with common bladder irritation.

Directions: Adults: Dissolve 2 – 3 tablets under tongue every 4 hours or as needed. Children 6 to 12 years old: ½ adult dose.

Warnings: Do not use if imprinted cap band is broken or missing. If symptoms persist for more than seven days or worsen, contact a licensed health care professional. As with any drug, if you are pregnant or nursing a baby, seek the advice of a licensed health care professional before using this product. Keep this and all medications out of the reach of children. In case of accidental overdose, contact a poison control center immediately. In case of emergency, the manufacturer may be contacted 24 hours a day, 7 days a week at 800/624-9659.

How Supplied: Bottles of 100 three-grain sublingual tablets (NDC 54973-2953-02). Bottles of 50 three-grain sublingual tablets (NDC 54973-2953-01). Store at room temperature.

HYLAND'S CALMS FORTÉ™ TABLETS

Active Ingredients: *Passiflora* (Passion Flower) 1X triple strength HPUS, *Avena Sativa* (Oat) 1X double strength HPUS,

Humulus Lupulus (Hops) 1X double strength HPUS, *Chamomilla* (Chamomile) 2X HPUS, *Calcarea Phosphorica* (Calcium Phosphate) 3X HPUS, *Ferrum Phosphorica* (Iron Phosphate) 3X HPUS, *Kali Phosphoricum* (Potassium Phosphate) 3X HPUS, *Natrum Phosphoricum* (Sodium Phosphate) 3X HPUS, *Magnesia Phosphoricum* (Magnesium Phosphate) 3X HPUS.

Inactive Ingredients: Lactose N.F.

Indications: Temporary symptomatic relief of simple nervous tension and insomnia.

Directions: Adults: As a relaxant: 1–2 tablets as needed, up to 3 times daily, preferably before meals. Tablets may be swallowed. In insomnia: 1 to 3 tablets ½ to 1 hour before retiring. Repeat as needed without danger of side effects. Children: As a relaxant: 1 tablet as needed, up to 3 times daily, preferably before meals. Tablets may be swallowed. In insomnia: 1 to 2 tablets ½ to 1 hour before retiring. Repeat as needed without danger of side effects.

Warning: Do not use if cap band is broken or missing. If symptoms persist for more than seven days or worsen, consult a licensed health care professional. As with any drug, if you are pregnant or nursing a baby, seek the advice of a licensed health care professional before using this product. Keep this and all medications out of the reach of children.

How Supplied: Bottles of 100 4-grain tablets (NDC 54973-1121-02), 50 4-grain tablets (NDC 54973-1121-01) and 32 5.5-grain caplets (NDC 54973-1121-48). Store at room temperature.

HYLAND'S COLD TABLETS WITH ZINC

Active Ingredients: Aconitum Napellus 6X, HPUS; Allium Cepa 6X, HPUS; Gelsemium Sempervirens 6X, HPUS; Zinc Gluconate 2X, HPUS.

Inactive Ingredients: Lactose, NF

Indications: Temporary symptomatic treatment for the relief of the common cold.

Directions: Dissolve 2 – 3 tablets under tongue every 4 hours or as needed. Children 6 to 12 years old: ½ adult dose.

Warnings: Do not use if imprinted cap band is broken or missing. If symptoms persist for more than seven days or worsen, contact a licensed health care professional. Discontinue if symptoms are accompanied by a high fever (over 101 °F) and contact a licensed health care professional. As with any drug, if you are pregnant or nursing a baby, seek the advice of a licensed health care professional before using this product. Keep this and all medications out of the reach of children. In case of accidental overdose, contact a poison control center im-

Continued on next page

Hyland's Cold w/Zinc—Cont.

mediately. In cases of emergency, the manufacturer may be contacted 24 hours a day, 7 days a week at 800/624-9659.

How Supplied: Bottles of 50 three-grain sublingual tablets (NDC 54973-3010-01). Store at room temperature.

HYLAND'S COLIC TABLETS

Active Ingredients: *Disocorea* (Wild Yam) 3X HPUS, *Chamomilla* (Chamomile) 3X HPUS, *Colocynthinum* (Bitter Apple) 3X HPUS.

Inactive Ingredients: Lactose N.F.

Indications: A homeopathic combination for the temporary relief of symptoms of colic and gas pains caused by irritating food, feeding too quickly, swallowing air and similar conditions during teething, colds and other minor upset periods in children.

Directions: For children up to 2 years of age: Dissolve 2 tablets under the tongue every 15 minutes for up to 8 doses until relieved; then every 2 hours as required. If you prefer, tablets may first be dissolved in a teaspoon of water and then given to the child. Children over 2 years: Dissolve 3 tablets under the tongue as above; or as recommended by a licensed health care professional. Colic Tablets are very soft and dissolve almost instantly under the tongue. If your baby has been crying or has been very upset, your baby may fall asleep after using this product. This is because pain has been relieved and your child can rest.

Warnings: Do not use if imprinted cap band is broken or missing. If symptoms persist for more than seven days or worsen, consult a licensed health care professional. As with any drug, if you are pregnant or nursing a baby, seek the advice of a licensed health care professional before using this product. Keep this and all medications out of the reach of children. In case of accidental overdose, contact a poison control center immediately. In cases of emergency, the manufacturer may be contacted 24 hours a day, 7 days a week at 800/624-9659

How Supplied: Bottles of 125—one grain sublingual tablets (NDC 54973-7502-1). Store at room temperature.

HYLAND'S EARACHE TABLETS

Active Ingredients: Pulsatilla (Passion Flower) 30C, HPUS; Chamomilla (Chamomile) 30C, HPUS; Sulphur 30C, HPUS; Calcarea Carbonica (Carbonate of Lime) 30C, HPUS; Belladonna 30C, HPUS; $(3 \times 10^{-60}$ % Alkaloids) and Lycopodium (Club Moss) 30C, HPUS.

Inactive Ingredients: Lactose NF

Indications: For the relief of symptoms of fever, pain, irritability and sleeplessness associated with earaches in children after diagnosis by a physician. If symptoms persist for more than 48 hours or if there is a discharge from the ear, discontinue use and contact your health care professional.

Directions: Dissolve 2–3 tablets under the tongue 3 times per day for 48 hours or until symptoms subside. If you prefer, tablets may be dissolved in a teaspoon of water and then given to the child. Earache Tablets are very soft and dissolve almost instantly under the tongue.

Warnings: Do not use if imprinted blisters are broken or damaged. If symptoms persist for more than 48 hours, or if there is a discharge from the ear, discontinue use and consult a licensed health care professional. As with any drug, if you are pregnant or nursing a baby, seek the advice of a licensed health care professional before using this product. Keep this and all medications out of the reach of children. In case of accidental overdose, contact a poison control center immediately. In cases of emergency, the manufacturer may be contacted 24 hours a day, 7 days a week at 800/624-9659.

How Supplied: Blister pack of 40 tablets (NDC 54973-7507-1). Store at room temperature.

HYLAND'S LEG CRAMPS WITH QUININE TABLETS

Active Ingredients: Cinchona Officinalis 3X, HPUS (Quinine), Viscum Album 3X, HPUS; Gnaphalium Polycephalum 3X, HPUS; Rhus Toxicodendron 6X, HPUS; Aconitum Napellus 6X, HPUS; Ledum Palustre 6X, HPUS; Magnesia Phosphorica 6X, HPUS.

Inactive Ingredients: Lactose N.F.

Indications: Hyland's Leg Cramps is a traditional homeopathic formula for the relief of symptoms of cramps and pains in lower back and legs often made worse by damp weather. Working without contraindications or side effects, Hyland's Leg Cramps stimulates your body's natural healing response to relieve symptoms. Hyland's Leg Cramps is safe for adults and can be used in conjuction with other medications.

Directions: Adults: Dissolve 2–3 tablets under tongue every 4 hours as needed.

Warnings: Do not use if imprinted cap band is missing or broken. If symptoms persist for more than seven days or worsen, contact a licensed health care professional. As with any drug, if you are pregnant or nursing a baby, seek the advice of a licensed health care professional before using this product. Do not use if pregnant, sensitive to quinine or under 12 years of age. Keep this and all medications out of the reach of children. In case of accidental overdose, contact a poi-

son control center immediately. In case of emergency, the manufacturer may be reached 24 hours a day, 7 days a week at 800-624-9659.

How Supplied: Bottles of 100 three-grain sublingual tablets (NDC 54973-2956-02), Bottles of 50 three-grain sublingual tablets (NDC 54973-2956-01). Store at room temperature.

HYLAND'S MOTION SICKNESS TABLETS

Active Ingredients: Nux Vomica 6X HPUS, Tabacum 6X HPUS, Petroleum 12X HPUS, Cocculus Indicus 30X HPUS.

Inactive Ingredients: Lactose NF

Indications: For the relief of symptoms of nausea and dizziness associated with or aggravated by motion. Useful for car sickness and sea sickness. Safe for adults and children and can be used in conjunction with other medications.

Directions: Adults: Dissolve 2–3 tablets under tongue every 4 hours or as needed. Children 6 to 12 years old: $^1/_2$ adult dose. Use no more than 6 times per day.

Warnings: Do not use if imprinted cap band is missing or broken. If symptoms persist for more than seven days or worsen, contact a licensed health care professional. As with any drug, if you are pregnant or nursing a baby, seek the advice of a licensed health care professional before using this product. Keep this and all medications out of the reach of children. In case of accidental overdose, contact a poison control center immediately.

How Supplied: Bottles of 50 three grain sublingual tablets (NDC 54973-9147-01). Store at room temperature.

HYLAND'S NERVE TONIC

Active Ingredients: Calcarea Phosphorica (Calcium Phosphate) 3X, HPUS; Ferrum Phosphorica (Iron Phosphate 3X, HPUS; Kali Phosphoricum (Potassium Phosphate) 3X, HPUS; Natrum Phosphoricum (Sodium Phosphate) 3X, HPUS; Magnesia Phosphoricum (Magnesium Phosphate) 3X, HPUS.

Inactive Ingredients: Lactose NF

Indications: Temporary symtomatic relief of simple nervous tension and stress.

Directions: Adults take 1 to 2 caplets before each meal and at bedtime. Children: ½ adult dose.

Warnings: Do not use if imprinted cap band is broken or missing. If symptoms persist for more than seven days or worsen, contact a licensed health care professional. As with any drug, if you are pregnant or nursing a baby, seek the advice of a licensed health care professional before using this product. Keep this and all medications out of the reach of children. In case of accidental overdose, contact a poison control center immediately. In cases of emergency, the manufacturer may be contacted 24 hours a day, 7 days a week at 800/624-9659.

How Supplied: Bottles of 32 caplets (NDC 54973-1129-68), Bottles of 500 tablets (NDC 54973-1129-1), Bottles of 1000 tablets (NDC 54973-1129-2)

HYLAND'S PMS

Active Ingredients: Viburnum Opulus 2X, HPUS; Caulophyllum Thalictroides 3X, HPUS; Cocculus Indicus 3X, HPUS; Gelsemium Sempervirens 3X, HPUS.

Inactive Ingredients: Lactose NF

Indications: Relief of symptoms of menstrual pain, cramping and irritability associated with menstrual period.

Directions: Adults: Dissolve 2 – 3 tablets under the tongue every 4 hours or as needed.

Warnings: Do not use if imprinted cap band is broken or missing. If symptoms persist for more than seven days or worsen, contact a licensed health care professional. As with any drug, if you are pregnant or nursing a baby, seek the advice of a licensed health care professional before using this product. Keep this and all medications out of the reach of children. In case of accidental overdose, contact a poison control center immediately. In cases of emergency, the manufacturer may be contacted 24 hours a day, 7 days a week at 800/624-9659.

How Supplied: Bottles of 100 three-grain sublingual tablets (NDC 54973-2957-02). Bottles of 50 three-grain sublingual tablets (NDC 54973-2957-01). Store at room temperature.

HYLAND'S POISON IVY/OAK TABLETS

Active Ingredients: Rhus Toxicodendron 6X, HPUS; Croton Tiglium 6X, HPUS; Xerophyllum 6X, HPUS

Inactive Ingredients: Lactose NF

Indications: A homeopathic combination for symptomatic treatment after contact with poison ivy or oak. Skin breaks out with red, swollen, intensely itching, burning, watery blisters, sometimes followed by oozing or crusting.

Directions: Adults: Dissolve 2 to 3 tablets under the tongue every 2 hours as needed, then 4 times per day. Children 6 to 12 years old: ½ adult dose.

Warnings: Do not use if imprinted cap band is broken or missing. If symptoms persist for more than seven days or worsen, contact a licensed health care professional. As with any drug, if you are pregnant or nursing a baby, seek the ad-

vice of a licensed health care professional before using this product. Keep this and all medications out of the reach of children. In case of accidental overdose, contact a poison control center immediately. In case of emergency, the manufacturer may be contacted 24 hours a day, 7 days a week at 800/624-9659.

How Supplied: Bottles of 50 three-grain sublingual tablets (NDC 54973-1130-01). Store at room temperature.

HYLAND'S TEETHING GEL

Active Ingredients: Calcarea Phosphorica (Calcium Phosphate) 12X, HPUS; Chamomilla (Chamomile) 6X, HPUS; Coffea Cruda (Coffee) 6X, HPUS; and Belladonna 6X, HPUS (Alkaloids 0.0000003%)

Inactive Ingredients: Deionized water, Vegetable Glycerin, Hydroxyethyl Cellulose, Methyl Paraben and Propyl Paraben.

Indications: A homeopathic combination for the temporary relief of symptoms of simple restlessness and wakeful irritability due to cutting teeth.

Directions: Apply to gums as necessary. If symptoms persist for more than seven days or worsen, discontinue use and contact your health care professional. Please note, if your baby has been crying or has been very upset, your baby may fall asleep after using this product because the pain has been relieved and your child can rest.

Warnings: Do not use if tube tip is broken or missing. If symptoms persist for more than seven days or if irritation persists, inflammation develops or fever or infection develop, discontinue use and consult a licensed health care professional. As with any drug, if you are pregnant or nursing a baby, seek the advice of a licensed health care professional before using this product. Keep this and all medications out of the reach of children. In case of accidental overdose, contact a poison control center immediately. In case of emergency, the manufacturer may be contacted 24 hours a day, 7 days a week at 800/624-9659.

How Supplied: Tubes of 1/3 OZ. (NDC 54973-7504-3). Store at room temperature.

HYLAND'S TEETHING TABLETS

Active Ingredients: *Calcarea Phosphorica* (Calcium Phosphate) 3X HPUS, *Chamomilla* (Chamomile) 3X HPUS, *Coffea Cruda* (Coffee) 3X HPUS, *Belladonna* 3X HPUS (Alkaloids 0.0003%).

Inactive Ingredients: Lactose N.F.

Indications: A homeopathic combination for the temporary relief of symptoms of simple restlessness and wakeful irritability due to cutting teeth.

Directions: Dissolve 2 to 3 tablets under the tongue 4 times per day. If you prefer, tablets may first be dissolved in a teaspoon of water and then given to the child. If the child is restless or wakeful, 2 tablets every hour for 6 doses or as recommended by a licensed health care professional. Teething Tablets are very soft and dissolve almost instantly under the tongue. Please note, if your baby has been crying or has been very upset, your baby may fall asleep after using this product because the pain has been relieved and your child can rest.

Warning: Do Not use if imprinted cap band is broken or missing. If symptoms persist for more than seven days, or if irritation persist, inflammation develops or fever or infection develop, discontinue use and consult a licensed health care professional. As with any drug, if you are pregnant or nursing a baby, seek the advice of a health care professional before using this product. Keep this and all medications out of the reach of children. In case of accidental overdose, contact a poison control center immediately. In case of emergency, the manufacturer may be contacted 24 hours a day, 7 days a week at 800/624-9659.

How Supplied: Bottles of 125—one grain sublingual tablets (NDC 54973-7504-01). Store at room temperature.

HYLAND'S VAGINITIS

Active Ingredients: Natrum Muriaticum 12X HPUS, Candida Albicans 30X HPUS, Kreosotum 12X HPUS, Carbolicum Acidum 12X HPUS.

Inactive Ingredients: Lactose NF

Indications: Relief of symptoms of vaginal itching and burning due to vaginal irritation or discharge after diagnosis by your doctor. Symptoms may be accompanied by clear to white vaginal discharge.

Directions: Adults: Dissolve 2–3 tablets under tongue every 4 hours or as needed.

Warnings: Do not use if imprinted cap band is missing or broken. If symptoms persist for more than seven days or worsen, contact a licensed health care professional. As with any drug, if you are pregnant or nursing a baby, seek the advice of a licensed health care professional before using this product. Keep this and all medications out of the reach of children. In case of accidental overdose, contact a poison control center immediately.

How Supplied: Bottles of 100 three grain sublingual tablets (NDC 54973-2962-02). Bottles of 50 three grain sub-

Continued on next page

Hyland's Vaginitis—Cont.

lingual tablets (NDC 54973-2962-01). Store at room temperature.

Thompson Medical Company, Inc.

**777 SO. FLAGLER DR.
WEST TOWER, SUITE 1500
WEST PALM BEACH
FLORIDA 33401**

Direct Inquiries to:
Consumer Services: (561) 820-9900
Fax: (561) 832-2297

ENCARE®

[en 'kar]
Vaginal Contraceptive Suppositories

Description: Encare is a safe and effective contraceptive in a convenient vaginal suppository form available without a prescription. Encare is reliable because it offers two-way protection: (1) Encare kills sperm on contact by releasing a premeasured dose of nonoxynol 9, the spermicide most recommended by doctors. (2) Encare gently disperses a physical barrier of protection against the cervix to help prevent pregnancy.
Encare is colorless and odorless.
It is an effective contraceptive in vaginal suppository form.

Active Ingredient: Each suppository contains 100 mg Nonoxynol 9.

Other Ingredients: Polyethylene Glycols, Sodium Bicarbonate, Sodium Citrate, Tartaric Acid.

Indications: Encare provides reliable protection against pregnancy.

Action: Encare is 100% free of hormones and free of the serious side effects associated with oral contraceptives.
Encare is convenient and easy to use. Women like Encare because each insert is individually wrapped and can be easily carried in a pocket or purse. Encare is approximately as effective as vaginal foam contraceptives in actual use, yet there is no applicator, so there is nothing to fill, remove, or clean. For added protection, Encare may be used in conjunc-

tion with other contraceptive methods, such as a condom or as a second application with a diaphragm.
Because Encare can be inserted as much as an hour before intercourse, it does not interfere with spontaneity. Encare has been used successfully by millions of women throughout Europe and America.

Special Warning: Spermicidal contraceptives should not be used during pregnancy. Some experts believe that there may be an increased risk of birth defects occurring in children whose mothers used a spermicidal contraceptive at the time of conception or during pregnancy. If you believe you may be pregnant, have a pregnancy test before using a spermicidal contraceptive. If you have used a spermicidal contraceptive after becoming pregnant, or used a spermicidal contraceptive when you became pregnant, discuss this issue with your doctor.

Cautions: If your doctor has told you that you should not become pregnant, consult your doctor as to which method, (including Encare), is best for you.

If you or your partner experience irritation, discontinue use. If irritation persists, consult your doctor. This product has not been shown to protect against HIV (AIDS) and other sexually transmitted diseases.

Do not take orally. **KEEP THIS AND ALL DRUGS OUT OF THE REACH OF CHILDREN.** In case of accidental ingestion, call a poison control center, emergency medical facility or a doctor immediately.

Keep away from excessive heat and moisture. Store at controlled room temperature: 15°C–30°C (59°–86°F).

Dosage and Administration: For best protection against pregnancy, it is essential to follow package instructions. At least 10 minutes before intercourse, place one Encare suppository with your fingertip as far as possible into the vagina, towards the small of your back. Best protection will occur when Encare is placed deep into the vagina. You may feel a sensation of warmth as Encare effervesces and distributes the spermicide, nonoxynol 9, within the vagina. This is a natural attribute of the active ingredient.

IMPORTANT: It is essential to insert Encare at least 10 minutes before intercourse. If one chooses, Encare can be inserted up to one hour before intercourse. If intercourse has not taken place within one hour after insertion, use a new Encare suppository. Use a new Encare suppository each time intercourse is repeated. Encare can be used safely and as frequently as needed.

Douching after use of Encare is not recommended, however, should you desire to do so, wait at least six hours after intercourse.

Instructions enclosed in package are in both English and Spanish.

How Supplied: Boxes of 12 and 18.

SLEEPINAL®
Night-time Sleep Aid Capsules and Softgels

(Diphenhydramine HCl)

Description: Sleepinal® is a nighttime sleep aid. When taken prior to bedtime, it aids in falling asleep and helps to relieve occasional sleeplessness.

Active Ingredient: Diphenhydramine HCl 50 mg.

Other Ingredients: Capsules: FD&C Blue No. 1, Gelatin, Lactose, Magnesium Stearate, Povidone, Talc.

Softgels: D&C Yellow No. 10, FD&C Green No. 3, Gelatin, Glycerin, Polyethylene Glycol 400, Povidone, Propylene Glycol, Purified Water, Sorbitol.

Indications: For relief of occasional sleeplessness.

Action: Sleepinal® is an antihistamine with anticholinergic and sedative action.

Warnings: Read before using. Do not exceed recommended dosage. Do not give to children under 12 years of age. **Do Not Use** with any other product containing diphenhydramine, including one applied topically. If sleeplessness persists continuously for more than 2 weeks, consult your doctor. Insomnia may be a symptom of serious underlying medical illness. Do not take this product, unless directed by a physician, if you have a breathing problem such as emphysema or chronic bronchitis, or if you have glaucoma or difficulty in urination due to the enlargement of the prostate gland. Avoid alcoholic beverages while taking this product. Do not take this product if you are taking sedatives or tranquilizers, without first consulting your doctor. As with any drug, if you are pregnant or nursing a baby, seek the advice of a health professional before using this product.

KEEP THIS AND ALL DRUGS OUT OF THE REACH OF CHILDREN.

In case of accidental overdose, seek professional assistance or contact a poison control center immediately.

Dosage and Administration: Capsules and Softgels: Adults and children 12 years of age and over: Oral dosage is one pill at bedtime if needed, or as directed by a doctor.

How to Store: Store in a dry place at controlled room temperature 15°–30° C (59°–86° F). Protect softgels from light, retain product in box until administered.

How Supplied: Capsules and Softgels: Sleepinal® is supplied in tamper-evident blister packages. Do not use if individual seals are broken. Packages of 16 and 32 capsules and 8 and 16 softgels.

Triton Consumer Products, Inc.
561 W. GOLF ROAD
ARLINGTON HEIGHTS, IL 60005

Direct Inquiries to:
Karen Shrader
(800) 942-2009

For Medical Emergencies Contact:
(800) 942-2009

MG 217® PSORIASIS/DANDRUFF MEDICATION
Ointment, Lotion, Solution, Shampoo

Active Ingredients: Ointment—Coal Tar Solution USP 10%. **Lotion**—Coal Tar Solution USP 5%. **Sal-Acid Ointment and Solution**—Salicylic acid 3%. **Tar Shampoo**—Coal Tar Solution USP 15%. **Tar-Free Shampoo**—Sulfur 5% and salicylic acid 3%.

Action/Uses: Relief for itching, scaling and flaking of psoriasis, seborrheic dermatitis and/or dandruff.

Warnings: For external use only. Avoid contact with eyes. If undue skin irritation occurs, discontinue use.

Administration: Ointment, Lotion, Solution—Apply to affected area one to four times daily. **Shampoo**—Use at least twice a week or as directed by a physician.

How Supplied: Ointment—3.8 oz. jars. **Lotion**—4 oz. bottles. **Sal-Acid Ointment/Solution**—2 oz. jars/bottles. **Shampoo**—4 oz. and 8 oz. bottles.

UAS Laboratories
5610 ROWLAND RD #110
MINNETONKA, MN 55343

Direct Inquiries To:
Dr. S.K. Dash: (612) 935-1707
Fax: (612) 935-1650

Medical Emergency Contact:
Dr. S.K. Dash: (612) 935-1707
Fax: (612) 935-1650

DDS®-ACIDOPHILUS
Capsule, Tablet & Powder free of dairy products, corn, soy, and preservatives

Description: DDS®-Acidophilus is the source of a special strain of Lactobacillus acidophilus free of dairy products, corn, soy and preservatives. Each capsule or tablet contains one billion viable DDS-1 L.acidophilus at the time of manufacturing. One gram of powder contains two billion viable DDS®- L.acidophilus.

CLEARBLUE EASY®

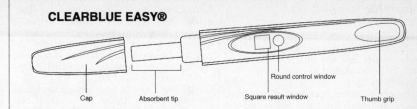

Cap — Absorbent tip — Round control window — Square result window — Thumb grip

Indications and Usages: An aid in implanting the gut with beneficial Lactobacillus acidophilus under conditions of digestive disorders, acne, yeast infections, and following antibiotic therapy.

Administration: One to two capsules or tablets twice daily before meals. One-fourth teaspoon powder can be substituted for two capsules or tablets.

How Supplied: Bottles of 100 capsules or tablets. 12 bottles per case. Powder is available in 2 oz. bottle; 12 bottles per case.

Storage: Keep refrigerated under 40°F.

EDUCATIONAL MATERIAL

DDS-Acidophilus
Booklet describing superior-strain Acidophilus without dairy products, corn, soy, or preservatives. Two billion viable DDS-L. acidopohilus per gram.

Unilever
Home & Personal Care USA
33 BENEDICT PLACE
GREENWICH, CT 06830

Direct Inquiries to:
Consumer Services
1-800-598-5005

"ALL" FREE CLEAR® with ALLERGEN FIGHTER™
Laundry Detergent

Ingredients: *Liquid*—Cleaning agents (anionic and nonionic surfactants), buffering agent, stabilizer and brightening agent. Contains no dyes or perfumes; *Powder*—Cleaning agents (anionic and nonionic surfactants), water softeners (sodium aluminosilicate and sodium carbonate), anti-redeposition agent, fabric whitener, washer protection agent (sodium silicate) and processing aids (sodium sulfate).

Description/Actions and Uses: "all" Free Clear with Allergen Fighter is a mild, gentle laundry detergent that is specially formulated for sensitive skin. "all" Free Clear with Allergen Fighter removes everyday allergens like dust mite

matter that can cling to fiber. This dermatologist tested formulation has been found to contain no known allergens. "all" Free Clear with Allergen Fighter provides excellent cleaning and stainlifting that will not harm the flame resistance of children's sleepwear.

Directions: Instruct patients to follow directions on back of "all" Free Clear with Allergen Fighter package.

How Supplied: 50 oz., 100 oz., 200 oz. Liquid; 42 load and 48 load Powder.
Shown in Product Identification Guide, page 523

Unipath Diagnostics Company
47 HULFISH STREET
SUITE 400
PRINCETON, NJ 08542

Direct Inquiries to:
1-800-321-EASY

CLEARBLUE EASY®
One Minute Pregnancy Test

INSTRUCTIONS FOR USE
A clear Yes or No in just one minute.
Please read this leaflet carefully before carrying out your test.
ClearBlue Easy® is an easy-to-use one-step pregnancy test which gives the user a clear, accurate result in just **one** minute. With ClearBlue Easy the user can test from the first day of her missed period and at any time of the day.
ClearBlue Easy has been shown to be more than 99% accurate in laboratory tests.
[See graphic above]
ClearBlue Easy is a rapid, one-step pregnancy test for home use, which detects the pregnancy hormone HCG (human chorionic gonadotropin) in the urine. This hormone is produced in increasing amounts during the first part of pregnancy. ClearBlue Easy uses sensitive monoclonal antibodies to detect the presence of this hormone from the first day of a missed period.
A negative result means that no pregnancy hormone was detected and the woman is probably not pregnant. If the menstrual period does not start within a week, she may have miscalculated the day her period was due. She should re-

Continued on next page

Clearblue Easy—Cont.

peat the test using another ClearBlue Easy test. If the second test gives a negative result and she still has not menstruated, she should see her doctor.

ClearBlue Easy is specially designed for easy use at home. However, if you have questions about the test, please call the ClearBlue Easy Helpline at 1-800-321-EASY Monday-Friday 8:30 a.m. to 5:00 p.m. EST.

Unipath LTD, Bedford, United Kingdom. Distributed by Unipath Diagnostics Company, Princeton, New Jersey 08542. ©1999 Unipath. All rights reserved

Shown in Product Identification Guide, page 523

CLEARPLAN EASY®
Ovulation Test

ClearPlan Easy Ovulation Test identifies the most fertile days in a woman's cycle, when she has the greatest chance of becoming pregnant. The ClearPlan Easy Ovulation Test is quick and simple to use:

- requires only one easy step
- 99% accurate in laboratory tests
- gives a clear result in just 3 minutes
- allows the user to test any time of day

ClearPlan Easy employs highly sensitive monoclonal antibody technology to accurately predict the onset of ovulation, and consequently, the best time each month for a woman to try to become pregnant. The test monitors the amount of LH in a woman's urine. Small amounts of LH are present during most of the menstrual cycle, but the level normally rises sharply about 24–36 hours before ovulation. ClearPlan Easy detects this LH surge so that a woman knows 24–36 hours before the time when she is most likely to become pregnant.

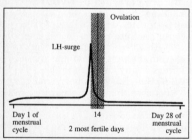

To use ClearPlan Easy, a woman simply holds the absorbent tip in her urine stream for 5 seconds only and then, after 3 minutes, reads the result. The results are ready by comparing the two lines in the Result Window. The line nearest the arrow is the Surge Line and the line farthest from the arrow is the Reference Line. When the Reference Line is present, it indicates that the test was conducted correctly. If the Surge Line is similar to or darker than the Reference Line, then the user has detected her LH surge. If the Surge Line is lighter than the Reference Line, the LH surge has not begun.

Each ClearPlan Easy kit contains 5 Test Sticks for 5 days of testing. If, because she has long or irregular cycles, or for any other reason, a woman does not detect her LH surge after 5 days of testing, she should continue testing with a second ClearPlan Easy kit.

ClearPlan Easy is specifically designed for easy use at home. However, if the user has questions about the test, she can call the ClearPlan Easy Helpline at 1-800-321-EASY Monday-Friday 8:30 a.m. to 5:00 p.m. EST.

Unipath Ltd., Bedford, UK. Distributed by Unipath Diagnostics Co., Princeton, New Jersey, 08542. ©1999 Unipath. All Rights Reserved.

Shown in Product Identification Guide, page 523

Upsher-Smith Laboratories, Inc.
**14905 23rd AVENUE N.
PLYMOUTH, MN 55447**

Direct inquiries to:
Professional Services
(612) 475-3023
Fax (612) 475-3410

AMLACTIN® 12% Moisturizing Lotion and Cream
[ăm-lăk-tĭn]
Cosmetic Lotion and Cream

Description: AMLACTIN® Moisturizing Lotion and Cream are special formulations of 12% lactic acid neutralized with ammonium hydroxide to provide a lotion or cream pH of 4.5–5.5. Lactic acid, an alpha-hydroxy acid, is a naturally occurring humectant for the skin. AMLACTIN® moisturizes and softens rough, dry skin.

How Supplied: 225g (8oz) plastic bottle: List No. 0245-0023-22
400g (14oz) plastic bottle: List No. 0245-0023-40
140g (4.9oz) tube: List No. 0245-0024-14

UNKNOWN DRUG?
Consult the
Product Identification Guide
(Gray Pages)
for full-color photos of
leading over-the-counter
medications

Wallace Laboratories
**P.O. BOX 1001
HALF ACRE ROAD
CRANBURY, NJ 08512**

Direct Inquiries to:
Wallace Laboratories
Div. of Carter-Wallace, Inc.
P.O. Box 1001
Cranbury, NJ 08512
(609) 655-6000

**For Medical Information, Contact:
Generally:
Professional Services**
800-526-3840

After Hours and Weekend Emergencies
609-655-6474

MALTSUPEX®
(malt soup extract)
Powder, Liquid, Tablets

Composition: MALTSUPEX is a non-diastatic extract from barley malt, which is available in powder, liquid, and tablet form. Each MALTSUPEX product has a gentle laxative action and promotes soft, easily passed stools.

Tablet: Each tablet contains 750 mg of Malt Soup Extract. Other ingredients: D&C Yellow No. 10, FD&C Red No. 40, flavor (artificial), hydroxypropyl methylcellulose, methylparaben, polyethylene glycol, povidone, propylparaben, simethicone emulsion, stearic acid, talc, titanium dioxide. Sodium content: Each tablet contains approximately 1 mg of sodium.

Powder: Each level scoop provides approximately 8 g of Malt Soup Extract. Sodium content: Each scoopful contains approximately 5 mg of sodium.

Liquid: Each tablespoonful ($^{1}/_{2}$ fl. oz.) contains approximately the equivalent of 16 g Malt Soup Extract Powder. Other ingredients: Potassium sorbate and sodium propionate. Sodium content: Each tablespoon contains approximately 36 mg of sodium.

EFFECTIVE, NON-HABIT-FORMING

Indications: For relief of occasional constipation. This product generally produces a bowel movement in 12 to 72 hours.

Warnings: Do not use laxative products when abdominal pain, nausea or vomiting are present unless directed by a physician. If constipation persists, consult a physician.

If you have noticed a sudden change in bowel habits that persists over a period of 2 weeks, consult a physician before using a laxative.

Keep this and all medications out of the reach of children. In case of accidental overdose, seek professional assistance or contact a poison control center immediately.

Laxative products should not be used for a period longer than one week unless di-

MALTSUPEX Powder

AGE	CORRECTIVE*	MAINTENANCE
12 years to ADULTS	Up to 4 scoops twice a day (Take a full glass [8 oz.] of liquid with each dose.)	2 to 4 scoops at bedtime
CHILDREN 6–12 years of age	Up to 2 scoops twice a day (Take a full glass [8 oz.] of liquid with each dose.)	
CHILDREN 2–6 years of age	1 scoop twice a day (Take a full glass [8 oz.] of liquid with each dose.)	
INFANTS under 2 years of age	Consult a doctor.	

* Full corrective dosage should be used for 3 or 4 days or until relief is noted. Then continue on maintenance dosage as needed. Use a clean, dry scoop to remove powder. Replace cover tightly to keep out moisture.

MALTSUPEX Liquid

AGE	CORRECTIVE*	MAINTENANCE
12 years to ADULTS	2 tablespoonfuls twice a day (Take a full glass [8 oz.] of liquid with each dose.)	1 to 2 tablespoonfuls at bedtime
CHILDREN 6–12 years of age	1 tablespoonful twice a day (Take a full glass [8 oz.] of liquid with each dose.)	
CHILDREN 2–6 years of age	$1/_2$ tablespoonful twice a day (Take a full glass [8 oz.] of liquid with each dose.)	
INFANTS under 2 years of age	Consult a doctor.	

* Full corrective dosage should be used for 3 or 4 days or until relief is noted. Then continue on maintenance dosage as needed. Use a clean, dry scoop to remove the liquid. Replace cover tightly after use.

rected by a physician. Rectal bleeding or failure to have a bowel movement after use of a laxative may indicate a serious condition. Discontinue use and consult a physician.

As with any drug, if you are pregnant or nursing a baby, seek the advice of a health professional before using this product.
MALTSUPEX Liquid only—Do not use this product if you are on a sodium-restricted diet unless directed by a physician. Maltsupex Liquid contains approximately 1.58 mEq (36 mg) of sodium per tablespoon.
Maltsupex Tablets contain approximately 0.02 mEq (0.46 mg) of sodium per tablet.
Each scoop of Maltsupex Powder contains approximately 0.22 mEq (5 mg) of sodium per scoop.
Note: Allow for carbohydrate content in diabetic diets and infant formulas.
Liquid: (67%, 14 g/tablespoon, or 56 calories/tablespoon)
Powder: (83%, 6 g or 24 calories per scoop)
Tablets: (Approximately 83%, 0.5 g or 2.5 calories per tablet)

Directions: General—Drink a full glass (8 ounces) of liquid with each dose. The recommended daily dosage of MALT-SUPEX may vary. Use the smallest dose that is effective and lower dosage as improvement occurs.
MALTSUPEX Powder—Each bottle contains a scoop. Each scoopful (which is the

equivalent of a standard measuring tablespoon) should be levelled with a knife.
MALTSUPEX Tablets: Adult Dosage: Start with four tablets (3 g) four times daily (with meals and at bedtime) and adjust dosage according to response, not to exceed 48 tablets (36 g) daily. Drink a full glass (8 oz.) of liquid with each dose.
Usual Dosage—Powder:
[See first table above]
Usual Dosage—Liquid:
[See second table above]
Preparation Tips: Powder—Add dosage to milk, water, or fruit juice and stir until dissolved. Mixing is easier if added to warm milk or warm water. May be flavored with vanilla or cocoa to make "malteds." Excellent with warm milk at bedtime. Also available in tablet and liquid forms.
Note: Although shade, texture, taste, and height of contents may vary between bottles, action remains the same.
Liquid: Mixing is easier if MALTSU-PEX Liquid is added to an ounce or two of warm water and stirred. Then add milk, water, or fruit juice and stir until dissolved. May be flavored with vanilla or cocoa to make "malteds." Excellent with warm milk at bedtime. Also available in tablet and powder forms.
Professional Labeling:
The dosage for children under 2 years of age is:
Powder: 2 to 3 level measuring teaspoonfuls, 3 to 4 times per day, in water, fruit juice, or formula.

Liquid: 1 to 2 measuring teaspoonfuls, 2 to 3 times per day, in water, fruit juice, or formula.

How Supplied: MALTSUPEX is supplied in 8 ounce (NDC 0037-9101-12) and 16 ounce (NDC 0037-9101-08) jars of MALTSUPEX Powder; 8 fluid ounce (NDC 0037-9051-12) and 1 pint (NDC 0037-9051-08) bottles of MALTSUPEX Liquid; and in bottles of 100 MALTSU-PEX Tablets (NDC 0037-9201-01).
Storage: Store at controlled room temperature 20°–25°C (68°–77°F). Protect MALTSUPEX powder and tablets from moisture.

MALTSUPEX **Powder** and **Liquid** are

Distributed by
WALLACE LABORATORIES
Division of Carter-Wallace, Inc.
Cranbury, New Jersey 08512

MALTSUPEX **Tablets** are

Manufactured by
WALLACE LABORATORIES
Division of Carter-Wallace, Inc.
Cranbury, New Jersey 08512

Rev. 8/97
Shown in Product Identification Guide, page 523

RYNA®
(Liquid)
RYNA–C®
(Liquid)　　　　　　　　　　　　　ℂ
RYNA–CX®
(Liquid)　　　　　　　　　　　　　ℂ

Description:
RYNA® (Liquid)—Each 5 mL (one teaspoonful) contains:
Chlorpheniramine maleate .... 2 mg
Pseudoephedrine hydrochloride .. 30 mg
Other ingredients: flavor (artificial), glycerin, malic acid, purified water, sodium benzoate, sorbitol in a clear, colorless to slightly yellow-colored, lemon-vanilla flavored demulcent base containing no sugar, dyes, or alcohol.
RYNA-C® (Liquid)—Each 5 mL (one teaspoonful) contains, in addition:
Codeine phosphate .... 10 mg
(WARNING: May be habit-forming)
Other ingredients: flavor (artificial), glycerin, malic acid, purified water, saccharin sodium, sodium benzoate, sorbitol in a clear, colorless to slightly yellow, cinnamon flavored demulcent base containing no sugar, dyes, or alcohol.
RYNA-CX® (Liquid)—Each 5 mL (one teaspoonful) contains:
Codeine phosphate .... 10 mg
(WARNING: May be habit-forming)
Pseudoephedrine hydrochloride .. 30 mg
Guaifenesin .... 100 mg
Other ingredients: flavors (artificial), glycerin, glycine, malic acid, povidone, propylene glycol, purified water, saccharin sodium, sorbitol in a clear, colorless to slightly yellow or straw-colored, cher-

Continued on next page

Ryna/Ryna-C/Ryna-CX—Cont.

ry-vanilla-menthol flavored demulcent base containing no sugar, dyes, or alcohol.

Actions: Chlorpheniramine maleate in RYNA and RYNA-C is an antihistamine that antagonizes the effects of histamine.

Codeine phosphate in RYNA-C and RYNA-CX is a centrally-acting antitussive that relieves cough.

Pseudoephedrine hydrochloride in RYNA, RYNA-C and RYNA-CX is a sympathomimetic nasal decongestant that acts to shrink swollen mucosa of the respiratory tract.

Guaifenesin in RYNA-CX is an expectorant, the action of which promotes or facilitates the removal of secretions from the respiratory tract. By increasing sputum volume and making sputum less viscous, guaifenesin facilitates expectoration of retained secretions.

Indications: RYNA: For the temporary relief of nasal congestion due to the common cold, hay fever, or other upper respiratory allergies. Temporarily relieves runny nose, and alleviates sneezing, itching of the nose or throat, and itchy, watery eyes due to hay fever, or other respiratory allergies such as allergic rhinitis.

RYNA-C: For the temporary relief of nasal congestion due to the common cold, hay fever, or other upper respiratory allergies. Temporarily relieves runny nose and alleviates sneezing, itching of the nose or throat, and itchy, watery eyes due to the common cold, hay fever, or other upper respiratory allergies. Temporarily relieves cough due to minor throat and bronchial irritation as may occur with a cold. Temporarily helps to control the cough reflex that causes coughing. Temporarily reduces the intensity of coughing. Controls the impulse to cough to help you sleep. Calms the cough control center and relieves coughing.

RYNA-CX: Temporarily relieves cough due to minor throat and bronchial irritation as may occur with the common cold. Temporarily helps to control the cough reflex that causes coughing. Temporarily reduces the intensity of coughing. Controls the impulse to cough to help you sleep. Calms the cough control center and relieves coughing. Helps loosen phlegm (mucus) and thin bronchial secretions to rid the bronchial passageways of bothersome mucus, drain bronchial tubes, and make coughs more productive. For the temporary relief of nasal congestion due to the common cold, hay fever, or other upper respiratory allergies.

Warnings:
For RYNA: Do not give this product to children taking other medication or to children under 6 years except under the advice and supervision of a doctor. **Do not exceed the recommended dosage.** If nervousness, dizziness or sleep-

lessness occur, discontinue use and call a doctor. If symptoms do not improve within 7 days or are accompanied by fever, consult a doctor. Do not take this product, unless directed by a doctor, if you have a breathing problem such as emphysema or chronic bronchitis, or if you have glaucoma, heart disease, high blood pressure, thyroid disease, diabetes, or difficulty in urination due to enlargement of the prostate gland. May cause excitability, especially in children. May cause drowsiness; alcohol, sedatives, and tranquilizers may increase drowsiness effect. Avoid alcoholic beverages while taking this product. Do not take this product if you are taking sedatives or tranquilizers, without first consulting your doctor. Use caution when driving a motor vehicle or operating machinery. As with any drug, if you are pregnant or nursing a baby, seek the advice of a health care professional before taking this product.

For RYNA-C and RYNA-CX:
Adults and children who have a chronic pulmonary disease or shortness of breath, or children who are taking other drugs, should not take this product unless directed by a doctor. Do not give this product to children under 6 years of age except under the advice and supervision of a doctor. A persistent cough may be a sign of a serious condition. If cough persists for more than one week, tends to recur, or is accompanied by fever, rash or persistent headache, consult a doctor. Do not take this product for persistent or chronic cough such as occurs with smoking, asthma, or emphysema, or if cough is accompanied by excessive phlegm (mucus) unless directed by a doctor. Do not take this product unless directed by a doctor if you have a breathing problem such as emphysema or chronic bronchitis, or if you have glaucoma, heart disease, high blood pressure, thyroid disease, diabetes, or difficulty in urination due to enlargement of the prostate gland. May cause or aggravate constipation. May cause marked drowsiness; alcohol, sedatives, and tranquilizers may increase the drowsiness effect. Avoid alcoholic beverages while taking this product. Do not take this product if you are taking sedatives or tranquilizers, without first consulting your doctor. Use caution when driving a motor vehicle or operating machinery. May cause excitability, especially in children. **Do not exceed recommended dosage.** If nervousness, dizziness or sleepiness occur, discontinue use and consult a doctor. If symptoms do not improve within 7 days or are accompanied by a fever, consult a doctor. As with any drug, if you are pregnant or nursing a baby, seek the advice of a health professional before using this drug.

For RYNA, RYNA-C and RYNA-CX:

Drug Interaction Precaution: Do **not** use this product if you are now taking a prescription monoamine oxidase inhibitor (MAOI) (certain drugs for depression, psychiatric or emotional conditions, or

Parkinson's disease), or for 2 weeks after stopping the MAOI drug. If you are uncertain whether your prescription drug contains an MAOI, consult a health professional before taking this product.

Dosage and Administration:
Adults and children 12 years of age and over: 2 teaspoonfuls every 4 to 6 hours, not to exceed 8 teaspoonfuls in 24 hours, or as directed by a doctor.
Children 6 to under 12 years: 1 teaspoonful every 4 to 6 hours, not to exceed 4 teaspoonfuls in 24 hours, or as directed by a doctor.
Children under 6 years of age: Consult a doctor.
RYNA-C and RYNA-CX:
A special measuring device should be used to give an accurate dose of these products to children under 6 years of age. Giving a higher dose than recommended by a doctor could result in serious side effects for the child.

How Supplied: RYNA: bottles of 4 fl oz (NDC 0037-0638-66).
RYNA-C: bottles of 4 fl oz (NDC 0037-0522-66) and one pint (NDC 0037-0522-68).
RYNA-CX: bottles of 4 fl oz (NDC 0037-0801-66) and one pint (NDC 0037-0801-68).

TAMPER-RESISTANT BAND ON CAP PRINTED "WALLACE LABORATORIES." DO NOT USE IF BAND IS MISSING OR BROKEN.

Storage: RYNA: Store at controlled room temperature 15°–30°C (59°–86°F).
RYNA-C and RYNA-CX: Store at controlled room temperature 15°–30°C (59°–86°F). Dispense in a tight, light-resistant container.

KEEP THESE AND ALL DRUGS OUT OF THE REACH OF CHILDREN. IN CASE OF ACCIDENTAL OVERDOSE, SEEK PROFESSIONAL ASSISTANCE OR CONTACT A POISON CONTROL CENTER IMMEDIATELY.

WALLACE LABORATORIES
Division of Carter-Wallace, Inc.
Cranbury, New Jersey 08512

Rev. 9/94

RYNA-C and RYNA-CX
Shown in Product Identification Guide, page 524

Warner-Lambert Company

Consumer Health Products Group
201 TABOR ROAD
MORRIS PLAINS, NJ 07950

Direct Inquiries to:
1-(800) 223-0182

For Consumer Product Information Call:
1-(800) 524-2854 – Celestial Seasonings Soothers (only)
1-(800) 223-0182

CELESTIAL SEASONINGS® SOOTHERS™ Herbal Throat Drops

Active Ingredients: Menthol and Pectin.

Inactive Ingredients: HARVEST CHERRY—Ascorbic Acid (Vitamin C); Cherry and Elderberry Juices; Citric Acid; Corn Syrup; Natural Flavoring; Oils of Angelica Root, Anise Star, Ginger, Lemon Grass, Sage and White Thyme; Sodium Ascorbate and Sucrose. **WILD MOUNTAIN BERRY QUINCE**—Ascorbic Acid (Vitamin C); Corn Syrup; Elderberry Juice; Natural Flavoring; Oils of Angelic Root, Anise Star, Ginger, Lemon Grass, Sage and White Thyme; Quince Juice, Sodium Ascorbate and Sucrose. **HONEY-LEMON CHAMOMILE**—Ascorbic Acid (Vitamin C); Chamomile Flower Extract; Citric Acid; Corn Syrup; Honey; Lemon Juice; Natural Flavoring; Oils of Angelica Root, Anise Star, Ginger, Lemon Grass, Sage and White Thyme; Sodium Ascorbate; Sucrose and Tea Extract. **SUNSHINE CITRUS**—Ascorbic Acid (Vitamin C); Beta Carotene; Citric Acid; Corn Syrup; Natural Flavoring; Oils of Angelica Root, Anise Star, Ginger, Lemon Grass, Sage and White Thyme; Orange Juice; Sodium Ascorbate, and Sucrose.

Indications: For temporary relief of occasional minor irritation, pain, sore mouth and sore throat. Provides temporary protection of irritated areas in sore mouth and sore throat.

Warnings: If sore throat is severe, persists for more than 2 days, is accompanied or followed by fever, headache, rash, nausea, or vomiting, consult a doctor promptly. If sore mouth symptoms do not improve in 7 days, see your dentist or doctor promptly. KEEP THIS AND ALL DRUGS OUT OF REACH OF CHILDREN.

Dosage and Administration: Adults and children 5 years and over: Dissolve 2 drops (one at a time) slowly in the mouth. May be repeated every 2 hours as needed or as directed by a dentist or doctor. Children under 5 years: Consult a dentist or doctor.

How Supplied: Celestial Seasonings Soothers Throat Drops are available in bags of 24 drops. They are available in four flavors: Harvest Cherry, Honey-Lemon Chamomile, Sunshine Citrus, Wild Mountain Berry Quince.

Shown in Product Identification Guide, page 524

CERTS® Cool Mint Drops with a Retsyn® Center
[*Surts cul mint drops*]

Ingredients: PEPPERMINT: Sugar, Modified Food Starch, Glucose Syrup, Artificial and Natural Flavoring*, Maltodextrin, Gum Arabic, Rice Starch, Magnesium Stearate, Blue 2 Lake, Partially Hydrogenated Cottonseed Oil*, and Copper Gluconate*.
FRESHMINT: Sugar, Modified Food Starch, Glucose Syrup, Artificial and Natural Flavoring*, Maltodextrin, Gum Arabic, Rice Starch, Magnesium Stearate, Blue 2 Lake, Yellow 5 Lake, Partially Hydrogenated Cottonseed Oil* and Copper Gluconate*.
CINNAMINT: Sugar, Modified Food Starch, Glucose Syrup, Artificial and Natural Flavoring* Mahodextrin, Gum Arabic, Rice Starch, Magnesium Stearate, Red 40 Lake, Partially Hydrogenated Cottonseed Oil* and Copper Gluconate*.
*RETSYN®: A combination of Partially Hydrogenated Cottonseed Oil, Copper Gluconate and Flavoring.

Description: Oval breath drop.

Directions: Take 1 mint as desired.

How Supplied: Certs® Cool Mint Drops with a Retsyn® Center are available in Peppermint, Freshmint and Cinnamint Flavors in slide-top cartons of about 27 pressed mints each.

Shown in Product Identification Guide, page 524

CERTS® Powerful Mints with Retsyn® Crystals
[*Surts pau wur ful mints*]

Ingredients: Sorbitol, Maltodextrin, Natural Flavoring* Aspartame, Magnesium Stearate, Partially Hydrogenated Cottonseed Oil*, Copper Gluconate* and Blue 1. PHENYLKETONURICS: CONTAINS PHENYLALANINE *Retsyn®.

Description: Breath Freshening Mint.

Directions: Take 1 tablet as desired.

How Supplied: Certs® Powerful Mints with Retsyn® Crystals are available in a Peppermint flavor in a credit card size vial of 50 tablets each.

Shown in Product Identification Guide, page 524

HALLS® JUNIORS SUGAR FREE Cough Suppressant Drops
[*Hols*]

Active Ingredient: Menthol 2.5 mg per drop.

Inactive Ingredients: ORANGE: Acesulfame Potassium, Aspartame, Eucalyptus Oil, Isomalt, Natural Flavoring and Yellow 6. GRAPE: Acesulfame Potassium, Aspartame, Blue 1, Eucalyptus Oil, Isomalt, Natural Flavoring and Red 40. PHENYLKETONURICS: CONTAINS 2 mg PHENYLALANINE PER DROP.

Indications: For temporary relief of minor throat irritation and coughs due to colds or inhaled irritants.

Warnings: A persistent cough may be a sign of a serious condition. If cough persists for more than 1 week, tends to recur, or is accompanied by fever, rash, or persistent headache, consult a doctor. Do not take this product for persistent or chronic cough such as occurs with smoking, asthma, or emphysema, or if cough is accompanied by excessive phlegm (mucus) unless directed by a doctor. If sore throat is severe, persists for more than 2 days, is accompanied or followed by fever, headache, rash, swelling, nausea, or vomiting, consult a doctor promptly. KEEP THIS AND ALL DRUGS OUT OF THE REACH OF CHILDREN.

Dosage and Administration: Adults and children 5 years and over: dissolve 2 drops (one at a time) slowly in mouth. Repeat every hour as needed or as directed by a doctor. Children under 5 years: consult a doctor.

Additional Information:
Exchange Information*:
2 Drops = Free Exchange
22 Drops = 2 Fruits
*The dietary exchanges are based on the *Exchange Lists for Meal Planning,* Copyright © 1989 by the American Diabetes Association, Inc. and the American Dietetic Association.

How Supplied: Halls Juniors Sugar Free Cough Suppressant Drops are available in Grape and Orange flavors in bags of 22 drops each.

Shown in Product Identification Guide, page 524

HALLS® MENTHO–LYPTUS® Cough Suppressant Drops
[*Hols*]

Active Ingredient: MENTHO-LYPTUS: Menthol 7 mg per drop. CHERRY: Menthol 7.6 mg per drop. HONEY-LEMON: Menthol 8.6 mg per drop. ICE BLUE PEPPERMINT: Menthol 12 mg per drop. SPEARMINT: 6 mg per drop.

Inactive Ingredients: MENTHO-LYPTUS: Eucalyptus Oil, Flavoring, Glucose Syrup and Sucrose. CHERRY: Blue 2, Eucalyptus Oil, Flavoring, Glucose Syrup, Red 40 and Sucrose. HONEY-LEMON: Beta Carotene, Eucalyptus Oil, Flavoring, Glucose Syrup and Sucrose. ICE BLUE PEPPERMINT: Blue 1, Eucalyptus Oil, Flavoring, Glucose Syrup and Sucrose. SPEARMINT: Beta

Continued on next page

Halls Mentho-Lyptus—Cont.

Carotene, Blue 1, Eucalyptus Oil, Flavoring, Glucose Syrup and Sucrose.

Indications: For temporary relief of minor throat irritation and coughs due to colds or inhaled irritants.

Warnings: A persistent cough may be a sign of a serious condition. If cough persists for more than 1 week, tends to recur, or is accompanied by fever, rash or persistent headache, consult a doctor. Do not take this product for persistent or chronic cough such as occurs with smoking, asthma, or emphysema, or if cough is accompanied by excessive phlegm (mucus) unless directed by a doctor. If sore throat is severe, persists for more than 2 days, is accompanied or followed by fever, headache, rash, swelling, nausea, or vomiting, consult a doctor promptly. KEEP THIS AND ALL DRUGS OUT OF THE REACH OF CHILDREN.

Dosage and Administration: Adults and children 5 years and over: dissolve 1 drop slowly in mouth. Repeat every hour as needed or as directed by a doctor. Children under 5 years: consult a doctor.

How Supplied: Halls Mentho-Lyptus Cough Suppressant Drops are available in single sticks of 9 drops each and in bags of 30. They are available in five flavors: Regular Mentho-Lyptus, Cherry, Honey-Lemon, Ice Blue Peppermint and Spearmint. Regular Mentho-Lyptus Cherry and Honey-Lemon flavors are also available in bags of 60 drops.

Shown in Product Identification Guide, page 524

HALLS® PLUS
Cough Suppressant/Throat Drops
[Hols]

Active Ingredients: Each drop contains Menthol 10 mg and Pectin.

Inactive Ingredients: MENTHO-LYPTUS®: Carrageenan, Eucalyptus Oil, Flavoring, Glucose Syrup, Glycerin and Sucrose. CHERRY: Blue 2, Carrageenan, Eucalyptus Oil, Flavoring, Glucose Syrup, Glycerin, Red 40 and Sucrose. HONEY-LEMON: Beta Carotene, Carrageenan, Eucalyptus Oil, Flavoring, Glucose Syrup, Glycerin, Honey and Sucrose.

Indications: For temporary relief of minor throat irritation and coughs due to colds or inhaled irritants. Provides temporary protection of irritated areas in sore throat.

Warnings: A persistent cough may be a sign of a serious condition. If cough persists for more than 1 week, tends to recur, or is accompanied by fever, rash, or persistent headache, consult a doctor. Do not take this product for persistent or chronic cough such as occurs with smoking, asthma, or emphysema, or if cough is accompanied by excessive phlegm (mu-

cous) unless directed by a doctor. If sore throat is severe, persists for more than 2 days, is accompanied or followed by fever, headache, rash, swelling, nausea, or vomiting, consult a doctor promptly. KEEP THIS AND ALL DRUGS OUT OF THE REACH OF CHILDREN.

Dosage and Administration: Adults and children 5 years and over: Dissolve 1 drop slowly in the mouth. Repeat every hour as needed or as directed by a doctor. Children under 5 years: consult a doctor.

How Supplied: Halls® Plus Cough Suppressant / Throat Drops are available in single sticks of 10 drops each and in bags of 25 drops. They are available in three flavors: Regular Mentho-Lyptus®, Cherry and Honey-Lemon.

Shown in Product Identification Guide, page 524

HALLS® SUGAR FREE
HALLS® SUGAR FREE SQUARES
MENTHO-LYPTUS®
Cough Suppressant Drops
[Hols]

Active Ingredient: Halls® Sugar Free: BLACK CHERRY and CITRUS BLEND: Menthol 5 mg per drop. MOUNTAIN MENTHOL: Menthol 5.8 mg per drop.
Halls® Sugar Free Squares: BLACK CHERRY: Menthol 5.8 mg per drop. MOUNTAIN MENTHOL: Menthol 6.8 mg per drop.

Inactive Ingredients: BLACK CHERRY: Acesulfame Potassium, Blue 1, Citric Acid, Eucalyptus Oil, Flavoring, Isomalt and Red 40. CITRUS BLEND: Acesulfame Potassium, Citric Acid, Eucalyptus Oil, Flavoring, Isomalt and Yellow 5 (Tartrazine). MOUNTAIN MENTHOL: Acesulfame Potassium, Eucalyptus Oil, Flavoring and Isomalt.

Indications: For temporary relief of minor throat irritation and coughs due to colds or inhaled irritants.

Warnings: A persistent cough may be a sign of a serious condition. If cough persists for more than 1 week, tends to recur, or is accompanied by fever, rash, or persistent headache, consult a doctor. Do not take this product for persistent or chronic cough such as occurs with smoking, asthma, or emphysema, or if cough is accompanied by excessive phlegm (mucus) unless directed by a doctor. If sore throat is severe, persists for more than 2 days, is accompanied or followed by fever, headache, rash, swelling, nausea, or vomiting, consult a doctor promptly. KEEP THIS AND ALL DRUGS OUT OF THE REACH OF CHILDREN.

Dosage and Administration: Adults and children 5 years and over: dissolve 1 drop slowly in mouth. Repeat every hour as needed or as directed by a doctor. Children under 5 years: consult a doctor.

Additional Information:
Halls® Sugar Free:
Exchange Information*:
1 Drop = Free Exchange
10 Drops = 1 Fruit
*The dietary exchanges are based on the *Exchange Lists for Meal Planning,* Copyright ©1989 by the American Diabetes Association, Inc. and the American Dietetic Association.

How Supplied: Halls® Sugar Free: Halls Sugar Free Mentho-Lyptus Cough Suppressant Drops are available in bags of 25 drops. They are available in three flavors: Black Cherry, Citrus Blend and Mountain Menthol. Halls® Sugar Free Squares: Halls® Sugar Free Squares Mentho-Lyptus Cough Suppressant Drops are available in single sticks of 9 drops each. They are available in two flavors: Blackcherry and Mountain Menthol.

Shown in Product Identification Guide, page 524

HALLS® Vitamin C Supplement Drops
[Hols]

Ingredients: ASSORTED CITRUS FLAVORS: Sugar, Glucose Syrup, Citric Acid, Sodium Ascorbate, Natural Flavoring, Ascorbic Acid, Color Added and Red 40.

Description: Halls® Vitamin C Supplement Drops are a delicious way to get 100% of the Daily Value of Vitamin C. Each drop provides 60 mg of Vitamin C (100% of the Daily Value).

Indication: Dietary Supplementation.

How Supplied: Halls® Vitamin C Supplement Drops are available in single sticks of 9 drops each and in bags of 30 drops. They are available in an all-natural citrus flavor assortment (lemon, sweet grapefruit and orange).

Shown in Product Identification Guide, page 524

Warner-Lambert
Consumer HealthCare
Warner-Lambert Company
201 TABOR ROAD
MORRIS PLAINS, NJ 07950

Direct Inquiries to:
1-(800) 223-0182

For Medical Information Contact:
1-(800) 223-0182
1-(800) 378-1783 (e.p.t)
1-(800) 337-7266 (e.p.t–Spanish)

ACTIFED® Cold & Allergy Tablets
[ăk 'tuh-fĕd]

Active Ingredients: Each tablet contains Pseudoephedrine Hydrochloride 60 mg and Triprolidine Hydrochloride 2.5 mg.

Inactive Ingredients: Corn Starch, Flavor, Hydroxypropyl Methylcellulose, Lactose, Magnesium Stearate, Polyethylene Glycol, Potato Starch, Povidone, Sucrose, and Titanium Dioxide.

Indications: Temporarily relieves nasal congestion due to the common cold. Temporarily dries runny nose and alleviates sneezing, itching of the nose or throat, and itchy, watery eyes due to hay fever or other upper respiratory allergies.

Directions: Adults and children 12 years of age and over: 1 tablet. Children 6 to under 12 years of age: $^1/_2$ tablet. Dosage may be repeated every 4 to 6 hours, not to exceed 4 doses in 24 hours, or as directed by a doctor. Children under 6 years of age: consult a doctor.

Warnings: Do not exceed recommended dosage. If nervousness, dizziness, or sleeplessness occur, discontinue use and consult a doctor. If symptoms do not improve within 7 days or are accompanied by fever, consult a doctor. Do not take this product, unless directed by a doctor, if you have heart disease, high blood pressure, thyroid disease, diabetes, a breathing problem such as emphysema or chronic bronchitis, or if you have glaucoma or difficulty in urination due to enlargement of the prostate gland. May cause excitability especially in children. May cause drowsiness; alcohol, sedatives, and tranquilizers may increase the drowsiness effect. Avoid alcoholic beverages while taking this product. Do not take this product if you are taking sedatives or tranquilizers, without first consulting your doctor. Use caution when driving a motor vehicle or operating machinery. As with any drug, if you are pregnant or nursing a baby, seek the advice of a health professional before using this product. **KEEP THIS AND ALL DRUGS OUT OF THE REACH OF CHILDREN.** In case of accidental overdose, seek professional assistance or contact a Poison Control Center immediately.

Drug Interaction Precaution: Do not use this product if you are now taking a prescription monoamine oxidase inhibitor (MAOI) (certain drugs for depression, psychiatric or emotional conditions, or Parkinson's disease), or for 2 weeks after stopping the MAOI drug. If you are uncertain whether your prescription drug contains an MAOI, consult a health professional before taking this product.

How Supplied: Boxes of 12, 24, 48, and 96 tablets.
Store at 59° to 77°F in a dry place and protect from light.
Shown in Product Identification Guide, page 524

ANUSOL®
Hemorrhoidal Suppositories/
Ointment
[ă 'nū-sŏl ″]

Description:
Anusol Suppositories: **Active Ingredient:** Topical Starch 51%. Also contains: Ben-

zyl Alcohol, Hydrogenated Vegetable Oil, Tocopheryl Acetate.
Anusol Ointment: **Active ingredients:** Pramoxine HCl 1%, Mineral Oil and Zinc Oxide 12.5%. Also contains: Benzyl Benzoate, Calcium Phosphate Dibasic, Cocoa Butter, Glyceryl Monooleate, Glyceryl Monostearate, Kaolin, Peruvian Balsam and Polyethylene Wax.

Actions: Anusol Suppositories and Anusol Ointment help to relieve burning, itching and discomfort arising from irritated anorectal tissues. They have a soothing, lubricant action on the intrarectal mucous membrane. Pramoxine Hydrochloride in Anusol Ointment is a rapidly acting local anesthetic for the skin and mucous membranes in the lower portion of the anal canal. Pramoxine HCl is also chemically distinct from procaine, cocaine, and dibucaine and can often be used in the patient previously sensitized to other surface anesthetics. Surface analgesia lasts for several hours.

Indications: Anusol Suppositories: Gives temporary relief from the itching, burning and discomfort associated with hemorrhoids and other anorectal disorders and provides a coating to protect irritated tissue.
Anusol Ointment: For relief of pain, soreness, burning and itching associated with hemorrhoids and anorectal disorders. Temporarily forms a protective coating over inflamed tissues to help prevent the drying of tissues. Anusol Ointment is to be applied externally or in the lower portion of the anal canal (The enclosed dispensing cap is designed to control dispersion of the ointment to the affected area in the lower portion of the anal canal only.)

Warnings: Anusol Ointment: If condition worsens or does not improve within 7 days, consult a physician. Certain persons can develop allergic reactions to ingredients in this product. If the symptom being treated does not subside or if redness, irritation, swelling, pain or other symptoms develop or increase, discontinue use and consult a phsyician. In case of bleeding, consult a physician promptly. Do not exceed the recommended daily dosage unless directed by a physician. Do not put this product into the rectum by using fingers or any mechanical device or applicator. KEEP THIS AND ALL DRUGS OUT OF THE REACH OF CHILDREN. In case of accidental ingestion seek professional assistance or contact a Poison Control Center immediately. Anusol Suppositories: Do not exceed recommended daily dosage unless directed by a physician. If condition worsens or does not improve within 7 days, consult a physician. In case of bleeding, consult a physician promptly. KEEP THIS AND ALL DRUGS OUT OF THE REACH OF CHILDREN. In case of accidental ingestion seek professional assistance or contact a Poison Control Center immediately. As with any drug, if you

are pregnant or nursing a baby, seek the advice of a health professional before using this product.

Directions: Anusol Suppositories: Adults—when practical, cleanse the affected area with mild soap and warm water and rinse thoroughly. Gently dry by patting or blotting with toilet tissue or a soft cloth before application of this product.
1. Detach one suppository from the strip of suppositories.
2. Remove wrapper before inserting into the rectum as follows: Hold suppository upright (with words "pull apart" at top) and carefully separate foil by inserting tip of fingernail at foil split.

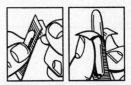

3. Peel foil slowly and evenly down both sides, exposing suppository.
4. Avoid excessive handling of suppository which is designed to melt at body temperature. If suppository seems soft, hold in foil wrapper under cold water for 2 or 3 minutes.
5. Insert one (1) suppository rectally up to six times daily or after each bowel movement.
Children under 12 years of age: consult a physician.

Anusol Ointment: Adults: When practical, cleanse the affected area with mild soap and warm water and rinse thoroughly. Gently dry by patting or blotting with toilet tissue or a soft cloth before application of this product. Apply externally to the affected area up to 5 times daily. To use dispensing cap, attach it to tube, lubricate well, then gently insert part way into the anul canal. Squeeze tube to deliver medication. Thoroughly cleanse dispensing cap after use. Children under 12 years of age: Consult a physician.

How Supplied: Anusol Suppositories— boxes of 12 or 24 in silver foil strips.

Suppositories: Do not store above 86°F or suppositories may melt.

Anusol Ointment—1-oz (28.3g) tubes with plastic applicator.

Ointment: Store at 59° to 77°F.

Shown in Product Identification Guide, page 524

Continued on next page

This product information was prepared in November 1998. On these and other Warner-Lambert Consumer Healthcare Products, detailed information may be obtained by addressing Warner-Lambert Consumer Healthcare Products, Morris Plains, NJ 07950 USA

ANUSOL HC-1
Hydrocortisone Anti-Itch Ointment
[ă 'nū-sŏl "]

Active Ingredient: Hydrocortisone Acetate (equivalent to 1% Hydrocortisone).

Inactive Ingredients: Diazolidinyl Urea, Methylparaben, Microcrystalline Wax, Mineral Oil, Propylene Glycol, Propylparaben, Sorbitan Sesquioleate and White Petrolatum.

Indications: For temporary relief of itching associated with minor skin irritations, rashes and for external anal itching. Other uses of this product should be only under the advice and supervision of a physician.

Warnings: For external use only. Avoid contact with the eyes. If condition worsens, or if symptoms persist for more than 7 days or clear up and occur again within a few days, stop use of this product and do not begin use of any other hydrocortisone product unless you have consulted a physician. Do not exceed the recommended daily dosage unless directed by a physician. In case of bleeding, consult a physician promptly. Do not put this product into the rectum by using fingers or any mechanical device or applicator. Do not use for treatment of diaper rash. Consult a physician. KEEP THIS AND ALL DRUGS OUT OF THE REACH OF CHILDREN. In case of accidental ingestion, seek professional assistance or contact a Poison Control Center immediately.

Directions: Adults: When practical, cleanse the affected area with mild soap and warm water and rinse thoroughly. Gently dry by patting or blotting with toilet tissue or a soft cloth before application of this product. Apply to affected area not more than 3 to 4 times daily. Children under 12 years of age: consult a physician.

How Supplied: Anusol HC-1 Ointment in 0.7 oz (19.8 g) tube. Store at 59° to 77°F.

Shown in Product Identification Guide, page 524

BENADRYL® Allergy
Ultratab™ Tablets and Kapseal® Capsules
[bĕ 'nă-drĭl]

Active Ingredients: Each Tablet/Capsule contains: Diphenhydramine Hydrochloride 25 mg.

Inactive Ingredients: Each Tablet contains: Candelilla Wax, Crospovidone, Dibasic Calcium Phosphate Dihydrate, D&C Red No. 27 Aluminum Lake, Hydroxypropyl Methylcellulose, Magnesium Stearate, Microcrystalline Cellulose, Polyethylene Glycol, Polysorbate 80, Pregelatinized Starch, Stearic Acid, and Titanium Dioxide.

Each Capsule contains: Lactose and Magnesium Stearate. The Kapseals capsule shell contains: D&C Red No. 28, FD&C Red No. 3, FD&C Red No. 40, FD&C Blue No. 1, Gelatin, Glyceryl Monooleate, and Titanium Dioxide.

Indications: Temporarily relieves runny nose and sneezing, itching of the nose or throat, and itchy, watery eyes due to hay fever or other upper respiratory allergies, and runny nose and sneezing associated with the common cold.

Directions: Follow dosage directions or use as directed by your doctor. Adults and children 12 years of age and over: 25 to 50 mg (1 to 2 tablets/capsules) every 4 to 6 hours. Not to exceed 12 tablets/capsules in 24 hours. Children 6 to under 12 years of age: 12.5 mg** to 25 mg (1 tablet/capsule) every 4 to 6 hours, not to exceed 6 tablets/capsules in 24 hours. Children under 6 years of age: consult your doctor.

** This dosage is not available in this package. Do not attempt to break tablet/capsule. This dosage is available in pleasant tasting Benadryl Allergy Liquid Medication.

Warnings: May cause excitability especially in children. Do not take this product, unless directed by a doctor, if you have a breathing problem such as emphysema or chronic bronchitis, or if you have glaucoma or difficulty in urination due to enlargement of the prostate gland. May cause marked drowsiness; alcohol, sedatives, and tranquilizers may increase the drowsiness effect. Avoid alcoholic beverages while taking this product. Do not take this product if you are taking sedatives or tranquilizers, without first consulting your doctor. Use caution when driving a motor vehicle or operating machinery. **Do not use any other products containing diphenhydramine while using this product.** As with any drug, if you are pregnant or nursing a baby, seek the advice of a health professional before using this product. KEEP THIS AND ALL DRUGS OUT OF THE REACH OF CHILDREN. In case of accidental overdose, seek professional assistance or contact a Poison Control Center immediately.

How Supplied: Benadryl tablets are supplied in boxes of 24 and 48, bottle of 100; capsules are supplied in boxes of 24 and 48.
Store at room temperature 15°–30° C (59°–86° F). Protect from moisture.

Shown in Product Identification Guide, page 524

BENADRYL® ALLERGY/COLD TABLETS
[bĕ 'nă-drĭl]

Active Ingredients: Each tablet contains: Diphenhydramine Hydrochloride 12.5 mg, Pseudoephedrine Hydrochloride 30 mg and Acetaminophen 500 mg.

Inactive Ingredients: Candelilla Wax, Croscarmellose Sodium, Hydroxypropyl Cellulose, Hydroxypropyl Methylcellulose, Magnesium Stearate, Microcrystalline Cellulose, Polyethylene Glycol, Pregelatinized Starch, Propylene Glycol, Sodium Starch Glycolate, Starch, Stearic Acid, Titanium Dioxide, and Zinc Stearate. Printed with edible blue ink.

Indications: For the temporary relief of minor aches, pains, headache, muscular aches, sore throat, fever, runny nose and sneezing, itching of the nose or throat, and itchy, watery eyes due to hay fever, and nasal congestion due to the common cold.

Directions: Follow dosage recommendations, or use as directed by your doctor. Adults and children 12 years of age and over: two (2) tablets every 6 hours while symptoms persist. Not to exceed 8 tablets in 24 hours. Children under 12 years of age: consult a doctor.

Warnings: Do not exceed recommended dosage. If nervousness, dizziness, or sleeplessness occur, discontinue use and consult a doctor. Do not take this product for more than 10 days. If symptoms do not improve or are accompanied by fever that lasts for more than 3 days, or if new symptoms occur, consult a doctor. If sore throat is severe, persists for more than 2 days, is accompanied or followed by fever, headache, rash, nausea, or vomiting, consult a doctor promptly. Do not take this product, unless directed by a doctor, if you have a breathing problem such as emphysema or chronic bronchitis, heart disease, high blood pressure, thyroid disease, diabetes, or if you have glaucoma or difficulty in urination due to enlargement of the prostate gland. May cause excitability especially in children. May cause marked drowsiness; alcohol, sedatives, and tranquilizers may increase the drowsiness effect. Avoid alcoholic beverages while taking this product. Do not take this product if you are taking sedatives or tranquilizers, without first consulting your doctor. Use caution when driving a motor vehicle or operating machinery. Do not use any other products containing diphenhydramine while using this product. As with any drug, if you are pregnant or nursing a baby, seek the advice of a health professional before using this product. KEEP THIS AND ALL DRUGS OUT OF THE REACH OF CHILDREN. In case of accidental overdose, seek professional assistance or contact a Poison Control Center immediately. Prompt medical attention is critical for adults as well as for children even if you do not notice any signs or symptoms.

Alcohol Warning: If you generally consume 3 or more alcohol-containing drinks per day, you should consult your physician for advice on when and how you should take Benadryl Allergy/Cold and other pain relievers.

Drug Interaction Precaution: Do not use this product if you are now taking a prescription monoamine oxidase inhibitor (MAOI) (certain drugs for depression, psychiatric or emotional conditions, or Parkinson's disease), or for 2 weeks after stopping the MAOI drug. If you are uncertain whether your prescription drug contains an MAOI, consult a health professional before taking this product.

How Supplied: Benadryl® Allergy/Cold tablets are supplied in boxes of 24 tablets. Store at room temperature (59°–86°F). Protect from moisture.

Shown in Product Identification Guide, page 525

BENADRYL® ALLERGY CHEWABLES
[bě 'nă-drĭl]

Active Ingredients: Each chewable tablet contains: Diphenhydramine Hydrochloride 12.5 mg.

Inactive Ingredients: Aspartame, Dextrates, D&C Red No. 27 Aluminum Lake, FD&C Blue No. 1 Aluminum Lake, Flavors, Magnesium Stearate, Magnesium Trisilicate, and Tartaric Acid.

Indications: Temporarily relieves runny nose and sneezing, itching of the nose or throat, and itchy, water eyes due to hay fever or other upper respiratory allergies, and runny nose and sneezing associated with the common cold.

Directions: Follow dosage recommendations, or use as directed by your doctor. Chew tablets thoroughly before swallowing. Adults and children 12 years of age and over: 2 to 4 tablets (25 to 50 mg) every 4 to 6 hours. Not to exceed 24 tablets in 24 hours. Children 6 to under 12 years of age: 1 to 2 tablets (12.5 to 25 mg) every 4 to 6 hours. Not to exceed 12 tablets in 24 hours. Children under 6 years of age: consult a doctor.

Warnings: May cause excitability especially in children. Do not take this product, unless directed by a doctor, if you have a breathing problem such as emphysema or chronic bronchitis, or if you have glaucoma or difficulty in urination due to enlargement of the prostate gland. May cause marked drowsiness; alcohol, sedatives, and tranquilizers may increase the drowsiness effect. Avoid alcoholic beverages while taking this product. Do not take this product if you are taking sedatives or tranquilizers, without first consulting your doctor. Use caution when driving a motor vehicle or operating machinery. **Do not use any other products containing diphenhydramine while using this product.** As with any drug, if you are pregnant or nursing a baby, seek the advice of a health professional before using this product. KEEP THIS AND ALL DRUGS OUT OF THE REACH OF CHILDREN. In case of accidental overdose, seek professional assistance or contact a Poison Control Center immediately. **Phenylketonurics: Contains Phenylalanine 4.2 mg. Per Tablet.**

How Supplied: Benadryl® Allergy Chewables are supplied in boxes of 24 tablets. Store between 59°–77°F. Protect from heat and humidity.

Shown in Product Identification Guide, page 524

BENADRYL®
Allergy/Congestion Tablets
[bě 'nă-drĭl]

Formally Benadryl Allergy Decongestant Tablets

Active Ingredients: Each tablet contains: Diphenhydramine Hydrochloride 25 mg and Pseudoephedrine Hydrochloride 60 mg.

Inactive Ingredients: Each tablet contains: Croscarmellose Sodium, Dibasic Calcium Phosphate Dihydrate, FD&C Blue No. 1 Aluminum Lake, Hydroxypropyl Methylcellulose, Microcrystalline Cellulose, Polyethylene Glycol, Polysorbate 80, Pregelatinized Starch, Stearic Acid, Titanium Dioxide and Zinc Stearate.

Indications: Temporarily relieves nasal congestion, runny nose and sneezing, itching of the nose or throat, and itchy, watery eyes due to hay fever or other upper respiratory allergies, and runny nose, sneezing, and nasal congestion associated with the common cold.

Directions: Follow dosage recommendation, or use as directed by your doctor. Adults and children 12 years of age and over: one (1) tablet every 4 to 6 hours, not to exceed 4 tablets in 24 hours. Children under 12 years of age: consult a doctor.

Warning: Do not exceed recommended dosage. If nervousness, dizziness, or sleeplessness occur, discontinue use and consult a doctor. If symptoms do not improve within 7 days or are accompanied by fever, consult a doctor. Do not take this product, unless directed by a doctor, if you have a breathing problem such as emphysema or chronic bronchitis, heart disease, high blood pressure, thyroid disease, diabetes, or if you have glaucoma or difficulty in urination due to enlargement of the prostate gland. May cause excitability especially in children. May cause marked drowsiness; alcohol, sedatives, and tranquilizers may increase the drowsiness effect. Avoid alcoholic beverages while taking this product. Do not take this product if you are taking sedatives or tranquilizers, without first consulting your doctor. Use caution when driving a motor vehicle or operating machinery. Do not use any other products containing diphenhydramine while using this product. As with any drug, if you are pregnant or nursing a baby, seek the advice of a health professional before using this product. KEEP THIS AND ALL DRUGS OUT OF THE REACH OF CHILDREN. In case of accidental overdose, seek professional assistance or contact a Poison Control Center immediately.

Drug Interaction Precaution: Do not use this product if you are now taking a prescription monoamine oxidase inhibitor (MAOI) (certain drugs for depression, psychiatric or emotional conditions, or Parkinson's disease), or for 2 weeks after stopping the MAOI drug. If you are uncertain whether your prescription drug contains an MAOI, consult a health professional before taking this product.

How Supplied: Benadryl Allergy/Congestion Tablets are supplied in boxes of 24.
Store at room temperature (59°–86° F). Protect from moisture.

Shown in Product Identification Guide, page 525

BENADRYL®
Allergy/Congestion Liquid Medication
[bě 'nă-drĭl]

Formally Benadryl Allergy Decongestion Liquid Medication

Active Ingredients: Each teaspoonful (5 mL) contains: Diphenhydramine Hydrochloride 12.5 mg and Pseudoephedrine Hydrochloride 30 mg.

Inactive Ingredients: Citric Acid, FD&C Blue No. 1, FD&C Red No. 40, Flavors, Glycerin, Poloxamer 407, Polysorbate 20, Purified Water, Saccharin Sodium, Sodium Benzoate, Sodium Chloride, Sodium Citrate and Sorbitol Solution.

Indications: Temporarily relieves nasal congestion, runny nose and sneezing, itching of the nose or throat, and itchy, watery eyes due to hay fever or other upper respiratory allergies, and runny nose, sneezing, and nasal congestion associated with the common cold.

Directions: Follow dosage recommendations below, or use as directed by your doctor.

Benadryl® Allergy/Congestion
Liquid Medication

AGE	DOSAGE
Children under 6 years of age	Consult a doctor.
Children 6 to under 12 years of age	One (1) teaspoonful every 4 to 6 hours. Not to exceed 4 teaspoonfuls in 24 hours.

Continued on next page

This product information was prepared in November 1998. On these and other Warner-Lambert Consumer Healthcare Products, detailed information may be obtained by addressing Warner-Lambert Consumer Healthcare Products, Morris Plains, NJ 07950 USA

Benadryl Allergy/Cong—Cont.

Adults and children 12 years of age and over	Two (2) teaspoonfuls every 4 to 6 hours. Not to exceed 8 teaspoonfuls in 24 hours.

Warnings: Do not exceed recommended dosage. If nervousness, dizziness, or sleeplessness occur, discontinue use and consult a doctor. If symptoms do not improve within 7 days or are accompanied by fever, consult a doctor. Do not take this product, unless directed by a doctor, if you have a breathing problem such as emphysema or chronic bronchitis, heart disease, high blood pressure, thyroid disease, diabetes, or if you have glaucoma or difficulty in urination due to enlargement of the prostate gland. May cause excitability especially in children. May cause marked drowsiness; alcohol, sedatives, and tranquilizers may increase the drowsiness effect. Avoid alcoholic beverages while taking this product. Do not take this product if you are taking sedatives or tranquilizers, without first consulting your doctor. Use caution when driving a motor vehicle or operating machinery. **Do not use any other products containing diphenhydramine while using this product.** As with any drug, if you are pregnant or nursing a baby, seek the advice of a health professional before using this product. KEEP THIS AND ALL DRUGS OUT OF THE REACH OF CHILDREN. In case of accidental overdose, seek professional assistance or contact a Poison Control Center immediately.

Drug Interaction Precaution: Do not use this product if you are now taking a prescription monoamine oxidase inhibitor (MAOI) (certain drugs for depression, psychiatric or emotional conditions, or Parkinson's disease), or for 2 weeks after stopping the MAOI drug. If you are uncertain whether your prescription drug contains an MAOI, consult a health professional before taking this product.

How Supplied: Benadryl Allergy/Congestion Liquid Medication is supplied in 4 fl. oz. bottles.
Store at room temperature (59°–86°F).
Protect from freezing.
Shown in Product Identification Guide, page 525

BENADRYL® Allergy Liquid Medication
[bĕ 'nă-drĭl]

Active Ingredient: Each teaspoonful (5 mL) contains Diphenhydramine Hydrochloride 12.5 mg.

Inactive Ingredients: Each teaspoonful (5 mL) contains: Citric Acid, D&C Red No. 33, FD&C Red No. 40, Flavors, Glycerin, Poloxamer 407, Purified Water, Sodium Benzoate, Sodium Chloride, Sodium Citrate, and Sugar.

Indications: Temporarily relieves runny nose and sneezing, itching of the nose or throat, and itchy, watery eyes due to hay fever or other upper respiratory allergies, and runny nose and sneezing associated with the common cold.

Directions: Follow dosage recommendations below, or use as directed by your doctor.

Benadryl® Allergy Liquid Medication

AGE	DOSAGE
Children under 6 years of age	Consult a doctor.
Children 6 to under 12 years of age	**1 to 2 teaspoonfuls (12.5 to 25 mg)** every 4 to 6 hours. Not to exceed 12 teaspoonfuls in 24 hours.
Adults and children 12 years of age and over	**2 to 4 teaspoonfuls (25 to 50 mg)** every 4 to 6 hours. Not to exceed 24 teaspoonfuls in 24 hours.

Warnings: May cause excitability especially in children. Do not take this product, unless directed by a doctor, if you have a breathing problem such as emphysema, or chronic bronchitis, or if you have glaucoma or difficulty in urination due to enlargment of the prostate gland. May cause marked drowsiness; alcohol, sedatives, and tranquilizers may increase the drowsiness effect. Avoid alcoholic beverages while taking this product. Do not take this product if you are taking sedatives or tranquilizers, without first consulting your doctor. Use caution when driving a motor vehicle or operating machinery. **Do not use any other products containing diphenhydramine while using this product.** As with any drug, if you are pregnant or nursing a baby, seek the advice of a health professional before using this product. KEEP THIS AND ALL DRUGS OUT OF THE REACH OF CHILDREN. In case of accidental overdose, seek professional assistance or contact a Poison Control Center immediately.

How Supplied: Benadryl Allergy Liquid Medication is supplied in 4 and 8 fluid ounce bottles.
Store at room temperature (59°–86°F).
Protect from freezing.
Shown in Product Identification Guide, page 524

BENADRYL® Allergy Sinus Headache Caplets & Gelcaps
[bĕ 'nă-drĭl]

Action: BENADRYL ALLERGY/SINUS HEADACHE is specially formulated to provide effective relief of your upper respiratory allergy symptoms complicated by sinus and headache problems. It combines the strength of BENADRYL to relieve your runny nose, sneezing, itchy, water eyes, itchy nose or throat, with a maximum strength NASAL DECONGESTANT to relieve nasal and sinus congestion, and a maximum strength non-aspirin PAIN RELIEVER to relieve sinus pain and headache.

Active Ingredients: Each caplet and gelcap contains Diphenhydramine Hydrochloride 12.5 mg, Pseudoephedrine Hydrochloride 30 mg and Acetaminophen 500 mg.

Inactive Ingredients: For Caplet: Candelilla Wax, Croscarmellose Sodium, D&C Yellow No. 10 Aluminum Lake, FD&C Blue No. 1 Aluminum Lake, FD&C Yellow No. 6 Aluminum Lake, Hydroxypropyl Cellulose, Hydroxypropyl Methylcellulose, Microcrystalline Cellulose, Polyethylene Glycol, Polysorbate 80, Pregelatinized Starch, Sodium Starch Glycolate, Starch, Stearic Acid, Titanium Dioxide, and Zinc Stearate. Printed with edible red ink.
For Gelcaps: Colloidal Silicon Dioxide, Croscarmellose Sodium, D&C Yellow No. 10 Aluminum Lake, FD&C Green No. 3 Aluminum Lake, Gelatin, Hydroxypropyl Methylcellulose, Polysorbate 80, Sodium Lauryl Sulfate, Stearic Acid, and Titanium Dioxide.

Indications: For the temporary relief of minor aches, pains, and headache, runny nose and sneezing, itching of the nose or throat, and itchy, watery eyes due to hay fever, and nasal congestion due to the common cold, hay fever, or other upper respiratory allergies. Helps decongest sinus openings and passages; temporarily relieves sinus congestion and pressure.

Warnings: Do not exceed recommended dosage. If nervousness, dizziness, or sleeplessness occur, discontinue use and consult a doctor. Do not take this product for more than 10 days. If symptoms do not improve or are accompanied by fever that lasts for more than 3 days, or if new symptoms occur, consult a doctor. Do not take this product, unless directed by a doctor, if you have a breathing problem such as emphysema or chronic bronchitis, heart disease, high blood pressure, thyroid disease, diabetes, or if you have glaucoma or difficulty in urination due to enlargement of the prostate gland. May cause excitability especially in children. May cause marked drowsiness; alcohol, sedatives, and tranquilizers may increase the drowsiness effect. Avoid alcoholic beverages while taking this product. Do not take this product if you are taking sedatives or tranquilizers, without first consulting your doctor. Use caution when driving a motor vehicle or operating machinery. Do not use any other products containing diphenhydramine while using this product. As with any drug, if you are pregnant or nursing a baby, seek the advice of a health professional before using this product. KEEP THIS AND ALL DRUGS OUT OF THE REACH OF CHILDREN. In case of accidental overdose, seek professional assistance or contact a Poison Control Center immediately. Prompt medical attention is critical for adults as well as for children even if you do not notice any signs or symptoms.

Alcohol Warning: If you generally consume 3 or more alcohol-containing drinks per day, you should consult your physician for advice on when and how you should take Benadryl Allergy/Sinus Headache and other pain relievers.

Drug Interaction Precaution: Do not use this product if you are now taking a prescription monoamine oxidase inhibitor (MAOI) (certain drugs for depression, psychiatric or emotional conditions, or Parkinson's disease), or for 2 weeks after stopping the MAOI drug. If you are uncertain whether your prescription drug contains an MAOI, consult a health professional before taking this product.

Directions: Adults and children 12 years of age and over: two (2) caplets or gelcaps every 6 hours while symptoms persist. Not to exceed 8 caplets or gelcaps in 24 hours. Children under 12 years of age: consult a doctor.

How Supplied: Benadryl Allergy Sinus Headache is available in boxes of 24 and 48 caplets, and box of 24 gelcaps. Store at room temperature, (59°–86°F). Protect from moisture.

Shown in Product Identification Guide, page 525

BENADRYL® Dye-Free Allergy Liqui-gels® Softgel
[bĕ 'nă-drĭl]

Active Ingredients: Each softgel contains: Diphenhydramine Hydrochloride 25 mg.

Inactive Ingredients: Gelatin, Glycerin, Polyethylene Glycol 400 and Sorbitol.

Indications: Temporarily relieves runny nose and sneezing, itching of the nose or throat, and itchy, watery eyes due to hay fever or other upper respiratory allergies, and runny nose and sneezing associated with the common cold.

Directions: Follow dosage recommendations below, or use as directed by your doctor.

Benadryl® Dye-Free Allergy
Liqui-Gels® Softgel

AGE	DOSAGE
Adults and children 12 years of age and over	25 to 50 mg (1 to 2 softgels) every 4 to 6 hours. Not to exceed 12 softgels in 24 hours.
Children 6 to under 12 years of age **See ** symbol below**	12.5** to 25 mg (1 softgel) every 4 to 6 hours. Not to exceed 6 softgels in 24 hours.
Children under 6 years of age	Consult a doctor.

**12.5 mg dosage strength is not available in this package. Do not attempt to break softgels. This dosage is available in bubble gum flavored Benadryl® Dye-Free Allergy Liquid Medication.

Warnings: May cause excitability especially in children. Do not take this product, unless directed by a doctor, if you have a breathing problem such as emphysema or chronic bronchitis, or if you have glaucoma or difficulty in urination due to enlargement of the prostate gland. May cause marked drowsiness; alcohol, sedatives, and tranquilizers may increase the drowsiness effect. Avoid alcoholic beverages while taking this product. Do not take this product if you are taking sedatives or tranquilizers, without first consulting your doctor. Use caution when driving a motor vehicle or operating machinery. **Do not use any other products containing diphenhydramine while using this product.** As with any drug, if you are pregnant or nursing a baby, seek the advice of a health professional before using this product. KEEP THIS AND ALL DRUGS OUT OF THE REACH OF CHILDREN. In case of accidental overdose, seek professional assistance or contact a Poison Control Center immediately.

How Supplied: Benadryl® Dye-Free Allergy Liqui-Gels® Softgels are supplied in boxes of 24.
Store at 59°–77°F. Protect from heat and humidity.

Liqui-Gels is a registered trademark of R.P. Scherer Corporation.

Shown in Product Identification Guide, page 525

BENADRYL® Dye-Free Allergy Liquid Medication
[bĕ 'nă-drĭl]
New Formula
New Dose
Bubble Gum Flavor

Active Ingredients: Each teaspoonful (5 mL.) contains Diphenhydramine Hydrochloride 12.5 mg.

Inactive Ingredients: Each teaspoonful (5 mL.) contains: Carboxymethylcellulose Sodium, Citric Acid, Flavor, Glycerin, Purified Water, Saccharin Sodium, Sodium Benzoate, Sodium Citrate, and Sorbitol Solution.

Indications: Temporarily relieves runny nose and sneezing, itching of the nose or throat, and itchy, watery eyes due to hay fever or other upper respiratory allergies, and runny nose and sneezing associated with the common cold.

Directions: Follow dosage recommendations below, or use as directed by your doctor.

Benadryl® Dye-Free Allergy
Liquid Medication
New Formula
New Dose

AGE	DOSAGE
Children under 6 years of age	Consult a doctor.
Children 6 to under 12 years of age	**1–2 Teaspoonfuls (12.5 to 25 mg)** every 4 to 6 hours. Not to exceed 12 teaspoonfuls in 24 hours.
Adults and children 12 years of age and over	**2–4 teaspoonfuls (25 to 50 mg)** every 4 to 6 hours. Not to exceed 24 teaspoonfuls in 24 hours.

Warnings: May cause excitability especially in children. Do not take this product, unless directed by a doctor, if you have a breathing problem such as emphysema or chronic bronchitis, or if you have glaucoma or difficulty in urination due to enlargement of the prostate gland. May cause marked drowsiness; alcohol, sedatives, and tranquilizers may increase the drowsiness effect. Avoid alcoholic beverages while taking this product. Do not take this product if you are taking sedatives or tranquilizers, without first consulting your doctor. Use caution when driving a motor vehicle or operating machinery. **Do not use any other products containing diphenhydramine while using this product.** As with any drug, if you are pregnant or nursing a baby, seek the advice of a health professional before using this product. KEEP THIS AND ALL DRUGS OUT OF THE REACH OF CHILDREN. In case of accidental overdose, seek professional assistance or contact a Poison Control Center immediately.

How Supplied: Benadryl Dye-Free Allergy Liquid Medication is supplied in 4 fl. oz. bottles.

Store at room temperature (59°–86°F).

Continued on next page

This product information was prepared in November 1998. On these and other Warner-Lambert Consumer Healthcare Products, detailed information may be obtained by addressing Warner-Lambert Consumer Healthcare Products, Morris Plains, NJ 07950 USA

Benadryl Dye-Free All.—Cont.

Protect from freezing.

Shown in Product Identification Guide, page 525

BENADRYL® Itch Relief Stick Extra Strength
Topical Analgesic/Skin Protectant
[bĕ 'nă-drĭl]

Active Ingredients: Diphenhydramine Hydrochloride 2%, Zinc Acetate 0.1%.

Inactive Ingredients: Alcohol 73.5% v/v, Glycerin, Povidone, Purified Water and Tromethamine.

Indications: For the temporary relief of itching and pain associated with insect bites, minor skin irritations and rashes due to poison oak, poison ivy or poison sumac. Dries the oozing and weeping of poison ivy, poison oak and poison sumac.

Warnings: FOR EXTERNAL USE ONLY. Do not use on chicken pox, measles, blisters, or on extensive areas of skin, except as directed by a physician. Avoid contact with the eyes. If condition worsens, or does not improve within 7 days or if symptoms persist for more than 7 days or clear up and occur again within a few days, discontinue use of this product and consult a physician. Do not use on children under 6 years of age without consulting a physician. **Do not use any other drugs containing diphenhydramine while using this product.** KEEP THIS AND ALL DRUGS OUT OF THE REACH OF CHILDREN. In case of accidental ingestion, seek professional assistance or contact a Poison Control Center immediately. Flammable. Keep away from fire or flame.

Directions: Adults and children 6 years of age and older: Apply to the affected area not more than 3 to 4 times daily. Children under 6 years of age: Consult a physician.

How Supplied: Benadryl® Itch Relief Stick is available in a .47 fl. oz (14 mL) dauber.

Shown in Product Identification Guide, page 525

BENADRYL® Itch Stopping Cream
Original Strength & Extra Strength
[bĕ 'nă-drĭl]

Active Ingredients:
Original Strength: Diphenhydramine Hydrochloride 1% and Zinc Acetate 0.1%.
Extra Strength: Diphenhydramine Hydrochloride 2% and Zinc Acetate 0.1%.

Inactive Ingredients: Cetyl Alcohol, Diazolidinyl Urea, Methylparaben, Polyethylene Glycol Monostearate 1000, Propylene Glycol, Propylparaben and Purified Water.

Indications: For the temporary relief of itching and pain associated with insect bites, minor skin irritations and rashes due to poison ivy, poison oak or poison sumac. Dries the oozing and weeping of poison ivy, poison oak and poison sumac.

Actions: Benadryl Itch Stopping Cream:
• Stops your itch at the source by blocking the histamine that causes itch.
• Provides local anesthetic itch and pain relief in a greaseless vanishing cream.
• Blocks the histamine hydrocortisone can't.
Original Strength:
• Contains 1% diphenhydramine hydrochloride - for itch relief that is appropriate for the whole family to use (ages 2 and up).
Extra Strength:
• Contains the maximum amount of diphenhydramine hydrochloride - for times when you need extra strength itch relief.

Warnings: FOR EXTERNAL USE ONLY.
Original Strength: Do not use on chicken pox, measles, blisters, or on extensive areas of skin, except as directed by a physician. Avoid contact with the eyes. If condition worsens, or does not improve within 7 days or if symptoms persist for more than 7 day or clear up and occur again within a few days, discontinue use of this product and consult a physician. Do not use on children under 2 years of age without consulting a physician. **Do not use any other drugs containing diphenhydramine while using this product.** KEEP THIS AND ALL DRUGS OUT OF THE REACH OF CHILDREN. In case of accidental ingestion, seek professional assistance or contact a Poison Control Center immediately.
Extra Strength: Do not use on chicken pox, measles, blisters or on extensive areas of skin, except as directed by a physician. Avoid contact with the eyes. If condition worsens, or does not improve within 7 days or if symptoms persist for more than 7 days or clear up and occur again within a few days, discontinue use of this product and consult a physician. Do not use on children under 12 years of age without consulting a physician. Do not use any other drugs containing diphenhydramine while using this product. KEEP THIS AND ALL DRUGS OUT OF THE REACH OF CHILDREN. In case of accidental ingestion, seek professional assistance or contact a Poison Control Center immediately.

Directions: Original Strength: Adults and children 2 years of age and older: Apply to affected area not more than 3 to 4 times daily. Children under 2 years of age: Consult a physician. Extra Strength: Adults and children 12 years of age and older: Apply to affected area not more than 3 to 4 times daily. Children under 12 years of age: Consult a physician.

How Supplied: Benadryl Itch Stopping Cream is available in 1 oz (28.3 g) Original Strength and 1 oz (28.3 g) Extra Strength tubes.

Shown in Product Identification Guide, page 525

BENADRYL® Itch Stopping Spray
Original Strength & Extra Strength
[bĕ 'nă-drĭl]

Active Ingredients:
Original Strength: Diphenhydramine Hydrochloride 1% and Zinc Acetate 0.1%.
Extra Strength: Diphenhydramine Hydrochloride 2% and Zinc Acetate 0.1%.

Inactive Ingredients: Alcohol up to 73.6% v/v, Glycerin, Povidone, Purified Water and Tromethamine.

Indications: For the temporary relief of itching and pain associated with insect bites, minor skin irritations and rashes due to poison ivy, poison oak or poison sumac. Dries the oozing and weeping of poison ivy, poison oak and poison sumac.

Warnings: FOR EXTERNAL USE ONLY.
Original Strength: Do not use on chicken pox, measles, blisters or on extensive areas of skin, except as directed by a physician. Avoid contact with the eyes. If condition worsens or does not improve within 7 days, or if symptoms persist for more than 7 days or clear up and occur again within a few days, discontinue use of this product and consult a physician. Do not use on children under 2 years of age without consulting a physician. **Do not use any other drugs containing diphenhydramine while using this product.** KEEP THIS AND ALL DRUGS OUT OF THE REACH OF CHILDREN. In case of accidental ingestion, seek professional assistance or contact a Poison Control Center immediately. Flammable. Keep away from fire or flame.
Extra Strength: Do not use on chicken pox, measles, blisters or on extensive areas of skin, except as directed by a physician. Avoid contact with the eyes. If condition worsens or does not improve within 7 days, or if symptoms persist for more than 7 days or clear up and occur again within a few days, discontinue use of this product and consult a physician. Do not use on children under 12 years of age without consulting a physician. Do not use any other drugs containing diphenhydramine while using this product. KEEP THIS AND ALL DRUGS OUT OF THE REACH OF CHILDREN. In case of accidental ingestion, seek professional assistance or contact a Poison Control Center immediately. Flammable. Keep away from fire or flame.

Directions: Original Strength: Adults and children 2 years of age and older: Apply to affected area not more than 3 to 4 times daily. Children under 2 years of age: Consult a physician. Extra

Strength: Adults and children 12 years of age and older: Apply to affected area not more than 3 to 4 times daily. Children under 12 years of age: Consult a physician.

How Supplied: Benadryl Itch Stopping Spray Original and Extra Strength is available in a 2 fl. oz. (59mL) pump spray bottle.

Shown in Product Identification Guide, page 525

BENADRYL® Itch Stopping Gel
Original Strength & Extra Strength
[bĕ 'nă-drĭl]

Active Ingredients:
Original Strength: Diphenhydramine Hydrochloride 1%.
Extra Strength: Diphenhydramine Hydrochloride 2%.

Inactive Ingredients: SD Alcohol 38B, Camphor, Citric Acid, Diazolidinyl Urea, Glycerin, Hydroxypropyl Methylcellulose, Methylparaben, Propylene Glycol, Propylparaben, Purified Water, and Sodium Citrate.

Indications: For the temporary relief of itching and pain associated with insect bites, minor skin irritations and rashes due to poison ivy, poison oak or poison sumac.

Actions: Original Strength: Benadryl Original Strength Gel stops your itch at the source by blocking the histamine that causes itch. It contains 1% diphenhydramine hydrochloride for itch relief appropriate for the whole family to use (ages 6 and up). It provides local anesthetic itch and pain relief. Benadryl Itch Stopping Gel blocks the histamine hydrocortisone can't!
Extra Strength: Benadryl Extra Strength Gel stops your itch at the source by blocking the histamine that causes itch. It contains the maximum amount of diphenhydramine hydrochloride for times when you need extra stength itch relief. It provides local anesthetic itch and pain relief. Benadryl Itch Stopping Gel blocks the histamine hydrocortisione can't!

Warnings: FOR EXTERNAL USE ONLY.
Do not use on chicken pox, measles, blisters or on extensive areas of skin, except as directed by a physician. Avoid contact with the eyes. If condition worsens, or if symptoms persist for more than 7 days or clear up and occur again within a few days, discontinue use of this product and consult a physician. **Do not use any other drugs containing diphenhydramine while using this product. KEEP THIS AND ALL DRUGS OUT OF THE REACH OF CHILDREN.** In case of accidental ingestion, seek professional assistance or contact a Poison Control Center immediately.

Directions: Original Strength: Shake well. Adults and children 6 years of age

and older: Apply to affected area not more than 3 to 4 times daily. Children under 6 years of age: Consult a physician.
Extra Strength: Shake well. Adults and children 12 years of age and older: Apply to affected area not more than 3 to 4 times daily. Children under 12 years of age: Consult a physician.

How Supplied: Benadryl Itch Stopping Gel is supplied in 4 fl. oz. (118mL) bottles in both Original and Extra.

Shown in Product Identification Guide, page 525

BENYLIN® Adult Formula
Cough Suppressant
[bĕ '-nă-lĭn]

Active Ingredient: Each teaspoonful (5 mL) contains: Dextromethorphan Hydrobromide 15 mg.

Inactive Ingredients: Caramel, Citric Acid, D&C Red No. 33, FD&C Red No. 40, Flavors, Glycerin, Poloxamer 407, Polysorbate 20, Purified Water, Saccharin Sodium, Sodium Benzoate, Sodium Carboxymethyl Cellulose, Sodium Citrate, and Sorbitol Solution.

Indication: Temporarily relieves cough due to minor throat and bronchial irritation occurring with the common cold.

Directions: Follow dosage recommendations below, or as directed by a doctor. Dosage may be repeated every 6 to 8 hours, not to exceed 4 doses in 24 hours.

Benylin® Adult Formula

AGE	DOSAGE
Adults and children 12 years of age and over	Two (2) teaspoonfuls
Children 6 to under 12 years of age	One (1) teaspoonful
Children 2 to under 6 years of age	One-half (½) teaspoonful
Children under 2 years of age	Consult a doctor

Warnings: A persistent cough may be a sign of a serious condition. If cough persists for more than 1 week, tends to recur, or is accompanied by fever, rash or persistent headache, consult a doctor. Do not take this product for persistent or chronic cough such as occurs with smoking, asthma, emphysema, or if cough is accompanied by excessive phlegm (mucus) unless directed by a doctor. As with any drug, if you are pregnant or nursing a baby, seek the advice of a health professional before using this product. KEEP THIS AND ALL DRUGS OUT OF THE

REACH OF CHILDREN. In case of accidental overdose, seek professional assistance or contact a Poison Control Center immediately.

Drug Interaction Precaution: Do not use this product if you are now taking a prescription monoamine oxidase inhibitor (MAOI) (certain drugs for depression, psychiatric or emotional conditions, or Parkinson's disease), or for 2 weeks after stopping the MAOI drug. If you are uncertain whether your prescription drug contains an MAOI, consult a health professional before taking this product. Store at room temperature 59–86°F.

How Supplied: Benylin Adult Formula is supplied in 4 oz. bottles.
Shown in Product Identification Guide, page 525

BENYLIN® Expectorant
Cough Suppressant/Expectorant
[bĕ '-nă-lĭn]

Active Ingredients: Each teaspoonful (5 mL) contains Guaifenesin 100 mg and Dextromethorphan Hydrobromide 5 mg.

Inactive Ingredients: Caramel, Citric Acid, D&C Red No. 33, Disodium Edetate, FD&C Red No. 40, Flavors, Poloxamer 407, Polyethylene Glycol, Propyl Gallate, Propylene Glycol, Purified Water, Saccharin Sodium, Sodium Benzoate, Sodium Chloride, Sodium Citrate, and Sorbitol Solution.

Indications: Temporarily relieves cough due to minor throat and bronchial irritation occurring with the common cold. Helps loosen phlegm (mucus) and thin bronchial secretions to drain bronchial tubes and make coughs more productive.

Directions: Follow dosage recommendations below, or as directed by a doctor. Dosage may be repeated every 4 hours, not to exceed 6 doses in 24 hours.

Benylin® Expectorant

AGE	DOSAGE
Adults and children 12 years of age and over	Four (4) teaspoonfuls
Children 6 to under 12 years of age	Two (2) teaspoonfuls

Continued on next page

This product information was prepared in November 1998. On these and other Warner-Lambert Consumer Healthcare Products, detailed information may be obtained by addressing Warner-Lambert Consumer Healthcare Products, Morris Plains, NJ 07950 USA

Benylin Expectorant—Cont.

Children 2 to under 6 years of age	One (1) teaspoonful
Children under 2 years of age	Consult a doctor

Warning: A persistent cough may be a sign of a serious condition. If cough persists for more than 1 week, tends to recur, or is accompanied by fever, rash, or persistent headache, consult a doctor. Do not take this product for persistent or chronic cough such as occurs with smoking, asthma, chronic bronchitis, or emphysema, or where cough is accompanied by excessive phlegm (mucus) unless directed by a doctor. As with any drug, if you are pregnant or nursing a baby, seek the advice of a health professional before using this product. **KEEP THIS AND ALL DRUGS OUT OF THE REACH OF CHILDREN.** In case of accidental overdose, seek professional assistance or contact a Poison Control Center immediately.

Drug Interaction Precaution: Do not use this product if you are now taking a prescription monoamine oxidase inhibitor (MAOI) (certain drugs for depression, psychiatric or emotional conditions, or Parkinson's disease), or for 2 weeks after stopping the MAOI drug. If you are uncertain whether your prescription drug contains an MAOI, consult a health professional before taking this product. Store at room temperature 59°–86°F.

How Supplied: Benylin Expectorant is available in 4 oz. bottles.

Shown in Product Identification Guide, page 525

BENYLIN® Multisymptom

[bĕ '-nă-lĭn]

Active Ingredients: Each teaspoonful (5 mL) contains Guaifenesin 100 mg, Pseudoephedrine Hydrochloride 15 mg, and Dextromethorphan Hydrobromide 5 mg.

Inactive Ingredients: Caramel, Citric Acid, D&C Red No. 33, Edetate Disodium, FD&C Red No. 40, Flavors, Poloxamer 407, Polyethylene Glycol 1450, Propyl Gallate, Propylene Glycol, Purified Water, Saccharin Sodium, Sodium Benzoate, Sodium Chloride, Sodium Citrate, and Sorbitol Solution.

Indications: Temporarily relieves cough due to minor throat and bronchial irritation and nasal congestion occurring with the common cold. Helps loosen phlegm (mucus) and thin bronchial secretions to drain bronchial tubes and make coughs more productive.

Directions: Follow dosage recommendations below, or use as directed by a doctor. Dosage may be repeated every 4 hours, not to exceed 4 doses in 24 hours.

Benylin® Multisymptom

AGE	DOSAGE
Adults and children 12 years and over	Four (4) teaspoonfuls
Children 6 to under 12 years of age	Two (2) teaspoonfuls
Children 2 to under 6 years of age	One (1) teaspoonful
Children under 2 years of age	Consult a doctor

Warnings: Do not exceed recommended dosage. If nervousness, dizziness, or sleeplessness occur, discontinue use and consult a doctor. If symptoms do not improve within 7 days or are accompanied by fever, consult a doctor. Do not take this product if you have heart disease, high blood pressure, thyroid disease, diabetes, or difficulty in urination due to enlargement of the prostate gland unless directed by a doctor. A persistent cough may be a sign of a serious condition. If cough persists for more than 1 week, tends to recur, or is accompanied by a fever, rash or persistent headache, consult a doctor. Do not take this product for persistent or chronic cough such as occurs with smoking, asthma, chronic bronchitis, or emphysema, or where cough is accompanied by excessive phlegm (mucus) unless directed by a doctor. As with any drug, if you are pregnant or nursing a baby, seek the advice of a health professional before using this product. **KEEP THIS AND ALL DRUGS OUT OF THE REACH OF CHILDREN.** In case of accidental overdose, seek professional assistance or contact a Poison Control Center immediately.

Drug Interaction Precaution: Do not use this product if you are now taking a prescription monoamine oxidase inhibitor (MAOI) (certain drugs for depression, psychiatric or emotional conditions, or Parkinson's disease), or for 2 weeks after stopping the MAOI drug. If you are uncertain whether your prescription drug contains an MAOI, consult a health professional before taking this product. Store at room temperature (59°–86°F).

How Supplied: Benylin Multisymptom is available in 4 oz bottles.

Shown in Product Identification Guide, page 525

BENYLIN® Pediatric Cough Suppressant

[bĕ '-nă-lĭn]

Active Ingredient: Each teaspoonful (5 mL) contains: Dextromethorphan Hydrobromide 7.5 mg.

Inactive Ingredients: Citric Acid, FD&C Blue No. 1, FD&C Red No. 40, Flavors, Glycerin, Poloxamer 407, Polysorbate 20, Purified Water, Saccharin Sodium, Sodium Benzoate, Sodium Carboxymethyl Cellulose, Sodium Citrate, and Sorbitol Solution.

Indications: Temporarily relieves cough due to minor throat and bronchial irritation occurring with the common cold.

Directions: Follow dosage recommendations below, or as directed by a doctor. Dosage may be repeated every 6 to 8 hours, not to exceed 4 doses in 24 hours.

Benylin® Pediatric

AGE	DOSAGE
Children under 2 years of age	Consult a doctor
Children 2 to under 6 years of age	One (1) teaspoonful
Children 6 to under 12 years of age	Two (2) teaspoonfuls
Adults and children 12 years of age and over	Four (4) teaspoonfuls

Warnings: A persistent cough may be a sign of a serious condition. If cough persists for more than 1 week, tends to recur, or is accompanied by fever, rash, or persistent headache, consult a doctor. Do not take this product for persistent or chronic cough such as occurs with smoking, asthma or emphysema, or if cough is accompanied by excessive phlegm (mucus) unless directed by a doctor. As with any drug, if you are pregnant or nursing a baby, seek the advice of a health professional before using this product. **KEEP THIS AND ALL DRUGS OUT OF THE REACH OF CHILDREN.** In case of accidental overdose, seek professional assistance or contact a Poison Control Center immediately.

Drug Interaction Precaution: Do not use this product if you are now taking a prescription monoamine oxidase inhibitor (MAOI) (certain drugs for depression, psychiatric or emotional conditions, or Parkinson's disease), or for 2 weeks after stopping the MAOI drug. If you are uncertain whether your prescription drug contains an MAOI, consult a health professional before taking this product.

Store at room temperature (59°–86°F).

How Supplied: Benylin Pediatric is supplied in 4 oz bottles.

Shown in Product Identification Guide, page 525

CALADRYL® Lotion
CALADRYL® Cream For Kids
CALADRYL® Clear Lotion
[că 'lă drĭl"]

Active Ingredients: Caladryl Lotion and Caladryl Cream For Kids: Calamine 8%, and Pramoxine Hydrochloride 1%. Caladryl Clear Lotion: Pramoxine Hydrochloride 1% and Zinc Acetate 0.1%.

Inactive Ingredients: Caladryl Lotion: SD Alcohol 38B, Camphor, Diazolidinyl Urea, Fragrance, Hydroxypropyl Methylcellulose, Methylparaben, Polysorbate 80, Propylene Glycol, Propylparaben, Purified Water and Xanthan Gum.
Caladryl Cream for Kids: Camphor, Cetyl Alcohol, Cyclomethicone, Diazolidinyl Urea, Fragrance, Methylparaben, Polysorbate 60, Propylene Glycol, Propylparaben, Purified Water, Sorbitan Monostearate and Soya Sterol.
Caladryl Clear Lotion: SD Alcohol 38B, Camphor, Citric Acid, Diazolidinyl Urea, Fragrance, Glycerin, Hydroxypropyl Methylcellulose, Methylparaben, Polysorbate 40, Propylene Glycol, Propylparaben, Purified Water and Sodium Citrate.

Indications: For the temporary relief of itching and pain associated with rashes due to poison ivy, poison oak or poison sumac, insect bites and minor irritations. Dries the oozing and weeping of poison ivy, poison oak and poison sumac.

Warnings: FOR EXTERNAL USE ONLY. Avoid contact with the eyes. If condition worsens or does not improve within 7 days, or if symptoms persist for more than 7 days or clear up and occur again within a few days, discontinue use of this product and consult a physician. KEEP THIS AND ALL DRUGS OUT OF THE REACH OF CHILDREN. In case of accidental ingestion, seek professional assistance or contact a Poison Control Center immediately.
Caladryl Clear Lotion: Do not use on children under 2 years of age without consulting a physician.

Directions: Before application, wash affected area of skin. Adults and children 2 years of age and older: Apply to affected area not more than 3 to 4 times daily. Children under 2 years of age: Consult a physician.
Additional instructions for only Lotion and Clear Lotion: SHAKE WELL.

How Supplied: Caladryl Cream for Kids—1.5 oz (42.5 g) tubes
Caladryl Clear Lotion—6 fl. oz. (177 mL) bottles
Caladryl Lotion—6 fl. oz. (177 mL) bottles
Shown in Product Identification Guide, page 525

---

e.p.t® PREGNANCY TEST

A woman can find out whether or not she is pregnant by testing any time of day and as early as the first day of her missed period.

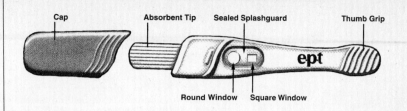

Cap — Absorbent Tip — Sealed Splashguard — Thumb Grip — ept — Round Window — Square Window

With just one easy step **e.p.t** gives clear results in just 3 minutes. **e.p.t Pregnancy Test.** The name more women trust™.
Before beginning the test. Please read the instructions carefully. For questions: Call toll-free 1-800-ept-1step (1-800-378-1783). Registered nurses are available 8:30 am – 5:00 pm EST weekdays to confidentially answer calls regarding **e.p.t.**
To use e.p.t
For in-vitro diagnostic use. (Not for internal use). Remove the **e.p.t.** test stick from its foil pouch just prior to use. [See graphic above]
Remove the purple cap to expose absorbent tip. Hold the test stick by its thumb grip. **Pointing the absorbent tip downward. Place the absorbent tip in the urine flow for just 5 seconds.**

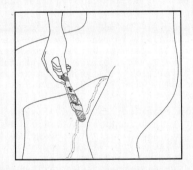

(If you prefer, **dip the absorbent tip into a clean container of urine for just 5 seconds.**)
Place the test stick of a flat surface with the windows facing up for at least 3 minutes. (If you wish, replace the cap to cover the absorbent tip.) You may notice a light pink color moving across the windows.
Important: **To avoid affecting the test result, wait at least 3 minutes before lifting the stick.**

To read the result.
Wait 3 minutes to read the result. A line will appear in the square window showing the test is complete. Be sure to read the result before 20 minutes have passed.

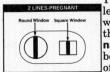

2 LINES-PREGNANT
Round Window — Square Window

Two distinct parallel lines, one in each window, indicate that you are **pregnant.** The lines can be different shades of pink and need not match the color in the illustration. Please see your doctor to discuss your pregnancy and the next steps. Early prenatal care is important to ensure the health of you and your baby.

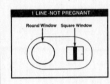

1 LINE -NOT PREGNANT
Round Window — Square Window

One line in the square window but none in the round window indicates that you are **not pregnant.** If your period does not start within a week, repeat the test. If you still get a negative result and your period has not started, please see your doctor.
Important: **If no line appears in the square window, the test result is invalid. Do not read the result. Call toll-free number 1-800-378-1783 (1-800-EPT-1STEP).**

Frequently Asked Questions
When can I use e.p.t?
e.p.t can be used any time of day as soon as you miss your period and any day thereafter.

How does e.p.t work?
e.p.t detects hCG (human Chorionic Gonadotropin), a hormone present in urine only during pregnancy. **e.p.t** can detect hCG in your urine as early as the first day your period is late.

What if the lines in the round and square windows are different shades of pink? As long as 2 parallel lines appear, one in each window, the result is positive, even if the two lines are different shades of pink.

What if I think the test result is incorrect? Following the instructions carefully should yield an accurate reading. If you think the result is incorrect, or if it is difficult to detect a line in the round window, repeat test after 2–3 days with a new **e.p.t** stick.

Are there any factors that can affect the test result? Yes. Certain drugs which contain hCG or are used in combination

Continued on next page

This product information was prepared in November 1998. On these and other Warner-Lambert Consumer Healthcare Products, detailed information may be obtained by addressing Warner-Lambert Consumer Healthcare Products, Morris Plains, NJ 07950 USA

E.P.T. Pregnancy Test—Cont.

with hCG (such as Humegon™, Pregnyl, Profasi, Pergonal, APL) and rare medical conditions. If you repeat the test and continue to get an unexpected result, contact your doctor.

Using **e.p.t** within 8 weeks of giving birth or having a miscarriage may cause a false positive result. The test may detect hCG still in your system from a previous pregnancy. You should ask your doctor for help in interpreting the result of your **e.p.t** test if you have recently been pregnant.

Factors which should not affect the test result include alcohol, analgesics (pain killers), antibiotics, birth control pills or hormone therapies containing clomiphene citrate (Clomid or Serophen). Store at room temperature 15°–30°C (59°–86°F). For in-vitro Diagnostic use. (Not for internal use.) KEEP OUT OF THE REACH OF CHILDREN.

Shown in Product Identification Guide, page 526

LISTERINE® Antiseptic
[lĭs 'tərēn]

Active Ingredients: Thymol 0.064%, Eucalyptol 0.092%, Methyl Salicylate 0.060% and Menthol 0.042%.

Inactive Ingredients: Water, Alcohol 26.9%, Benzoic Acid, Poloxamer 407, Sodium Benzoate and Caramel.

Indications: To help prevent and reduce plaque and gingivitis/For bad breath.

Actions: Listerine® Antiseptic has been shown to help prevent and reduce supragingival plaque accumulation and gingivitis when used in a conscientiously applied program of oral hygiene and regular professional care. Its effect on periodontitis has not been determined. Listerine is the only leading nonprescription mouthrinse that has received the American Dental Association's Council on Scientific Affairs Seal of Acceptance for helping to prevent and reduce plaque above the gumline and gingivitis.

Directions: Rinse full strength for 30 seconds with 20 ml (²/₃ fl. ounce or 4 teaspoonfuls) morning and night. If bad breath persists, see your dentist.

Warnings: Do not administer to children under twelve years of age. Keep this and all drugs out of the reach of children. Do not swallow. In case of accidental overdose, seek professional assistance or contact a poison control center immediately.

How Supplied: Listerine® Antiseptic is supplied in 250 ml, 500 ml, 1.0 liter and 1.5 liter bottles, as well as 3 fl. oz. bottles. It is also available to professionals in 3 fl. oz. bottles and in gallons.

Shown in Product Identification Guide, page 526

COOL MINT LISTERINE®
[lĭs 'tərēn]

Active Ingredients: Thymol 0.064%, Eucalyptol 0.092%, Methyl Salicylate 0.060% and Menthol 0.042%.

Inactive Ingredients: Water, Alcohol 21.6%, Sorbitol Solution, Flavor, Poloxamer 407, Benzoic Acid, Sodium Saccharin, Sodium Benzoate and FD&C Red No. 3.

Indications: To help prevent and reduce plaque and gingivitis/For bad breath.

Actions: Cool Mint Listerine® Antiseptic has been shown to help prevent and reduce supragingival plaque accumulation and gingivitis when used in a conscientiously applied program of oral hygiene and regular professional care. Its effect on periodontitis has not been determined. Listerine is the only leading nonprescription mouthrinse that has received the American Dental Association's Council on Scientific Affairs Seal of Acceptance for helping to prevent and reduce plaque above the gumline and gingivitis.

Directions: Rinse full strength for 30 seconds with 20 ml (²/₃ fl. ounce or 4 teaspoonfuls) morning and night. If bad breath persists, see your dentist.

Warnings: Do not administer to children under twelve years of age. Keep this and all drugs out of the reach of children. Do not swallow. In case of accidental overdose, seek professional assistance or contact a poison control center immediately.

How Supplied: Cool Mint Listerine® Antiseptic is supplied in 250 ml, 500 ml, 1.0 liter and 1.5 liter bottles, as well as 3 and 58 fl. oz. bottles. It is also available to professionals in gallon bottles.

Shown in Product Identification Guide, page 526

FRESHBURST LISTERINE®
[lĭs 'tərēn]

Active Ingredients: Thymol 0.064%, Eucalyptol 0.092%, Methyl Salicylate 0.060% and Menthol 0.042%.

Inactive Ingredients: Water, Alcohol 21.6%, Sorbitol Solution, Flavor, Poloxamer 407, Benzoic Acid, Sodium Saccharin, Sodium Benzoate, D&C Yellow No. 10 and FD&C Green No. 3.

Indications: To help prevent and reduce plaque and gingivitis/For bad breath.

Actions: FreshBurst Listerine® Antiseptic has been shown to help prevent and reduce supragingival plaque accumulation and gingivitis when used in a conscientiously applied program of oral hygiene and regular professional care. Its effect on periodontitis has not been determined. Listerine is the only leading nonprescription mouthrinse that has re-

ceived the American Dental Association's Council on Scientific Affairs Seal of Acceptance for helping to prevent and reduce plaque above the gumline and gingivitis.

Directions: Rinse full strength for 30 seconds with 20 ml (²/₃ fl. ounce or 4 teaspoonfuls) morning and night. If bad breath persists, see your dentist.

Warnings: Do not administer to children under twelve years of age. Keep this and all drugs out of the reach of children. Do not swallow. In case of accidental overdose, seek professional assistance or contact a poison control center immediately.

How Supplied: FreshBurst Listerine® antiseptic is supplied in 250 ml, 500 ml, 1.0 liter and 1.5 liter bottles, as well as 3 fl. oz. bottles. It is also available to professionals in gallon bottles.

Shown in Product Identification Guide, page 526

LISTERMINT®
Alcohol-Free Mouthrinse
[lĭs 'tər mĭnt]

Ingredient: Water, Glycerin, Poloxamer 335, PEG 600, Flavors, Sodium Lauryl Sulfate, Sodium Benzoate, Sodium Saccharin, Benzoic Acid, Zinc Chloride, D&C Yellow No. 10, FD&C Green No. 3.

Indications: Freshens breath; contains no fluoride.

Directions: Rinse with 30 ml (1 fl. oz.) for 30 seconds to freshen breath in the morning and after meals as needed.

Warnings: Do not swallow. Keep out of reach of children.

How Supplied: Listermint® is supplied to consumers in a 32 fl. oz. bottle and is available to professionals in 3 fl. oz. bottles and in gallons.

Shown in Product Identification Guide, page 526

LUBRIDERM® Advanced Therapy Creamy Lotion
[lū brĭ dĕrm]

Composition: Contains Water, Cetyl Alcohol, Glycerin, Mineral Oil, Cyclomethicone, Propylene Glycol Dicaprylate/Dicaprate, PEG-40 Stearate, Isopropyl Isostearate, Emulsifying Wax, Lecithin, Carbomer 940, Diazolidinyl Urea, Titanium Dioxide, Sodium Benzoate, BHT, Tri(PPG-3 Myristyl Ether) Citrate, Disodium EDTA, Retinyl Palmitate, Tocopheryl Acetate, Sodium Pyruvate, Iodopropynyl Butylcarbamate, Fragrance, Sodium Hydroxide, Xanthan Gum.

Actions and Uses: Lubriderm Advanced Therapy's nourishing, rich and creamy formula helps heal extra-dry skin. Its unique combination of nutrient enriched moisturizers penetrate dry skin leaving you with soft, smooth and comfortable skin. This non-greasy feeling lotion absorbs quickly and is non-comedogenic.

Administration and Dosage: Smooth Lubriderm on hands and body every day.

Precautions: For external use only.

How Supplied: Available in 6, 10, 16 fl. oz plastic bottles.

Shown in Product Identification Guide, page 526

LUBRIDERM® BATH AND SHOWER OIL
[lū brĭ dĕrm]

Composition: Contains Mineral Oil, PPG-15 Stearyl Ether, Oleth-2, Nonoxynol-5, Fragrance, D&C Green No. 6.

Actions and Uses: Lubriderm Bath and Shower Oil is a unique, freshly scented formula created for dermatologists to help replenish moisture to dry skin. It disperses instantly in water. With regular use, your skin feels noticeably softer and smoother, and appears more healthy looking.

Administration and Dosage: Remove foil seal before using. Use one or two capfuls in the bath. For shower or sponge bath, apply all over your body by hand or with a sponge and rinse.

Precautions: Avoid getting in eyes; if this occurs, flush with clear water. When using any bath and shower oil, take precautions against slipping. For external use only.

How Supplied: Available in 8 fl. oz. plastic bottles.

Shown in Product Identification Guide, page 526

LUBRIDERM® Daily UV Lotion w/Sunscreen
[lū brĭ dĕrm]

Composition: Octyl Methoxycinnamate 7.5%, Octyl Salicylate 4%, Oxybenzone 3%. Also contains: Purified Water, C12-15 Alkyl Benzoate, Cetearyl Alcohol (and) Ceteareth-20, Cetyl Alcohol, Glyceryl Monostearate, Propylene Glycol, Petrolatum, Diazolidinyl Urea, Triethanolamine, Disodium EDTA, Xanthan Gum, Acrylates/C10-30 Alkyl Acrylate Crosspolymer, Tocopheryl Acetate, Iodopropynyl Buthylcarbamete, Fragrance, Carbomer.

Actions and Uses: Lubriderm Daily UV Lotion's unique formula combines daily moisturization with dermatologist-recommended SPF 15 sun protection. This non-greasy feeling lotion moisturizes dry skin and protects against the damaging rays of the sun—so your skin can feel clean, smooth and protected every day.

Administration and Dosage: Apply liberally as often as necessary. Children under 6 months of age: consult a doctor.

Precautions: For external use only. Avoid contact with the eyes. If contact occurs, rinse eyes thoroughly with water. Discontinue use if signs of irritation or rash appear. If irritation or rash persists, consult a doctor. Keep out of reach of children. In case of accidental ingestion, seek professional assistance or contact a Poison Control Center immediately.

How Supplied: Available in 6, 10, 16 fl. oz plastic bottles.

Shown in Product Identification Guide, page 526

LUBRIDERM®
Dry Skin Care Lotion
[lū brĭ dĕrm]

Composition: Scented—Contains Water, Mineral Oil, Petrolatum, Lanolin, Sorbitol Solution, Stearic Acid, Lanolin Alcohol, Cetyl Alcohol, Glyceryl Stearate/PEG-100 Stearate, Triethanolamine, Dimethicone, Propylene Glycol, Tri(PPG-3 Myristyl Ether) Citrate, Disodium EDTA, Methylparaben, Ethylparaben, Propylparaben, Fragrance, Xanthan Gum, Butylparaben, Methyldibromo Glutaronitrile.

Fragrance Free—Contains Water, Mineral Oil, Petrolatum, Lanolin, Sorbitol Solution, Stearic Acid, Lanolin Alcohol, Cetyl Alcohol, Glyceryl Stearate/PEG-100 Stearate, Triethanolamine, Dimethicone, Propylene Glycol, Tri(PPG-3 Myristyl Ether) Citrate, Disodium EDTA, Methylparaben, Ethylparaben, Propylparaben, Xanthan Gum, Butylparaben, Methyldibromo Glutaronitrile.

Actions and Uses: Lubriderm Lotion is an oil-in-water emulsion indicated for use in softening, soothing and moisturizing dry chapped skin. Lubriderm's water-based formula penetrates dry skin and effectively moisturizes without leaving a greasy feel. Lubriderm helps heal and protect skin from dryness, absorbs rapidly for a clean, natural feel and is non-comedogenic so it won't clog pores.

Administration and Dosage: Apply to hands and body every day. Particularly effective when used after showering or bathing.

Precautions: For external use only.

How Supplied:
Scented: Available in 1, 6, 10 and 16 fl. oz. plastic bottles, and a 2.5 fl. oz. tube.
Fragrance Free: Available in 1, 6, 10 and 16 fl. oz. plastic bottles, and a 2.5 fl. oz. tube.

Shown in Product Identification Guide, page 526

LUBRIDERM®
Seriously Sensitive® Lotion
[lū brĭ dĕrm]

Composition: Contains Water, Butylene Glycol, Mineral Oil, Petrolatum, Glycerin, Cetyl Alcohol, Propylene Glycol Dicaprylate/Dicaprate, PEG-40 Stearate, C11-13 Isoparaffin, Glyceryl Stearate, Tri (PPG-3 Myristyl Ether) Citrate, Emulsifying Wax, Dimethicone, DMDM Hydantoin, Methylparaben, Carbomer 940, Ethylparaben, Propylparaben, Titanium Dioxide, Disodium EDTA, Sodium Hydroxide, Butylparaben, Xanthan Gum.

Action and Uses: Lubriderm Seriously Sensitive Lotion's unique combination of emollients provides sensitive dry skin with the moisture it needs while helping to create a protective layer. It is noncomedogenic, 100% lanolin free, fragrance free, and dye free so its appropriate for skin that is sensitive to these ingredients. It is lightweight, nongreasy, and absorbs quickly.

Administration and Dosage: Apply to hands and body everyday. Particularly effective when used after showering or bathing.

Precautions: For external use only.

How Supplied: Available in 1, 6, 10, and 16 fl. oz. plastic bottles.

Shown in Product Identification Guide, page 526

NEOSPORIN® Ointment
[nē 'uh-spō 'rŭn]

Each Gram Contains: Polymyxin B Sulfate 5,000 units, Bacitracin Zinc 400 units and Neomycin 3.5 mg. Also contains a base of Cocoa Butter*, Cottonseed Oil*, Olive Oil*, Sodium Pyruvate*, Tocopheryl Acetate* and White Petrolatum. *U.S. Patent # 5,652,274

Indications: First aid to help prevent infection in minor cuts, scrapes, and burns.

Directions: Clean the affected area. Apply a small amount of this product (an amount equal to the surface area of the tip of a finger) on the area 1 to 3 times daily. May be covered with a sterile bandage.

Warnings: For external use only. Do not use in the eyes or apply over large areas of the body. In case of deep or puncture wounds, animal bites, or serious burns, consult a physician. Stop use and consult a physician if the condition persists or gets worse, or if a rash or other allergic reaction develops. Do not use if you are allergic to any of the ingredients. Do not use longer than 1 week unless di-

Continued on next page

This product information was prepared in November 1998. On these and other Warner-Lambert Consumer Healthcare Products, detailed information may be obtained by addressing Warner-Lambert Consumer Healthcare Products, Morris Plains, NJ 07950 USA

Neosporin Ointment—Cont.

rected by a physician. KEEP THIS AND ALL DRUGS OUT OF THE REACH OF CHILDREN. In case of accidental ingestion, seek professional assistance or contact a Poison Control Center immediately.

How Supplied: Tubes, $^1/_2$ oz (14.2 g) (with applicator tip), 1 oz (28.3 g), $^1/_{31}$ oz (0.9 g) foil packets packed 10 per box (Neo To Go™) or 144 per box.
Store at 59° to 77°F.

Shown in Product Identification Guide, page 526

NEOSPORIN® + PAIN RELIEF MAXIMUM STRENGTH Cream
[nē "uh-spō 'rŭn]

Each Gram Contains: Polymyxin B Sulfate 10,000 units, Neomycin 3.5 mg, and Pramoxine Hydrochloride 10 mg. Also contains: Emulsifying Wax, Methylparaben 0.25% (added as a preservative), Mineral Oil, Poloxamer 188, Propylene Glycol, Purified Water, and White Petrolatum.

Indications: First aid to help prevent infection and provide temporary relief of pain or discomfort in minor cuts, scrapes, and burns.

Directions: Adults and children 2 years of age and older: Clean the affected area. Apply a small amount of this product (an amount equal to the surface area of the tip of a finger) on the area 1 to 3 times daily. May be covered with a sterile bandage. Children under 2 years of age: Consult a physician.

Warnings: For external use only. Do not use in the eyes or apply over large areas of the body. In case of deep or puncture wounds, animal bites, or serious burns, consult a physician. Stop use and consult a physician if the condition persists or gets worse, or if symptoms persist for more than 1 week or clear up and occur again within a few days, or if a rash or other allergic reaction develops. Do not use if you are allergic to any of the ingredients. Do not use longer than 1 week unless directed by a physician. KEEP THIS AND ALL DRUGS OUT OF THE REACH OF CHILDREN. In case of accidental ingestion, seek professional assistance or contact a Poison Control Center immediately.

How Supplied: $^1/_2$ oz (14.2 g) tubes. Store at 59° to 77°F.

Shown in Product Identification Guide, page 526

NEOSPORIN® + PAIN RELIEF MAXIMUM STRENGTH Ointment
[nē "uh-spō 'rŭn]

Each Gram Contains: Polymyxin B Sulfate 10,000 units, Bacitracin Zinc 500 units, Neomycin 3.5 mg, and Pramoxine Hydrochloride 10 mg, in a custom blend of White Petrolatum.

Indications: First aid to help prevent infection and provide temporary relief of pain or discomfort in minor cuts, scrapes, and burns.

Directions: Adults and children 2 years of age and older: Clean the affected area. Apply a small amount of this product (an amount equal to the surface area of the tip of a finger) on the area 1 to 3 times daily. May be covered with a sterile bandage. Children under 2 years of age: Consult a physician.

Warnings: For external use only. Do not use in the eyes or apply over large areas of the body. In case of deep or puncture wounds, animal bites, or serious burns, consult a physician. Stop use and consult a physician if the condition persists or gets worse, or if symptoms persist for more than 1 week or clear up and occur again within a few days, or if a rash or other allergic reaction develops. Do not use if you are allergic to any of the ingredients. Do not use longer than 1 week unless directed by a physician. KEEP THIS AND ALL DRUGS OUT OF THE REACH OF CHILDREN. In case of accidental ingestion, seek professional assistance or contact a Poison Control Center immediately.

How Supplied: $^1/_2$ oz (14.2 g) and 1 oz (28.3 g) tubes.
Store at 59° to 77°F.

Shown in Product Identification Guide, page 526

NIX® Creme Rinse Permethrin Lice Treatment
[nĭks]

Each Fluid Ounce Contains: Active Ingredient: permethrin 280 mg (1%). Also contains: balsam canada, cetyl alcohol, citric acid, FD&C Yellow No. 6, fragrance, hydrolyzed animal protein, hydroxyethylcellulose, polyoxyethylene 10 cetyl ether, propylene glycol, stearalkonium chloride, water, isopropyl alcohol 5.6 g (20%), methylparaben 56 mg (0.2%), and propylparaben 22 mg (0.08%).

Product Benefits: Nix Creme Rinse kills lice and their unhatched eggs with usually only one application. Nix protects against head lice reinfestation for 14 days. The creme rinse formula leaves hair manageable and easy to comb.

Indications: For the treatment of head lice.

Directions for Use: Nix Creme Rinse should be used after hair has been washed with your regular shampoo, rinsed with water and towel dried. A sufficient amount should be applied to saturate hair and scalp (especially behind the ears and on the nape of the neck). Leave on hair for 10 minutes but no longer. Rinse with water. A single application is usually sufficient. If live lice are observed seven days or more after the first application of this product, a second treatment should be given. For proper head lice management, remove nits with the nit comb provided.

Head lice live on the scalp and lay small white eggs (nits) on the hair shaft close to the scalp. The nits are most easily found on the nape of the neck or behind the ears. All personal headgear, scarfs, coats, and bed linen should be disinfected by machine washing in hot water and drying, using the hot cycle of a dryer for at least 20 minutes. Personal articles of clothing or bedding that cannot be washed may be dry-cleaned, sealed in a plastic bag for a period of about 2 weeks, or sprayed with a product specifically designed for this purpose. Personal combs and brushes may be disinfected by soaking in hot water (above 130°F) for 5 to 10 minutes. Thorough vacuuming of rooms inhabited by infected patients is recommended.
Shake well before using.

Warnings: For external use only. Keep out of eyes when rinsing hair. Adults and children: Close eyes and do not open eyes until product is rinsed out. If product gets into the eyes, immediately flush with water. Do not use near the eyes or permit contact with mucous membranes, such as inside the nose, mouth, or vagina, as irritation may occur. Children: Also protect children's eyes with a washcloth, towel, or other suitable material or method. This product should not be used on children less than 2 months of age. Itching, redness, or swelling of the scalp may occur. If skin irritation persists or infection is present or develops, discontinue use and consult a doctor. Consult a doctor if infestation of eyebrows or eyelashes occurs. This product may cause breathing difficulty or an asthmatic episode in susceptible persons. As with any drug, if you are pregnant or nursing a baby, seek the advice of a health professional before using this product. Keep this and all drugs out of the reach of children. In case of accidental ingestion, seek professional assistance or contact a Poison Control Center immediately.

Professional Labeling:
Indications: For the treatment of head lice. For prophylactic use during head lice epidemics.

Warnings: For external use only. Keep out of eyes when rinsing hair. Adults and children: Close eyes and do not open eyes until product is rinsed out. If product gets into the eyes, immediately flush with water. Do not use near the eyes or permit contact with mucous membranes, such as inside the nose, mouth, or vagina, as irritation may occur. Children: Also protect children's eyes with a washcloth, towel, or other suitable material or method. This product should not be used on pediatric patients less than 2 months of age. Itching, redness, or swelling of the scalp may occur. If skin irritation persists or infection is present or develops, discontinue use and consult a doctor. Consult a doctor if infestation of eyebrows or eyelashes occurs. This product may cause breathing difficulty or an asthmatic episode in susceptible persons. As with any drug, if you are pregnant or nursing a baby, seek the advice of a health professional before using this product. Keep this and all drugs out of the reach of children. In case of accidental ingestion, seek professional assistance or contact a Poison Control Center immediately.

Dosage and Administration
Treatment
Nix Creme Rinse should be used after hair has been washed with patient's regular shampoo, rinsed with water and towel dried. A sufficient amount should be applied to saturate hair and scalp (especially behind the ears and on the nape of the neck). Leave on hair for 10 minutes but no longer. Rinse with water. A single application is usually sufficient. If live lice are observed seven days or more after the first application of this product, a second treatment should be given. For proper head lice management, remove nits with the nit comb provided.

Head lice live on the scalp and lay small white eggs (nits) on the hair shaft close to the scalp. The nits are most easily found on the nape of the neck or behind the ears. All personal headgear, scarfs, coats, and bed linen should be disinfected by machine washing in hot water and drying, using the hot cycle of a dryer for a least 20 minutes. Personal articles of clothing or bedding that cannot be washed may be dry-cleaned, sealed in a plastic bag for a period of about 2 weeks, or sprayed with a product specifically designed for this purpose. Personal combs and brushes may be disinfected by soaking in hot water (above 130°F) for 5 to 10 minutes. Thorough vacuuming of rooms inhabited by infected patients is recommended.

Prophylaxis
Prophylactic use of Nix Creme Rinse is only recommended for individuals exposed to head lice epidemics in which at least 20% of the population at an institution are infested and for immediate household members of infested individuals. Casual use is strongly discouraged. The method of application of Nix Creme Rinse for prophylaxis is identical to that described above for treatment of a lice infestation except nit removal is not required.

Directions for Use
One application of Nix Creme Rinse has been shown to protect greater than 95% of patients against reinfestation for at least two weeks. In epidemic settings, a second prophylactic application is recommended two weeks after the first because the life cycle of a head louse is approximately four weeks.

How Supplied: Bottles of 2 fl. oz. (59 mL) with nit removal comb and Family

Pack of 2 bottles, 2 fl. oz. (59 mL) each, with two nit removal combs. Store at 15° to 25°C (59° to 77°F).
Shown in Product Identification Guide, page 526

POLYSPORIN® Ointment
[pŏl 'ē-spō 'rŭn]

Each Gram Contains: Polymyxin B Sulfate 10,000 units and Bacitracin Zinc 500 units in a special White Petrolatum Base.

Indications: First aid to help prevent infection in minor cuts, scrapes, and burns.

Directions: Clean the affected area. Apply a small amount of this product (an amount equal to the surface area of the tip of a finger) on the area 1 to 3 times daily. May be covered with a sterile bandage.

Warnings: For external use only. Do not use in the eyes or apply over large areas of the body. In case of deep or puncture wounds, animal bites, or serious burns, consult a physician. Stop use and consult a physician if the condition persists or gets worse, or if a rash or other allergic reaction develops. Do not use if you are allergic to any of the ingredients. Do not use longer than 1 week unless directed by a physician. KEEP THIS AND ALL DRUGS OUT OF THE REACH OF CHILDREN. In case of accidental ingestion, seek professional assistance or contact a Poison Control Center immediately

How Supplied: Tubes, $\frac{1}{2}$ oz (14.2 g) with applicator tip, 1 oz (28.3 g); $\frac{1}{32}$ oz (0.9 g) foil packets packed in cartons of 144.
Store at 59° to 77°F.
Shown in Product Identification Guide, page 526

POLYSPORIN® Powder
[pŏl 'ē-spō 'rŭn]

Each Gram Contains: Polymyxin B Sulfate 10,000 units and Bacitracin Zinc 500 units in a Lactose Base.

Indications: First aid to help prevent infection in minor cuts, scrapes, and burns.

Directions: Clean the affected area. Apply a light dusting of the powder on the area 1 to 3 times daily. May be covered with a sterile bandage.

Warnings: For external use only. Do not use in the eyes or apply over large areas of the body. In case of deep or puncture wounds, animal bites, or serious burns, consult a physician. Stop use and consult a physician if the condition persists or gets worse, or if a rash or other allergic reaction develops. Do not use if you are allergic to any of the ingredients. Do not use longer than 1 week unless di-

rected by a physician. KEEP THIS AND ALL DRUGS OUT OF THE REACH OF CHILDREN. In case of accidental ingestion, seek professional assistance or contact a Poison Control Center immediately.

How Supplied: 0.35 oz (10 g) shaker-vial.

Store at 15° to 25°C (59° to 77°F). Do not store under refrigeration.
Shown in Product Identification Guide, page 526

ROLAIDS® Antacid Tablets
Original Peppermint, Spearmint, Cherry and
Assorted Fruit flavors

Active Ingredients: Calcium Carbonate 550 mg and Magnesium Hydroxide 110 mg per tablet.

Inactive Ingredients: Peppermint and Spearmint flavors: Flavoring, Light Mineral Oil, Magnesium Stearate, Microcrystalline Cellulose, Polyethylene Glycol, Pregelatinized Starch, Silicon Dioxide and Sucrose.
Cherry flavor: Flavoring, Light Mineral Oil, Magnesium Stearate, Microcrystalline Cellulose, Polyethylene Glycol, Pregelatinized Starch, Red 27 Lake, Silicon Dioxide and Sucrose.
Assorted Fruit flavors: Color (Blue 1 Lake, Red 27 Lake, Yellow 5 Lake [Tartrazine] and Yellow 6 Lake), Flavoring, Light Mineral Oil, Magnesium Stearate, Microcrystalline Cellulose, Polyethylene Glycol, Pregelatinized Starch, Silicon Dioxide and Sucrose.

Indications: For the relief of heartburn, sour stomach or acid indigestion and upset stomach associated with these symptoms.

Actions: Rolaids® provides rapid neutralization of stomach acid. Each tablet has an acid-neutralizing capacity of 14.7 mEq and the ability to maintain the pH of stomach contents at 3.5 or greater for a significant period of time. Each tablet provides 22% of the adult nutritional Daily Value for calcium and 11% of the adult nutritional Daily Value for magnesium. Each tablet contains less than 1 mg of sodium and is considered to be dietetically sodium free.

Warnings: Do not take more than 12 tablets in a 24 hour period or use the maximum dosage of this product for more than 2 weeks except under the advice and supervision of a physician. KEEP THIS AND ALL DRUGS OUT OF THE REACH OF CHILDREN.

Continued on next page

This product information was prepared in November 1998. On these and other Warner-Lambert Consumer Healthcare Products, detailed information may be obtained by addressing Warner-Lambert Consumer Healthcare Products, Morris Plains, NJ 07950 USA

Rolaids—Cont.

Drug Interaction Precaution: Antacids may interact with certain prescription drugs. If you are presently taking a prescription drug, do not take this product without checking with your physician or other health professional.

Dosage and Administration: Chew 1 to 4 tablets as symptoms occur. Repeat hourly if symptoms return, or as directed by a physician.

How Supplied: Rolaids® is available in 12-tablet rolls, 3-packs containing three 12-tablet rolls and in bottles containing 75, 150, or 300 tablets.
Shown in Product Identification Guide, page 527

SINUTAB® Non-Drying Liquid Caps
[sĭn 'ū tăb]

Active Ingredients: Each liquid cap contains: Pseudoephedrine Hydrochloride 30 mg., Guaifenesin 200 mg.

Inactive Ingredients: FD&C Blue No. 1, Gelatin, Glycerin, Polyethylene Glycol 400, Povidone, Propylene Glycol, and Sorbitol. Printed with edible white ink.

Indications: Temporarily relieves nasal congestion associated with sinusitis. Helps loosen phlegm (mucus) and thin bronchial secretions to drain bronchial tubes.

Dosage and Administration: Adults and children 12 years of age and over: swallow 2 liquid caps every 4 hours, not to exceed 8 liquid caps in 24 hours, or as directed by a doctor. Children under 12 years of age: consult a doctor.

Warnings: Do not exceed recommended dosage. If nervousness, dizziness, or sleeplessness occur, discontinue use and consult a doctor. If symptoms do not improve within 7 days or are accompanied by fever, consult a doctor. Do not take this product if you have heart disease, high blood pressure, thyroid disease, diabetes, or difficulty in urination due to enlargement of the prostate gland unless directed by a doctor. A persistent cough may be a sign of a serious condition. If cough persists for more than 1 week, tends to recur, or is accompanied by a fever, rash, or persistent headache, consult a doctor. Do not take this product for persistent or chronic cough such as occurs with smoking, asthma, chronic bronchitis, or emphysema, or where cough is accompanied by excessive phlegm (mucus) unless directed by a doctor. As with any drug, if you are pregnant or nursing a baby, seek the advice of a health professional before using this product.
KEEP THIS AND ALL DRUGS OUT OF THE REACH OF CHILDREN. In case of accidental overdose, seek professional assistance or contact a Poison Control Center immediately.

Drug Interaction Precaution: Do not use this product if you are now taking a prescription monoamine oxidase inhibitor (MAOI) (certain drugs for depression, psychiatric or emotional conditions, or Parkinson's disease), or for 2 weeks after stopping the MAOI drug. If you are uncertain whether your prescription drug contains an MAOI, consult a health professional before taking this product.

How Supplied: Sinutab® Non-Drying supplied in a box of 24 liquid caps.
Store at 59°–77°F. Protect from heat and humidity.
Shown in Product Identification Guide, page 527

SINUTAB® Sinus Allergy Medication, Maximum Strength Formula, Tablets and Caplets
[sĭn 'ū tăb]

Active Ingredients: Each tablet/caplet contains: Acetaminophen 500 mg., Chlorpheniramine Maleate 2 mg., Pseudoephedrine Hydrochloride 30 mg.

Inactive Ingredients: Croscarmellose Sodium, Crospovidone, D&C Yellow No. 10 Aluminum Lake, FD&C Yellow No. 6 Aluminum Lake, Microcrystalline Cellulose, Povidone, Pregelatinized Starch and Stearic Acid. May also contain Calcium Stearate, Candelilla Wax, Carnauba Wax, Hydroxypropyl Cellulose, Hydroxypropyl Methylcellulose, Polyethylene Glycol, Polysorbate 80, Titanium Dioxide and Zinc Stearate. See package for complete listing.

Indications: For the temporary relief of minor aches, pains and headache and nasal congestion associated with sinusitis. Temporarily relieves runny nose, sneezing itching of the nose or throat, and itchy, watery eyes due to hay fever or other upper respiratory allergies.

Dosage: Adults and children 12 years of age and over: 2 tablets or caplets every 6 hours while symptoms persist, not to exceed 8 tablets or caplets in 24 hours, or as directed by a doctor. Children under 12 years of age: consult a doctor.

Warnings: Do not exceed recommended dosage. If nervousness, dizziness, or sleeplessness occur, discontinue use and consult a doctor. Do not take this product for more than 10 days. If symptoms do not improve or are accompanied by fever that lasts for more than 3 days, or if new symptoms occur, consult a doctor. Do not take this product, unless directed by a doctor, if you have heart disease, high blood pressure, thyroid disease, diabetes, a breathing problem such as emphysema or chronic bronchitis, or if you have glaucoma or difficulty in urination due to enlargement of the prostate gland. May cause excitability especially in children. May cause drowsiness; alcohol, sedatives, and tranquilizers may increase the drowsiness effect. Avoid alco-

holic beverages while taking this product. Do not take this product if you are taking sedatives or tranquilizers, without first consulting your doctor. Use caution when driving a motor vehicle or operating machinery. As with any drug, if you are pregnant or nursing a baby, seek the advice of a health professional before using this product. **KEEP THIS AND ALL DRUGS OUT OF THE REACH OF CHILDREN.** In case of accidental overdose, seek professional assistance or contact a Poison Control Center immediately. Prompt medical attention is critical for adults as well as for children even if you do not notice any signs or symptoms.

Alcohol Warning: If you generally consume 3 or more alcohol-containing drinks per day, you should consult your physician for advice on when and how you should take Sinutab Sinus Allergy and other pain relievers.

Drug Interaction Precaution: Do not use this product if you are now taking a prescription monoamine oxidase inhibitor (MAOI) (certain drugs for depression, psychiatric or emotional conditions, or Parkinson's disease), or for 2 weeks after stopping the MAOI drug. If you are uncertain whether your prescription drug contains an MAOI, consult a health professional before taking this product.

How Supplied: Sinutab® Sinus Allergy Medication, Maximum Strength Formula, Caplets and Tablets are supplied in child-resistant blister packs in boxes of 24 tablets or caplets.

Store at 59° to 77°F in a dry place.
Shown in Product Identification Guide, page 527

SINUTAB® Sinus Medication, Maximum Strength Without Drowsiness Formula, Tablets and Caplets
[sĭn 'ū tăb]

Active Ingredients: Each tablet/caplet contains: Acetaminophen 500 mg., Pseudoephedrine Hydrochloride 30 mg.

Inactive Ingredients: Croscarmellose Sodium, Crospovidone, FD&C Yellow No. 6 Aluminum Lake, Microcrystalline Cellulose, Povidone, Pregelatinized Starch and Stearic Acid. May also contain: Calcium Stearate, Candelilla Wax, Carnauba Wax, D&C Yellow No. 10 Aluminum Lake, Hydroxypropyl Cellulose, Hydroxypropyl Methylcellulose, Polyethylene Glycol, Polysorbate 80, Titanium Dioxide, and Zinc Stearate. See package for complete listing.

Indications: For the temporary relief of minor aches, pains, and headache and nasal congestion associated with sinusitis.

Dosage: Adults and children 12 years of age and over: 2 tablets or caplets every 6 hours while symptoms persist, not to exceed 8 tablets or caplets in 24 hours, or as directed by a doctor. Children under 12 years of age: consult a doctor.

Warnings: Do not exceed recommended dosage. If nervousness, dizziness, or sleeplessness occur, discontinue use and consult a doctor. Do not take this product for more than 10 days. If symptoms do not improve or are accompanied by fever that lasts for more than 3 days, or if new symptoms occur, consult a doctor. Do not take this product if you have heart disease, high blood pressure, thyroid disease, diabetes, or difficulty in urination due to enlargement of the prostate gland unless directed by a doctor. As with any drug, if you are pregnant or nursing a baby, seek the advice of a health professional before using this product. **KEEP THIS AND ALL DRUGS OUT OF THE REACH OF CHILDREN.** In case of accidental overdose, seek professional assistance or contact a Poison Control Center immediately. Prompt medical attention is critical for adults as well as for children even if you do not notice any signs or symptoms.

Alcohol Warning: If you generally consume 3 or more alcohol-containing drinks per day, you should consult your physician for advice on when and how you should take Sinutab Sinus and other pain relievers.

Drug Interaction Precaution: Do not use this product if you are now taking a prescription monoamine oxidase inhibitor (MAOI) (certain drugs for depression, psychiatric or emotional conditions, or Parkinson's disease), or for 2 weeks after stopping the MAOI drug. If you are uncertain whether your prescription drug contains an MAOI, consult a health professional before taking this product.

How Supplied: Sinutab® Sinus Medication, Maximum Strength Without Drowsiness Formula, Caplets and Tablets are supplied in child-resistant blister packs in boxes of 24 tablets or caplets and in boxes of 48 caplets.
Store at room temperature (59°–86°F).
Shown in Product Identification Guide, page 527

SUDAFED® 12 Hour Tablets*
[sū 'duh-fĕd]
*Capsule-shaped Tablets

Description: Sudafed 12 Hour is a long acting nasal decongestant providing temporary relief of nasal and sinus congestion due to a cold, allergy, or sinusitis for up to 12 hours. Sudafed 12 Hour helps clear nasal congestion and release sinus pressure to restore freer breathing without drowsiness.

Active Ingredient: Each coated extended-release tablet contains Pseudoephedrine Hydrochloride 120 mg.

Inactive Ingredients: Carnauba Wax, Hydroxypropyl Methylcellulose, Magnesium Stearate, Microcrystalline Cellulose, Polyethylene Glycol, Povidone, and Titanium Dioxide. Printed with edible blue ink.

Indications: For temporary relief of nasal congestion due to the common cold, hay fever, or other upper respiratory allergies, and nasal congestion associated with sinusitis. Promotes nasal and/or sinus drainage; temporarily relieves sinus congestion and pressure. Temporarily restores freer breathing through the nose.

Directions: Adults and children 12 years and over—One tablet every 12 hours, not to exceed two tablets in 24 hours. Sudafed 12 Hour is not recommended for children under 12 years of age.

Warnings: Do not exceed recommended dosage. If nervousness, dizziness, or sleeplessness occur, discontinue use and consult a doctor. If symptoms do not improve within 7 days or are accompanied by fever, consult a doctor. Do not take this product if you have heart disease, high blood pressure, thyroid disease, diabetes, or difficulty in urination due to enlargement of the prostate gland unless directed by a doctor. As with any drug, if you are pregnant or nursing a baby, seek the advice of a health professional before using this product. **KEEP THIS AND ALL DRUGS OUT OF THE REACH OF CHILDREN.** In case of accidental overdose, seek professional assistance or contact a Poison Control Center immediately.

Drug Interaction Precaution: Do not use this product if you are now taking a prescription monoamine oxidase inhibitor (MAOI) (certain drugs for depression, psychiatric or emotional conditions, or Parkinson's disease), or for 2 weeks after stopping the MAOI drug. If you are uncertain whether your prescription drug contains an MAOI, consult a health professional before taking this product.

How Supplied: Boxes of 10 and 20. Store at 15° to 25°C (59° to 77°F) in a dry place and protect from light.
Shown in Product Identification Guide, page 527

SUDAFED® 24 Hour Tablets Non-Drowsy
[sū 'duh-fĕd]

Description: Sudafed 24 Hour is specially formulated to provide relief for 24 hours with a one tablet, once daily dosage. Each Sudafed 24 Hour tablet releases an outer coating of medication immediately and then continues to work by releasing medication at a precisely controlled rate for 24 hours of relief. Sudafed 24 Hour contains a nasal decongestant that provides relief without drowsiness.

Active Ingredient: Each Sudafed 24 Hour tablet contains a total of 240 mg pseudoephedrine hydrochloride, 60 mg immediate release and 180 mg controlled release.

Inactive Ingredients: Cellulose, cellulose acetate, hydroxypropyl cellulose,

hydroxypropyl methylcellulose, magnesium stearate, polyethylene glycol, polysorbate 80, povidone, sodium chloride, and titanium dioxide.

Indications: Provides temporary relief of nasal congestion due to the common cold, hay fever, or other upper respiratory allergies, and nasal congestion associated with sinusitis; reduces swelling of nasal passages; shrinks swollen membranes; relieves sinus pressure, and temporarily restores freer breathing through the nose.

Directions: Adults and children 12 years of age and over: Take just one tablet with fluid every 24 hours. **DO NOT EXCEED ONE TABLET IN 24 HOURS.** SWALLOW EACH TABLET WHOLE; DO NOT DIVIDE, CRUSH, CHEW OR DISSOLVE THE TABLET. The tablet does not completely dissolve and may be seen in the stool (this is normal). Not for use in children under 12 years of age.

Warnings: DO NOT EXCEED RECOMMENDED DOSAGE. If nervousness, dizziness, or sleeplessness occur, discontinue use and consult a physician. Do not take this product for more than 7 days. If symptoms do not improve or are accompanied by fever, consult a physician. Do not take this product if you have heart disease, high blood pressure, thyroid disease, diabetes, or difficulty in urination due to enlargement of the prostate gland, unless directed by a physician.
Rarely, tablets of this kind may cause bowel obstruction (blockage), usually in people with severe narrowing of the bowel (esophagus, stomach or intestine). If you have had obstruction or narrowing of the bowel, do not take this product without consulting your physician. Contact your physician if you experience persistent abdominal pain or vomiting. As with any drug, if you are pregnant or nursing a baby, seek the advice of a health professional before using this product. **KEEP THIS AND ALL DRUGS OUT OF THE REACH OF CHILDREN.** In case of accidental overdose, seek professional assistance or contact a Poison Control Center immediately.

Drug Interaction Precaution: Do not use this product if you are now taking a prescription monoamine oxidase inhibitor (MAOI) (certain drugs for depression, psychiatric or emotional conditions, or Parkinson's disease), or for 2 weeks after stopping the MAOI drug. If you are uncertain whether your prescription

Continued on next page

This product information was prepared in November 1998. On these and other Warner-Lambert Consumer Healthcare Products, detailed information may be obtained by addressing Warner-Lambert Consumer Healthcare Products, Morris Plains, NJ 07950 USA

Sudafed 24 Hour—Cont.

drug contains an MAOI, consult a health professional before taking this product.

How Supplied: Box of 5 tablets. Store in a dry place between 4° and 30°C (39° and 86°F). **BLISTER PACKAGED FOR YOUR PROTECTION. DO NOT USE IF INDIVIDUAL SEALS ARE BROKEN.**
Shown in Product Identification Guide, page 527

SUDAFED® Nasal Decongestant Tablets 30 mg.
[sū 'duh-fĕd]

Description: Sudafed Nasal Decongestant tablets provide temporary, maximum strength relief of nasal and sinus congestion due to a cold, allergy, or sinusitis. Sudafed Nasal Decongestant helps clear nasal congestion and relieve sinus pressure to restore freer breathing without drowsy or overdrying side effects.

Active Ingredient: Each tablet contains Pseudoephedrine Hydrochloride 30 mg.

Inactive Ingredients: Acacia, Corn Starch, FD&C Red No. 40 Aluminum Lake, FD&C Yellow No. 6 Aluminum Lake, Magnesium Stearate, Pharmaceutical Glaze, Polysorbate 60, Povidone, Sodium Benzoate, Stearic Acid, Sucrose, and Titanium Dioxide. May also contain: Candelilla Wax, Carnauba Wax, Dibasic Calcium Phosphate, Hydroxypropyl Methylcellulose, Lactose Monohydrate, Poloxamer 407, Polyethylene Glycol, Polyethylene Oxide, Potato Starch, Propylene Glycol, Silicon Dioxide, Sodium Lauryl Sulfate and Talc. See package for complete listing. Printed with edible black ink.

Indications: For the temporary relief of nasal congestion due to the common cold, hay fever or other upper respiratory allergies, and nasal congestion associated with sinusitis. Helps decongest sinus openings and passages; temporarily relieves sinus congestion and pressure. Temporarily restores freer breathing through the nose.

Directions: To be given every 4 to 6 hours. Do not exceed 4 doses in 24 hours. Adults and children 12 years of age and over: 2 tablets. Children 6 to under 12 years of age: 1 tablet. Children 2 to under 6 years of age: use Children's Sudafed Liquid. Children under 2 years of age: consult a doctor.

Warnings: Do not exceed recommended dosage. If nervousness, dizziness or sleeplessness occur, discontinue use and consult a doctor. If symptoms do not improve within 7 days or are accompanied by fever, consult a doctor. Do not take this product if you have heart disease, high blood pressure, thyroid disease, diabetes, or difficulty in urination due to enlargement of the prostate gland unless directed by a doctor. As with any drug, if you are pregnant or nursing a baby, seek the advice of a health professional before using this product. **KEEP THIS AND ALL DRUGS OUT OF THE REACH OF CHILDREN.** In case of accidental overdose, seek professional assistance or contact a Poison Control Center immediately.

Drug Interaction Precaution: Do not use this product if you are now taking a prescription monoamine oxidase inhibitor (MAOI) (certain drugs for depression, psychiatric or emotional conditions, or Parkinson's disease), or for 2 weeks after stopping the MAOI drug. If you are uncertain whether your prescription drug contains an MAOI, consult a health professional before taking this product.

How Supplied: Boxes of 24, 48 and 96. Store at 15° to 25°C (59°–77°F) in a dry place and protect from light.
Shown in Product Identification Guide, page 527

CHILDREN'S SUDAFED®
Cold & Cough Liquid
[sū 'duh-fĕd]

Description: Children's Sudafed Cold and Cough Liquid provides temporary relief for a child's stuffy nose and coughing due to the common cold. It also comes in a great tasting cherry-berry flavor that makes it easy to give to children.

Active Ingredients: Each teaspoonful (5 mL) contains Pseudoephedrine Hydrochloride 15 mg and Dextromethorphan Hydrobromide 5 mg.

Inactive Ingredients: Carboxymethylcellulose Sodium, Citric Acid, D&C Red No. 33, FD&C Red No. 40, Flavors, Glycerin, Poloxamer 407, Polyethylene Glycol 1450, Purified Water, Saccharin Sodium, Sodium Benzoate, Sodium Chloride, Sodium Citrate and Sorbitol Solution.

Indications: For the temporary relief of nasal congestion due to the common cold; temporarily quiets cough due to minor throat and bronchial irritation occurring with a cold or inhaled irritants. Suppresses cough impulses without narcotics.

Directions: Follow dosage recommendations below, or as directed by a doctor. Dosage may be repeated every 4 hours, not to exceed 4 doses in 24 hours.

Children's Sudafed®
Cold & Cough Liquid

AGE	DOSAGE
Children under 2 years of age	Consult a doctor
Children 2 to under 6 years of age	One (1) teaspoonful
Children 6 to under 12 years of age	Two (2) teaspoonfuls
Adults and children 12 years of age and over	Four (4) teaspoonfuls

Warnings: Do not exceed recommended dosage. If nervousness, dizziness, or sleeplessness occur, discontinue use and consult a doctor. If symptoms do not improve within 7 days or are accompanied by fever, consult a doctor. Do not take this product if you have heart disease, high blood pressure, thyroid disease, diabetes, or difficulty in urination due to enlargement of the prostate gland unless directed by a doctor. A persistent cough may be a sign of a serious condition. If cough persists for more than 1 week, tends to recur, or is accompanied by fever, rash, or persistent headache, consult a doctor. Do not take this product for persistent or chronic cough such as occurs with smoking, asthma or emphysema, or if cough is accompanied by excessive phlegm (mucus) unless directed by a doctor. As with any drug, if you are pregnant or nursing a baby, seek the advice of a health professional before using this product. **KEEP THIS AND ALL DRUGS OUT OF THE REACH OF CHILDREN.** In case of accidental overdose, seek professional assistance or contact a Poison Control Center immediately.

Drug Interaction Precaution: Do not use this product if you are now taking a prescription monoamine oxidase inhibitor (MAOI) (certain drugs for depression, psychiatric or emotional conditions, or Parkinson's disease), or for 2 weeks after stopping the MAOI drug. If you are uncertain whether your prescription drug contains an MAOI, consult a health professional before taking this product.

How Supplied: Sudafed Children's Cold and Cough Liquid is supplied in 4 fl. oz. bottles.
Store at 15° to 25°C (59° to 77°F) and protect from light.
Shown in Product Identification Guide, page 527

CHILDREN'S SUDAFED®
Nasal Decongestant Chewables
[sū ' duh-fĕd]

Description: Children's Sudafed Nasal Decongestant Chewables provides temporary relief for a child's stuffy nose and head due to a cold, allergy, or sinusitis. It also comes in a wonderful orange flavor chewable tablet that makes it easy to give to children.

Active Ingredient: Each chewable tablet contains Pseudoephedrine Hydrochloride 15 mg.

Inactive Ingredients: Ascorbic Acid, Aspartame, Carnauba Wax, Citric Acid, Crospovidone, FD&C Yellow No. 6 Aluminum Lake, Flavors, Hydroxypropyl Methylcellulose, Magnesium Stearate, Mannitol, Microcrystalline Cellulose, Sodium Chloride, Tartaric Acid.

Indications: For the temporary relief of nasal congestion due to the common cold, hay fever or other upper respiratory allergies, and nasal congestion associated with sinusitis. Promotes nasal and/or sinus drainage; temporarily relieves sinus congestion and pressure.

Directions: Do not exceed 4 doses in a 24-hour period. Children 6 to under 12 years of age: 2 chewable tablets every 4 to 6 hours. Children 2 to under 6 years of age: 1 chewable tablet every 4 to 6 hours. Children under 2 years of age: consult a doctor.

Warnings: Do not exceed recommended dosage. If nervousness, dizziness, or sleeplessness occur, discontinue use and consult a doctor. If symptoms do not improve within 7 days or are accompanied by fever, consult a doctor. Do not give this product to a child who has heart disease, high blood pressure, thyroid disease, or diabetes unless directed by a doctor. **KEEP THIS AND ALL DRUGS OUT OF THE REACH OF CHILDREN.** In case of accidental overdose, seek professional assistance or contact a Poison Control Center immediately. **Phenylketonurics: Contains Phenylalanine 0.78 mg Per Tablet.**

Drug Interaction Precaution: Do not give this product to a child who is taking a prescription monoamine oxidase inhibitor (MAOI) (certain drugs for depression, psychiatric or emotional conditions), or for 2 weeks after stopping the MAOI drug. If you are uncertain whether your child's prescription drug contains an MAOI, consult a health professional before giving this product.

How Supplied: Box of 24 chewable tablets. Store at 59° to 77°F in a dry place and protect from light.

Shown in Product Identification Guide, page 527

SUDAFED® CHILDREN'S NASAL DECONGESTANT LIQUID MEDICATION
[sū 'duh-fĕd]

Description: Children's Sudafed Nasal Decongestant Liquid provides temporary relief for a child's stuffy nose and head due to a cold or allergy. It also comes in a wonderful grape flavor that makes it easy to give to children.

Active Ingredient: Each teaspoonful (5 mL) contains Pseudoephedrine Hydrochloride 15 mg.

Inactive Ingredients: Citric Acid, Edetate Disodium, FD&C Red No. 40, FD&C Blue No. 1, Flavors, Glycerin, Poloxamer 407, Polyethylene Glycol 1450, Povidone K-90, Purified Water, Saccharin Sodium, Sodium Benzoate, Sodium Citrate and Sorbitol Solution.

Indications: For the temporary relief of nasal congestion due to the common cold, hay fever or other upper respiratory allergies, and nasal congestion associated with sinusitis. Promotes nasal and/or sinus drainage; temporarily relieves sinus congestion and pressure.

Directions: Follow dosage recommendations below. Dosage may be repeated every 4 to 6 hours, not to exceed 4 doses in 24 hours.

Sudafed® Children's Nasal Decongestant Liquid Medication

Age	Dosage
Children under 2 years of age	Consult a doctor
Children 2 to under 6 years of age	One (1) teaspoonful
Children 6 to under 12 years of age	Two (2) teaspoonfuls
Adults and children 12 years of age and over	Four (4) teaspoonfuls

Warnings: Do not exceed recommended dosage. If nervousness, dizziness, or sleeplessness occur, discontinue use and consult a doctor. If symptoms do not improve within 7 days or are accompanied by fever, consult a doctor. Do not take this product if you have heart disease, high blood pressure, thyroid disease, diabetes, or difficulty in urination due to enlargement of the prostate gland unless directed by a doctor. As with any drug, if you are pregnant or nursing a baby, seek the advice of a health professional before using this product. **KEEP THIS AND ALL DRUGS OUT OF THE REACH OF CHILDREN.** In case of accidental overdose, seek professional assistance or contact a Poison Control Center immediately.

Drug Interaction Precaution: Do not use this product if you are now taking a prescription monoamine oxidase inhibitor (MAOI) (certain drugs for depression, psychiatric or emotional conditions, or Parkinson's disease), or for 2 weeks after stopping the MAOI drug. If you are uncertain whether your prescription drug contains an MAOI, consult a health professional before taking this product.

How Supplied: Sudafed Children's Nasal Decongestant is supplied in 4 fl. oz. bottles
Store at 59° to 77°F and protect from light.

Shown in Product Identification Guide, page 527

SUDAFED® Cold & Allergy Tablets
[sū 'duh-fĕd]

Description: Sudafed Cold & Allergy provides temporary, maximum strength relief of nasal congestion and allergy symptoms. Sudafed Cold & Allergy helps dry a runny nose and relieve sneezing, and itchy, watery eyes due to allergies.

Active Ingredients: Each tablet contains: Chlorpheniramine Maleate 4 mg. and Pseudoephedrine Hydrochloride 60 mg.

Inactive Ingredients: May contain: Candelilla Wax, Crospovidone, Lactose Monohydrate, Hydroxypropyl Methylcellulose, Magnesium Stearate, Microcrystalline Cellulose, Poloxamer 407, Polyethylene Glycol, Polyethylene Oxide, Potato Starch, Povidone, Pregelatinized Corn Starch, Silicon Dioxide, Sodium Lauryl Sulfate, Stearic Acid and Titanium Dioxide. See package for complete listing.

Indications: For the temporary relief of runny nose, sneezing and nasal congestion due to the common cold. For the temporary relief of runny nose, sneezing, itching of the nose or throat, itchy, watery eyes, and nasal congestion due to hay fever (allergic rhinitis).

Directions: To be given every 4 to 6 hours. Do not exceed 4 doses in 24 hours, or as directed by a doctor. Adults and children 12 years of age and over: 1 tablet. Children 6 to under 12 years of age: $1/_2$ tablet. Children under 6 years of age: consult a doctor.

Warnings: Do not exceed recommended dosage. If nervousness, dizziness, or sleeplessness occur, discontinue use and consult a doctor. If symptoms do not improve within 7 days or are accompanied by fever, consult a doctor. Do not take this product, unless directed by a doctor, if you have a breathing problem such as emphysema or chronic bronchitis, heart disease, high blood pressure, thyroid disease, diabetes, or if you have glaucoma or difficulty in urination due to enlargement of the prostate gland. May cause excitability especially in children. May cause drowsiness; alcohol, sedatives, and tranquilizers may increase the drowsiness effect. Avoid alcoholic beverages while taking this product. Do not take this product if you are taking sedatives or tranquilizers, without first consulting your doctor. Use caution when driving a motor vehicle or operating machinery. As with any drug, if you are pregnant or nursing a baby, seek the advice of a health professional before using this product. **KEEP THIS AND ALL DRUGS OUT OF THE REACH OF CHILDREN.** In case of accidental overdose, seek professional assistance or contact a Poison Control Center immediately.

Continued on next page

This product information was prepared in November 1998. On these and other Warner-Lambert Consumer Healthcare Products, detailed information may be obtained by addressing Warner-Lambert Consumer Healthcare Products, Morris Plains, NJ 07950 USA

Sudafed Cold/Allergy—Cont.

Drug Interaction Precaution: Do not use this product if you are now taking a prescription monoamine oxidase inhibitor (MAOI) (certain drugs for depression, psychiatric or emotional conditions, or Parkinson's disease), or for 2 weeks after stopping the MAOI drug. If you are uncertain whether your prescription drug contains an MAOI, consult a health professional before taking this product.

How Supplied: Boxes of 24 tablets. Store at 15° to 25° C (59°–77°F) in a dry place and protect from light.

Shown in Product Identification Guide, page 528

SUDAFED® Cold & Cough Liquid Caps

[sū 'duh-fĕd]

Description: Sudafed Cold & Cough Liquid Caps provide temporary relief of colds and coughs. Sudafed Cold & Cough helps clear nasal and chest congestion and relieve sinus pressure while relieving headaches, fever, body aches, coughs and sore throats due to colds without drowsy or overdrying side effects.

Active Ingredients: Each liquid cap contains: Acetaminophen 250 mg, Guaifenesin 100 mg, Pseudoephedrine Hydrochloride 30 mg, and Dextromethorphan Hydrobromide 10 mg.

Inactive Ingredients: D&C Yellow No. 10, FD&C Red No. 40, Gelatin, Glycerin, Polyethylene Glycol 400, Povidone, Propylene Glycol, Purified Water, and Sorbitol. Printed with edible white ink.

Indications: For the temporary relief of nasal congestion, minor aches, pains, headache, muscular aches, sore throat, and fever associated with the common cold. Temporarily relieves cough occurring with a cold. Helps loosen phlegm (mucus) and thin bronchial secretions to drain bronchial tubes and make coughs more productive.

Directions: Adults and children 12 years of age and over: 2 liquid caps every 4 hours, while symptoms persist, not to exceed 8 liquid caps in 24 hours, or as directed by a doctor. Children under 12 years of age: consult a doctor.

Warnings: Do not exceed recommended dosage. If nervousness, dizziness, or sleeplessness occur, discontinue use and consult a doctor. Do not take this product for more than 10 days. A persistent cough may be a sign of a serious condition. If symptoms do not improve of if cough persists for more than 7 days, tends to recur, or is accompanied by rash, persistent headache, fever that lasts for more than 3 days, or if new symptoms occur, consult a doctor. Do not take this product for persistent or chronic cough such as occurs with smoking, asthma, chronic bronchitis, or emphysema, or where cough is accompanied by excessive phlegm (mucus) unless directed by a doctor. If sore throat is severe, persists for more than 2 days, is accompanied or followed by fever, headache, rash, nausea, or vomiting, consult a doctor promptly. Do not take this product if you have heart disease, high blood pressure, thyroid disease, diabetes, or difficulty in urination due to enlargement of the prostate gland unless directed by a doctor. As with any drug, if you are pregnant or nursing a baby, seek the advice of a health professional before using this product. **KEEP THIS AND ALL DRUGS OUT OF THE REACH OF CHILDREN.** In case of accidental overdose, seek professional assistance or contact a Poison Control Center immediately. Prompt medical attention is critical for adults as well as for children even if you do not notice any signs or symptoms.

Alcohol Warning: If you generally consume 3 or more alcohol-containing drinks per day, you should consult your physician for advice on when and how you should take Sudafed Cold & Cough Liquid Caps and other pain relievers.

Drug Interaction Precaution: Do not use this product if you are now taking a prescription monoamine oxidase inhibitor (MAOI) (certain drugs for depression, psychiatric or emotional conditions, or Parkinson's disease), or for 2 weeks after stopping the MAOI drug. If you are uncertain whether your prescription drug contains an MAOI, consult a health professional before taking this product.

How Supplied: Boxes of 10 and 20. Store at 15° to 25°C (59°–77°F) in a dry place and protect from light.

Shown in Product Identification Guide, page 528

SUDAFED® COLD & SINUS Liquid Caps

[sū 'duh-fed]

Description: Sudafed Cold & Sinus temporarily relieves cold symptoms and sinus pain. Sudafed Cold & Sinus contains Sudafed's maximum strength nasal decongestant to help clear nasal congestion and relieve sinus pressure, plus a pain reliever to alleviate the headache, fever, sore throat, and body aches for relief without drowsy or overdrying side effects.

Active Ingredients: Each liquid cap contains: Acetaminophen 325 mg and Pseudoephedrine Hydrochloride 30 mg.

Inactive Ingredients: FD&C Blue No. 1, FD&C Red No. 40, Gelatin, Glycerin, Pharmaceutical Glaze, Polyethylene Glycol, Povidone, Purified Water, Sodium Acetate, Sorbitol Special, and Titanium Dioxide.

Indications: For the temporary relief of nasal congestion, minor aches, pains, headache, muscular aches, sore throat, and fever due to the common cold. Temporarily relieves nasal congestion associated with sinusitis. Reduces swelling of nasal passages; shrinks swollen membranes. Promotes nasal and/or sinus drainage; temporarily relieves sinus congestion and pressure. Temporarily restores freer breathing through the nose.

Directions: Adults and children 12 years of age and over: 2 liquid caps every 4 to 6 hours, while symptoms persist, not to exceed 8 liquid caps in 24 hours, or as directed by a doctor. Children under 12 years of age: consult a doctor.

Warnings: Do not exceed recommended dosage. If nervousness, dizziness, or sleeplessness occur, discontinue use and consult a doctor. Do not take this product for more than 10 days. If symptoms do not improve or are accompanied by fever that lasts for more than 3 days, or if new symptoms occur, consult a doctor. If sore throat is severe, persists for more than 2 days, is accompanied or followed by fever, headache, rash, nausea, or vomiting, consult a doctor promptly. Do not take this product if you have heart disease, high blood pressure, thyroid disease, diabetes, or difficulty in urination due to enlargement of the prostate gland unless directed by a doctor. As with any drug, if you are pregnant or nursing a baby, seek the advice of a health professional before using this product. **KEEP THIS AND ALL DRUGS OUT OF THE REACH OF CHILDREN.** In case of accidental overdose, seek professional assistance or contact a Poison Control Center immediately. Prompt medical attention is critical for adults as well as for children even if you do not notice any signs or symptoms.

Alcohol Warning: If you generally consume 3 or more alcohol-containing drinks per day, you should consult your physician for advice on when and how you should take Sudafed Cold & Sinus Liquid Caps and other pain relievers.

Drug Interaction Precaution: Do not use this product if you are now taking a prescription monoamine oxidase inhibitor (MAOI) (certain drugs for depression, psychiatric or emotional conditions, or Parkinson's disease), or for 2 weeks after stopping the MAOI drug. If you are uncertain whether your prescription drug contains an MAOI, consult a health professional before taking this product.

How Supplied: Boxes of 10 and 20 liquid caps. Store at 15° to 25°C (59° to 77°F) in a dry place and protect from light.

Shown in Product Identification Guide, page 527

SUDAFED® NON-DRYING SINUS LIQUID CAPS

[sū 'duh-fĕd]

Description: Sudafed Non-Drying Sinus provides temporary, maximum strength relief of nasal congestion and sinus pressure due to sinusitis, colds, or allergies. Sudafed Non-Drying Sinus contains ingredients that help clear nasal congestion, relieve sinus pressure without overdrying sensitive nasal tissue or causing drowsiness and temporarily relieves chest congestion.

Active Ingredients: Each liquid cap contains Guaifenesin 200 mg. and Pseudoephedrine Hydrochloride 30 mg.

Inactive Ingredients: FD&C Blue No. 1, Gelatin, Glycerin, Polyethylene Glycol 400, Povidone, Propylene Glycol and Sorbitol. Printed with edible white ink.

Indications: For the temporary relief of nasal congestion associated with sinusitis. Promotes nasal and/or sinus drainage; temporarily relieves sinus congestion and pressure. Helps loosen phlegm (mucus) and thin bronchial secretions to rid the bronchial passageways of bothersome mucus and make coughs more productive.

Directions: Adults and children 12 years of age and over: swallow 2 liquid caps every 4 hours, not to exceed 8 liquid caps in 24 hours, or as directed by a doctor. Children under 12 years of age: consult a doctor.

Warnings: Do not exceed recommended dosage. If nervousness, dizziness, or sleeplessness occur, discontinue use and consult a doctor. If symptoms do not improve within 7 days or are accompanied by fever, consult a doctor. Do not take this product if you have heart disease, high blood pressure, thyroid disease, diabetes, or difficulty in urination due to enlargement of the prostate gland unless directed by a doctor. A persistent cough may be a sign of a serious condition. If cough persists for more than 1 week, tends to recur, or is accompanied by a fever, rash, or persistent headache, consult a doctor. Do not take this product for persistent or chronic cough such as occurs with smoking, asthma, chronic bronchitis, or emphysema, or where cough is accompanied by excessive phlegm (mucus) unless directed by a doctor. As with any drug, if you are pregnant or nursing a baby, seek the advice of a health professional before using this product. **KEEP THIS AND ALL DRUGS OUT OF THE REACH OF CHILDREN.** In case of accidental overdose, seek professional assistance or contact a Poison Control Center immediately.

Drug Interaction Precaution: Do not use this product if you are now taking a prescription monoamine oxidase inhibitor (MAOI) (certain drugs for depression, psychiatric or emotional conditions, or Parkinson's disease), or for 2 weeks after stopping the MAOI drug. If you are uncertain whether your prescription drug contains an MAOI, consult a health professional before taking this product.

How Supplied: Sudafed Non-Drying Sinus is supplied in boxes of 24 liquid caps.

Store at 15° to 25°C (59° to 77°F) in a dry place and protect from light.
Shown in Product Identification Guide, page 528

SUDAFED® Severe Cold Formula Caplets and Tablets
[sū 'duh-fĕd]

Description: Sudafed Severe Cold Formula contains maximum strength ingredients to temporarily relieve the worst cold symptoms. Sudafed Severe Cold Formula helps clear nasal congestion and relieve sinus pressure while relieving headaches, fever, body aches, coughs and sore throats due to colds without drowsy or overdrying side effects.

Active Ingredients: Each coated caplet/tablet contains: Acetaminophen 500 mg, Pseudoephedrine Hydrochloride 30 mg, and Dextromethorphan Hydrobromide 15 mg.

Inactive Ingredients: May contain: Candelilla or Carnauba Wax, Crospovidone, Hydroxypropyl Methylcellulose, Magnesium Stearate, Microcrystalline Cellulose, Poloxamer 407 NF, Polyethylene Glycol, Polyethylene Oxide NF, Povidone, Pregelatinized Corn Starch, Silicon Dioxide, Sodium Lauryl Sulfate NF, Stearic Acid and Titanium Dioxide. See package for complete listing.

Indications: For the temporary relief of nasal congestion, minor aches, pains, headache, muscular aches, sore throat, and fever associated with the common cold. Temporarily relieves cough occurring with a cold.

Directions: Adults and children 12 years of age and over: 2 caplets or tablets every 6 hours, while symptoms persist, not to exceed 8 caplets or tablets in 24 hours, or as directed by a doctor. Children under 12 years of age: consult a doctor.

Warnings: Do not exceed recommended dosage. If nervousness, dizziness, or sleeplessness occur, discontinue use and consult a doctor. Do not take this product for more than 10 days. A persistent cough may be a sign of a serious condition. If symptoms do not improve or if cough persists for more than 7 days, tends to recur, or is accompanied by rash, persistent headache, fever that lasts for more than 3 days, or if new symptoms occur, consult a doctor. Do not take this product for persistent or chronic cough such as occurs with smoking, asthma or emphysema, or if cough is accompanied by excessive phlegm (mucus) unless directed by a doctor. If sore throat is severe, persists for more than 2 days, is accompanied or followed by fever, headache, rash, nausea, or vomiting, consult a doctor promptly. Do not take this product if you have heart disease, high blood pressure, thyroid disease, diabetes, or difficulty in urination due to enlarge-

ment of the prostate gland unless directed by a doctor. As with any drug, if you are pregnant or nursing a baby, seek the advice of a health professional before using this product. **KEEP THIS AND ALL DRUGS OUT OF THE REACH OF CHILDREN.** In case of accidental overdose, seek professional assistance or contact a Poison Control Center immediately. Prompt medical attention is critical for adults as well as for children even if you do not notice any signs or symptoms.

Alcohol Warning: If you generally consume 3 or more alcohol-containing drinks per day, you should consult your physician for advice on when and how you should take Sudafed Severe Cold Formula and other pain relievers.

Drug Interaction Precaution: Do not use this product if you are now taking a prescription monoamine oxidase inhibitor (MAOI) (certain drugs for depression, psychiatric or emotional conditions, or Parkinson's disease), or for 2 weeks after stopping the MAOI drug. If you are uncertain whether your prescription drug contains an MAOI, consult a health professional before taking this product.

How Supplied: Boxes of 12 and 24 caplets; boxes of 12 tablets.
Store at 15° to 25°C (59°–77°F) in a dry place and protect from light.
Shown in Product Identification Guide, page 527

SUDAFED® Sinus Caplets and Tablets
[sū 'duh-fĕd]

Description: Sudafed Sinus contains Sudafed's maximum strength decongestant and a maximum strength pain reliever to temporarily relieve sinus symptoms. Sudafed Sinus helps clear nasal congestion and relieve sinus pressure while relieving sinus headaches due to sinusitis, allergies or colds without drowsy or overdrying side effects.

Active Ingredients: Each coated caplet/tablet contains: Acetaminophen 500 mg and Pseudoephedrine Hydrochloride 30 mg.

Inactive Ingredients: Caplets and Tablets contain Crospovidone, FD&C Yellow No. 6 Aluminum Lake, Hydroxypropyl Methylcellulose, Microcrystalline Cellulose, Polyethylene Glycol, Polysor-

Continued on next page

This product information was prepared in November 1998. On these and other Warner-Lambert Consumer Healthcare Products, detailed information may be obtained by addressing Warner-Lambert Consumer Healthcare Products, Morris Plains, NJ 07950 USA

Sudafed Sinus—Cont.

bate 80, Povidone, Pregelatinized Starch, Stearic Acid and Titanium Dioxide.

May also contain: Carnauba Wax or Candelilla Wax, Calcium Stearate, Magnesium Stearate and Croscarmellose Sodium. See package for complete listing.

Indications: For the temporary relief of nasal congestion associated with sinusitis. Helps decongest sinus openings and passages; temporarily relieves sinus congestion and pressure. Temporarily relieves headache, minor aches, and pains. Temporarily restores freer breathing through the nose.

Directions: Adults and children 12 years and over: 2 caplets or tablets every 6 hours, while symptoms persist, not to exceed 8 caplets or tablets in 24 hours, or as directed by a doctor. Children under 12 years of age: consult a doctor.

Warnings: Do not exceed recommended dosage. If nervousness, dizziness, or sleeplessness occur, discontinue use and consult a doctor. Do not take this product for more than 10 days. If symptoms do not improve or are accompanied by fever that lasts for more than 3 days, or if new symptoms occur, consult a doctor. Do not take this product if you have heart disease, high blood pressure, thyroid disease, diabetes, or difficulty in urination due to enlargement of the prostate gland unless directed by a doctor. As with any drug, if you are pregnant or nursing a baby, seek the advice of a health professional before using this product. **KEEP THIS AND ALL DRUGS OUT OF THE REACH OF CHILDREN.** In case of accidental overdose, seek professional assistance or contact a Poison Control Center immediately. Prompt medical attention is critical for adults as well as for children even if you do not notice any signs or symptoms.

Alcohol Warning: If you generally consume 3 or more alcohol-containing drinks per day, you should consult your physician for advice on when and how you should take Sudafed Sinus and other pain relievers.

Drug Interaction Precaution: Do not use this product if you are now taking a prescription monoamine oxidase inhibitor (MAOI) (certain drugs for depression, psychiatric or emotional conditions, or Parkinson's disease), or for 2 weeks after stopping the MAOI drug. If you are uncertain whether your prescription drug contains an MAOI, consult a health professional before taking this product.

How Supplied: Box of 24.
Store at 15° to 25°C (59° to 77°F) in a dry place and protect from light.
Shown in Product Identification Guide, page 528

TUCKS®
Pre-moistened Hemorrhoidal/Vaginal Pads
[tŭks]

Active Ingredients: Soft pads are pre-moistened with a solution containing Witch Hazel 50%.

Inactive Ingredients: Water, Glycerin, Alcohol, Propylene Glycol, Sodium Citrate, Diazolidinyl Urea, Citric Acid, Methylparaben, Propylparaben.

Indications: For the temporary relief of external itching, burning and irritation associated with hemorrhoids.

Other Uses:
Hygienic Wipe: Tucks Pads are effective for everyday personal hygienic use on outer rectal and vaginal areas. Used in place of toilet tissue, Tucks Pads gently and thoroughly remove irritation-causing matter. They are especially handy during menstrual periods.
Moist Compress: For additional relief, Tucks Pads can be folded and used as a compress on inflamed tissue. Tucks Pads are particularly helpful in relieving discomfort following childbirth, rectal or vaginal surgery.

Directions: For external use only. *As a hemorrhoidal treatment* —Adults: When practical, cleanse the affected area with mild soap and warm water and rinse thoroughly. Gently dry by patting or blotting with toilet tissue or soft cloth before application of this product. Gently apply to affected area by patting and then discard. Can be used up to six times daily or after each bowel movement. Children under 12 years of age: consult a physician.
As a hygienic wipe —Use as a wipe instead of toilet tissue.
As a moist compress —For soothing relief, fold pad and place in contact with irritated tissue. Leave in place for 5 to 15 minutes. Repeat as needed.

Warnings: If condition worsens or does not improve within 7 days, consult a physician. Do not exceed recommended daily dosage unless directed by a physician. In case of bleeding, consult a physician promptly. Do not put this product in the rectum by using fingers or any mechanical device or applicator. **Keep this and all drugs out of the reach of children.** In case of accidental ingestion, seek professional assistance or contact a Poison Control Center immediately.

How Supplied: Jars of 40 and 100 pads. Also available Tucks Take-Alongs®; individual foil-wrapped towelettes.
Shown in Product Identification Guide, page 528

ZANTAC® 75
Ranitidine Tablets 75 mg
Acid Reducer
[zan ' tak]

Active Ingredient: Each tablet contains: 84 mg ranitidine hydrochloride (equivalent to 75 mg ranitidine).

Inactive Ingredients: Hydroxypropyl methylcellulose, magnesium stearate, microcrystalline cellulose, synthetic red iron oxide, titanium dioxide and triacetin. Zantac 75 tablets are sodium and sugar free.

Uses:
• For **relief** of heartburn associated with acid indigestion and sour stomach.
• For **prevention** of heartburn associated with acid indigestion and sour stomach brought on by certain foods and beverages.

Directions:
• For **relief** of symptoms, swallow 1 tablet with a glass of water.
• To **prevent** symptoms, swallow 1 tablet with a glass of water **30 to 60 minutes before** eating food or drinking beverages that cause heartburn.
• Can be used up to twice daily (up to 2 tablets in 24 hours).
• This product should not be given to children under 12 years old unless directed by a doctor.

Warnings:
• **Allergy Warning:** Do not use if you are allergic to Zantac (ranitidine hydrochloride) or other acid reducers.
• Do not use with other acid reducers.
• Do not take the maximum daily dose for more than 14 consecutive days, unless directed by your doctor.
• If you have trouble swallowing or persistent abdominal pain, see your doctor promptly. You may have a serious condition that may need different treatment.
• As with any drug, if you are pregnant or nursing a baby, seek the advice of a health professional before using this product.
• Keep this and all drugs out of the reach of children.
• In case of accidental overdose, seek professional assistance or contact a poison control center immediately.

Read the Label: Read the directions, consumer information leaflet and warnings before use. Keep the carton. It contains important information.

How Supplied: Zantac 75 is available in convenient blister packs in boxes of 4, 10, 20 and 30 tablets, and in bottles of 60, 80 and 90 count. Store between 2°C and 30°C (30°F and 86°F). Avoid excessive heat or humidity.

Zantac is a registered trademark of the Glaxo Wellcome group of companies.

Questions or Comments? Call us Toll-Free at 1-800-223-0182 weekdays between 9:00 am and 5:00 pm EST.
Shown in Product Identification Guide, page 528

**IF YOU SUSPECT
AN INTERACTION...**
The 1,800-page
PDR Companion Guide™ can help.
Use the order form
in the front of this book.

Wellness International Network, Ltd.
5800 DEMOCRACY DRIVE
PLANO, TX 75024

Direct Inquiries to:
Director, Product Development
(972) 245-1097
FAX: (972) 389-3060

BIO-COMPLEX 5000™
Gentle Foaming Cleanser

Uses: BIO-COMPLEX 5000™ Gentle Foaming Cleanser, with alpha-hydroxy acids, aloe vera and botanical infusions, is an advanced cleansing gel designed for all skin types. BIO-COMPLEX 5000 Gentle Foaming Cleanser protects the skin and works to restore elasticity while gently removing surface impurities, make-up and pollution.

Ingredients: Aloe Vera Gel, Infusion of Sage, Infusion of Chamomile, Ammonium Lauryl Sulfate, Lauramidopropyl Betaine, Glycerin, Lauramide DEA, Cetyl Betaine, Tocopherol, Citric Acid, Lactic Acid, Malic Acid, Ascorbic Acid, Methylchloroisothiazolinone, Methylisothiazolinone, Propylparaben, Methylparaben.

Directions: Splash warm water onto face. Place a small amount of gel on fingertips. Apply evenly to face and neck in circular motions, massaging skin gently but thoroughly. Rinse completely and pat dry with a soft towel.

How Supplied: 8 fluid ounce/236 ml. bottle.

BIO-COMPLEX 5000™
Revitalizing Conditioner

Uses: BIO-COMPLEX 5000™ Revitalizing Conditioner, with vitamins, antioxidants, and sunscreen, helps restore moisture to dried-out, heat-styled hair. This advanced conditioner contains silkening agents which enhance the hair as well as detangle it after shampooing. Hair is left clean, soft, manageable, and protected against styling aids and environmental elements. BIO-COMPLEX 5000 Revitalizing Conditioner is excellent for all hair types, especially damaged or over-processed hair.

Ingredients: Water, Stearyl Alcohol, Propylene Glycol, Stearamidopropyl Dimethalymine, Cyclomethicone, Polyquaternium - 11, Stearalkonium Chloride, Cetearyl Alcohol, PEG - 40 Hydrogenated Castor Oil, Citric Acid, Tocopherol, Ascorbic Acid, Retinyl Palmitate, Octyl Methoxycinnamate, Awapuhi Fragrance, Ceteth - 20, Soluble Animal Keratin, Imidazolidinyl Urea, Propylparaben, Methylparaben.

Directions: After shampooing with BIO-COMPLEX 5000™ Revitalizing Shampoo, apply to wet hair. Massage through hair, paying special attention to the ends. Leave on 2–3 minutes. Rinse thoroughly. Towel dry and style as usual.

How Supplied: 12 fluid ounce bottle.

BIO-COMPLEX 5000™
Revitalizing Shampoo

Uses: BIO-COMPLEX 5000™ Revitalizing Shampoo, with vitamins, antioxidants, and sunscreen, cleanses and moisturizes hair for excellent manageability. Specially formulated with the essence of awapuhi, a Hawaiian ginger plant extract known for its healing qualities, this formula contains the mildest blend of surfactants and a wealth of natural conditioning ingredients to provide body, luster and healthier-looking hair.

Ingredients: Water, Ammonium Lauryl Sulfate, Tea Lauryl Sulfate, Cetyl Betaine, Lauramide DEA, Cocamidopropyl Betaine, Glycerin, Ascorbic Acid, Tocopherol, Retinyl Palmitate, Citric Acid, Hydrolyzed Wheat Protein, Awapuhi Fragrance, Octyl Methoxycinnamate, PEG - 7 Glyceryl Cocoate, Methylchloroisothiazolinone, Methylisothiazolinone, Caramel.

Directions: Apply a small amount to wet hair and massage gently into scalp, creating a generous lather. Rinse and repeat if necessary. To further intensify this reconstructive process, follow with BIO-COMPLEX 5000™ Revitalizing Conditioner.

How Supplied: 12 fluid ounce bottle.

STEPHAN™ BIO-NUTRITIONAL
Daytime Hydrating Creme

Uses: Hypo-allergenic STEPHAN™ BIO-NUTRITIONAL Daytime Hydrating Creme hydrates the skin and preserves the moisture level of the upper layers of the epidermis. It is an excellent day cream for both men and women who wish to combat the visible signs of aging skin, the appearance of wrinkles or lines, and the inelastic look of facial features and contours. These light emulsions are absorbed rapidly, leaving an invisible protective film which hydrates the epidermis, regulates moisture levels and leaves skin feeling supple and soft.

Ingredients: Purified Water, Stearic Acid, Isodecyl Neopentanoate, Isostearyl Stearoyl Stearate, DEA-Cetyl Phosphate, C12-15 Alkyl Benzoate, Tocopherol, Aloe Barbadensis Gel, Squalane, Cetyl Esters, Benzophenone-3, Dimethicone, Fragrance, Carbomer, Triethanolamine, Imidazolidinyl Urea, Propylparaben, Methylparaben, Annatto.

Directions: Apply evenly on a completely cleansed face and neck. May be used around the eye area, avoiding direct contact with the eyes. Suitable for all skin types. For best results, use in conjunction with the complete STEPHAN BIO-NUTRITIONAL Skin Care line.

Warnings: For external use only. Avoid contact with eyes.

How Supplied: Net Wt. 1.75 oz.

STEPHAN™ BIO-NUTRITIONAL
Eye-Firming Concentrate

Uses: Hypo-allergenic STEPHAN™ BIO-NUTRITIONAL Eye-Firming Concentrate is specially formulated to revitalize the delicate area around the eyes. This non-oily fluid pampers sensitive eyes while reducing the look of puffiness and dark circles, and smoothing and softening the appearance of fine lines in the eye area.

Ingredients: Purified Water, Cornflower Extract, Methylsilanol Hydroxyproline Aspartate, Methyl Gluceth-20, Dimethicone Copolyol, PEG-30 Glyceryl Laurate, Horsetail Extract, Panthenol, Propylene Glycol, Carbomer, Disodium EDTA, Triethanolamine, Xanthan Gum, Diazolidinyl Urea, Methylparaben, Propylparaben.

Directions: Apply in the morning, or any time of the day, in small quantities to the skin around the eyes with light, tapping motions, avoiding direct contact with the eyes. In the evening, apply gently to the entire eye contour area. For best results, use in conjunction with the complete STEPHAN BIO-NUTRITIONAL Skin Care line.

Warnings: For external use only. Avoid direct contact with eyes.

How Supplied: 1 fl. oz.

STEPHAN™ BIO-NUTRITIONAL
Nightime Moisture Creme

Uses: Hypo-allergenic STEPHAN™ BIO-NUTRITIONAL Nightime Moisture Creme is a heavier, richer cream for mature, dry or sun-damaged skin. This advanced formula is excellent for dehydrated skin, promoting suppleness and moisture, while improving the appearance of fine lines and wrinkles.

Ingredients: Purified Water, Caprylic/Capric Triglyceride, Propylene, Glycol/Dicaprylate/Dicaprate, Stearic Acid, Polysorbate 60, Cetyl Alcohol, Octyl Palmitate, Beeswax, Sorbitan Stearate, Canola Oil, Avocado Oil, Safflower Oil, Squalane, Lecithin (Liposomes), Soluble Collagen, Dimethicone, Bisabolol, Aloe Barbadensis Gel, Fragrance, C12–15 Alkyl Benzoate, Hydroxyethylcellulose, Octyl Methoxycinnamate, Disodium EDTA, Sodium Borate, Benzophenone-3, Allantoin, Potassium Sorbate, Phenoxyethanol, Methylparaben, Propylparaben, Butylparaben, Ethylparaben, D&C Yellow No. 10, Caramel.

Continued on next page

Stephan Nightime—Cont.

Directions: In the evening, apply by lightly massaging onto a thoroughly cleansed face and neck. Avoid direct contact with eyes. For drier skin, it may be used during the day as a moisturizer, under make-up or after sun bathing. For best results, use in conjunction with the complete STEPHAN BIO-NUTRITIONAL Skin Care line.

Warning: For external use only. Avoid contact with eyes.

How Supplied: Net Wt. 1.75 oz.

STEPHAN™ BIO-NUTRITIONAL
Refreshing Moisture Gel

Uses: Hypo-allergenic STEPHAN™ BIO-NUTRITIONAL Refreshing Moisture Gel is specially formulated to refine pores and promote a clear, clean and smooth-looking complexion. It is designed to deeply cleanse and super-stimulate the skin. This gel is suitable for all skin types, especially problem areas. A quick "pick-me-up," STEPHAN BIO-NUTRITIONAL Refreshing Moisture Gel immediately restores the radiant, firm and youthful appearance of the face while acting as a cumulative, revitalizing beauty treatment.

Ingredients: Water, Propylene Glycol, Glycerin, Hydroxyethylcellulose, Sugar Cane Extract, Citrus Extract, Apple Extract, Green Tea Extract, Hydrolyzed Wheat Protein, Tissue Respiratory Factors, Panthenol, Aloe Vera Gel, Laureth-4, Magnesium Aluminum Silicate, Tetrasodium EDTA, Benzophenone-3, Imidazolidinyl Urea, Methylchloroisothiazolinone, Methylisothiazolinone, Methylparaben, Propylparaben, Phenethyl Alcohol, FD&C Yellow No. 10, FD&C Red No. 40, FD&C Yellow No. 5.

Directions: After thoroughly cleansing in the morning or evening, apply a liberal layer to the face, neck and eye area, avoiding eye contact. Remove after 20–30 minutes with warm water. Suitable for all skin types. For best results, use in conjunction with the complete STEPHAN BIO-NUTRITIONAL Skin Care line.

Warnings: For external use only. Avoid contact with eyes.

How Supplied: Net Wt. 1.75 oz.

STEPHAN™ BIO-NUTRITIONAL
Ultra Hydrating Fluid

Uses: Hypo-allergenic STEPHAN™ BIO-NUTRITIONAL Ultra Hydrating Fluid is a complete treatment formulated to soften fine lines and preserve youthful-looking, radiant skin. By utilizing ingredients focused on revitalization, STEPHAN BIO-NUTRITIONAL Ultra Hydrating Fluid possesses a progressive firming effect, helping to combat the aged look of skin due to external negative conditions.

Ingredients: Purified Water, Methyl Gluceth-20, Dimethicone Copolyol, Peg-30 Glyceryl Laurate, Panthenol Sugar Cane Extract, Citrus Extract, Apple Extract, Green Tea Extract, Live Yeast Cell Derivative, Laureth-4, Plant Pseudocollagen, Hydrolyzed Wheat Protein, Methylchloroisothiazolinone, Methylisothiazolinone, Methylsilanol Hydroxyproline Aspartate, Phenethyl Alcohol, 2-Bromo-2-Nitropropane-1, 3-Diol, Xanthan Gum, Disodium EDTA, Methylparaben, Propylparaben.

Directions: Gently apply all over the face, neck and eye contour area, preferably in the morning. Use as a part of a regular daily skin care routine or as an occasional preventive treatment. For best results, use in conjunction with the complete STEPHAN BIO-NUTRITIONAL Skin Care line.

Warnings: For external use only. Avoid direct contact with eyes.

How Supplied: 1 fl. oz.

Whitehall-Robins Healthcare
American Home Products Corporation
FIVE GIRALDA FARMS
MADISON, NJ 07940

Direct Inquiries to:
Whitehall Consumer Product Information 800-322-3129
Robins Consumer Product Information 800-762-4672

ADVIL®
[ad 'vĭl]
Ibuprofen Tablets, USP
Ibuprofen Caplets
(Oval-Shaped Tablets)
Ibuprofen Gel Caplets
(Oval-Shaped Gelatin Coated Tablets)

WARNING: ASPIRIN-SENSITIVE PATIENTS. Do not take this product if you have had a severe allergic reaction to aspirin, e.g.— asthma, swelling, shock or hives, because even though this product contains no aspirin or salicylates, cross-reactions may occur in patients allergic to aspirin.

Active Ingredient: Each tablet or caplet contains Ibuprofen 200 mg.

Inactive Ingredients: Tablets and Caplets Acetylated Monoglyceride, Beeswax and/or Carnauba Wax, Croscarmellose Sodium, Iron Oxides, Lecithin, Methylparaben, Microcrystalline Cellulose, Pharmaceutical Glaze, Povidone, Propyl-paraben, Silicon Dioxide, Simethicone, Sodium Benzoate, Sodium Lauryl Sulfate, Starch, Stearic Acid, Sucrose, Titanium Dioxide. Gel Caplets Croscarmellose Sodium, FD&C Red 40, FD&C Yellow 6, Gelatin, Glycerin, Hydroxypropyl Methylcellulose, Iron Oxides, Lecithin, Pharmaceutical Glaze, Propyl Gallate, Silicon Dioxide, Simethicone, Sodium Lauryl Sulfate, Starch, Stearic Acid, Titanium Dioxide, Triacetin.

Indications: For the temporary relief of minor aches and pains associated with the common cold, headache, toothache, muscular aches, backache, for the minor pain of arthritis, for the pain of menstrual cramps and for reduction of fever.

Dosage and Administration: Adults: Take one tablet or caplet every 4 to 6 hours while symptoms persist. If pain or fever does not respond to one tablet or caplet, two tablets or caplets may be used but do not exceed six tablets or caplets in 24 hours unless directed by a doctor. The smallest effective dose should be used. Take with food or milk if occasional and mild heartburn, upset stomach, or stomach pain occurs with use. Consult a doctor if these symptoms are more than mild or if they persist. Children: Do not give this product to children under 12 years of age except under the advice and supervision of a doctor.

Warnings: Do not take for pain for more than 10 days or for fever for more than 3 days unless directed by a doctor. If pain or fever persists or gets worse, if new symptoms occur, or if the painful area is red or swollen, consult a doctor. These could be signs of serious illness. If you are under a doctor's care for any serious condition, consult a doctor before taking this product. As with aspirin and acetaminophen, if you have any condition which requires you to take prescription drugs or if you have had any problems or serious side effects from taking any nonprescription pain reliever, do not take this product without first discussing it with your doctor. **IF YOU EXPERIENCE ANY SYMPTOMS WHICH ARE UNUSUAL OR SEEM UNRELATED TO THE CONDITION FOR WHICH YOU TOOK IBUPROFEN, CONSULT A DOCTOR BEFORE TAKING ANY MORE OF IT.** Although ibuprofen is indicated for the same conditions as aspirin and acetaminophen, it should not be taken with them except under a doctor's direction. Do not combine this product with any other ibuprofen-containing product. As with any drug, if you are pregnant or nursing a baby, seek the advice of a health professional before using this product. **IT IS ESPECIALLY IMPORTANT NOT TO USE IBUPROFEN DURING THE LAST 3 MONTHS OF PREGNANCY UNLESS SPECIFICALLY DIRECTED TO DO SO BY A DOCTOR BECAUSE IT MAY CAUSE PROBLEMS IN THE UNBORN CHILD OR COMPLICATIONS DURING DELIVERY.** Keep this and all drugs out of the reach of children. In case of accidental overdose, seek professional assistance or contact a poison control center immediately.

How Supplied: Coated tablets in bottles of 8, 24, 50 (non-child resistant size), 100, 165 and 250. Coated caplets in bottles of 24, 50 (non-child resistant size), 72 (E-Z Cap) 100, 165, and 250. Coated tablets in thermoform packaging of 8.
Gel caplets in bottles of 8, 24, 50, 100, 165 and 250.

Storage: Store at room temperature; avoid excessive heat (40°C, 104°F).

Advil® Liqui-Gels
Solubilized ibuprofen capsules, 200 mg

ADVIL® Cold and Sinus
Ibuprofen/Pseudoephedrine HCl Caplets* and Tablets
Pain Reliever/Fever Reducer/Nasal Decongestant

---

*Oval-Shaped tablets

WARNING: ASPIRIN-SENSITIVE PATIENTS. Do not take this product if you have had a severe allergic reaction to aspirin, eg, asthma, swelling, shock or hives, because even though this product contains no aspirin or salicylates, cross-reactions may occur in patients allergic to aspirin.

Indications: For temporary relief of symptoms associated with the common cold, sinusitis or flu, including nasal congestion, headache, fever, body aches, and pains.

Directions: *Adults:* Take 1 caplet or tablet every 4 to 6 hours while symptoms persist. If symptoms do not respond to 1 caplet or tablet, 2 caplets or tablets may be used, but do not exceed 6 caplets or tablets in 24 hours unless directed by a doctor. The smallest effective dose should be used. Take with food or milk if occasional and mild heartburn, upset stomach, or stomach pain occurs with use. Consult a doctor if these symptoms are more than mild or if they persist. *Children:* Do not give this product to children under 12 years of age except under the advice and supervision of a doctor.

Warnings: Do not take for colds for more than 7 days or for fever for more than 3 days unless directed by a doctor. If the cold or fever persists or gets worse, or if new symptoms occur, consult a doctor. These could be signs of serious illness. As with aspirin and acetaminophen, if you have any condition which requires you to take prescription drugs or if you have had any problems or serious side effects from taking any nonprescription pain reliever, do not take this product without first discussing it with your doctor. IF YOU EXPERIENCE ANY SYMPTOMS WHICH ARE UNUSUAL OR SEEM UNRELATED TO THE CONDITION FOR WHICH YOU TOOK THIS PRODUCT,

CONSULT A DOCTOR BEFORE TAKING ANY MORE OF IT. If you are under a doctor's care for any serious condition, consult a doctor before taking this product.
Do not exceed recommended dosage. If nervousness, dizziness, or sleeplessness occur, discontinue use and consult a doctor. Do not take this product if you have high blood pressure, heart disease, diabetes, thyroid disease or difficulty in urination due to enlargement of the prostate gland, except under the advice and supervision of a doctor.
Drug Interaction Precaution: Do not use if you are now taking a prescription monoamine oxidase inhibitor (MAOI) (certain drugs for depression, psychiatric or emotional conditions, or Parkinson's disease), or for 2 weeks after stopping the MAOI drug. If you are uncertain whether your prescription drug contains an MAOI, consult a health professional before taking this product. Do not combine this product with other non-prescription pain relievers. Do not combine this product with any other ibuprofen-containing product. As with any drug, if you are pregnant or nursing a baby, seek the advice of a health professional before using this product.
IT IS ESPECIALLY IMPORTANT NOT TO USE THIS PRODUCT DURING THE LAST 3 MONTHS OF PREGNANCY UNLESS SPECIFICALLY DIRECTED TO DO SO BY A DOCTOR BECAUSE IT MAY CAUSE PROBLEMS IN THE UNBORN CHILD OR COMPLICATIONS DURING DELIVERY. Keep this and all drugs out of the reach of children. In case of accidental overdose, seek professional assistance or contact a poison control center immediately.

Active Ingredients: Each caplet or tablet contains Ibuprofen 200 mg and Pseudoephedrine HCl 30 mg.

Inactive Ingredients: Carnauba or Equivalent Wax, Croscarmellose Sodium, Iron Oxides, Methylparaben, Microcrystalline Cellulose, Propylparaben, Silicon Dioxide, Sodium Benzoate, Sodium Lauryl Sulfate, Starch, Stearic Acid, Sucrose, Titanium Dioxide.

How Supplied: Advil® Cold and Sinus is an oval-shaped tan-colored caplet or tan-colored tablet. The caplet is supplied in blister packs of 20 and 40. The tablet is available in blister packs of 20.

Storage: Store at room temperature; avoid excessive heat (40°C, 104°F).

CHILDREN'S ADVIL®
Oral Suspension
Junior Strength Advil Tablets
Pediatric Advil Drops
[ad ' vil]
Ibuprofen

Oral Suspension

Description: Children's Advil® Ibuprofen Oral Suspension is an alcohol-free, fruit-flavored liquid specially devel-

oped for children. Each 5 mL (teaspoon) contains ibuprofen 100 mg. Each Junior Strength Advil Coated Tablet contains ibuprofen 100 mg. Each 2.5 mL (½ teaspoon) of Pediatric Advil Drops contains ibuprofen 100 mg.

Inactive Ingredients (Children's Advil Oral Suspension, Pediatric Advil Drops): Artificial flavors, Carboxymethylcellulose Sodium, Citric Acid, Edetate Disodium, FD&C Red No. 40, FD&C Blue No. 1 (grape flavor only) Glycerin, Microcrystalline Cellulose, Polysorbate 80, Purified Water, Sodium Benzoate, Sorbitol Solution, Sucrose, Xanthan Gum.

Inactive Ingredients (Junior Strength Advil Tablets): Acetylated monoglycerides, Carnauba Wax, Colloidal Silicon Dioxide, Croscarmellose Sodium, Iron Oxides, Methylparaben, Microcrystalline Cellulose, Povidone, Pregelatinized Starch, Propylene Glycol, Propylparaben, Shellac, Sodium Benzoate, Starch, Stearic Acid, Sucrose, and Titanium Dioxide.

Indications: Children's Advil® Ibuprofen Oral Suspension, Junior Strength Advil Tablets, and Pediatric Advil Drops are indicated for the temporary relief of fever, and minor aches and pains due to colds, flu, sore throat, headaches and toothaches. One dose lasts 6–8 hours.

WARNINGS:
ASPIRIN SENSITIVE CHILDREN:
- Although this product dose not contain aspirin, it may cause a severe reaction in people allergic to aspirin
- Do not give to children who have had any of the following reactions to any pain reliever/fever reducer: allergic reaction, difficulty breathing, shock, asthma, hives, or swelling.

CALL YOUR DOCTOR IF:
- Your child is under a doctor's care for any serious condition or is taking any other drug.
- Your child has problems or serious side effects from taking fever reducers or pain relievers.
- Your child does not get any relief within first day (24 hours) of treatment or pain or fever gets worse.
- Stomach upset gets worse or lasts.
- Redness or swelling is present in the painful area.
- Sore throat is severe, lasts for more than two days or occurs with fever, headache, rash, nausea or vomiting.
- Any new symptoms appear.

DO NOT USE:
- With any other product that contains ibuprofen, or any other pain reliever/fever reducer, unless directed by a doctor.
- For more than 3 days for fever or pain unless directed by a doctor.
- For stomach pain unless directed by a doctor.
- If your child is dehydrated (significant fluid loss) due to continued vomiting, diarrhea or lack of fluid intake.
- CHILDREN'S ADVIL ORAL SUSPENSION: If plastic bottle wrap imprinted "CHILDREN'S ADVIL SAFETY SEALED" is broken or missing; JUNIOR STRENGTH ADVIL: if

Continued on next page

Children's Advil—Cont.

carton is open or foil seal imprinted "SEALED FOR YOUR PROTECTION" under cap is broken or missing when purchased; PEDIATRIC ADVIL DROPS: If breakable ring on bottle cap is separated.

IMPORTANT:
- Keep this and all drugs out of the reach of children. In case of accidental overdose, seek professional assistance or contact a poison control center immediately.
- If stomach upset occurs while taking this product, give with food or milk.

Directions (Children's Advil Oral Suspension): Shake well before using. Find right dose on chart. If possible, use weight to dose; otherwise, use age. Measure dose with cup provided. Do not discard the measuring cup. Repeat dose every 6–8 hours, if needed. Do not use more than 4 times a day. If stomach upset occurs while taking this product, give with food or milk.

DOSING CHART

WEIGHT (lb.)	AGE (yr.)	DOSE (tsp.)
Under 24	Under 2	Consult a Doctor
24–35	2–3	1 tsp.
36–47	4–5	1½ tsp.
48–59	6–8	2 tsp.
60–71	9–10	2½ tsp.
72–95	11	3 tsp.

Directions (Junior Strength Advil Tablets): Find right dose on chart below. If possible, use weight to dose; otherwise use age. Repeat dose every 6–8 hours, if needed.

Do not use more than 4 times a day.

DOSING CHART

Weight (lb.)	Age (yr.)	Dose (tablets)
Under 48	Under 6	Consult a Doctor
48–71	6–10	2
72–95	11	3

Directions (Pediatric Advil Drops): This product is intended for use in children ages 2–3 years. If possible, use weight to dose. Otherwise, use age. Measure dose with the dosing device provided. Repeat dose every 6–8 hours, if needed. Do not use more than 4 times a day. If stomach upset occurs while taking this product, give with food or milk.

DOSING CHART

Weight (lb)	Age (yr)	Dose (mL)
Under 24	Under 2	Consult Doctor
24–35	2–3	2.5 mL

Store at controlled room temperature 15°–30°C (59°–86°F).

How Supplied (Children's Advil Oral Suspension): bottles of 2 fl. oz. and 4 fl. oz. Also available as a grape-flavored liquid.
Junior Strength Advil: Coated tablets in bottles of 24.
Pediatric Advil Drops: bottles of ½ fl. oz. in grape and fruit flavors.

Maximum Strength ANBESOL® Gel and Liquid
[an 'ba-sol "]
Oral Anesthetic
BABY ANBESOL®
Original and Grape Flavors
Oral Anesthetic Gel

Description: Anbesol is an oral anesthetic which is available in a Maximum Strength gel and liquid. Baby Anbesol, available in gel, is an anesthetic and is alcohol-free. Baby Anbesol is available in original and grape flavors.
The Maximum Strength formulations contain Benzocaine 20%.
The Baby Anbesol Gels contain Benzocaine 7.5%.

Indications: Maximum Strength Anbesol is indicated for the temporary relief of pain associated with toothache, canker sore, minor dental procedures, or minor injury or irritation of the mouth and gums caused by dentures or orthodontic appliances. Baby Anbesol Gels are indicated for the temporary relief of sore gums due to teething in infants and children 4 months of age and older.

Warnings: Do not use for more than 7 days unless directed by a doctor/dentist. If sore mouth symptoms do not improve in 7 days; if irritation, pain or redness persists or worsens; or if swelling, rash or fever develops, see your doctor/dentist promptly. Do not exceed recommended dosage. Do not use this product if you have a history of allergy to local anesthetics such as procaine, butacaine, benzocaine, or other "caine" anesthetics. If these symptoms persist, consult your doctor. Avoid contact with eyes. Keep this and all drugs out of the reach of children. In case of accidental overdose, seek professional assistance or contact a poison control center immediately.

Dosage and Administration: Maximum Strength Anbesol: Gel—To open tube, cut tip on score mark with scissors. Liquid—Wipe liquid on with cotton, cotton swab, or fingertip.
Adults and children 2 years of age and older: Apply to the affected area on or within the mouth up to 4 times daily or as directed by a doctor/dentist. Children under 12 years of age should be supervised in the use of this product. Children under 2 years of age: Consult a doctor/dentist.
For gel only: For denture irritation, apply thin layer to affected area and do not reinsert dental work until irritation/pain is relieved. Rinse mouth well before reinserting. If irritation/pain persists, contact your doctor/dentist.

Baby Anbesol and Grape Baby Anbesol: To open tube, cut tip on score mark with scissors. Apply to the affected area not more than 4 times daily or as directed by a doctor/dentist. For infants under 4 months of age there is no recommended dosage or treatment except under the advice and supervision of a doctor/dentist.

Inactive Ingredients:
Gel Inactive Ingredients: Carbomer 934P, D&C Yellow No. 10, FD&C Blue No. 1, FD&C Red No. 40, Flavor, Glycerin, Methylparaben, Phenylcarbinol, Polyethylene Glycol, Propylene Glycol, Saccharin.
Liquid: D&C Yellow No. 10, FD&C Blue No. 1, FD&C Red No. 40, Flavor, Methylparaben, Phenylcarbinol, Polyethylene Glycol, Propylene Glycol, Saccharin.
Original Baby Gel: Carbomer 934P, D&C Red #33, Disodium EDTA, Flavor, Glycerin, PEG-8, Saccharin, Water.
Grape Baby Gel: Benzoic Acid, Carbomer 934P, D&C Red #33, Disodium EDTA, FD&C Blue #1, Flavor, Glycerin, Methylparaben, PEG-8, Propylparaben, Saccharin, Water.

How Supplied: All Gels in .25 oz (7.1 g) tubes, Maximum Strength Liquid in .31 fl oz (9 mL) bottle.

AXID® AR
[ak ' sid]
Nizatidine

Active Ingredient: Nizatidine 75 mg per tablet.

Inactive Ingredients: Colloidal Silicon Dioxide, Hydroxypropylmethylcellulose, Synthetic Iron Oxides, Magnesium Stearate, Microcrystalline Cellulose, Polyethylene Glycol, Pregelatinized Starch, Propylene Glycol, Corn Starch, Titanium Dioxide.

Product Benefits: Taken right before eating or up to 60 minutes before eating, one tablet of AXID® AR prevents heartburn, acid indigestion, and sour stomach caused by food and beverages. Unlike antacids which neutralize acid after symptoms have occurred, AXID AR reduces the production of acid in the stomach so you can prevent symptoms. AXID AR also relieves heartburn, acid indigestion and sour stomach.

Action: The stomach normally produces acid especially following eating and drinking. Sometimes, acid backing up into the esophagus can cause a burning pain and discomfort, commonly known as heartburn.
In clinical studies AXID AR was significantly better than placebo in preventing and relieving heartburn symptoms.
[See graphic at top of next page]

Use: For relief and/or prevention of heartburn, acid indigestion and sour stomach brought on by consuming food and beverages.

Benefit of AXID AR Compared to Placebo

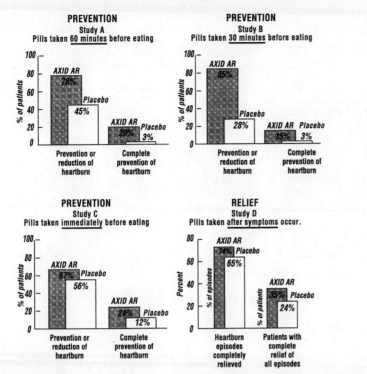

PREVENTION
Study A
Pills taken 60 minutes before eating

PREVENTION
Study B
Pills taken 30 minutes before eating

PREVENTION
Study C
Pills taken immediately before eating

RELIEF
Study D
Pills taken after symptoms occur.

How to help avoid symptoms:
- Avoid lying down flat or bending over soon after eating.
- Avoid eating late at night or right before bedtime.
- If you are overweight, lose weight.
- If you smoke, stop or cut down.
- Eat slowly and do not eat big meals.
- Elevate the head of your bed
- Avoid wearing tight fitting clothing around your stomach.
- Avoid certain foods or beverages more likely to cause heartburn, such as rich, spicy, fried foods, chocolate, caffeine, alcohol; even some fruits and vegetables.

Warnings: While the symptoms of heartburn are common, you should see your doctor promptly if:
- You have trouble swallowing or persistent abdominal pain. You may have a serious condition that may need different treatment.
- You have taken the maximum dosage (2 tablets per 24 hours) for 2 weeks continuously.

Important:
- As with any drug, if you are pregnant or nursing a baby, seek the advice of a health professional before using this product.
- This product should not be given to children under 12 years old unless directed by a doctor.
- Keep this and all drugs out of the reach of children.
- In case of accidental overdose, seek professional assistance or contact a poison control center immediately.

Directions: To prevent heartburn, take one tablet with a full glass of water right before eating or up to 60 minutes before consuming food and beverages that you expect to cause symptoms. For relief of symptoms, take one tablet with a full glass of water. AXID AR can be used up to twice daily (up to 2 tablets in 24 hours); the maximum daily dosage.

How Supplied: AXID AR Acid Reducer is available in boxes of 6 individual packets and bottles of 12, 18, 30, and 50 tablets.
Store at 20°–25° C (68°–77°F). Protect from light. Replace cap tightly after opening bottle. The bottle is sealed with printed foil under cap. Do not use if foil is open or torn.

DIMETAPP® Cold & Allergy
[di 'mě-tap]
Chewable Tablets
Quick Dissolve Tablets

Description: Each Dimetapp Cold & Allergy chewable tablet and each Dimetapp Cold & Allergy Quick Dissolve grape-flavored instantly dissolving tablet contains:
Brompheniramine Maleate,
USP .... 1 mg
Phenylpropanolamine Hydrochloride,
USP .... 6.25 mg

Inactive Ingredients (chewable tablets): Aspartame, Citric Acid, Crospovidone, D&C Red 30 Lake, D&C Red 7 Lake, FD&C Blue 1 Lake, Flavor, Glycine, Magnesium Stearate, Mannitol, Microcrystalline Cellulose, Pregelatinized Starch, Silicon Dioxide, Sorbitol, Stearic Acid. Quick Dissolve tablet: Aspartame, FD&C Blue 2, FD&C Red 40, Flavors, Gelatin, Glycine, Mannitol.

Indications: For temporary relief of nasal congestion due to the common cold, hay fever, or other upper respiratory allergies or associated with sinusitis. Temporarily relieves runny nose, sneezing, and itchy, watery eyes due to hay fever (allergic rhinitis). Temporarily restores freer breathing through the nose.

Warnings: Do not to give this product to children who have a breathing problem such as chronic bronchitis, or who have glaucoma, high blood pressure, heart disease, diabetes, or thyroid disease, without first consulting the child's physician. This product may cause drowsiness: sedatives and tranquilizers may increase the drowsiness effect. Do not give this product to children who are taking sedatives or tranquilizers without first consulting the child's physician. May cause excitability, especially in children.
Do not exceed recommended dosage. If nervousness, dizziness, or sleeplessness occur, discontinue use and consult a doctor. If symptoms do not improve within 7 days, or are accompanied by a fever, consult a physician. As with any drug, if you are pregnant or nursing a baby, seek the advice of a health professional before using this product.

Drug Interaction Precaution: Do not give this product to a child who is taking a prescription monoamine oxidase inhibitor (MAOI) (certain drugs for depression, psychiatric or emotional conditions) or for 2 weeks after stopping the MAOI drug. If you are uncertain whether your child's prescription drug contains an MAOI, consult a health professional before taking this product.
KEEP THIS AND ALL DRUGS OUT OF THE REACH OF CHILDREN. IN CASE OF ACCIDENTAL OVERDOSE, SEEK PROFESSIONAL ASSISTANCE OR CONTACT A POISON CONTROL CENTER IMMEDIATELY.
Phenylketonurics: Each chewable tablet contains phenylalanine, 8 mg per tablet. Each Quick Dissolve tablet contains phenylalanine, 2.10 mg per tablet.

Directions: Children 6 to under 12 years of age: 2 chewable or Quick Dissolve tablets every 4 hours. Children under 6: Consult a physician. DO NOT EXCEED 6 DOSES IN A 24-HOUR PERIOD.

Professional Labeling: The suggested dosage for children age 2 to under 6 years, only when the child is under the care of a physician, is 1 tablet every 4 hours, not to exceed 6 doses in a 24-hour period.

How Supplied: Chewable tablets: Purple tablet scored on one side and engraved with AHR 2290 on the other in bottles of 24 tablets. **Quick Dissolve:** 10 instantly dissolving tablets.

Continued on next page

Dimetapp Cold/Allergy—Cont.

Store at Controlled Room Temperature, Between 20°C and 25°C (68°F and 77°F).

DIMETAPP Cold and Fever Suspension
[dī 'mĕ-tap]

Description: Nasal Decongestant, Antihistamine, Pain reliever-Fever reducer Alcohol Free

Active Ingredients: Each 5 mL (1 teaspoonful) contains: Acetaminophen, USP, 160 mg; Pseudoephedrine Hydrochloride, USP, 15 mg; Brompheniramine Maleate, USP, 1 mg.

Inactive Ingredients: Carboxymethylcellulose Sodium, Citric Acid, D&C Red 33, Disodium Edetate, FD&C Blue 1, Flavors, Glycerin, High Fructose Corn Syrup, Maltol, Methylparaben, Microcrystalline Cellulose, Polysorbate 80, Potassium Sorbate, Propylene Glycol, Propylparaben, Sorbitol, Sucrose, Water, Xanthan Gum.

Indications: For temporary relief of nasal congestion, minor aches, pains, headache and sore throat and to reduce fever associated with a cold or sinusitis. Temporarily relieves runny nose and sneezing, itching of the nose or throat and itchy, watery eyes due to hay fever or other upper respiratory allergies.

Warnings: Do not give this product to children who have a breathing problem such as chronic bronchitis, or who have high blood pressure, heart disease, diabetes, thyroid disease, or glaucoma unless directed by a physician. May cause drowsiness; sedatives and tranquilizers may increase the drowsiness effect. Do not give this product to children who are taking sedatives or tranquilizers without first consulting the child's physician. May cause excitability, especially in children. **Do not exceed recommended dosage.** If nervousness, dizziness or sleeplessness occur, discontinue use and consult a doctor. If symptoms do not improve within 7 days or are accompanied by a fever, consult a doctor. If sore throat is severe, persists for more than 2 days, is accompanied or followed by fever, headache, rash, nausea or vomiting, consult a physician promptly. Do not give this product for pain for more than 5 days or for fever for more than 3 days unless directed by a doctor. If pain or fever persists, or gets worse, if new symptoms occur or if redness or swelling is present, consult a physician because these could be signs of a serious condition.

Drug Interaction Precaution: Do not give this product to a child who is taking a prescription monoamine oxidase inhibitor (MAOI) (certain drugs for depression, psychiatric or emotional conditions, or Parkinson's disease), or for 2 weeks after stopping the MAOI drug. If you are uncertain whether your child's prescription drug contains an MAOI, consult a health professional before giving this product.

Directions: Shake Well Before Using. Children 6 to under 12: two teaspoonfuls every 4 hours (or as directed by a physician). Do Not Exceed 4 Doses in a 24-hour Period. Children under 6 years: consult a physician.
KEEP THIS AND ALL DRUGS OUT OF THE REACH OF CHILDREN. IN CASE OF ACCIDENTAL OVERDOSE, SEEK PROFESSIONAL ASSISTANCE OR CONTACT A POISON CONTROL CENTER IMMEDIATELY, PROMPT MEDICAL ATTENTION IS CRITICAL FOR ADULTS AS WELL AS CHILDREN EVEN IF YOU DO NOT NOTICE ANY SIGNS OR SYMPTOMS.

Storage: Store at Controlled Room Temperature, Between 20°C and 25°C (68°F and 77°F).

How Supplied: 4 oz bottle with dosage cup.

DIMETAPP® Decongestant Pediatric Drops
[dī 'mĕ-tap]

Description: Nasal Decongestant (Pseudoephedrine Hydrochloride)

Active Ingredients: Each 0.8 mL (1 dropperful) contains: 7.5 mg Pseudoephedrine Hydrochloride, USP.

Inactive Ingredients: Caramel, Citric Acid, FD&C Blue 1, D&C Red 33, Flavors, Glycerin, High Fructose Corn Syrup, Maltol, Menthol, Polyethylene Glycol, Propylene Glycol, Sodium Benzoate, Sorbitol, Sucrose, Water.

Indications: For temporary relief of nasal congestion due to the common cold, hay fever, other upper respiratory allergies or associated with sinusitis.

Warnings: Do not exceed recommended dosage. If nervousness, dizziness, or sleeplessness occur, discontinue use and consult a physician. If symptoms do not improve within 7 days or are accompanied by a fever, consult a physician. Do not give this product to a child who has heart disease, high blood pressure, thyroid disease, or diabetes, unless directed by a physician.

Drug Interaction Precaution: Do not give this product to a child who is taking a prescription monoamine oxidase inhibitor (MAOI) (certain drugs for depression, psychiatric or emotional conditions), or for 2 weeks after stopping the MAOI drug. If you are uncertain whether your child's prescription drug contains an MAOI, consult a health professional before giving this product.
KEEP THIS AND ALL DRUGS OUT OF THE REACH OF CHILDREN. IN CASE OF ACCIDENTAL OVERDOSE, SEEK PROFESSIONAL ASSISTANCE OR CONTACT A POISON CONTROL CENTER IMMEDIATELY.

Directions: Children 2 to 3 years: Two dropperfuls (1.6 mL) every 4–6 hours (or as directed by a physician). Children under 2: Consult a physician. DO NOT EXCEED 4 DOSES IN A 24-HOUR PERIOD. Take by mouth only. Not for nasal use.
Store at Controlled Room Temperature, between 20°C and 25°C (68°F and 77°F).

How Supplied: $^1/_2$ oz (15 mL) bottle with dropper.

DIMETAPP® DM ELIXIR
DIMETAPP® Cold & Cough
Liqui-Gels®
Maximum Strength
[dī 'mĕ-tap]

Description: Each 5 mL (1 teaspoonful) of DIMETAPP DM Elixir contains:

Brompheniramine Maleate, USP	2 mg
Phenylpropanolamine Hydrochloride, USP	12.5 mg
Dextromethorphan Hydrobromide, USP	10.0 mg

Each Dimetapp Cold & Cough Liqui-Gel Maximum Strength contains:

Brompheniramine Maleate	4 mg
Phenylpropanolamine Hydrochloride	25 mg
Dextromethorphan Hydrobromide	20 mg

Inactive Ingredients (DIMETAPP DM Elixir): Citric Acid, FD&C Blue 1, FD&C Red 40, Flavors, Glycerin, Propylene Glycol, Saccharin Sodium, Sodium Benzoate, Sorbitol, Water.

Inactive Ingredients (DIMETAPP COLD & COUGH LIQUI-GEL) MAXIMUM STRENGTH: FD&C Red 40, Gelatin, Glycerin, Mannitol, Pharmaceutical Glaze, Polyethylene Glycol, Povidone, Propylene Glycol, Sorbitan, Sorbitol, Titanium Dioxide, Water.

Indications: Temporarily relieves cough due to minor throat and bronchial irritation as may occur with a cold. For temporary relief of nasal congestion due to the common cold, hay fever or other upper respiratory allergies or associated with sinusitis. Temporarily relieves runny nose, sneezing, itching of the nose or throat and itchy, watery eyes due to allergic rhinitis (hay fever). Temporarily restores freer breathing through the nose.

Warnings: Do not take this product if you have a breathing problem such as emphysema or chronic bronchitis or persistent or chronic cough such as occurs with smoking or asthma, or cough that is accompanied by excessive phlegm (mucus) unless directed by a physician. Likewise, if you have high blood pressure, heart disease, diabetes, thyroid disease, glaucoma, or difficulty in urination due to enlargement of the prostate gland, do not take this product unless directed by a physician.

May cause marked drowsiness; alcohol, sedatives and tranquilizers may increase the drowsiness effect. Avoid alcoholic beverages while taking this product. Do not take this product if you are taking sedatives or tranquilizers without first consulting your physician. Use caution when driving a motor vehicle or operating machinery. May cause excitability, especially in children.

Do not exceed the recommended dosage. If nervousness, dizziness or sleeplessness occur, discontinue use and consult a physician. A persistent cough may be a sign of a serious condition. If cough or other symptoms persist, do not improve within 7 days, tend to recur, or are accompanied by fever, rash or persistent headache, consult a physician. As with any drug, if you are pregnant or nursing a baby, seek the advice of a health professional before using this product. KEEP THIS AND ALL DRUGS OUT OF THE REACH OF CHILDREN. IN CASE OF ACCIDENTAL OVERDOSE, SEEK PROFESSIONAL ASSISTANCE OR CONTACT A POISON CONTROL CENTER IMMEDIATELY.

Drug Interaction Precaution: Do not use this product if you are now taking a prescription monoamine oxidase inhibitor (MAOI) (certain drugs for depression, psychiatric or emotional conditions, or Parkinson's disease) or for 2 weeks after stopping the MAOI drug. If you are uncertain whether your prescription drug contains an MAOI, consult a health professional before taking this product.

Directions (DIMETAPP DM ELIXIR): Adults and children 12 years of age and over: Two teaspoonfuls every 4 hours; children 6 to under 12 years: one teaspoonful every 4 hours. DO NOT EXCEED 6 DOSES IN A 24-HOUR PERIOD. Children under 6 years: consult a physician.

Professional Labeling (DIMETAPP DM ELIXIR): The suggested dosage for children age 2 to under 6 years, only when the child is under the care of a physician, is $1/2$ teaspoonful every 4 hours, not to exceed 6 doses in a 24-hour period. The dosage for children under 2 years should be determined by the physician on the basis of the patient's weight, physical condition, or other appropriate consideration. Dimetapp DM Elixir is contraindicated in neonates (children under the age of one month).

Directions (DIMETAPP COLD & COUGH LIQUI-GELS MAXIMUM STRENGTH): Adults and children 12 years of age and over: one softgel every 4 hours. Children under 12: Consult a physician. DO NOT EXCEED 6 LIQUI-GELS IN A 24-HOUR PERIOD.

How Supplied (DIMETAPP DM ELIXIR): Red, grape-flavored liquid in bottles of 4 fl oz, 8 fl oz. Not a USP Elixir.

How Supplied (DIMETAPP COLD & COUGH LIQUI-GELS MAXIMUM STRENGTH): Blister packs of 12's. Liqui-Gels is a registered trademark of R.P. Scherer International Corporation. Store at Controlled Room Temperature, Between 20°C and 25°C (68°F and 77°F)

DIMETAPP® Tablets and Liqui-Gels®
[dī ' mĕ-tap]
Maximum Strength
DIMETAPP® Extentabs®
DIMETAPP® Elixir

Description: Each **Dimetapp** Tablet or Liquigel® contains:

Brompheniramine
Maleate, USP .... 4 mg
Phenylpropanolamine
Hydrochloride, USP .... 25 mg

Each **Dimetapp Extentabs®**Tablet contains:

Brompheniramine Maleate,
USP .... 12 mg
Phenylpropanolamine
Hydrochloride, USP .... 75 mg

Each 5 mL (1 teaspoonful) of **Dimetapp Elixir** contains:

Brompheniramine
Maleate, USP .... 2 mg
Phenylpropanolamine
Hydrochloride, USP .... 12.5 mg

Inactive Ingredients: Tablets: Corn Starch, FD&C Blue 1 Aluminum Lake, Magnesium Stearate, Microcrystalline Cellulose. Liqui-Gels: D&C Red 33, Gelatin, Glycerin, Mannitol, Pharmaceutical Glaze, Polyethylene Glycol, Povidone, Propylene Glycol, Sorbitan, Sorbitol, Titanium Dioxide, Water. Extentabs: Acacia, Acetylated Monoglycerides, Calcium Sulfate, Carnauba Wax, Citric Acid, Edible Ink, FD&C Blue 1, Gelatin, Hydrogenated Castor Oil, Magnesium Stearate, Magnesium Trisilicate, Pharmaceutical Glaze, Polysorbates, Povidone, Silicon Dioxide, Stearyl Alcohol, Sucrose, Titanium Dioxide, White Wax. May also contain Wheat Flour. Elixir: Citric Acid, FD&C Blue 1, FD&C Red 40, Flavors, Glycerin, Saccharin Sodium, Sodium Benzoate, Sorbitol, Water.

Indications: For temporary relief of nasal congestion due to the common cold, hay fever or other upper respiratory allergies or associated with sinusitis. Temporarily relieves runny nose, sneezing, and itchy, watery eyes due to allergic rhinitis (hay fever). Temporarily restores freer breathing through the nose.

Warnings: Do not take take this product, unless directed by a physician, if you have a breathing problem such as emphysema or chronic bronchitis, or if you have high blood pressure, heart disease, diabetes, thyroid disease, glaucoma, or difficulty in urination due to enlargement of the prostate gland. This product may cause drowsiness; alcohol, sedatives and tranquilizers may increase the drow-

siness effect. Avoid alcoholic beverages while taking this product. Do not take this product if you are taking sedatives or tranquilizers without first consulting your physician. Use caution when driving a motor vehicle or operating machinery. May cause excitability, especially in children. **Do not exceed the recommended dosage.** If nervousness, dizziness or sleeplessness occur, discontinue use and consult a physician. If symptoms do not improve within 7 days or are accompanied by fever, consult a physician. Do not take this product if you are hypersensitive to any of the ingredients.

As with any drug, if you are pregnant or nursing a baby, seek the advice of a health professional before using this product.

KEEP THIS AND ALL DRUGS OUT OF THE REACH OF CHILDREN. IN CASE OF ACCIDENTAL OVERDOSE, SEEK PROFESSIONAL ASSISTANCE OR CONTACT A POISON CONTROL CENTER IMMEDIATELY.

Drug Interaction Precaution: Do not use this product if you are now taking a prescription monoamine oxidase inhibitor (MAOI) (certain drugs for depression, psychiatric or emotional conditions, or Parkinson's disease) or for 2 weeks after stopping the MAOI drug. If you are uncertain whether your prescription drug contains an MAOI, consult a health professional before taking this product.

Directions: Tablets: Adults and children 12 years of age and over: one tablet every 4 hours. Children 6 to under 12 years: one-half tablet every 4 hours. DO NOT EXCEED 6 DOSES IN A 24-HOUR PERIOD. Liqui-Gels: Adults and children 12 years of age and over: one softgel every 4 hours. Children under 12 years: consult a physician. DO NOT EXCEED 6 SOFTGELS IN A 24-HOUR PERIOD.

Extentabs: Do not give Extentabs to children under 12 years, except under the advice and supervision of a physician. Adults and children 12 years of age and over: one tablet every 12 hours. DO NOT EXCEED 1 TABLET EVERY 12 HOURS OR 2 TABLETS IN A 24-HOUR PERIOD. Elixir: Adults and children 12 years of age and over: 2 teaspoonfuls every 4 hours; children 6 to under 12 years: 1 teaspoonful every 4 hours; DO NOT EXCEED 6 DOSES IN A 24-HOUR PERIOD. Children under 6 years: consult a physician.

Professional Labeling (Elixir): The suggested dosage for children age 2 to under 6 years, only when the child is under the care of a physician, is ½ teaspoonful every 4 hours, not to exceed 6 doses in a 24-hour period. The dosage for children under 2 years should be determined by the physician on the basis of the patient's weight, physical condition, or other appropriate consideration. Dimetapp Elixir is contraindicated in neonates (children under the age of one month).

Continued on next page

Dimetapp—Cont.

How Supplied: <u>Tablets:</u> Blue, scored compressed tablets engraved AHR and 2254 in consumer packages of 24 (individually packaged).
<u>Liqui-Gels:</u> Purple Liquigel imprinted AHR and 2255 in consumer packages of 12 (individually packaged).
Liqui-Gels is a registered trademark of R.P. Scherer International Corporation.
<u>Extentabs:</u> Pale blue sugar-coated tablets monogrammed DIMETAPP AHR in bottles of 100, 500; Dis-Co® Unit Dose Packs of 100; and blister packs of 12 tablets, 24 tablets and 48 tablets.
Dimetapp Extentabs® Tablets are the A. H. Robins Company's uniquely constructed extended action tablets.
<u>Elixir:</u> Purple, grape-flavored liquid in bottles of 4 fl oz and 8 fl oz. Not a USP elixir.

Store at Controlled Room Temperature, between 20°C and 25°C (68°F and 77°F).

ORUDIS® KT™
[Orūdĭs]

Description: Pain Reliever/Fever Reducer.

Active Ingredients: Each tablet or caplet contains ketoprofen 12.5 mg.

Inactive Ingredients: Cellulose, D&C Yellow 10 Lake, FD&C Blue 1 Lake, Iron Oxide, Pharmaceutical Glaze, Povidone, Silica, Sodium Benzoate, Sodium Lauryl Sulfate, Starch, Stearic Acid, Sugar, Titanium Dioxide, Wax. Contains FD&C Yellow 5 Lake (Tartrazine) as a color additive.

Indications: Temporarily relieves minor aches and pains associated with the common cold, headache, toothache, muscular aches, backache, minor pain of arthritis and menstrual cramps. Temporarily reduces fever.

Warnings: **Do not take this product if you have had asthma, hives or any other allergic reaction after taking any pain reliever/fever reducer. Ketoprofen could cause similar reactions in patients allergic to other pain relievers/fever reducers.** As with any drug, if you are pregnant or nursing a baby, seek the advice of a health professional before using this product. **IT IS ESPECIALLY IMPORTANT NOT TO USE KETOPROFEN DURING THE LAST 3 MONTHS OF PREGNANCY UNLESS SPECIALLY DIRECTED TO DO SO BY A DOCTOR BECAUSE IT MAY CAUSE PROBLEMS IN THE UNBORN CHILD OR COMPLICATIONS DURING DELIVERY.**
If you generally consume 3 or more alcohol-containing drinks per day, you should talk to your doctor for advice on when and how you should take ORUDIS® KT™ or other pain relievers.
Do not use: with any other pain reliever/

fever reducer, with any other product containing ketoprofen, for more than 3 days for fever or for more than 10 days for pain. **Ask a doctor <u>before</u> use if:** the painful area is red or swollen, you take other drugs on a regular basis, you are under a doctor's care for any continuing medical condition or you have had problems or side effects with any pain reliever/fever reducer. **Ask a doctor <u>after</u> use if:** symptoms continue or worsen, new or unexpected symptoms occur or stomach pain occurs with use of this product.
Keep this and all drugs out of the reach of children. In case of accidental overdose, seek professional assistance or contact a poison control center immediately.

Directions: Take with a full glass of **water** or other **liquid**. **Adults:** Take 1 tablet every 4–6 hours. If pain or fever does not get better in 1 hour, you may take 1 more tablet. With experience, some people may find they need 2 tablets for the first dose. The smallest effective dose should be used. **Do not take more than:** 2 tablets in any 4–6 hour period; 6 tablets in any 24 hour period. **Children:** Do not give to children under age 16 unless directed by a doctor.
Store at room temperature. Avoid excessive heat 98°F (37°C).

How Supplied: Coated tablets in bottles of 24, 50, 100
Coated caplets in bottles of 24, 50, 100
ORUDIS is a registered trademark of RHONE-POULENC. KT and the appearance of the green ORUDIS KT tablet are trademarks of WHITEHALL-ROBINS HEALTHCARE.
If you have questions or comments, please call 1-800-Orudis2.

PREPARATION H®
[prep-e 'rā-shen-āch]
Hemorrhoidal Ointment and Cream
PREPARATION H®
Hemorrhoidal Suppositories

Description: Preparation H is available in ointment, cream and suppository product forms. The **Ointment** contains Petrolatum 71.9%, Mineral Oil 14%, Shark Liver Oil 3% and Phenylephrine HCl 0.25%.
The **Cream** contains Petrolatum 18%, Glycerin 12%, Shark Liver Oil 3% and Phenylephrine HCl 0.25%.
The **Suppositories** contain Cocoa Butter 85.5%, Shark Liver Oil 3%, and Phenylephrine HCL 0.25%.

Indications: Preparation H Ointment, Suppositories and Cream, temporarily shrink hemorrhoidal tissue and give temporary relief of the itching, burning and discomfort associated with hemorrhoids.

Warnings: In case of bleeding, or if condition worsens or does not improve within 7 days, consult a doctor promptly. Do not exceed the recommended daily dosage unless directed by a doctor. Keep this and all drugs out of the reach of chil-

dren. In case of accidental ingestion, seek professional assistance or contact a poison control center immediately. As with any drug, if you are pregnant or nursing a baby, seek the advice of a health professional before using this product.
Ointment/Cream/Suppository: Do not use this product if you have heart disease, high blood pressure, thyroid disease, diabetes, or difficulty in urination due to enlargement of the prostate gland unless directed by a doctor.
Ointment: Do not use this product with an applicator if the introduction of the applicator into the rectum causes additional pain. Consult a doctor promptly.
Cream: Do not put this product into the rectum by using fingers or any mechanical device or applicator.

Drug Interaction Precaution: Ointment/Cream/Suppository—Do not use this product if you are presently taking a prescription drug for high blood pressure or depression, without first consulting your doctor.

Dosage and Administration:
Ointment/Cream/Suppositories—
ADULTS—When practical, cleanse the affected area by patting or blotting with an appropriate cleansing tissue. Gently dry by patting or blotting with toilet tissue or a soft cloth before application of this product.
Children under 12 years of age: consult a doctor.

Ointment—Apply to the affected area up to 4 times daily, especially at night, in the morning or after each bowel movement. Regular application and lubrication with Preparation H Ointment provide continual therapy for relief of hemorrhoidal symptoms. FOR INTRA-RECTAL USE: Before applying, remove protective cover from applicator. Attach applicator to tube. Lubricate applicator well, then gently insert applicator into the rectum. Thoroughly cleanse applicator after each use and replace protective cover. Also apply ointment to external area.

Cream—Apply externally to the affected area up to 4 times daily, especially at night, in the morning, or after each bowel movement. Preparation H Cream is to be applied externally or in the lower portion of the anal canal only. The enclosed dispensing cap is designed to control dispersion of the cream to the affected area in the lower portion of the anal canal. Before applying, remove protective cover from dispensing cap. Attach cap to tube. Lubricate dispensing cap well, then gently insert dispensing cap part way into the anus. Thoroughly cleanse dispensing cap after each use and replace protective cover. Regular application and lubrication with Preparation H Cream provides continual therapy for relief of hemorrhoidal symptoms.
Suppositories—Detach one suppository from the strip. Remove foil wrapper before inserting into the rectum as follows: Hold suppository with rounded end up. Carefully separate foil by inserting tip of

fingernail at end marked "peel down". Peel foil slowly and evenly down both sides, exposing suppository. Remove exposed suppository from wrapper. Insert one suppository into the rectum up to 4 times daily, especially at night, in the morning or after each bowel movement. Regular application and lubrication with Preparation H Suppositories provide continual therapy for relief of hemorrhoidal symptoms.

Inactive Ingredients: Ointment— Beeswax, Benzoic Acid, BHA, Corn Oil, Glycerin, Lanolin, Lanolin Alcohol, Methylparaben, Paraffin, Propylparaben, Thyme Oil, Tocopherol, Water.
Cream—BHA, Carboxymethylcellulose Sodium, Cetyl Alcohol, Citric Acid, Edetate Disodium, Glyceryl Oleate, Glyceryl Stearate, Lanolin, Methylparaben, Propyl Gallate, Propylene Glycol, Propylparaben, Simethicone, Sodium Benzoate, Sodium Lauryl Sulfate, Stearyl Alcohol, Tocopherol, Xanthan Gum, Water.
Suppositories—Methylparaben, Propylparaben, Starch.

How Supplied: Ointment: Net Wt. 1 oz and 2 oz **Cream:** Net wt. 0.9 oz and 1.8 oz **Suppositories:** 12's, 24's and 48's.
Store at room temperature or in cool place but not over 80° F.

PREPARATION H® HYDROCORTISONE 1%
[prep-e 'ra-shen-ach]
Anti-Itch Cream

Description: Preparation H® Hydrocortisone 1% is an antipruritic cream containing 1% Hydrocortisone.

Indications: For the temporary relief of external anal itch and itching associated with minor skin irritations and rashes. Other uses of this product should be only under the advice and supervision of a doctor.

Warnings: For external use only. Avoid contact with the eyes. If condition worsens, or if symptoms persist for more than 7 days or clear up and occur again within a few days, stop use of this product and do not begin use of any other hydrocortisone product unless you have consulted a doctor. Do not exceed the recommended daily dosage unless directed by a doctor. In case of bleeding, consult a doctor promptly. Do not put this product into the rectum by using fingers or any mechanical device or applicator. Do not use for the treatment of diaper rash; consult a doctor. Keep this and all drugs out of the reach of children. In case of accidental ingestion, seek professional assistance or contact a Poison Control Center immediately.

Directions: Adults: When practical, cleanse the affected area by patting or blotting with an appropriate cleansing tissue. Gently dry by patting or blotting with toilet tissue or soft cloth before application of this product. Apply to affected area not more than 3 to 4 times daily.
Children under 12 years of age: consult a doctor.

Inactive Ingredients: BHA, Cellulose Gum, Cetyl Alcohol, Citric Acid, Disodium EDTA, Glycerin, Glyceryl Oleate, Glyceryl Stearate, Lanolin, Methylparaben, Petrolatum, Propyl Gallate, Propylene Glycol, Propylparaben, Simethicone, Sodium Benzoate, Sodium Lauryl Sulfate, Stearyl Alcohol, Water, Xanthan Gum.

How Supplied: Available in Net Wt. 0.9 oz tube. Store at room temperature or in cool place but not over 80°F. If cellophane tear strip is missing or if cellophane wrap is broken or missing when purchased, do not use.

PRIMATENE®
[prīm 'a-tēn]
Mist
(Epinephrine Inhalation Aerosol Bronchodilator)

Description: Primatene Mist contains Epinephrine 5.5 mg/mL.

FDA approved uses.

Indications: For temporary relief of shortness of breath, tightness of chest, and wheezing due to bronchial asthma. Eases breathing for asthma patients by reducing spasms of bronchial muscles.

Directions: Inhalation dosage for adults and children 12 years of age and over, and children 4 to under 12 years of age: Start with one inhalation, then wait at least 1 minute. If not relieved, use once more. Do not use again for at least 3 hours. The use of this product by children should be supervised by an adult. Children under 4 years of age: Consult a physician. Each inhalation delivers 0.22 mg of epinephrine.

Warnings: Do not use this product unless a diagnosis of asthma has been made by a physician. Do not use this product if you have heart disease, high blood pressure, thyroid disease, diabetes, or difficulty in urination due to enlargement of the prostate gland unless directed by a physician. As with any drug, if you are pregnant or nursing a baby, seek the advice of a health professional before using this product. Do not use this product if you have ever been hospitalized for asthma or if you are taking any prescription drug for asthma unless directed by a physician. Keep this and all drugs out of the reach of children. In case of accidental overdose, seek professional assistance or contact a poison control center immediately. **DO NOT CONTINUE TO USE THIS PRODUCT BUT SEEK MEDICAL ASSISTANCE IMMEDIATELY IF SYMPTOMS ARE NOT RELIEVED WITHIN 20 MINUTES OR BECOME WORSE. DO NOT USE THIS PRODUCT MORE FREQUENTLY OR AT HIGHER DOSES THAN RECOMMENDED UNLESS DIRECTED BY A PHYSICIAN. EXCESSIVE USE MAY CAUSE NERVOUSNESS AND RAPID HEART BEAT AND, POSSIBLY, ADVERSE EFFECTS ON THE HEART.**

Drug Interaction Precaution: Do not use this product if you are now taking a prescription monoamine oxidase inhibitor (MAOI) (certain drugs for depression, psychiatric or emotional conditions, or Parkinson's disease), or for 2 weeks after stopping the MAOI drug. If you are uncertain whether your prescription drug contains an MAOI, consult a health professional before taking this product.

Caution: Contents under pressure. Do not puncture or throw container into incinerator. Using or storing near open flame or heating above 120° F (49° C) may cause bursting. Store at room temperature 59° F to 86° F (15° C to 30° C).

Directions For Use of Mouthpiece: The Primatene Mist mouthpiece, which is enclosed in the Primatene Mist 15 mL size (not the refill size), should be used for inhalation only with Primatene Mist.
1. Take plastic cap off mouthpiece. (For refills, use mouthpiece from previous purchase.)
2. Take plastic mouthpiece off bottle.
3. Place other end of mouthpiece on bottle.
4. Turn bottle upside down. Place thumb on bottom of mouthpiece over circular button and forefinger on top of vial. Empty the lungs as completely as possible by exhaling.
5. Place mouthpiece in mouth with lips closed around opening. Inhale deeply while squeezing mouthpiece and bottle together. Release immediately and remove unit from mouth. Complete taking the deep breath, drawing the medication into your lungs and holding breath as long as comfortable.
6. Exhale slowly keeping lips nearly closed. This helps distribute the medication in the lungs.
7. Replace plastic cap on mouthpiece.

Care of the Mouthpiece:
The Primatene Mist mouthpiece should be washed once daily with soap and hot water, and rinsed thoroughly. Then it should be dried with a clean, lint-free cloth.
If the unit becomes clogged and fails to spray, please send the clogged unit to:
Whitehall Laboratories
5 Giralda Farms
Madison, N.J. 07940

Inactive Ingredients: Alcohol 34%, Ascorbic Acid, Fluorocarbons (Propellant), Water. Contains No Sulfites.

Warning: Contains CFC 12, 114, substances which harm public health and environment by destroying ozone in the upper atmosphere.

How Supplied:
$\frac{1}{2}$ Fl oz (15 mL) With Mouthpiece.
$\frac{1}{2}$ Fl oz (15 mL) Refill
$\frac{3}{4}$ Fl oz (22.5 mL) Refill

Continued on next page

PRIMATENE®
[prĭm 'a-tēn]
Tablets

Description: Primatene Tablets contain Ephedrine Hydrochloride 12.5 mg, USP, Guaifenesin, USP 200 mg.

Indications: For temporary relief of shortness of breath, tightness of chest, and wheezing due to bronchial asthma. Eases breathing for asthma patients by reducing spasms of bronchial muscles and helps loosen phlegm (mucus) and thin bronchial secretions to rid bronchial passageways of bothersome mucus and make coughs more productive.

Warnings: Do not use this product unless a diagnosis of asthma has been made by a doctor. Do not use this product if you have heart disease, high blood pressure, thyroid disease, diabetes or difficulty in urination due to enlargement of the prostate gland unless directed by a doctor. Do not use this product if you have ever been hospitalized for asthma or if you are taking any prescription drug for asthma unless directed by a doctor. **DRUG INTERACTION PRECAUTION:** Do not use this product if you are now taking a prescription monoamine oxidase inhibitor (MAOI) (certain drugs for depression, psychiatric or emotional conditions or Parkinson's disease), or for 2 weeks after stopping the MAOI drug. If you are uncertain whether your prescription drug contains an MAOI, consult a health professional before taking this product. Do not continue to use this product but seek medical assistance immediately if symptoms are not relieved within 1 hour or become worse. Some users of this product may experience nervousness, tremor, sleeplessness, nausea, and loss of appetite. If these symptoms persist or become worse, consult your doctor. Do not take this product for persistent or chronic cough such as occurs with smoking, asthma, chronic bronchitis, or emphysema, or where cough is accompanied by excessive phlegm (mucus) unless directed by a doctor. A persistent cough may be a sign of a serious condition. If cough persists for more than one week, tends to recur, or is accompanied by fever, rash, or persistent headache, consult a doctor. As with any drug, if you are pregnant or nursing a baby, seek the advice of a health professional before using this product. Keep this and all drugs out of the reach of children. In case of accidental overdose, seek professional assistance or contact a poison control center immediately. Intentional abuse of this product can be harmful or fatal.

Directions: Adults and children 12 years of age and over: 2 tablets initially then two every 4 hours, as needed, not to exceed 12 tablets in 24 hours. Do not exceed recommended dosage unless directed by a doctor. For children under 12 years of age, consult a doctor.

Inactive Ingredients:
Crospovidone, D&C Yellow 10 Lake, FD&C Yellow 6 Lake, Magnesium Stearate, Microcrystalline Cellulose, Povidone, Silicon Dioxide.

How Supplied: Available in 24 and 60 tablet thermoform blister cartons.
Store at room temperature, between 20°C and 25°C (68°F to 77°F).

ROBITUSSIN® COLD
COLD & COUGH LIQUI-GELS®
[ro "bĭ-tuss 'ĭn]

Description: Each Softgel contains:
Guaifenesin, USP .... 200 mg
Pseudoephedrine Hydrochloride,
   USP .... 30 mg
Dextromethorphan Hydrobromide,
   USP .... 10 mg

Inactive Ingredients: FD&C Blue 1, FD&C Red 40, Gelatin, Glycerin, Mannitol, Pharmaceutical Glaze, Polyethylene Glycol, Povidone, Propylene Glycol, Sorbitan, Sorbitol, Titanium Dioxide, Water.

Indications: Temporarily relieves cough due to minor throat and bronchial irritation and nasal congestion due to the common cold, hay fever or other upper respiratory allergies, or associated with sinusitis. Helps loosen phlegm (mucus) and thin bronchial secretions to make coughs more productive.

Warnings: Do not take this product for persistent or chronic cough such as occurs with smoking, asthma, chronic bronchitis, emphysema, or if cough is accompanied by excessive phlegm (mucus), unless directed by a physician. Likewise, if you have heart disease, high blood pressure, thyroid disease, diabetes, or difficulty in urination due to enlargement of the prostate gland, do not take this product unless directed by a physician.
Do not exceed the recommended dosage. If nervousness, dizziness or sleeplessness occur, discontinue use and consult a physician. A persistent cough may be a sign of a serious condition. If cough or other symptoms persist, do not improve within 7 days, tend to recur, or are accompanied by fever, rash, or persistent headache, consult a physician.
As with any drug, if you are pregnant or nursing a baby, seek the advice of a health professional before using this product.
KEEP THIS AND ALL DRUGS OUT OF THE REACH OF CHILDREN. IN CASE OF ACCIDENTAL OVERDOSE, SEEK PROFESSIONAL ASSISTANCE OR CONTACT A POISON CONTROL CENTER IMMEDIATELY.

Drug Interaction Precaution: Do not use this product if you are now taking a prescription monoamine oxidase inhibitor (MAOI) (certain drugs for depression, psychiatric or emotional conditions, or Parkinson's disease) or for 2 weeks after stopping the MAOI drug. If you are

uncertain whether your prescription drug contains an MAOI, consult a health professional before taking this product.

Directions: Follow dosage below: DO NOT EXCEED 4 DOSES IN A 24-HOUR PERIOD. Adults and children 12 years of age and over: swallow two Softgels every 4 hours. Children 6 to under 12 years: swallow one Softgel every 4 hours. Children under 6–consult your doctor.

How Supplied: Red Liquigel imprinted AHR and 8600 in consumer packages of 12 and 20 (individually packaged).
Store at Controlled Room Temperature, between 20°C and 25°C (68°F and 77°F) Liqui-Gels and Liquigel are registered trademarks of R.P. Scherer International Corporation.

ROBITUSSIN® COLD
COLD COUGH & FLU LIQUI-GELS®
[ro "bĭ-tuss 'ĭn]

Description: Pain Reliever, Fever Reducer, Cough Suppressant, Nasal Decongestant, Expectorant.

Active Ingredients: Acetaminophen 250 mg, Guaifenesin 100 mg, Pseudoephedrine HCl 30 mg, Dextromethorphan HBr 10 mg

Inactive Ingredients: D&C Yellow #10, FD&C Red #40, Gelatin, Glycerin, Mannitol, Polyethylene Glycol, Povidone, Propylene Glycol, Sorbitan, Sorbitol, Water

Indications: For the temporary relief of minor aches and pains, headache, muscular aches and sore throat associated with cold or flu, and to reduce fever. Temporarily relieves cough due to minor throat and bronchial irritation and nasal congestion as may occur with a cold. Helps loosen phlegm (mucus) and thin bronchial secretions to make coughs more productive.

Warnings: Do not take this product for persistent or chronic cough such as occurs with smoking, asthma, chronic bronchitis, emphysema, or if cough is accompanied by excessive phlegm (mucus), unless directed by a doctor. Likewise, if you have heart disease, high blood pressure, thyroid disease, diabetes, or difficulty in urination due to enlargement of the prostate gland, do not take this product unless directed by a doctor.

Alcohol Warning: If you generally consume 3 or more alcohol-containing drinks per day you should consult your physician for advice on when and how you should take this product or any other acetaminophen-containing product.
Do not exceed recommended dosage. If nervousness, dizziness, or sleeplessness occur, discontinue use and consult a doctor. Do not take this product for more than 7 days (adults) or 5 days (children under 12) or for fever for more than 3 days unless directed by a doctor.

If pain or fever persists or gets worse, if new symptoms occur, or if redness or swelling is present, consult a doctor because these could be signs of a serious condition. If sore throat is severe, persists for more than 2 days, is accompanied or followed by fever, headache, rash, nausea, or vomiting, consult a doctor promptly. A persistent cough may be a sign of a serious condition. If cough or other symptoms persist, do not improve within 7 days, tend to recur, or are accompanied by fever, rash, or persistent headache, consult a doctor.

As with any drug, if you are pregnant or nursing a baby, seek the advice of a health professional before using this product.

Drug Interaction Precaution: Do not use this product if you are now taking a prescription monoamine oxidase inhibitor (MAOI) (certain drugs for depression, psychiatric or emotional conditions, or Parkinson's disease), or for 2 weeks after stopping the MAOI drug. If you are uncertain whether your prescription drug contains an MAOI, consult a health professional before taking this product.

Directions: Follow dosage below: Do not exceed 4 doses in a 24-hour period. Adult Dose (and children 12 yrs. and over): Swallow 2 Softgels every 4 hrs. Child Dose: (6 yrs. to under 12 yrs.): Swallow 1 Softgel every 4 hrs. Children under 6—Consult your doctor. KEEP THIS AND ALL DRUGS OUT OF THE REACH OF CHILDREN. IN CASE OF ACCIDENTAL OVERDOSE, SEEK PROFESSIONAL ASSISTANCE OR CONTACT A POISON CONTROL CENTER IMMEDIATELY. PROMPT MEDICAL ATTENTION IS CRITICAL FOR ADULTS AS WELL AS CHILDREN EVEN IF YOU DO NOT NOTICE ANY SIGNS OR SYMPTOMS.

How Supplied: Blister Packs of 12's and 20's

Storage: Store at Controlled Room Temperature, Between 20°C and 25°C (68°F and 77°F).

ROBITUSSIN® COUGH DROPS
[ro "bǐ-tuss 'ĭn]
Menthol Eucalyptus, Cherry, and Honey-Lemon Flavors

Active Ingredients: Each cough drop contains:
Menthol Pectin and Eucalyptus and *Cherry:*
Menthol .... 7.4 mg
Honey-Lemon:
Menthol .... 10 mg

Inactive Ingredients:
Menthol Eucalyptus: Corn Syrup, Eucalyptus Oil, Sucrose
Cherry: Corn Syrup, Eucalyptus Oil, FD & C Red #40, Flavors, Methylparaben, Propylparaben, Sodium Benzoate, Sucrose

Honey-Lemon: Corn Syrup, D & C Yellow #10 Aluminum Lake, Eucalyptus Oil, FD&C Yellow #6, Flavors, Honey, Methylparaben, Povidone, Propylparaben, Sodium Benzoate, Sucrose

Indications: Temporarily relieves coughs and minor throat irritations due to colds or inhaled irritants and protects irritated areas of sore throat.

Warnings: Patients with the following conditions are warned not to use these products unless directed by a physician: sore throat that lasts more than 2 days, or persistent or chronic cough such as occurs with smoking, asthma, or emphysema, or if cough is accompanied by excessive phlegm (mucus).

A persistent cough or sore throat may be a sign of a serious condition. Patients are warned to consult a physician if cough persists for more than one week, tends to recur, or is accompanied by fever, rash, or persistent headache, or if sore throat is severe, persistent or accompanied by fever, headache, nausea, or vomiting.

As with any drug, women who are pregnant or nursing a baby should seek the advice of a health professional before using these products.

Directions: Adults and children 4 years and over: allow cough drop to dissolve slowly in the mouth. May be repeated every hour, as needed, or as directed by a physician. Children under 4 years: as directed by physician.

How Supplied: All 3 flavors of Robitussin Cough Drops are available in bags of 25 drops and sticks of 9 drops.

ROBITUSSIN® COLD SEVERE CONGESTION LIQUI-GELS® ROBITUSSIN®-PE
[ro "bǐ-tuss 'ĭn]

Description: Each Robitussin Severe Congestion Liquigel® contains:
Guaifenesin, USP .... 200 mg
Pseudoephedrine Hydrochloride,
    USP .... 30 mg

Each teaspoonful of Robitussin-PE (5 mL) contains:
Guaifenesin, USP .... 100 mg
Pseudoephedrine Hydrochloride,
    USP .... 30 mg

Inactive Ingredients Robitussin Severe Congestion Liqui-Gels: FD&C Green 3, Gelatin, Glycerin, Mannitol, Pharmaceutical Glaze, Polyethylene Glycol, Povidone, Propylene Glycol, Sorbitan, Sorbitol, Titanium Dioxide, Water.
Robitussin-PE: Citric Acid, FD&C Red 40, Flavors, Glucose, Glycerin, High Fructose Corn Syrup, Maltol, Propylene Glycol, Saccharin Sodium, Sodium Benzoate, Water.

Indications: For the temporary relief of nasal congestion due to the common cold, hay fever or other upper respiratory allergies, or associated with sinusitis.

Helps loosen phlegm (mucus) and thin bronchial secretions to make coughs more productive.

Warnings: Do not take this product for persistent or chronic cough such as occurs with smoking, asthma, chronic bronchitis, emphysema, or if cough is accompanied by excessive phlegm (mucus), unless directed by a physician. Likewise, if you have heart disease, high blood pressure, thyroid disease, diabetes, or difficulty in urination due to enlargement of the prostate gland, do not take this product unless directed by a physician.

Do not exceed the recommended dosage. If nervousness, dizziness or sleeplessness occur, discontinue use and consult a physician. A persistent cough may be a sign of a serious condition. If cough or other symptoms persist, do not improve within 7 days, tend to recur, or are accompanied by fever, rash, or persistent headache, consult a physician.

As with any drug, if you are pregnant or nursing a baby, seek the advice of a health professional before using this product.
KEEP THIS AND ALL DRUGS OUT OF THE REACH OF CHILDREN. IN CASE OF ACCIDENTAL OVERDOSE, SEEK PROFESSIONAL ASSISTANCE OR CONTACT A POISON CONTROL CENTER IMMEDIATELY.

Drug Interaction Precaution: Do not use this product if you are now taking a prescription monoamine oxidase inhibitor (MAOI) (certain drugs for depression, psychiatric or emotional conditions or Parkinson's disease) or for 2 weeks after stopping the MAOI drug. If you are uncertain whether your prescription drug contains an MAOI, consult a health professional before taking this product.

Directions Robitussin Severe Congestion Liqui-Gels: DO NOT EXCEED 4 DOSES IN A 24-HOUR PERIOD. Adults and children 12 years of age and over: swallow two Softgels every 4 hours. Children 6 to under 12 years: swallow one Softgel every 4 hours. Children under 6, consult a physician.

Directions Robitussin-PE: Dosage cup provided. DO NOT EXCEED 4 DOSES IN A 24-HOUR PERIOD. Adults and children 12 years and over: 2 teaspoonfuls every 4 hours; children 6 years to under 12 years, 1 teaspoonful every 4 hours; children 2 years to under 6 years, ½ teaspoonful every 4 hours; children under 2 years—consult your doctor.

How Supplied: Aqua Liquigel imprinted AHR and 8501 in consumer packages of 12 and 20 (individually packaged). Liqui-Gels and Liquigel are registered trademarks of R.P. Scherer International Corporation. Robitussin-PE (orange-red) in bottles of 4 fl oz, and 8 fl oz. Store at Controlled Room Temperature, between 20°C and 25°C (68°F and 77°F).

Continued on next page

ROBITUSSIN®
[ro "bĭ-tuss 'ĭn]
(Guaifenesin Syrup, USP)

Active Ingredients: Each teaspoonful (5 mL) contains:
Guaifenesin, USP .... 100 mg
Alcohol-Free Cough Formula

Inactive Ingredients: Caramel, Citric Acid, FD&C Red 40, Flavors, Glucose, Glycerin, High Fructose Corn Syrup, Saccharin Sodium, Sodium Benzoate, Water.

Indications: Helps loosen phlegm (mucus) and thin bronchial secretions to make coughs more productive.

Professional Labeling: Helps loosen phlegm and thin bronchial secretions in patients with stable chronic bronchitis.

Warnings: Do not take this product for persistent or chronic cough such as occurs with smoking, asthma, chronic bronchitis, emphysema, or where cough is accompanied by excessive phlegm (mucus) unless directed by a physician.
A persistent cough may be a sign of a serious condition. If cough persists for more than one week, tends to recur, or is accompanied by a fever, rash, or persistent headache, consult a physician.
Do not take this product if you are hypersensitive to any of the ingredients. As with any drug, if you are pregnant or nursing a baby, seek the advice of a health professional before using this product.
KEEP THIS AND ALL DRUGS OUT OF THE REACH OF CHILDREN. IN CASE OF ACCIDENTAL OVERDOSE, SEEK PROFESSIONAL ASSISTANCE OR CONTACT A POISON CONTROL CENTER IMMEDIATELY.

Directions: Follow dosage below. Dosage cup provided. **Do Not Exceed Recommended Dosage**. Adults and children 12 years and over: 2–4 teaspoonfuls every 4 hours; children 6 years to under 12 years: 1–2 teaspoonfuls every 4 hours. Children 2 years to under 6 years: $^1/_2$–1 teaspoonful every 4 hours. Children under 2 years—consult your doctor.

How Supplied: Robitussin (wine-colored) in bottles of 4 fl oz, 8 fl oz, 16 fl oz. Store at Controlled Room Temperature, between 20°C and 25°C (68°F and 77°F).

ROBITUSSIN®–CF
[ro "bĭ-tuss 'ĭn]

Active Ingredients: Each teaspoonful (5 mL) contains:
Guaifenesin, USP .... 100 mg
Phenylpropanolamine
  Hydrochloride, USP .... 12.5 mg
Dextromethorphan
  Hydrobromide, USP .... 10 mg

Inactive Ingredients: Citric Acid, FD&C Red 40, Flavors, Glycerin, Propylene Glycol, Saccharin Sodium, Sodium Benzoate, Sorbitol, Water.

Indications: Temporarily relieves cough due to minor throat and bronchial irritation and nasal congestion as may occur with a cold. Helps loosen phlegm (mucus) and thin bronchial secretions to make coughs more productive.

Warnings: Do not take this product for persistent or chronic cough such as occurs with smoking, asthma, chronic bronchitis, emphysema, or if cough is accompanied by excessive phlegm (mucus) unless directed by a physician. Likewise, if you have heart disease, high blood pressure, thyroid disease, diabetes, or difficulty in urination due to enlargement of the prostate gland, do not take this product unless directed by a physician.
Do not exceed the recommended dosage. If nervousness, dizziness, or sleeplessness occur, discontinue use and consult a doctor. A persistent cough may be a sign of a serious condition. If cough or other symptoms persist, do not improve within 7 days, tend to recur, or are accompanied by fever, rash, or persistent headache, consult a physician. As with any drug, if you are pregnant or nursing a baby, seek the advice of a health professional before using this product.
KEEP THIS AND ALL DRUGS OUT OF THE REACH OF CHILDREN. IN CASE OF ACCIDENTAL OVERDOSE, SEEK PROFESSIONAL ASSISTANCE OR CONTACT A POISON CONTROL CENTER IMMEDIATELY.

Drug Interaction Precaution: Do not use this product if you are now taking a prescription monoamine oxidase inhibitor (MAOI) (certain drugs for depression, psychiatric or emotional conditions, or Parkinson's disease) or for 2 weeks after stopping the MAOI drug. If you are uncertain whether your prescription drug contains an MAOI, consult a health professional before taking this product.

Directions: Follow dosage below: Dosage cup provided. DO NOT EXCEED 6 DOSES IN A 24-HOUR PERIOD. Adults and children 12 years and over: 2 teaspoonfuls every 4 hours; children 6 years to under 12 years, 1 teaspoonful every 4 hours; children 2 years to under 6 years, $^1/_2$ teaspoonful every 4 hours; children under 2 years—consult your doctor.

How Supplied: Robitussin-CF (red-colored) in bottles of 4 fl oz, 8 fl oz, and 12 fl oz.
Store at Controlled Room Temperature, between 20°C and 25°C (68°F and 77°F).

ROBITUSSIN®-DM
[ro "bĭ-tuss 'ĭn]

Active Ingredients: Each teaspoonful (5 mL) contains:
Guaifenesin, USP .... 100 mg
Dextromethorphan Hydrobromide,
  USP .... 10 mg

Inactive Ingredients: Citric Acid, FD&C Red 40, Flavors, Glucose, Glycerin, High Fructose Corn Syrup, Saccharin Sodium, Sodium Benzoate, Water.

Indications: Temporarily relieves cough due to minor throat and bronchial irritation as may occur with a cold and helps loosen phlegm (mucus) and thin bronchial secretions to make coughs more productive.

Warnings: Do not take this product for persistent or chronic cough such as occurs with smoking, asthma, chronic bronchitis, emphysema, or if cough is accompanied by excessive phlegm (mucus) unless directed by a physician.
A persistent cough may be a sign of a serious condition. If cough persists for more than one week, tends to recur, or is accompanied by a fever, rash, or persistent headache, consult a physician.
Do not take this product if you are hypersensitive to any of the ingredients. As with any drug, if you are pregnant or nursing a baby, seek the advice of a health professional before using this product.
KEEP THIS AND ALL DRUGS OUT OF THE REACH OF CHILDREN. IN CASE OF ACCIDENTAL OVERDOSE, SEEK PROFESSIONAL ASSISTANCE OR CONTACT A POISON CONTROL CENTER IMMEDIATELY.

Drug Interaction Precaution: Do not use this product if you are now taking a prescription monoamine oxidase inhibitor (MAOI) (certain drugs for depression, psychiatric or emotional conditions, or Parkinson's disease) or for 2 weeks after stopping the MAOI drug. If you are uncertain whether your prescription drug contains an MAOI, consult a health professional before taking this product.

Directions: Follow dosage below or use as directed by a doctor. Dosage cup provided. DO NOT EXCEED 6 DOSES IN A 24-HOUR PERIOD. Adults and children 12 years and over: 2 teaspoonfuls every 4 hours; children 6 years to under 12 years, 1 teaspoonful every 4 hours; children 2 years to under 6 years, $^1/_2$ teaspoonful every 4 hours; children under 2 years—consult your doctor.

How Supplied: Robitussin-DM (cherry-colored) in bottles of 4 fl oz, 8 fl oz, 12 fl oz, 16 fl oz and single doses: 6 premeasured doses—$^1/_3$ fl oz each.
Store at Controlled Room Temperature, between 20°C and 25°C (68°F and 77°F).

ROBITUSSIN® MAXIMUM STRENGTH COUGH SUPPRESSANT
ROBITUSSIN® PEDIATRIC COUGH SUPPRESSANT
[ro "bĭ-tuss 'ĭn]

Description: Each 5 mL (1 teaspoonful) of Robitussin Maximum Strength Cough Suppressant contains:

Dextromethorphan
  Hydrobromide, USP .... 15 mg

Age	Weight	Dose
Under 2 yrs.	Under 24 lbs.	Consult doctor
2 to under 6 yrs.	24–47 lbs.	1 Teaspoonful
6 to under 12 yrs.	48–95 lbs.	2 Teaspoonfuls
12 yrs. and older	96 lbs. and over	4 Teaspoonfuls

Description: Each 5 mL (1 teaspoonful) of Robitussin Pediatric Cough Suppressant contains:

Dextromethorphan
   Hydrobromide, USP .... 7.5 mg

Inactive Ingredients (Robitussin Maximum Strength Cough Suppressant): Alcohol 1.4%, Citric Acid, FD&C Red 40, Flavors, Glycerin, Glucose, High Fructose Corn Syrup, Saccharin Sodium, Sodium Benzoate, Water.

Inactive Ingredients (Robitussin Pediatric Cough Suppressant): Citric Acid, FD&C Red 40, Flavors, Glycerin, Propylene Glycol, Saccharin Sodium, Sodium Benzoate, Sorbitol, Water.

Indications: Temporarily relieves cough due to minor throat and bronchial irritation as may occur with a cold.

Warnings: Do not take this product for persistent or chronic cough such as occurs with smoking, asthma, emphysema, or if cough is accompanied by excessive phlegm (mucus) unless directed by a physician.
A persistent cough may be a sign of a serious condition. If cough persists for more than one week, tends to recur, or is accompanied by fever, rash, or persistent headache, consult a physician. Do not take this product if you are hypersensitive to any of its ingredients.
As with any drug, if you are pregnant or nursing a baby, seek the advice of a health professional before using this product.
KEEP THIS AND ALL DRUGS OUT OF THE REACH OF CHILDREN. IN CASE OF ACCIDENTAL OVERDOSE, SEEK PROFESSIONAL ASSISTANCE OR CONTACT A POISON CONTROL CENTER IMMEDIATELY.

Drug Interaction Precaution: Do not use this product if you are now taking a prescription monoamine oxidase inhibitor (MAOI) (certain drugs for depression, psychiatric or emotional conditions, or Parkinson's disease) or for 2 weeks after stopping the MAOI drug. If you are uncertain whether your prescription drug contains an MAOI, consult a health professional before taking this product.

Directions: Follow dosage recommendations below or use as directed by a doctor. Repeat every 6–8 hours as needed. DO NOT EXCEED 4 DOSES IN A 24-HOUR PERIOD. Robitussin Maximum Strength Cough Suppressant Adults and children 12 years and over: 2 teaspoonfuls every 6–8 hours, in medicine cup. Children under 12 years: consult your doctor.

Professional Labeling: Children 6 years to under 12 years, 1 teaspoonful every 6–8 hours; children 2 years to under 6 years, $1/2$ teaspoonful every 6–8 hours.

Do not exceed 4 doses in a 24-hour period.
Tamper-Evident Bottle Cap. If Breakable Ring Is Separated, Do Not Use.
Robitussin Pediatric Cough Suppressant Dosage: choose by weight, if known; if weight is no known, choose by age.
[See table above]

How Supplied: Robitussin Maximum Strength (dark red-colored) in bottles of 4 and 8 fl oz.

How Supplied: Robitussin Pediatric (cherry-colored) in bottles of 4 fl oz.
Store at Controlled Room Temperature, between 20°C and 25°C (68°F and 77°F).

ROBITUSSIN® MAXIMUM STRENGTH COUGH& COLD
ROBITUSSIN® PEDIATRIC COUGH & COLD FORMULA
[ro "bĭ-tuss 'ĭn]

Description: Each teaspoonful (5 mL) of Robitussin Maximum Strength Cough & Cold contains:
Dextromethorphan Hydrobromide,
   USP .... 15 mg
Pseudoephedrine Hydrochloride,
   USP .... 30 mg

Description: Each 5 mL (1 teaspoonful) of Robitussin Pediatric Cough & Cold Formula contains:
Dextromethorphan Hydrobromide,
   USP .... 7.5 mg
Pseudoephedrine Hydrochloride,
   USP .... 15 mg

Inactive Ingredients (Robitussin Maximum Strength Cough & Cold): Alcohol 1.4%, Citric Acid, FD&C Red 40, Flavors, Glycerin, Glucose, High Fructose Corn Syrup, Saccharin Sodium, Sodium Benzoate, Water.

Inactive Ingredients (Robitussin Pediatric Cough & Cold Formula): Citric Acid, FD&C Red 40, Flavors, Glycerin, Propylene Glycol, Saccharin Sodium, Sodium Benzoate, Sorbitol, Water.

Indications: Temporarily relieves cough due to minor throat and bronchial irritation and nasal congestion as may occur with a cold.

Warnings: Do not take this product for persistent or chronic cough such as occurs with smoking, asthma, emphysema, or if cough is accompanied by excessive phlegm (mucus) unless directed by a physician. Likewise, if you have heart disease, high blood pressure, thyroid disease, diabetes, or difficulty in urination due to enlargement of the prostate gland, do not take this product unless directed by a physician.

Do not exceed the recommended dosage. If nervousness, dizziness, or sleep-

lessness occur, discontinue use and consult a doctor. A persistent cough may be a sign of a serious condition. If cough or other symptoms persist, do not improve within 7 days, tend to recur, or are accompanied by fever, rash, or persistent headache, consult a physician.
As with any drug, if you are pregnant or nursing a baby, seek the advice of a health professional before using this product.
KEEP THIS AND ALL DRUGS OUT OF THE REACH OF CHILDREN. IN CASE OF ACCIDENTAL OVERDOSE, SEEK PROFESSIONAL ASSISTANCE OR CONTACT A POISON CONTROL CENTER IMMEDIATELY.

Drug Interaction Precaution: Do not use this product if you are now taking a prescription monoamine oxidase inhibitor (MAOI) (certain drugs for depression, psychiatric or emotional conditions, or Parkinson's disease) or for 2 weeks after stopping the MAOI drug. If you are uncertain whether your prescription drug contains an MAOI, consult a health professional before taking this product.

Directions: Follow dosage recommendations below or use as directed by a doctor. Repeat every 6 hours as needed. DO NOT EXCEED 4 DOSES IN A 24-HOUR PERIOD. Robitussin Maximum Strength Cough & Cold. Adults and children 12 years and over: 2 teaspoonfuls every 6 hours in medicine cup. Children under 12 years: consult your doctor.
Robitussin Pediatric Cough & Cold Formula Dosage: choose by weight, if known; if weight is not known, choose by age.
[See table at top of next page]

How Supplied Robitussin Maximum Strength Cough & Cold: Red syrup in bottles of 4 fl oz and 8 fl oz.
How Supplied: Robitussin Pediatric Cough & Cold formula (bright red) in bottles of 4 fl oz and 8 fl oz.
Store at Controlled Room Temperature, Between 20°C and 25°C (68°F and 77°F).

ROBITUSSIN® COLD NIGHT-TIME LIQUIGELS
[ro "bĭ-tuss 'ĭn]

Description: Cough Suppressant, Nasal Decongestant, Antihistamine, Pain Reliever-Fever Reducer

Active Ingredients: Acetaminophen 325 mg, Pseudoephedrine HCl 30 mg, Dextromethorphan HBr 15 mg, Doxylamine Succinate 6.25 mg.

Inactive Ingredients: D&C Green 5, D&C Yellow 10, FD&C Green 3, FD&C Yellow 6, Gelatin, Glycerin, Mannitol, Pharmaceutical Glaze, Polyethylene Glycol, Povidone, Propylene Glycol, Sodium Acetate, Sorbitan, Sorbitol, Titanium Dioxide, Water

Indications: For the temporary relief of minor aches and pains, headache,

Continued on next page

Robitussin Night-Time—Cont.

muscular aches and sore throat associated with cold or flu, and to reduce fever. Temporarily relieves cough due to minor throat and bronchial irritation and nasal congestion as may occur with a cold. Temporarily relieves runny nose, and sneezing, itching of the nose or throat, and itchy, watery eyes due to hay fever or other upper respiratory allergies (allergic rhinitis).

Warnings: Do not take this product for persistent or chronic cough such as occurs with smoking, asthma, chronic bronchitis, emphysema, or if cough is accompanied by excessive phlegm (mucus), unless directed by a doctor. Likewise, if you have heart disease, high blood pressure, thyroid disease, diabetes, or difficulty in urination due to enlargement of the prostate gland, do not take this product unless directed by a doctor.

Alcohol Warning: Avoid alcoholic beverages while taking this product. If you generally consume 3 or more alcohol-containing drinks per day, you should consult your physician for advice on when and how you should take this product or any other acetaminophen-containing product.

May cause marked drowsiness; alcohol, sedatives, and tranquilizers may increase the drowsiness effect. Do not take this product if you are taking sedatives or tranquilizers, without first consulting your doctor. Use caution when driving a motor vehicle or operating machinery. May cause excitability especially in children.

Do not exceed recommended dosage. If nervousness, dizziness or sleeplessness occur, discontinue use and consult a doctor. Do not take this product for more than 7 days or for fever for more than 3 days unless directed by a doctor.

If pain or fever persists or gets worse, if new symptoms occur, or if redness or swelling is present, consult a doctor because these could be signs of a serious condition. If sore throat is severe, persists for more than 2 days, is accompanied or followed by fever, headache, rash, nausea, or vomiting, consult a doctor promptly. A persistent cough may be a sign of a serious condition. If cough or other symptoms persist for more than one week without improvement, tend to recur, or are accompanied by fever, rash or persistent headache, consult a doctor. As with any drug, if you are pregnant or nursing a baby, seek the advice of a health professional before using this product.

Drug Interaction Precaution: Do not use this product if you are now taking a prescription monoamine oxidase inhibitor (MAOI) (certain drugs for depression, psychiatric or emotional conditions, or Parkinson's disease), or for 2 weeks after stopping the MAOI drug. If you are uncertain whether your prescription drug contains an MAOI, consult a health professional before taking this product.

Robitussin® Cough & Cold

Age	Weight	Dose
Under 2 yrs.	Under 24 lbs.	Consult doctor
2 to under 6 yrs.	24–47 lbs.	1 Teaspoonful
6 to under 12 yrs.	48–95 lbs.	2 Teaspoonfuls
12 yrs. and older	96 lbs. and over	4 Teaspoonfuls

Directions: Follow dosage below: Do not exceed 4 doses in a 24-hour period. Adult Dose (and children 12 yrs. and over): Swallow 2 Softgels every 6 hrs. Not recommended for children under 12 years of age
KEEP THIS AND ALL DRUGS OUT OF THE REACH OF CHILDREN. IN CASE OF ACCIDENTAL OVERDOSE, SEEK PROFESSIONAL ASSISTANCE OR CONTACT A POISON CONTROL CENTER IMMEDIATELY. PROMPT MEDICAL ATTENTION IS CRITICAL FOR ADULTS AS WELL AS CHILDREN EVEN IF YOU DO NOT NOTICE ANY SIGNS OR SYMPTOMS.

Storage: Store at Controlled Room Temperature, Between 20°C and 25°C (68°F and 77°F).

How Supplied: Blister Pack of 12's Blister Pack of 20's

ROBITUSSIN PEDIATRIC DROPS

[ro "bĭ-tuss 'ĭn]

Description: Nasal Decongestant/Cough Suppressant/Expectorant

Active Ingredients: Each 2.5 mL contains Guaifenesin, USP 100 mg, Pseudoephedrine Hydrochloride, USP 15 mg, Dextromethorphan Hydrobromide, USP 5 mg in a pleasant tasting berry flavored syrup.

Inactive Ingredients: Citric Acid, FD&C Red 40, Flavors, Glycerin, High Fructose Corn Syrup, Menthol, Polyethylene Glycol, Propylene Glycol, Saccharin Sodium, Sodium Benzoate, Sodium Carboxymethylcellulose, Sorbitol, Water.

Indications: Temporarily relieves cough due to minor throat and bronchial irritation, and nasal congestion due to a cold. Helps loosen phlegm (mucus) and thin bronchial secretions to make coughs more productive.

Warnings: Do not give this product for persistent or chronic cough such as occurs with asthma, or where cough is accompanied by excessive phlegm (mucus) unless directed by a physician. Likewise, do not give this product to a child who has heart disease, high blood pressure, thyroid disease, or diabetes, unless directed by a physician.

Do not exceed recommended dosage. If nervousness, dizziness or sleeplessness occur, discontinue use and consult a physician. A persistent cough may be a sign of a serious condition. If cough or other symptoms persist, do not improve within 7 days, tend to recur, or are accompanied by fever, rash, or persistent headache, consult a physician

Drug Interaction Precaution: Do not give this product to a child who is

taking a prescription monoamine oxidase inhibitor (MAOI) (certain drugs for depression, psychiatric or emotional conditions), or for 2 weeks after stopping the MAOI drug. If you are uncertain whether your child's prescription drug contains an MAOI, consult a health professional before giving this product.
KEEP THIS AND ALL DRUGS OUT OF THE REACH OF CHILDREN. IN CASE OF ACCIDENTAL OVERDOSE, SEEK PROFESSIONAL ASSISTANCE OR CONTACT A POISON CONTROL CENTER IMMEDIATELY.

Directions: Follow recommended dosage below or use as directed by a doctor. Repeat every 4 hours. Do Not Exceed 4 Doses in a 24-Hour Period.

Dosage: Choose by weight. (If weight is not known, choose by age):

Age	Weight	Dose
Under 2 yrs.	Under 24 lbs.	Consult doctor
2–under 6 yrs.	24–47 lbs.	2.5 mL

Store at Controlled Room Temperature, between 20°C and 25°C (68°F and 77°F).

How Supplied: 1 oz bottle with dosing syringe.

J.B. Williams Company, Inc.

**65 HARRISTOWN ROAD
GLEN ROCK, NJ 07452**

Address Inquiries to:
Consumer Affairs: (800) 254-8656
(201) 251-8100
FAX: (201) 251-8097

For Medical Emergency Contact:
(800) 254-8656

CĒPACOL®/CĒPACOL MINT

[sē 'pə-cŏl]
Antiseptic Mouthwash/Gargle

Ingredients: Cēpacol Antiseptic Mouthwash: Ceepryn® (cetylpyridinium chloride) 0.05%. Also contains: Alcohol 14%, Edetate Disodium, FD&C Yellow No. 5 (tartrazine) as a color additive, Flavors, Glycerin, Polysorbate 80, Saccharin, Sodium Biphosphate, Sodium Phosphate, and Water.
Cēpacol Antiseptic Mint Mouthwash: Ceepryn® (cetylpyridinium chloride) 0.05%. Also contains: Alcohol 14.5%, D&C Yellow No. 10, FD&C Green No. 3,

Flavor, Glucono Delta-Lactone, Glycerin, Poloxamer 407, Sodium Saccharin, Sodium Gluconate, and Water.

Actions: Cēpacol/Cēpacol Mint is an effective antiseptic mouthwash/gargle. It kills germs that cause bad breath for a fresher, cleaner mouth.

Cēpacol/Cēpacol Mint has a low surface tension, approximately $1/2$ that of water. This property is the basis of the spreading action in the oral cavity as well as its foaming action. Cēpacol/Cēpacol Mint leaves the mouth feeling fresh and clean and helps provide soothing, temporary relief of dryness and minor mouth irritations.

Uses: Recommended as a mouthwash and gargle for daily oral care; as an aromatic mouth freshener to provide a clean feeling in the mouth; as a soothing, foaming rinse to freshen the mouth.

Used routinely before dental procedures, helps give patient confidence of not offending with mouth odor. Often employed as a foaming and refreshing rinse before, during, and after instrumentation and dental prophylaxis. Convenient as a mouth-freshening agent after taking dental impressions. Helpful in reducing the unpleasant taste and odor in the mouth following gingivectomy.

Used in hospitals as a mouthwash and gargle for daily oral care. Also used to refresh and soothe the mouth following emesis, inhalation therapy, and intubations, and for swabbing the mouths of patients incapable of personal care.

Warning: In case of accidental ingestion seek professional assistance or contact a poison control center immediately. Do not use in children under 6 years of age. Children over 6 should be supervised when using Cēpacol. Keep out of reach of children.

Directions: Rinse vigorously before or after brushing or any time to freshen the mouth. Cēpacol/Cēpacol Mint leaves the mouth feeling refreshingly clean.

Use full strength every two or three hours as a soothing, foaming gargle, or as directed by a physician or dentist. May also be mixed with warm water.

Product label directions are as follows: Rinse or gargle full strength before or after brushing or as directed by a physician or dentist.

How Supplied: Cēpacol/Cēpacol Mint Antiseptic Mouthwash: 12 oz, 24 oz, and 32 oz. 4 oz trial size.
Shown in Product Identification Guide, page 528

CĒPACOL® Maximum
[sē ′pə-cŏl]
Strength Sore Throat Spray; Cherry and Cool Menthol Flavors.

Ingredients:
Cherry: Active Ingredient:
Dyclonine Hydrochloride 0.1%. Also contains: Cetylpyridinium Chloride, D&C Red No. 33, Dibasic Sodium Phosphate,

FD&C Yellow No. 6, Flavors, Glycerin, Phosphoric Acid, Poloxamer, Potassium Sorbate, Sorbitol, and Water.
Cool Menthol: Active Ingredient: Dyclonine Hydrochloride 0.1%. Also contains: Cetylpyridinium Chloride, Dibasic Sodium Phosphate, FD&C Blue No. 1, Flavors, Glycerin, Phosphoric Acid, Poloxamer, Potassium Sorbate, Polysorbate 20, Sodium Saccharin, Sorbitol and Water.

Indications: For temporary relief of occasional minor sore throat pain and sore mouth. Also, for temporary relief of pain due to canker sores, minor irritation or injury to the mouth and gums, minor dental procedures, dentures or orthodontic appliances.

Directions: Adults: Spray 4 times into throat or affected area (children 2 to 12 years of age: spray 2–3 times) and swallow. Repeat as needed up to 4 times daily or as directed by a physician or dentist. Children 2 to 12 years of age should be supervised in product use. Children under 2 years: Consult physician or dentist.

Warnings: If sore throat is severe, persists for more than 2 days, is accompanied or followed by fever, headache, rash, nausea, or vomiting, consult a physician promptly. If sore mouth symptoms do not improve in 7 days, or if irritation, pain, or redness persists or worsens, see your dentist or physician promptly. Do not exceed recommended dosage. Keep this and all drugs out of the reach of children. In case of accidental overdose, seek professional assistance or contact a Poison Control Center immediately. As with any drug, if you are pregnant or nursing a baby, seek the advice of a health professional before using this product.
Store at room temperature. Do not freeze.

How Supplied: Available in Cherry and Cool Menthol flavors in 4 fl. oz. (118 mL) plastic bottles with pump sprayer.
Shown in Product Identification Guide, page 528

CĒPACOL®
[sē ′pə-cŏl]
Sore Throat Lozenges
Regular Strength Original Mint,
Regular Strength Cherry,
Maximum Strength Mint,
Maximum Strength Cherry.
Sugar Free Maximum Strength Cool Mint
Sugar Free Maximum Strength Cherry
Oral Anesthetic

Ingredients: (per lozenge)

Regular Strength Original Mint: Active Ingredient: Menthol 2 mg. Also contains: Cetylpyridinium Chloride (Ceepryn®), D&C Yellow No. 10, FD&C Yellow No. 6, Flavor, Glucose, and Sucrose.

Regular Strength Cherry: Active Ingredient: Menthol 3.6 mg. Also con-

tains: Cetylpyridinium Chloride (Ceepryn®), D&C Red No. 33, FD&C Red No. 40, Flavor, Glucose, and Sucrose.

Maximum Strength Mint: Active Ingredients: Benzocaine 10 mg., Menthol 2 mg. Also contains: Cetylpyridinium Chloride (Ceepryn®), D&C Yellow No. 10, FD&C Yellow No. 6, Flavor, Glucose, and Sucrose.

Maximum Strength Cherry: Active Ingredients: Benzocaine 10 mg., Menthol 3.6 mg. Also contains: Cetylpyridinium Chloride (Ceepryn®), D&C Red No. 33, FD&C Red No. 40, Flavor, Glucose, and Sucrose.

Sugar Free Maximum Strength Cool Mint: Active Ingredients: Benzocaine 10 mg., Menthol 2.5 mg. Also contains: Acesulfame Potassium, Cetylpyridinium Chloride (Ceepryn®), D&C Yellow No. 10, FD&C Yellow No. 6, Flavor, Isomalt, Maltitol, and Propylene Glycol.

Sugar Free Maximum Strength Cherry: Active Ingredients: Benzocaine 10 mg., Menthol 4.5 mg. Also contains: Acesulfame Potassium, Cetylpyridinium Chloride (Ceepryn®), D&C Red No. 33, FD&C Red No. 40, Flavor, Isomalt, Maltitol, and Propylene Glycol.

Actions: Menthol provides a mild anesthetic effect and cooling sensation for symptomatic relief of occasional minor sore throat pain and minor throat irritations. Benzocaine in the Maximum Strength lozenges provides an anesthetic effect for additional symptomatic relief of minor sore throat pain.

Indications: For temporary relief of occasional minor sore throat pain and dry, scratchy throat.

Warnings: If sore throat is severe, persists for more than 2 days, is accompanied or followed by fever, headache, rash, nausea, or vomiting, consult a physician promptly. Do not administer to children under 6 years of age unless directed by physician or dentist. Keep this and all drugs out of the reach of children. In case of accidental overdose, seek professional assistance or contact a Poison Control Center immediately. As with any drug, if you are pregnant or nursing a baby, seek the advice of a health professional before using this product.

Directions: Adults and children 6 years of age and older: Dissolve 1 lozenge in the mouth every 2 hours as needed or as directed by a physician or dentist. For children under 6 years, consult a physician or dentist.

How Supplied:

Trade package: 18 lozenges in 2 pocket packs of 9 each.
Sugar Free Maximum Strength: 16 lozenges in 2 pocket packs of 8 each.

Institutional package: Regular Strength Original Mint and Maximum

Continued on next page

Cepacol Lozenges—Cont.

Strength Mint: 648 lozenges in 72 blisters of 9 each.
Store at room temperature, below 86°F (30°C). Protect contents from humidity.

Shown in Product Identification Guide, page 528

CĒPACOL® VĪRACTIN®

[sē 'pə-cŏl] [vī 'rak-tin]
Cold Sore and Fever Blister Treatment; Gel and Cream Formulas

Ingredients:

Gel: Active Ingredient: Tetracaine HCl 2%. Also contains: Ethoxydiglycol, Eucalyptus Oil, Hydroxyethyl Cellulose, Maleated Soybean Oil, Methylparaben, Propylparaben, Sodium Lauryl Sulfate, Water.

Cream: Active Ingredient: Tetracaine 2%. Also contains: Chloroxylenol, Eucalyptus Oil, Hydrochloric Acid, Lauramide DEA, Methylparaben, Sodium Borate, Sodium Lauryl Sulfate, Steareth-2, Steareth-21, Stearic Acid, Water, White Wax.

Indications: For the temporary relief of pain and itching associated with cold sores and fever blisters.

Directions: Adults and children 2 years of age and older: apply to affected area not more than 3 to 4 times daily. Children under 2 years of age: Consult a doctor.

Warnings: For external use only. Avoid contact with eyes. If contact occurs, rinse eyes thoroughly with water. If condition worsens, or symptoms persist for more than 7 days, or clear up and occur again within a few days, discontinue use of this product and consult a doctor. Do not use in large quantities, particularly over raw surfaces or blistered areas. Keep this and all drugs out of the reach of children. In case of accidental ingestion, seek professional assistance or contact a Poison Control Center immediately. Store at room temperature. Do not freeze.

How Supplied: Available in Gel and Cream formulas in 0.25 oz. (7.1 g) tubes.

Shown in Product Identification Guide, page 529

CHILDREN'S CĒPACOL® SORE THROAT FORMULA

[sē' pə-cŏl]
Pain Reliever, Nasal Decongestant, Fever Reducer
Grape and Cherry Flavor Liquids

Active Ingredients: Each teaspoon (5 mL) contains Acetaminophen USP 160 mg and Pseudoephedrine Hydrochloride USP 15 mg.
Also contains (Grape Flavor): Benzoic Acid, Carboxymethyl Cellulose, Cetylpyridinium Chloride (Ceepryn®), Citric Acid, FD&C Blue No. 1, FD&C Red No. 40, Flavor, Glycerin, PEG-8, Polysorbate 20, Propylene Glycol, Purified Water, Saccharin Sodium, Sodium Benzoate, and Sorbitol.
Also contains (Cherry Flavor): Benzoic Acid, Carboxymethyl Cellulose, Cetylpyridinium Chloride (Ceepryn®), Citric Acid, D&C Red No. 33, FD&C Red No. 40, Flavor, Glycerin, PEG-8, Polysorbate 20, Propylene Glycol, Purified Water, Saccharin Sodium, Sodium Benzoate, and Sorbitol.

AGE (yr)	WEIGHT (lb)	DOSE (teaspoon)
Under 2	Under 24	Consult doctor
2–5	24–47	1
6–11	48–95	2
12 and Over	Over 95	4

Indications: For temporary relief of sore throat pain, other minor aches and pains, and nasal congestion due to a cold or flu. Promotes nasal and/or sinus drainage; temporarily relieves sinus congestion and pressure. Reduces fever.

Directions: Follow dosage recommendations below, or as directed by a doctor. Dosages may be repeated every 4–6 hours, not to exceed 4 doses in 24 hours. For accurate dosing, use the enclosed dosage cup.
SHAKE WELL BEFORE USING.
[See table above]
Store at room temperature.

Warnings: If sore throat is severe, persists for more than 2 days, is accompanied or followed by fever, headache, rash, nausea, or vomiting, consult a doctor promptly. Do not take for pain or nasal congestion for more than 5 days or for fever for more than 3 days unless directed by a physician. If pain or fever persists or gets worse, if new symptoms occur, or if redness or swelling is present, consult a physician because these could be signs of a serious condition. Do not exceed recommended dosage. If nervousness, dizziness, or sleeplessness occur, discontinue use and consult a doctor. KEEP THIS AND ALL MEDICINES OUT OF THE REACH OF CHILDREN. Do not use with other products containing acetaminophen. In case of accidental overdose, contact a physician or poison control center immediately. Prompt medical attention is critical even if you do not notice any signs or symptoms.
Do not take product if you have heart disease, high blood pressure, thyroid disease, diabetes, or difficulty in urination due to enlargement of the prostate gland unless directed by a physician. As with any drug, if you are pregnant or nursing a baby, seek the advice of a health professional before using this product.

Drug Interaction Precaution: Do not take this product if you are now taking a prescription monoamine oxidase inhibitor (MAOI) (certain drugs for depression, psychiatric or emotional conditions, or Parkinson's disease), or for 2 weeks after stopping the MAOI drug. If you are uncertain whether your prescription drug contains an MAOI, consult a health professional before taking this product.

How Supplied: Available in Grape and Cherry flavors in 4 fl. oz. (118 mL) plastic bottles with dosage cup.

Shown in Product Identification Guide, page 528

Wyeth-Ayerst Pharmaceuticals

Division of American Home Products Corporation
P.O. BOX 8299
PHILADELPHIA, PA 19101

Direct General Inquiries to:
(610) 688-4400

For Professional Services
(For example: Sales representative information, product pamphlets, educational materials):
800-395-9938

For Medical Product Information Contact:
Medical Affairs
Day: (800) 934-5556 (8:30 AM to 4:30 PM, Eastern Standard Time, Weekdays only)
Night: (610) 688-4400 (Emergencies only; non-emergencies should wait until the next day)

Wyeth-Ayerst Tamper-Resistant/Evident Packaging

Statements alerting consumers to the specific type of Tamper-Resistant/Evident Packaging appear on the bottle labels and cartons of all Wyeth-Ayerst over-the-counter products. This includes plastic cap seals on bottles, individually wrapped tablets or suppositories, and sealed cartons. This packaging has been developed to better protect the consumer.

AMPHOJEL®

[am 'fo-jel]
Antacid
(aluminum hydroxide gel)
ORAL SUSPENSION • TABLETS

Composition: *Suspension*—Peppermint flavored —Each teaspoonful (5 mL) contains 320 mg aluminum hydroxide [Al(OH)$_3$] as a gel, and not more than 0.10 mEq of sodium. The inactive ingredients present are calcium benzoate, glycerin, hydroxypropyl methylcellulose, menthol, peppermint oil, potassium butylparaben, potassium propylparaben, saccharin, simethicone, sorbitol solution, and water. *Tablets* are available in 0.3 and 0.6 g strengths. Each contains, respectively, the equivalent of 300 mg and 600 mg aluminum hydroxide as a dried gel. The inactive ingredients present are artificial and natural flavors, cellulose, hydrogenated vegetable oil, magnesium stearate, polacrilin potassium, saccharin, starch, and talc. The 0.3 g (5 grain) strength is equivalent to about 1 teaspoonful of the suspension and the 0.6 g (10 grain) strength is equivalent to about 2 teaspoonfuls. Each 0.3 g tablet contains 0.08 mEq of sodium and each 0.6 g tablet contains 0.13 mEq of sodium.

Indications: For temporary relief of heartburn, upset stomach, sour stomach, and/or acid indigestion.

Directions: *Suspension* —Two teaspoonfuls (10 ml) to be taken five or six times daily, between meals and on retiring or as directed by a physician. Medication may be followed by a sip of water if desired. *Tablets* —Two tablets of the 0.3 g strength, or one tablet of the 0.6 g strength, five or six times daily, between meals and on retiring or as directed by a physician. It is unnecessary to chew the 0.3 g tablet before swallowing with water. After chewing the 0.6 g tablet, sip about one-half glass of water.

Warnings: Do not take more than 12 teaspoonfuls (60 ml) of suspension, or more than twelve (12) 0.3 g tablets, or more than six (6) 0.6 g tablets in a 24-hour period or use this maximum dosage for more than two weeks except under the advice and supervision of a physician. May cause constipation. Prolonged use of aluminum-containing antacids in patients with renal failure may result in or worsen dialysis osteomalacia. Elevated tissue aluminum levels contribute to the development of dialysis encephalopathy and osteomalacia syndromes. Also, a number of cases of dialysis encephalopathy have been associated with elevated aluminum levels in the dialysate water. Small amounts of aluminum are absorbed from the gastrointestinal tract and renal excretion of aluminum is impaired in renal failure. Prolonged use of aluminum-containing antacids in such patients may contribute to increased plasma levels of aluminum. Aluminum is not well removed by dialysis because it is bound to albumin and transferrin, which do not cross dialysis membranes. As a result, aluminum is deposited in bone, and dialysis osteomalacia may develop when large amounts of aluminum are ingested orally by patients with impaired renal function. As with any drug, if you are pregnant or nursing a baby, seek the advice of a health professional before using this product.

Drug Interaction Precaution: Antacids may interact with certain prescription drugs. Do not use this product if you are presently taking a prescription antibiotic containing any form of tetracycline. If you are presently taking a prescription drug, do not take this product without checking with your physician. Keep tightly closed and store at room temperature, Approx. 77°F (25°C). Suspension should be shaken well before use. Avoid freezing. Keep this and all drugs out of the reach of children.

How Supplied: *Suspension* —Peppermint flavored; bottles of 12 fluid ounces. *Tablets* —a convenient auxiliary dosage form—0.3 g (5 grain) bottles of 100; 0.6 g (10 grain), bottles of 100. Manufactured by: Wyeth Laboratories A Wyeth-Ayerst Company Philadelphia, PA 19101
Shown in Product Identification Guide, page 529

Professional Labeling: Consult *1999 Physicians' Desk Reference.*

CEROSE® DM
[*se-ros 'DM*]
Antihistamine/Nasal Decongestant/ Cough Suppressant

Description: Each teaspoonful (5 mL) contains 15 mg dextromethorphan hydrobromide, 4 mg chlorpheniramine maleate, and 10 mg phenylephrine hydrochloride. Alcohol 2.4%. The inactive ingredients present are artificial flavors, citric acid, edetate disodium, FD&C Yellow 6, glycerin, saccharin sodium, sodium benzoate, sodium citrate, sodium propionate, and water.

Indications: For the temporary relief of cough due to minor throat and bronchial irritation as may occur with the common cold or with inhaled irritants. Temporarily relieves nasal congestion, runny nose, and sneezing due to the common cold, hay fever, or other upper respiratory allergies.

Directions: Adults and children 12 years of age and over: One teaspoonful every four hours as needed. Children 6 to under 12 years of age: One-half teaspoonful every four hours as needed. Do not exceed six doses in a 24-hour period. Consult a physician for use in children under 6 years of age.

Warnings: May cause marked drowsiness; alcohol, sedatives, and tranquilizers may increase the drowsiness effect. Avoid alcoholic beverages while taking this product. Do not take this product if you are taking sedatives or tranquilizers, without first asking your doctor. Use caution when driving a motor vehicle or operating machinery. May cause excitability, especially in children. Do not take this product if you have heart disease, high blood pressure, thyroid disease, diabetes, a breathing problem such as emphysema or chronic bronchitis, glaucoma, or difficulty in urination due to enlargement of the prostate gland unless directed by a doctor. Do not take this product for persistent or chronic cough such as occurs with smoking, asthma, or emphysema, or if cough is accompanied by excessive phlegm (mucus) unless directed by a doctor. A persistent cough may be a sign of a serious condition. If cough or other symptoms persist for more than one week without improvement, tend to recur, or are accompanied by fever, rash, or persistent headache, consult a doctor. **Do not exceed recommended dosage.** Do not take this product for more than 7 days. If nervousness, dizziness, or sleeplessness occur, discontinue use and consult a doctor. As with any drug, if you are pregnant or nursing a baby, seek the advice of a health professional before using this product. Keep this and all drugs out of the reach of children. In case of accidental overdose, seek professional assistance or contact a Poison Control Center immediately.

Drug Interaction Precaution: Do not use this product if you are now taking a prescription monoamine oxidase inhibitor (MAOI) (certain drugs for depression, psychiatric or emotional conditions, or Parkinson's disease), or for 2 weeks after stopping the MAOI drug. If you are uncertain whether your prescription drug contains an MAOI, consult a health professional before taking this product.

How Supplied: Cases of 12 bottles of 4 fl. oz.; bottles of 1 pint.

Keep tightly closed—Store at room temperature, below 77° F (25° C).
Manufactured by:
Wyeth Laboratories
A Wyeth-Ayerst Company
Philadelphia, PA 19101
Shown in Product Identification Guide, page 529

DONNAGEL®
[*don 'nă-jel*]
Liquid and Chewable Tablets

Each tablespoon (15 mL) of **Donnagel Liquid** contains: 600 mg Attapulgite, Activated, USP.

Inactive Ingredients: Alcohol 1.4%, Benzyl Alcohol, Carboxymethylcellulose Sodium, Citric Acid, FD&C Blue 1, Flavors, Magnesium Aluminum Silicate, Methylparaben, Phosphoric Acid, Propylene Glycol, Propylparaben, Saccharin Sodium, Sorbitol, Titanium Dioxide, Water, Xanthan Gum.

Each **Donnagel Chewable** Tablet contains: 600 mg Attapulgite, Activated, USP.

Continued on next page

Donnagel—Cont.

Inactive Ingredients: D&C Yellow 10 Aluminum Lake, FD&C Blue 1 Aluminum Lake, Flavors, Magnesium Stearate, Mannitol, Saccharin Sodium, Sorbitol, Water.

Indications: Donnagel is indicated for the symptomatic relief of diarrhea. It reduces the number of bowel movements, improves consistency of loose, watery bowel movements and relieves cramping.

Warnings: Patients are told that diarrhea may be serious. They are warned not to use this product for more than 2 days, or in the presence of fever, or in children under 3 years of age unless directed by a doctor.

This product should not be taken by patients who are hypersensitive to any of the ingredients. As with any drug, women who are pregnant or nursing a baby should seek the advice of a health professional before using this product. KEEP THIS AND ALL DRUGS OUT OF THE REACH OF CHILDREN. IN CASE OF ACCIDENTAL OVERDOSE, SEEK PROFESSIONAL ASSISTANCE OR CONTACT A POISON CONTROL CENTER IMMEDIATELY.

Dosage and Administration: Full recommended dose should be administered at the first sign of diarrhea and after each subsequent bowel movement, NOT TO EXCEED 7 DOSES IN A 24-HOUR PERIOD.

[See table below]

How Supplied: Donnagel Liquid (green suspension) in 4 fl. oz. (NDC 0008-0888-02), and 8 fl. oz. (NDC 0008-0888-04).

Donnagel Chewable Tablets (light-green, flat-faced, beveled-edged, round tablets with darker green flecks; one side engraved "W", obverse engraved Donnagel) in consumer blister packages of 18 (NDC 0008-0889-02.)

Store at controlled room temperature, between 20°C and 25°C (68°F and 77°F).

Manufactured by:

Wyeth Laboratories

A Wyeth-Ayerst Company

Philadelphia, PA 19101

Shown in Product Identification Guide, page 529

Zila Pharmaceuticals, Inc.
5227 NORTH 7th STREET PHOENIX, AZ 85014-2800

Direct Inquiries to:
Jerry Kaster,
Vice President of Marketing:
(602) 266-6700
World Wide Web Address
www.zila.com

ZILACTIN® Medicated Gel
ZILACTIN®-L Liquid
ZILACTIN®-B Medicated Gel with Benzocaine

Description: Zilactin Medicated Gel stops pain and speeds healing of canker sores, fever blisters and cold sores. Zilactin forms a tenacious, occlusive film which holds the medication in place while controlling pain. Intra-orally, the film can last up to 6 hours, usually allowing pain-free eating and drinking. Extra-orally, the film will last much longer.

Zilactin-L is a non film-forming liquid that treats and relieves the pain, itching and burning of developing and existing cold sores and fever blisters. Zilactin-L is specially formulated to treat the initial signs of tingling, itching or burning that signal an oncoming cold sore or fever blister. Zilactin-L can often prevent developing cold sores or fever blisters from breaking out. If a lesion does occur, Zilactin-L will significantly reduce the size and the duration of the outbreak.

Zilactin-B is a medicated gel containing benzocaine that forms a smooth, flexible and occlusive film on the oral mucosa. It's specially formulated to control pain and shield the mouth sores, canker sores, cheek bites and gum sores that occur from dental appliances from the environment of the mouth. The film can last up to 6 hours. *Clinical studies on the effectiveness of Zila's products are available on request.*

Active Ingredients: Zilactin—Benzyl Alcohol (10%); **Zilactin-L**—Lidocaine (2.5%); **Zilactin-B**—Benzocaine (10%);

Application: Zilactin: FOR USE IN THE MOUTH AND ON LIPS. Apply every four hours for the first three days and then as needed. Dry the affected area. Apply a thin coat of Zilactin and allow 60 seconds for the gel to dry into a film. Outside the mouth, Zilactin forms a transparent film. Inside the mouth, the film is white.

Zilactin-L: FOR USE ON THE LIPS AND AROUND THE MOUTH. Apply every 1-2 hours for the first three days and then as needed. For maximum effectiveness use at first signs of tingling or itching. Moisten a cotton swab with several drops of Zilactin-L. Apply on lip area where symptoms are noted or directly on existing cold sore or fever blister and allow to dry for 15 seconds.

Zilactin-B: FOR USE IN THE MOUTH. Apply every four hours for the first three days and then as needed. Dry the affected area. Apply a thin coat of Zilactin-B and allow 60 seconds for the gel to dry into a film.

Warning: A mild, temporary stinging sensation may be experienced when applying Zilactin, Zilactin-L or Zilactin-B to an open cut, sore or blister. This may be minimized by first applying ice for a minute before application of the medication. **Do not peel off protective film.** Attempting to peel off film may result in skin irritation or tenderness. To remove film, first apply another coat of Zilactin-B to film, and immediately wipe the area with a gauze pad or tissue. DO NOT USE IN OR NEAR EYES. In the event of accidental contact with the eye, flush with water immediately and continuously for ten minutes. Seek immediate medical attention if pain or irritation persists. For temporary relief only. As with all medications, keep out of the reach of children. Do not use Zilactin-L or Zilactin-B if you have a history of allergy to local anesthetics such as benzocaine, lidocaine or other "caine" anesthetics.

How Supplied: Zila products are non-prescription and carried by most drug wholesalers, retail chains and independent pharmacies. Each product is available to physicians and dentists directly from Zila in single use packages.

For further information call or write:

Zila Pharmaceuticals, Inc.
5227 N. 7th Street, Phoenix, AZ 85014-2800, (602) 266-6700

U.S. patent numbers 4,285,934; 4,381,296; and 5,081,158

Shown in Product Identification Guide, page 529

ZILACTIN® BABY
Medicated Gel
Alcohol-Free

Description: Zilactin-Baby medicated gel is uniquely formulated to temporarily relieve sore gums caused by teething in infants and children 4 months of age and older. The extra strength level of medication in Zilactin-Baby begins relieving the discomfort of teething pain in seconds. This specially developed gel combines a

	Liquid	Chewable Tablets
Adults	2 Tablespoons	2 Tablets
Children		
12 years and over	2 Tablespoons	2 Tablets
6 to under 12 years	1 Tablespoon	1 Tablet
3 to under 6 years	1/2 Tablespoon	1/2 Tablet
Under 3 years	Consult Physician	

Liquid should be shaken well. Tablets should be chewed thoroughly and swallowed.

pleasant grape flavor with an advanced ingredient that imparts a cooling sensation.

Active Ingredient: Benzocaine (10%)

Inactive Ingredients: PEG-8, PEG-75, Glycerin, Water, Potassium Acesulfame, Flavor, Menthyl Lactate, Glycine, Methylparaben, Propylparaben, Sorbic Acid.

Directions: Wash hands. Apply small amount to the affected gum area with fingertip or cotton applicator. Apply to affected area not more than 4 times daily or as directed by a dentist or physician. For infants under 4 months of age, there is no recommended dosage or treatment except under the advice and supervision of a physician.

Warning: DO NOT USE THIS PRODUCT FOR MORE THAN 7 DAYS UNLESS DIRECTED BY A DENTIST OR PHYSICIAN. If sore mouth symptoms do not improve in 7 days, or if irritation, pain, rash or fever develops, see a dentist or physician promptly. Do not exceed the recommended dosage. Do not use this product if there is a history of allergy to topical anesthetics such as procaine, butacaine, benzocaine or other "caine" anesthetics. Fever and nasal congestion are not symptoms of teething and may indicate the presence of infection. If these symptoms persist consult your physician. Keep this and all drugs out of the reach of children. In case of accidental overdose, seek professional assistance or contact a Poison Control Center immediately.

Shown in Product Identification Guide, page 529

EDUCATIONAL MATERIAL

Samples and literature are available to medical professionals on request.

DIETARY SUPPLEMENT INFORMATION

This section presents information on natural remedies and nutritional supplements marketed under the Dietary Supplement Health and Education Act of 1994. It is made possible through the courtesy of the manufacturers whose products appear on the following pages. The information concerning each product has been prepared, edited, and approved by professional staff of the manufacturer.

Products to be found in this section include vitamins, minerals, herbs and other botanicals, amino acids, other substances intended to supplement the diet, and concentrates, metabolites, constituents, extracts, and combinations of these ingredients. The descriptions of these products are designed to provide all information necessary for informed use, including, when applicable, active ingredients, inactive ingredients, actions, warnings, cautions, interactions, symptoms and treatment of oral overdosage, dosage and directions for use, and how supplied.

Descriptions in this section must be in full compliance with the Dietary Supplement Health and Education Act, which permits claims regarding a product's effect on the structure or functioning of the body, but forbids claims regarding a product's ability to treat, diagnose, cure, or prevent any specific disease. Descriptions of products marketed under the act do not receive formal evaluation or approval from the Food and Drug Administration.

In compiling this section, the publisher has emphasized the necessity of describing products comprehensively. The descriptions seen here include all information made available by the manufacturer. The publisher does not warrant or guarantee any product described here, and does not perform any independent analysis of the information provided. Inclusion of a product in this book does not represent an endorsement, and the publisher does not necessarily advocate the use of any product listed.

AdvoCare International, L.L.C.

2727 REALTY ROAD
SUITE 134
CARROLLTON, TX 75006

Direct inquiries to:
Medical/Scientific Advisory Board
(972) 478-4500
Fax: (972) 831-8830

ADVANTIN

Uses: Advantin, a high-potency, all-natural mixture of standardized botanical extracts blended into a whole papaya base, is scientifically designed to support improved digestion and absorption of nutrients. With optimized digestion, energy levels increase, skin tone improves, joints move more smoothly and heartburn and other gastrointestinal discomforts subside.

With improved fat and protein digestion, more nutrients are absorbed from food, beverages and dietary supplements. Higher nutrient uptake helps people to eat less food and make better food choices, making Advantin an important part of a weight management program. Advantin supports the body's production and release of digestive enzymes. Standardized ginger extract is combined with natural digestive enzymes to help calm the stomach and increase the efficiency of digestion. Curcumin extract contains a revolutionary new botanical fraction loaded with powerful antioxidants to help protect the delicate intestinal cell lining from free radical damage.

Advantin is also beneficial in allowing the joints and muscles to move more smoothly. Boswellia extract, along with curcumin extract, contains powerful elements to help reduce inflammation and water build-up (edema).

Directions: Take one Advantin capsule immediately before a meal. For best results, take Advantin two or three times every day. Advantin is appropriate for anyone 12 years of age and older.

Ingredients: One capsule provides 200 mg of Ginger extract (standardized), 150 mg of Boswellia extract (standardized), 100 mg of Curcumin (standardized), 50 mg of whole Papaya powder, 50 mg of Papain and 50 mg of Bromelain.

How Supplied: One bottle contains 60 capsules.

ANTIOXIDANT BOOSTER

Uses: Antioxidant Booster helps protect against free radical damage and oxidation of LDL cholesterol.

Free radicals are extremely destructive chemical species in our bodies which are now strongly linked to an increased risk of a variety of serious diseases, as well as premature aging. Oxidized LDL cholesterol has received a great deal of current biomedical research attention, and is thought to be one of the main factors contributing to increased risk of heart disease and strokes.

Antioxidant Booster's unique formulation provides essential materials for the body's own internal antioxidant enzyme systems. The minerals zinc, manganese and selenium, are in highly bioavailable forms for maximum potency.

Antioxidant Booster contains a unique and scientifically based blend of phytochemicals to further protect body tissues against the hazards of free radical damage. These phytochemicals contain compounds known as "flavones", some of the most active of which are found in green tea, ginkgo biloba and silymarin. Antioxidant Booster contains natural vitamin E, beta-carotene and both water- and fat-soluble forms of vitamin C, thus giving a more complete spectrum of protection than products just containing ascorbic acid (vitamin C).

Directions: Take two caplets of Antioxidant Booster daily, with food, to enhance the body's protection against free radicals.

Ingredients: Two caplets provide the following: 250IU of Vitamin E (D-alpha tocopheryl succinate), 1000 mg of Vitamin C (ascorbic acid and ascorbyl palmitate), 15,000 IU of Betacarotene, 50mcg of Selenium (Selenomethionine), 5 mg of Zinc (OptiZinc), 1 mg of Manganese (Amino acid chelate), 50 mg of Green Tea Extract (Standardized), 50 mg of Silymarin (Standardized milk thistle extract) and 100 mg of Grape Seed Flavonoids (Activin).

How Supplied: Each bottle contains 60 caplets.

BODYLEAN
Protein Mix

Uses: BodyLean is an exceptional source of high protein combined with muscle enhancing nutrients. BodyLean is designed to optimize muscle mass during times of intensive exercise such as weight lifting. BodyLean may also be used in a weight management program, or for anyone seeking to increase their protein intake.

BodyLean provides a full 50 grams of protein in each serving. The highest grade proteins available are used for easy digestion and maximum utilization by the body.

The exceptional protein profile of BodyLean is further enhanced with free-form branched chain amino acids (BCAAs). During intensive physical activity, muscles selectively lose BCAAs, and supplementation with BCAAs may help spare muscle breakdown and replenish muscle losses quickly.

During weight loss, protein is essential for muscle strength and to maintain muscle mass. Diets rich in carbohydrates and plant foods often lack enough protein to sustain muscle while losing body fat.

Directions: Blend or shake three heaping scoops of Body Lean powder into at least 16 fluid ounces of any beverage of choice.

Ingredients: Metabolically Balanced Protein Isolate™ (containing total milk protein, calcium sodium caseinate, whey protein concentrate, soy protein concentrate, branched chain amino acids [L-leucine, L-isoleucine, L-valine], fructose, natural and artificial flavors, magnesium oxide, ascorbic acid, adrenal extract, acesultame potassium, pyridoxine hydrochloride, calcium pantothenate, niacin, manganese sulfate, papain, bromelain, thiamine hydrochloride, riboflavin, biotin and cyanocobalamin.

How Supplied: One can contains 10 servings of 75 grams each. One box contains 15 packets containing 37.5 grams each (25 grams of protein per serving).

BRITE-LIFE
Metabolic Nutrition

Uses: Brite-Life is a gentle yet powerful blend of standardized herbal extracts and vitamins designed to enhance a positive mood and feelings of well-being.

Brite-Life contains the important mood-boosting herb St. John's Wort. St. John's Wort has been found to help alleviate depression through its influence on brain serotonin levels. Serotonin is also involved in weight management. Higher serotonin levels are linked to appetite suppression. Lower serotonin levels are associated with obesity. Brite-Life uses the highest potency, standardized St. John's Wort extract to give brain chemistry maximum support.

Directions: *Take one caplet two times a day, 30 minutes before meals, as a natural dietary supplement.*

Ingredients: *One caplet contains 300 mg of St. John's Wort extract (standardized), 100 mg of Pyridoxine (HCl), 250 mg of Green Orange extract (standardized), 50 mg of German Chamomile extract (standardized) and 100 mg of Guarana extract (standardized).*

How Supplied: *One bottle contains 60 caplets.*

CARDIOPTIMA

Uses: CardiOptima is a heart-healthy drink mix rich in the most potent blend of antioxidants, blood vessel protectors and cardiac tonics. This pleasant-tasting product provides nutritional support for the prevention of oxidized LDL cholesterol and sticky platelets, thereby dramatically decreasing the liklihood of cardiovascular disease.

CardiOptima contains a proprietary blend of antioxidant mineral ascorbates, vitamin E and ActiVin™ grape seed extract which work together to support cardiovascular function. Also features Coenzyme Q-10, taurine and selected amino acids to prevent LDL deposition on arterial walls.

Complementary vitamins, minerals and herbs also assist the body in clearing homocysteine, a metabolic by-product identified as a cardiovascular risk factor.

Directions: Drink one or more glasses of CardiOptima daily on an empty stomach any time of the day or night.

Ingredients: One serving of CardiOptima 100 mg L-methionine, 600 mg L-lysine, 400 mg Taurine, 100 mg L-proline, 10mg Coenzyme Q-10, 20 mg L-carnitine and 100 mg Activin™ Grape Seed Extract as well as dextrose, fructose, 1000 mg vitamin C (potassium/calcium ascorbates), Krebs Cycle Mineralized Substrates ™ (citric acid, magnesium citrate, calcium citrate, 300 IU D-alpha tocopheryl succinate (vitamin E), gum arabic, beet powder, food flavoring, magnesium sulfate, inositol hexanicotinate, pyridoxine hydrochloride, Phytocardia Complex™ (hibiscus flower powder, hawthorn berry powder, Golden Root extract), folic acid and cyanocobalamin.

How Supplied: Each box contains 15 packets, each having a net weight of 26 grams.

COLD SEASON NUTRITION BOOSTER

Uses: Cold Season Nutrition Booster is a potent immune-boosting formula designed to augment resistance to colds and flu. Contains a mixture of standardized herbal extracts traditionally used to boost a depressed immune system. Cold Season Nutrition Booster contains large quantities of these key herbals, providing maximum efficacy.

Echinacea is widely known for its immune boosting properties, and the standardized extract contained in the product provides the most potent echinacea available. Golden seal extract complements the benefits of echinacea.

Astragalus is widely used in Chinese herbal medicine as an immune booster. Shiitake mushroom also enjoys great popularity in Asia as a major immune support.

Directions: Take Cold Season Nutrition Booster at the first sign of a cold or flu. Consume Cold Season Nutrition Booster for 7 to 10 days, then go off of the formula for 4 to 7 days.

Ingredients: Each capsule contains 200 mg of echinacea extract (standardized), 50 mg astragalus extract (standardized), 25 mg golden seal extract (standardized), 100 mg shiitake mushroom extract (standardized), 10 mg elderberry extract (standardized), 50 mg thymus extract and 50 mg quercetin.

COREPLEX
Metabolic Nutrition

Uses: *CorePlex is a premier multi-nutrient supplement including vitamins, minerals and complementary pytochemicals.*
CorePlex supplies the body with all known essential vitamins and minerals (except iron) in a metabolically optimizing formula. CorePlex is nutritionally proportioned for maximum potency and support of metabolic nutrition, balancing each nutrient against the others for maximum absorption and utilization. CorePlex contains mineral chelates such as OptiZinc™ (zinc monomethionine), ChromeMate™, (niacin-bound chromium) and selenomethionine for highest bioavailability. Most leading multiple vitamin/mineral products contain ionic forms of minerals such as zinc oxide and chromium chloride, which are much more poorly absorbed than the chelated minerals used in CorePlex.

Directions: Take three CorePlex daily as the cornerstone of the AdvoCare nutrition program. Take CorePlex with food, either in the morning or at noon.

Warning: Keep out of reach of children.

Ingredients: Three caplets provide 2,500 IU of vitamin A (palmitate), 12,500 IU of vitamin A (beta carotene), 600 mg of vitamin C, 400 IU of vitamin D (ergocalciferol), 150 IU of vitamin E (d-alpha tocopheryl succinate), 9 mg thiamine, 10.2 mg riboflavin, 20 mg niacin, 100 mg niacinamide, 40 mg panothenic acid, 12 mg pyridoxine (HCl), 36 mcg vitamin B-12 (cyanocobalamin), 400 mcg folic acid, 300 mcg biotin, 6 mg inositol, 60mg choline, 150 mg calcium# 200 mg magnesium#, 15 mg zinc, 150 mcg iodine (Kelp), 80 mcg selenium (Selenomethionine), 4 mg Manganese#, 100 mcg Chromium (Chromemate), 50 mcg Molybdenum#, 2 mg copper#, 100 mg potassium#, 300 mcg Boron#, 50 mcg Vanadium (BMOV), 100 mg Phosphorus#, 500 mcg silicon#, 150 mcgcoenzyme Q10, 2 mg Octacosanol, 2 mg RNA, 50 mg odorless garlic, 5 mg L-Glutathione, 5 mg Gamma Oryzanol, 100 mg Citrus Bioflavonoids, 5 mg red wine polyphenolss (Standardized), 5 mg Milk Thistle (Standardized), 10 mg Ginkgo Biloba (Standardized) and 100 mg L-Methionine.
#: Amino acid chelate or complex

INTELLEQ

Uses: InteleQ is a formula providing nutritional support for mental alertness, which containing a proprietary blend of biochemical building blocks.
Phospholipids are key to brain function and are converted to the biochemicals used by nerve and brain cells. The standardized phospholipid complex contains a unique mixture of choline and phosphatidylserine, a most sophisticated mixture based on the latent breakthroughs in nutrition research.

Ginkgo Biloba has been used for over 5000 years as a mental tonic and is among the top selling herbal extracts in Europe.

Rhodiola is a botanical widely used in eastern Europe, Asia and Tibet. Some studies have found that Rhodiola helps to increase memory in human subjects. Brahm IQ™ is a standardized extract of Bacopa monniera, shown in both human and animal studies to increase short-term and long-term memory.

Directions: Take one (1) to two (2) capsules per day with a meal, preferably early in the day.

Ingredients: Two capsules contain 150 mg of phospholipid complex (standardized), 100 mg of ginkgo biloba extract (standardized), 10 mg grape seed anthocyanidins (Activin™), 700 mcg boron (amino acid complex), 20 mg niacin, 1000 mcg RNA, 200 mg taurine, 100 mg choline (bitartrate) 60 mg vitamin C (potassium ascorbate), 500 mg Bacopa extract (BrahmIQ™).

MACRO-MINERAL COMPLEX

Uses: Macro-Mineral Complex is a comprehensive formulation which incorporates the full spectrum of bone-building nutrients in highly bioavailable forms.

The chelated calcium complex offers absorption which is superior to typical calcium supplements (which use the relatively poorly absorbed calcium carbonate). The forms of magnesium and complementary trace elements in Macro-Mineral Complex are also in the chelated form, thus speeding these bone-building nutrients into the body at the highest absorption rate.

The balance between calcium and magnesium is critical. Taking calcium by itself can actually drain the body of magnesium, which could result in muscle cramps, irritability, depression and other serious conditions. Macro-Mineral Complex uses a 1 to 1 calcium to magnesium ratio to perfectly balance these two key minerals.

Directions: Take two to six caplets daily, preferably with meals or at bedtime.

Ingredients: *Two caplets contain 220 mg calcium (amino acid chelate and hydroxyapatite), 220 mg magnesium (amino acid chelate and magnesium ascorbate), 2 mg zinc (OptZinc™), 600 mcg silicon (amino acid complex), 1 mg manganese (amino acid chelate), 400 mcg boron (amino acid complex), 200 mcg cooper (amino acid chelate), 40 IU vitamin D (ergocalciferol), 120 mg vitamin C (magnesium ascorbate), 12 mg pyridoxine (HCl), 500 mg potassium bicarbonate, 100 mg shave grass extract, 50 mg green tea extract and 20 mg ginger extract.*

Continued on next page

Macro-Mineral—Cont.

How Supplied: *One bottle contains 120 caplets.*

METABOLIC NUTRITION SYSTEM

Uses: *Metabolic Nutrition System Yellow*—Optimum foundational nutrients for metabolic support. Includes Acto-Therm which provides gentle support for thermogenesis and energy production. *Metabolic Nutrition System Red*—Maximum appetite suppression plus optimum levels of nutrients. Includes ActoTherm (see above) and OptiTherm, a 75 mg. sustained release phenylpropanolamine caplet.
Metabolic Nutrition System Orange—Energy and a heightened sense of well-being. Includes Thermo-E, which provides a proprietary combination of ephedra alkoloids and other adrenergic boosting herbs for maximum thermogenesis and weight management.
Metabolic Nutrition System Blue—Complete-spectrum nutrients plus Brite-Life, containing St. John's Wort, an herbal mood enhancer.
Every ingredient in the components of Metabolic Nutrition has been specifically selected based on the latest, most advanced scientific research studies from around the world.
Each of the four versions of Metabolic Nutrition System contain the following components:
CorePlex™ is a premier multinutrient supplement containing the complete spectrum of vitamins and minerals, phytochemical antioxidants, and complementary herbal concentrates. (See complete list of ingredients for CorePlex in this section).
LipoTrol™ is a natural formula designed to help control appetite and encourage proper metabolism of fats. The formula contains standardized Garcinia extract, standardized tulsi extract, taurine, L-carnitine, beta sitosterol, zinc (monomethionine-OptiZinc™), standardized gymnema sylvestre extract, pyridoxine (HCl), vanadium (BMOV), chromium (polynicotinate-ChromeMate™).
OmegaPlex™ is an exceptional source of the omega-3 fatty acids, eicosapentaenoic acid (EPA) and docosahexaenoic acid (DHA) for maximum cardiovascular support.
MetaBoost™ is a blend of nutrients and phytochemicals formulated to support the endocrine system. The formula includes potassium/magnesium/sodium ascorbates, desiccated pituitary extract, desiccated adrenal extract, iodine, guarana extract and Siberian ginseng extract.

PERFECT MEAL

Uses: Perfect Meal features a proprietary mixture of whole proteins, amino acids, peptides, digestive enzymes, and whole vegetable powders, as well as simple and complex carbohydrates, plus a full spectrum of vitamins and minerals. Easy-to-digest proteins and high-energy, easily absorbed peptides help build strong, powerful muscles and maximize metabolic function—essential for general well-being during weight loss.

Directions: Perfect Meal is designed to replace a lunch or dinner meal as part of a comprehensive weight loss program which also includes sensible food choices, plenty of water and regular physical activity.

Ingredients: One 170-calorie serving provides PM Ultra Protein complex (modified casein, soy protein powder, whey protein concentrate, di-/tri-peptides), fructose, maltodextrin, cocoa powder, purified cellulose, canola oil, hydrolyzed guar gum, L-lysine monohydrochloride, potassium chloride, L-glutamine, calcium carbonate, magnesium oxide, soy lecithin, dicalcium phosphate, natural and artificial flavors, carrot powder, oat grass powder, Lactobacillus acidophilus, acesulfame, medium chain triglycerides, papain, bromelain, rice syrup solids, choline citrate, ascorbic acid, vitamin E acetate, inositol, ferrous fumarate, niacinamide, zinc oxide, calcium pantothenate, vitamin A palmitate, copper sulfate, manganese sulfate, vitamin D, pyridoxine hydrochloride, riboflavin, thiamine mononitrate, chromium polynicotinate, folic acid, biotin, sodium selenite, sodium molybdate, potassium iodide, vitamin K and cyanocobalamin.

How Supplied: One can contains fourteen 45-gram servings.

PERFORMANCE GOLD

Uses: Performance Gold is an energy-enhancing formulation supplying key nutritional support for building muscle and endurance. The herbal extracts which comprise Performance Gold are called adaptogens. They help the body adapt to physical and mental stress. The enzyme-hydrolyzed whey protein is a source of easily absorbable peptides (protein fragments) which accelerate the positive benefits of the herbal extracts.
One of the key herbal extracts is Golden Root. Research has shown that Golden Root helps bring oxygen to tissues, which is vital for optimal performance. During exercise, the muscle and the brain suffer from lowered oxygen status, which brings on fatigue. Golden Root helps oxygenate the body, allowing lengthier, more rigorous exercise as well as quicker recovery.

Directions: Take one or two caplets 60 minutes before exercise or between meals.

Warning: This product is not intended for persons under 18, or for pregnant or lactating women.

Ingredients: Two caplets contain 100 mg of moomiyo, 25 mg of Golden Root extract (Standarized), 50 mg Siberian ginseng extract (Standarized), 500 mg of inosine and 1000 mg of enzyme-hydrolyzed whey protein.

PERFORMANCE OPTIMIZER SYSTEM

Uses: *Performance Optimizer System is a family of three interlocking nutritional formulas designed to enhance physical performance, promote peak muscle physiology and speed post-exercise recovery.*
Peak physical performance depends on a series of physiological processes including body and muscle fueling, hydration, support of anabolic and energy systems, and proper rest and recovery. AdvoCare's Performance Optimizer System addresses the metabolic needs of the active person.
Performance Optimizer System 1 supports anabolic physiology, enhancing the production of muscle. Muscle production is essential to anyone seeking to lose weight and perform at top physical levels.
Performance Optimizer System 2 supports the body's ability to make muscle protein and heal micro-tears that occur in muscle fiber during physical exercise. The unique blend of high quality dietary proteins combined with sports-enhancing glucose polymers and other unique carbohydrates provides energy and structural support for building strength. The inclusion of branched chain amino acids (BCAAs), creatine, medium chain triglycerides and digestive enzymes results in a superior formulation.
Performance Optimizer System 3 is an advanced sports drink which includes B-vitamins to support aerobic and anaerobic body energy pathways, as well as co-enzyme Q-10 and PAK, two natural energy compounds for extensive energy support for muscles, brain and body. By combining both quick-acting and "time-released" carbohydrates, the energy effects are both immediate and sustained. This beverage also contains glutamine, a key amino acid which helps buffer lactic acid buildup in muscles during exercise-and also supports keener mental function. Glutamine has also been shown to increase plasma bicarbonate which helps eliminate acids from the muscles and bloodstream. Isotonicity of POS 3 assures rapid gastric emptying for quick and effective rehydration and replenishment of electrolytes.

Directions: Performance Optimizer System 1 is designed to be taken at bedtime, preferably on an empty stomach. performance Optimizer System 2 should be used immediately after exercise to aid recovery and healing of muscles. Performance Optimizer System 3 should be consumed to provide rapid re-hydration as well as sustained energy.

Ingredients: Three caplets of Performance Optimizer System 1 contain 100 mg of moomiyo, 1200 mg of L-arginine, 600 mg of L-ornithine, 200 mg of oatgrass extract, 50 mg of nettles extract, 25 mg of Siberian ginseng extract, 50 mg of Ashwaganda extract, 5 mg of zinc (Opti-Zinc™), 500 mcg of copper (amino acid chelate), 150 mg of magnesium (amino acid chelate), 200 mcg vanadium (BMOV), 100 mg of saw palmetto extract, 20 mg of niacin, 50 mg of rantarin and 50 mg of wild yam extract.

One serving of Performance Optimizer System 2 contains 12 g of protein, 36 g of carbohydrate, 3 g of fat, 50 mcg of choline, 50 mg of inositol, 200 mcg of vanadium, 250 mcg of boron, 150 mcg of gamma oryzanol, 25 mg of L-carnitine, 100 mg of inosine, 1 mg of silicon, 2000 mg of creatine, 250 mg of methionine, 200 mg of L-leucine, 100 mg of L-valine, 100 mg of L-isoleucine as well as glucose polymers, fructose, modified casein, soy protein powder, cocoa powder, soy lecithin, MyoForce™ (creatine monohydrate, creatine phosphate, Siberian ginseng), carob powder, canola oil, dicalcium phosphate, corn syrup solids, branched chain amino acids (leucine, isoleucine, valine), natural and artificial flavors, medium chain triglycerides, magnesium oxide, calcium carbonate, DL-methionine, silicon dioxide, guar gum, xanthan gum, ascorbic acid, potassium chloride, rice syrup solids, fructooligosaccharides, citrus pectin, inositol, zinc gluconate, L-carnitine hydrochloride, calcium pantothenate, niacinamide, vitamin E succinate, beta carotene, manganese sulfate, ferrous fumarate, selenomethionine, calcium borate copper gluconate, pyridoxine hydrochloride, riboflavin, thiamine hydrochloride, vanadyl sulfate, chromium polynicotinate (ChromeMate™), vitamin D, papain, bromelain, gamma oryzanol, folic acid, choline dihydrogen citrate, biotin, sodium molybdate, dibencozide, cyanocobalamin, potassium iodide.

One serving of Performance Optimizer System 3 contains fructose, glucose polymers, magnesium/sodium/potassium citrates, citric acid, dextrose, tricalcium phosphate, natural flavors, ascorbic acid, potassium chloride, pyridoxine alpha ketoglutarate, creatine monohydrate/creatine phosphate, beta carotene, salt, l-glutamine, niacinamide, calcium pantothenate, riboflavin, thiamine hydrochloride, chromium polynicotinate (ChromeMate™), l-glutathione, coenzyme Q-10.

How Supplied: A bottle of Performance Optimizer System 1 contains 90 caplets.
One can of Performance Optimizer System 2 contains fifteen 60-gram servings.
One can of Performance Optimizer System 3 contains thirty 15-gram servings.

PROBIOTIC RESTORE

Uses: Restore contains more than two billion freeze-dried, beneficial lactic microflora, the consumption of which promotes optimal digestion, absorption of nutrients and elimination of wastes. Additionally, this product can ease constipation by supporting normal intestinal function.

Directions: Take one to three capsules per day with water, preferably on an empty stomach, 30 minutes or more before a meal. For children, capsules may be opened and contents mixed with water or fruit juice.

Ingredients: Lactobacillus acidophilus, Bifidobacterium bifidus, fructooligosaccharides, moomiyo, zinc monomethionine (OptiZinc™), vitamin A (beta–carotene and palmitate), aloe vera juice powder.

How Supplied: Each bottle contains 90 capsules

PROMOTION

Uses: ProMotion contains compounds that provide both lubrication and protection to the articular surfaces of the bone, promoting ease of motion. At the same time, ProMotion nourishes these tissues with the key biochemical building block for cartilage synthesis, essential for joint function.

ProMotion contains glucosamine HCl, a newly available and readily absorbed form of this vital biochemical. Glucosamine is one of the major building blocks of articular cartilage and of synovial fluid, the lubricating and cushioning material in joints. Glucosamine is found in high concentrations in hyaluronic acid and glycosaminoglycans, a group of compounds that are responsible for proper hydration and moisture retention throughout the body.

In several recent studies, glucosamine was shown to have a positive effect on both joint mobility and joint inflammatory conditions. In these studies, glucosamine relieved the most overt symptoms of osteoarthrosis, including tenderness, pain, and restricted movement, outperforming aspirin, ibuprofen, and naproxen in alleviating these symptoms. The glucosamine selected for ProMotion is a 100% pure, natural form for maximum bioactivity.

ProMotion also contains grape proanthocyanidins, phytochemicals that possess powerful antioxidant activity as well as potent protection against breakdown of cartilage.

These polyphenols are a subclass of flavonoids which have been shown in scores of scientific studies to be anti-inflammatory, anti-allergic, and to increase capillary strength. Proanthocyanidins have a particular affinity for collagen, protecting it from free radical attack and the inflammation that often accompanies this errant process.

Recent research has validated the ability of proanthocyanidins to inhibit hyaluronidase. Hyaluronidase is an enzyme that hydrolyzes and depolymerizes hyaluronic acid, the cementing substance of the body. This enzyme is involved in allergic reactions, inflammation, and capillary leakage. Proanthocyanidins have been shown to arrest the activity hyaluronidase, preventing the damage that this enzyme can inflict.

Directions: Take three (3) capsules per day, preferably with meals. ProMotion can be taken all at once or divided throughout the day, as desired.

Ingredients: *Three capsules contain 1500 mg of glucosamine HCl, 25 mg proanthocyanidins (wine grape seed), and 25 mg manganese sulfate.*

How Supplied: *One bottle contains 90 capsules.*

SPARK!
Nutritional Beverage Mix

Uses: Spark is a stimulating powdered beverage mix containing NeuroActives™, which are natural promoters of brain biochemistry. An array of vitamins, minerals and other factors are presented for efficient production of neuro-energy. The NeuroActives in Spark also work to help reduce appetite. Unlike many other energy drinks, Spark does not over stimulate and overburden body energy systems, but rather supports their activities with specific nutrients and neuro-precursor compounds. Spark provides endocrine support for energy without the let-down feeling often associated with non-nutritional artificial stimulants.

Directions: Blend one level scoop (15 grams) into 8 ounces of chilled or warm water or beverage of choice, 2 or 3 times a day or as desired.

Warning: Phenylketonuries: Contains phenylalanine. Children and pregnant or lactating women should consult a physician prior to use. Not for use by persons who are abnormally sensitive to caffeine or choline.

Ingredients: One serving contains 10 mg of L-carnitine, 200 mg of taurine, 50 mg of GABA, 100 mg of L-glycine, 500 mg of L-pheylalanine, 2 mg of RNA, 100 mg of ubiquinone, 500 mg of choline, 120 mg of caffeine, as well as fructose, maltodextrin, citric acid, ascorbic acid, natural flavor, calcium pantothenate, vitamin A (beta carotene, palmitate), niacinamide, vitamin E succinate, acesulfame, niacin, pyridoxine hydrochloride, zinc monomethionine (OptiZinc™), riboflavin, thiamine hydrochloride, copper amino acid chelate, chromium polynicotinate (ChromeMate™) and cyanocobalamin.

How Supplied: One can contains thirty 15-gram powdered servings.

Continued on next page

SYSTEM 3-4-3: Metabolic Cleansing System

The booklet enclosed with each System 3-4-3 box gives a day-by-day guide on how to use each component.

Ingredients:

FIBER 10—Fiber Blend (psyllium husk, guar gum, carboxymethyl cellulose, citrus pectin, butternut bark powder), fructose, beta-carotene, citric acid, natural and artificial flavors, acesulfame, fructooligosaccharides, papaya powder, prune powder, ascorbic acid, digestive enzyme complex (protease, lipase, cellulase), rhubarb root extract, black walnut hull extract, licorice root extract, Lactobacillus acidophilus, Bifidobacterium bifidus.

HERBAL CLEANSE—Three tablets contain: 3-4-3 Herbal Cleanse Complex (Green Kamut juice powder, Burdock Root extract, Cranberry juice powder, Senna extract, Astragalus extract, Echinacea extract, Odorless Garlic, Milk Thistle extract, Beet Root powder, Shisandra extract), Ascorbic Acid, Taurine, Niacin/Niacinamide, Pantothenic Acid, Zinc Monomethionine, Pyridoxine, Riboflavin, Thiamine, Inositol, Folic Acid, Biotin, Vitamin B-12 (cyanocobalamin).

RESTORE—Two capsules contain: Lactobacillus acidophilus, Bifodobacterium bifidus, Fructooligosaccharides, Aloe vera powder, Moomiyo, Zinc Monomethionine, Beta-Carotene, Vitamin A (palmitate).

Use System 3-4-3

* at the start of a healthy weight loss program
* if you are among the 80 million people who suffer from constipation
* after you have finished using antibiotics
* as part of a sports training and rehabilitation program
* if you have recurring colds or flus
* if you have fatigue, irritability, or experience mood swings
* if you have problems losing body fat
* as part of a comprehensive health promotion program

Uses: System 3-4-3 is a ten-day routine formulated to cleanse and rejuvenate the internal system. System 3-4-3 helps rid the body of toxins, enhancing energy levels, improving skin tone and assisting in weight management.

Directions: Take the Herbal Cleanse Tablets for the first seven days, take Fiber-10 for the first three days and, subsequently, on days eight through ten, and take ProBiotic Restore on days four through ten.

Warning: System 3-4-3 is not intended for use by pregnant or breast-feeding women, or for children. If you are ill, consult a health care professional before starting System 3-4-3. This product contains senna. Read and follow directions carefully. Do not use if you have or develop diarrhea, loose stools or abdominal pain. Consult your physician if you have frequent diarrhea. If you are taking medication, or have a medical condition, consult your physician before using this product.

AkPharma Inc.

P.O. BOX 111
PLEASANTVILLE, NJ
08232-0111

Direct Inquiries To:
Elizabeth Klein: (609) 645-5100
FAX: (609) 645-0767

Medical Emergency Contact:
Alan E. Kligerman: (609) 645-5100

PRELIEF®

PRODUCT OVERVIEW

Key Facts: Prelief is AkPharma's brand name for calcium glycerophosphate. It is used to remove acid from acidic foods and beverages when acidic foods are to be avoided for more tolerable ingestion. Prelief tablets are swallowed with the food or beverage. Prelief granulate is added to each serving of acidic food or beverage.

Major Uses: Helps neutralize the acid in acidic foods such as spaghetti and pizza sauce, citrus and other fruit drinks, coffee, wine, beer and colas.

Safety Information: Prelief is made from an FDA Generally Recognized as Safe (GRAS)[1] dietary supplement ingredient and is also listed as a food ingredient in the US Government Food Chemicals Codex (FCC)[2]

PRODUCT INFORMATION

Prelief®

Description: Prelief Tablets: Each tablet contains 333 mg of calcium glycer-ophosphate. The tablets also contain 0.5% magnesium stearate as a processing aid. Two or three tablets should be swallowed with the food or beverage. (See chart)

Prelief Granulate: Each packet contains 333 mg of calcium glycerophosphate. Add 2 packets of granulate to each serving of acidic food or beverage. Except for alcoholic beverages, the granulate dissolves rapidly in the acidic food or beverage. An additional 1–2 tablets or packets may be needed on foods that may be particularly high in acid. (See chart)

Each tablet or packet of granulate supplies 6% (65 mg) of the US Recommended Daily Allowance (USRDA) for calcium and 5% (50 mg) of the USRDA for phosphorus. No sodium; no aluminum; no sugar.

---

[1]reference 21 CFR §184.1201
[2]reference Food Chemicals Codex, 3rd Edition, pp 51–52

Reasons for Use: Prelief is a dietary supplement for use with acidic foods and beverages. It is a dietary intervention used to reduce the acid of these ingestibles for persons who identify acid discomfort with the ingestion of acidic foods and beverages.

Action: Prelief neutralizes the acid found in a large number of foods which many people find cause them discomfort. **See Table.**

Usage: 2 tablets or 2 granulate packets per serving of acidic food or beverage.

How Supplied: Prelief is supplied in both tablet form (30, 60 and 120 tablet bottle sizes and 24 tablets in 12–2 tablet packets), and granulate form (36 packets).

Kosher: Prelief is Kosher and Pareve.

Use Limitations: None, except as may apply below.

Adverse Reactions: None known

Toxicity: None known

Typical Food Acid Reduction by Prelief

Product	1 Packet or 1 Tablet	2 Packets or 2 Tablets	3 Packets or 3 Tablets
Pepsi Cola® – 8 oz.	98%	99.8%	–
Mott's® 100% Apple Juice – 4 oz.	49.8%	74.9%	90%
Tropicana® Orange Juice – 4 oz.	20.6%	36.9%	60%
Coors Light® Beer – 12 oz.	80.1%	95%	96.8%
Monty's Hill® Chardonnay – 4 oz.	37%	60.1%	80%
Ireland® Coffee – 6 oz.	93.7%	96.8%	98%
Tetley® Iced Tea – 8 oz.	99%	99.5%	–
Seven Seas® Red Wine & Vinegar Salad Dressing – 31 gm	90%	95%	98%
Old El Paso® Thick'n Chunky Salsa Medium – 2 Tbsp	80.1%	95%	97.5%
Heinz® Tomato Ketchup – 1 Tbsp.	68.4%	87.4%	92.1%
Kraft® Original Barbeque Sauce 2 Tbsp.	60.2%	80%	90%
Ragu® Old World Style Traditional Sauce – 125 gm	20.6%	36.9%	60.2%
Dannon® Strawberry Lowfat Yogurt (fully mixed) – 116 gm	49.9%	68.4%	80.1%
Grapefruit Sections – 150 gm	36.9%	50%	68.3%
Sauerkraut – 2 Tbsp.	60.3%	80%	92.1%
Red Cabbage – 130 gm	49.7%	68.3%	74.8%

Lead Content: Conforms with California Prop. 65 on lead content, to 15 tablets per day and 30 packets of granulate per day.

Interactions with Drugs: Calcium may interfere with efficacy of some medications. If a medication is being taken, check with physician, pharmacist or other health professional about the possible interactions of calcium with that medication. No other drug interactions known.

Precautions: People who have been advised by their physician not to take calcium, phosphorus or glycerin/glycerol should consult with their physician before using Prelief.

Prelief is classified as a dietary supplement, not a drug.

For more information and samples, please write or call toll-free 1-800-994-4711.

[See table at bottom of previous page]

Shown in Product Identification Guide, page 503

Bayer Corporation
Consumer Care Division

36 Columbia Road
P.O. Box 1910
Morristown, NJ 07962-1910

Direct Inquiries to:
Consumer Relations
(800) 331-4536
www.bayercare.com

For Medical Emergency Contact:
Bayer Corporation
Consumer Care Division
(800) 331-4536

FERGON®
Ferrous Gluconate
Iron Supplement

Description: Fergon Tablets are for use as a dietary iron supplement.

Directions For Use: Adults take one tablet daily, with food.

	Amount Per Serving	% Daily Value
Iron	27 mg	150

Use: Daily dietary supplement

Ingredients: Each tablet contains 240 mg Ferrous Gluconate equal to approximately 27 mg elemental Iron. Also contains: Sucrose, Corn Starch, Talc, Magnesium Stearate, Silica Gel, Hydroxypropyl Methylcellulose, Titanium Dioxide, Polyethylene Glycol, FD&C Yellow #5 Aluminum Lake (Tartrazine), FD&C Blue #1 Aluminum Lake, Polysorbate 80.

Warning: Accidental overdose of iron-containing products is a leading cause of fatal poisoning in children under 6. Keep this product out of the reach of children. In case of accidental overdose, call a doctor or poison control center immediately.

If you are pregnant of nursing a baby, seek the advice of a doctor before using this product.

Do not use this product if safety seal bearing Bayer Corporation under cap is torn or missing.

How Supplied: Bottles of 100 Tablets with child-resistant caps.

Shown in Product Identification Guide, page 504

FLINTSTONES® Original Children's Chewable Multivitamin Supplement

BUGS BUNNY™ Plus Iron Chewable Children's Multivitamin Plus Iron Supplement

FLINTSTONES® Plus Iron Chewable Children's Multivitamin Plus Iron Supplement

Amount Per Tablet	% Daily Value for Children 2–3 Years of Age	% Daily Value for Adults and Children 4 or more Years of Age
Vitamin A 2500 IU	100	50
Vitamin C 60 mg	150	100
Vitamin D 400 IU	100	100
Vitamin E 15 IU	150	50
Thiamin (B_1) 1.05 mg	150	70
Riboflavin (B_2) 1.2 mg	150	70
Niacin 13.5 mg	150	67
Vitamin B_6 1.05 mg	150	52
Folic Acid 300 mcg	150	75
Vitamin B_{12} 4.5 mcg	150	75
Iron (elemental) 15 mg	150	83

FLINTSTONES® Original Children's Chewable Vitamins provide the same quantities of vitamins, but do not provide iron.

Use: Dietary supplement.

Serving Size: For adults and children two years and older chew one tablet daily. Chew one tablet daily.

Warning
For Bugs Bunny Only: Phenylketonurics: Contains Phenylalanine.
FOR IRON CONTAINING SUPPLEMENTS ONLY:

WARNING: Accidental overdose of iron-containing products is a leading cause of fatal poisoning in children under 6. Keep this product out of the reach of children. In case of accidental overdose, call a doctor or poison control center immediately.

KEEP OUT OF REACH OF CHILDREN. CHILD RESISTANT CAP
Do not use this product if safety seal bearing Bayer Corporation under cap is torn or missing.

How Supplied: Flintstones are supplied in bottles of 60 and 100, Bugs Bunny in bottles of 60 with child-resistant caps.

Shown in Product Identification Guide, page 504

FLINTSTONES® COMPLETE
Children's Chewable Multivitamin/ Multimineral Supplement
BUGS BUNNY™ COMPLETE
Children's Chewable Multivitamin/ Multimineral Supplement (Sugar Free)

Vitamin Ingredients: Each supplement provides the ingredients listed in the chart below:
[See table at bottom of next page]

Use: Dietary Supplement.
Serving Size: 2–3 years of age: Chew one-half tablet daily. Over 4 years of age: Chew one tablet daily.

Warning: Phenylketonurics: Contains Phenylalanine.

WARNING: Accidental overdose of iron-containing products is a leading cause of fatal poisoning in children under 6. Keep this product out of the reach of children. In case of accidental overdose, call a doctor or poison control center immediately.

KEEP OUT OF REACH OF CHILDREN. CHILD RESISTANT CAP
Do not use this product if safety seal bearing Bayer Corporation under cap is torn or missing.

How Supplied: Bottles of 60's with child-resistant caps.
Shown in Product Identification Guide, page 504

FLINTSTONES® PLUS CALCIUM
Children's Chewable Multivitamin Plus Calcium Supplement

Ingredients: Calcium Carbonate, Sorbitol, Starch, Sodium Ascorbate, Natural

Continued on next page

Flintstones Plus Cal.—Cont.

and Artificial Flavors (including fruit acids), Stearic Acid, Gelatin, Magnesium Stearate, Vitamin E Acetate, Niacinamide, Artificial Colors (including FD&C Yellow #6), Aspartame* (a sweetener), Riboflavin, Pyridoxine Hydrochloride, Thiamine Mononitrate, Vitamin A Acetate, Monoammonium Glycyrrhizinate, Folic Acid, Beta Carotene, Vitamin D, Vitamin B$_{12}$.

Amount Per Tablet	% Daily Value for Children 2–3 Years of Age	% Daily Value for Adults and Children 4 or more Years of Age
Vitamin A 2500 IU	100	50
Vitamin C 60 mg	150	100
Vitamin D 400 IU	100	100
Vitamin E 15 IU	150	50
Thiamin (B$_1$) 1.05 mg	150	70
Riboflavin (B$_2$) 1.2 mg	150	70
Niacin 13.5 mg	150	67
Vitamin B$_6$ 1.05 mg	150	52
Folic Acid 300 mcg	150	75
Vitamin B$_{12}$ 4.5 mcg	150	75
Calcium 200 mg	25	20

Use: Dietary supplement.

Serving Size: For adults and children 2 years and older chew one tablet daily.

Warning: Phenylketonurics: contains phenylalanine

KEEP OUT OF REACH OF CHILDREN.

CHILD RESISTANT CAP

Do not use this product if safety seal bearing Bayer Corporation under cap is torn or missing.

How Supplied: Bottle of 60 Tablets with child-resistant caps.

Shown in Product Identification Guide, page 504

Directions for Use: 2 & 3 years of age —**Chew** one-half tablet daily. Adults and children 4 years of age and older—**Chew** one tablet daily.

Supplement Facts

Serving Size: $^1/_2$ tablet (2 & 3 years of age); 1 tablet (4 years of age and older)

Amount Per Tablet	% Daily Value for Children 2 & 3 Years of Age ($^1/_2$ Tablet)	% Daily Value for Adults and Children 4 Years of Age and older (1 Tablet)
Vitamin A 5000 IU	100	100
Vitamin C 60 mg	75	100
Vitamin D 400 IU	50	100
Vitamin E 30 IU	150	100
Thiamin (B$_1$) 1.5 mg	107	100
Riboflavin (B$_2$) 1.7 mg	106	100
Niacin 20 mg	111	100
Vitamin B$_6$ 2 mg	143	100
Folic Acid 400 mcg	100	100
Vitamin B$_{12}$ 6 mcg	100	100
Biotin 40 mcg	13	13
Pantothenic Acid 10 mg	100	100
Calcium 100 mg	6	10
Iron (elemental) 18 mg	90	100
Phosphorus 100 mg	6	10
Iodine 150 mcg	107	100
Magnesium 20 mg	5	5
Zinc 15 mg	94	100
Copper 2 mg	100	100

FLINTSTONES® Plus Extra C
Children's Chewable Multivitamin Supplement
BUGS BUNNY™ With Extra C
Children's Chewable Multivitamin Supplement
(Sugar Free)

Vitamin Ingredients: Each multivitamin supplement contains the ingredients listed in the chart below:

Amount Per Tablet	% Daily Value for Children 2–3 Years of Age	% Daily Value for Adults and Children 4 or more Years of Age
Vitamin A 2500 IU	100	50
Vitamin C 250 mg	625	417
Vitamin D 400 IU	100	100
Vitamin E 15 IU	150	50
Thiamin (B$_1$) 1.05 mg	150	70
Riboflavin (B$_2$) 1.2 mg	150	70
Niacin 13.5 mg	150	67
Vitamin B$_6$ 1.05 mg	150	52
Folic Acid 300 mcg	150	75
Vitamin B$_{12}$ 4.5 mcg	150	75

Use: Dietary supplement.

Serving Size: One tablet daily for adults and children two years and older; chew one tablet daily.

Warning

For Bugs Bunny Only: Phenylketonurics: Contains Phenylalanine.

KEEP OUT OF REACH OF CHILDREN.

CHILD RESISTANT CAP

Do not use this product if safety seal bearing Bayer Corporation under cap is torn or missing.

How Supplied: Flintstones in bottles of 60's & 100's, Bugs Bunny in bottles of 60 with child-resistant caps.

Shown in Product Identification Guide, page 504

ONE-A-DAY® 50 PLUS
Multivitamin/Multimineral Supplement For Adults

Description: ONE-A-DAY 50 Plus is scientifically balanced to meet the changing nutritional needs of adults over 50. This special formula is complete with all of the essential vitamins including more than 100% of the key nutrients important for mature adults, including Antioxidants, B Vitamins, and Essential Trace Minerals.

Directions For Use: Adults take one tablet daily with food.

VITAMINS	AMOUNT PER SERVING		% DAILY VALUE
Vitamin A	5000	IU	100
Vitamin C	120	mg	200
Vitamin D	400	IU	100
Vitamin E	60	IU	200
Vitamin K	20	mcg	25
Thiamin (B₁)	4.5	mg	300
Riboflavin (B₂)	3.4	mg	200
Niacin	20	mg	100
Vitamin B₆	6	mg	300
Folic Acid	400	mcg	100
Vitamin B₁₂	30	mcg	500
Biotin	30	mcg	10
Pantothenic Acid	15	mg	150

MINERALS	AMOUNT PER SERVING		% DAILY VALUE
Calcium (elemental)	120	mg	12
Iodine	150	mcg	100
Magnesium	100	mg	25
Zinc	22.5	mg	150
Selenium	105	mcg	150
Copper	2	mg	100
Manganese	4	mg	200
Chromium	180	mcg	150
Molybdenum	90	mcg	120
Chloride	34	mg	1
Potassium	37.5	mg	1

Use: Dietary supplement

Ingredients: Calcium Carbonate, Magnesium Hydroxide, Niacinamide Ascorbate, Potassium Chloride, Ascorbic Acid, Vitamin E Acetate, Gelatin, Zinc Sulfate, Starch, Modified Cellulose Gum, Cellulose, Calcium Silicate, Citric Acid, Calcium Pantothenate, Dextrin, Titanium Dioxide, Manganese Sulfate, Zinc Oxide, Pyridoxine Hydrochloride, Cupric Sulfate, Thiamine Mononitrate, Riboflavin, Vitamin A Acetate, Chromium Chloride, Artificial Color (FD&C Yellow #5 [Tartrazine], FD&C Yellow #6), Beta Carotene, Folic Acid, Sodium Selenate, Sodium Molybdate, Potassium Iodide, Phytonadione, Vitamin B₁₂, Biotin, Vitamin D.

KEEP OUT OF REACH OF CHILDREN CHILD RESISTANT CAP

Do not use this product if safety seal bearing Bayer Corporation under cap is torn or missing.

How Supplied: Bottles of 50's and 80's with child-resistant caps.

Shown in Product Identification Guide, page 505

ONE-A-DAY® ANTIOXIDANT
Antioxidant Supplement
Complete Antioxidant Group Plus
Essential Trace Minerals

Ingredients: Ascorbic Acid, Vitamin E Acetate, Gelatin, Glycerin, Soybean Oil, Selenium Yeast, Lecithin, Zinc Oxide, Vegetable Oil (Partially Hydrogenated Cottonseed and Soybean Oils), Yellow Wax (Beeswax, Yellow) Manganese Sulfate, Beta Carotene, Cupric Oxide, Titanium Dioxide, Artificial Colors including FD&C Yellow #5 (Tartrazine).

VITAMINS	AMOUNT PER SERVING		% DAILY VALUE
Vitamin A (100% as beta-carotene)	5000	IU	100
Vitamin C	250	mg	417
Vitamin E	200	IU	667

MINERALS	AMOUNT PER SERVING		% DAILY VALUE
Zinc	7.5	mg	50
Selenium	15	mcg	21
Copper	1	mg	50
Manganese	1.5	mg	75

Directions for Use: Adults take one softgel capsule daily with food. To preserve quality and freshness, keep bottle tightly closed and store at room temperature.

Use: Dietary supplement.
ONE-A-DAY ANTIOXIDANT may reduce the risk of harmful cell damage attributed to free radicals. Antioxidant Vitamins (C, E, and Beta Carotene) may neutralize the effects of free radicals (oxidants) which may be a cause of harmful cell damage.

KEEP OUT OF REACH OF CHILDREN
CHILD RESISTANT CAP

Do not use this product if safety seal bearing Bayer Corporation under cap is torn or missing.

How Supplied: Bottle of 50 softgels.

Shown in Product Identification Guide, page 505

ONE-A-DAY® BONE STRENGTH
Dietary Supplement

Ingredients: Calcium Carbonate, Cellulose, Maltodextrin, Soy Extract, Hydroxypropyl Methylcellulose, Talc, Croscarmellose Sodium, Acacia, Starch, Silicon Dioxide, Titanium Dioxide, Magnesium Stearate, Hydroxypropyl Cellulose, Polysorbate 80, FD&C Yellow #6 Lake, Polyethylene Glycol, FD&C Blue #1 Lake, FD&C Red #40 Lake, Cholecalciferol.

One tablet of One-A-Day Bone Strength provides:

	AMOUNT PER SERVING		% DAILY VALUE
Vitamin D	100	IU	25
Calcium (precipitated)	500	mg	50

Soy
Standardized
Extract
(*Glycine max*
or spp.)
(bean)   28 mg   *
*Daily Value not established.

Use: Dietary Supplementation

Dosage and Administration: Take one to two tablets daily, with food.

Warnings: Do not exceed four tablets per day. Keep out of the reach of children.
Child Resistant Cap
Do not use this product if safety seal bearing *Sealed For Your Protection* under cap is torn or missing.

How Supplied: Bottles of 60 with child-resistant caps.

Shown in Product Identification Guide, page 505

ONE-A-DAY® CALCIUM PLUS
Calcium Supplement with
Vitamin D and Magnesium

Use: Dietary supplement.

Ingredients: Calcium Carbonate, Sorbitol, Magnesium Carbonate, Maltodextrin, Xylitol, Starch, Stearic Acid, Aspartame* (a sweetener), Natural and Artificial Flavors, Magnesium Stearate, Polyethylene Glycol, Gelatin, Polydextrose, Poloxamer 407, Docusate Sodium, Vitamin D₃.
*PHENYLKETONURICS: CONTAINS PHENYLALANINE.

Each Tablet Contains

VITAMINS:	AMOUNT PER SERVING		% DAILY VALUE
Vitamin D	100	IU	25

MINERALS:	AMOUNT PER SERVING		% DAILY VALUE
Calcium (elemental)	500	mg	50
Magnesium (elemental)	50	mg	12.5

Directions For Use: Adults and children 12 years of age or older take one to two chewable tablets daily (with food), or as recommended by your doctor, to supplement your normal dietary intake.
Two tablets provide 1,000 mg of elemental calcium, 100% of the Recommended Daily Value for adults and children 12 years of age or older.
Special Note for Pregnant and Lactating Women: Three tablets provide 1,500 mg of elemental calcium (125% of the Recommended Daily Value).

Actions: ONE-A-DAY Calcium Plus aids in the prevention of the bone disease osteoporosis*. This high potency formula contains 500 mg of the most concentrated form of Calcium, plus Vitamin D and Magnesium, in a fruit flavored chewable tablet. Calcium is essential for building

Continued on next page

One-A-Day Calcium—Cont.

and maintaining strong and healthy bones. Vitamin D is necessary for optimal absorption and utilization of calcium by the body. Magnesium is necessary for strong teeth and bones.

KEEP OUT OF REACH OF CHILDREN CHILD RESISTANT CAP

Do not use this product if safety seal bearing Bayer Corporation under cap is torn or missing.

How Supplied: Bottles of 60 Chewable Tablets.

*Osteoporosis is a reduction in the amount of bone mass, related to bone fractures later in life. This disease affects middle-aged and older individuals. Those at increased risk of developing osteoporosis include: white and Asian women during their teen, young adult, menopausal and post-menopausal years; as well as those individuals with a family history of the disease; and the elderly. A lifetime of regular exercise and healthy diet with adequate calcium intake will help build and maintain good bone health and may reduce the risk of osteoporosis later in life.

Adequate calcium intake is important, but daily intakes above 2,000 mg are not likely to provide any additional benefit.

Shown in Product Identification Guide, page 505

ONE-A-DAY® CHOLESTEROL HEALTH
Dietary Supplement

Ingredients: Dicalcium Phosphate, Cellulose, dl-alpha Tocopheryl Acetate, Soy Extract, Gelatin, Lecithin, Croscarmellose Sodium, Hydroxypropyl Methylcellulose, Polyethylene Glycol, Silicon Dioxide, Garlic Powder, Calcium Silicate, Magnesium Stearate, Titanium Dioxide, Hydroxypropyl Cellulose, FD&C Yellow #6 Lake, FD&C Red #40 Lake, FD&C Blue #1 Lake, Polysorbate 80.
Two tablets of One-A-Day Cholesterol Health provides:

	AMOUNT PER SERVING	% DAILY VALUE
Vitamin E	200 IU	667
Lecithin	100 mg	*
Garlic (*Allium* (bulb sativum) (freeze-dried) (bulb)	30 mg	*
Soy Standardized Extract (*Glycine max* or spp.) (bean)	140 mg	*

*Daily Value not established.

Use: Dietary Supplementation

Dosage and Administration: Take two tablets daily, with food.

Warnings: Keep out of the reach of children.

Child Resistant Cap: Do not use this product if safety seal bearing *Sealed For Your Protection* under cap is torn or missing.

How Supplied: Bottles of 30 with child-resistant caps.

Shown in Product Identification Guide, page 505

ONE-A-DAY® COLD SEASON
Dietary Supplement

Ingredients: Ascorbic Acid, Zinc Gluconate, Starch, Echinacea Extract, Cellulose, Hydroxypropyl Methylcellulose, Stearic Acid, Silicon Dioxide, Titanium Dioxide, Magnesium Stearate, Propylene Glycol, FD&C Yellow #5 Lake (Tartrazine), FD&C Yellow #6 Lake.
One tablet of One-A-Day Cold Season provides:

	AMOUNT PER SERVING	% DAILY VALUE
Vitamin C	500 mg	883
Zinc	7.5 mg	50
Echinacea Standardized Extract *Echinacea purpurea*) (whole plant and root)	50 mg	*

*Daily Value not established.

Use: Dietary Supplementation

Dosage and Administration: Take one to two tablets daily, with food.

Warnings: Do not use this product for more than 2 weeks. Not for chronic administration. **Caution:** This product is **not** recommended for people with autoimmune problems. Keep out of the reach of children.

Children Resistant Cap

Do not use this product if safety seal bearing *Sealed For Your Protection* under cap is torn or missing.

How Supplied: Bottles of 30 with child-resistant caps.

Shown in Product Identification Guide, page 505

ONE-A-DAY® ENERGY FORMULA
Dietary Supplement

Ingredients: Calcium Carbonate, American Ginseng Extract, Cellulose, Maltodextrin, Nicotinic Acid, Hydroxypropyl Methylcellulose, Croscarmellose Sodium, d-Calcium Pantothenate, Crospovidone, Stearic Acid, Silicon Dioxide, Pyridoxine Hydrochloride, Titanium Dioxide, Magnesium Stearate, Starch, Thiamine Mononitrate, Acacia, Hydroxypropyl Cellulose, Polyethylene Glycol,

---

FD&C Yellow #6 Lake, Chromium Picolinate, FD&C Blue #1 Lake, Folic Acid, Polysorbate 80.
One tablet of One-A-Day Energy Formula provides:

	AMOUNT PER SERVING	% DAILY VALUE
Thiamin (B_1)	2.25 mg	150
Niacin	20 mg	100
Vitamin B_6	3 mg	150
Folic Acid	200 mcg	50
Pantothenic Acid	10 mg	100
Chromium (as Picolinate)	100 mcg	83
American Ginseng Standardized Extract (*Panax quinquefolius*) (root)	200 mg	*

*Daily Value not established.

Use: Dietary Supplementation

Dosage and Administration: Take one tablet daily, with food.

Warnings: Seek the advice of a health professional before using this product if you are: pregnant or nursing a baby; taking medication for high blood pressure. Keep out of the reach of children.

Child Resistant Cap

Do not use this product if safety seal bearing *Sealed For Your Protection* under cap is torn or missing.

How Supplied: Bottles of 30 with child-resistant caps.

Shown in Product Identification Guide, page 505

ONE–A–DAY® Essential Multivitamin Supplement 100% USRDA of 11 Essential Vitamins in a small easy-to-swallow tablet.

Ingredients: Calcium Carbonate, Ascorbic Acid, Gelatin, Vitamin E Acetate, Starch, Niacinamide, Calcium Pantothenate, Calcium Silicate, Hydroxypropyl Methylcellulose, Pyridoxine Hydrochloride, Artificial Color, Vitamin A Acetate, Riboflavin, Thiamine Mononitrate, Folic Acid, Beta Carotene, Vitamin B_{12}, Vitamin D.

VITAMINS	AMOUNT PER SERVING	% DAILY VALUE
Vitamin A	5000 IU	100
Vitamin C	60 mg	100
Vitamin D	400 IU	100
Vitamin E	30 IU	100
Thiamin (B_1)	1.5 mg	100
Riboflavin (B_2)	1.7 mg	100
Niacin	20 mg	100
Vitamin B_6	2 mg	100
Folic Acid	400 mcg	100
Vitamin B_{12}	6 mcg	100
Pantothenic Acid	10 mg	100

Use: Dietary supplement.

Dosage and Administration: Adults one tablet daily, with food.
KEEP OUT OF REACH OF CHILDREN.
CHILD RESISTANT CAP
Do not use this product if safety seal bearing Bayer Corporation under cap is torn or missing.

How Supplied: Bottles of 75's and 130's with child-resistant caps.
Shown in Product Identification Guide, page 505

ONE-A-DAY® GARLIC SOFTGELS
Garlic Supplement

Description: One-A-Day GARLIC SOFTGELS are specially formulated to provide 600 mg of concentrated garlic, the equivalent of one fresh garlic clove, in each odor-free softgel capsule. One-A-Day Garlic Softgels provide the benefits of garlic without the unpleasant after-odor typical of fresh garlic.

	Amount Per Serving	% Daily Value
Garlic Oil Macerate	600 mg	*

* Daily Value not established

Ingredients: Garlic Oil Macerate, Gelatin, Glycerin, Sorbitol, Xylose.

Use: Dietary supplement

Directions For Use: Adults take one softgel capsule daily with a meal, alone or with your One-A-Day everyday multivitamin. Do not chew. Swallow whole with liquid to ensure maximum strength and fresh breath. To preserve quality and freshness, keep bottle tightly closed and store at room temperature.
KEEP OUT OF REACH OF CHILDREN
CHILD RESISTANT CAP
Do not use this product if safety seal bearing Bayer Corporation under cap is torn or missing.

How Supplied: Bottles of 45 softgels
Shown in Product Identification Guide, page 505

ONE-A-DAY® MAXIMUM
Multivitamin/Multimineral Supplement

Ingredients: Dicalcium Phosphate, Magnesium Hydroxide, Potassium Chloride, Cellulose, Ferrous Fumarate, Zinc Sulfate, Calcium Carbonate, Niacinamide Ascorbate, Gelatin, Vitamin E Acetate, Ascorbic Acid, Modified Cellulose Gum, Hydroxypropyl Methylcellulose, Citric Acid, Tablet Lubricant, Calcium Pantothenate, Niacinamide, Manganese Sulfate, Artificial Color, Cupric Sulfate, Pyridoxine Hydrochloride, Sodium Metasilicate, Vitamin A Acetate, Riboflavin, Thiamine Mononitrate, Sodium Borate, Beta Carotene, Folic Acid, Sodium Molybdate, Potassium Iodide, Chromium Chloride, Sodium Selenate, Phytonadione, Biotin, Sodium Metavanadate, Stannous Chloride, Nickelous Sulfate, Vitamin B12, Vitamin D.

VITAMINS	AMOUNT PER SERVING		% DAILY VALUE
Vitamin A	5000	IU	100
Vitamin C	60	mg	100
Vitamin D	400	IU	100
Vitamin E	30	IU	100
Vitamin K	25	mcg	31
Thiamin (B$_1$)	1.5	mg	100
Riboflavin (B$_2$)	1.7	mg	100
Niacin	20	mg	100
Vitamin B$_6$	2	mg	100
Folic Acid	400	mcg	100
Vitamin B$_{12}$	6	mcg	100
Biotin	30	mcg	10
Pantothenic Acid	10	mg	100

MINERALS	AMOUNT PER SERVING		% DAILY VALUE
Calcium (elemental)	162	mg	16
Iron	18	mg	100
Phosphorus	109	mg	11
Iodine	150	mcg	100
Magnesium	100	mg	25
Zinc	15	mg	100
Selenium	20	mcg	29
Copper	2	mg	100
Manganese	3.5	mg	175
Chromium	65	mcg	54
Molybdenum	160	mcg	213
Chloride	72	mg	2
Potassium	80	mg	2
Boron	150	mcg	*
Nickel	5	mcg	*
Silicon	2	mg	*
Tin	10	mcg	*
Vanadium	10	mcg	*

---

*Daily Value not established

Use: Dietary supplementation.

Dosage and Administration: Adults: Take one tablet daily, with food.

> **Warning:** Accidental overdose of iron-containing products is a leading cause of fatal poisoning in children under 6. Keep this product out of the reach of children. In case of accidental overdose, call a doctor or poison control center immediately.

CHILD RESISTANT CAP
Do not use this product if safety seal bearing Bayer Corporation under cap is torn or missing.

How Supplied: Bottles of 60 and 100 with child-resistant caps.
Shown in Product Identification Guide, page 505

ONE-A-DAY® MEMORY & CONCENTRATION
Dietary Supplement

Ingredients: Calcium Carbonate, Choline Bitartrate, Cellulose, Ginkgo Biloba Leaf Extract, Maltodextrin, Hydroxypropyl Methylcellulose, Polyethylene Glycol, Silicon Dioxide, Croscarmellose Sodium, Magnesium Stearate, Crospovidone, Titanium Dioxide, FD&C Yellow #5 Lake (Tartrazine), Pyridoxine Hydrochloride, Hydroxypropyl Cellulose, Resin, FD&C Yellow #6 Lake, Polysorbate 80, Cyanocobalamin.
One tablet of One-A-Day Memory & Concentration provides:

	AMOUNT PER SERVING	% DAILY VALUE
Vitamin B6	1 mg	50
Vitamin B12	3 mcg	50
Choline	60 mg	*
Ginkgo Standardized Extract (Ginkgo biloba) (Leaf)	60 mg	*

*Daily Value not established.

Use: Dietary Supplementation

Dosage and Administration: Adults (18 years and older): Take one to two tablets daily, with food.

Warnings: Do not take this product without first consulting a health professional, if you are: Taking a prescription monoamine oxidase inhibitor (MAOI) (certain drugs for depression, psychiatric or emotional conditions, or Parkinson's disease) or for two weeks after stopping the MAOI drug. If you are pregnant or nursing a baby, seek the advice of a health professional before using this product. Keep out of the reach of children.

Child Resistant Cap
Do not use this product if safety seal bearing *Sealed For Your Protection* under cap is torn or missing.

How Supplied: Bottles of 60 with child-resistant caps.
Shown in Product Identification Guide, page 505

ONE-A-DAY® MENOPAUSE HEALTH
Dietary Supplement

Ingredients: Calcium Carbonate, Starch, Cellulose, Soy Extract, Maltodextrin, Hydroxypropyl Methylcellulose, Talc, di-alpha Tocopheryl Acetate, Gelatin, Polyethylene Glycol, Lecithin, Croscarmellose Sodium, Black Cohosh Extract, Titanium Dioxide, Acacia, Magnesium Stearate, Silicon Dioxide, Hydroxypropyl Cellulose, Pharmaceutical Glaze, Polysorbate 80, FD&C Yellow #6 Lake, FD&C Yellow #5 Lake (Tartrazine).
One tablet of One-A-Day Menopause provides:

	AMOUNT PER SERVING	% DAILY VALUE
Vitamin E	15 IU	50
Calcium (precipitated)	250 mg	25

Continued on next page

One-A-Day Menopause—Cont.

Lecithin	15 mg	*
Black Cohosh Standardized Extract (*Cimicifuga racemosa*) (root)	10 mg	*
Soy Standardized Extract (*Glycine max* or spp.) (bean)	42 mg	*

*Daily Value not established.

Use: Dietary Supplementation

Dosage and Administration: Adults: Take one to two tablets daily, with food.

Warnings: Consult your health care professional if you are taking any prescription antihypertensive medication. If you are pregnant or nursing a baby, seek the advice of a health professional before using this product. Keep out of the reach of children.

Child Resistant Cap

Do not use this product if safety seal bearing *Sealed For Your Protection* under cap is torn or missing.

How Supplied: Bottles of 60 with child-resistant caps.

Shown in Product Identification Guide, page 505

ONE-A-DAY® MEN'S MULTIVITAMIN/MULTIMINERAL SUPPLEMENT

Description: ONE-A-DAY Men's is scientifically balanced to meet the unique nutritional needs of men. This special formula provides essential vitamins and minerals plus higher levels of the key nutrients that help keep men healthy, including extra C, E, and B Vitamins.

Ingredients: Magnesium Hydroxide, Niacinamide Ascorbate, Potassium Chloride, Zinc Sulfate, Gelatin, Vitamin E Acetate, Ascorbic Acid, Modified Cellulose Gum, Cellulose, Calcium Pantothenate, Calcium Silicate, Manganese Sulfate, Dextrin, Citric Acid, Povidone, Dicalcium Phosphate, Cupric Sulfate, Pyridoxine Hydrochloride, Thiamine Mononitrate, Riboflavin, Vitamin A Acetate, Artificial Color (FD&C Yellow #6, FD&C Yellow #5 [Tartrazine]), Chromium Chloride, Beta Carotene, Folic Acid, Sodium Selenate, Potassium Iodide, Sodium Molybdate, Vitamin B_{12}, Vitamin D.

VITAMINS	AMOUNT PER SERVING		% DAILY VALUE
Vitamin A	5000	IU	100
Vitamin C	90	mg	150
Vitamin D	400	IU	100
Vitamin E	45	IU	150
Thiamin (B_1)	2.25	mg	150
Riboflavin (B_2)	2.55	mg	150
Niacin	20	mg	100
Vitamin B_6	3	mg	150
Folic Acid	400	mcg	100

Vitamin B_{12}	9	mcg	150
Pantothenic Acid	10	mg	100

MINERALS	AMOUNT PER SERVING		% DAILY VALUE
Iodine	150	mcg	100
Magnesium	100	mg	25
Zinc	15	mg	100
Selenium	87.5	mcg	125
Copper	2	mg	100
Manganese	3.33	mg	167
Chromium	150	mcg	125
Molybdenum	75	mcg	100
Chloride	34	mg	1
Potassium	37.5	mg	1

Use: Dietary Supplement.

KEEP OUT OF REACH OF CHILDREN

CHILD RESISTANT CAP

Directions for Use: Adults take one tablet daily with food.

Do not use this product if safety seal bearing Bayer Corporation under cap is torn or missing.

How Supplied: Bottles of 60's & 100's with child-resistant caps.

Shown in Product Identification Guide, page 505

ONE-A-DAY® PROSTATE HEALTH
Dietary Supplement

Ingredients: Saw Palmetto Berry Extract, Gelatin, Glycerin, Zinc Gluconate, Pumpkin Seed Oil Extract, Vegetable Oil, Beeswax, Lecithin, Titanium Dioxide, FD&C Red #40, FD&C Yellow #6, FD&C Blue #1, FD&C Yellow #5 (Tartrazine)

Two softgels of One-A-Day Prostate Health provides:

	AMOUNT PER SERVING	% DAILY VALUE
Zinc	15 mg	100
Pumpkin Seed Oil Standardized Extract	80 mg	*
Saw Palmetto Standardized Extract (*Serenoa repens*) (berry)	320 mg	*

*Daily Value not established.

Use: Dietary Supplementation

Dosage and Administration: Take two softgels daily, with food.

Warnings: If you are experiencing urinary problems, or are being treated for prostate problems, consult your doctor. Keep out of the reach of children.

Child Resistant Cap

Do not use this product if safety seal bearing *Sealed For Your Protection* under cap is torn or missing.

How Supplied: Bottles of 30 with child-resistant caps.

Shown in Product Identification Guide, page 505

ONE-A-DAY® TENSION & MOOD
Dietary Supplement

Ingredients: Dicalcium Phosphate, St. John's Wort Extract, Cellulose, Kava Kava Extract, Ascorbic Acid, Croscarmellose Sodium, Hydroxypropyl Methylcellulose, Lecithin, Stearic Acid, Niacin, Silicon Dioxide, Magnesium Stearate d-Calcium Pantothenate, Titanium Dioxide, Pharmaceutical Glaze, Polyethylene Glycol, Thiamine Mononitrate, Startch, Hydroxylpropyl Cellulose, FD&C Yellow #5 Lake (Tartazine), FD&C Yellow #6 Lake, Polysorbate 80, Folic Acid, FD&C Blue #1 Lake, FD&C Red #40 Lake.

One tablet of One-A-Day Tension & Mood provides:

	AMOUNT PER SERVING	% DAILY VALUE
Vitamin C	60 mg	100
Thiamin (B1)	1.125 mg	75
Niacin	10 mg	50
Folic Acid	100 mcg	25
Pantothenic Acid	5 mg	50
Lecithin	15 mg	*
Kava Kava Standardized Extract (*Piper methysticum*) (rhizome and root)	100 mg	*
St. John's Wort Standardized Extract (*Hypericum perforatum*) (leaves and flowers)	225 mg	*

*Daily Value not established.

Use: Dietary Supplementation

Dosage and Administration: Adults (18 years and older): Take one to two tablets daily with food.

Warnings: Do not exceed two tablets per 24 hours. Do not take this product without first consulting a health professional, if you are: Taking a prescription monoamine oxidase inhibitor (MAOI) (certain drugs for depression, psychiatric or emotional conditions, or Parkinson's disease) or for two weeks after stopping the MAOI drug; Taking sedatives or tranquilizers (May cause drowsiness. Alcohol, sedatives and tranquilizers may increase the drowsiness effect. Avoid alcoholic beverages while taking this product); Taking any prescription medication; or if you are pregnant or nursing a baby. Use caution when driving a motor vehicle or operating machinery. St. John's Wort may cause skin sensitivity to light; increased heart rate; convulsions; or shortness of breath. Keep out of the reach of children.

Child Resistant Cap
Do not use this product if safety seal bearing *Sealed For Your Protection* under cap is torn or missing.

How Supplied: Bottles of 30 with child-resistant caps.
Shown in Product Identification Guide, page 505

ONE-A-DAY® WOMEN'S
Multivitamin/Multimineral Supplement

Description: ONE-A-DAY Women's is scientifically balanced to meet the unique nutritional needs of women. This special formula provides 100% Daily Value of 11 essential vitamins plus Calcium and Iron, the two minerals women need most, and Zinc.

Ingredients: Calcium Carbonate, Starch, Ferrous Fumarate, Ascorbic Acid, Gelatin, Vitamin E Acetate, Modified Cellulose Gum, Niacinamide, Dextrin, Zinc Oxide, Titanium Dioxide, Calcium Pantothenate, Pyridoxine Hydrochloride, Vitamin A Acetate, Riboflavin, Thiamine Mononitrate, Beta Carotene, Artificial Color (FD&C Yellow #5 [Tartrazine], FD&C Yellow #6), Folic Acid, Vitamin D, Vitamin B_{12}.

VITAMINS	AMOUNT PER SERVING		% DAILY VALUE
Vitamin A	5000	IU	100
Vitamin C	60	mg	100
Vitamin D	400	IU	100
Vitamin E	30	IU	100
Thiamine (B_1)	1.5	mg	100
Riboflavin (B_2)	1.7	mg	100
Niacin	20	mg	100
Vitamin B_6	2	mg	100
Folic Acid	400	mcg	100
Vitamin B_{12}	6	mcg	100
Pantothenic Acid	10	mg	100

MINERALS	AMOUNT PER SERVING		% DAILY VALUE
Calcium	450	mg	45
Iron	27	mg	150
Zinc	15	mg	100

Use: Dietary supplement.

Dosage and Administration: Adults take one tablet daily with food.

> **Warning:** Accidental overdose of iron-containing products is a leading cause of fatal poisoning in children under 6. Keep this product out of the reach of children. In case of accidental overdose, call a doctor or poison control center immediately.

KEEP OUT REACH OF CHILDREN
CHILD RESISTANT CAP
Do not use this product if safety seal bearing Bayer Corporation under cap is torn or missing.

How Supplied: Bottles of 60 and 100 with child-resistant caps.
Shown in Product Identification Guide, page 505

Beach Pharmaceuticals
Division of Beach Products, Inc.
5220 SOUTH MANHATTAN AVE.
TAMPA, FL 33611

Direct Inquiries to:
Richard Stephen Jenkins, Exec. V.P.:
(813) 839-6565

BEELITH Tablets
MAGNESIUM SUPPLEMENT with PYRIDOXINE HCL
Each tablet supplies 362 mg (30 mEq) of magnesium and 25 mg of pyridoxine hydrochloride.

Description: Each tablet contains magnesium oxide 600 mg and pyridoxine hydrochloride (Vitamin B_6) 25 mg equivalent to Vitamin B_6 20 mg. Each tablet yields 362 mg of magnesium and supplies 90% of the Adult U.S. Recommended Daily Allowance (RDA) for magnesium and 1000% of the Adult RDA for Vitamin B_6.

Inactive Ingredients: D&C Yellow No. 10, FD&C Yellow No. 6, hydroxypropylmethylcellulose, magnesium stearate, microcrystalline cellulose, polyethylene glycol, sodium starch glycolate, titanium dioxide, and water.

Indications: As a dietary supplement for patients with magnesium and/or Vitamin B_6 deficiencies resulting from malnutrition, alcoholism, magnesium depleting drugs, chemotherapy, and inadequate nutritional intake or absorption. Also, increases urinary magnesium levels.

Dosage: One tablet daily or as directed by a physician.

Drug Interaction Precaution: Do not take this product if you are presently taking a prescription drug without consulting your physician or other health professional.

Warnings: If you have kidney disease, take only under the supervision of a physician. Excessive dosage may cause laxation. **KEEP OUT OF THE REACH OF CHILDREN.** As with any drug, if you are pregnant or nursing a baby, seek the advice of a health professional before using this product.

How Supplied: Golden yellow, film-coated tablet with the letters **BP** and the number **132** imprinted on each tablet. Packaged in bottles of 100 (NDC 0486-1132-01) tablets.

Block Drug Company, Inc.
257 CORNELISON AVENUE
JERSEY CITY, NJ 07302

Direct Inquiries to:
Lori Hunt
(201) 434-3000 Ext. 1308

For Medical Emergencies Contact:
Consumer Affairs/Block
(201) 434-3000 Ext. 1308

BEANO®
[bēan ō]
Food Enzyme Dietary Supplement

PRODUCT INFORMATION

Description:
Beano drops: each 5 drop dosage follows Food Chemical Codex (FCC) standards for activity and contains 150 GalU (galactosidase units) of alpha-D-galactosidase derived from *Aspergillus niger* mold. The enzyme is in a liquid carrier of water and sorbitol. Add about 5 drops on the first bite of food serving, but remember a normal meal has 2-3 servings of the problem foods.
Beano tablets: each tablet follows Food Chemical Codex (FCC) standards for activity and contains 150 GalU (galactosidase units) of alpha-D-galactosidase derived from *Aspergillus niger* mold. The enzyme is in a carrier of cellulose gel, mannitol, invertase, potato starch, magnesium stearate, gelatin, colloidal silica. 3 tablets swallowed, chewed, or crumbled onto food should be enough for a normal meal of 3 servings of problem foods (1 tablet per serving). Beano® will hydrolyze complex sugars, raffinose, stachyose and verbascose, into the simple sugars - glucose, galactose and fructose, and the easily digestible disaccharide, sucrose. (Sucrose hydrolysis happens simultaneously with normal digestion.) In some cases, more enzyme than 5 drops or 3 tablets will be required, and this is a function of the quantity of food eaten, the levels of alpha-linked sugars in the food, and the gas-producing propensity of the person.

Action: Hydrolysis converts raffinose, stachyose and verbascose into their monosaccharide components: glucose, galactose, fructose and sucrose. Raffinose yields sucrose + galactose; stachyose yields sucrose + galactose; verbascose yields glucose + fructose + galactose.

Indications: Helps stop flatulence and/or bloat before starting from a variety of grains, cereals, nuts, seeds, and vegetables containing the sugars raffinose, stachyose and/or verbascose. This includes all or most legumes and all or most cruciferous vegetables. Examples of such foods are oats, wheat, beans of all

Continued on next page

Beano—Cont.

kinds, chickpeas, peas, lentils, peanuts, soy-content foods, broccoli, brussel sprouts, cabbage, carrots, corn, leeks, onions, parsnips, squash. Note: Most vegetables and beans also contain fiber, which is gas productive in some people, but usually far less so than the alpha-linked sugars. Beano® has no effect on fiber.

Usage: About 5 drops per food serving or 3 tablets per meal (1 tablet per serving) of 3 servings of problem foods; higher levels depending on symptoms.

Adverse Reactions: Reports to date include gastroenterological symptoms, such as cramping and diarrhea as well as allergic-type reactions including rash and pruritus. Rare reports of more serious allergic reactions have been received.

Precautions: Galactosemics should not use without physician's advice, since one of the breakdown sugars is galactose.

How Supplied: Beano® is supplied in both a liquid form (30 and 75 serving sizes, at 5 drops per serving), and a tablet form (12, 30, 60, and 100 tablet sizes as well as 24 tablets in packets of 2). These statements have not been evaluated by the Food and Drug Administration. This product is not intended to diagnose, treat, cure or prevent any disease.
For more information and free samples, please write or call toll-free 1-800-257-8650.

Bristol-Myers Products

(A Bristol-Myers Squibb Company)
345 PARK AVENUE
NEW YORK, NY 10154

Direct Inquiries to:
Bristol-Myers Products Division
Consumer Affairs Department
1350 Liberty Avenue
Hillside, NJ 07207

Questions or Comments?
1-(800) 468-7746

THERAGRAN-M
High Potency Multi-Vitamins with Minerals

Composition:
Nutrition Facts
Serving Size 1 caplet

Amount Per Caplet	% Daily Value
Vitamin A 5000 IU	100%
20% as Beta Carotene	
Vitamin C 90 mg	150%
Vitamin D 400 IU	100%
Vitamin E 30 IU	100%
Vitamin K 28 mcg	*

Thiamin 3 mg	200%
Riboflavin 3.4 mg	200%
Niacin 20 mg	100%
Vitamin B₆ 3 mg	150%
Folate 400 mcg	100%
Vitamin B₁₂ 9 mcg	150%
Biotin 30 mcg	10%
Pantothenic Acid 10 mg	100%
Calcium 40 mg	4%
Iron 18 mg	100%
Phosphorus 31 mg	3%
Iodine 150 mcg	100%
Magnesium 100 mg	25%
Zinc 15 mg	100%
Selenium 21 mcg	*
Copper 2 mg	100%
Manganese 3.5 mg	*
Chromium 26 mcg	*
Molybdenum 32 mcg	*
Chloride 7.5 mg	*
Potassium 7.5 mg	Less than 1%

*Daily Value not established

Each caplet also contains 5 mcg nickel, 2 mg silicon, 150 mcg boron, 10 mcg tin, and 10 mcg vanadium.

Description:
• **Theragran-M, a complete formula** with over 20 vitamins and minerals, helps you meet your daily nutritional requirements.
• Theragran-M contains **antioxidant vitamins,** such as beta carotene (a source of Vitamin A) and Vitamins C and E. Studies suggest that daily consumption of antioxidant-rich fruits and vegetables may play an important role in maintaining good health.
• Theragran-M gives you more **B1, B2, and C** than other leading multivitamin/multimineral formulas. Your body doesn't store these vitamins.
• Theragran-M caplets are coated to make them **easy to swallow**
• Theragran-M is **thoroughly tested** to assure potency and reliability.

*USP: Theragran-M meets the USP standards of strength, quality, and purity for Oil- and Water-soluble Vitamins with Minerals Tablets.

Ingredients: Magnesium oxide, calcium phosphate, microcrystalline cellulose, ascorbic acid[1], dl-alpha tocopheryl acetate[2], ferrous fumarate, crospovidone, niacinamide[2], zinc oxide, povidone, hydroxypropyl methylcellulose, potassium chloride, calcium pantothenate[2], vitamin A acetate[2], beta carotene, manganese sulfate, vitamin D3[2], cupric sulfate, pyridoxine hydrochloride[2], silica gel, triacetin, polyethylene glycol, magnesium stearate, riboflavin[2], phytonadione, thiamin mononitrate[2], stearic acid, biotin[1], sodium borate, Red 40 Lake, Blue 2 Lake, cyanocobalamin[1], folic acid[1], potassium citrate, sodium citrate, potassium iodide, titanium dioxide, chromic chloride, sodium molybdate[1], sodium selenate[1], sodium metavanadate, nickelous sulfate, stannous chloride.

[1]USP Method 2; [2]USP Method 3

Directions
One caplet daily

Warning: Accidental overdose of iron-containing products is a leading cause of fatal poisoning in children under 6. Keep this product out of reach of children. In case of accidental overdose, call a doctor or poison control center immediately.

Store at room temperature; avoid excessive heat.

How Supplied: Dark red coated caplets embossed with T-M on one side. Available in bonus packaging of 100 plus 30 caplets. Guide, page 306
Shown in Product Identification Guide, page 507

J. R. Carlson Laboratories, Inc.
15 COLLEGE DR.
ARLINGTON HEIGHTS, IL 60004-1985

Direct Inquiries to:
Customer Service
(847) 255-1600
FAX: (847) 255-1605

For Medical Emergency Contact:
Customer Service
(847) 255-1600
FAX: (847) 255-1605

ACES®
Vitamin, Antioxidants

Description: ACES provides four natural antioxidant nutrients.

Two Soft Gels Contain:	% U.S. RDA
Beta-Carotene (Pro-Vitamin A) 10,000 IU	200%
Vitamin C (Calcium Ascorbate) 1,000 mg	1667%
Vitamin E (d-Alpha Tocopherol) 400 IU	1333%
Selenium (L-Selenomethionine) 100 mcg	

RDA: Recommended Daily Allowance - Adults

The nutrients in ACES are: Beta-Carotene (Pro-vitamin A) derived from tiny sea plants or algae (D. salina) grown in the fresh ocean waters off southern Australia; Vitamin C provided as the gentle, buffered calcium ascorbate; Vitamin E 100% natural-source from soy, the most biologically active form; and Selenium, organically bound with the essential nutrient methionine to promote assimilation.

How Supplied: In bottles of 50, 90, 200, and 360.
Also available as ACES (R) plus ZINC.

E-GEMS®
Vitamins, Antioxidants

Description: 100% natural-source vitamin E (d-alpha tocopheryl acetate) soft gels. Available in 8 strengths: 30IU, 100IU, 200IU, 400IU, 600IU, 800IU, 1000IU, 1200IU.

How Supplied: Supplied in a variety of bottle sizes. Also in creams, ointments, spray, and more.

TRI-B

Description: Tri-B is an nutritional supplement designed to help maintain normal blood levels of Homocysteine. Based upon research in popular medical journals, plasma Homocysteine levels may be involved in the hardening and stiffening of the arteries. Tri-B contains three prominent B Vitamins, B-12, B-6 and Folic Acid.
One Small Tablet contains:
Vitamin B-12 (Cobalamin Concentrate)
                                        400mcg
Vitamin B-6 (Pyridoxine HCL)   25mg
Folate (Folic Acid)   800mcg

How Supplied: Supplied in bottles of 120 and 360

EDUCATIONAL MATERIAL
"Don't be fooled" is a free 5 page consumer brochure on the difference between natural and synthetic vitamin E. "Help your body fight free radicals" is a free 4 page consumer brochure explaining antioxidants.

Cooke Pharma
1404 OLD COUNTRY ROAD
BELMONT, CA 94002

Direct Inquiries to:
Customer Service Dept.
(888) 808-6838

HEARTBAR™
L-arginine-enriched
Medical Food

Description: The HeartBar™ is a formulation of nutrients and vitamins for the dietary management of vascular disease. These ingredients are placed in a convenient and pleasant-tasting nutrition bar. The major active ingredient in the HeartBar is L-arginine, which is an amino acid required for the production of nitric oxide (NO). Each 50g bar contains L-arginine (3.3 g) and other amino acids, folate (200 µcg) and other B-complex vitamins, antioxidant vitamins E (200 IU) and C (250 mg), niacin (25 mg) and phytoestrogens. These nutrients are combined in a fruit, fiber, and soy protein-based nutrition bar. One HeartBar contains 13 g of protein, 27 g of carbohydrate (20 g of sugars, 3 g of fiber), 3 g of fat (1 g saturated fat, 0 mg of cholesterol), and is 190 calories.

Composition (original flavor): High fructose corn syrup, soy protein isolate, fructose, toasted soy pieces, raisins, vanilla cookie pieces, L-arginine HCl, natural and artificial flavors, oat fiber, DL-alpha-tocopherol acetate, sodium ascorbate, dipotassium phosphate, niacinamide, cyanocobalamin, pyridoxine hydrochloride, folic acid.

Clinical Background: The major active ingredient of the HeartBar, L-arginine, is a semi-essential amino acid, and is the precursor for endothelium-derived nitric oxide (NO). NO is a potent vasodilator, and a major regulator of vasomotion and blood pressure. In addition, NO inhibits platelet aggregation, vascular smooth muscle proliferation and adherence of leukocytes to the vessel wall, key processes in atherosclerosis and restenosis.
Endothelium-derived NO activity is reduced in patients with cardiovascular disease; this abnormality contributes to insufficient blood flow, elevated blood pressure, as well as progression of disease. L-arginine has been shown to enhance the synthesis of NO. In humans, L-arginine improves vasodilation, enhances coronary and peripheral blood flow, and inhibits platelet aggregation.
The usual dietary intake of L-arginine is about 5 g/day, which in some cardiovascular conditions, may not be sufficient intake to maintain healthy NO levels. Two HeartBar/day provides an additional 6.6 g of L-arginine. The other active ingredients of the HeartBar contribute to the production of, or help prevent the breakdown of NO further augmenting the activity of NO.
The HeartBar has been tested clinically in several patient populations and shown to be effective in improving blood flow. In individuals with total cholesterol over 230 mg/dl (n=39), two HeartBars per day restored flow-mediated vasodilation to normal within two weeks. In patients with peripheral arterial disease secondary to atherosclerosis (n=39), 2 HeartBars/day improved pain-free walking distance by 66% (compared to placebo of 18%). In addition to this improvement in physical function, these patients experienced an improvement in quality of life scores as measured by the SF-36 Medical Outcomes Survey.

Pharmacokinetics: Following the administration of 1 HeartBar (3.0 g L-arginine), plasma arginine levels rise from 18 µg/ml to a peak of 28 µg/ml within one hour of ingestion. Arginine levels are maintained above those of individuals on an arginine-free diet for at least 8 hours after ingestion. A similar pattern of arginine levels is observed following the ingestion of a single HeartBar after a week of b.i.d. use. These arginine levels compare favorably with L-arginine administration by capsular form.

Precautions:
Diabetics
The HeartBar contains 190 calories, 27g of carbohydrate (20g of sugars) and 3 g of

fat. Diabetics should monitor their blood glucose carefully while initiating regular use of the HeartBar.

Renal Failure Patients
The HeartBar contains 13 g of protein. This amount of protein should be considered when determining total daily protein load.

Allergies
The base of the bar is of soy protein, which is generally considered hypoallergenic. However, the original flavor contains vanilla cookie pieces that contain wheat flour. Therefore, individuals with allergies to wheat products should be cautious.

Sepsis
The hypotension associated with sepsis is, in-part, mediated by excessive NO production. Such patients should not be given HeartBar.

Adverse Reactions: No serious adverse reactions have been demonstrated or reported in clinical trials or in the HeartBar Safety-In-Use study.

Minor adverse reactions are infrequent, generally related to gastrointestinal disturbances and appear unrelated to the L-arginine in the bar (Adverse events were just as common in the group given placebo bar). In a two-week study of the HeartBar, 4 of 41 individuals reported increased flatulence that resolved after several days of bar use. One of 41 individuals complained of increased frequency of bowel movements and soft stools. In a 10-week study of the HeartBar, 2 of 41 individuals reported dry mouth. A change in bowel habits was reported by 1 individual in each of the placebo and HeartBar groups.

The bar is not indicated for individuals with diabetic retinopathy, neoplastic disease or inflammatory arthritis.

Administration:
Symptomatic or High-Risk Population
One HeartBar twice daily
At-risk Population
One HeartBar daily

How Supplied: Individually wrapped bars, cartons of 16 and cases of 64.

Original Flavor	
Individual Bars	NDC 63535-10102
By Carton	NDC 63535-10103

Berry Flavor	
Individual Bars	NDC 63535-10202
By Carton	NDC 63535-10203

References: Lucher, TF *et al*. Annu Rev Med, 44: 395-418, 1993.

Moncada, S. *et al*. FASEB J, 13: 1319-1330, 1995.

Cooke, JP and Dzau, VJ, Annu Rev Med, 48: 489-509, 1997.

Maxwell, AJ and Cooke, JP, Curr Opin Nephrol Hypertens, 7: 63-70, 1998.

Shown in Product Identification
Guide, page 507

Fleming & Company
1600 FENPARK DR.
FENTON, MO 63026

Direct Inquiries to:
Tom Fleming
(314) 343-8200
FAX (314) 343-9865

MAGONATE TABLETS
MAGONATE LIQUID
Magnesium Gluconate
(Dihydrate)
MAGONATE NATAL LIQUID
Isotomic Solution of Magnesium
Gluconate

Active Ingredients: Each tablet contains magnesium gluconate (dihydrate) 500mg (27mg of Mg^{++} or 2.2 mEq/tablet). Each 5cc of Magonate Liquid contains magnesium gluconate (dihydrate) 1000mg (54mg of Mg^{++} or 4.4 mEq/tsp). Each 5cc of Magonate Natal Liquid contains 326mg magnesium gluconate (dihydrate) or 17.6mg of Mg^{++}).

Indications: For all patients in negative magnesium balance.

Precaution: Excessive dosage may cause loose stools.

Dosage and Administration: (Magonate is recommended during and for three weeks after a course in chemotherapy, then monitored regularly.)
Infants—The recommended dosage is .87 mEq/kg/day.
Adults and children over 12 yrs.—one or two tablets or $^1/_2$ to 1 teaspoon of liquid t.i.d. Under 12 yrs.—one tablet or $^1/_2$ teaspoon of liquid t.i.d. Dosage may be increased in severe cases.

How Supplied: Magonate Tablets are supplied in bottles of 100 and 1000 tablets. Magonate Liquid is supplied in pints. Magonate Natal Liquid is supplied in pints.

General Nutrition Corp. (GNC)
300 SIXTH AVENUE
PITTSBURGH, PA 15222

Direct Inquiries to:
Customer Resources (888) 462-2548

KIDS MULTIBITE™ PLUS MINERALS
Chewable Multivitamin For Kids
All natural flavors and colors
No aspartame

Directions: As a dietary supplement, chew one tablet daily followed by a liquid.

Supplement Facts
Serving Size One Tablet

Amount Per Serving			% Daily Value
Calories	10		
Total Carbohydrates	2	g	1%†
Sugars	2	g	*
Vitamin A (20% as beta-Carotene, 80% as Acetate)	5000	IU	100%
Vitamin C (as Ascorbic Acid)	120	mg	200%
Vitamin D (as Cholecalciferol)	400	IU	100%
Vitamin E (as dl-alpha Tocopheryl Acetate)	30	IU	100%
Thiamin (Vitamin B-1) (as Thiamin Mononitrate)	5	mg	333%
Riboflavin (Vitamin B-2)	5	mg	294%
Niacin (as Niacinamide)	20	mg	100%
Vitamin B-6 (as Pyridoxine Hydrochloride)	5	mg	250%
Folic Acid	400	mcg	100%
Vitamin B-12 (as Cyanocobalamin)	10	mcg	166%
Biotin	100	mcg	33%
Pantothenic Acid (as Calcium d-Pantothenate)	15	mg	150%
Calcium (as Calcium Carbonate, Ascorbate and Citrate)	25	mg	2%
Iron (as Ferrous Fumarate)	10	mg	55%
Iodine (as Kelp)	70	mcg	46%
Magnesium (as Magnesium Oxide)	12	mg	3%
Zinc (as Zinc Gluconate and Citrate)	5	mg	33%
Selenium (as L-Selenomethionine)	2	mcg	2%
Copper (as Copper Gluconate)	200	mcg	10%
Manganese (as Manganese Gluconate)	1	mg	50%
Chromium (as Hydrolyzed Protein Chelate)	10	mcg	8%
Molybdenum (as Molybdenum Yeast)	2	mcg	2%
High Choline Soya Lecithin	10	mg	*
Inositol	10	mg	*
para-Aminobenzoic Acid (PABA)	5	mg	*

†Percent Daily Value based on a 2000 calorie diet.
*Daily Value not established.

WARNING: Accidental overdose of iron-containing products is a leading cause of fatal poisoning in children under 6. Keep this product out of reach of children. In case of accidental overdose, call a doctor or poison control center immediately.

Other Ingredients: Fructose, Mannitol, Natural Flavors, Natural Annatto Color.
No Starch, No Artificial Colors, No Artificial Flavors, No Preservatives, Sodium Free, No Wheat, No Gluten, No Dairy, No Aspartame.

How Supplied: 30 tablets
CODE 119211

PLATINUM YEARS®
Superior Nutrition for Adults
Over 50
Nutraseal™ Coating

Directions: As a dietary supplement, take two tablets daily with food.

Supplement Facts

Amount Per Serving			% Daily Value
Vitamin A (67% as beta-Carotene; 33% as Acetate)	15000	IU	300%
Vitamin C (as Ascorbic Acid)	250	mg	417%
Vitamin D (as Cholecalciferol)	400	IU	100%
Vitamin E (as d-alpha Tocopheryl Succinate)	100	IU	333%
Vitamin K (as Phytonadione)	10	mcg	13%
Thiamin (Vitamin B-1) (as Thiamin Mononitrate)	35	mg	2333%
Riboflavin (Vitamin B-2)	35	mg	2059%
Niacin	35	mg	175%
Vitamin B-6 (as Pyridoxine Hydrochloride)	35	mg	1750%
Folic Acid	400	mcg	100%
Vitamin B-12 (as Cyanocobalamin)	30	mcg	500%
Biotin	30	mcg	10%
Pantothenic Acid (as Calcium d-Pantothenate)	20	mg	200%
Calcium (as Calcium Carbonate)	200	mg	20%
Iron (as Ferronyl)	10	mg	56%
Phosphorus (as Dicalcium Phosphate)	35	mg	4%
Iodine (as Potassium Iodide)	30	mcg	20%
Magnesium (as Magnesium Oxide)	100	mg	25%
Zinc (as Zinc Oxide)	15	mg	100%
Selenium (as Selenium Yeast)	25	mcg	36%
Copper (as Cupric Sulfate)	2	mg	100%
Manganese (as Manganese Sulfate)	3	mg	150%
Chromium (as GTF Chromium Yeast)	100	mcg	83%
Molybdenum (as Molybdenum Yeast)	25	mcg	33%
Chloride (as Potassium Chloride)	72	mg	2%
Potassium (as Potassium Chloride)	80	mg	2%

Silica (as Sodium Metasilicate)	10	mcg	*
Nickel (as Nickel Sulfate)	5	mcg	*
Inositol	50	mcg	*
Choline (as Choline Bitartrate)	50	mcg	*
para-Aminobenzoic Acid (PABA)	50	mcg	*
Citrus Bioflavonoids Complex	50	mg	*
Coenzyme Q-10 Powder	75	mcg	*
Lecithin Powder	50	mg	*
Superoxide Dismutase	50	units	*

*Daily Value not established.

Other Ingredients: Cellulose, Titanium Dioxide (Natural Mineral Whitener), Vegetable Acetoglycerides, Caramel Color, Ethyl Vanillin.
No Sugar, No Artificial Colors, No Preservatives, No Wheat, No Gluten, No Soy, No Dairy.

How Supplied: 90 Tablets

> **WARNING: Accidental overdose of iron-containing products is a leading cause of fatal poisoning in children under 6. Keep this product out of reach of children. In case of accidental overdose, call a doctor or poison control center immediately.**

CODE 138311

WOMEN'S PRE-NATAL FORMULA WITHOUT IRON
Multiple Vitamin and Mineral Formula For Pregnant and Lactating Women

DIRECTIONS: As a dietary supplement, take two tablets daily.

Supplement Facts
Serving Size Two Tablets

Amount Per Serving			%Daily Value*
Vitamin A (100% as beta-Carotene)	10000	IU	125%
Vitamin C (as Ascorbic Acid)	150	mg	250%
Vitamin D (as Cholecalciferol)	400	IU	100%
Vitamin E (as dl-alpha Tocopheryl Acetate)	50	IU	167%
Thiamin (Vitamin B-1) (as Thiamin Mononitrate)	25	mg	1470%
Riboflavin (Vitamin B-2)	25	mg	1250%
Niacin (as Niacinamide)	40	mg	200%
Vitamin B-6 (as Pyridoxine Hydrochloride)	50	mg	2000%
Folic Acid	800	mcg	100%

Vitamin B-12 (as Cyanocobalamin)	25	mcg	312%
Biotin	50	mcg	17%
Pantothenic Acid (as Calcium d-Pantothenate)	25	mg	250%
Calcium (as Calcium Carbonate)	300	mg	23%
Phosphorus (as Dicalcium Phosphate)	50	mg	3%
Iodine (as Kelp)	150	mcg	100%
Magnesium (as Magnesium Oxide)	150	mg	33%
Zinc (as Zinc Gluconate)	15	mg	100%
Selenium (as Selenium Yeast)	25	mcg	†
Manganese (as Manganese Gluconate)	10	mg	†
Chromium (as GTF Chronium Yeast)	25	mcg	†
Potassium (as Potassium Citrate)	10	mg	†
Choline (as Choline Bitartrate)	10	mg	†
Inositol	10	mcg	†
para-Aminobenzoic Acid (PABA)	15	mg	†

*Percent Daily Values for pregnant or lactating women.
†Daily Value not established.

OTHER INGREDIENTS: Cellulose, Food Glaze, Rose Hips.

How Supplied: 60 Tablets

Lederle Consumer Health

A Division of Whitehall-Robins Healthcare
FIVE GIRALDA FARMS
MADISON, NJ 07940

Direct Inquiries to:
Lederle Consumer Product Information
(800) 282-8805

CALTRATE® 600
CALTRATE® 600 + D
[căl-trāte]

Description: HIGH POTENCY CALCIUM SUPPLEMENT WITHOUT/WITH VITAMIN D, NATURE'S MOST CONCENTRATED FORM OF CALCIUM®
NO SUGAR, NO SALT, NO LACTOSE, NO PRESERVATIVES, TABLET SHAPE SPECIALLY DESIGNED FOR EASIER SWALLOWING
Can help Prevent Osteoporosis: "It's Never Too Late For Caltrate.™"
CALTRATE® 600 and CALTRATE® 600 + D are dietary supplements that meet USP standards for purity, potency and dissolution.

NUTRITION FACTS
Serving Size 1 Tablet

		EACH TABLET CONTAINS	% DAILY VALUE
CALTRATE® 600	Calcium 600 mg		60%
CALTRATE® 600 + D	Vitamin D 200 IU		50%
	Calcium 600 mg		60%

Ingredients: CALTRATE® 600: Calcium Carbonate, Maltodextrin, Soy Polysaccharide, Powdered Cellulose, Mineral Oil, Hydroxypropyl Methylcellulose, Starch, Titanium Dioxide, Polysorbate 80, Sodium Lauryl Sulfate, Acacia, Stearic Acid, Magnesium Stearate, and Crospovidone.
CALTRATE® 600 + D: Calcium Carbonate, Maltodextrin, Soy Polysaccharide, Powdered Cellulose, Mineral Oil, Hydroxypropyl Methylcellulose, Starch, Titanium Dioxide, Sodium Lauryl Sulfate, Gelatin, Sucrose, Edible Fat, FD&C Yellow #6 Aluminum Lake, Acacia, Stearic Acid, Magnesium Stearate, Crospovidone, Vitamin D (Cholecalciderol), dl-Alpha Tocopherol.

Warnings: KEEP OUT OF REACH OF CHILDREN.

Dosage and Administration: RECOMMENDED INTAKE
One or two tablets daily or as directed by your physician.

How Supplied: Caltrate 600, Bottle of 60
Caltrate 600 + D
Bottles of 60, 120
Store at Room temperature.
© 1997

CALTRATE® 600 Plus™ Chewables
[căl-trāte]
Calcium Carbonate

Nutrient Enriched Calcium Supplement With Vitamin D & Minerals Contains the most concentrated form of calcium you can buy
No Salt, No Lactose, No Preservatives
Can help Prevent Osteoporosis. "It's Never Too Late For Caltrate.™"

EACH TABLET CONTAINS:
Calories 10   % Daily Value†

Vitamin D	200 IU	50%
Calcium	600 mg	60%
Magnesium	40 mg	10%
Zinc	7.5 mg	50%
Copper	1 mg	50%
Manganese	1.8 mg	90%
Boron	250 mcg	*
Sodium	0 mg	0%
Sugars	2 g	0%

* Daily Value not established.
† Percent daily value is based on a 2000 calorie diet.

Continued on next page

Caltrate 600 Plus—Cont.

Recommended Intake: One or two tablets daily or as directed by your physician.

Warnings: Keep out of the reach of children.

Ingredients:
Assorted Fruit Flavors (• Cherry • Orange • Fruit Punch): Dextrose, Calcium Carbonate, Mineral Oil, Magnesium Stearate, Magnesium Oxide, Maltodextrin, Adipic Acid, Modified Food Starch, Cellulose, Zinc Oxide, Manganese Sulfate, Sodium Borate, Natural and Artificial Flavors, Sucrose, FD&C Red #40, Cupric Oxide, FD&C Yellow #6, FD&C Blue #2, Gelatin, Vitamin D, Crospovidone, Stearic Acid

Spearmint Flavor: Dextrose, Calcium Carbonate, Mineral Oil, Magnesium Stearate, Magnesium Oxide, Maltodextrin, Cellulose, Zinc Oxide, Modified Food Starch, Manganese Sulfate, Contains color additives including FD&C Yellow #5 (Tartrazine), Sodium Borate, Sucrose, Cupric Oxide, FD&C Blue #1, Natural Spearmint Flavor, Gelatin, Vitamin D, Crospovidone, Stearic Acid

How Supplied:
Bottles of 60 with Assorted Fruit Flavors Also available in bottles of 60 as, Caltrate® Plus Tablets No Sugar, No Salt, No Lactose, No Preservatives: Tablet Shape Specially Designed for Easier Swallowing.
Store at Room Temperature.
© 1996

CENTRUM®
[sĕn-trŭm]
High Potency Multivitamin-Multimineral Dietary Supplement, Advanced Formula From A to Zinc®

Supplement Facts
Serving Size 1 Tablet

Each Tablet Contains	%DV
Vitamin A 5000 IU (40% as Beta Carotene)	100%
Vitamin C 60 mg	100%
Vitamin D 400 IU	100%
Vitamin E 30 IU	100%
Vitamin K 25 mcg	31%
Thiamin 1.5 mg	100%
Riboflavin 1.7 mg	100%
Niacin 20 mg	100%
Vitamin B$_6$ 2 mg	100%
Folic Acid 400 mcg	100%
Vitamin B$_{12}$ 6 mcg	100%
Biotin 30 mcg	10%
Pantothenic Acid 10 mg	100%
Calcium 162 mg	16%
Iron 18 mg	100%
Phosphorus 109 mg	11%
Iodine 150 mcg	100%
Magnesium 100 mg	25%
Zinc 15 mg	100%
Selenium 20 mcg	29%
Copper 2 mg	100%
Manganese 2 mg	100%
Chromium 120 mcg	100%
Molybdenum 75 mcg	100%
Chloride 72 mg	2%
Potassium 80 mg	2%
Nickel 5 mcg	*
Tin 10 mcg	*
Silicon 2 mg	*
Vanadium 10 mcg	*
Boron 150 mcg	*

*Daily Value (%DV) not established.

Suggested Use: Adults, 1 tablet daily.

Warning: Accidental overdose of iron-containing products is a leading cause of fatal poisoning in children under 6. Keep this product out of reach of children. In case of accidental overdose, call a doctor or a Poison Control Center immediately.

Ingredients: Calcium Phosphate, Magnesium Oxide, Potassium Choride, Microcrystalline Cellulose, Ascorbic Acid (Vit. C), Ferrous Fumarate, Calcium Carbonate, Gelatin, dl-alpha Tocopheryl Acetate (Vit. E), Crospovidone, Niacinamide, Zinc Oxide, Hydroxypropyl Methylcellulose, Starch, Titanium Dioxide, Calcium Pantothenate, Silicon Dioxide, Manganese Sulfate, Sucrose, Magnesium Stearate, Pyridoxine Hydrochloride (Vit. B$_6$), Cupric Oxide, Riboflavin (Vit. B$_2$), Thiamin Mononitrate (Vit. B$_1$), Vitamin A Acetate/Vitamin D, Triethyl Citrate, Beta Carotene, Lactose, Polysorbate 80, Chromium Chloride, Borates, Folic Acid, Glucose, Potassium Iodide, Sodium Molybdate, Sodium Selenate, FD&C Yellow 6, Phytonadione (Vit. K), Biotin, Sodium Metavanadate, Nickelous Sulfate, Stannous Chloride and Cyanocobalamin (Vit. B$_{12}$).

Nutrition Facts

Serving Size:	Children 2–4 Years Old $^1/_2$ tablet		Adults and Children Over 4 Years Old 1 tablet	
	Amount Per Serving % Daily Value		Amount Per Serving % Daily Value	
Vitamin A (20% as Beta Carotene)	2500 IU	100%	5000 IU	100%
Vitamin C	30 mg	75%	60 mg	100%
Vitamin D	200 IU	50%	400 IU	100%
Vitamin E	15 IU	150%	30 IU	100%
Vitamin K	5 mcg	*	10 mcg	13%
Thiamin	0.75 mg	107%	1.5 mg	100%
Riboflavin	0.85 mg	106%	1.7 mg	100%
Niacin	10 mg	111%	20 mg	100%
Vitamin B$_6$	1 mg	143%	2 mg	100%
Folic Acid	200 mcg	100%	400 mcg	100%
Vitamin B$_{12}$	3 mcg	100%	6 mcg	100%
Biotin	22.5 mcg	15%	45 mcg	15%
Pantothenic Acid	5 mg	100%	10 mg	100%
Calcium	54 mg	7%	108 mg	11%
Iron	9 mg	90%	18 mg	100%
Phosphorous	25 mg	3%	50 mg	5%
Iodine	75 mcg	107%	150 mcg	100%
Magnesium	20 mg	10%	40 mg	10%
Zinc	7.5 mg	94%	15 mg	100%
Copper	1 mg	100%	2 mg	100%
Manganese	0.5 mg	*	1 mg	50%
Chromium	10 mcg	*	20 mcg	17%
Molybdenum	10 mcg	*	20 mcg	27%

*Daily Value not established.

How Supplied: Light peach, engraved CENTRUM C1.
Bottles of 60, 180
Combopack†
†Bottles of 100 plus 30
Liquid in bottles of 8 oz.
Store at Room Temperature.

CENTRUM® HERBALS:
CENTRUM ECHINACEA
CENTRUM GARLIC
CENTRUM GINKGO BILOBA
CENTRUM GINSENG
CENTRUM SAW PALMETTO
CENTRUM ST. JOHN'S WORT

See Whitehall-Robins Healthcare

CENTRUM® Kids™ Complete
[sĕn-trŭm]
Shamu and his Crew®
Children's Chewable Vitamin/Mineral Formula

[See table below]

Ingredients: Sugar, Calcium Phosphate, Mannitol, Calcium Carbonate, Magnesium Oxide, Ascorbic Acid (Vit. C), Mono- and Diglycerides, Microcrystalline Cellulose, Modified Food Starch, Gelatin, dl-alpha Tocopheryl Acetate (Vit. E), FD&C Yellow #6, Niacinamide, Zinc Oxide, Iron Carbonyl, Natural and Artificial Flavors, Calcium Pantothenate, Citric Acid, Malic Acid, (Food) Starch, Guar Gum, FD&C Red #40, FD&C Blue #2, Carragenan, Vitamin A Acetate/Vitamin D, Aspartame**, Magnesium Sterate,

Silicon Dioxide, Partially Hydrogenated Coconut Oil, Pyridoxine Hydrochloride (Vit. B_6), Cupric Oxide, Riboflavin (Vit. B_2), Thiamin Mononitrate (Vit. B_1), Dextrose, Manganese Sulfate, Beta Carotene, Folic Acid, Lactose, Acacia, Potassium Iodide, Biotin, Sodium Molybdate, Chromium Chloride, Phytonadione (Vit. K) and Cyanocobalamin (Vit. B_{12}).

Contains Aspartame. **Phenylketonurics: Contains Phenylalanine.

Warnings: CLOSE TIGHTLY AND KEEP OUT OF REACH OF CHILDREN. CONTAINS IRON, WHICH CAN BE HARMFUL OR FATAL TO CHILDREN IN LARGE DOSES. IN CASE OF ACCIDENTAL OVERDOSE, SEEK PROFESSIONAL ASSISTANCE OR CONTACT A POISON CONTROL CENTER IMMEDIATELY.

Recommended Intake: Children 2 to 4 years of age, chew approximately one-half tablet daily. Adults and children over 4 years of age, chew one tablet daily.

How Supplied: Assorted Flavors—Uncoated Tablet—Bottle of 60
Also available as: Centrum® Kids™ + Extra C (250 mg); and as: Centrum® Kids™ + Extra Calcium (200 mg).
Store at Room Temperature.
© 1998
Sea World Characters ©1998 Sea World, Inc. All Rights Reserved.
Shamu and his Crew® are trademarks and copyrights of Sea World, Inc.
CENTRUM® KIDS™, the color spectrum design and all other marks and indicia are trademarks and copyrights of American Cyanamid Company. Centrum® Kids™ is a dietary supplement

---

CENTRUM® SILVER®
Multivitamin/Multimineral Dietary Supplement for Adults
50+
Iron-Free Formula
From A to Zinc®

Supplement Facts
Serving Size 1 Tablet

Each Tablet Contains	%DV
Vitamin A 5000 IU	100%
(50% as Beta Carotene)	
Vitamin C 60 mg	100%
Vitamin D 400 IU	100%
Vitamin E 45 IU	150%
Thiamin 1.5 mg	100%
Riboflavin 1.7 mg	100%
Niacinamide 20 mg	100%
Vitamin B_6 3 mg	150%
Folic Acid 400 mcg	100%
Vitamin B_{12} 25 mcg	416%
Biotin 30 mcg	10%
Pantothenic Acid 10 mg	100%
Calcium 200 mg	20%
Phosphorus 48 mg	5%
Iodine 150 mcg	100%
Magnesium 100 mg	25%
Zinc 15 mg	100%
Copper 2 mg	100%
Potassium 80 mg	2%
Vitamin K 10 mcg	13%
Selenium 20 mcg	29%
Manganese 2.0 mg	100%
Chromium 150 mcg	125%
Molybdenum 75 mcg	100%
Chloride 72 mg	2%
Nickel 5 mcg	*
Silicon 2 mg	*
Vanadium 10 mcg	*
Boron 150 mcg	*

*Daily Value (% DV) not established.

Recommended Intake:
Adults, 1 tablet daily.

Warning: Keep out of the reach of children.

Ingredients: Calcium Carbonate, Calcium Phosphate, Magnesium Oxide, Potassium Chloride, Microcrystalline Cellulose, Ascorbic Acid (Vit. C), Gelatin, dl-Alpha Tocopheryl Acetate (Vit. E), Starch, Crospovidone, Hydroxypropyl Methylcellulose, Niacinamide, Zinc Oxide, Calcium Pantothenate, Silicon Dioxide, Titanium Dioxide, Manganese Sulfate, Sucrose, Magnesium Stearate, Pyridoxine Hydrochloride (Vit. B_6), Cupric Oxide, Riboflavin (Vit. B_2), Beta Carotene, Triethyl Citrate, Thiamin Mononitrate (Vit. B_1), Vitamin A Acetate/Vitamin D, Lactose, Polysorbate 80, Chromium Chloride, Borates, Folic Acid, Potassium Iodide, Glucose, Sodium Molybdate, Sodium Selenate, Biotin Cyanocobalamin (Vit. B_{12}), Sodium Metavanadate, Nickelous Sulfate, Phytonadione (Vit. K), FD&C Blue 2, FD&C Red 40 and FD&C Yellow 6.

How Supplied: Bottle of 60
Bottle of 100
Store at Room Temperature.
© 1995

Leiner Health Products
901 E. 233rd STREET
CARSON, CA 90745-6204

Direct Inquiries to:
Sandra Jean, M.S.
Ph: (310) 835-8400
Fax: (310) 835-6615

YOUR LIFE® Healthy Legs™

Description: *Your Life® Healthy Legs™* is a unique blend of herbal and plant ingredients in a sustained release formulation designed to help maintain normal circulation in the legs and maintain normal structure and permeability of leg veins.*
Serving Size: 1 caplet
Suggested Use: 1 caplet 2 times per day
Ingredients per Caplet:
[See table at bottom of next page]

General Description: A unique blend of five herbal ingredients in a convenient, sustained release caplet.
How and Why It Works
Horsechestnut Seed Extract: The main active principles in HCSE are thought to be escin, esculin, and proanthocyanidin A_2. Escin is a saponin that has antiedema, antiinflammatory, and vasoprotective properties. Escin is used in medicine to treat venous disease and has been successfully used to alleviate fluid pressure in the brain due to head trauma, meningitis, cerebral tumors, or encephalitis. Escin is also used to prevent edemas in surgery. Esculin is a coumarin glycoside that improves capillary permeability and fragility, and has been used to treat venous peripheral diseases, including hemorrhoids. Proanthocyanidin A_2 has antioxidant properties and has been demonstrated to stimulate venous healing under conditions of impaired capillary permeability and fragility.
Ginger: The principles in ginger responsible for its biologic activity are believed to be the sesquiterpenes (eg, zingiberene and zingiberol) and the nonvolatile pungent ketones (eg, gingerols, shogaols, and zingerone). These compounds have been shown to have antioxidant activity and to stimulate chemical modulators and messengers of vascular tone, blood formulation, and muscle contraction, which suggests an indirect role of ginger in promoting circulation.
Gotu Kola: Recent experimental evidence suggests gotu kola may affect various parameters associated with venous structure and circulation. Triterpenoids from gotu kola (astiatic acid, madecassic acid, and asiaticoside) have demonstrated activity on connective tissue metabolism and have been shown to stimulate collagen synthesis in human fibroblasts and promote wound healing in animal models. Madecassol, a gotu kola triterpenoid preparation, has been used clinically to promote normal collagen synthesis in the prevention of unsightly surgical scars and in the treatment of skin ulcers. Gotu kola triterpenoids have also been utilized as a therapy for inflammatory skin lesions in leprosy. A recent in vitro screening of medicinal plants indicated that gotu kola inhibited angiotensin-converting enzyme (ACE). ACE is the rate-limiting step in the formation of angiotensin II, which increases vascular smooth muscle contraction and peripheral resistance and is associated with extracellular fluid accumulation and hypertension. These data, although indirect, may suggest a vasoprotective role for gotu kola that needs further clarification.
Citrus Bioflavonoids: Flavonoids exert a variety of biological effects that promote vessel integrity and maintain circulatory health. Flavonoids may scavenge free radicals and prevent them from inhibiting vasodilators (including nitric oxide and prostacyclin) and inducing vascu-

Continued on next page

Your Life Healthy Legs—Cont.

lar injury. Flavonoids may modulate nerve responses involved in venous contraction during blood flow. Evidence suggests platelet aggregation and adhesion, which contribute to thrombosis or abnormal blood clotting and inadequate circulation, are inhibited by flavonoids. Modulation of arachidonic acid metabolism and intracellular signaling within platelets may in part be responsible for the antiaggregatory and vasoprotective effect of flavonoids. Some researchers have even identified flavonoids in citrus that have successfully reduced blood pressure in hypertensive rats. When orally ingested, the flavonoid troxerutin was readily taken up by vessel walls in patients with chronic venous insufficiency suggesting a potential mechanism for the improvement in venous tone associated with flavonoid treatment.

Grape Seed Extract: The effects of grape seed extract on vascular health are similar to those of flavonoids. Proanthocyanidins found in grape seed scavenge oxygen radicals, which are associated with free radical-mediated vascular injury. Proanthocyanidins also have antiaggregatory effects, which probably involve arachidonic acid metabolism. Furthermore, proanthocyanidins may bind to and protect proteins that make up vascular structures, as well as inhibit proteolytic enzymes (eg, elastase and collagenase) that catalyze the breakdown of fibrous components (eg, elastin, collagen) of vessel walls and compromise vascular integrity.

Summary: Your Life® Healthy Legs™ contains a unique blend of HCSE and plant extracts that may help promote circulatory health. Clinical evidence supports the use of HCSE in conditions such as varicose veins and chronic venous insufficiency. Limited investigations suggest HCSE supplementation may be of benefit in normal subjects for alleviating leg-swelling common during orthostatic stress (eg, long air flights). Flavonoids supplied in the citrus bioflavonoid powder and grape seed extracts may support vein health by decreasing capillary permeability and fragility. Flavonoids may also function as antioxidants and help protect blood vessels from free radical injury. Indirect evidence suggests gotu kola and ginger extracts may positively influence circulation, perhaps by modulating platelet aggregation and parameters involved in connective tissue metabolism and blood vessel contraction.

Safety: There are no known safety concerns with the use of the herbal ingredients in Your Life® Healthy Legs™ when taken as recommended. The clinical evidence reviewed here tested the efficacy and safety of a standardized HCSE delivered in a delayed-released capsule. This preparation was well tolerated with no more side effects being reported with HCSE treatment than with placebo. The Commission E Monograph lists no special notes of warning or caution on use, and indicates no known interaction with other drugs or any known restriction for use during pregnancy and lactation. Potential side effects listed include isolated cases of itching, nausea, and gastric complaints. Providing HCSE in a sustained release formulation may minimize the potential for gastric upset. There are anecdotal reports of side effects (muscle twitching, weakness, vomiting, diarrhea, and stupor) in children eating horsechestnut seeds or drinking infusions made from the leaves of the horsechestnut tree. High-dose intravenous escin therapy (340–510 µg/kg body weight) has resulted in renal impairment and acute renal failure in patients following cardiac surgery. The efficacious HCSE dose noted in the German Commission E Monograph for treatment of venous disorders, and heaviness, swelling, cramping, pain, or itching in the legs is 100 mg escin, corresponding to 250–312.5 mg HCSE twice daily in delayed release form.

The ESCOP Monograph on ginger lists no restriction on use in adults and children over 6 years old with dosages of ginger ranging from 500–2000 mg per day. No contraindications or special warnings are listed. Heartburn may be an undesirable effect and toxic overdose is not believed possible. As a standard precaution, medical advice is recommended with use during pregnancy and lactation. The German Commission E monograph listed a possible contraindication in individuals with gallstones and warns ginger should not be used for morning sickness during pregnancy. Otherwise, no toxicity is noted.

Clinical trials that examined effectiveness in circulatory disorders have reported gotu kola extracts in doses up to 120 mg per day were well tolerated with no side effects observed. The amount of gotu kola supplied in this product is expected to be safe.

Citrus bioflavonoids and grape seed extract are very safe at the levels supplied in this product. The amount of flavonoids provided by these ingredients is lower than typical dietary intakes, which are estimated to range from 500–1000 mg per day and have been safely consumed for years.

Who Would or Should Use the Product

1. *Primary target consumer group:* healthy adults who desire the benefits of a dietary supplement designed to help maintain normal leg circulatory health as they age.
2. *Secondary target consumer group:* adults who are prone to fragile veins or capillaries may benefit from regular supplementation with HCSE.

Who Should Not Use the Product

There are no specific contraindications known for the ingredients present in the product. However, individuals under medical care and/or taking prescription medicines should consult their physician before taking Your Life® Healthy Legs™ or other dietary supplements. Likewise, pregnant or lactating women should seek medical advice before using herbal supplements.

How Supplied: 50 Caplets
References available upon request.
Shown in Product Identification Guide, page 508

YOUR LIFE® Osteo Joint™

Your Life® Osteo Joint™ provides nutrients essential for maintaining healthy joints, connective tissue, cartilage, and bone; and promotes optimal joint flexibility, function, and range of motion.*
Serving Size: 1 caplet
Suggested Use: 3 caplets daily, preferably with meals
Ingredients per Caplet:
[See table at top of next page]

General Description: A special blend of glucosamine sulfate, standardized devil's claw extract, methylsulfonylmethane, and lecithin in a base of rice starch.

How and Why It Works

Glucosamine Sulfate: Glucosamine is *essential* for normal glycosaminoglycan synthesis, which begins with the synthesis of a core protein pool that is transported to specialized compartments within secretory cells such as cartilage cells. Next, sugar residues, including glucosamines, are added to the core protein, followed by the rapid addition of an extremely large number of long glycosaminoglycan chains. The addition of sulfur to the aminosugar residues occurs almost simultaneously in cartilage cells and in cells from which connective tissue is developed (fibroblasts). Thus, one hypothesis for enhanced cartilage repair is to provide sufficient glucosamine to ensure rapid synthesis of glycosaminoglycans. Enhanced synthesis of glycosaminoglycans and proteoglycans may then be able to overcome the degradation that occurs during joint disease and after injury.

Glucosamine may also offer other health benefits. It has been suggested that the health benefit of oral glucosamine in osteoarthritis—a disease characterized by a net loss of joint cartilage and an increase in the amount of enzymes that break down proteoglycans—may be due to increased synthesis of cartilage pro-

NUTRIENT	AMOUNT	% DAILY VALUE
Horsechestnut Seed Extract (*Aesculus hippocastanum*)(seed) (standardized to 18% escin)	300 mg	+
Ginger Root Powder (*Zingiber officinale*)(root)	100 mg	+
Gotu Kola Powder (*Centella asiatica*)(herb)	33 mg	+
Citrus Bioflavonoids Powder (*Citrus* spp.) (Fruit)	15 mg	+
Grape Seed Extract (*Vitis vinifera*)(seed)	2 mg	+
+Daily Value not established		

NUTRIENT	AMOUNT	% DAILY VALUE
Glucosamine Sulfate	500 mg	+
Devil's Claw Extract (*Harpagophytum procumbens*)(root) (5% harpagoside)	40 mg	+
Methylsulfonylmethane	25 mg	+
Lecithin	25 mg	+

+Daily Value not established.

teoglycans. Ingested glucosamine may likewise enhance heparan sulfate production in endothelial cells of blood vessels thereby acting to reduce artery-clogging damage. A similar glucosamine-mediated increase in heparan sulfate production in certain types of skin cells may provide a therapeutic benefit for psoriasis.

Glucosamine may also have clinical value in postsurgical wound healing. Normal hyaluronic acid synthesis is a function of glucosamine availability. Rapid production of hyaluronic acid by fibroblasts in the early stages of wound healing may be crucial as hyaluronic acid stimulates the migration and division of mesenchymal and epithelial cells. Epithelial cells are the cells that form the epidermis of the skin and the surface layer of mucous and serous (secreting) membranes; mesenchymal cells are cells that give rise to various tissues including connective tissues such as cartilage and bone. Thus, consuming adequate amounts of glucosamine during the first few days after surgery or trauma may enhance hyaluronic acid production in the wound, promote swifter healing, and possibly diminish complications related to scarring.

Devil's Claw: The antiinflammatory, analgesic, antiarrhythmic, and hypotensive effects of devil's claw, harpagoside (the main iridoid found in devil's claw), and harpagogenin (a harpagoside derivative) have been investigated. Intravenous and intraperitoneal administration of aqueous extracts of devil's claw root, harpagoside, and harpagogenin have demonstrated antiinflammatory activity in animal models. However, results from oral administration have been inconsistent. Evidence suggests that this inconsistency may be a result of degradation of the active compounds in devil's claw by gastric juice.

Although a mechanism of action has not been established for the antiinflammatory effect of devil's claw, evidence suggests that it is unlike that of nonsteroidal antiinflammatory drugs (NSAIDs); that is, devil's claw does not affect eicosanoid production. Eicosanoids are metabolic products of the fatty acid arachidonic acid, many of which (eg, prostaglandins and leukotrienes) are directly involved in inflammation. The main iridoid glycoside, harpagoside, does not appear to contribute to the antiinflammatory effect of devil's claw; however, it does appear to contribute, in part, to the peripheral analgesic effect of devil's claw. Extracts of devil's claw have also exhibited various cardiac effects in animal models—arterial blood pressure reduc-

tion in rats, decreased heart rate in rabbits, and a protective effect against arrhythmias in rats. The cardiac effects of devil's claw have been attributed to the iridoids, flavonoids, and triterpenes (ie, harpagoside, harpagide, luteolin and kaempeferol, and ursolic acid).

Methylsulfonylmethane (MSM): Sulfur, whether from MSM or other sources, has many functions in the body. It is an essential component of 3 vitamins (ie, thiamin, biotin, and pantothenic acid) and 3 amino acids (ie, cystine, cysteine, and methionine) found in all proteins in the body. The sulfur in cysteine is necessary for the proper structure and function of enzymes. It is also necessary for proteins involved in the transfer of energy (oxidative phosphorylation). Sulfur is also a component of the anticoagulant heparin and the antioxidant glutathione. Of particular importance to joint health is sulfur's role as an essential component of chondroitin sulfate, a primary glycosaminoglycan found in bone and cartilage.

Lecithin: Dietary lecithin contributes to the body's stores of choline—a necessary precursor to cell membrane phospholipids. Phospholipids have a strong affinity for both water-soluble and fat-soluble substances. This property makes them effective structural materials in the body. Large concentrations of phospholipids are found in combination with protein in cell membranes, where they facilitate the passage of fat in and out of cells, and in the blood, where they also function in the transport of fats (as part of lipoproteins). Phospholipids also appear to play a critical role in generating second messengers for cell membrane signal transduction. This process involves a cascade of reactions that translate an external cell stimulus such as a hormone or growth factor into a change in cell transport, metabolism, growth, function, or gene expression. Disruptions in phospholipid metabolism can interfere with this process.

A limited number of studies have reported a lecithin-mediated increase in the absorption and/or utilization of certain nutrients in animal models. Kimura et al demonstrated improved absorption in rats of a lecithin-dispersed form of vitamin E (d-alpha-tocopherol acetate) compared to nonlecithin-dispersed forms. Boccio et al demonstrated increased bioavailability and stability of iron (ferrous sulfate) from milk in a mouse model. Microencapsulating the iron in fluid milk with lecithin resulted in a 46% increase in iron bioavailability compared to regular fluid milk. Thus, microencapsulation prevented the inter-

action of iron with other ingredients in milk that may have inhibited its absorption. Igarashi et al demonstrated increased cell membrane affinity of the antioxidant superoxide dismutase when chemically attached to lecithin, compared to unmodified superoxide dismutase.

Summary

Glucosamine: The clinical efficacy of glucosamine has been established for the treatment of degenerative joint conditions. Glucosamine administration has been shown to offer symptomatic relief—reducing pain/swelling and improving joint flexibility/restricted function—of osteoarthritis. In addition, glucosamine helps rebuild damaged cartilage by providing an essential nutrient for the production of the glycosaminoglycans found in cartilage, which are necessary for structural and functional integrity.

Devil's Claw: Although animal and in vitro studies are inconsistent with regard to the pharmacologic effects of devil's claw, the few published clinical trials involving oral administration of devil's claw for symptomatic relief of arthritis show promise. Based on a limited number of open-label and double-blind studies, oral administration of powdered devil's claw (2010 mg/day) and extracts of devil's claw (2400–9000 mg/day) have been shown to be efficacious for symptomatic relief of arthritis (ie, reduced pain, greater mobility, and improved strength) and were well tolerated. However, oral administration of a lower dose of devil's claw extract (1230 mg/day) did not show the same therapeutic benefits in a small, open-label study. Although this preliminary research is encouraging, more clinical trails involving larger patient populations and longer duration are needed to verify the potential beneficial effects of devil's claw for symptomatic relief of arthritic symptoms.

Methylsulfonylmethane (MSM): MSM is a bioavailable source of sulfur. Sulfur has many functions in the body. It is an essential component of 3 vitamins (ie, thiamin, biotin, and pantothenic acid) and 3 amino acids (ie, cystine, cysteine, and methionine) found in all proteins in the body. The sulfur in cysteine is necessary for the proper structure and function of enzymes. It is also necessary for proteins involved in the transfer of energy (oxidative phosphorylation). Sulfur is a component of the anticoagulant heparin and the antioxidant glutathione. Of particular importance of joint health is sulfur's role as an essential component of chondroitin sulfate, a primary glycosaminoglycan found in bone and cartilage.

Lecithin: Dietary lecithin, also known as phosphatidylcholine, is a phospholipid. It is widely distributed in foods and is an approved food additive. Dietary lecithin serves as a contributor to the body's stores of choline—a necessary precursor to cell membrane phospholipids. Large concentrations of phospholipids are

Continued on next page

Your Life Osteo-Joint—Cont.

found in cell membranes, where they facilitate the passage of fat in and out of cells, and in the blood, where they also function in the transport of fats (as part of lipoproteins). Dietary lecithin has also been shown to enhance absorption and/or utilization of certain nutrients in animal studies, but clinical data are lacking.

Safety: No safety problems have been observed with oral dosages of glucosamine sulfate at levels up to 1500 mg/day. Devil's claw is contraindicated with gastric and duodenal ulcers, and patients with gallstones should use devil's claw only after consultation with a physician. Devil's claw may also interact with antiarrhythmic medications. No data are available for devil's claw with regard to its use during pregnancy and lactation; thus, this product should not be used during pregnancy and lactation. Mild gatrointestinal disturbances may occur in sensitive individuals with devil's claw, especially at higher doses. No toxicity has been reported for MSM. The amount of lecithin found in this product is known to be safe.

Who Would or Should Use the Product

1. *Primary target consumer group(s):* consumers who desire symptomatic relief of pain and inflammation associated with degenerative joint conditions such as arthritis, and who would like to rebuild damaged cartilage and maintain healthy cartilage.
2. *Secondary target consumer group(s):* consumers who desire symptomatic relief of pain and inflammation associated with joint injury, and who would like to rebuild damaged cartilage and maintain healthy cartilage.
3. *Tertiary target consumer group(s):* healthy consumers who would like to ensure an adequate intake of nutrients important for joint health.

Who Should Not Use the Product

Pregnant and nursing women should not use this product, nor should people with gastric or duodenal ulcers. People taking medication for arrythmia and those with gallstones should use this product only after consultant with a physician.

How Supplied: 50 Caplets
References available upon request.
Shown in Product Identification Guide, page 508

UNKNOWN DRUG?
Consult the
Product Identification Guide
(Gray Pages)
for full-color photos of
leading over-the-counter
medications

Lichtwer Pharma U.S., Inc.

FOSTER PLAZA 9
750 HOLIDAY DRIVE
PITTSBURGH, PA 15220

Direct Inquiries to:
(412) 928-9334
Fax: (412) 928-9655
Direct Healthcare Professional inquiries/clinical study requests/professional sample requests to:
1 (800) 837-3203
Email: lpusinc@aol.com
For more consumer information call:
1 (800) 92PROOF
Website: www.lichtwer.com

GINKAI® Ginkgo Biloba
30 Standardized Tested Tablets
Unique "LI 1370" Formulation
Dietary Supplement

Description: Improves Memory And Concentration*

• Independent researchers have documented that Lichtwer Pharma's unique Ginkai formulation "LI 1370" has been proven in some of the most well designed clinical studies on Ginkgo Biloba extracts. **Ginkai** was shown in these studies to improve the blood flow to the brain. When the brain receives more oxygen, it becomes more active and quicker to respond. Memory and concentration are improved, helping patients maintain their mental edge. The effects of taking Ginkai were observed at a clinically relevant level after 6 weeks of use.
• Contains 50mg per tablet of highly purified and concentrated (50:1) Ginkgo Biloba "LI 1370" (processed from the Ginkgo leaf).
• Standardized to 25% ginkgo flavonoids and 6% terpenoids in their proven ratio.
• Standardized using the HPLC and Gas Chromatography methods ensuring the same high quality extract in each tablet.

Contents: Each tablet contains 50 mg Ginkgo Biloba "LI 1370" dried leaf extract (50:1) standardized to 25% ginkgo flavonoids and 6% terpenoids, and lactose, microcrystalline cellulose, citric acid, magnesium silicate, hydroxy propylmethyl cellulose, magnesium stearate, silicum dioxide, castor oil, stearic acid.

Suggested Serving: Take 1 tablet, three times with water at meal-times.

Cautions: Blister pack ensures freshness, safety and convenience. Do not use if blister is broken. Keep in a cool, dry place out of reach of children. If you are pregnant, nursing a baby or administrating to children, seek the advice of a health professional before using this product.
Product of Germany. Packaged in the U.S.
Distributed by Lichtwer Pharma U.S., Inc., Pittsburgh, PA 15220.

*This statement has not been evaluated by the Food and Drug Administration. This product is not intended to diagnose, treat, cure or prevent any disease.
Shown in Product Identification Guide, page 509

KIRA® St. John's Wort
45 Standardized Tested Tablets
Special Extract (LI 160) Dietary Supplement

Description: Promotes a Healthy Emotional Balance and Well-Being*
Supports Healthy Motivation and Self-Esteem*
Kira St. John's Wort is standardized to ensure an optimum, proven effective amount of special Hypericum extract (LI 160) in every tablet (0.3% hypericin hyperforin and flavonoids).
Kira is non-habit forming. It does not have a sedative effect and has no interactions with alcohol. No interaction with caffeine has been observed and its safety profile also supports longer term use.
Kira is free from preservatives, yeast and gluten.
Kira has been proven effective in over 23 clinical studies on real people, more than any other brand.
The exclusive LI 160 formula in **Kira** is the leading prescription St. John's Wort product in Germany.

Contents: Each tablet contains 300mg dried Hypericum Perforatum (St. John's Wort) special extract "LI 160" from upper parts of flower and leaves of the plant including ingredients hyperforin, flavonoids and 0.3% hypericin. Binders and coating: sucrose, lactose, talc, powdered cellulose, hydroxypropyl methylcellulose, polyethylene glycol, castor oil, magnesium stearate, polyvinylpyrrolidone (pvp), silicon dioxide, gelatin, titanium dioxide, carnauba wax.

Suggested Serving: Take 1 tablet, 3 times daily with water at mealtimes.

Cautions: Blister pack ensures freshness, safety and convenience. Do not use if blister is broken. Keep in a cool, dry place. As with other supplements, keep out of reach of children. If you are taking prescription medicine, are pregnant, nursing a baby, or administering to children under the age of 12, consult a health professional before using this product. When taking Hypericum, use caution in exposing skin to excessive sunlight.

How Supplied: 45 Tablets, Net. wt. 1.2 oz (34 g).
*These statements have not been evaluated by the Food and Drug Administration. This product is not intended to diagnose, treat, cure or prevent any disease. Results observed after two weeks. Product of Germany. Packaged in the US.
Distributed by Lichtwer Pharma U.S., Inc. Pittsburgh, PA 15220
Shown in Product Identification Guide, page 509

KWAI® Odor Free Garlic
90 and 180 Count
Standardized and Tested Tablets
Dietary Supplement

Description: Clinically Proven To Lower Cholesterol* Kwai has been repeatedly proven to lower cholesterol in more published human clinical studies than any other garlic supplement brand. In fact, some garlic brands may rely on Kwai's testing to support their own garlic claims. Kwai is recognized in the world's foremost medical journals, because Kwai has the quality, the research, and the proof. Kwai has been proven in over 30 clinical studies.

- Easy to swallow.
- Take 2 Kwai tablets 3 times daily to maintain a consistent level of garlic in your system.
- Contains all the components of garlic cloves. Each standardized tablet yields 600 mcg of allicin and contains 100 mg of concentrated dried garlic, equivalent to 300 mg of fresh garlic.
- Suitable for diabetics. $^1/_2$ calorie per tablet.
- Over 100 quality control procedures.

Contents: Each tablet contains **Core**-100 mg dried garlic clove powder.
Core binders and coating layer-Lactose, powdered cellulose, silicon dioxide, magnesium stearate, sucrose, magnesium silicate (mineral source), hydroxypropyl methylcellulose, gelatin, bees wax.
The garlic powder used in Kwai undergoes analytical testing to standardize the allicin yield. The tablet coating ensures the freshness and intensity of the garlic component and delivers an odor-free product.
Suggested Serving: Take 2 tablets, 3 times daily with liquid, ideally with meals. Do not chew but swallow whole to ensure maximum breath freshness.
Why 3 Times A Day Is Better Than Once A Day.
Like vitamin C and other natural substances, garlic's qualities are short-lived, lasting only about 4 to 6 hours. To maintain a consistent level of garlic in the body, you should take it at regular intervals during the day rather than in one large amount. That's why we suggest Kwai® 3 times a day.

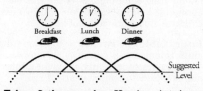

Taken 3 times a day, Kwai maintains a consistent high level of garlic in your system for 24 hours. Taken once a day, garlic products wear off in just a few hours.

Cautions: Blister pack ensures product freshness, safety, and convenience. Do not use if seal or blister is broken. Keep in a cool dry place out of reach of children.
Product of Germany. Packaged in the U.S. Distributed by Lichtwer Pharma U.S., Inc., Pittsburgh, PA 15220.

Guaranteed Odor Free. Kwai's special scientific coating protects the concentrated garlic and releases it well down the digestive tract to prevent any odor, as long as tablet is not broken or chewed before swallowing. In the event you are not satisfied, a full refund of your purchase price will be made if you send the unused portion and your receipt to the name and address below. Only one refund per household is allowed. Kwai Guarantee-P.O. Box 16345, Pittsburgh, PA 15242-0345.
*This statement has not been evaluated by the Food and Drug Administration. Kwai is not intended to diagnose, treat, cure or prevent disease. If you have a disease or health related condition that requires the lowering of cholesterol, consult your doctor. Results observed after 12 weeks of usage.
Shown in Product Identification Guide, page 509

Matol Botanical International, Ltd.
1111, 46th AVENUE
LACHINE QUEBEC,
CANADA H8T 3C5

Direct Inquiries to:
Ph: (800) 363-3890
website: www.matol.com

BIOMUNE OSF PLUS
Dietary supplement for immune system support

Description: Biomune OSF Plus is an immune system support product for all ages. Biomune OSF Plus is a combination of a special extract of bovine colostrum and whey with the herb Astragalus. The exclusive extract of colostrum/whey is prepared using patented and proprietary processes unique to the nutritional industry. Astragalus is a traditional Chinese herb that has been used for centuries, initially in the Orient, then throughout the world and is known for its immune enhancing properties.
Biomune OSF Plus has been tested in clinical trials and has been proven to be very effective in consistently and dramatically increasing Natural Killer (NK) cell activity. Medical research has shown that low NK cell activity is present in most illness.
Summary of the clinical study: *The Use of Dialyzable Bovine Colostrum Extract in Conjunction with a Holistic Treatment Model for Natural Killer Cell Stimulation in Chronic Illness by Jesse A. Stoff, MD, MFHOM, FACLM.*
The study consisted of 107 patients with an average treatment time of 13.2 months. The youngest participant was 17 years and the oldest was 83 years. The average initial NK cell activity was 18 Lytic Units and the average final NK

cell activity was 246 Units. All patients in the study greatly improved, went into remission or recovered. Conclusions: The Study Group demonstrated that stimulation of NK activity paralleled restored resistance to illness and recovery from illness. NK cell function is a well-regulated activity, subject to both inhibitory and excitatory control. The complete clinical study on Biomune OSF Plus by Dr. Stoff is available upon request.

Use: Dietary Supplement

Directions for Use: Take one capsule daily for maintenance and one or two capsules every 2–3 hours when additional immune support is needed. The product can be taken daily for maintenance or as above for extended periods of time. There is no known toxicity.

How Supplied: One bottle contains 30 capsules.
Shown in Product Identification Guide, page 509

McNeil Consumer Healthcare
Division of McNeil-PPC, Inc.
FORT WASHINGTON, PA 19034

Direct Inquiries to:
Consumer Affairs Department
Fort Washington, PA 19034
(215) 233-7000

LACTAID® Original Strength Caplets
(lactase enzyme)

LACTAID® Extra Strength Caplets
(lactase enzyme)

LACTAID® ULTRA Caplets and Chewable Tablets
(lactase enzyme)

Description: Each *LACTAID® Original Strength Caplet* contains 3000 FCC (Food Chemical Codex) units of lactase enzyme (derived from *Aspergillus oryzae*).
Each *LACTAID® Extra Strength Caplet* contains 4500 FCC units of lactase enzyme (derived from *Aspergillus oryzae*).
Each *LACTAID® ULTRA Caplet* contains 9000 FCC units of lactase enzyme (derived from *Aspergillus oryzae*).
Each *LACTAID® ULTRA Chewable Tablet* contains 9000 FCC units of lactase enzyme (derived from *Aspergillus oryzae*).
LACTAID® is the original lactase dietary supplement that makes milk and dairy foods more digestible. *LACTAID®* lactase enzyme hydrolyzes lactose into two digestible simple sugars: glucose and galactose. *LACTAID® Caplets* are taken orally for *in vivo* hydrolysis of lactose.

Continued on next page

Lactaid Caplets—Cont.

Actions: *LACTAID® Caplets/Chewable Tablets* work to naturally replenish lactase enzyme that aids in dairy food digestion. Lactase enzyme hydrolyzes lactose sugar (a double sugar) into its simple sugar components, glucose and galactose.

Indications: Lactose intolerance, suspected from gastrointestinal discomfort (ie, gas, bloating, flatulence, cramps, and diarrhea) after drinking milk or ingesting other dairy foods such as cheese and ice cream.

Directions: These convenient, portable caplets are easy to swallow or chew and can be used with milk or any dairy food. **Original Strength:** Swallow or chew 3 caplets with the first bite of dairy food. For best results, you may have to adjust the number of caplets up or down. Take no more than 6 caplets at a time. **Extra Strength:** Swallow or chew 2 caplets with first bite of dairy food. For best results, you may have to adjust the number of caplets up or down. Take no more than 4 caplets at a time. **Ultra Caplets:** Swallow 1 caplet with the first bite of dairy food. For best results, you may have to adjust the number of caplets up or down. Take no more than 2 caplets at a time. **Ultra Chewables:** Chew and swallow 1 chewable tablet with your first bite of dairy food. If you suffer from severe digestive discomfort, you may have to take more than one tablet but no more than two at a time. Don't be discouraged if at first Lactaid does not work to your satisfaction. Because the degree of enzyme deficiency naturally varies from person to person and from food to food, you may have to adjust the number of caplets/chewable tablets up or down to find your own level of comfort. Since Lactaid Caplets/chewable tablets work only on the food as you eat it, use them every time you enjoy dairy foods.

Warnings: Consult your doctor: If you experience any symptoms which are unusual or seem unrelated to the condition for which you took this product. Do not use if carton is open or if printed plastic neckwrap is broken or if single serve packet is open.
LACTAID® Ultra Chewable Tablets: Contains Phenylalanine 0.49 mg/tablet

Ingredients: *LACTAID® Original Strength Caplets:* Mannitol, Cellulose, Lactase Enzyme (3,000 FCC Lactase units/Caplet), Magnesium Stearate, Dextrose, Sodium Citrate.
LACTAID® Extra Strength Caplets: Lactase Enzyme (4,500 FCC Lactase units/Caplet), Mannitol, Cellulose, Dextrose, Sodium Citrate, Magnesium Stearate.
LACTAID® ULTRA Caplets: Cellulose, Lactase Enzyme (9,000 FCC Lactase units/Caplet), Dextrose, Sodium Citrate, Magnesium Stearate, Colloidal Silicon Dioxide.
LACTAID® ULTRA Chewable Tablets: Mannitol, Cellulose, Sodium Citrate, Dextrose, Magnesium Stearate, Flavor, Citric Acid, Acesulfame K, Aspartame.

How Supplied: *LACTAID® Original Strength Caplets* are available in bottles of 60, and 120 counts. *LACTAID® Extra Strength Caplets* are available in bottles of 24, and 50 counts. *LACTAID® ULTRA Caplets* are available in single serve packets of 12, 32 and 60 counts. *LACTAID® Ultra Chewable Tablets* are available in bottles of 12 and 32 counts. Store at or below room temperature (below 77°F) but do not refrigerate. Keep away from heat.
LACTAID® Caplets and *LACTAID® Ultra Chewable Tablets* are certified kosher from the Orthodox Union.
Also available: 70% lactose reduced Lactaid Milk and 100% lactose-free Lactaid Milk.

*Shown in Product Identification
Guide, page 509*

LACTAID® Drops
(lactase enzyme)

Description: *LACTAID®* is the original dairy digestive supplement that makes milk more digestible. *LACTAID®* lactase enzyme hydrolyzes lactose into two digestible simple sugars: glucose and galactose. *LACTAID® Drops* are added to milk for *in vitro* hydrolysis of lactose. *LACTAID® Drops* contain sufficient lactase enzyme (derived from *Kluyveromyces lactis*) to hydrolyze lactose in milk.

Actions: *LACTAID® Drops* are a liquid form of the natural lactase enzyme that makes milk more digestible. The lactase enzyme hydrolyzes the lactose sugar (a double sugar) into its simple sugar components, glucose and galactose.

Indications: Lactose intolerance, suspected from gastrointestinal discomfort (ie. gas, bloating, cramps, and diarrhea) after drinking milk.

Directions: *LACTAID® Drops* are a liquid form of the natural lactase enzyme that makes milk more digestible. To use, add *LACTAID® Drops* to a quart of milk, shake gently and refrigerate for 24 hours. We recommend starting with 5–7 drops per quart of milk but because sensitivity to lactose can vary, you may have to adjust the number of drops you use. If you are still experiencing discomfort after consuming milk with 5–7 *LACTAID® Drops* per quart, you may want to add 10 drops per quart or even 15 drops per quart. Lactaid can be used with any kind of milk: whole, 1%, 2%, non-fat, skim, powdered and chocolate milk.

Warnings: If you experience any symptoms which are unusual or seem unrelated to the condition for which you took this product, consult a doctor before taking any more of it. Do not use if carton is opened or if printed plastic bodywrap is broken.

Ingredients: Glycerin, Water, Lactase Enzyme

How Supplied: *LACTAID® Drops* are available in .22 fl. oz. (7 mL), (30 quart supply). Store at or below room temperature (below 77°F). Refrigerate after opening.
Lactaid Drops are certified kosher from the Orthodox Union.
Also available: 70% lactose reduced Lactaid Milk and 100% lactose-free Lactaid Milk.

*Shown in Product Identification
Guide, page 509*

Mission Pharmacal Company
**10999 IH 10 WEST
SUITE 1000
SAN ANTONIO, TX 78230-1355**

Direct Inquiries to:
PO Box 786099
San Antonio, TX 78278-6099
TOLL FREE: (800) 292-7364
(210) 696-8400
FAX: (210) 696-6010
**For Medical Information Contact:
In Emergencies:**
George Alexandrides
(830) 249-9822
FAX: (830) 816-2545

CITRACAL®Ⓤ
[*sit'ra-cal*]
Ultradense™ Calcium Citrate Dietary Supplement

Ingredients: Calcium (as Ultradense™ calcium citrate) 200 mg, polyethylene glycol, croscarmellose sodium, HPMC, color added, magnesium silicate, magnesium stearate.

Sensitive Patients: CITRACAL® contains no wheat, barley, yeast or rye; is sugar, dairy and gluten free and contains no artificial colors.

One Tablet Provides: 200 mg calcium (elemental), equaling 20% of the U.S. recommended daily value for adults and children 4 or more years of age.

Four Tablets Provide: 800 mg calcium (elemental), equaling 80% of the U.S. recommended daily value for adults and children 4 or more years of age.

Directions: Take 1 to 2 tablets twice daily or as recommended by a physician, pharmacist or health professional.

Warning: Keep out of reach of children.

How Supplied: CITRACAL® is supplied as white, nearly oval shaped, coated tablets in bottles of 100 UPC 0178-0800-01, and bottles of 200 UPC 0178-0800-20.
Store at room temperature.
Ⓤ=Kosher Parvae approved by Orthodox Union.

CITRACAL® Caplets + D ⓤ

[sit ' ra-cal]
Ultradense™ Calcium Citrate Dietary Supplement

Ingredients: CITRACAL® Caplets + D are supplied in an ultra-dense caplet formulation, each containing calcium (as Ultradense™ calcium citrate) 315 mg, polyethylene glycol, croscarmellose sodium, HPMC, color added, magnesium silicate, magnesium stearate, vitamin D_3 (200IU).

Directions: Take 1 to 2 caplets two times daily or as recommended by a physician, pharmacist or health professional.

Warning: Keep out of reach of children.

How Supplied: CITRACAL® Caplets + D are available in bottles of 60 UPC 0178-0815-60, and bottles of 120 UPC 0178-0815-12.
Store at room temperature.
ⓤ= Kosher Parvae approved by Orthodox Union.

CITRACAL® LIQUITAB® ⓤ

[sit ´ ra-cal]
Calcium Citrate Dietary Supplement

Ingredients: CITRACAL® LIQUITAB® is supplied as effervescent tablets each containing calcium (as calcium citrate) 500 mg, citric acid, adipic acid, saccharin sodium, orange flavor, cellulose gum, aspartame.
This product contains NutraSweet®.
Phenylketonurics: Contains 6 mg phenylalanine per tablet.

Directions: Take 1 tablet dissolved in a glass of water, one to two times daily, or as recommended by a physician, pharmacist or health professional.

Warning: Keep out of reach of children.

How Supplied: CITRACAL® LIQUITAB® is available in bottles of 30 tablets. UPC 0178-0811-30.
Store at room temperature.
ⓤ=Kosher Parvae approved by Orthodox Union.

Natrol

**21411 PRAIRIE STREET
CHATSWORTH, CA 91311**

Direct Inquiries to:
(818) 739-6000
Fax: (818) 739-6001

KAVATROL FORMULA

Directions: Take 1 capsule 3 times per day, preferably before a meal or on an empty stomach.

Each Capsule contains: Kava Root (*P. Methysticum*) Extract (30% Kavalactones) 200mg in an exclusive base of complementary herbs, Passion Flower (*P. Incarnata*), Chamomile Flower (*M. Chamomilla*), Hops Flowers (*H. Lupulus*) and Schizandra Fruit (*S. Chinensis*)

Singh NN, Ellis CR, Singh YN. A double-blind, placebo controlled study of the effects of kava (Kavatrol) on daily stress and anxiety in adults.
Study Purpose: Ethnographic studies in the South Pacific have extolled the virtues of kava—a native drink in the South Pacific Polynesian Islands—for reducing daily stress and anxiety as well as inducing a general state of relaxation without any side effects. The effectiveness and safety of the kava drink as evaluated in a number of clinical trials in Europe confirm the findings from the ethnographic studies. However, the number of double-blind, placebo-controlled, clinical studies with adults in the general population is limited. Clinical studies suggest that the pharmacological activity of kava is comparable to the benzodiazepines, but does not have the untoward effects associated with the benzodiazepines; it is not addictive and does not lead to dose tolerance. Current research suggests that kava can be used in a safe and effective manner at therapeutic doses of up to 400 mg of kava-lactones per day. The purpose of our study was to investigate the effectiveness and safety of kava (in capsule form) in a general population of adults with daily stress and nonclinical levels of anxiety.
Research Questions: We asked the following questions: (1) What is the efficacy of kava in a population of adults who have elevated levels of daily stress? (2) What is the efficacy of kava in a population of adults who have elevated levels of anxiety? (3) What are the side effects of kava?
Methods: This was a randomized, double-blind, placebo-controlled, fixed-dose study of kava using a parallel groups design. Sixty individuals (28 males and 32 females; mean age, 37 years) from the general population who had elevated levels of daily stress and anxiety participated in a 4-week trial. Each subject received either two capsules of kava twice a day (experimental group) or two capsules of placebo twice a day (control group). A nonprescription, commercially available brand of kava (Kavatrol) was used. Kavatrol is produced from dried kava roots in a multistage extraction process. The extract is packaged in 200-mg capsules, with 60-mg kava-lactones in each capsule. Therefore, each dose of kava contained 120-mg kava-lactones in 2 × 200-mg capsules. Data collected at baseline included scores on the SCL-90 (a measure of psychopathology), medical history including previous treatments for nonclinical anxiety and daily stress, sociodemographics, Daily Stress Inventory (DSI), State-Trait Anxiety Inventory (STAI), Untoward Effects Checklist, and vital signs (blood pressure, heart rate, and respiratory rate). Efficacy data on the DSI and STAI were collected once each week, on the same day, for 4 weeks. Adverse effects data were collected daily on the Untoward Effects Checklist.
Results: This was a repeated measures, double-blind study. The subjects were assigned either to Kavatrol or to placebo, and the effects of Kavatrol and placebo were assessed over a 4-week period. The dependent measures included five content clusters on the DSI and two major factors on the STAI. The results showed that daily stress due to interpersonal problems, personal competency, cognitive stressors, environmental hassles, and varied stressors was significantly reduced ($P<.0001$) only for those subjects who were in the Kavatrol group. Overall, daily stress summed for each week decreased only for those subjects who were in the Kavatrol group. Furthermore, state anxiety significantly decreased ($P<.0001$) only for those subjects who were in the Kavatrol group. No significant difference was found in trait anxiety—a fairly fixed attribute among humans—for the subjects in the Kavatrol and placebo groups. When compared with baseline levels, none of the subjects experienced a worsening in any of the 27 side effects as a consequence of taking Kavatrol or placebo capsules.
Discussion And Conclusion: Our study showed that Kavatrol reduced daily stress and nonclinical levels of anxiety in adults when compared with baseline and placebo conditions. This is the first study to show that kava reduces stress associated with the daily hassles of life. In this study, the commercially available Kavatrol brand of kava was used and it was found that overall stress decreased as a function of the time a person was on the herbal product. Greater reductions were evident with longer use of Kavatrol. State anxiety was significantly reduced on a moderate dose of Kavatrol without any untoward side effects. Kava products may offer an alternative to benzodiazepines in the reduction of daily stress and anxiety states in adults. Given that the pharmacological activity of kava is comparable to the benzodiazepines—but without their untoward effects (ie, it is not addictive and does not lead to dose tolerance)—Kavatrol may produce an alternative treatment for daily stress and anxiety.

Shown in Product Identification Guide, page 513

Niche Pharmaceuticals, Inc.

200 N. OAK
P.O. BOX 449
ROANOKE, TX 76262

Direct inquiries to:
Stephen Brandon
(817) 491-2770
Fax (817) 491-3533

MAG-TAB® SR
[măg-tăb]
(Magnesium L-lactate dihydrate)
Sustained release Magnesium
Supplement

Description: Mag-Tab SR is a sustained release oral magnesium supplement. Each pale yellow caplets contain 7mEq (84 Mg) magnesium as magnesium L-lactate dihydrate (835 Mg in a patented, sustained release wax matrix formulation).

Indications/Uses: As a dietary supplement, Mag-Tab SR, is indicated for patients with, or at risk for, magnesium deficiency. Hypomagnesemia and/or magnesium deficiency can result from inadequate nutritional intake or absorption, magnesium depleting drugs such as diuretics, or alcoholism.

Warnings: Patients with renal disease should not take magnesium supplements without the advice and direct supervision of a physician. Excessive dosage of magnesium can cause loose stools or diarrhea.

Dosage: As a dietary supplement, take 1 or 2 caplets b.i.d. or as directed by a physician.

How Supplied: Mag-Tab SR is available for oral administration as uncoated yellow caplets, in bottles of 60 and 100.

UniFiber®
[uni fi 'ber]
(Powdered Cellulose)
3 grams Fiber per tablespoon

Description: UniFiber is an all natural insoluble bulk fiber supplement that promotes normal bowel function by adding needed bulk to the diet. UniFiber contains powdered cellulose 75%, water 5%, corn syrup 19%, and xanthan gum 1%. UniFiber mixes easily with liquids or soft foods, and is tasteless, non-gelling, and pleasant to take. One tablespoon of UniFiber provides 3 grams of concentrated dietary fiber.

Nutrition Information: Each 4 gram (1T) serving of UniFiber contains 3 grams of fiber equivalent to the amount of fiber in one large bran muffin, 4 calories, 0% fat, 0% cholesterol, 0% protein, and is free of all electrolytes.

Indication/Uses: As a dietary supplement, UniFiber is indicated for patients needing a concentrated source of fiber to help maintain and promote normal bowel function. Because UniFiber is electrolyte free and contains no excitoxins, it is an ideal fiber supplement for patients on a restricted diet, such as the OB patient, kidney patients on dialysis, diabetic patients, and the elderly.

Contraindications: Intestinal obstruction or fecal impaction.

Dosage:
Adults: Stir one tablespoon into a glass with 3 or 4 ounces of fruit juice, milk, or water; or mix with soft foods such as applesauce, mashed potatoes, or pudding. Can be taken up to 3 times daily if needed, or as recommended by a doctor. Generally produces effect in 12 – 72 hours.
Tube Feedings: Mix one tablespoon in 30 – 60 cc of water.
Children (6 to 12 years): ½ dose 2 or 3 times daily.

How Supplied: UniFiber is available over the counter in powder containers of 5 oz (36 servings), 9 oz (64 servings), or 16 oz (114 servings).

Novartis Consumer Health, Inc.

560 MORRIS AVE.
SUMMIT, NJ 07901-1312

Direct Product Inquiries to:
Consumer & Professional Affairs
(800) 452-0051
Fax: (800) 635-2801
Or write to above address.

SLOW FE®
Slow Release Iron Tablets

Description: SLOW FE supplies ferrous sulfate for the treatment of iron deficiency and iron deficiency anemia with a significant reduction in the incidence of the common side effects of oral iron preparations. The wax matrix delivery system of SLOW FE is designed to maximize the release of ferrous sulfate in the duodenum and the jejunum where it is best tolerated and absorbed. SLOW FE has been clinically shown to be associated with a lower incidence of constipation, diarrhea and abdominal discomfort when compared to an immediate release iron tablet[1] and a leading sustained release iron capsule.[2]

Formula: Each tablet contains 160 mg. dried ferrous sulfate USP, equivalent to 50 mg. elemental iron. Also contains cetostearyl alcohol, FD&C Blue No. 2 aluminum lake, hydroxypropyl methylcellulose, lactose, magnesium stearate, polysorbate 80, talc, titanium dioxide, yellow iron oxide.

Dosage: ADULTS—one or two tablets daily or as recommended by a physician. A maximum of four tablets daily may be taken. CHILDREN—one tablet daily. Tablets must be swallowed whole.

Warning: Accidental overdose of iron-containing products is a leading cause of fatal poisoning in children under 6. Keep this product out of reach of children. In case of accidental overdose, call a doctor or poison control center immediately.

Warning: The treatment of any anemic condition should be under the advice and supervision of a physician. As oral iron products interfere with absorption of oral tetracycline antibiotics, these products should not be taken within two hours of each other. As with any drug, if you are pregnant or nursing a baby, seek the advice of a health professional before using this product.
Blister packaged for your protection. Do not use if individual seals are broken.

How Supplied: Child-resistant blister packages of 30, 60, and 90.
Do Not Store Above 30°C (86°F). Protect From Moisture.
Tablets made in Great Britain
Novartis Consumer Health, Inc.
Summit, NJ 07901–1312

References
1. Brock C et al. Adverse effects of iron supplementation: A comparative trial of a wax-matrix iron preparation and conventional ferrous sulfate tablets. *Clin Ther.* 1985; 7:568-573.
2. Brock C, Curry H. Comparative incidence of side effects of a wax-matrix and a sustained-release iron preparation. *Clin Ther.* 1985; 7:492-496.
Shown in Product Identification Guide, page 514

SLOW FE® WITH FOLIC ACID
(Slow Release Iron, Folic Acid)

Description: Slow Fe + Folic Acid delivers 50 mg. elemental iron (160 mg. dried ferrous sulfate) plus 400 mcg. folic acid using the unique wax matrix delivery system described above (for SLOW FE® Slow Release Iron Tablets).
Provides women of childbearing potential with the daily target level of folic acid to reduce the risk of neural tube birth defects. These birth defects are rare, but serious, and occur within 28 days of conception, often before a woman knows she's pregnant.

Formula: Each tablet contains: Active Ingredients: 160 mg. dried ferrous sulfate, USP (equivalent to 50 mg. elemental iron) and 400 mcg. folic acid. Inactive Ingredients: cetostearyl alcohol, hydroxypropyl methylcellulose, lactose, magnesium stearate, polysorbate 80, talc, titanium dioxide, yellow iron oxide.

Dosage: ADULTS—One or two tablets once a day or as recommended by a physician. A maximum of two tablets daily may be taken. CHILDREN UNDER 12—Consult a physician. Tablets must be swallowed whole.

Warning: The treatment of any anemic condition should be under the advice and supervision of a physician. As oral iron products interfere with absorption of oral tetracycline antibiotics, these products should not be taken within two hours of each other. Intake of folic acid from all sources should be limited to 1000 mcg. per day to prevent the masking of Vitamin B_{12} deficiencies. Should you become pregnant while using this product, consult a physician as soon as possible about good prenatal care and the continued use of this product. If you are already pregnant or nursing a baby, seek the advice of a health care professional before using this product.

> **Warning:** Accidental overdose of iron-containing products is a leading cause of fatal poisoning in children under 6. Keep this product out of reach of children. In case of accidental overdose, call a doctor or poison control center immediately.

How Supplied: Blister packages of 20 supplied in Child-Resistant packaging. Do not store above 30°C (86°F). Protect from moisture.
Tablets made in Great Britain
Novartis Consumer Health, Inc.
Shown in Product Identification Guide, page 514

CHILDREN'S CHEWABLE SUNKIST® VITAMINS + EXTRA C 60 TABLETS

Nutrition Facts
Serving Size 1 Tablet

Amount Per Tablet
Calories 5
Total Carbohydrate 1 g

Amount Per Tablet	% Daily Value for Children 2–4 Years of Age	% Daily Value for Adults and Children 4 or more Years of Age
Vitamin A 2500 I.U.	100%	50%
Vitamin C 250 mg	630%	420%
Vitamin D 400 I.U.	100%	100%
Vitamin E 15 I.U.	150%	50%
Vitamin K 5 mcg	*	*
Thiamin 1.1 mg	160%	70%
Riboflavin 1.2 mg	150%	70%
Niacin 15 mg	160%	70%
Vitamin B_6 1 mg	140%	50%
Folate 0.3 mg	150%	80%
Vitamin B_{12} 5 mcg	170%	80%

*Daily Value not established.

Amount Per Tablet	% Daily Value for Children 2–4 Years of Age	% Daily Value for Adults and Children 4 or More Years of Age
Vitamin A 5000 I.U.	100%	100%
Vitamin C 60 mg	80%	100%
Vitamin D 400 I.U.	50%	100%
Vitamin E 30 I.U.	150%	100%
Vitamin K 10 mcg	*	*
Thiamin 1.5 mg	110%	100%
Riboflavin 1.7 mg	110%	100%
Niacin 20 mg	110%	100%
Vitamin B_6 2 mg	140%	100%
Folate 0.4 mg	100%	100%
Vitamin B_{12} 6 mcg	100%	100%
Biotin 40 mcg	15%	15%
Pantothenic Acid 10 mg	100%	100%
Calcium 100 mg	6%	10%
Iron 18 mg	90%	100%
Phosphorus 78 mg	4%	8%
Iodine 150 mcg	110%	100%
Magnesium 20 mg	5%	6%
Zinc 10 mg	60%	60%
Copper 2.0 mg	100%	100%
Manganese 1 mg	*	*

* Daily Value not established.

Ingredients: Sorbitol, Sodium Ascorbate, Ascorbic Acid, Natural Flavors, Mono & Diglycerides, Starch, Stearic Acid, Hydrolyzed Protein, Vitamin E Acetate, Niacinamide, Aspartame Hydrogenated Vegetable Oils, Magnesium Stearate, FD&C Yellow #6, Calcium Silicate, Silica, FD&C Red #40, Vitamin A Palmitate, Cellulose, FD&C Yellow #5, Gelatin, Riboflavin, Thiamin, Vitamin B_6, Sucrose, Ascorbyl Palmitate, Folic Acid, Beta Carotene, Vitamin D, Vitamin K, Vitamin B_{12}.

Directions: Adults and children 2 years and older—Chew one tablet daily. PHENYLKETONURICS: CONTAINS PHENYLALANINE

How Supplied: Bottles of 60 tablets. Store at controlled room temperature, 15°–30°C (59°–86°F). Protect from moisture.
Manufactured for and distributed by Novartis Consumer Health, Inc., Summit, NJ 07901-1312 under a trademark license from Sunkist Growers, Inc.
Sunkist® is a registered trademark of Sunkist Growers, Inc., Sherman Oaks, CA 91423©
Shown in Product Identification Guide, page 514

SUNKIST® CHILDREN'S CHEWABLE MULTIVITAMINS— COMPLETE WITH CALCIUM, IRON & MINERALS

Nutrition Facts
Serving Size $1/2$ Tablet or 1 Tablet, depending on age (see Directions)
Servings Per Container 120 $1/2$-tablet servings or 60 single-tablets servings
Amount Per Tablet
Sodium 8 mg
Total Carbohydrate less than 1g
[See table above]

Ingredients: Sorbitol, Dicalcium Phosphate, Mono & Diglycerides, Ferrous Fumarate, Natural Flavors, Stearic Acid, Carrageenan, Starch, Sodium Ascorbate, Vitamin E, Magnesium Oxide, Hydrolyzed Protein, Ascorbic Acid, Niacinamide, Citric Acid, FD&C Yellow #6, Zinc Oxide, Gelatin, Magnesium Stearate, FD&C Red #40, Calcium Pantothenate, FD&C Yellow #5, Aspartame, Silica, Calcium Silicate, Vitamin A Palmitate, Cellulose, Manganese Sulfate, Vitamin B_6, Cupric Oxide, Riboflavin, Hydrogenated Vegetable Oils, Thiamin, Sucrose, Ascorbyl Palmitate, Folic Acid, Beta Carotene, Potassium Iodide, Biotin, Calcium Stearate, Vitamin K, Vitamin D, Vitamin B_{12}.
PHENYLKETONURICS: CONTAINS PHENYLALANINE

Directions: Ages 2 to 4 years—Chew one-half tablet daily. Ages 4 years and older—Chew one tablet daily.

Warning: Close tightly and keep out of reach of children. Contains iron, which can be harmful or fatal to children in large doses. In case of accidental overdose, seek professional assistance or contact a poison control center immediately.

How Supplied: Bottles of 60 tablets. Store at controlled room temperature, 15°–30°C (59°–86°F). Protect from moisture.
Manufactured for and distributed by Novartis Consumer Health, Inc., Summit, NJ 07901-1312 under a trademark license from Sunkist Growers, Inc.

Continued on next page

Information on Novartis Consumer Health, Inc., products appearing on these pages is effective as of November 1998.

Sunkist Children's—Cont.

Sunkist® is a registered trademark of Sunkist Growers, Inc. Sherman Oaks, CA 91423.©

Shown in Product Identification Guide, page 514

SUNKIST® VITAMIN C
Citrus Complex
Chewable Tablets

Description: All Sunkist Vitamin C chewable tablets have a delicious orange flavor unlike any other Vitamin C tablet. Each 60 mg chewable tablet contains 100% of the U.S. RDA* of Vitamin C. Each 250 mg chewable tablet contains 417% of the U.S. RDA* of Vitamin C. Each 500 mg chewable tablet contains 833% of the U.S. RDA* of Vitamin C.

Sunkist Vitamin C chewable tablets do not contain artificial flavors or colors.

*U.S. Recommended Daily Allowance for adults and children over 4 years of age.

Indication: Dietary supplementation.

How Supplied: 60 mg Chewable Tablets—Rolls of 11.
250 mg and 500 mg Chewable Tablets—Bottles of 60.
Store at controlled room temperature 15°–30°C (59°–86°F).
Manufactured for and distributed by Novartis Consumer Health, Inc., Summit, NJ 07901-1312 under a trademark license from Sunkist Growers, Inc.
Sunkist® is a registered trademark of Sunkist Growers, Inc., Sherman Oaks, CA 91423.©

Shown in Product Identification Guide, page 514

Novogen, Inc
1 LANDMARK SQUARE
STAMFORD, CONNECTICUT
06901

Direct Inquiries to:
Tollfree (877)-TRINOVIN
        (874-6684)
Fax: (203) 327-0011
website: www.novogen.com.
promensil@novogen.com

PROMENSIL
A dietary supplement of isoflavone plant estrogens.

Description: Dry concentrated extract of *Trifolium pratense* (Red clover). Standardized to 40mg of bioavailable isoflavone plant estrogens. Contains the four main dietary estrogenic isoflavones at a standardized ratio.
biochanin A *(4',methoxy-5,7-dihydroxy-isoflavone)*
formononetin *(4'-methoxy-7-hydroxy-isoflavone)*
genistein *(4',5,7-trihydroxyisoflavone)*
daidzein *(4',7-dihydroxyisoflavone)*

Composition:
Dietary Ingredients: Isoflavone plant estrogens are hetrocyclic plant diphenols with similar chemical structure to the body's own steroidal estrogens.
Other Ingredients: Dicalcium hydrogen phosphate, Microcrystalline, Hydroxpropyll methyl cellulose, Magnesium stearate, Mixed tocopherols, Silica, Soy polysaccharide, Natural Colors.
FREE OF sugar, yeast, milk derivatives, wheat and cornstarch, gluten, preservatives, artificial colors and flavors.

Key Facts: Promensil is made from red clover, the richest natural source of isoflavones. Isoflavones, natural plant estrogens are abundant in legumes such as clover, beans and soy. They provide a supplement to the body's own decreasing supply of estrogens before during and after menopause. One Promensil tablet per day provides 40mg of natural plant estrogens- eight times more than an American woman typically consumes during a day.

Major Uses: Promensil is recommended as a dietary supplement for women concerned about maintaining healthy estrogen levels to preserve physical and emotional well-being as the body's own estrogen levels decline in midlife.*

Precautions: Not recommended for pregnant or lactating women or children under the age of 15 years. Contact your doctor before taking this or any supplement if you are already taking a prescription medicine.
In clinical trials no adverse reactions were found at the recommended intake. No weight change was seen in a double blind placebo controlled 12 week study. Promensil did not induce changes in uterine wall thickness in menopausal trial subjects.

Pharmacokinetics: Following oral administration, peak plasma levels are achieved in 5 hours. All four isoflavones are present in plasma post-challenge. After oral administration, the terminal half-life is between 9 and 12 hours. The kinetics of plasma levels for all 4 isoflavones are similar. Isoflavones are conjugated by the liver and excreted as glucuronides and sulphonates largely in the urine with lesser amounts in the bile.

Absorption, bioavailability: The isoflavone plant estrogens are either absorbed intact or undergo fermentation by gut flora. Lative importance of these two processes varies between individuals. Biochanin A is converted partially to genistein and formononetin to daidzein; the genistein and daidzein then either are absorbed intact or undergo further degradation to various metabolites. The metabolic conversion of biochanin to genistein and formononetin to daidzein is 45 to 50%. The principal further metabolic products the isoflavan, equol (7-hydroxy-3-(4'-hydroxyphenol)chroman), O-desmethylangolensin and 6-hydroxy-O-desmethylangolensin which then are absorbed.

Safety Data: *Human studies: Safety* data has been gathered from placebo-controlled trials involving peri-menopausal women. Four tablets per day (160mg of isoflavones) have shown no adverse or intolerance reactions. There were no significant changes in serum biochemical (total protein, albumin, ALP, AST, GGT, bilirubin) parameters and haematological (haemoglobin, WBC, platelet levels) parameters over a 12 week period. Vaginal ultrasound was performed on women (treated with one Promensil tablet daily) both before and after to determine endometrial thickness; no evidence of endometrial thickening was detected.

Directions for Use: Adults one tablet daily with food.
Presentation: Coated 500mg tablets. Each tablet contains 40mg of standardised isoflavones plant estrogens.
Storage: Store in a cool dry place below 85° F. Shelf life is greater than 2 years.
Poisons Schedule: None. *Trifolium pratense* is an approved human foodstuff (GRAS 21 CFR 182.10) and is a traditional herb for human use.

Supplements Facts
Serving Size 1 Tablet
Servings Per Container 30
Each tablet Contains
Isoflavone Phytoestrogens 40mg*
(as red clover leaf extract)

*Daily Value not Established.
These statements have not been evaluated by the food and Drug Administration. This product is not intended to treat, cure, or prevent any disease
Distributed in North America by:
Novogen Inc., 1 Landmark Square, Stamford, CT 06901 USA
www.novogen.com
Email: promensil@novogen.com
Shown in Product Identification Guide, page 516

Numark Laboratories, Inc.
164 NORTHFIELD AVENUE
EDISON, NJ 08837

Direct Inquiries to:
Consumer Services
Phone (800) 331-0221
Fax (732) 225-0066

LIPOFLAVONOID® Nutritional Supplement
with Eriodictyol Glycoside, Vitamin B Complex, and Lemon Bioflavonoids

Suggested Use: Nutritional Supplement for improved circulation in the inner ear.

Three Caplets daily provide:		% U.S RDA*
Vitamin C	300 mg	500%
Thiamine (B1)	1 mg	67%
Riboflavin (B2)	1 mg	59%
Niacin (Niacinamide)	10 mg	50%
Vitamin B6 (Pyridoxine HCl)	1 mg	50%
Vitamin B12 (Cyanocobalamin)	5 mcg	83%
Panthothenic Acid	5 mg	50%
Choline	334 mg	**
Bioflavonoids***	300 mg	**
Inositol	334 mg	**

* Percentage of U.S. Recommended Daily Allowance for Adults.
** U.S. RDA has not been established.
***Contains the flavor Eridictyol Glycoside.

Ingredients: Choline Bitartrate, Dibasic Calcium Phosphate, Microcrystalline Cellulose, Inositol, Ascorbic Acid, Lemon Bioflavonoids complex, Croscarmellose Sodium, Stearic Acid, Niacinamide, Calcium Pantothenate, Silica, Ethyl Vanillin, Pyridoxine HCl, Thiamine Mononitrate, Riboflavin, Cyanocobalamin, Pharmaceutical Glaze, Hydroxypropyl Methylcellulose, Methylcellulose, FD&C Red #40 Lake, FD&C Blue #1 Lake, FD&C Yellow #6 Lake (Sunset Yellow), and Titanium Dioxide.

Recommended Intake: Three caplets daily. For best results use for at least six (6) months.

Caution: If you are pregnant or nursing a baby, seek the advice of a health professional before using this product. **Keep out of reach of children.**

Pharmanex, Inc.

a wholly owned subsidiary of Nu Skin Enterprises, Inc., PROVO, UT 84601

Direct Inquiries to:
Michael Chang, Ph.D. or
Joseph Chang, Ph.D.
1-800-800-0260 or 1-801-345-1000
FAX: 801-345-1999

Medical Emergency Contact:
Michael Chang, Ph.D. or Joseph Chang, Ph.D.
1-800-800-0260 or 1-801-345-1000

Pharmanex is a science-based, natural healthcare company that develops and markets a line of clinically-supported and standardized proprietary natural healthcare products (listed below) as well as a line of Premium Quality Selfcare Botanical Extracts—ranging from Cranberry, Echinacea and Garlic to Kava, Saw Palmetto, Valerian, etc. Each highly concentrated, scientifically standardized extract is formulated to provide clinically supported dosages that guarantee optimal levels of the key health promoting compounds in their proper ratios. For a full list of dietary supplement products and scientific support documents call toll free: **1-800-800-0260**.

BIO GINKGO 27/7® Extra Strength
[bī 'ō-gǐng 'ko]
Ginkgo biloba leaf Extract
Dietary Supplement

Description: BioGinkgo 27/7 Extra Strength is an all-natural, standardized extract of the leaves of *Ginkgo biloba* trees for use as a dietary supplement to improve blood circulation to the brain and extremities, improve cognitive functions and conserve mental sharpness, and protect the body from oxidative cellular damage caused by free radicals.* *Ginkgo biloba* extract (GBE) is primarily used to affect the age-related relatively slow decline in cognitive functions.* There have been several controlled clinical trials designed to test the effectiveness of GBE in mitigating symptoms such as: difficulties of concentration and memory, absent mindedness, confusion, lack of energy, tiredness and decreased physical performance.*
GBE is one of the most widely used botanicals in the world and the focus of extensive scientific research, including over 300 published studies and reports to its credit. Twenty years of research led to the development of a standardized, concentrated extract from the leaves—with a scientifically-supported composition of 22 to 27% flavonoid glycoside content and 5 to 7% terpene lactone content as specified by European health authority standards for phytomedicines.
BioGinkgo 27/7 Extra Strength (27% ginkgo flavone glycosides and 7% terpene lactones) contains significantly greater levels of the identified active constitutents than the standard 24/6 strength formulation. BioGinkgo 27/7 is specifically enriched to provide higher levels of ginkgolide B than other standardized GBE products. Ginkgolides are potent Platelet Activating Factor (PAF) antagonists, and ginkgolide B is the most potent PAF antagonist. Ginkgolide B has been demonstrated to produce beneficial effects in promoting blood circulation.* In a bioavailability study in rabbits published in *Planta Medica* (Li C.L. and Wong Y.Y., December, 1997) comparing BioGinkgo 27/7 to another commercially available GBE, BioGinkgo 27/7 reached higher levels of plasma concentration of anti-PAF components, and manifested a faster onset and longer duration of action of anti-PAF activity over a 12-hour period.

Ingredients: BioGinkgo 27/7 is a standardized 50:1 extract of *Ginkgo biloba* leaf supplied in 60 mg green-colored coated tablets. Other ingredients include: lactose anhydrous, microcrystalline cellulose, corn starch, sodium starch glycolate, Opadry® colors (which contain added colors, including the Lakes of Yellow 5 and Blue 1), colloidal silicon dioxide, and magnesium stearate.

Benefits of *Ginkgo biloba* extract (GBE)
GBE promotes healthy blood flow: A meta-analysis of several controlled clinical studies shows that GBE helps to maintain normal blood circulation in the body, including the brain and the extremities (arms, legs, eyes, inner ear, etc.) without a "borrowing" effect on adjacent areas of normal flow.* GBE promotes efficient circulation by helping to maintain the elasticity of arteries and capillaries.* Terpene lactones specific to GBE inhibit PAF, which may contribute to circulation blockage.* Ginkgolide B binds to PAF receptors.*
GBE improves memory and enhances cognitive function: GBE increases the rate at which information is transmitted between nerve cells by increasing blood flow to the brain and the Central Nervous System (CNS).* Also, by inhibiting PAF-induced platelet aggregation and reducing the resulting viscosity or "stickiness" of the blood, the ginkgolides increase cerebral blood flow and contribute to the improvement in cognitive function seen after GBE treatment.*
GBE promotes eye health: The macular area of the retina is responsible for fine reading, and is particularly sensitive to damage by lipid free radicals.* GBE may promote eye health in the elderly through its protective antioxidant properties.*

Recommended Use: As a dietary supplement, take one 60 mg tablet bid. Allow from 2 weeks up to 12 weeks for optimum benefits to manifest.

Safety: GBE appears to be well tolerated at prescribed doses. Adverse reactions include mild gastrointestinal discomfort, and rare reports of allergic skin reactions. Some people may experience a mild, transient headache for the first two or three days of use.

Warnings: BioGinkgo 27/7 has not been evaluated in children and should only be used by adults. Pregnant or breast feeding mothers should consult a physician prior to use. Consult a physician if using concurrently with anticoagulant or NSAID medications.

How Supplied: BioGinkgo 27/7 tablets of 60 mg each are supplied in 60 count boxes or bottles (30 day supply). For order information, call toll free 1-800-800-0260.
Shown in Product Identification Guide, page 518

BIO ST. JOHN'S™
[bī'ō-sānt jŏnz]
Enhanced St. John's wort (Hypericum) Extract
Dietary Supplement

Description: Bio St. John's [Patent Pending] combines two of nature's most

Continued on next page

Bio St. John's—Cont.

effective botanicals in a unique formulation that helps promote vitality, stamina and a healthy emotional balance.* It consists of a complementary combination of a standardized extract of the herb St. John's wort (Hypericum perforatum), together with a proprietary strain of the Cordyceps sinensis mushroom (CordyMax Cs-4®). St. John's wort is highly regarded and widely used in Europe as a safe, effective mood-promoting supplement.* Numerous clinical studies suggest that St. John's wort influences mood and helps people to maintain a positive mental outlook.* CordyMax Cs-4 helps to reduce fatigue and increase stamina and resistance to stress while providing important protective and stabilizing benefits for numerous bodily systems, including the cardiovascular, respiratory, hepatic and nervous systems.*

Ingredients: Bio St. John's [Patent Pending], at the recommended 4 capsules/day, contains clinically supported dosages of CordyMax Cs-4 mycelium (1500 mg/day) standardized to adenosine and mannitol content, and St. John's wort extract (900 mg/day) standardized to 0.3% hypericin within a complex or other natural compounds.

Scientific Support: Animal and in vitro studies with St. John's wort extract have shown that it positively effects modulation of the functions and availability of serotonin and other neurotransmitters at nerve synapses and regulation of the expression of neurotransmitter receptors.* Its mechanism of action is incompletely understood—it is a weak MAOI and has not been demonstrated to act as an MAOI in vivo. In clinical studies, St. John's wort extract:
• Stabilizes mood and promotes a positive mental outlook*
• Improves sleep patterns in older individuals*
• Moderates seasonal mood changes*
A systematic meta-analysis of 23 randomized clinical trials (including a total of 1757 outpatients) concluded that St. John's wort extract preparations were 2.67 times more effective in the placebo controlled trials. Dropouts due to side effects were rare in the Hypericum treated group (0.8%). (Linde K. et al., 1996, British Medical Journal, 313:253–8)

The other ingredient in Bio St. John's is CordyMax Cs-4® (Patent Pending). CordyMax Cs-4 is an exclusive mycelial strain of Cordyceps sinensis (Berk.) Sacc., a traditional Chinese mushroom that has been demonstrated in pre-clinical and clinical studies to act as a general tonic to:
• Improve energy, vitality and endurance*
• Elevate energy states (ATP) in organs*
• Have calming and stress-relieving effects*
• Optimize cardiac, respiratory, immune, liver and kidney functions*
• Optimize blood lipid metabolism and promote healthy blood lipid profiles*
• Provide a positive benefit for sexuality*

(See CordyMax Cs-4 section for additional information)

Recommended Use: As a dietary supplement, the recommended clinically supported dosage is 2 capsules bid with food and drink. It typically takes 4 to 6 weeks to achieve optimal results.

Safety: Toxicological studies in animals indicate that the toxicity of St. John's wort extracts is quite low. No mutagenic activity has been found. A potential for erythema exists for fair-skinned patients taking doses greater than 1800 mg/day who are exposed to UV-A or UV-B. The most common side effects reported in one study of 3250 patients were gastrointestinal symptoms (0.6%), allergic reactions (0.5%) and fatigue (0.4%). (Woelk, H et al., 1994, Journal of Geriatric Psychiatry Neurology, 7:S34–38) No negative influences on performance or ability to drive have been reported. (See CordyMax Cs-4 section for safety information regarding this ingredient.)

Warnings: Keep out of reach of children. Pregnant and breast-feeding mothers should consult a physician prior to use. Patients on prescription medications for clinical depression should consult a physician before using St. John's wort extract as a dietary supplement. St. John's wort extract has been reported to significantly prolong narcotic-induced sleeping times and to antagonize the effects of reserpine. Hypericin causes a reduction in barbiturate-induced sleeping times. (See CordyMax Cs-4 section for warnings regarding this ingredient.)

How Supplied: Bio St. John's capsules (600 mg each) are supplied in 120 count (30 day supply) boxes or bottles. For order information, call toll free 1-800-800-0260. Clear gelatin capsules are USP quality and are designed to disintegrate within 30 minutes after ingestion.

CHOLESTIN™
[kō lĕs 'tĭn]
Monascus purpureus Went
(Red Yeast Rice)
Dietary Supplement

Description: Dietary supplementation with Cholestin (Patent Pending) is recommended for healthy adult males and postmenopausal women concerned about maintaining healthy blood cholesterol levels, and who—in consultation with their physicians—have determined that dietary supplementation rather than medical treatment is appropriate to achieve desirable cholesterol levels.* Cholestin is intended for use as part of a cholesterol maintenance program that includes a healthy diet restricted in saturated fat and cholesterol, and other appropriate measures including regular exercise. **Cholestin is not recommended for treating a disease, and this product should not be substituted for prescribed medications.**

Cholestin has been rigorously evaluated in terms of its pharmacology and toxicity, and in clinical studies to confirm its safety and beneficial effects. It naturally contains HMG-CoA reductase inhibitors, including mevinolin, and unsaturated fatty acids. Thirty-three clinical trials in China and two in the U.S., including one at UCLA School of Medicine confirm its efficacy and safety; 17 were controlled, 18 were open label. In one major randomized multicenter clinical trial involving 446 hyperlipidemic patients with baseline total serum cholesterol levels >230 mg/dL, after 8 weeks of treatment, Monascus was found to promote the health of all lipid levels.* In total, more than 1,000 men and women with elevated lipid levels were given the proprietary ingredient in Cholestin at daily doses of 0.6 to 2.4 g/day for 8 weeks. For clinical results, refer to the references listed below or call Pharmanex at 1-800-800-0260 for reprints and product information.

• Wang J, et al., "Multicenter Clinical Trial of the Serum Lipid-lowering Effects of a Monascus purpureus (Red Yeast) rice preparation from traditional Chinese medicine," Current Therapeutic Research, 1997; 58(12):964–978.
• Heber D, et al., "Cholesterol-lowering effects of a proprietary Chinese red yeast rice dietary supplement," FASEB Journal, 1998; 12(4):A206.

Ingredients: Each capsule of Cholestin (Patent Pending) contains 600 mg of scientifically-standardized Monascus purpureus Went yeast fermented on premium rice. Among the key constituents found in Cholestin is a mixture of natural metabolites which resemble well-characterized HMG-CoA reductase inhibitors, including mevinolin, as well as significant levels of unsaturated fatty acids. Yeast in final product is inactive.

Recommended Use: As a dietary supplement, take two 600 mg capsules bid, or take all 4 capsules after dinner; take with food to minimize the risk of digestive tract discomfort. **Do not take more than four capsules in any 24-hour period, unless recommended by a physician. Immediately discontinue use if you experience any unexplained muscle pain, tenderness, or weakness, especially if accompanied by flu symptoms.**

Safety: Based on foreign and U.S. clinical studies involving thousands of subjects, only a small number of individuals reported slight discomfort in the digestive tract; otherwise, no adverse effects were observed during eight week study periods. Additionally, there were no clinically significant changes in laboratory tests for liver and kidney functions or in routine blood tests. Cholestin was also shown to be safe in acute and long-term animal toxicity studies where there were no adverse reactions at doses up to 50 times the normal human dose over 3 to 4 months.

Warnings: Keep out of reach of children.

- **Do not use if you are pregnant, can become pregnant, or are breast feeding.** Not to be used by anyone under 20 years of age. Consult with a physician if you are taking any medication or if you are under physician supervision for cholesterol control.
- One of the natural constituents in Cholestin (mevinolin) in much higher doses has been associated with some rare but serious side effects. Do not take Cholestin if: you are at risk for liver disease, have active liver disease or any history of liver disease; you consume more than 2 drinks of alcohol per day; you have a serious infection; you have undergone an organ transplantation; you have a serious disease or physical disorder or have recently undergone major surgery.

How Supplied: Cholestin capsules of 600 mg each are supplied in 120 count (30 day supply) boxes or bottles. For order information, call toll free 1-800-800-0260.

Shown in Product Identification Guide, page 518

CORDYMAX Cs-4®
Cordyceps sinensis mushroom mycelia
[kord 'ə-măk sē ěs fōr, kord' ə-seps sĭ-něn-sĭs]
Dietary Supplement

Description: CordyMax Cs-4 (Patent Pending) is a dietary supplement used to reduce fatigue, and to promote vitality and healthy lung function.* It is an exclusive fermentation product derived from the mycelia of the principal fungal strain (*Paecilomyces hepiali* Chen Cs-4) isolated from the *Cordyceps sinensis* mushroom. CordyMax has been profiled extensively by chemical and pharmacological methods, and is recognized as having activity most similar to wild *Cordyceps sinensis*. In humans and animals, CordyMax substantially increases the serum levels of the enzyme superoxide dismutase (SOD). This enhancement of the enzyme's proven ability to scavenge the free radicals associated with age-related oxidative cellular damage may explain the traditional use of the mushroom as a dietary supplement to improve vitality, energy, and quality of life.* Scientific studies also indicate that supplementation with CordyMax CS-4 may:
(1) Reduce oxidative stress by scavenging oxygen-free radicals in mitochondria;* (2) Promote efficient utilization of oxygen and promote healthy lung function;* (3) Elevate energy states (ATP) in organs;* (4) Redistribute blood flow to essential organs;* (5) Improve liver and kidney functions through metabolizing and excreting toxic substances;* (6) Provide a positive benefit for sexuality.*

Ingredients: Each capsule of CordyMax Cs-4 contains 525 mg of the fermentation product of mycelia (*Paecilomyces hepiali* Chen, Cs-4) isolated from the mushroom *Cordyceps sinensis* (Berk.) Sacc., and is scientifically standardized by HPLC method to contain a minimum of 0.14% adenosine and no less than 5% mannitol (an indicator of polysaccharide content).

Recommended Use: As a dietary supplement, take two 525 mg capsules bid or tid with water or food. Optimal results typically take 3 to 6 weeks.

Safety: With the exception of one case of allergic skin reaction, no other adverse reactions have been reported. During clinical trials in China, some subjects noted a mild sensation of thirst, and one subject noted slight nausea. All subjects considered these effects quite tolerable. No CNS effects have been reported. No contraindications were identified based on Chinese human studies. CordyMax is non-mutagenic and non-teratogenic.

Warnings: CordyMax has not been evaluated in children and should only be used by adults. Pregnant and breast feeding mothers should consult a physician prior to use. Consult a physician prior to use if taking a prescription medication.

How Supplied: CordyMax CS-4 capsules of 525 mg each are supplied in 120 count (30 day supply) boxes or bottles. For order infomation, call toll free 1-800-800-0260.

TĒGREEN 97®
[tē 'grēn 97]
Green tea polyphenol extract
Dietary Supplement

Description: Tēgreen 97 is a standardized, caffeine-free polyphenol extract of the fresh leaves of the tea plant *Camellia sinensis*. The major components of Tēgreen are polyphenols, which have proven free radical scavenging and antioxidant properties.* The polyphenols with the most active antioxidant activity are the catechins, specifically epigallocatechin gallate (EGCg) and epigallocatechin (EGC).* Using the Ames test, researchers at Kansas University found the EGCg component of Tēgreen to be approximately 80 times more effective than Vitamin C, 10 times more effective than Vitamin E and twice as effective as the antioxidant compound in red wine at protecting cells from DNA degradation. The dietary supplement use of green tea polyphenols (especially the catechin EGCg) may help: (1) block the formation of toxic compounds, including nitrosamines* (2) suppress the activation of free radicals* (3) detoxify or trap free radicals* (4) inhibit spontaneous and photo-enhanced lipid peroxidation* (5) inhibit the enzyme urokinase.*

Ingredients:
Tēgreen Polyphenolic Profile
Total polyphenols ≥97%
Catechins fraction ≥65%
EGCg ≥38% Epigallocatechin gallate
ECG ≥15% Epicatechin gallate
EGC ≥6% Epigallocatechin

Caffeine-free formula, containing less than <0.5% (1.25 mg) caffeine per capsule.

Scientific Support: The ingestion of green tea polyphenols promotes general well-being by affecting a very broad spectrum of functions. In large-scale epidemiological studies in Asia (totaling more than 100,000 people for study periods up to 10 years), daily consumption of 4 or more cups of a green tea beverage was associated with significant overall health benefits, even after adjustments were made for potential confounding factors including age, tobacco and alcohol use, and body weight.

In addition to providing direct protection from the oxidative effects of toxic free radicals, green tea polyphenols may also enhance the body's natural resistance to environmental toxins and stresses by increasing the activity of certain antioxidant and detoxifying enzymes, including glutathione peroxidase, glutathione reductase, glutathione S-transferase, catalase, and quinone reductase in some cells and tissues.*

Recommended Use: As a dietary supplement, take one 250 mg capsule qd with food. Each capsule provides the green tea polyphenols typically found in about 4 cups of high-quality brewed green tea.

Safety: Not known to be associated with any significant side effects or toxicity. Since Tēgreen contains only minimal amounts of caffeine (approximately 3 mg), it should not produce the stimulant effect in some people caused by the consumption of caffeine-containing beverages.

Warnings: Tēgreen has not been evaluated in children and should only be used by adults. Pregnant or breast feeding mothers should consult a physician prior to use.

How Supplied: Tēgreen capsules are supplied in 30 count (30 day supply) boxes or bottles. For order information, call toll free 1-800-800-0260.

Standardized Botanical Extracts
For a full list of dietary supplements, and product information, call toll free 1-800-800-0260.

1. **Coenzyme Q10 with Vitamin E,** 30 softgels. Promotes healthy heart function.*
2. **Cranberry fruit extract,** 30 capsules. Promotes healthy urinary tract and kidney health and pH (acidic) level.*
3. **Echinacea purpurea root extract,** 60 capsules. Supports the body's immune system.*
4. **Feverfew leaf extract,** 30 capsules. Promotes cerebral blood vessel tone and proper balance of serotonin.*
5. **Garlic powder (odor control),** 30 caplets. Supports cardiovascular health.*
6. **Ginseng, Panax Root Extract,** 60 capsules. Enhances vitality and well-being.*

Continued on next page

Tegreen 97—Cont.

7. **Hawthorn flower and leaf extract,** 60 capsules. Helps maintain healthy heart function by stimulating cardio blood flow.*
8. **Kava Kava root extract,** 30 softgels. Promotes relaxation of mind and body (including the muscles).*
9. **Saw palmetto berry extract,** 60 softgels. Promotes prostate health and normal urinary function.*
10. **Vitex fruit extract,** 30 capsules. Nutritional support during monthly cycles.*

STORAGE/SHELF LIFE

For all Pharmanex dietary supplements:

Storage: Store in a dry, cool place. Avoid excessive heat. Protect from light.

Shelf Life: Expiration date and lot code number is imprinted on bottom of box or bottle.

---

*These statements have not been evaluated by the Food and Drug Administration. These products are not intended to diagnose, treat, cure or prevent any disease.

EDUCATIONAL MATERIALS

For more information and copies of scientific support papers for Pharmanex Natural Healthcare Products: Call toll free 800-800-0260 or FAX # 801-345-1999, M–F, 8am–5pm, Mountain Time. **Website: www.pharmanex.com**

Pharmaton Natural Health Products Division of Boehringer Ingelheim Pharmaceuticals, Inc.

900 RIDGEBURY ROAD RIDGEFIELD, CT 06877

Direct Inquiries to:
Consumer Affairs
(800) 203-2916
FAX: (203) 798-5771

For Medical Emergency Contact:
Marvin Wetter, M.D.: (203) 798-4361

GINKOBA™
Ginkgo Biloba Extract
[Gĭn-kō-bă]

GINKOBA—Standardized Ginkgo Biloba Extract (50:1).

Over 30 years of extensive research results have shown that GINKOBA is a safe and natural way to supplement your diet. No other extract of the Ginkgo Biloba tree meets the standards of the one in GINKOBA.

NUTRITION FACTS:
Serving Size: 1 tablet
Each Tablet contains:
Calories: 0   Calories from Fat 0

	% Daily Value*
Total Fat 0g	0%
Cholesterol 0mg	0%
Sodium 0mg	0%
Total Carbohydrate 0g	0%
Protein 0g	0%

* Percent Daily Values are based on a 2,000 calorie diet.

Ingredients: Each GINKOBA tablet contains 40 mg of concentrated (50:1) extract from the leaves of the *Ginkgo Biloba* tree. The extract in GINKOBA is precisely standardized to 24% Ginkgo flavonoid glycosides along with other key constituents (Ginkgolides and Bilobalides) in their proven ratios.

Also Contains: Hydroxypropyl methyl cellulose, lactose, talc, polyethylene glycol, magnesium stearate, titanium dioxide, synthetic iron oxides.

Suggested Use: When taken as directed, GINKOBA is a natural way to enhance your mental focus. GINKOBA will help you maintain an overall feeling of healthy well-being, reducing normal forgetfulness and improving concentration.

Recommended Adult Intake: Adults over 12 years old should take one tablet, swallowed whole, with water three times daily at mealtimes.

Cautions: As with other supplements, please keep this product out of the reach of children. In case of accidental overdose, seek the advice of a professional immediately. If you are taking a prescription medicine, are pregnant or lactating, please contact your doctor before taking GINKOBA. No information is available on the use of ginkgo biloba extract in children under the age of 12 years old.
The statements presented on this package have not been evaluated by the Food and Drug Administration. This product is not intended to diagnose, treat, cure or prevent any disease. Store at room temperature and avoid excessive heat above 40°C (104°F) to maintain optimal freshness.

Shown in Product Identification Guide, page 518

GINSANA®
G115 Ginseng Extract
[Gin-sa-na]

GINSANA Capsules — Standardized G115® Ginseng Extract (4%).
GINSANA Chewy Squares—Standardized G115® Ginseng Extract.

No other ginseng extract meets the quality standards of the one in GINSANA. Over 25 years of extensive research has shown that GINSANA is a safe and beneficial way to supplement your diet.

NUTRITION FACTS:
Serving Size: 1 capsule
Each Capsule contains:
Calories: 5   Calories from Fat 0

	% Daily Value*
Total Fat 0g	0%
Cholesterol 0mg	0%
Sodium 0mg	0%
Total Carbohydrate 0g	0%
Protein 0g	0%

* Percent Daily Values are based on a 2,000 calorie diet.

Supplement Facts
Serving Size: 1 Square
Amount Per Square: Standardized G115® Ginseng Extract (Panax Ginseng, C.A. Meyer) (root) 50 mg*
* Daily Value not established

Ingredients: Each GINSANA capsule contains 100 mg of highly standardized, concentrated ginseng extract from the roots of the highest quality Korean Panax Ginseng, C.A. Meyer. This special standardization insures a consistent level of the eight most effective ginsenosides in their proven ratios.

Also contains: Sunflower oil, gelatin, glycerin, lecithin, beeswax, chlorophyll.

Ingredients: Each GINSANA Chewy Square contains 50 mg of highly standardized, concentrated ginseng extract from the roots of the highest quality Korean Panax Ginseng, C.A. Meyer.

Also contains: Sucrose, glucose, palm kernel oil, gelatin, citric acid, ascorbic acid, lecithin, natural flavoring and coloring.

Suggested Use: When taken as directed, GINSANA is a natural way to enhance your physical endurance by improving your body's ability to utilize oxygen more efficiently. GINSANA will help you maintain your natural energy and an overall feeling of healthy well-being.

Recommended Adult Intake/Capsules: Adults over 12 years old should take two soft gelatin capsules, swallowed whole, with water in the morning or one capsule in the morning and one in the afternoon. Research on doses above 200 mg per day does not substantiate any better effectiveness. Optimal effectiveness has been shown with 4 weeks of continuous use.

Recommended Adult Intake/Chewy Squares: Adults over 12 years old should take up to four GINSANA Chewy Squares daily.

Precautions: As with other vitamins and supplements, please keep

this product out of the reach of children. No serious or significant adverse reactions or drug interactions have been reported to date. However, as with any supplement, contact your doctor if you are taking a prescription medicine, are pregnant or lactating. There have been rare reports of mild allergic skin reactions with the use of the extract in this product. In case of accidental overdose, seek the advice of a professional immediately.

The statements presented on this package have not been evaluated by the Food and Drug Administration. This product is not intended to diagnose, treat, cure or prevent any disease. Store at room temperature and avoid excess heat above 40°C (104°F) to maintain optimal freshness.

Shown in Product Identification Guide, page 518

MOVANA™
[mō-vă-nă]
Advanced St. John's Wort
Hyperforin-Rich Formula
Dietary Supplement For Mood Support

St. John's Wort extract is clinically proven to enhance emotional well-being by promoting normal levels of neurotransmitters responsible for maintaining positive emotions. However, all St. John's Wort products are not alike. Researchers have identified a component of St. John's Wort called hyperforin that is a key ingredient responsible for its effectiveness. Hyperforin can degrade rapidly, often compromising a product's efficacy. But in MOVANA the hyperforin is stabilized to ensure potency and effectiveness. This process is such a breakthrough that the extract in MOVANA (WS-5572) has patents pending around the world. MOVANA is safe and there are no sedative side effects.

Suggested Use: Use MOVANA™ regularly, as directed below, to maintain normal emotional balance, a healthy good mood and a sense of well-being even during times of stress, and low-light seasons. MOVANA™ helps maintain a healthy motivation and a positive outlook on life.

Recommended Adult Intake: Adults (12 years and older) should take one tablet 3 times per day. Like most herbal supplements, MOVANA™ takes time to work; optimal effectiveness has been shown in as little as 2 weeks with continued use. Doses above 900 mg per day have not shown any greater effectiveness.

Precautions: As with vitamins and other supplements, please keep this product out of the reach of children. No serious side effects have been reported to date. However, if you are taking a prescription medicine, are pregnant or lactating, consult your physician. If you have fair and sensitive skin avoid prolonged direct sunlight, as photosensitivity may occur. There have been rare re-

ports (<1%) of gastrointestinal disturbances, allergic reactions, or fatigue. In case of accidental overdose, seek the advice of a healthcare professional immediately.

These statements have not been evaluated by the Food and Drug Administration. This product is not intended to diagnose, treat, cure, or prevent any disease.

Questions about Movana?
For more information about MOVANA™, visit us at our web site http://www.Movana.com or write to:
Pharmaton Natural Health Products
900 Ridgebury Road
Ridgefield, CT 06877

How Supplied:

SUPPLEMENT FACTS:	
Serving Size: 1 Tablet	
Amount Per Tablet	
Standardized WS-5572 St. John's Wort Extract (flower & leaves) Stabilized Hyperforin content, minimum 3%	300mg*
*Daily value not established	

Other Ingredients: Microcrystalline Cellulose, Corn Starch, Croscarmellose Sodium, Hydroxypropyl Methylcellulose, PEG-4000, Magnesium Stearate, Silicon Dioxide, Ascorbic Acid, Synthetic Iron Oxide, Titanium Dioxide, Talc, Vanillin. Contains no artificial stimulants, caffeine, or sugar.

Store in a cool dry place. Avoid excessive moisture and heat (above 86° F).

Shown in Product Identification Guide, page 518

VENASTAT—Backed by Decades of Clinical Research and Worldwide Experience

The all-natural horse chestnut seed extract in VENASTAT is one of the most researched natural health products in the world. The international research on horse chestnut seed extract includes over 40 clinical trials. This research, combined with years of worldwide patient experience, has demonstrated that VENASTAT is a safe way to supplement your dietary regimen.
VENASTAT—Sustained Release Standardized Horse Chestnut Seed Extract. 50mg (16%) The Horse Chestnut Seed Extract used in VENASTAT is Aesculin free and has been shown through extensive research to be a safe and beneficial way to supplement your diet for optimal leg vein health. The standardized extract in VENASTAT has been used for more than 1 million patient years around the world with no serious side effects that can be related to its use.

Suggested Use: When taken as directed, VENASTAT is a natural way to support leg vein health and protect against lower leg swelling by maintaining the circulation in the leg veins. VENASTAT will help you maintain good venous blood flow in your legs.

Recommended Adult Intake: Adults over 12 years old should take one Supro Cap every 12 hours swallowed whole with water. Research shows that effectiveness is reached after 4 to 6 weeks of use and sustained with continuous use.

Precautions: As with other vitamins and supplements, please keep this product out of the reach of children. Do not take this product if you have kidney or liver problems, or if you have had a stroke or heart disease, without advice from a physician. Also, if you are pregnant or nursing a baby consult your physician before use. Discontinue use and see a physician if gastric irritation, nausea or rapid heartbeat occurs.

SUPPLEMENT FACTS:	
Serving Size: 1 Supro Cap	
Amount per Supro Cap:	
Sustained Release Pellets of Standardized Horse Chestnut Seed Extract (seed) as Triterpene glycosides calculated as Escin (16%)	300 mg*
*Daily value not established	

Other Ingredients: Dextrin, gelatin, copolyvidone, talc, polymethacrylic acid derivitives, titanium dioxide, dibutyl phthalate, synthetic iron oxide.

The statements presented on this package have not been evaluated by the Food and Drug Administration. This product is not intended to diagnose, treat, cure or prevent any disease.

Store at room temperature and avoid excessive heat above 40°C (104°F) to maintain optimal freshness.

Shown in Product Identification Guide, page 519

VITASANA™
DAILY DIETARY SUPPLEMENT

VITASANA is the first scientifically formulated and clinically tested ginseng multivitamin combination. VITASANA is a unique formula of essential vitamins and minerals you need for good nutrition, plus GINSANA's exclusive G115 ginseng extract for the vitality that's an integral part of your total health. VITASANA is the first multivitamin/ginseng supplement in an easy to swallow Gelcap dosage form.

Continued on next page

Vitasana—Cont.

Recommended Adult Intake: Adults over 12 years old should take two Gelcaps in the morning or one gelcap in the morning and one in the afternoon. Optimal effectiveness has been clinically seen after 4 weeks of continuous use.

The statements presented on this package have not been evaluated by the Food and Drug Administration. This product is not intended to diagnose, treat, cure or prevent any disease.

Supplement Facts
Serving Size 2 Gelcaps

Each Serving Contains			% Daily Value
Vitamin A	4000	IU	
(as beta carotene)			80%
Vitamin C	120	mg	
(as ascorbic acid)			200%
Vitamin D	400	IU	
(as cholecalciferol)			100%
Vitamin E	30	IU	
(as dl-alpha tocopherol)			100%
Vitamin B1	2.4	mg	
(as thiamine mononitrate)			160%
Vitamin B2	3.4	mg	
(riboflavin)			200%
Vitamin B3	30	mg	
(niacinamide)1			50%
Vitamin B6	4	mg	
(as pyridoxine HCl)			200%
Folic Acid	400	mcg	100%
Vitamin B12	2	mcg	
(as cobalamin conc.)			33%
Calcium	200	mg	
(as calcium phosphate)			20%
Iron	18	mg	
(as ferrous sulfate)			100%
Phosphorus	160	mg	
(as calcium phosphate)			16%
Magnesium	20	mg	
(as magnesium oxide)			5%
Zinc	2	mg	
(as zinc sulfate)			13.3%
Copper	2	mg	
(as copper sulfate)			100%
Manganese	2	mg	
(as manganese sulfate)			100%
Potassium	16	mg	
(as potassium chloride)			0.5%

Standardized G115 Ginseng Extract 80 mg (from Panax Ginseng C.A. Meyer) (root)*

*Daily Value not established

Other Ingredients: Microcrystalline Cellulose, Povidone, Croecarmellose Sodium, Magnesium Stearate, Colloidal Silica, Hydroxypropyl mentyl cellulose, Ethylcellulose, Dibutyl Sebecate, Vanillin powder, Polyethylene Glycol.

Warning: Close tightly and keep out of reach of children. Contains iron, which can be harmful or fatal to children in large doses. In case of accidental overdose, seek professional assistance or contact a Poison Control Center Immediately.
Store at room temperature and avoid excessive heat above 40° C (104° F) to maintain optimal freshness.
Shown in Product Identification Guide, page 519

Pharmavite
**15451 SAN FERNANDO MISSION BLVD.
MISSION HILLS, CA 91345**

Direct Inquiries to:
Nature's Resource Brand Group
800-423-2405
(FAX) 818-837-6129

Medical Emergency Contact:
800-423-2405, ext. 2281

ECHINACEA HERB
Echinacea purpurea

Active Ingredients: Each capsule contains 380 mg of whole *Echinacea purpurea* herb.

Suggested Use: To stimulate natural resistance by boosting the immune system.

Recommended Intake: Take one to three capsules three times daily with water at mealtimes.

Warnings: Keep out of reach of children. Not recommended for individuals with auto-immune conditions. Do not use this product if you are allergic to flowers or of the daisy family (composite flowers).

How Supplied: Capsule, bottles of 100 and 240. Store at room temperature.

GINKGO BILOBA LEAF STANDARDIZED EXTRACT

Active Ingredients: Each capsule contains 40 mg of concentrated (50:1) Ginkgo biloba leaf extract standardized to 24% Ginkgo flavone glycosides along with the important terpene lactones (Ginkgolides and Bilobalide), supplied in a base of Alfalfa leaves.

Suggested Use: Increases peripheral circulation, thereby enhancing blood flow to the arms, legs and brain.

Recommended Intake: Take one capsule three times daily with water at mealtimes.

Warnings: Keep out of reach of children.

How Supplied: Capsules, bottles of 50 and 75. Store at room temperature.

SAW PALMETTO STANDARDIZED EXTRACT
Serona repens

Active Ingredients: Each capsule contains 80 mg of a liposterolic extract of Saw Palmetto berries standardized to contain between 85% and 95% fatty acids and sterols.

Suggested Use: Helps maintain proper urinary function in mature men.

Recommended Intake: Take two caplets, two times daily with water at mealtimes.

Warnings: Keep out of reach of children.

How Supplied: Capsule, bottle of 50. Store at room temperature.

ST. JOHN'S WORT HERB
Standardized Extract
Hypericum perforatum

Active ingredients: Each capsule contains 150 mg of concentrated St. John's wort herb extract standardized to .2% hypericin.

Suggested Use: May help to enhance mood.

Recommended intake: Take two capsules two to three times daily with water at mealtimes.

Warnings: Keep out of reach of children. Do not use if you are pregnant, lactating or taking antidepressant medication. Limit the exposure to the sun as St. John's wort may cause increased photosensitivity in fair skinned individuals. Discontinue use in the event of a rash.

How Supplied: Capsules, bottles of 50 and 100. Store at room temperature.

STANDARDIZED VALERIAN ROOT
Valerina officinalis

Active Ingredients: Each capsule contains 530 mg of whole Valeriana officinalis root.

Suggested Use: Natural support to enhance night time rest.

Recommended Intake: Take one or two capsules with water one hour prior to bedtime.

Warnings: Keep out of reach of children. Do not drive or operate heavy equipment while taking this product.

How Supplied: Capsule, bottle of 100. Store at room temperature.

UNKNOWN DRUG?
Consult the
Product Identification Guide
(Gray Pages)
for full-color photos of
leading over-the-counter
medications

PhytoPharmica
825 CHALLENGER DRIVE
GREEN BAY, WI 54311

Direct Inquiries To:
Doctors and Pharmacists,
call 1-800-553-2370
Consumers, call 1-800-644-0799

CELLULAR FORTÉ WITH IP-6™

Cellular Forté with IP-6™
Dramatically increases natural killer
cell activity Cellular Forté provides the
exact ratio of IP-6 (inositol hexaphos-
phate) and inositol needed for healthy
cellular growth. It is the only patented
combination available.
The result of 15 years of research, Cellular Forté with IP-6 is the only product
endorsed by discoverer and patent-
holder Dr. A. Shamsuddin, M.D., Ph.D.
This specially formulated supplement is
available in North America exclusively
from PhytoPharmica.
Patent no. 5,082,833.
120 hard shell capsules, or 240 hard
shell capsules for convenience.

Recommendations: Two capsules
twice per day, once before breakfast and
once between meals, as an addition to the
regular diet. Best taken on an empty
stomach.
Each capsule contains:
IP-6 (Rice) .... 400 mg
Inositol (Rice) .... 110 mg
Contains no sugar, salt, yeast, wheat,
gluten, corn, soy, dairy products, coloring, flavoring, or preservatives.

ESBERITOX™
Dietary supplement to nutritionally
support and stimulate the immune
system*

Description: Esberitox delivers
uniquely powerful immune system support. It's preferred over single-herb echinacea products because it's made with an
herbal combination that's more effective
and addresses a broader range of immune functions than echinacea alone.
That combination includes the key components of two echinacea extracts—Echinacea purpurea and pallida (purple
coneflower), with Thuja (white cedar),
and Baptisia (wild indigo).

Recommendations: Adults and chil-
dren over 12 years of age, take three tab-
lets, three times per day. Ages 8–12, take
two tablets, three times per day. Age 7
and younger, take one tablet, three times
per day. Tablet can be chewed.
Each tablet contains:
Baptisia Tinctoria (Root) Extract
(Wild Indigo Root) .... 10 mg
Echinacea Purpurea and Pallida (1:1)
(Root) extract
(Purple Coneflower Root) .... 7.5 mg
Thuja Occidentalis (Leaf) Extract
(White Cedar Leaf) .... 2 mg

Contains no salt, yeast, wheat, gluten,
corn, soy, dairy products (except lactose),
coloring, flavoring or preservatives.
Esberitox can be used anytime to fortify
the immune system, but is especially important when optimum support is desired.

How Supplied: 100 Tablets
Esberitox is produced by Schaper and
Brümmer of Germany, makers of
Remifemin™. Esberitox's proprietary
formula is now available in the United
States exclusively from PhytoPharmica.
*This statement has not been evaluated
by the Food and Drug Administration.
This product is not intended to diag-
nose, treat, cure or prevent any disease.
Shown in Product Identification
Guide, page 519

REMIFEMIN™
Nutritional support for women
experiencing menopause

Remifemin is the original standardized
black cohosh extract that provides important nutritional support for women
experiencing menopause.
Remifemin is backed by 40 years of extensive research and decades of successful use in Europe and now America. This
all-natural product is recommended by
some of the most respected names in
health care, such as Jan de Vries, Ph.D.,
and Michael Murray, N.D.
Most women enjoy remarkable benefits
within four to eight weeks of use.
18552 in 120 tablets and 18556 in 60 tab-
lets

Recommendations: One tablet in the
morning and one tablet in the evening.
As part of a good health program, we encourage you to see your health care practitioner on a regular basis. If you are
pregnant or considering becoming pregnant, seek the advice of your health care
practitioner before using this product.
Each tablet contains: Standardized
Cimicifuga racemosa (black cohosh) root
and rhizome extract corresponding to 20
mg of Cimicifuga racemosa. Each tablet
is standardized for triterpene glycosides
content (calculated as 27-deoxyactein.)
Contains no sugar, salt, yeast, wheat,
gluten, corn, soy, dairy products (except
lactose), coloring, flavoring, or preservatives.
Remifemin™: The natural choice for
women experiencing menopause:
Remifemin has been used successfully by
millions of women. This remarkable
plant extract has been available in Europe for 40 years and has quickly grown
in popularity throughout America.
Produced by Schaper and Brümmer, a
German manufacturing company,
Remifemin is a standardized, clinically
studied extract of black cohosh. Since
the 1950s, Schaper and Brümmer has
been the leading researcher of black cohosh.
Does not affect hormone lev-
els: Clinical research has shown that

the unique black cohosh extract in
Remifemin does not change hormone levels in the body.
Standardized extract: Remifemin
delivers a consistent level of the key compounds in black cohosh. This standardization ensures that you will get optimum natural benefits from this extraordinary extract.
Widely recommended: Remifemin is
recognized throughout Europe and the
United States as the ideal dietary supplement for women experiencing menopause. It is highly endorsed by health experts like Dr. Varro Tyler, Ph.D.; Dr. Jan
de Vries, Ph.D.; and Dr. Michael T. Murray, N.D.
Most women enjoy a dramatically improved sense of well-being within 4 to 8
weeks of using Remifemin.
Manufactured in Germany by Shaper
and Brümmer GmbH & Co. KG

Now available! Remifemin™ Plus Nutritional Support for women experienc-
ing menopause, plus the support of St.
John's Wort for emotional well-being.*
Remifemin™ Plus combines the benefits
of Remifemin with the additional sup-
port of a specially prepared, clinically
studied extract of St. John's Wort.
*This statement has not been evaluated
by the Food & Drug Administration.
This product is not intended to diagnose,
treat, cure or prevent any disease.
Exclusively distributed in North America
by
PhytoPharmica.
Green Bay, Wisconsin 54311 • Product of
Germany
Sold through physicians' offices and
pharmacies
© PhytoPharmica 1998
Visit us at www.PhytoPharmica.com
Shown in Product Identification
Guide, page 519

Procter & Gamble
P. O. BOX 5516
CINCINNATI, OH 45201

Direct Inquiries to:
Charles Lambert
(800) 358-8707

For Medical Emergencies:
Call Collect: (513) 558-4422

METAMUCIL® DIETARY FIBER SUPPLEMENT
[met uh-mū sil]
(psyllium husk)
Also see Metamucil Fiber Laxative in
Nonprescription Drugs section

Description: Metamucil contains
psyllium husk (from the plant *Plantago*
ovata), a concentrated source of soluble
fiber which can be used to increase one's
dietary fiber intake. When used as part

Continued on next page

Metamucil—Cont.

of a diet low in saturated fat and cholesterol, 7g per day of soluble fiber from psyllium husk (the amount in 3 doses of Metamucil) may reduce the risk of heart disease by lowering cholesterol. Each dose contains approximately 3.4 grams of psyllium husk (or about 2.3 grams of soluble fiber). A listing of ingredients and nutrition information is available in the listing of Metamucil Fiber Laxative in the Nonprescription Drug section. Metamucil Smooth Texture Sugar-Free Regular Flavor contains no sugar and no artificial sweeteners. Metamucil Smooth Texture Sugar-Free Orange Flavor contains aspartame (phenylalanine content of 25 mg per dose). Metamucil powdered products are gluten-free.

Actions: Metamucil Dietary Fiber Supplement can be used as a concentrated source of soluble fiber to increase the dietary intake of fiber. Diets low in saturated fat and cholesterol that include 7g per day of soluble fiber from psyllium husk, as in Metamucil, may reduce the risk of heart disease by lowering cholesterol.

Claims: Clinical studies have shown that 7 grams of soluble fiber from psyllium husk, the amount in three doses of Metamucil, may help reduce the risk of heart disease when part of a diet low in saturated fat and cholesterol. For laxative indications and directions for use, see **Metamucil Fiber Laxative** in the Nonprescription Drugs Section.

Contraindications: Intestinal obstruction, fecal impaction, allergy to any component.

Warnings: Patients are advised they should consult a doctor before using this product if they have abdominal pain, nausea, vomiting or rectal bleeding, if they have noticed a sudden change in bowel habits that persists over a period of two weeks, or if they are considering use of Metamucil as part of a cholesterol-lowering program. If taking Metamucil for contipation relief, patients are advised to consult a physician if constipation persists for longer than one week, as this may be a sign of a serious medical condition. **Patients are cautioned that taking this product without adequate fluid may cause it to swell and block the throat or esophagus and may cause choking. They should not take the product if they have difficulty in swallowing. If they experience chest pain, vomiting, or difficulty in swallowing or breathing after taking this product, they are advised to seek immediate medical attention.** Psyllium products may cause allergic reaction in people sensitive to inhaled or ingested psyllium. Keep out of the reach of children. In case of accidental overdose, seek professional assistance or contact a poison control center immediately.

Precaution: Notice to Health Care Professionals: To minimize the potential for allergic reaction, health care professionals who frequently dispense powdered psyllium products should avoid inhaling airborne dust while dispensing these products. Handling and Dispensing: To minimize generating airborne dust, spoon product from the canister into a glass according to label directions.

Dosage and Administration: The usual adult dosage is one rounded teaspoon, or tablespoon, depending on the product version. Some versions are available in single-dose packets. For children under 12 consult a docutor. The appropriate dose should be mixed with 8 oz. of liquid (e.g., cool water, fruit juice, milk) following the label instructions. **The product should be taken with at least 8 oz. (a full glass) of water or other fluid. Taking this product without enough liquid may cause choking (see warnings).** Metamucil can be taken three times per day.

This product, like other bulk fibers, may affect how well medicines work. If you are taking a prescription medicine by mouth, take this product at least 2 hours before or 2 hours after the prescribed medicine. As your body adjusts to increased fiber intake, you may experience changes in bowel habits or minor bloating.

How Supplied: Powder: canisters and cartons of single-dose packets. For complete ingredients and sizes for each version, see Metamucil Table 1, page 725, Nonprescription Drug section.

Shown in Product Identification Guide, page 519

Real Health Laboratories, Inc.
1424 30TH STREET
SAN DIEGO, CA 92154

Direct Inquiries to:
Consumer Product Information Center
(800) 565-6656

THE PROSTATE FORMULA™
1,100 mg tablets
Dietary Supplement

Description: Dietary supplementation with THE PROSTATE FORMULA™ is recommended for healthy adult males concerned about maintaining a healthy prostate and healthy urogenital functioning. Prior to beginning supplementation, a physician must determine that dietary supplementation, alone or as an adjunct to medical treatment, is needed for healthy prostate and urogenital functioning.* THE PROSTATE FORMULA™ is intended to support prostate health in aging adult males and is to be used as a part of a healthy life style, including proper diet and exercise. Scientific studies have demonstrated the ingredients in THE PROSTATE FORMULA™ benefit maintenance of a healthy prostate and proper urogenital functioning.

These ingredients provide prostate-specific nutrients and help maintain proper cell growth in the periuritheral region of the prostate gland, contributing to free urine flow.* As men age, the estrogen/androgen ratio increases, which may impact quality of life. Although the mechanisms behind the changes observed in the biochemistry of the prostate gland remain poorly understood, numerous studies indicate that one fundamental enzymatic conversion may contribute to morphological changes in the prostate gland. This reaction is the conversion of testosterone to dihydrotestosterone (DHT), which is catalyzed by 5-alpha-reducatase. Testosterone is secreted by the Leydig cells in the testes. It then crosses the plasma membrane of stromal cells in the prostate gland. 5-alpha-reductase, located in the nuclear membrane of the stromal cells, reduces testosterone to dihydrotestosterone. This potent androgen induces mRNA transcription for cytokines such as fibroblast growth factor and transforming growth factor beta. An autocrine effect then causes stromal cells to grow, and a paracrine effect causes prostatic epithelial tissues to grow. Estrogen also contributes to the population of DHT receptors in the stromal cell nuclei. These changes can be balanced by governing the activity of 5-alpha-reductase.* THE PROSTATE FORMULA™ contains ingredients scientifically shown to keep 5-alpha-reductase in balance.*

Ingredients: Three tablets of THE PROSTATE FORMULA™ contain 320 milligrams of Saw Palmetto Berry Powder, 300 milligrams of *Pygeum africanum* Bark Powder, 100 milligrams of *Urtica dioica* powder, 100 mg of Pumpkin Seed Powder, 5 mg Zinc from Zinc Picolinate (20% D.V.), 250 mg of Lysine from Lysine HCl, 250 mg of L-Glutamic Acid Base, 250 mg of Glycine, 50 mg of Vitamin B_6 from Pyridoxine HCl (2,500% D.V.), 200 IU Vitamin D from cholecalciferol (50% D.V.), and 100 IU of Vitamin E (333% D.V.). Tablets are coated with white titanium dioxide using an aqueous process. Coating is flavored with natural peppermint oil.

Recommended Use: As a dietary supplement, it is recommended a 1,000 mg tablet of THE PROSTATE FORMULA™ be taken three times per day. THE PROSTATE FORMULA™ should be taken with meals or a snack to minimize the risk of minor stomach irritation. The product should be used consistently for a minimum of 90–120 days for product benefits to be realized. Continued use is recommended for optimal benefits.

Warnings: Keep out of reach of children.
• **Consult your physician before using THE PROSTATE FORMULA™, especially if you are taking other medications.**

Adverse Effects: Based on corporate historical data, only a small number of individuals have reported minor stomach discomfort; otherwise, no adverse effects have been observed during the product's five year history.

How Supplied: White, standard oval tablets of THE PROSTATE FORMULA™, 1,100 mg each, are supplied in 400 CC white HDPE bottles, with cotton, white vertical ridged cap, inner pressure safety seal, and heat-sealed safety neck band in 270 count. The bottle is placed in an individual consumer box, and sealed at each end with safety tabs. THE PROSTATE FORMULA™ can be purchased at major drug stores, and grocery stores with pharmacies, in the OTC aisle, near the laxative section.

Storage: Store in a dry, cool place. Protect from light. Avoid excessive heat.

Shelf Life: The expiration date is printed on the bottom or the side of the product bottle, and on the exterior bottom of the individual consumer box.

Quality Assurance: THE PROSTATE FORMULA™ is manufactured in USFDA registered manufacturing plants. In addition to pre-process and in-process controls, Real Health Laboratories, Inc. contracts a USFDA registered analytical chemistry laboratory and microbiology laboratory to test for safety, potency and disintegration, using USP and AOAC methodology on each lot manufactured. Each lot of product undergoes this analytical chemistry and microbiological testing.

Mandatory FDA Disclaimer

*These statements have not been evaluated by the Food and Drug Administration. This product is not intended to diagnose, treat, cure or prevent any disease.

Shown in Product Identification Guide, page 519

THE VASORECT FORMULA™
710 mg capsules
Dietary Supplement

Description: Dietary supplementation with THE VASORECT FORMULA™ is recommended for healthy adult males concerned about maintaining healthy erectile and cardiovascular functioning. The product may also be used by adult females with the same concerns. The erectile process involves a number of biochemical events that ultimately lead to erection required for intromission. THE VASORECT FORMULA™ was designed to benefit the biochemical reactions required for erection. Sexual arousal causes the parasympathetic nervous system to release acetylcholine (ACh). ACh binds to endothelial cell receptors lining the arterioles that supply the corpus cavernosum with blood upon arousal. Ca^{2+} helps the enzyme, nitric oxide synthase (NOS), to derive nitric oxide (NO) from arginine. NO diffuses to smooth muscle cells of the arterioles supplying the cor-

pus cavernosum. NO stimulates the enzyme guanylate cyclase, by binding to that enzyme's heme group, and converts cytosolic guanosine 5'-triphosphate (GTP) to guanosine 3',5'-cyclic monophosphate (cGMP). cGMP relaxes the arterioles (cGMP relaxation) of the corpus cavernosum, allowing blood engorgement of the erectile tissues. The increase in the available free arginine can contribute to the erectile process by providing the substrate for NO. This is particularly important when considering the instability of NO and its very short lifetime of just a few seconds, at which time it is converted to nitrite or nitrate and excreted from the body. The formula also contains calcium, an essential part of the vasodilation process. Cardiovascular health is of utmost concern to American men and women. In addition to the ability of THE VASORECT FORMULA™ to contribute to the vascular aspect of the erectile process, it provides the arginine required for vasodilator tone that contributes to the healthy functioning of the entire cardiovascular system. The cardiovascular system has numerous regulators, but its healthy function relies heavily on the endothelium-derived NO/cGMP mechanism for regulating blood pressure and blood flow throughout the body. Arginine is an essential part of this process, contributing to the available NO required for homeostatic control of the vasculature. This is accomplished throughout the body in the same biochemical fashion as the erectile process described above, involving the smooth muscle cells lining the penis blood vessels. Anticohesiveness of cardiovascular endothelial tissue is essential in maintaining normal blood flow, and this anticohesiveness is associated with high levels of NO in those tissues. THE VASORECT FORMULA™ provides the free arginine required to contribute to these healthy states.

Ingredients: 4 capsules of THE VASORECT FORMULA™ contain 2,500 mg of Arginine free base, USP grade, and 50 mg of Calcium (5% DV) from calcium carbonate, USP grade.

Recommended Use: As a dietary supplement, take one to four capsules of THE VASORECT FORMULA™ per day. Regular use is recommended for optimal benefits.

Warnings: Keep out of reach of children.
- **Consult your physician before using THE VASORECT FORMULA™, especially if you are taking other medications.**
- **DO NOT use this product if you are using nitrate drugs, such as nitroglycerin in sublingual, skin patch, ointment, or other form.**
- **This product should not be used by pregnant or lactating women, or women who are planning to become pregnant.**
- **Keep out of reach of children. Product intended for use by adults 18 years of age and older.**

Adverse Effects: Arginine is registered as a GRAS substance in The Code of Federal Regulations, Title 21, Volume 3, Parts 170–199 Rev. 4/1/98. No reports of serious adverse events were located at the time of print.

How supplied: 710 mg opaque 00 capsules containing 625 mg of arginine free base, calcium carbonate & magnesium stearate. Bottled in 225 cc white HDPE bottle, cotton, desiccant, white vertical ridged cap, inner pressure sensitive safety seal, clear printed perforated neck band, product label, lot number, expiration date (2 year shelf life under proper storage conditions).

Storage: Product should be stored in a cool dry place. Keep lid closed when not in use. Keep away from direct light and heat.

Shelf Life: The expiration date is printed on the bottom or the side of the product bottle, and on the exterior of the product box.

Quality Assurance: THE VASORECT FORMULA™ is manufactured in USFDA registered manufacturing plants. In addition to pre-process and in-process controls, Real Health Laboratories, Inc. contracts a USFDA registered analytical chemistry laboratory and microbiology laboratory to test for safety, potency and disintegration, using USP and AOAC methodology on each lot manufactured. Each lot of finished product undergoes this analytical chemistry and microbiological testing.

Mandatory FDA Disclaimer

Statements in this entry have not been evaluated by the Food and Drug Administration. This product is not intended to diagnose, treat, cure or prevent any disease.

Shown in Product Identification Guide, page 519

Rexall Sundown, Inc.
6111 BROKEN SOUND PARKWAY, NW BOCA RATON, FL 33487-2745

Direct Inquiries to:
1-888-VITAHELP (848-2435)

OSTEO BI-FLEX®

Description: Osteo-Bi-Flex is an exclusive patented formula combining Glucosamine HCl and Chondroitin Sulfate. This nutritional combination of ingredients helps in maintaining healthy, mobile joint function and connective tissues. Osteo Bi-Flex is available in regular strength and maximum strength, in tablet and softgel dosage forms.

Active Ingredients: Each regular strength tablet contains 250 mg Glucosamine HCl and 200 mg Chondroitin Sul-

Continued on next page

Osteo Bi-Flex—Cont.

fate. Each maximum strength tablet contains 500 mg Glucosamine HCl and 400 mg Chondroitin Sulfate.

Also contains: Dextrose direct compression, cellulose, red beet juice powder, croscarmellose sodium, silica, and magnesium stearate.

Suggested use: Cartilage rebuilding and regeneration is a normal function of the body. As our bodies age, the ability to produce some of the nutrients necessary for cartilage building declines. Our bodies also produce enzymes which can be a factor in cartilage breakdown. Chondroitin Sulfate inhibits this enzyme activity, thereby enhancing the production and maintenance of healthy new cartilage and connective tissues. Glucosamine, a naturally occuring amino-sugar found in the body, plays an important role in the maintenance and repair of cartilage, including cartilage adversely affected by aging and physical stress. Osteo Bi-Flex's combination of Glucosamine HCl and Chondroitin Sulfate provides an important nutritional approach for healthy points and cartilage.

Recommended Adult Intake:

Regular strength:

Initial 60 Days: Six tablets should be taken daily (three in the morning, three in the evening), with food.

After 60 Days (maintenance level): Three to six tablets per day, according to individual needs, with food.

Maximum strength:

Initial 60 Days: Three tablets should be taken daily, with food.

After 60 Days (maintenance level): One to three tablets per day, according to individual needs, with food.

For children, consult your healthcare practitioner.

Note: If you are allergic to shellfish, please consult your healthcare professional before taking this product.

Shown in Product Identification Guide, page 519

---

sigma-tau Consumer Products

A division of sigma-tau Pharmaceuticals, Inc.
GAITHERSBURG, MARYLAND 20877

Direct Medical Inquiries to:
Toll Free (888) 818–5448
or (301) 948–5450
Fax: (301) 948–5452
Email: info@sigmatau.com

Direct Product Orders to:
Toll Free: (877) PROXEED (776–9333)
Web: www.proxeed.com

PROXEED™
[*prox'-ēde*]
dietary supplement
promotes optimum sperm quality

Description: PROXEED is a dietary supplement specifically formulated to optimize sperm quality. Sperm quality refers to motility, rapid linear progression, count, concentration and morphology.

Suggested Use: To optimize sperm quality.

Active Ingredients: L-carnitine fumarate, fructose, acetyl-L-carnitine HCl, citric acid
Levocarnitine (L-carnitine) is a carrier molecular for medium and long-chain fatty acids and is essential in the transportation of these fatty acids into the mitochondria where they can be utilized for β-oxidation. Levocarnitine is a component of both seminal plasma and sperm cells, and it plays a critical role in sperm maturation and potential sperm motility[1–3].
Fructose is one of the major energy-yielding substrates present in seminal fluid[4].
Acetyl-L-carnitine is the acetyl ester of levocarnitine and occurs naturally in the body. When converted to acetyl-CoA, it can enter the Krebs Cycle, be converted to acetoacetate (a ketone body) or be used for fatty acid synthesis. Additionally, acetyl-L-carnitine is important for membrane stabilization, is the most prominent form of carnitine in sperm[5–7], serves as a circulating energy source for sperm[5–7], plays an important role in sperm maturation and metabolism[5–7] and provides the primary fuel for sperm motility[4–5, 8].
Citric acid is a key intermediate in the Kreb's Cycle.

Inactive Ingredients: mannitol, artificial flavorings, saccharin

Supplement Facts:

Serving Size 1 Packet
Serving Per Container 30

	Amount Per Serving	% Daily Value
Calories	8	<1%*
Total Carbohydrate	2g	<1%*
Sugars	2g	**
L-carnitine	1g	**
Acetyl-L-carnitine	.5g	**

---

* Percent daily values based on a 2,000 calorie diet.
**Daily Value not established.

Clinical Findings: Among healthy couples taking longer than expected to conceive, poor sperm quality is a contributing factor for nearly 40% of all cases[5]. PROXEED's primary ingredients are levocarnitine and acetyl-L-carnitine. In eight clinical trials, levocarnitine and acetyl-L-carnitine have been proven to provide the nutritional support needed for sperm's production of energy and optimum sperm quality[2–3, 5, 8–12].

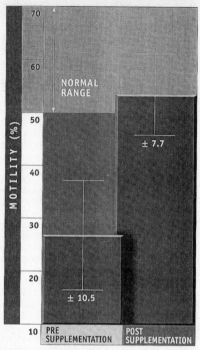

Sperm motility was normalized after 3 months of supplementation.
[Vitali, G, *et al*, *Drugs Experimental Clinical Research* 1995; 21(4): 157–159]

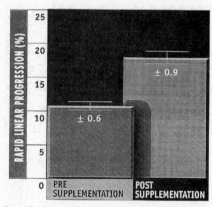

Rapid linear progression of sperm showed an 80% improvement after 4 months of supplementation.
[Costa, M, *et al*, *Andrologia* 1994; 26: 155–159]
[See graph at top of next column.]
There has been only limited data on whether the ingredients in PROXEED have a measurable effect on sperm morphology.

Bioavailability/Pharmacokinetics:
Levocarnitine and acetyl-L-carnitine have oral bioavailabilities of between 5 and 15% in healthy adults. Clinical studies have shown that oral doses of 3g per day (total) of carnitines are appropriate to optimize sperm quality[2, 8, 12]. To achieve the appropriate dose, it is necessary for PROXEED to be provided as a powder formulation.
The oral half-lives of levocarnitine and acetyl-L-carnitine are approximately

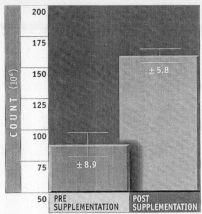

Sperm count nearly doubled after 3 months of supplementation, approaching normal levels.
[Vitali, G, *et al, Drugs Experimental Clinical Research* 1995; 21(4): 157–159]

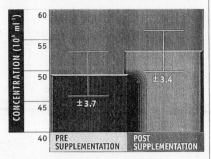

Sperm concentration improved after 4 months of supplementation.
[Vitali, G, *et al, Drugs Experimental Clinical Research* 1995; 21(4): 157–159]
3–4 hours. As a result, the total daily dose should be divided b.i.d., and spaced 8 or more hours apart to maintain elevated blood levels of levocarnitine and acetyl-L-carnitine.

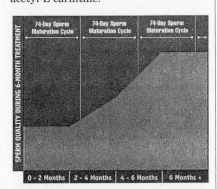

On average, sperm require 74 days to mature, and up to 30 additional days to become capable of fertilization. Initial results should be seen within 3 months and continued improvement—leading to optimum results—within 6 months.

Precautions: As with all supplements, please keep this product out of the reach of children, and consult with your physician before use if you are taking any medications.

Contraindications: none known.

Drug Interactions: none known.

Dosage and Administration: Take two packets of PROXEED per day, one packet in the morning and one packet in the evening. Mix each packet with at least 4 ounces (120ml) of water or other beverage. Initial results should be seen within 3 months and continued improvement—leading to optimum results—within 6 months. Patients who miss a dose should continue with the next dose. Double dosing is not necessary.

PROXEED is designed for long-term administration and should be taken as long as attempting to conceive.

How Supplied: PROXEED is available in single dose packets packaged 30 per box. PROXEED's powder formulation allows for the necessary ingredients in the amounts shown to be effective in clinical trials. To order PROXEED, visit the web site: WWW.PROXEED.COM or call toll-free (877) PROXEED (776–9333).

PROXEED is manufactured for sigma-tau Pharmaceuticals, Inc., Gaithersburg, Maryland 20877. Product of Italy. PROXEED is a trademark of sigma-tau HealthScience S.p.A. Patent Pending. All rights reserved.

References:
1. Jeulin, C, *et al,* Role of Free L-carnitine and Acetyl-L-carnitine in Post-Gonadal Maturation of Mammalian Spermatozoa. *Human Reproduction Update* 1996; 2(2): 87–102
2. Vitali, G, *et al,* Carnitine Supplementation in Human Idiopathic Asthenospermia: Clinical Results. *Drugs Experimental Clinical Research* 1995; 21(4): 157–159
3. Loumbakis, P, *et al,* Effect of L-carnitine in Patients with Asthenospermia; 12th Congress of the European Association of Urology, Sept. 1–4, 1996. *Paris in European Urology* 1996; 30(2): 225, Abstract 954
4. Golan, R, *et al,* Influence of Various Substrates on the Acetylcarnitine: Carnitine Ratio in Motile and Immotile Human Spermatozoa. *Reproduction and Fertility* 1986; 78: 287–293
5. Moncada, ML, *et al,* Effect of Acetylcarnitine Treatment in Oligoasthenospermic Patients. *Acta Europaea Fertilitatis* 1992; 23(5): 221–224
6. Bartellini, M, *et al,* L-carnitine and Acetylcarnitine in Human Sperm with Normal and Reduced Motility. *Acta Europaea Fertilitatis* 1987; 19(1): 29–31
7. Kohengkul, S, *et al,* Levels of L-carnitine and L-O-acetylcarnitine in Normal and Infertile Human Semen: A Lower Level of L-O-acetylcarnitine in Infertile Semen. *Fertility and Sterility* 1977; 28(12): 1333–1336
8. Costa, M, *et al,* L-carnitine in Idiopathic Asthenozoospermia: A Multicenter Study. *Andrologia* 1994; 26: 155–159
9. Campaniello, E, *et al,* Carnitine Administration in Asthenospermia; 4th International Congress of Andrology, Firenze, May 14–18, 1989. Abstract
10. Muller-Tyl, E, *et al,* Effects of Carnitine on Sperm Count and Motility. *Fertilitat* 1988; 4(1): 1–4
11. Micic, S, *et al,* Does L-carnitine Administered In Vivo Improve Sperm Motility? *ARTA* 1995; 7: 127–130
12. Micic, S, Effects of L-carnitine on Sperm Motility and Number in Infertile Men; 16th World Congress on Fertility and Sterility, San Francisco, Oct. 4–9, 1998. Abstract

pxd-pdr-1
12/98
Shown in Product Identification Guide, page 521

SmithKline Beecham Consumer Healthcare, L.P.
POST OFFICE BOX 1467
PITTSBURGH, PA 15230

For Medical Information Contact:
(800) 245-1040 (Consumer Inquiries)
(800) 378-4055 (Healthcare Professional Inquiries)

Direct Healthcare Professional Sample Requests to:
(800) BEECHAM

OS-CAL® CHEWABLE
Calcium Supplement

Description: Calcium supplement to help reduce the risk of osteoporosis. Osteoporosis affects middle-aged and older persons, especially Caucasian and Asian women, and those whose families tend to have fragile bones in later years. A lifetime of regular exercise and eating a healthful diet that includes enough calcium, especially during teen and early adult years, builds & maintains good bone health & may reduce the risk of osteoporosis in later life.
Adequate calcium intake is important, but daily intakes above 2000mg are not likely to provide any additional benefit.
Supplement Facts
Serving Size 1 Tablet

Each tablet Contains	% Daily Value
Calories 5	
Calcium 500mg	50%

Ingredients: Calcium carbonate, dextrose monohydrate, maltodextrin, microcrystalline cellulose, magnesium stearate, artificial flavors, sodium chloride.

Directions: One tablet two to three times a day with meals, or as recommended by your physician.

Continued on next page

Os-Cal Chewable—Cont.

How Supplied: Bottle of 60 tablets
Store at room temperature.
Keep out of reach of children.
*Shown in Product Identification
Guide, page 522*

OS-CAL® 250 + D
Calcium with Vitamin D Supplement

Description: Calcium supplement to help reduce the risk of osteoporosis (see below*). Also contains Vitamin D.

Supplement Facts
Serving Size 1 Tablet

Each tablet Contains	% Daily Value
Calcium 250mg	25%
Vitamin D 125 IU	31%

Ingredients: Oyster shell powder, talc, corn syrup solids, hydroxypropyl methylcellulose, corn starch. Contains less than 1% of calcium stearate, polysorbate 80, titanium dioxide, polyethylene glycol, Vitamin D, propyl paraben and methyl paraben (preservative), simethicone, yellow 10 lake, blue 1 lake, carnauba wax, edetate sodium.

Directions: One tablet three times a day with meals, or as recommended by your physician.

How Supplied: Bottle of 100 and 240 tablets
Store at room temperature.
Keep out of reach of children.
*Osteoporosis affects middle-aged and older persons, especially Caucasian and Asian women, and those whose families tend to have fragile bones in later years. A lifetime of regular exercise and eating a healthful diet that includes enough calcium, especially during teen and early adult years, builds & maintains good bone health & may reduce the risk of osteoporosis in later life.
Adequate calcium intake is important, but daily intakes above 2000mg are not likely to provide any additional benefit.
*Shown in Product Identification
Guide, page 522*

OS-CAL® 500
Calcium Supplement

Description: Calcium supplement to help reduce the risk of osteoporosis. Osteoporosis effects middle-aged and older persons, especially Caucasian and Asian women, and those whose families tend to have fragile bones in later years. A lifetime of regular exercise and eating a healthful diet that includes enough calcium, especially during teen and early adult years, builds & maintains good bone health & may reduce the risk of osteoporosis in later life.

Adequate calcium intake is important, but daily intakes above 2000mg are not likely to provide any additional benefit.

Supplement Facts
Serving Size 1 Tablet

Each table Contains	% Daily Value
Calcium 500mg	50%

Ingredients: Oyster shell powder, talc, corn syrup solids, hydroxypropyl methylcellulose, corn starch. Contains less than 1% of sodium starch glycolate, calcium stearate, polysorbate 80, titanium dioxide, polyethylene glycol, propyl paraben and methyl paraben (preservative), polydextrose, triacetin, yellow 10 lake, blue 1 lake, carnauba wax.

Directions: One tablet two to three times a day with meals, or as recommended by your physician.

How Supplied: Bottles of 75 and 160 tablets
Store at room temperature.
Keep out of reach of children.
*Shown in Product Identification
Guide, page 522*

OS-CAL® 500 + D
Calcium with Vitamin D Supplement

Description: Calcium supplement with to help reduce the risk of osteoporosis (see below*). Also contains Vitamin D.

Supplement Facts
Serving Size 1 Tablet

Each tablet Contains	% Daily Value
Calcium 500mg	50%
Vitamin D 200 IU	50%

Ingredients: Oyster shell powder, talc, corn syrup solids, hydroxypropyl methylcellulose, corn starch. Contains less than 1% of sodium starch glycolate, calcium stearate, polysorbate 80, titanium dioxide, polyethylene glycol, Vitamin D, propyl paraben and methyl paraben (preservative), polydextrose, triacetin, yellow 10 lake, blue 1 lake, carnauba wax.

Directions: One tablet two to three times a day with meals, or as recommended by your physician.

How Supplied: Bottle of 75 and 160 tablets
Store at room temperature.
Keep out of reach of children.
*Osteoporosis affects middle-aged and older persons, especially Caucasian and Asian women, and those whose families tend to have fragile bones in later years. A lifetime of regular exercise and eating a healthful diet that includes enough calcium, especially during teen and early adult years, builds & maintains good bone health & may reduce the risk of osteoporosis in later life.
Adequate calcium intake is important, but daily intakes above 2000mg are not likely to provide any additional benefit.
*Shown in Product Identification
Guide, page 522*

Sunpower Nutraceutical Inc.
**18003 SKY PARK CIRCLE
SUITE G
IRVINE, CA 92614**

Direct Inquiries to:
Ph: (949) 833-8899

PRODUCT LISTING

Descriptions: Sunpower Nutraceutical System combined vitamins, minerals, special formulated herbs, Pycnogenol® and proprietary Traditional Chinese Medicines (TCM) from S.P. Pharmaceutical Inc. (S.P.) which manufactured at GMP facility and under FDA Act and U.S. Pharmacopeia quality, purity and potency standards.
Time-released, Double-layered tablets are made by advanced manufacturing techniques which allows nutrients to be released slowly for better absorption during digestion.

Sunpower Product Overview:
Sun Liver™: contains vitamins, minerals, Pycnogenol® and S.P. Pro-Liver Pill to help to fight free radical damage, and provide nutrients essential for healthy liver function.
*Shown in Product Identification
Guide, page 523*

Sun Cardio™: contains CoQ10, OPC, Ginkgo Biloba, Red Wine Extract and S.P. Pro-Cardio Pill to help maintain normal cardiovascular system.

Power Circulation™: contains Ginkgo Biloba, Barley Grass, Lecithin and S.P. Pro-Circulation Pill to help maintain a healthy blood circulatory system.

Power Arthritis™: contains Glucosamine, Chondroitin, Wild Yam, Propolis and S.P. Pro-Joint Pill to provide essential nutrients for bone, joint, ligament and cartilage function.

Power Lasting™: contains Yohimbe, Damiana, Saw Palmetto, Gotu Kola, Sarsaparilla Root, and S.P. Pro-Long Pill to help maintain normal kidney and sexual function and enhance endurance.

Sun Beauty™ 1: contains Alfalfa, St. John's Wort, Cranberry, Royal Jelly, and S.P. Beauty I Pill to help establish healthy hormonal rhythms and basic immunity.

Sun Beauty™ 2: contains Alfalfa, Selenium, Green Tea, Uva Ursi Leaves, Cranberry, and S.P. Beauty II Pill to support and balance a woman's vitality and healthy immunity during the menstrual cycle.

Sun Beauty™ 3: contains chromium, Burdock Root, Fo-Ti, Black Cohoshe, Red Clover, Chaste Tree Berries, and S.P. Beauty III Pill to support general well-being during menopause and post-menopause.

Thompson Medical Company, Inc.

777 SO. FLAGLER DR.
WEST TOWER, SUITE 1500
WEST PALM BEACH
FLORIDA 33401

Direct Inquiries to:
Consumer Services: (561) 820-9900
Fax: (561) 832-2297

NATURE'S REWARD™ CALCI COMPLEX
Dietary Supplement

Description: Nature's Reward™ Calci Complex contains eight vitamins and minerals plus a unique herbal blend to help maintain strong and healthy bones. Calci Complex contains calcium, magnesium and phosphorous to help maintain strong and healthy bones, vitamin D and boron to help increase the absorption of calcium and folic acid to help support a healthy heart.*

*These statements have not been evaluated by the Food and Drug Administration. This product is not intended to diagnose, treat, cure or prevent any disease.

SUPPLEMENT FACTS:
Serving Size: 2 Caplets

	Amount Per Serving	% Daily Value
Vitamin D (as cholecalciferol)	200 IU	50%
Vitamin C (ascorbic acid)	60 mg	100%
Folic Acid	400 mcg	100%
Calcium (as calcium carbonate, phosphate and citrate)	500 mg	50%
Phosphorus (as calcium phosphate)	100 mg	10%
Magnesium (as magnesium oxide, carbonate and citrate)	250 mg	60%
Zinc (as zinc citrate)	7.5 mg	50%

	Amount Per Serving	% Daily Value
Ginseng Root Standardized Extract (Panax ginseng) (4% ginsenosides)	100 mg.	†
Ginkgo Leaf Standardized Extract (Ginkgo biloba) (24% flavonoids)	60 mg.	†
Garlic Standardized (Allium sativum) (bulb)	300 mg.	†

† Daily value not established.

Herbal blend Valencia orange bioflavonoids, horsetail herb standardized extract (provides 30 mg silica), fennel seed	150 mg	†
Boron (as boron chelate)	1 mg	†

†Daily value not established.

Other Ingredients: Cellulose, fractionated vegetable oil, silica, polysorbate 80.

Suggested Use: As a dietary supplement, take two Calci Complex caplets daily, preferably with a meal.
Important: This product is not intended for children. Do not take this product if you are pregnant or nursing a baby. If you have a medical condition or are taking any prescription medication, consult your doctor before using this product.
How to Store: Store at controlled room temperature 59°–86°F (15°–30°C).

How Supplied: Nature's Reward Calci Complex is supplied in tamper-evident blister packages. Do not use if individual seals are broken. Package contains 30 caplets.

NATURE'S REWARD™ GINKOGIN®
[gǐng-kō-jǐn]
Standardized Extracts of Ginkgo Biloba, Ginseng and Garlic
Dietary Supplement

Nature's Reward™ Ginkogin® combines three of the top herbal supplements into one formula. Ginkogin® contains all-natural sources of standardized extracts of ginkgo biloba, ginseng and garlic.
- **Ginkgo biloba**—a dietary supplement commonly used to help restore memory. Regular use of Ginkgo biloba may help restore age-related memory loss.* Ginkogin contains the same daily level of standardized Ginkgo biloba extract as the leading Ginkgo biloba supplement.
- **Ginseng**—a dietary supplement commonly used to help improve physical endurance. Athletes taking ginseng on a regular basis have experienced increased stamina and the ability to exercise longer.* Ginkogin contains the same level of standardized ginseng as the leading ginseng supplement.

- **Garlic**—a dietary supplement commonly used to help maintain healthy cholesterol levels.* Each daily dose is equal to eating a whole clove of garlic, but Ginkogin leaves no garlicky smell on your breath.

*These statements have not been evaluated by the Food and Drug Administration. This product is not intended to diagnose, treat, cure or prevent any disease.

SUPPLEMENT FACTS:
Serving Size: 1 Caplet
[See table above]

Other Ingredients: Dicalcium Phosphate, Microcrystalline Cellulose, Hydroxypropyl Methylcellulose Phthlate, Croscarmellose Sodium, Stearic Acid, Silica, Magnesium Stearate, Triacetin, Shellac, FD&C Yellow No. 6 Aluminum Lake, FD&C Blue No. 1 Aluminum Lake, FD&C Red No. 40 Aluminum Lake, Titanium Dioxide.

Suggested Use: As a dietary supplement, take one Ginkogin caplet two times a day.
Important: This product is not intended for children. Do not take this product if you are pregnant or nursing a baby. If you have a medical condition or are taking any prescription medication, consult your doctor before using this product.
How to Store: Store at controlled room temperature 59°–86°F (15°–30°C).

How Supplied: Ginkogin is supplied in tamper-evident blister packages. Do not use if individual seals are broken. Package contains 30 caplets.

NATURE'S REWARD™ HEART WISE™
Dietary Supplement
Standardized Extracts

Description: Nature's Reward™ Heart Wise™ contains seven herbs and vitamins combined in a unique formula to support good heart health. Heart Wise™ contains folic acid, vitamins B-6 and B-12 to help maintain healthy cardiovascular function, vitamin E to help support a healthy heart and hawthorn extract, which may help maintain a healthy circulatory system.*

Continued on next page

Heart Wise—Cont.

*These statements have not been evaluated by the Food and Drug Administration. This product is not intended to diagnose, treat, cure or prevent any disease.

SUPPLEMENT FACTS:
Serving Size: 2 Caplets

	Amount Per Serving	% Daily Value
Vitamin E (100% as natural d-alpha tocopherol succinate)	100 IU	335%
Vitamin B-6 (as pyridoxine hydrochloride)	3 mg	150%
Folic Acid	400 mcg	100%
Vitamin B-12 (as cyanocobalamin)	6 mcg	100%
Herbal blend Hawthorn standardized extract (2.2% flavonoids, supplying 10 mg total flavonoids) (fruit and/or leaf and flower), green tea leaf standardized extract (36% polyphenols), standardized resveratrol (provides 2 mg resveratrol from *Polygonum cuspidatum* root and red wine grape concentrate)	600 mg	†

†Daily value not established.

Other Ingredients: Dicalcium phosphate, cellulose, fractionated vegetable oil, silica.

Suggested Use: As a dietary supplement, take two Heart Wise caplets daily, preferably with a meal.
Important: This product is not intended for children. Do not take this product if you are pregnant or nursing a baby. If you have a medical condition or are taking any prescription medication, consult your doctor before using this product.
How to Store: Store at controlled room temperature 59°–86°F (15°–30°C).

How Supplied: Nature's Reward™ Heart Wise™ is supplied in tamper-evident blister packages. Do not use if individual seals are broken. Package contains 30 caplets.

NATURE'S REWARD™ PRIME OF LIFE™
Dietary Supplement
Standardized Extracts

Description: Nature's Reward™ Prime of Life™ is a unique multi-herbal, multi-vitamin/mineral formula that is specially formulated for a woman's nutritional needs during and after menopause. Prime of Life™ contains calcium, as well as Vitamin D, Magnesium and Zinc which help insure the proper absorption of calcium. It also contains isoflavones which are a good source of soy that may help maintain a natural hormone balance and Black Cohosh extract which is an important nutrient for women of menopausal age.*

*These statements have not been evaluated by the Food and Drug Administration. This product is not intended to diagnose, treat, cure or prevent any disease.

SUPPLEMENT FACTS:
Serving Size: 2 Caplets

	Amount Per Serving	% Daily Value
Vitamin D (as cholecalciferol)	200 IU	50%
Vitamin E (as di-alpha tocopheryl acetate)	30 IU	100%
Vitamin K (as phylloquinone)	80 mcg	100%
Thiamin (as thiamin mononitrate)	1.5 mg	100%
Riboflavin	1.7 mg	100%
Niacin (as niacinamide)	20 mg	100%
Vitamin B-6 (as pyridoxine hydrochloride)	2 mg	100%
Folic Acid	400 mcg	100%
Vitamin B-12 (as cyanocobalamin)	6 mcg	100%
Pantothenic Acid (as calcium pantothenate)	10 mg	100%
Calcium (as calcium carbonate)	400 mg	40%
Magnesium (as magnesium oxide and magnesium carbonate)	200 mg	50%
Zinc (as zinc citrate)	10 mg	65%
Manganese (as manganese gluconate)	2 mg	100%
Panax ginseng root standardized extract (4% ginsenosides)	200 mg	†
Soybean tofu and kudzu root standardized concentrate (20% daidzein and genistein isoflavones)	100 mg	†
Don quai root (Angelica sinensis)	100 mg	†
Chaste berry (Vitex agnus-castus)	50 mg	†
Black cohosh root standardized extract (5% triterpene glycosides, as 27-deoxyactein) (Cimicifuga racemosa)	20 mg	†
Boron (as boron chelate)	1 mg	†

†Daily value not established.

Other Ingredients: Cellulose, fractionated vegetable oil, silica, polysorbate 80.

Suggested Use: As a dietary supplement, take two Prime of Life™ caplets daily, preferably with a meal.
Important: This product is not intended for children. Do not take this product if you are pregnant or nursing a baby. If you have a medical condition or are taking any prescription medication, consult your doctor before using this product.
How to Store: Store at controlled room temperature 59°–86°F (15°–30°C).

How Supplied: Nature's Reward™ Prime of Life™ is supplied in tamper-evident blister packages. Do not use if individual seals are broken. Package contains 30 caplets.

Wakunaga Consumer Products
**23501 MADERO
MISSION VIEJO, CA 92691**

Direct Inquiries to:
(800) 527-5200

GINKGO-GO!®
Dietary Supplement

Active Ingredient: Each caplet—Ginkgo Biloba Extract 50:1 (120 mg).

Suggested Use: As a dietary supplement, take one caplet daily with food for enhancement of memory, alertness and mental acuity.

How Supplied: Boxes of 15 caplets.

KYOLIC®
Odor Modified Garlic Supplement

Active Ingredient: Each caplet contains 600 mg Aged Garlic Extract™.

Suggested Use: As a dietary supplement, take 1 or more caplets daily with food to promote healthy circulation.

How Supplied: Boxes of 30 Caplets.
Shown in Product Identification Guide, page 523

PROBIATA®
Probiotic Dietary Supplement

Active Ingredient: L. acidophilus

Suggested Use: Take one tablet, twice daily with meals. Replenishes healthy intestinal flora to avoid disorders such as diarrhea, constipation and yeast discomfort caused by antibiotic usage.

How Supplied: Bottles of 30 tablets.
Shown in Product Identification Guide, page 523

Warner-Lambert Consumer HealthCare

Warner-Lambert Company
201 TABOR ROAD
MORRIS PLAINS, NJ 07950

Direct Inquiries to:
1-(800) 223-0182

For Medical Information Contact:
1-(800) 223-0182
1-(800) 378-1783 (e.p.t)
1-(800) 337-7266 (e.p.t–Spanish)

QUANTERRA™ Mental Sharpness
Ginkgo biloba Herbal Supplement
[Quən-tər-ə]

Herbal Ingredient: 60 mg Ginkgo biloba extract per tablet standardized to 24% flavone glycosides and 6% terpene lactones.

Uses: Promotes and maintains mental sharpness, concentration, and focus.* Promotes circulation to the brain and extremeties.*

Supplement Facts
Serving Size: 2 Tablets
Servings Per Container: 14

	Amount Per 1 Tablet	Amount Per 2 Tablets
Ginkgo biloba (leaves) dried extract	60 mg†	120 mg†

†Daily value not established

Note: 28 servings per container in 56 count size.

Other Ingredients: Lactose, Microcrystalline Cellulose, Maize Starch, Hydroxypropyl Methylcellulose, Croscarmellose Sodium, Polyethylene Glycol, Magnesium Stearate, Silicon Dioxide, Artificial Color, Talc, Ferric Oxide, Dimethicone.
This product contains an all-natural herbal extract with no added salt or caffeine.

Directions: Adults: take one tablet two times a day with water (in the morning and evening). You may take up to 2 tablets 2 times a day with water. Results have been noted as early as 4 weeks when taken as directed. **Quanterra MENTAL SHARPNESS** is designed for continuous long-term use.

Warnings: Keep this and all herbal supplements out of the reach of children. As with any supplement, contact your doctor if you are currently taking prescription medicine, or are pregnant or nursing a baby.

How Supplied: Available in 28-tablet box or 56-tablet box.
Store in a cool, dry place.

*These statements have not been evaluated by the Food and Drug Administration. This product is not intended to diagnose, treat, cure, or prevent any disease.

Shown in Product Identification Guide, page 527

QUANTERRA™ Prostate
Saw Palmetto Herbal Supplement
[Quən-tər-ə]

Herbal Ingredient: 160 mg standardized saw palmetto extract.

Uses: Helps maintain healthy urinary flow and supports male prostate health.*

Supplement Facts
Serving Size: 1 Softgel
Servings Per Container: 28

	Amount Per Serving	% Daily Value
Saw Palmetto (Serenoa repens) berry dried extract	160 mg	†

†Daily value not established

Other Ingredients: Gelatin, Glycerol, Ferric Oxide. This product contains an all-natural herbal extract with no added sugar, starch, salt stimulants or caffeine.

Directions: For Male Adults: take one softgel two times a day with water (in the morning and evening with meals). Results have been noted as early as 4 weeks when taken as directed. **Quanterra PROSTATE** is designed for continuous long-term use.

Warnings: If you are receiving medical treatment, or taking medications for a prostate problem, or are experiencing symptoms of a prostate problem such as painful, frequent or difficult urination, consult your physician. Keep this and all herbal supplements out of the reach of children. As with any supplement, contact your doctor if you are currently taking prescription medicine.

How Supplied: Available in a 28-softgel box.
Store in a cool, dry place.

*These statements have not been evaluated by the Food and Drug Administration. This product is not intended to diagnose, treat, cure, or prevent any disease.

Shown in Product Identification Guide, page 527

Wellness International Network, Ltd.

5800 DEMOCRACY DRIVE
PLANO, TX 75024

Direct Inquiries to:
Director, Product Development
(972) 245-1097
FAX: (972) 389-3060

BIOLEAN®
Herbal & Amino Acid Food Supplement

Uses: BIOLEAN® is a unique combination of Chinese herbal extracts and pharmaceutical-grade amino acids specifically designed to help raise overall health, participate in individual life extension programs, and enhance athletic performance. It has been shown to be extremely effective in promoting the healthy loss of excess body fat while helping to maintain lean body mass and potent energy levels. BIOLEAN, when used as a daily nutritional supplement, has also been shown to stimulate immune function in individuals with blunted sympathetic nervous systems, especially overweight and obese persons. It acts as a positive stimulator to immune functions involved in protection from environmental and dietary carcinogens.
Components in BIOLEAN are known to cause fat loss through thermogenic activity and altered fuel metabolism resulting from sympathomimetic response to stimulation of beta receptors in adipose and muscle cells. The positive immune response, though not completely understood, is at least partially attributable to beta stimulation in adipocytes and the adaptogenic and tonifying activity of certain of the herbal extracts. This has been demonstrated in their long history of use in traditional Chinese herbal medicine as well as current scientific research which points to, among other possibilities, the extremely potent antioxidant properties found in some of the component plants, most notably in Green Tea and Schizandrae extracts. BIOLEAN may increase athletic performance and endurance through three pathways: 1) increased oxygen uptake in the lungs as a result of expanding bronchial passages; 2) enhanced mental acuity and response resulting from sympathetic nervous system stimulus; and 3) increasing the employment of fatty acids as fuel in muscle mitochondria while simultaneously sparing muscle glycogen and nitrogen.
The herbal extracts in BIOLEAN are produced in a unique and exclusive process which is proprietary to this product. Instead of creating extracts based on a set quantity of one particular active within many which may be present in

Continued on next page

Biolean—Cont.

any particular plant, BIOLEAN components are concentrated to maintain the natural and complete spectrum of biologically active factors, in the same ratio presented by the unprocessed plant.

Directions: Adults take one white capsule and one to three tablets with low-calorie food mid to late morning. If using BIOLEAN for the first time, take one capsule and one tablet on days 1 and 2, one capsule and two tablets on days 3 and 4, and one capsule and three tablets beginning day 5. Needs vary with the individual. Some persons may require less than three tablets daily or wish to spread the taking of the tablets throughout morning and early afternoon to achieve optimum results. Do not exceed recommended daily amounts. It is recommended that you drink at least eight glasses of water daily.

Warnings: Phenylketonurics: Contains Phenylalanine. Not for use by children. Consult your physician before using this product if you are taking asthma medications, appetite suppressing drugs, anti-depressants or cardiovascular medication. Do not consume if you are pregnant or lactating, or have high blood pressure, cardiovascular disease, arrhythmias, diabetes, prostatic hypertrophy, glaucoma, hyperthyroidism, psychosis or thyroid disease. If symptoms of allergy develop, discontinue use. It is recommended that you minimize your caffeine intake while consuming this product. Do not consume on the same day that you consume BIOLEAN Free.

Ingredients: *Capsules:* 400 mg. of the following mix: L-Phenylalanine, L-Tyrosine, L-Carnitine. *Tablets:* 650 mg. of the following herbal mix: Ma Huang, Green Tea, Schizandrae Berry, Rehmannia Root, Hawthorne Berry, Jujube Seed, Alisma Root, Angelicae Dahuricae Root, Epemidium, Poria Cocos, Rhizoma Rhei, Stephania Root, Angelicae Sinensis Root, Codonopsis Root, Eucommium Bark, Notoginseng Root.

How Supplied: One box contains 28 packets, one capsule and three tablets per packet.

BIOLEAN Accelerator®
Herbal & Amino Acid Formulation

Uses: BIOLEAN Accelerator® is a unique combination of Chinese herbal extracts and pharmaceutical grade amino acids specifically designed to complement both BIOLEAN® and BIOLEAN Free® by extending and accelerating their actions. BIOLEAN and BIOLEAN Free are, in the traditional view of Chinese herbal medicine, strong Yang blends. This means that they are energy or heat-producing at their core. The addition of the amino acids and certain of the herbal components lends a very definite restorative or Yin element, as well.

BIOLEAN Accelerator is a strong Yin herbal formula, intended to augment the lesser replenishing Yin elements of the other two herbal and amino acid supplements. Though the physiological actions of many herbs are complex and not totally understood, the formula in BIOLEAN Accelerator extends the adaptogenic, thermogenic, restorative and detoxifying results experienced with BIOLEAN and BIOLEAN Free, with an emphasis on the restorative and adaptogenic effects. The herbal formula is a combination of tonifiers traditionally used in China for the lungs, liver and kidneys.

Directions: For maximum effectiveness, use in conjunction with original BIOLEAN or BIOLEAN Free. (Do not consume BIOLEAN and BIOLEAN Free on the same day.) Take one tablet in the morning with original BIOLEAN or BIOLEAN Free. BIOLEAN Accelerator™ may also be taken in the afternoon with or without additional BIOLEAN or BIOLEAN Free if desired. Maximum absorption will be attained if taken with low-calorie food.

Warnings: Phenylketonurics: Contains Phenylalanine. Not for use by children. Consult your physician before using this product if you are taking appetite suppressing drugs or antidepressants, or if you are pregnant or lactating. If symptoms of allergy develop, discontinue use.

Ingredients: Each tablet contains 250 mg. herbal mix (Black Sesame Seed, Raw Chinese Foxglove Root, Chinese Wolfberry Fruit, Achyranthes Root, Cornelian Cherry Fruit, Chinese Yam, Eclipta Herb, Rose Hips, Privet Fruit, Mulberry Fruit-Spike, Polygonati Rhizome, Cooked Chinese Foxglove Root, Poria Cocos, Cuscuta Seed, Foxnut Seed, Alisma Rhizome, Moutan Bark, Phellodendron Bark, Anemarrhena Rhizome, Schisandra Berry, Royal Jelly), L-Tyrosine, L-Phenylalanine.

How Supplied: One bottle contains 56 tablets.

BIOLEAN Free®
Herbal & Amino Acid Food Supplement

Uses: BIOLEAN Free® is a strategic blend of herbs, spices, vitamins, minerals and amino acids specifically formulated to enhance fat utilization and energy production through various metabolic pathways. It has been shown to reduce body fat through its thermogenic effects and to enhance both physical and mental performance.

Thermogenesis refers to the body's ability to convert substrates such as proteins, fats and carbohydrates into heat energy. This is carried out most efficiently in the Brown Adipose Tissue of our body which uses fatty acids as its preferred fuel. Other fat cells, namely White Adipose Tissue, are concerned primarily with the storage of fat rather than its conversion to energy. The thermogenic pathway is complex and relies upon a series of reactions to occur. BIOLEAN Free utilizes many compounds which act at various locations in this pathway to ensure the maximum efficiency of the thermogenic process. Quebracho is one of these very special compounds. This South American plant contains quebrachine, aspidiospermine and other alkaloids that possess the ability to block alpha-2 adrenergic receptors in the body. This produces an enhanced sympathetic nervous system effect which, in turn, increases lipolysis (fat breakdown) within fat cells. The fatty acids released by this process can then be transported into the mitochondria to be used as a fuel. Ginger, cinnamon, horseradish, turmeric, cayenne and mustard are spices that stimulate thermogenesis in different ways. Some stimulate lipid mobilization in adipose tissue; others raise the resting metabolic rate; and some increase cAMP levels by inducing more beta receptors on fat cells and by increasing the concentration of adenylate cyclase. cAMP increases the breakdown of triglycerides to free fatty acids which are later used as fuel by the mitochondria in the cell. Methylxanthines (such as those found in green tea and yerba maté) also increase cAMP levels, but do this by inhibiting the enzyme, phosphodiesterase. These compounds have been noted to increase mental alertness, improve vitality, satisfy the appetite and increase energy. In addition to its methylxanthine content, green tea has recently been shown to possess strong antioxidant properties. Yerba maté is a plant that has been shown to produce the positive effects above without causing the insomnia seen with other methylxanthine-containing plants (such as coffee and kola nut). BIOLEAN Free also contains vitamin B-3, vitamin B-6, chromium and vanadium, which aid in the proper metabolism of fats, proteins and carbohydrates. L-tyrosine also aids in metabolism and promotes satiety through hypothalamic release of CCK. Methionine is a precursor of L-carnitine which aids in the transport of fatty acids into the mitochondria for thermogenesis. Other herbs have been utilized in BIOLEAN Free. Ginseng and ho shou wu possess adaptogenic properties. Adaptogens help the body adapt to physiological and environmental stresses. Ginseng accomplishes this through its stabilizing effect on the hypothalamic-pituitary-adrenal-sympathetic nervous system. It can mediate an increased adrenal response to stress.

Ho shou wu has a stabilizing effect on the endocrine system and has restorative properties. It is also an antioxidant with a high flavonoid content. *Centella asiatica* contains asiaticoside and has been shown to increase activity levels and ease the body's ability to overcome fatigue when taken with ginseng and cayenne. Individually, *centella* has been shown to increase memory and mental acuity in studies abroad. Uva ursi contains the glycoside arbutin and promotes urinary health and body strength through its purifying effects. Ginkgo biloba is a tree whose leaves have been used for centuries as an herbal medicine. It contains flavonoids and is therefore a strong antioxidant. It reduces the tendency of platelets to stick together by inhibiting Platelet Activating Factor. It has been shown to increase blood flow to the heart, brain and other organs.

Directions: Adults (18 years and older) may take 4 caplets in the mid to late morning with a low-calorie food. Needs may vary with each individual. Some persons may require less than 4 caplets, or may prefer taking 3 caplets mid morning and 1 additional caplet mid afternoon to achieve optimum results. Do not exceed recommended daily amounts. It is recommended that you drink at least eight glasses of water daily.

Warnings: Not for use by children, pregnant women or lactating women. Consult your physician before using this product if you are taking appetite suppressing drugs or cardiovascular medication. Consult your physician if you have hypertension, heart disease, arrhythmias, prostatic hypertrophy, glaucoma, liver disease, renal disease or diabetes. Do not use if you have hyperthyroidism, psychosis, Parkinson's Disease, or are taking Monoamine oxidase inhibitors. BIOLEAN Free should not be taken on the same day as original BIOLEAN®. It is recommended that you minimize your caffeine intake while consuming this product. If allergic symptoms develop, discontinue use. Store in a cool, dry place. Keep out of reach of children.

Ingredients: Each caplet contains the following: Standardized botanical extracts containing 720 mg of the following mixture: Green Tea, Yerba Maté, Korean Ginseng, Uva Ursi, Quebracho. Non-irradiated pure herbs and spices containing 360 mg of the following mixture: Jamaican Ginger, Ceylon Cinnamon, Chinese Horseradish, Alleppy Turmeric, Nigerian Cayenne, English Mustard, *Centella Asiatica,* Ho Shou Wu, Ginkgo Biloba. Also included are 125 mg of L-Tyrosine, 25 mg of Methionine, 25 mg of Potassium (citrate), 10 mg of Vitamin B-3, 4 mg of Vitamin B-6, 100 mcg of Chromium Chelavite™, 100 mcg of Vanadium.

How Supplied: One box contains 28 packets, four tablets per packet.

BIOLEAN LipoTrim®
All-Natural Dietary Supplement

Uses: LipoTrim® is a highly active, synergistic combination of garcinia cambogia extract and chromium polynicotinate specifically created for use with the other products in the BIOLEAN® System. The method of action is by inhibition of lipogenesis and regulation of blood glucose levels. Serum glucose derived from dietary carbohydrates and not immediately converted to energy or glycogen tends to be converted into fat stores and cholesterol. In individuals with excess body fat stores or slow basal metabolism, this tendency is thought to be higher. The garcinia cambogia extract present in LipoTrim is verified by HPLC analysis to be no less that 50%(-) hydroxycitrate (HCA). HCA inhibits ATP-citrate lyase which retards Acetyl CoA synthesis, severely restricting conversion of excess glucose into fatty acids and cholesterol. Animal studies have shown a post-meal fatty acid synthesis reduction of 40–80% for an 8–12 hour period. When glucose to fat/cholesterol conversion is retarded, glycogen conversion continues, increasing liver stores and causing satiety signals to be sent to the brain resulting in appetite suppression. In situations of intense physical exercise, increased glycogen stores have been shown to result in enhanced endurance and recovery. By restricting the activity of insulin, chromium has been shown to exhibit a regulating effect on blood glucose levels thus extending the benefits of HCA.

Directions: As a dietary supplement, take one capsule three times daily, 30 minutes before each meal. LipoTrim should be used in conjunction with a healthy diet and exercise plan.

Warnings: Do not consume if you are pregnant or lactating. Not for use by young children. Consult your physician before using this product if your diet consists of less than 1,000 calories per day.

Ingredients: CitriMax™* (garcinia cambogia), ChromeMate®* (chromium polynicotinate).

How Supplied: One bottle contains 84, easy-to-swallow capsules.

---

*CitriMax™ is a trademark of Inter-Health.
ChromeMate® is a registered trademark of InterHealth.

FOOD FOR THOUGHT™
Choline-Enriched Nutritional Drink

Uses: By utilizing scientifically established "smart nutrients", Food For Thought™ is a great-tasting citrus beverage ideal for work, school or anytime peak mental performance is desired.

Choline, a member of the B-complex family, is determined to be one of the few substances that possesses the ability to penetrate the blood-brain barrier—a protectant of the brain from the onslaught of chemicals taken into the body each day—and go directly into the brain cells to produce acetylcholine.

The most abundant neurotransmitter in the body, acetylcholine is the primary neurotransmitter between neurons and muscles. It is vital because of its role in motor behavior (muscular movement) and memory. Acetylcholine helps control muscle tone, learning, and primitive drives and emotions, while also controlling the release of the pituitary hormone vasopressin—which is involved in learning and in the regulation of urine output. Studies show that low levels of acetylcholine can contribute to lack of concentration and forgetfulness, and may interfere with sleep patterns.

Food For Thought further enhances its effectiveness through the utilization of essential vitamins—required for promoting the synthesis of brain neurotransmitters—with a unique blend of minerals. The brain uses vitamins B3 and B6 to convert the amino acid L-tryptophan into the mood- and sleep-regulating neurotransmitter serotonin, while vitamins B1, B5, B6, and C and the minerals zinc and calcium are required for the production of acetylcholine.

Directions: Add 6 ounces of chilled water or fruit juice to one packet of mix. Stir briskly. Consume 1–2 times per day. Keep in a cool, dry place. For maximum results, combine this product with one serving of Winrgy™.

Warnings: Not for use by children, pregnant or lactating women. Persons taking medications should seek medical advice before taking this product. Persons with ulcers or a history of ulcers should consult their physician before using a choline supplement. Do not consume more than four servings per day. Avoid the use of antacids containing aluminum with this product.

Ingredients: Fructose, Choline Bitartrate, Calcium Pantothenate, Natural Flavor, Glycine, Ascorbic Acid, Vitamin E Acetate, Niacinamide, Lysine, Silicon Dioxide, Zinc Gluconate, Chromium Aspartate, Niacin, Magnesium Gluconate, Pyridoxine Hydrochloride, Thiamin Mononitrate, Riboflavin, Copper Gluconate, Vitamin B12.

How Supplied: One box contains 28 packets of drink mix. Serving size equals one packet.

STEPHAN™ Clarity
Nutritional Supplement

Uses: STEPHAN™ Clarity, designed for use by both men and women, contains selected tissue proteins in the form of nutrients important to memory and concentration.

This is achieved by utilizing such ingredients as lecithin and glutamic acid. Lecithin is a popular supplement widely embraced for the treatment and prevention of memory loss. Known for properties that have been scientifically proven to increase the firing of neurons in the nervous system, glutamic acid is an amino acid which influences the body by serving as brain fuel. It also metabolizes sugars and fats, as well as detoxifies.

Ginkgo biloba, a third primary ingredient in STEPHAN™ Clarity, is a special

Continued on next page

Stephan Clarity—Cont.

additive which increases the flow of blood to the brain and is noted for improving concentration and learning ability. Recently, a study published in the *Journal of the American Medical Association* demonstrated that ginkgo biloba extract improves mental performance in dementias for individuals with Alzheimer's disease and multi-infarct dementia. It was also reported to stabilize and – in 20% of the cases – improve the subjects' functioning for periods of six months to a year.

Together with the support of carefully selected vitamins, minerals, amino acids, and herbs, STEPHAN™ Clarity is a natural and effective way to better one's health.

Directions: Take one to two capsules per day.

Warnings: Phenylketonurics: Contains Phenylalanine.

Ingredients: Lecithin, Bee Pollen, Glutamic Acid, Vitamin C, Ribonucleic Acid, Ginkgo Biloba (as 8:1 extract), Aspartic Acid, Vitamin E, Vitamin B-3, Leucine, Arginine, Lysine, Phenylalanine, Serine, Valine, Proline, Isoleucine, Alanine, Glycine, Threonine, Tyrosine, Vitamin B-5, Vitamin B-1, Histidine, Methionine, Cysteine, Adenosine Triphosphate, Vitamin B-6, Vitamin B-2, Vitamin A, Folic Acid, Biotin, Vitamin D-3, Vitamin B-12.

How Supplied: One bottle contains 60 easy-to-swallow capsules.

DHEA Plus™
Pharmaceutical-Grade Formulation

Uses: By utilizing the latest and most advanced breakthrough applications in age management, DHEA Plus™ uniquely combines dehydroepiandrosterone (DHEA), Bioperine® and ginkgo biloba leaf to safely and effectively aid the body.

These age management factors are mainly attributed to the properties of DHEA, a natural substance obtained from the barbasco root, also known as Mexican Wild Yam, which is synthesized in a pharmaceutical laboratory to be utilized for specific health applications. Once supplemental DHEA is orally consumed, it is quickly absorbed into the bloodstream through the intestines and binds to a sulfate compound which creates DHEA-S. DHEA-S is the ultimate substance for which the body uses to manufacture hormones. Natural DHEA levels, abundant in the bloodstream and present at an even higher level in the tissues of the brain, are known to decline with age in both sexes. Scientific research proves that adequate levels of DHEA in the body can actually slow the aging process. Further studies have shown that it often prevents, improves

and, many times, reverses conditions such as cancer, heart disease, memory loss, obesity and osteoporosis.

Bioperine, a pure piperine extract, enhances the body's natural thermogenic activity and is another important ingredient in DHEA Plus. Thermogenesis is the metabolic process that generates energy at the cellular level. While thermogenesis plays an integral role in our body's ability to properly utilize daily foods and nutrients in the body, it also sets in motion the mechanisms that lead to digestion and subsequent gastrointestinal absorption.

Known for possessing antioxidant activity, or flavonoid effects, ginkgo biloba proves to decrease platelet aggregation and increase vasodilation which appears to extend blood flow to the peripheral arteries and the brain. Some improvement in cognitive abilities has been noted as well as inhibition of lipid peroxidation, thereby stabilizing the cell wall against free-radical attack.

Directions: Adults take one capsule daily with food.

Warnings: This product should only be consumed by adults and is not intended for use by children. Do not consume if you are pregnant or lactating. Consult your physician before using this product if you are taking prescription medications. Persons with a history of prostate cancer should seek medical advice before using this product.

Ingredients: Dehydroepiandrosterone (DHEA), Bioperine*, Ginkgo Biloba.

How Supplied: One bottle contains 60 capsules.

---

*Bioperine is a registered trademark of Sabinsa Corporation.

MASS APPEAL™
Amino Acid & Mineral Workout Supplement

Uses: Utilizing natural compounds which mimic the beneficial effects of anabolic steroids, Mass Appeal™ is specifically formulated to enhance athletic performance without the harmful side effects of steroids.

Among Mass Appeal's scientifically researched and proven ingredients is creatine, a naturally occurring substance which functions as a storage molecule for high-energy phosphate – the ultimate source of muscular energy known as adenosine triphosphate, or ATP. More than 95 percent of the body's total amount of creatine is contained within the muscles, with type II muscle fibers (fibers that generate large amounts of force) possessing greater initial levels and higher rates of utilization. Unlike other artificial aids used to enhance performance, creatine monohydrate saturates the muscle cells and causes a muscle "cell volumizing" effect by beneficially forcing water molecules inside the mus-

cle cell. This promotes an increase in muscle growth by helping muscles form new proteins faster while slowing down the destructive breakdown of muscle cells during exercise. Studies show that creatine loading not only improves performance during short-duration, high intensity and intermittent exercises, but it accelerates energy recovery and reduces muscle fatigue by reducing lactic acid build-up as well.

Found in high concentrations within muscle cells and proteins throughout the body, the branched chain amino acids (BCAAs) L-leucine, L-valine and L-isoleucine are also incorporated into Mass Appeal's scientifically engineered formulation. BCAAs increase protein synthesis and can be oxidized inside muscle cells as ATP, a protein-sparing effect which indirectly increases anabolism by reducing the muscle's need to burn its own proteins during bodybuilding or strenuous exercise. When dietary intake of these amino acids is inadequate, muscle protein is broken down into its individual amino acid constituents and utilized in other essential metabolic reactions within the body. Through supplementation, the catabolic breakdown of muscle can be minimized and the muscle tissue preserved.

Alpha-ketoglutaric acid and the amino acid L-glutamine also protect against muscle catabolism by assisting muscle protein synthesis and preserving the body's natural stores of glutamine in the muscle.

Another major contributor to the Mass Appeal™ formulation is the amino acid inosine. By increasing hemoglobin's affinity for binding oxygen within red blood cells, inosine supplementation enables red blood cells to carry more oxygen as they travel from the lungs to the muscles.

Vanadyl sulfate, known for its vasodilator effects, has been shown to markedly increase the blood flow to muscle cells. Researchers also believe that this mineral not only contributes to increased efficiency in the metabolic pathways controlled by the body's insulin, but also triggers certain glucose transporters much in the same way insulin does. This results in increased glucose transport into the muscle tissue, increased glycogen storage, and decreases the breakdown of muscle protein as an energy source.

Directions: Adults (18 years and older) may take a loading dose of 3 packets in the morning and 2 packets in the late afternoon for one week. This dose may be repeated every three months. Following one week of the loading dose, begin the maintenance dose of 1 packet daily two hours after exercise. Needs may vary with each individual.

For individuals desiring enhanced effects, increase the loading dose to 3 to 4 packets, three times per day (morning, afternoon and evening). Following one week of this enhanced loading dose, begin the enhanced maintenance dose of 2 packets in the morning and 2 packets in the late afternoon. It is recommended that one maintain a low-fat, high-protein diet; drink at least eight glasses of water per day; and engage in 30 to 60 minutes of aerobic and anaerobic exercise three to four times per week. For optimal effects, take in conjunction with Phyto-Vite®, Pro-Xtreme™ and Sure2Endure™.

Warning: Not for use by children, pregnant women or lactating women. Consult your physician before using this product if you have any medical conditions. Do not take if you have kidney disease, muscle disease or are on a protein-restricted diet. Discontinue immediately if allergic symptoms develop. Keep out of the reach of children. Store in a cool, dry place.

Active Ingredients: Creatine Monohydrate (2,500 mg), L-Glutamine (150 mg), Phosphate-Bonded Inosine (300 mg), Vanadyl Sulfate (5 mg), and Branched Chain Amino Acid Complex with Keto Analogs (300 mg).

How Supplied: One box contains 28 packets, four tablets per packet.

PRO-XTREME™
Nutritional Meal Replacement Drink

Uses: The need for protein in the human diet has been increasingly studied, especially in the last decade. As a result of this research, several factors regarding the optimal daily requirements and sources of protein have become very clear. Even the current government published RDIs, which are based solely on minimal needs for survival, have increased to .6–.8 grams per kilogram of body weight per day.

Current clinical findings however indicate that an RDI necessary to maintain optimum health for even a sedentary adult are closer to double that. Circumstances including illness, fat-loss diets, regular exercise, accelerated adolescent growth, or chronic mental or emotional stress indicate requirements 2–3 times that. Competitive or strength athletes, post surgical patients or any situation causing wasting disease such as chemotherapy, HIV, burn trauma or radiation therapy can increase the metabolic need for protein by a factor of up to 6 times the official government RDIs.

Furthermore, these figures represent protein which has been absorbed and made available to the tissues of the body and *not* merely that which has been consumed. This is a distinction current clinical research has recognized as *critical* to proper understanding of the need for protein in the human diet.

Before protein can be absorbed and utilized it must first be digested. Following digestion the free amino acids and di and tripeptides that result from protein breakdown are absorbed at the surface of the small intestine. The process of digestion and absorption requires several steps and is most efficient in the upper portion or proximal section of the jejunum (small intestine). In order for absorption of dietary protein to occur, it must first be reduced from larger oligo and polypeptides to di and tripeptides, the smallest protein fragments consisting of only two or three peptide-bonded amino acids, and free amino acids. Di and tripeptides have been clearly shown to be preferential over free forms. This process must occur fast enough and at a rate high enough to take advantage of the proximal transporters, those that specialize in di and tripeptides and which are in abundance only in this short section of upper intestinal bowel. Once protein has passed this lumenal area, relatively no further protein breakdown or absorption occurs. The balance moves on relatively unchanged into the colon, where it is definitely a negative health factor causing minimal gas and gastrointestinal distress, and when experienced chronically, can lead to colon disease and malignancy. It is now generally believed to be the number one factor responsible for the world's highest rate of colon cancer experienced in the U.S.

Pro-Xtreme™ is specifically engineered based on a new profile for protein in optimum human metabolism arising from these new clinical findings. With an exceptionally high di and tripeptide content of 40 percent, Pro-Xtreme™ not only promotes increased nitrogen retention—thereby minimizing the negative effects of increased protein intake or reduced caloric intake—but it works in harmony with natural gastrointestinal activity to produce maximum absorption as well.

Because of the fat content and the density of the bolus, meals containing tissue-source protein are released from the stomach and travel through the intestines at a rate which is naturally slower and more conducive to efficient digestion and absorption. The problems begin when too much tissue protein is consumed or the process of digestion and absorption is incomplete. It is estimated that at best only 30–35% of the protein consumed in an average protein-containing meal is absorbed allowing the balance of now detrimental undigested protein to pass into the colon.

In the case of liquid protein supplements, the problem is one not only of excessive amounts of protein being consumed but also the speed at which the bolus travels throughout the jejunum. Liquid meals, especially those with insufficient soluble fiber, have decreased transit time, leaving less time for digestion and absorption. Consequently, even in individuals with normal gastrointestinal function, liquid forms of whole proteins generally result in equally incomplete and oftentimes less absorption than their tissue food counterparts.

Pro-Xtreme™ utilizes sequentially hydrolyzed whey protein isolates of the highest quality to insure complete and rapid absorption of the highest levels of essential and branched-chain amino acids (BCAAs) in the preferred smallest peptide bonded form. These features, coupled with its industry-leading lowest average molecular weight, soluble-fiber content and delicious vanilla-cappuccino flavor, offer a primary source of protein that may be used any time a protein supplement is desired.

The combination and sequencing of amino acids in whey protein also results in increased tissue storage of glutathione, a stable tripeptide whose antioxidant activity is known to improve immune function. And, although whey protein naturally contains 5 to 7 percent of glutamine, the formula for Pro-Xtreme™ incorporates additional gram amounts of L-glutamine to its list of highly evolved ingredients as well. This extra step is designed to promote anticatabolic effects in skeletal muscle while focusing on gastrointestinal and immune function improvement. Glutamine and the critical BCAA leucine are deemed indispensable for the healthy functioning of other tissues and metabolic processes. By maintaining a rich supply of BCAAs, Pro-Xtreme™ proves protein sparing within muscle and offers the highest biological value possible.

Pro-Xtreme™ is formulated specifically for use with the other products in the BIOLEAN® System.

Directions: Add 1 packet (40 grams) Pro-Xtreme™ to 1 cup (8 ounces) cold water and stir. There is no need for blending or shaking. Pro-Xtreme™ may also be mixed with lowfat or non-fat milk, milk substitutes or blended with ice for a delicious and nourishing dessert.

Warning: Phenylketonurics: Contains phenylalanine.

Ingredients: Hydrolyzed Whey Protein Isolate, Medium Chain Triglycerides, Maltodextrin, Natural Flavorings, Fructose, Psyllium Fiber, Glutamine, Dutch Process Cocoa, Aspartame.

How Supplied: One box contains 14 packets. Serving size equals one packet.

SATIETE™
Herbal and Amino Acid Supplement

Uses: With its synergistic blend of herbs and amino acids, Satiete™ addresses many of today's health concerns by ensuring maximum nutritional support.

One such ingredient is 5-HTP (5-Hydroxytryptophan). 5-HTP is an amino acid derivative and the immediate precursor to serotonin, a neurotransmitter involved in regulating mood, sleep, appetite, energy level and sensitivity to pain. Like drugs known as selective serotonin reuptake inhibitors (SSRI's), 5-HTP enhances the activity of serotonin, a hormone produced by the brain that is involved in mood, sleep, and appetite. Low levels of serotonin are associated with

Continued on next page

Satiete—Cont.

depression, anxiety, and sleep disorders. SSRI's prevent the brain cells from using up serotonin too quickly, thereby causing a deficiency. 5-HTP increases the cell's production of serotonin, which boosts serotonin levels.

L-5-HTP is a standardized extract of Griffonia simplicifolia (containing greater than 95% anhydrous 5-HTP), and the focus of an ABC Prime Time Live report that aired on June 17, 1998. The news segment explored claims that 5-HTP can help alleviate the effects of a variety of conditions, including depression, anxiety, insomnia, and obesity.

The diverse physiological functions of serotonin in the body include actions as a neurotransmitter, a regulator of smooth muscle function in the cardiovascular and gastrointestinal system, and a regulator of platelet function. Serotonin is involved in numerous central nervous system actions such as regulating mood, sleep and appetite. In the gastrointestinal system, serotonin stimulates gastric motility. Serotonin also stimulates platelet aggregation.

As a precursor to serotonin, 5-HTP helps to normalize serotonin activity in the body. Considerable research has been conducted regarding the activity of 5-HTP. Some of the clinical studies are summarized below:

Mood—Dysregulation of serotonin metabolism in the central nervous system has been shown to affect mood. 5-HTP helps to normalize serotonin levels and, thereby, positively affect mood. In a double-blind study using objective assessments of mood, researchers in Zurich reported significant improvements in mood with 5-HTP. Likewise, in a double-blind, multi-center study in Germany, researchers reported significant improvements in both objective and self-assessment indices of mood.

Sleep—Many studies have shown that depletion of serotonin results in insomnia, which is reversed by administration of 5-HTP. Likewise, Soulairac and Lambinet reported that 100 mg of 5-HTP resulted in significant improvement for people who complained of trouble sleeping. Futhermore, serotonin is metabolized to the hormone melatonin, which is known to help regulate the sleep cycle; by increasing serotonin levels with 5-HTP, melatonin levels are also increased.

Appetite—Food intake is thought to suppress appetite through the production of serotonin from the amino acid tryptophan. Because it is an intermediary in the conversion process of tryptophan to serotonin, 5-HTP may reduce appetite in a similar manner as food intake, but without the calories. In a recent double-blind placebo-controlled study, subjects taking 5-HTP lost significant weight compared to control subjects. A reduction in carbohydrate intake and early satiety were seen in the 5-HTP group.

Another key ingredient in the Satiete formulation is Gymnema sylvestre, whose active ingredient "gymnemic acid" affects the taste buds in the oral cavity as the acid prevents the taste buds from being activated by any sugar molecules in the food; and the absorptive surface of the intestines where the acid prevents the intestine from absorbing sugar molecules. Practically speaking, this creates a reduced appetite for sweet tasting food, as well as reducing the metabolic effect of sugar by reducing its digestion in the intestines thus reducing the blood sugar level. In experimental and clinical trials, Gymnema sylvestre has been successful in treating both insulin-dependent and non-insulin dependent diabetics without reducing the blood sugar level to below the normal blood sugar levels, an effect seen with the use of insulin oral hypoglycemic sulphony lurea compounds. Due to its non-toxic nature and sweetness-suppression activity, Gymnema sylvestre can play a role in treating conditions caused by excessive sugar intake. Not only may diabetics benefit from it, conditions like obesity, hypoglycemia, anemia and osteoporosis can also be treated using Gymnema sylvestre.

Vanadyl sulfate, because of its insulin-like properties and its ability to improve cell responsiveness, is being used by progressive alternative physicians and natural healers to treat diabetes. Studies show that vanadyl is very effective in normalizing blood sugar levels and controlling conditions such as insulin resistance, or Type II diabetes.

Magnesium, malic acid and St. John's Wort are also combined in Satiete's proven formulation. Magnesium is a key mineral cofactor for many anaerobic as well as aerobic reactions that generate energy, and has an oxygen-sparing effect. It is essential for the cell's mitochondria "powerhouses" to function normally, being involved in both the production and utilization of ATP.

Malic Acid has an oxygen-sparing effect and there are a number of indications that malic acid is a very critical molecule in controlling mitochondrial function. Malate is a source of energy from the Krebs cycle and is the only metabolite of the cycle which falls in concentration during exhaustive physical activity. Depletion of malate has also been linked to physical exhaustion. By giving malic acid and magnesium as dietary supplements, flexibility to use aerobic and anaerobic energy sources can be enhanced and energy production can be boosted. Lab studies show that many patients with fibromyalgia (or with chronic fatigue) have low magnesium levels. Magnesium supplementation enhances the treatment of both conditions. Its benefits appear to result, at least in part, from its positive impact on serotonin function.

Combining 5-HTP with St. John's Wort Extract (0.3% hypericin context), malic acid, and magnesium, is part of an overall fibromyalgia treatment plan providing excellent results, due in large measure to its improvement of sleep quality and mood.

Directions: Start by taking one hypoallergenic tablet three times per day 30 to 60 minutes before meals. If needed after two weeks of use, increase the dosage to two tablets, three times per day. Do not exceed nine tablets daily without medical supervision.

Warning: If you are taking MAO inhibitor drugs, tricyclic antidepressants, SSRI antidepressants (Prozac, Paxil, Zoloft) or prescription diet drugs, do not take this product without medical supervision. If you suffer from liver or kidney disease, serious gastrointestinal disorders or carcinoid syndrome, do not take this product without medical supervision. If gastrointestinal upset develops and persists, reduce dosage, take only with large meals or discontinue use. As with any product, pregnant or lactating women should first consult their doctor.

Ingredients: Three enteric-coated tablets contain: 150 mg of Griffonia Seed Extract (95% minimum naturally occurring L-5HTP; 99 mg of Gymnema Sylvestre; 1980 mcg of Vanadyl Sulfate; 19.5 mg of Vitamin B-2, 19.5 mg of Niacinamide; 165 mg of Magnesium (Oxide); 19.5 mg of Vitamin B-1; 19.5 mg of Vitamin B-6; 300 mg of Malic Acid; 150 mg of St. John's Wort Extract (0.3% hypericin content); 60 mg of Ginkgo Biloba Extract (24% ginkgo flavonglycosides and 6% bilobalides); 300 mcg of Vitamin B-12; and 99 mcg of Folic Acid.

How Supplied: One bottle contains 84 tablets.

STEPHAN™ Elasticity Nutritional Supplement

Uses: A nutritional food supplement for men and women, STEPHAN™ Elasticity contains a scientifically balanced mixture of specific tissue proteins established as important for skin tone and texture.

Utilizing such scientifically respected ingredients as vitamin A and selenium, STEPHAN™ Elasticity is also supported by various other vitamins, minerals and amino acids dedicated to epidermal appearance.

Due to its antioxidant properties, vitamin A has been dubbed the "skin vitamin." It is commonly used as a means of preventing premature aging of the skin. In addition, synthetic derivatives of vitamin A are often used to treat acne and psoriasis.

Selenium is also considered beneficial to the skin. It was recently reported that low blood selenium in the context of low blood vitamin A increases the risk for certain types of skin cancer.

Directions: Take one capsule per day.

Warning: Phenylketonurics: Contains Phenylalanine.

Ingredients: Equisetum Arvense, Protein Isolates (Alanine, Arginine, Aspartic Acid, Cysteine, Glutamic Acid, Glycine,

Histidine, Isoleucine, Leucine, Lysine, Methionine, Phenylalanine, Proline, Serine, Threonine, Tyrosine, Valine), Fucus, Vitamine E (Dl-Alpha), Zinc (Amino Acid Chelate), Vitamin C, Ribonucleic Acid, Calcium (Amino Acid Chelate), Magnesium (Amino Acid Chelate), Iron (Amino Acid Chelate), Manganese (Amino Acid Chelate), Selenium (Amino Acid Chelate), Chromium (Amino Acid Chelate), Adenosine Triphosphate, Vitamin A (Acetate).

How Supplied: One bottle contains 60 easy-to-swallow capsules.

STEPHAN™ Elixir
Nutritional Supplement

Uses: Formulated with an exclusive blend of specific proteins, STEPHAN™ Elixir is ideal for both men and women. These tissue proteins are supported by vitamins, minerals, amino acids and herbs recognized as important for general health and well-being.

Among the scientifically researched and proven ingredients utilized in STEPHAN™ Elixir are vitamin E and cysteine. Vitamin E protects against the ravages of aging in several ways. It is essential for the normal functioning of the body and is especially important for normal neurological functions in humans. It also serves as a potent antioxidant and has been dubbed the body's "first line of defense" against free-radical attack by helping to guard against free radicals, the type of cellular damage that has been linked to the initiation of cancer and heart disease.

Cysteine has also been found to inactivate free radicals and thus protect and preserve the cells. This sulfur-containing amino acid is a precursor of glutathione, a tripeptide, that is claimed to safeguard the body against various toxins and pollutants, therefore extending the life span.

Directions: Take one capsule per day.

Warnings: Phenylketonurics: Contains Phenylalanine.

Ingredient: Soya Isolate (Alanine, Arginine, Aspartic Acid, Cysteine, Glutamic Acid, Glycine, Histidine, Isoleucine, Leucine, Lysine, Methionine, Phenylalanine, Proline, Serine, Threonine, Tyrosine, Valine), Bee Pollen, Vitamin C, Malic Acid, Ginkgo Biloba (8:1 extract), Citric Acid, Ribonucleic Acid, Vitamin E, Vitamin B-3, Zinc (Amino Acid Chelate), Iron (Amino Acid Chelate), Calcium Pantothenate, Vitamin B-1, Vitamin B-5, Adenosine Triphosphate, Vitamin B-6, Vitamin B-2, Vitamin A, Folic Acid, Selenium (Amino Acid Chelate), Biotin, Vitamin D-3, Vitamin B-12.

How Supplied: One bottle contains 60 easy-to-swallow capsules.

STEPHAN™ Essential
Nutritional Supplement

Uses: STEPHAN™ Essential is a nutritional food supplement which contains specific tissue proteins supported by vitamins, minerals, herbs and amino acids that are proactive to cardiovascular and circulatory management. L-carnitine, vitamin E and linoleic acid are only some of these very important components.

Scientifically researched and a major contributor to the effects of STEPHAN™ Essential, L-carnitine is necessary for the transport of long-chain fatty acids into the mitochondria, the metabolic furnaces of the cells. These fatty acids prove a major source for the production of energy in the heart and skeletal muscles, structures that are particularly vulnerable to L-carnitine deficiency. Appropriate levels of L-carnitine in the body have been shown to protect against cardiovascular disease, muscle disease, diabetes and kidney disease.

While vitamin E has proven beneficial in serving to boost the immune system and protect against cardiovascular disease, it has also been established as an important therapy for disorders related to neurologic symptoms. Omega 3–Oil, another important addition to STEPHAN™ Essential, can lower serum cholesterol levels and decrease platelet stickiness, proving beneficial in the prevention of coronary heart disease.

STEPHAN™ Essential may be consumed by both men and women.

Directions: Take one to two capsules per day.

Warnings: Phenylketonurics: Contains Phenylalanine.

Ingredients: Bee Pollen, L-Carnitine, Omega 3 Oil, Glutamic Acid, Ribonucleic Acid, Aspartic Acid, Vitamin E, Leucine, Arginine, Lysine, Magnesium (Amino Acid Chelate), Phenylalanine, Serine, Valine, Proline, Isoleucine, Alanine, Glycine, Threonine, Tyrosine, Histidine, Methionine, Cysteine, Adenosine Triphosphate, Selenium (Amino Acid Chelate).

How Supplied: One bottle contains 60 easy-to-swallow capsules.

STEPHAN™ Feminine
Nutritional Supplement

Uses: Specifically designed for women, STEPHAN™ Feminine contains selected tissue proteins supported by vitamins, minerals and amino acids regarded as important to the ever-changing female body. This is achieved through such scientifically researched ingredients as magnesium and boron.

STEPHAN™ Feminine utilizes magnesium as an important ingredient responsible for regulating the flow of calcium between cells. Studies reveal that women with high-calcium diets report fewer PMS symptoms including less irritability and depression, as well as fewer headaches, backaches and cramps. Magnesium thus ensures individuals are receiving maximum benefits from calcium intake.

Researchers also report many promising results on the effects of dietary boron. Conclusions show that supplementary boron markedly reduces the excretion of both calcium and magnesium while increasing production of an active form of estrogen and testosterone.

Directions: Take one to two capsules per day.

Warnings: Phenylketonurics: Contains Phenylalanine.

Ingredients: Magnesium Oxide, Glutamic Acid, Ribonucleic Acid, Aspartic Acid, Vitamin E, Leucine, Arginine, Lysine, Phenylalanine, Serine, Valine, Proline, Isoleucine, Alanine, Glycine, Threonine, Tyrosine, Histidine, Methionine, Cysteine, Boron (Amino Acid Chelate), Adenosine Triphosphate, Selenium.

How Supplied: One bottle contains 60 easy-to-swallow capsules.

STEPHAN™ Flexibility
Nutritional Supplement

Uses: A nutritional supplement for both men and women, STEPHAN™ Flexibility is rich with exclusive proteins which are supported by vitamins, minerals and amino acids recognized as beneficial to the health of joint and soft tissues.

Glycine, an amino acid, is one very significant ingredient utilized in STEPHAN™ Flexibility. In a pilot study investigating the possibility of glycine's effect on spastic control, a 25% improvement was noted on subjects with chronic multiple sclerosis. Furthermore, all patients benefited to some degree, and no toxicity or other adverse side effects were noted.

Another important amino acid in STEPHAN Flexibility is L-histidine. Reports suggest that supplementary L-histidine may actually boost the activity of suppressor T cells. Because rheumatoid arthritis is one of the many autoimmune diseases in which T-cell activity is subnormal, these conclusions lend further support that L-histidine may prove beneficial in its treatment.

Vitamin E can also be found in STEPHAN Flexibility because of its ability to relieve muscular cramps. According to one popular study, supplemental vitamin E caused remarkable relief from persistent nocturnal leg and foot cramps in 82% of the 125 patients tested.

Directions: Take one to two capsules per day.

Warnings: Phenylketonurics: Contains Phenylalanine.

Ingredients: Vitamin C, Ribonucleic Acid, Vitamin E, Vitamin B-3, Glutamic Acid, Zinc (Amino Acid Chelate), Calcium (Amino Acid Chelate), Aspartic Acid, Bee Pollen, Leucine, Arginine, Lysine, Vitamin B-5, Vitamin B-1, Phenylalanine,

Continued on next page

Stephan Flexibility—Cont.

Serine, Valine, Proline, Isoleucine, Alanine, Glycine, Threonine, Tyrosine, Histidine, Cysteine, Adenosine Triphosphate, Vitamin B-6, Boron (Amino Acid Chelate), Vitamin B-2, Methionine, Vitamin A, Folic Acid, Selenium (Amino Acid Chelate), Biotin, Vitamin D-3, Vitamin B-12.

How Supplied: One bottle contains 60 easy-to-swallow capsules.

STEPHAN™ Lovpil
Nutritional Supplement

Uses: STEPHAN™ Lovpil is a nutritional food supplement for men and women of all ages that is formulated with vitamins, minerals, herbs, amino acids and selected proteins recognized as important for general health and sexual vitality.

Damiana, typically thought of as an aphrodisiac by those who are familiar with its effects, is an important ingredient utilized in STEPHAN Lovpil. A major herbal remedy in Mexican medical folklore, damiana is often used for the treatment of both impotency and sterility. However, its proven stimulating properties of male virility and libido make it an ideal addition to STEPHAN Lovpil's formulation.

A number of scientific studies have shown a direct relationship between low sperm count and diets deficient in arginine. Well established as being significant to normal sperm production, arginine is, therefore, an important contributor to STEPHAN Lovpil.

A third imperative ingredient is vitamin C. Scientific studies have uncovered that ascorbic acid may actually protect human sperm from oxidative DNA damage, which could in turn help prevent birth defects.

Directions: Take one capsule per day.

Warnings: Phenylketonurics: Contains Phenylalanine.

Ingredients: Calcium Carbonate, Vitamin C, Damiana Powder, Ribonucleic Acid, Soya Isolate (Isoleucine, Phenylalanine, Leucine, Threonine, Lysine, Methionine, Valine, Alanine, Glycine, Histidine, Arginine, Proline, Aspartic Acid, Serine, Cysteine, Tyrosine, Glutamic Acid), Zinc (Amino Acid Chelate), Manganese (Amino Acid Chelate), Adenosine Triphosphate, Vitamin A (Acetate), Folic Acid, Vitamin D (Cholecalciferol), Selenium (Methionine), Vitamin B12.

How Supplied: One bottle contains 60 easy-to-swallow capsules.

STEPHAN™ Masculine
Nutritional Supplement

Uses: A nutritional food supplement formulated for the adult male,

STEPHAN™ Masculine contains a special blend of nutrients with vitamins, minerals, herbs and amino acids.

Scientifically researched ingredients have been carefully selected to help ensure STEPHAN™ Masculine's effectiveness. Zinc is one such ingredient. Proven to be closely interrelated with the male sex hormone, testosterone, zinc deficiency often results in regression of the male sex glands, decreased sexual interest, mental lethargy, emotional problems and even poor appetite. It has been found that in males with only a mild zinc deficiency, zinc supplementation was accompanied by increased sperm count and plasma testosterone.

Selenium proves an important proponent of STEPHAN™ Masculine as well. Men in particular need this special mineral due to the fact that almost half of their body's supply is concentrated in the testicles and portions of the seminal ducts. Selenium is an antioxidant that helps protect cells from the kind of damage that could initiate the growth of cancerous tumors.

Directions: Take one to two capsules per day.

Ingredients: L-Histidine, Calcium (Carbonate), Bee Pollen, Parsley, Ribonucleic Acid, Zinc (Amino Acid Chelate), Magnesium (Amino Acid Chelate), Adenosine Triphosphate.

How Supplied: One bottle contains 60 easy-to-swallow capsules.

PHYTO-VITE®
Advanced Antioxidant, Vitamin and
Chelated Mineral Formulation

Uses: Phyto-Vite® is a state-of-the-art nutritional supplement providing chelated minerals, vitamins and a diverse group of antioxidants. It was formulated to meet the nutritional needs of our society where studies estimate only 9% consume foods in the quantities necessary to protect against the oxidative damage caused by free radicals.

The antioxidant coverage provided by Phyto-Vite is both comprehensive and diverse. First, it includes optimal amounts of vitamins A, C, and E as well as the pro-vitamins alpha and beta carotene. Vitamin A, in addition to its antioxidant capabilities, is also felt to improve immune function, protein synthesis, RNA synthesis and steroid hormone synthesis. In this product, vitamin A is derived from two sources: retinyl palmitate and lemongrass. Additional vitamin A activity is provided by the alpha and beta carotene found in *Dunaliella salina*. These carotenoids are strong antioxidants in their own right; however, they can also be converted to vitamin A. This occurs only when the body is deficient in this vitamin. Consequently, vitamin A toxicity cannot be caused by alpha or beta carotene. Vitamin C has long been associated with wound healing, collagen

formation, and maintaining the structural integrity of capillaries, cartilage, dentine and bone. Its antioxidant effects are felt to play a major role in the prevention of cardiovascular disease and some cancers. Phyto-Vite utilizes esterified vitamin C which has been shown to provide a quicker uptake and a decreased rate of excretion when compared with conventional vitamin C. This allows for higher, more sustained levels of this vitamin in the body. Phyto-Vite also contains 400 I.U. of vitamin E, from natural sources. The antioxidant effects of vitamin E have been shown to stabilize cell membranes, increase HDL cholesterol, and decrease platelet aggregation.

Many flavonoids are incorporated into Phyto-Vite. These substances possess antioxidant activity themselves and also potentiate the effects of vitamins C and E. This later effect is produced by decreasing the degradation of vitamin C and E into inactive metabolites. Ginkgo biloba has flavonoid activity as well as other significant effects. Among these are a decrease in platelet aggregation and an increase in vasodilation which appears to increase blood flow to the peripheral arteries and the brain. Some improvement in cognitive abilities has been noted. It also helps to inhibit lipid peroxidation, thereby stabilizing the cell wall against free radical attack.

A phytonutrient blend has been incorporated into Phyto-Vite to further enhance its antioxidant effects. Phytonutrient is a term given to the thousands of chemical compounds found in fruits and vegetables. Some of these compounds, including sulforaphane in broccoli and isothiocyanate in cabbage, have been shown to inhibit cancer in laboratory animals and human cell cultures. Others have shown great promise in aiding the cardiovascular system. Currently, much research is ongoing to isolate and identify more of these compounds, but it has already been clearly established that phytonutrients work best when the entire plant source is used rather than just the isolated compound. The phytonutrients found in Phyto-Vite are obtained from alfalfa (lutein), broccoli (indoles), cabbage (isothiocyanates), cayenne (capsanthin and capsorubin), green onion (thioallyl compounds), parsley (chlorophyll), spirulina (gamma linolenic acid), tomato (lycopene), soy isoflavones (genistein, lecithin and daidzein), aged garlic concentrate, and Pure-Gar-A-8000™ (allicin).

The antioxidant minerals copper, zinc, manganese and selenium have also been incorporated into Phyto-Vite. These minerals have been chelated via a patented process in which the mineral is wrapped within an amino acid. Once inside the body, the minerals can then be utilized in the millions of metabolic reactions that take place in the body. With this process, overall mineral absorption can approach 95% instead of the 5 to 10% absorption seen with other mineral supplements.

Phyto-Vite also provides two antioxidant enzymes (catalase and peroxidase). These help to reduce the body's free radical burden by neutralizing free radicals in the pharynx or stomach.

There are three other features that make Phyto-Vite unique among supplements. First, a small amount of canola oil was included to aid in the proper absorption of fat soluble vitamins, even on an empty stomach. Canola oil also provides essential fatty acids. Second, the product is formed into prolonged-release tablets which allow flexibility in dosing frequency. It can be taken all at once or staggered throughout the day. Dissolution testing has been performed to insure that the product will dissolve properly. Lastly, Phyto-Vite tablets are covered with a Betacoat™. This is a beta carotene coating that is designed to provide antioxidant coverage to the tablet itself. This helps to protect the integrity and activity of the product.

Directions: As a dietary supplement take six tablets per day with eight ounces of liquid. Tablets may be taken all at once or staggered throughout the day.

Warnings: If pregnant or lactating, consult physician before using.

Ingredients: Vitamin A (5,000 IU), Alpha and Beta Carotene (20,000 IU), Vitamin C (500 mg), Vitamin E (400 IU), Citrus Bioflavonoids with Hesperidin (50 mg), Rutin and Quercetin (50 mg), Bilberry Standardized Extract (10 mg), Grape Seed Proanthocyanidins (5 mg), Red Grape Polyphenols (5 mg), Ginkgo Biloba Standardized Extract (20 mg), Copper (2 mg), Zinc (15 mg), Manganese (5 mg), Selenium (200 mcg), Catalase and Peroxidase Enzymes (3,500 units), Phytonutrient Blend (800 mg), Vitamin B-1 (15 mg), Vitamin B-2 (17 mg), Vitamin B-3 (100 mg), Vitamin B-5 (75 mg), Vitamin B-6 (20 mg), Vitamin B-12 (60 mcg), Biotin (300 mcg), Folic Acid (400 mcg), Choline (50 mg), Inositol (50 mg), PABA (25 mg), Vitamin D-3 (400 IU), Vitamin K (70 mcg), Boron (1 mg), Calcium (500 mg), Magnesium (400 mg), Phosphorus (250 mg), Chromium (200 mcg), Iodine (150 mcg), Iron (4 mg), Potassium (70 mg), Essential Fatty Acids (100 mg).

How Supplied: One bottle contains 180 Betacoat™ tablets.

STEPHAN™ Protector
Nutritional Supplement

Uses: STEPHAN™ Protector is a nutritional food supplement that combines specific proteins, vitamins, minerals and amino acids recognized as important for the health of areas associated with the human immune system.

Among these specially selected and scientifically researched ingredients are astragalus, kelp and arginine. Known for its strengthening effects of both the immune and digestive systems, astragalus can be combined with other herbs to increase phagocytosis, interferon production and the number of macrophages. It, in combination, enhances T-cell transformation and functions as an adaptogen to relieve stress-induced immune system suppression.

Research clearly indicates that kelp supplies dozens of important nutrients for improved cardiovascular health and is used to balance the thyroid gland. Arginine stimulates the thymus gland and promotes production of lymphocytes, crucial for immunity, in that gland. The arginine lymphocytes are not only produced in better quantity, but they have also proven more active and effective in fighting illness.

STEPHAN™ Protector may be used by men and women of all ages.

Directions: Take one capsule per day.

Warnings: Phenylketonurics: Contains Phenylalanine.

Ingredients: Bee Pollen, Astragalus, Kelp, Glutamic Acid, Ribonucleic Acid, Aspartic Acid, Leucine, Arginine, Lysine, Phenylalanine, Serine, Proline, Valine, Isoleucine, Alanine, Glycine, Threonine, Tyrosine, Histidine, Methionine, Cysteine, Adenosine Triphosphate.

How Supplied: One bottle contains 60 easy-to-swallow capsules.

STEPHAN™ Relief
Nutritional Supplement

Uses: Designed for both men and women, STEPHAN™ Relief has been formulated with a special combination of nutrients, vitamins, minerals, amino acids and herbs which are recognized as important to the digestive and excretory systems.

Parsley, one of the ingredients found in STEPHAN™ Relief and a member of the carrot family, can be used as a carminative and an aid to digestion. While the root has a mild diuretic property, parsley has also been reported, in large doses, to lower blood pressure.

A second important ingredient in STEPHAN™ Relief is psyllium. This gel-forming fiber is used in many bulk laxatives to promote bowel regularity. In recent years, because of its ability to lower cholesterol, psyllium has gained widespread popularity and can be found in some ready-to-eat cereals.

Directions: Take one to two capsules per day.

Ingredients: Fucus, Parsley (extract 4:1), Psyllium, Leucine, Isoleucine, Valine, Bee Pollen, Ribonucleic Acid, Calcium Pantothenate, Adenosine Triphosphate.

How Supplied: One bottle contains 60 easy-to-swallow capsules.

SLEEP-TITE™
Herbal Sleep Aid

Uses: Sleep-Tite™ is a non-addicting herbal sleep aid formulated to promote a deeper, more restorative sleep without the use of pharmaceutically synthesized hormones. With the body's overall health, and proper functioning, dependent upon efficient sleep patterns in order to achieve cellular, organ, tissue and emotional repair, this powerful tool's primary function is to rejuvenate and restore by assisting the body in initiating and maintaining sleep.

Sleep-Tite is a blend of 10 highly effective, all-natural herbs. California poppy, passion flower, valerian, kava kava and skullcap have been used for centuries as a remedy for insomnia because of their calming effects and ability to relieve muscle tension. Hops and celery seed produce a generalized calming effect and are especially helpful for indigestion, gastrointestinal and smooth muscle relaxation. Chamomile also has a relaxing effect on the body and the gastrointestinal tract, but with the added benefit of producing anti-inflammatory effects on joints. Feverfew has been used as a treatment for fever, migraines and arthritic complaints dating back to ancient Greece. A study published in *Lancet* demonstrated that feverfew inhibited the body's production of prostaglandin and serotonin. These biochemicals can cause inflammation, fever and the vasoactive response that triggers migraine headaches.

By utilizing this unique blend of herbs to aid in the effective initiation and maintenance of sleep patterns, Sleep-Tite can be consumed by adults, thereby promoting physical and emotional well-being in a safe, active manner.

Directions: Adults (18 years and older) may take two Sleep-Tite caplets approximately 30 to 60 minutes prior to bedtime. Needs may vary with each individual. Some persons may require less than two caplets to achieve optimum results. Do not exceed recommended nightly amounts.

Warnings: Not for use by children, pregnant women or lactating women. Consult your physician before using this product if you have any medical condition or are taking antidepressant, sedative or hypnotic medications. Do not take this product if using Monoamine Oxidase (M.A.O.) Inhibitors. This product may cause drowsiness and should not be taken with alcohol or while operating a vehicle or other machinery. If allergic symptoms develop, discontinue use. Store in a cool, dry place. Keep out of reach of children.

Ingredients: European Valerian Rhizome and Root 4:1 Extract (*Valerian officinalis*), Fijian Kava Kava Root 5:1 Extract (*Piper methysticum*), American Hops Strobiles 4:1 Extract (*Humulus lupulus*), Central American Passion Flower Herb 4:1 Extract (*Passiflora incarnata*), Argentine Chamomile Flower 5:1 Extract (*Matricaria chamomilla*), California Poppy Herb 5:1 Extract (*Eschscholzia californica*), Chinese Fu Ling Sclero-

Continued on next page

Sleep-Tite—Cont.

tium 5:1 Extract (*Poria cocos*), Israeli Feverfew Herb 5:1 Extract (*Tanacetum parthenium*), Celery Seed 4:1 Extract (*Apium graveolens*), American Skullcap Herb (*Scutellaria lateriflora*).

How Supplied: One box contains 28 packets. Two caplets per packet.

STEPHAN™ Tranquility Nutritional Supplement

Uses: Designed for both men and women, STEPHAN™ Tranquility is a nutritional food supplement which contains a blend of vitamins, minerals and amino acids recognized as important to areas involved in stress management.

Myo-Inositol is among these specially researched ingredients. It has long been claimed to lower blood concentrations of triglycerides and cholesterol, as well as to generally protect against cardiovascular disease. In addition, Myo-Inositol intake can influence the phosphatidylinositol levels in the membranes of brain cells. Compounds derived from this process could conceivably have some beneficial effect on insomnia and anxiety proving a safer alternative than most to treat these common problems.

Another key ingredient used in STEPHAN Tranquility is valerian root, a folk remedy used throughout the years for several disorders including insomnia, hysteria, palpitations, nervousness and menstrual problems. Valerian root contains valepotriates which are said to be the source of its sedative effects. Studies reveal that valeranon, an essential oil component of this herb, produces a pronounced smooth-muscle effect on the intestine.

Directions: Take one to two capsules per day.

Warnings: Phenylketonurics: Contains Phenylalanine.

Ingredients: Lecithin, Choline Bitartrate, Myo-Inositol, Vitamin C, Valerian (As 4:1 extract), Ribonucleic Acid, Vitamin E, Vitamin B-3, Glutamic Acid, Aspartic Acid, Calcium (Amino Acid Chelate), Leucine, Arginine, Lysine, Phenylalanine, Serine, Valine, Proline, Isoleucine, Alanine, Glycine, Threonine, Tyrosine, Vitamin B-5, Vitamin B-1, Histidine, Magnesium, Methionine, Cysteine, Adenosine Triphosphate, Vitamin B-6, Vitamin B-2, Vitamin A, Folic Acid, Biotin (Amino Acid Chelate), Vitamin D-3, Vitamin B-12.

How Supplied: One bottle contains 60 easy-to-swallow capsules.

SURE2ENDURE™
Herbal, Vitamin & Mineral Workout Supplement

Uses: Attaining peak physical and athletic performance can be an elusive and time-consuming endeavor. It requires a conditioning process whereby the body's endurance, stamina and ability to recover are enhanced. Sure2Endure™ is formulated to aid in this process through an innovative blend of herbs, vitamins and minerals.

Among these specially selected ingredients is ciwujia (*Radix Acanthopanax senticosus*). Used in traditional Chinese medicine for almost 1,700 years to treat fatigue and boost the immune system, ciwujia has been shown to improve overall performance in aerobic exercise, endurance activities and weight lifting without any stimulant effects. According to a recent study, ciwujia increases fat metabolism during exercise by shifting toward the use of fat as an energy source instead of carbohydrates. In addition, the caffeine-free herb improves endurance by reducing lactic acid build-up in the muscles. This process delays the muscle fatigue which often leads to muscle pain and cramps.

Sure2Endure™ also provides antioxidant coverage and enzyme cofactors. Vitamins C and E address the otherwise high levels of free radicals generated from the oxidation of fuel substrates during exercise, while vitamins B1, B2, B6 and B12 aid in proper carbohydrate metabolism and serve as cofactors in numerous biochemical reactions in the body. Ciwujia has been credited with antioxidant properties as well.

Since tissue stress and damage are often the result of strenuous exercise, it is important to maintain proper integrity and recovery of connective tissue. Glucosamine, one of the basic constituents making up joint cartilage, is another special additive to Sure2Endure™. This substance enhances the synthesis of cartilage cells and protects against destructive enzymes. It stabilizes cell membranes and intercellular collagen thereby protecting cartilage during rest, exercise and recovery.

The anti-inflammatory activities of bromelain and boswellia further prove beneficial to the health of joint and soft tissues.

Directions: Adults (18 years and older) take 3 tablets one hour prior to exercise. Needs may vary with each individual. For optimum performance, use in conjunction with BIOLEAN® or BIOLEAN Free™ one hour before exercise. Phyto-Vite® may be taken with this product to maximize the antioxidant effect necessary with exercise. Pro-Xtreme™ and Mass Appeal™ may also be consumed for maximum effectiveness.

Warning: Not for use by children, pregnant women or lactating women. Consult your physician before using this product if you have any medical conditions. Discontinue immediately if allergic symptoms develop. Keep out of the reach of children. Store in a cool, dry place.

Active Ingredients: Proprietary Endurance, Stamina and Recovery Blend: Ciwujia Standardized Extract (900 mg of *Acanthopanax Seticosus* Root containing 0.8% Eleutherosides), Magnesium L-Aspartate, Potassium L-Aspartate; Proprietary Joint and Connective Tissue Enhancers Blend: *Boswellia Serrata* Extract containing 40% Boswellic Acid, Bromelain (600 GDU/g), Glucosamine Hydrochloride; Vitamin C (500 mg); Vitamin E (100 IU); Vitamin B1 (10 mg); Vitamin B2 (12 mg); Vitamin B6 (15 mg); Vitamin B12 (20 mcg); and Chromium Chelavite™ (200 mcg).

How Supplied: One box contains 28 packets, three tablets per packet.

WINRGY™
Nutritional Drink with Vitamin C

Uses: Through nutrients in the diet, nerves are able to send signals throughout the body called neurotransmitters. One such neurotransmitter, noradrenaline, provides individuals with the necessary alertness and energy required in day-to-day activity. A unique blend of vitamins and minerals important to the creation of noradrenaline has been incorporated into Winrgy™, making it a delicious, nutritional alternative to coffee and cola.

Studies reveal that vitamin B2 helps the body release energy from protein, carbohydrates and fat, while vitamin B12 is given to combat fatigue and alleviate neurological problems, including weakness and memory loss. Another important component of Winrgy, vitamin B3 (niacin), works with both thiamin and riboflavin in the metabolism of carbohydrates and is essential for providing energy for cell tissue growth. Niacin has also proven to dilate blood vessels and thereby increase the blood flow to various organs of the body, sometimes resulting in a blush of the skin and a healthy sense of warmth.

Unlike caffeine, Winrgy offers the raw materials necessary to continue the production of noradrenaline and is ideal for anytime performance is required.

Directions: Add 6 ounces of chilled water or fruit juice to one packet of mix. Stir briskly. Consume 1–2 times per day. Keep in a cool, dry place. For maximum results, combine this product with one serving size of Food For Thought.™

Warnings: Phenylketonurics: Contains Phenylalanine. Not for use by children, pregnant or lactating women. Persons taking medications should seek medical advice before taking this product. Do not consume more than four servings per day. Avoid the use of antacids containing aluminum with this product.

Ingredients: Fructose, L-Phenylalanine, Natural Flavor, Citric Acid, Taurine, Glycine, Ascorbic Acid, Caffeine, Niacinamide, Vitamin E Acetate, Calcium Pantothenate, Silicon Dioxide, Potassium Aspartate, Manganese Aspartate, Chromium Aspartate, Pyridoxine Hydrochloride, Zinc Gluconate, Riboflavin, Thiamin Mononitrate, Copper Gluconate, Folic Acid, Vitamin B12.

How Supplied: One box contains 28 packets. Serving size equals one packet.

Whitehall-Robins Healthcare American Home Products Corporation

**FIVE GIRALDA FARMS
MADISON, NJ 07940**

Direct Inquiries to:
Whitehall-Robins (and) Lederle Consumer Product Information 800-322-3129

CENTRUM® HERBALS
CENTRUM ECHINACEA
CENTRUM GARLIC
CENTRUM GINKGO BILOBA
CENTRUM GINSENG
CENTRUM SAW PALMETTO
CENTRUM ST. JOHN'S WORT

What Makes Centrum Herbals Different
Herbs are complex plants made up of many natural active ingredients which work together in the body to produce a beneficial effect. The most important part of choosing an herbal supplement is insuring that the natural active ingredients in the herb are present in the final product each and every time.
Centrum Herbals provide this benefit because:
• Centrum, using the PharmaPrint™ process, has identified the key components in the herb which are responsible for its beneficial effects, then insures that these natural actives are consistently present in each dose. Many brands, even if they are standardized, guarantee only marker compounds which may have no activity.
• Centrum Herbals are tested to insure the natural activity of the herb is preserved in each capsule.
• Only Centrum Herbals use this patent-pending technology.

CENTRUM ECHINACEA

This natural product is derived from the flowers and the root of the echinacea, or purple coneflower, plant which is native to North America. It is traditionally used during the winter months and has been shown in numerous clinical studies to:
• Help support immune system function and the body's natural defenses.*

Supplement Facts	
Serving Size: 1 Capsule	
Amount Per Capsule	
Echinacea Extract (flower & root) *Echinacea purpurea*	100 mg†
Standardized to contain (based on extract weight):	
Total Phenols (marker)	3.0%†
Cichoric acid (natural active)	†
Isobutyl alkylamides (natural active)	†
Assay used to confirm bioactivity: 15-lipoxygenase enzymatic assay	
†Daily value not established.	

OTHER INGREDIENTS: DIBASIC CALCIUM PHOSPHATE, CELLULOSE, LACTOSE MONOHYDRATE, HYDROXYPROPYL CELLULOSE, ETHYLCELLULOSE, CASTOR OIL, GELATIN, SILICON DIOXIDE, SODIUM LAURYL SULFATE, PROPYLENE GLYCOL, TITANIUM DIOXIDE.

Directions: Adults: Take one capsule two times daily with a full glass of water. For best results take consistently each day, when needed, for a maximum of eight weeks.

Specific Precautions: If you suspect or have a known allergy to the daisy family (Asteraceae) do not use this product. Individuals with autoimmune disease should consult their health care practitioner before use. As with any supplement, if you are taking a prescription medication, or if you are pregnant or are nursing a baby, contact your physician before using this product.

Shown in Product Identification Guide, page 528

CENTRUM GARLIC

This natural product is derived from fresh garlic bulbs. It is carefully harvested, dried, and concentrated to preserve the beneficial ingredients. Recent clinical studies have shown garlic's ability to:
• Help maintain healthy cholesterol levels and healthy blood pressure.*

Supplement Facts	
Serving Size: 1 Capsule	
Amount Per Capsule	
Garlic Powder (bulb) *Allium sativum*	300 mg†
Standardized to contain:	
Alliin (marker) (Allicin potential 45%)	1300 mcg†
γ-Glutamyl-S-allyl-cysteine (natural active)	†
γ-Glutamyl-S-trans-1-propenyl-cysteine (natural active)	†
γ-Glutamyl-phenylalanine (natural active)	†

Assay used to confirm bioactivity: Angiotensin converting enzyme assay	
† Daily value not established.	

OTHER INGREDIENTS: HYDROXYPROPYL CELLULOSE, HYDROXYPROPYL METHYLCELLULOSE PHTHALATE, CASTOR OIL, GELATIN, SILICON DIOXIDE, SODIUM LAURYL SULFATE, PHARMACEUTICAL GLAZE, RIBOFLAVIN, FD&C BLUE NO. 1, LECITHIN, SIMETHICONE.

Directions: Adults: Take one capsule two times daily with a full glass of water. Take consistently each day with food for best results.

Shown in Product Identification Guide, page 528

CENTRUM GINKGO BILOBA

This natural product is derived from the leaves of the Ginkgo Biloba tree. It has been shown in clinical studies to:
• Help maintain normal mental alertness, concentration, and memory.*

Supplement Facts	
Serving Size: 1 Capsule	
Amount Per Capsule	
Ginkgo Biloba Extract (leaf) *Ginkgo biloba*	60 mg†
Standardized to contain (based on extract weight):	
Ginkgo flavone glycosides (marker)	24.0%†
Terpene lactones (marker)	6.0%†
Ginkgolide A (natural active)	†
Ginkgolide B (natural active)	†
Amentoflavone (natural active)	†
Assay used to confirm bioactivity: $GABA_{Bdz}$ Central binding assay	
†Daily value not established.	

OTHER INGREDIENTS: SUCROSE, CELLULOSE, LACTOSE MONOHYDRATE, DIBASIC CALCIUM PHOSPHATE, HYDROXYPROPYL CELLULOSE, ETHYLCELLULOSE, CASTOR OIL, FLAVOR EXTRACTIVES OF ST.

Continued on next page

Centrum Ginkgo Biloba—Cont.

JOHN'S BREAD, GLUCOSE, CARAMEL COLOR, GELATIN, SILICON DIOXIDE, SODIUM LAURYL SULFATE, PROPYLENE GLYCOL, TITANIUM DIOXIDE.

Directions: Adults: Take one capsule two times daily with a full glass of water. Take consistently each day for best results.

Specific Precautions: May cause headache or stomach upset.

Shown in Product Identification Guide, page 528

CENTRUM GINSENG

This natural product is derived from the root of the ginseng plant. It has been shown in clinical studies to:
• Help your body generate the energy it needs and may enhance physical performance.*

Supplement Facts	
Serving Size: 1 Capsule	
Amount Per Capsule	
Ginseng Extract (root)	
Panax ginseng	100 mg†
Standardized to contain (based on extract weight):	
Total ginsenosides (marker)	7.0%†
Ginsenoside Rb1 (natural active)	†
Ginsenoside Rg1 (natural active)	†
GABA (natural active)	†
Assay used to confirm bioactivity: Phospholipase A_2 enzymatic assay	
† Daily value not established.	

OTHER INGREDIENTS: DIBASIC CALCIUM PHOSPHATE, CELLULOSE, LACTOSE, MONOHYDRATE, HYDROXYPROPYL CELLULOSE, ETHYLCELLULOSE, CASTOR OIL, GELATIN, SILICON DIOXIDE, SODIUM LAURYL SULFATE, PROPYLENE GLYCOL, TITANIUM DIOXIDE.

Directions: Adults: Take one capsule two times daily (morning and afternoon) with a full glass of water. Take consistently each day for best results.

Shown in Product Identification Guide, page 528

CENTRUM SAW PALMETTO

This natural product is derived from the berries of the saw palmetto plant, native to North America. It has been shown in clinical studies to:
• Help maintain prostate health and normal urine flow.*

Supplement Facts	
Serving Size: 1 Softgel	
Amount Per Softgel	
Saw Palmetto Extract (berry)	
Serenoa repens	160 mg†
Standardized to contain (based on extract weight):	
Total fatty acids (marker)	80%†
Linolenic acid (natural active)	†
Lauric acid, ethyl ester (natural active)	†
Linoleic acid, ethyl ester (natural active)	†
Assay used to confirm bioactivity: Adrenergic α_{1B} binding assay	
† Daily value not established.	

OTHER INGREDIENTS: CORN OIL, YELLOW WAX, GELATIN, PROPYLENE GLYCOL, HYDROXYPROPYL METHYLCELLULOSE, TITANIUM DIOXIDE, CARMINE.

Directions: Adults: Take one softgel two times daily with a full glass of water. Take consistently each day for best results.

Specific Precautions: May cause stomach upset. If stomach upset occurs, try taking with food.

Shown in Product Identification Guide, page 528

CENTRUM ST. JOHN'S WORT

This natural product is derived from the flowers and leaves of the St. John's Wort plant. It has been shown in clinical studies to:
• Help maintain healthy emotional balance and a positive outlook.*

Supplement Facts	
Serving Size: 1 Capsule	
Amount Per Capsule	
St. John's Wort Extract (flower & leaves)	
Hypericum perforatum	300 mg†
Standardized to contain (based on extract weight):	
Total Hypericin compounds (marker)	0.3%†
Hyperforin (marker)	†
Quercetin (natural active)	†
Amentoflavone (natural active)	†
GABA & Proline (natural actives)	†
Assay used to confirm bioactivity: Muscarinic M1 binding assay	
† Daily value not established.	

OTHER INGREDIENTS: DIBASIC CALCIUM PHOSPHATE, MALTODEXTRIN, CELLULOSE, LACTOSE MONOHYDRATE, SILICON DIOXIDE, HYDROXYPROPYL CELLULOSE, ETHYLCELLULOSE, CASTOR OIL, GELATIN, SODIUM LAURYL SULFATE, PROPYLENE GLYCOL, TITANIUM DIOXIDE.

Directions: Adults: Take one capsule two times daily with a full glass of water. Take consistently each day for a minimum of two weeks for best results.

Specific Precautions: While using this product, avoid excessive exposure to sun.

Overall Precautions: Use only as directed. Do not exceed recommended dosage. As with any supplement, if you are taking a prescription medication, or if you are pregnant or are nursing a baby, contact your physician before using this product. **Keep this and all dietary supplements out of the reach of children.** Store in a cool dry place. Avoid temperatures above 86°F.

*THESE STATEMENTS HAVE NOT BEEN EVALUATED BY THE FOOD AND DRUG ADMINISTRATION. THIS PRODUCT IS NOT INTENDED TO DIAGNOSE, TREAT, CURE, OR PREVENT ANY DISEASE.

Shown in Product Identification Guide, page 528

UNKNOWN DRUG?
Consult the
Product Identification Guide
(Gray Pages)
for full-color photos of
leading over-the-counter
medications

Youngevity
4951 AIRPORT PARKWAY,
   SUITE 500
DALLAS, TEXAS 75001

Direct Inquiries to:
1-800-469-6864

TURN BACK THE HANDS OF TIME
NATURALLY STIMULATES THE RELEASE OF
HGH

6 CAPSULES CONTAIN: 4850 mg.

ANTI-AGING PROPRIETARY BLEND:

L-Lysine HCL, L-Arginine, L-Ornithine,
L-Glutamine, L-Tyrosine,
Kelp Plant, Glycine, GABA,
The Vilcabamba Mineral Essence,
Vitamin B_6, Manganese, and Chromium.

"THE VILCABAMBA MINERAL ESSENCE®"

**13 Anti-Aging Patented Amino Acid
Chelated Minerals** – Potassium,
Calcium, Magnesium, Zinc, Chromium,
Selenium, Iron, Copper, Molybdenum,
Vanadium, Iodine, Cobalt, & Manganese.

Warning: Do not use if you are
pregnant or nursing.

Directions: Take 6 capsules daily, on
an empty stomach –
2 capsules upon awakening & 4 capsules
before bedtime.

How Supplied: 180 capsules

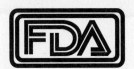

U.S. FOOD AND DRUG ADMINISTRATION

Professional and Consumer Information Numbers

Medical Product Reporting Programs

MedWatch (24 hour service) 800-332-1088
Reporting of problems with drugs, devices, biologics (except vaccines), medical foods, dietary supplements.

Vaccine Adverse Event Reporting System (24 hour service) 800-822-7967
Reporting of vaccine-related problems.

Mandatory Medical Device Reporting 301-594-3886
Reporting required from User facilities regarding device-related deaths and serious injuries.

Veterinary Adverse Drug Reaction Program 888-FDA-VETS
Reporting of adverse drug events in animals.

Medical Advertising Information 800-238-7332
Inquiries from health professionals regarding product promotion.

USP Medication Errors 800-233-7767
Reporting of medication errors or near-errors to help avoid future problems through improvement in product names and packaging.

Information for Health Professionals

Center for Drugs Information Branch 301-827-4573
Information on human drugs including hormones.

Center for Biologics Executive Secretariat 301-827-2000
Information on biological products including vaccines and blood.

Center for Devices and Radiological Health 301-443-4190
Automated request for information on medical devices and radiation-emitting products.

Office of Orphan Products Development 301-827-3666
Information on products for rare diseases.

Office of Health Affairs, Medicine Staff 301-827-6630
Information for health professionals on FDA activities.

General Information

General Consumer Inquiries 800-532-4440
Consumer information on regulated products/issues.   **Local: 301-827-4420**

Freedom of Information 301-827-6567
Requests for publicly available FDA documents.

Office of Public Affairs 301-827-6250
Interviews/press inquiries on FDA activities.

Seafood Hotline (24 hour service) 800-332-4010
Prerecorded message/request information (English/Spanish).

POISON CONTROL CENTERS

Many centers in this directory are certified members of the American Association of Poison Control Centers (AAPCC). Certified centers are marked by an asterisk after the name. They must meet certain criteria: for example, serve a large geographic area; be open 24 hours a day and provide direct dialing or toll-free access; be supervised by a medical director; and have registered pharmacists or nurses available to answer questions from healthcare professionals and the public.

Centers in each state are listed alphabetically by city. "TTY" numbers are reserved for the hearing impaired, and "TTD" numbers reach a telecommunication device for the deaf.

ALABAMA

BIRMINGHAM
Regional Poison Control Center, The Children's Hospital of Alabama (*)
1600 7th Ave. South
Birmingham, AL 35233-1711
Business: 205-939-9720
Emergency: 205-933-4050
            205-939-9201
            800-292-6678(AL)
Fax: 205-939-9245

TUSCALOOSA
Alabama Poison Center, Tuscaloosa (*)
2503 Phoenix Dr.
Tuscaloosa, AL 35405
Business: 205-345-0600
Emergency: 205-345-0600
            800-462-0800(AL)
Fax: 205-759-7994

ALASKA

ANCHORAGE
Anchorage Poison Center, Providence Hospital
P.O. Box 196604
3200 Providence Dr.
Anchorage, AK 99519-6604
Business: 907-562-2211
            ext. 3633
Emergency: 907-261-3193
            800-478-3193(AK)
Fax: 907-261-3645

FAIRBANKS
Fairbanks Poison Control Center
1650 Cowles St.
Fairbanks, AK 99701
Business: 907-456-7182
Emergency: 907-456-7182
Fax: 907-458-5553

ARIZONA

PHOENIX
Samaritan Regional Poison Center (*)
Good Samaritan Regional Medical Center
Ancillary-1
1111 East McDowell Rd.
Phoenix, AZ 85006
Business: 602-495-4884
Emergency: 602-253-3334
            800-362-0101(AZ)
Fax: 602-256-7579

TUCSON
Arizona Poison and Drug Information Center (*)
Arizona Health Sciences Center
1501 North Campbell Ave.
Rm. #1156
Tucson, AZ 85724
Emergency: 520-626-6016
            800-322-0101(AZ)
Fax: 520-626-2720

ARKANSAS

LITTLE ROCK
Arkansas Poison and Drug Information Center, College of Pharmacy - UAMS
4301 West Markham St.
Slot 522-2
Little Rock, AR 72205
Business: 501-661-6161
Emergency: 800-376-4766(AR)

CALIFORNIA

FRESNO
California Poison Control System-Fresno (*)
Valley Children's Hospital
3151 North Millbrook, IN31
Fresno, CA 93703
Business: 209-241-6040
Emergency: 800-876-4766(CA)
Fax: 209-241-6050

SACRAMENTO
California Poison Control System-Sacramento (*)
UCDMC-HSF Room 1024
2315 Stockton Blvd.
Sacramento, CA 95817
Business: 916-734-3415
Emergency: 800-876-4766(CA)
Fax: 916-734-7796

SAN DIEGO
California Poison Control System-San Diego (*)
UCSD Medical Center
200 West Arbor Dr.
San Diego, CA 92103-8925
Emergency: 800-876-4766(CA)

COLORADO

DENVER
Rocky Mountain Poison and Drug Center (*)
8802 East 9th Ave.
Denver, CO 80220-6800
Business: 303-739-1100
Emergency: 303-739-1123
            800-332-3073(CO)
Fax: 303-739-1119

CONNECTICUT

FARMINGTON
Connecticut Regional Poison Center (*)
University of Connecticut Health Center
263 Farmington Ave.
Farmington, CT 06030
Emergency: 800-343-2722(CT)
Fax: 203-679-1623

DELAWARE

PHILADELPHIA, PA
The Poison Control Center
3600 Market St.
Suite 220
Philadelphia, PA 19104
Emergency: 800-722-7112(PA)
            215-386-2100

DISTRICT OF COLUMBIA

WASHINGTON, DC
**National Capital
Poison Center (*)**
3201 New Mexico Ave., NW
Suite 310
Washington, DC 20016
Business: 202-362-3867
Emergency: 202-625-3333
TTY: 202-362-8563
Fax: 202-362-8377

FLORIDA

JACKSONVILLE
**Florida Poison Information
Center-Jacksonville (*)
University Medical Center
University of Florida Health
Science Center-Jacksonville**
655 W. 8th St.
Jacksonville, FL 32209
Emergency: 904-549-4480
800-282-3171(FL)
Fax: 904-549-4063

MIAMI
**Florida Poison Information
Center-Miami (*)
University of Miami,
School of Medicine
Department of Pediatrics**
P.O. Box 016960 (R-131)
Miami, FL 33101
Emergency: 305-585-5253
800-282-3171(FL)
Fax: 305-242-9762

TAMPA
**The Florida Poison
Information Center
Tampa General Hospital**
P.O. Box 1289
Tampa, FL 33601
Emergency: 813-253-4444
(Tampa)
800-282-3171(FL)
Fax: 813-253-4443

GEORGIA

ATLANTA
**Georgia Poison Center (*)
Hughes Spalding Children's
Hospital, Grady Health System**
80 Butler St. SE
P.O. Box 26066
Atlanta, GA 30335-3801
Emergency: 404-616-9000
800-282-5846(GA)
Fax: 404-616-6657

MACON
**Regional Poison
Control Center,
Medical Center of
Central Georgia**
777 Hemlock St.
Macon, GA 31201
Poison Ctr: 912-633-1427
Fax: 912-633-5082

IDAHO

(DENVER, CO)
**Rocky Mountain Poison
& Drug Center**
8802 E. 9th Ave.
Denver, CO 80220-6800
Emergency: 800-860-0620(ID)
303-739-1123

ILLINOIS

CHICAGO
Illinois Poison Center
222 South Riverside Plaza
Suite 1900
Chicago, IL 60606
Business: 312-906-6136
Emergency: 800-942-5969
Fax: 312-803-5400

URBANA
**ASPCA/National Animal
Poison Control Center**
1717 Philo Rd., Suite 36
Urbana, IL 61802
Business: 217-337-5030
Fax: 217-337-0599

INDIANA

INDIANAPOLIS
**Indiana Poison Center (*)
Methodist Hospital of Indiana**
I-65 at 21st St.
Indianapolis, IN 46206-1367
Emergency: 317-929-2323
800-382-9097(IN)
Fax: 317-929-2337

IOWA

SIOUX CITY
Iowa Poison Center
2720 Stone Park Blvd.
Sioux City, IA 51104
Business: 712-277-2222
Emergency: 800-352-2222(IA)
Fax: 712-279-7852

KANSAS

KANSAS CITY
**Mid-America Poison
Control Center,
University of Kansas
Medical Center**
3901 Rainbow Blvd.
Room B-400
Kansas City, KS 66160-7231
Business & 913-588-6633
Emergency: 800-332-6633(KS)
Fax: 913-588-2350

TOPEKA
**Stormont-Vail Regional
Medical Center
Emergency Department**
1500 S.W. 10th
Topeka, KS 66604-1353
Business: 913-354-6000
Emergency: 913-354-6100
Fax: 913-354-5004

KENTUCKY

LOUISVILLE
**Kentucky Regional
Poison Center**
Medical Towers S.
Suite 572
234 E. Gray St.
Louisville, KY 40202
Business: 502-629-7264
Emergency: 502-589-8222
Fax: 502-629-7277

LOUISIANA

MONROE
**Louisiana Drug and Poison
Information Center (*)
Northeast Louisiana University**
Sugar Hall
Monroe, LA 71209-6430
Business: 318-342-1710
Emergency: 800-256-9822(LA)
Fax: 318-342-1744

MAINE

PORTLAND
**Maine Poison Center
Maine Medical Center**
22 Bramhall St.
Portland, ME 04102
Business: 207-871-2950
Emergency: 800-442-6305(ME)
Fax: 207-871-6226

MARYLAND

BALTIMORE
Maryland Poison Center (*)
20 North Pine St.
Baltimore, MD 21201
Business: 410-706-7604
Emergency: 410-706-7701
800-492-2414(MD)
Fax: 410-706-7184

MASSACHUSETTS

BOSTON
**Massachusetts Poison Control
System (*)**
300 Longwood Ave.
Boston, MA 02115
Emergency: 617-232-2120
800-682-9211(MA)
Fax: 617-738-0032

MICHIGAN

DETROIT
**Poison Control Center (*)
Children's Hospital
of Michigan**
4160 John R. Harper
Office Bldg.
Suite 616
Detroit, MI 48201
Business: 313-745-5335
Emergency: 313-745-5711
800-764-7661(MI)
Fax: 313-745-5493

GRAND RAPIDS
**Spectrum Health Regional
Poison Center (*)**
1840 Wealthy SE
Grand Rapids, MI 49506-2968
Business: 616-774-5329
Emergency: 800-764-7661(MI)
Fax: 616-774-7204

MINNESOTA

MINNEAPOLIS
**Hennepin Regional Poison
Center (*) Hennepin County
Medical Center**
701 Park Ave.
Minneapolis, MN 55415
Business: 612-347-3144
Emergency: 800-764-7661(MN)
612-347-3141
Fax: 612-904-4289

**Minnesota Regional
Poison Center (*)**
8100 34th Ave. South
P.O. Box 1309
Minneapolis, MN 55440-1309
Business: 612-851-8100
Emergency: 612-221-2113
          800-222-1222(MN)
Fax: 612-851-8166

MISSISSIPPI

HATTIESBURG
**Poison Center,
Forrest General Hospital**
400 South 28th Ave.
Hattiesburg, MS 39401
Business: 601-288-4221
Emergency: 601-288-2100

JACKSON
**Mississippi Regional Poison
Control, University of
Mississippi Medical Center**
2500 North State St.
Jackson, MS 39216
Business: 601-984-1675
Emergency: 601-354-7660
Fax: 601-984-1676

MISSOURI

KANSAS CITY
**Poison Control Center,
Children's Mercy Hospital**
2401 Gillham Rd.
Kansas City, MO 64108
Business: 816-234-3053
Emergency: 816-234-3430
Fax: 816-234-3421

ST. LOUIS
**Cardinal Glennon
Children's Hospital
Regional Poison Center (*)**
1465 South Grand Blvd.
St. Louis, MO 63104
Emergency: 800-366-8888(MO)
          314-772-5200
Fax: 314-577-5355

MONTANA

(DENVER, CO)
**Rocky Mountain Poison
and Drug Center (*)**
8802 East 9th Ave.
Denver, CO 80220-6800
Emergency: 800-525-5042(MT)
Fax: 303-739-1119

NEBRASKA

OMAHA
The Poison Center (*)
8301 Dodge St.
Omaha, NE 68114
Emergency: 402-354-5555
          (Omaha)
          800-955-9119
          (NE & WY)

NEVADA

(DENVER, CO)
**Rocky Mountain Poison
and Drug Center (*)**
8802 East 9th Ave.
Denver, CO 80220-6800
Emergency: 800-446-6179(NV)
          303-739-1123
Fax: 303-739-1119

RENO
**Poison Center,
Washoe Medical Center**
77 Pringle Way
Reno, NV 89520
Business: 702-328-4129
Emergency: 702-328-4129
Fax: 702-328-5555

NEW HAMPSHIRE

LEBANON
**New Hampshire Poison
Information Center,
Dartmouth-Hitchcock
Medical Center**
1 Medical Center Dr.
Lebanon, NH 03756
Emergency: 603-650-5000
          (ask for Poison Center)
          800-562-8236(NH)
Fax: 603-650-8986

NEW JERSEY

NEWARK
**New Jersey Poison Information
and Education System (*)**
201 Lyons Ave.
Newark, NJ 07112
Emergency: 800-764-7661(NJ)
Fax: 973-705-8098

PHILLIPSBURG
**Warren Hospital
Poison Control Center**
185 Roseberry St.
Phillipsburg, NJ 08865
Business: 908-859-6768
Emergency: 908-859-6767
          800-962-1253(NJ)
Fax: 908-859-6812

NEW MEXICO

ALBUQUERQUE
**New Mexico Poison and
Drug Information Center (*)
University of New Mexico**
Health Sciences Library,
Rm. 125
Albuquerque, NM 87131-1076
Emergency: 505-272-2222
          800-432-6866(NM)
Fax: 505-277-5892

NEW YORK

BUFFALO
**Western New York Regional
Poison Control Center
Children's Hospital of Buffalo**
219 Bryant St.
Buffalo, NY 14222
Business: 716-878-7657
Emergency: 716-878-7654
          800-888-7655
          (NY Western Regions Only)

MINEOLA
**Long Island Regional Poison
Control Center (*)
Winthrop University Hospital**
259 First St.
Mineola, NY 11501
Emergency: 516-542-2323
Fax: 516-739-2070

NEW YORK
**New York City
Poison Control Center (*)
NYC Dept. of Health**
455 First Ave., Room 123
New York, NY 10016
Business: 212-447-8154
Emergency: 212-340-4494
          212-POISONS
          212-447-2205
Fax: 212-447-8223

ROCHESTER
**Finger Lakes Regional Poison
Center (*) University of
Rochester Medical Center**
601 Elmwood Ave.
Box 321
Rochester, NY 14642
Business: 716-273-4155
Emergency: 716-275-3232
          800-333-0542(NY)
Fax: 716-244-1677

SLEEPY HOLLOW
**Hudson Valley Regional Poison
Center (*) Phelps Memorial
Hospital Center**
701 N. Broadway
Sleepy Hollow, NY 10590
Emergency: 914-366-3030
          800-336-6997(NY)
Fax: 914-353-1050

SYRACUSE
**Central New York
Poison Control Center (*)
SUNY Health Science Center**
750 East Adams St.
Syracuse, NY 13210
Business: 315-464-7073
Emergency: 315-476-4766
          800-252-5655(NY)
Fax: 315-464-7077

NORTH CAROLINA

ASHEVILLE
**Western North Carolina
Poison Control Center,
Memorial Mission Hospital**
509 Biltmore Ave.
Asheville, NC 28801
Emergency: 704-255-4490
          800-542-4225(NC)
Fax: 704-255-4467

CHARLOTTE
**Carolinas Poison Center
Carolinas Medical Center**
5000 Airport Center Pkwy.
Suite B
P.O. Box 32861
Charlotte, NC 28232
Business: 704-355-3054
Emergency: 704-355-4000
          800-848-6946(NC)

NORTH DAKOTA

FARGO

**North Dakota Poison
Information Center,
Meritcare Medical Center**
720 North 4th St.
Fargo, ND 58122
Business: 701-234-6062
Emergency: 701-234-5575
         800-732-2200(ND)
Fax: 701-234-5090

OHIO

CINCINNATI

**Cincinnati Drug & Poison
Information Center
and Regional Poison
Control System (*)**
2368 Victory Pkwy.
Suite 300
Cincinnati, OH 45206
Emergency: 513-558-5111
         800-872-5111(OH)
Fax: 513-558-5301

CLEVELAND

**Greater Cleveland
Poison Control Center**
11100 Euclid Ave.
Cleveland, OH 44106
Emergency: 216-231-4455
         888-231-4455
Fax: 216-844-3242

COLUMBUS

**Central Ohio
Poison Center (*)**
700 Children's Dr.
Columbus, OH 43205-2696
Business: 614-722-2635
Emergency: 614-228-1323
         800-682-7625(OH)
Fax: 614-221-2672

**Greater Dayton Area
Hospital Association
at Central Ohio Poison Center**
700 Children's Dr.
Columbus, OH 43205
Business: 614-722-2635
Emergency: 937-222-2227
         800-762-0727(OH)

TOLEDO

**Poison Information
Center of NW Ohio,
Medical College of
Ohio Hospital**
3000 Arlington Ave.
Toledo, OH 43614
Business: 419-383-3897
Emergency: 419-381-3897
         800-589-3897(OH)
Fax: 419-381-6066

OKLAHOMA

OKLAHOMA CITY

**Oklahoma Poison Control
Center, University of
Oklahoma and Children's
Hospital of Oklahoma**
940 Northeast 13th St.
Oklahoma City, OK 73104
Business: 405-271-5454
         800-764-7661(OK)
TDD: 405-271-1122
Fax: 405-271-1816

OREGON

PORTLAND

**Oregon Poison Center (*)
Oregon Health
Sciences University**
3181 S.W. Sam Jackson Park Rd.
Portland, OR 97201
Emergency: 503-494-8968
         800-452-7165(OR)
Fax: 503-494-4980

PENNSYLVANIA

HERSHEY

**Central Pennsylvania
Poison Center (*)
University Hospital
Milton S. Hershey
Medical Center**
Hershey, PA 17033
Emergency: 800-521-6110(PA)
         717-531-6111
Fax: 717-531-6932

PHILADELPHIA

The Poison Control Center (*)
3600 Market St., Suite 220
Philadelphia, PA 19104-2641
Business: 215-590-2003
Emergency: 215-386-2100
         800-722-7112(PA)
Fax: 215-590-4419

PITTSBURGH

Pittsburgh Poison Center (*)
3705 Fifth Ave.
Pittsburgh, PA 15213
Business: 412-692-5600
Emergency: 412-681-6669
Fax: 412-692-7497

RHODE ISLAND

PROVIDENCE

**Lifespan Poison Center
Rhode Island Hospital**
593 Eddy St.
Providence, RI 02903
Emergency: 401-444-5727
Fax: 401-444-8062

SOUTH CAROLINA

COLUMBIA

**Palmetto Poison Center,
College of Pharmacy,
University of South Carolina**
Columbia, SC 29208
Business: 803-777-7909
Emergency: 803-777-1117
         800-922-1117(SC)
Fax: 803-777-6127

SOUTH DAKOTA

ABERDEEN

**Poison Control Center,
St. Luke's Midland Regional
Medical Center**
305 South State St.
Aberdeen, SD 57401
Business: 605-622-5000
Emergency: 605-622-5100
         800-592-1889
         (SD, MN, ND, WY)

TENNESSEE

MEMPHIS

Southern Poison Center
875 Monroe Ave.
Suite 104
Memphis, TN 38163
Business: 901-448-6800
Emergency: 901-528-6048
         800-288-9999(TN)
Fax: 901-448-5419

NASHVILLE

**Middle Tennessee
Poison Center (*)
The Center for Clinical
Toxicology, Vanderbilt
University Medical Center**
1161 21st Ave. South
501 Oxford House
Nashville, TN 37232-4632
Business: 615-936-0760
Emergency: 615-936-2034
         800-288-9999(TN)
Fax: 615-936-2046

TEXAS

DALLAS

North Texas Poison Center (*)
5201 Harry Hines Blvd.
P.O. Box 35926
Dallas, TX 75235
Business: 214-590-6625
Emergency: 800-764-7661(TX)
Fax: 214-590-5008

GALVESTON

**Southeast Texas
Poison Center (*)
The University of Texas
Medical Branch**
301 University Ave.
Galveston, TX 77555-1175
Emergency: 409-765-1420
         800-764-7661(TX)
Fax: 409-772-3917

TEMPLE

**Central Texas
Poison Center (*)
Scott & White
Memorial Hospital**
2401 South 31st St.
Temple, TX 76508
Business: 254-724-4636
Emergency: 800-764-7661(TX)
         254-724-7401
Fax: 254-724-1731

UTAH

SALT LAKE CITY

**Utah Poison
Control Center (*)**
410 Chipeta Way
Suite 230
Salt Lake City, UT 84108
Emergency: 801-581-2151
         800-456-7707(UT)
Fax: 801-581-4199

VERMONT

BURLINGTON
Vermont Poison Center,
Fletcher Allen Health Care
111 Colchester Ave.
Burlington, VT 05401
Business: 802-656-2721
Emergency: 802-658-3456
Fax: 802-656-4802

VIRGINIA

CHARLOTTESVILLE
Blue Ridge Poison Center (*)
Blue Ridge University of
Virginia Medical Center
Box 437
Charlottesville, VA 22908
Emergency: 804-924-5543
                 800-451-1428(VA)
Fax: 804-971-8657

RICHMOND
Virginia Poison Center,
Virginia Commonwealth
University
P.O. Box 980522
Richmond, VA 23298-0522
Emergency: 800-552-6337(VA)
                 804-828-9123
Fax: 804-828-5291

WASHINGTON

SEATTLE
Washington Poison Center (*)
155 N.E. 100th St.
Suite 400
Seattle, WA 98125-8012
Business: 206-517-2351
Emergency: 206-526-2121
                 800-732-6985(WA)
Fax: 206-526-8490

WEST VIRGINIA

CHARLESTON
West Virginia
Poison Center (*)
3110 MacCorkle Ave. S.E.
Charleston, WV 25304
Business: 304-347-1212
Emergency: 304-348-4211
                 800-642-3625(WV)
Fax: 304-348-9560

WISCONSIN

MADISON
Poison Control Center,
University of Wisconsin
Hospital and Clinics
600 Highland Ave.
F6-133
Madison, WI 53792
Business: 608-262-7537
Emergency: 608-262-3702
                 800-815-8855(WI)

MILWAUKEE
Children's Hospital
Poison Center,
Children's Hospital
of Wisconsin
9000 W. Wisconsin Ave.
P.O. Box 1997
Milwaukee, WI 53201
Business: 414-266-2000
Emergency: 414-266-2222
                 800-815-8855(WI)
Fax: 414-266-2820

WYOMING

(OMAHA, NE)
The Poison Center (*)
8301 Dodge St.
Omaha, NE 68114
Emergency: 402-354-5555
                 (Omaha)
                 800-955-9119
                 (WY & NE)

DRUG INFORMATION CENTERS

For additional information on overdosage, adverse reactions, drug interactions, and any other medication problem, specialized drug information centers are strategically located throughout the nation. Use the directory that follows to find the center nearest you. Listings are alphabetical by state and city.

ALABAMA

BIRMINGHAM
Drug Information Service
University of
Alabama Hospital
619 S. 20th Street
1720 Jefferson Tower
Birmingham, AL 35233-6860
Mon.-Fri. 8 AM-5 PM
Tel: 205-934-2162
Fax: 205-934-3501

Global Drug
Information Center
Samford University
McWhorter School
of Pharmacy
800 Lakeshore Drive
Birmingham, AL 35229-7027
Mon.-Fri. 8 AM-5 PM
Tel: 205-870-2659
Fax: 205-414-4012

HUNTSVILLE
Huntsville Hospital Drug
Information Center
101 Sivley Road
Huntsville, AL 35801
Mon.-Fri. 8 AM-5 PM
Tel: 256-517-8288
Fax: 256-517-6558

ARIZONA

TUCSON
Arizona Poison and Drug
Information Center
Arizona Health
Sciences Center
University Medical Center
1501 N. Campbell Ave.
Room 1156
Tucson, AZ 85724
7 days/week, 24 hours
Tel: 520-626-6016
      800-362-0101 (AZ)
Fax: 520-626-2720

CALIFORNIA

LOS ANGELES
Los Angeles Regional
Drug and Poison
Information Center
LAC & USC Medical Center
1200 N. State Street
Room 1107 A & B
Los Angeles, CA 90033
7 days/week, 24 hours
Tel: 213-226-2622
      800-777-6476 (CA)
Fax: 213-226-4194
Poison Control Hotline:
      213-222-3212

SAN DIEGO
Drug Information
Analysis Service
Veterans Administration
Medical Center
3350 La Jolla Village Drive
San Diego, CA 92161
Mon.-Fri. 8 AM-4:30 PM
Tel: 619-552-8585
Fax: 619-552-7582

Drug Information Center
U.S. Naval Hospital
34800 Bob Wilson Drive
San Diego, CA 92134-5000
Mon.-Fri. 8 AM-4 PM
Tel: 619-532-8414

Drug Information Service
University of California
San Diego Medical Center
135 Dickinson Street
San Diego, CA 92103-8925
Mon.-Fri. 9 AM-5 PM
Tel: 900-288-8273
      619-543-6222
Fax: 619-692-1867

STANFORD
Drug Information Center
University of California
Stanford Health
Stanford Campus
300 Pasteur Drive
Room 80301
Stanford, CA 94305
Mon.-Fri. 9 AM-4 PM
Tel: 650-723-6422
Fax: 650-725-5028

COLORADO

DENVER
Rocky Mountain Drug
Consultation Center
8802 E. 9th Avenue
Denver, CO 80220
Mon.-Fri. 8 AM-4:30 PM
Tel: 303-893-3784
      900-370-3784
      (Outside Denver
      County, $1.99
      per minute)

Drug Information Center
University of Colorado
Health Science Center
4200 E. 9th Avenue,
Box C239
Denver, CO 80262
Mon.-Fri. 8:30 AM-4:30 PM
Tel: 303-315-8489
Fax: 303-270-3353

CONNECTICUT

FARMINGTON
Drug Information Service
University of Connecticut
Health Center
263 Farmington Ave.
Farmington, CT 06030
Mon.-Fri. 8 AM-4:30 PM
Tel: 860-679-3783

HARTFORD
Drug Information Center
Hartford Hospital
P.O. Box 5037
80 Seymour Street
Hartford, CT 06102
Mon.-Fri. 8:30 AM-5 PM
Tel: 860-545-2221
      860-545-2961
      (main pharmacy)
      after hours
Fax: 860-545-2415

NEW HAVEN
Drug Information Center
Yale-New Haven Hospital
20 York Street
New Haven, CT 06504
Mon.-Fri. 8:15 AM-4:45 PM
Tel: 203-688-2248
Fax: 203-737-4229

DISTRICT OF COLUMBIA

Drug Information Center
Washington Hospital Center
110 Irving St., NW,
Room B147
Washington, DC 20010
Mon.- Fri. 7:30 AM-4 PM
Tel: 202-877-6646
Fax: 202-877-8925

Drug Information Service
Howard University Hospital
2041 Georgia Ave. NW
Washington, DC 20060
Mon.-Fri. 9 AM-5 PM
Tel: 202-865-1325
Fax: 202-745-3731

FLORIDA

GAINESVILLE

**Drug Information &
Pharmacy Resource Center
Shands Hospital at
University of Florida**
P.O. Box 100316
Gainesville, FL 32610-0316
Mon.-Fri. 9 AM- 5 PM
Tel: 352-395-0408
　　　(for healthcare
　　　professionals only)
Fax: 352-338-9860

JACKSONVILLE

**Drug Information Service
University Medical Center**
655 W. 8th Street
Jacksonville, FL 32209
Mon.-Fri. 8 AM-5 PM
Tel: 904-549-4095
Fax: 904-549-4272

MIAMI

**Drug Information
Center (119)
Miami VA Medical Center**
1201 NW 16th Street
Miami, FL 33125
Mon.-Fri. 7:30 AM-4:30 PM
Tel: 305-324-3237
Fax: 305-324-3394

TALLAHASSEE

**Drug Information
Education Center
Florida Agricultural and
Mechanical University**
Honor House Room 205
Tallahassee, FL 32307
Tel: 850-488-5239
　　　850-599-3064
　　　800-451-3181

GEORGIA

ATLANTA

**Emory University Hospital
Dept. of Pharmaceutical
Services-Drug Information**
1364 Clifton Rd. NE
Atlanta, GA 30322
Mon.-Fri. 8:30 AM-5 PM
Tel: 404-712-4640
Fax: 404-712-7577

**Drug Information Service
Northside Hospital**
1000 Johnson Ferry Road NE
Atlanta, GA 30342
Mon.-Fri. 9 AM-4 PM
Tel: 404-851-8676
Fax: 404-851-8682

AUGUSTA

**Drug Information Center
University of Georgia
Medical College of GA**
Room BIW201
1120 15th Street
Augusta, GA 30912-5600
Mon.-Fri. 8:30 AM-5 PM
Tel: 706-721-2887
Fax: 706-721-3827

IDAHO

POCATELLO

**Idaho Drug Information
Service**
MFU 3 Box 8092
Pocatello, ID 83209
Mon.-Fri. 8 AM-5 PM
Tel: 208-236-4689
Fax: 208-236-4687

ILLINOIS

CHICAGO

**Drug Information Center
Northwestern
Memorial Hospital**
250 E. Superior Street
Wesley 153
Chicago, IL 60611
Mon.-Fri. 8 AM-5 PM
Tel: 312-908-7573
Fax: 312-908-7956

Saint Joseph Hospital
2900 N. Lake Shore Drive
Chicago, IL 60657
8 AM-5 PM
Tel: 312-665-3140
Fax: 312-665-3462

**Drug Information Services
University of Chicago**
5841 S. Maryland Ave.
MC 0010
Chicago, IL 60637
Mon.-Fri. 8 AM-5 PM
Tel: 773-702-1388
Fax: 773-702-6631

**Drug Information Center
University of Illinois
at Chicago**
Room C300, MC 883
1740 W. Taylor St.
Chicago, IL 60612
Mon.-Fri. 8 AM-4 PM
Tel: 312-996-0209
Fax: 312-413-4146

HARVEY

**Drug Information Center
Ingalls Memorial Hospital**
1 Ingalls Drive
Harvey, IL 60426
Mon.-Fri. 8 AM-4:30 PM
Tel: 708-333-2300
Fax: 708-210-3108

HINES

**Drug Information Service
Hines Veterans
Administration Hospital**
Inpatient Pharmacy (119B)
P.O. Box 5000
Hines, IL 60141-5000
Mon.-Fri. 8 AM-4:30 PM
Tel: 708-343-7200

PARK RIDGE

**Drug Information Center
Lutheran General Hospital**
1775 Dempster St.
Park Ridge, IL 60068
Mon.-Fri. 7:30 AM-4 PM
Tel: 847-696-8128

INDIANA

INDIANAPOLIS

**Drug Information Center
St. Vincent Hospital
and Health Services**
2001 W. 86th St.
P.O. Box 40970
Indianapolis, IN 46260
Mon.-Fri. 8 AM-4 PM
Tel: 317-338-3200
Fax: 317-338-3041

**Indiana University Medical
Center/Pharmacy**
Dept. OH1451
550 N. University Blvd.
Indianapolis, IN 46202
Mon.-Fri. 8 AM-4:30 PM
Tel: 317-274-0353
Fax: 317-274-2327

IOWA

DES MOINES

**Regional Drug
Information Center
Mercy Hospital
Medical Center**
400 University Ave.
Des Moines, IA 50314
Mon.-Fri. 8 AM-6 PM
Tel: 515-247-3286
　　　(answered 7
　　　days/week,
　　　24 hours)
Fax: 515-247-3966

IOWA CITY

**Drug Information Center
University of Iowa
Hospitals and Clinics**
200 Hawkins Dr.
Iowa City, IA 52242
Mon.-Fri. 8 AM-5 PM
Tel: 319-356-2600
Fax: 319-356-4545

SIOUX CITY

Iowa Poison Center
2720 Stone Park Blvd.
Sioux City, IA 51104
Tel: 712-277-2222
　　　800-352-2222 (IA)
Fax: 712-279-7852

KANSAS

KANSAS CITY

**Drug Information Center
University of Kansas
Medical Center**
3901 Rainbow Blvd.
Kansas City, KS 66160
Mon.-Fri. 8 AM-6 PM
Tel: 913-588-2328
Fax: 913-588-2350

KENTUCKY

LEXINGTON

**Drug Information Center
Chandler Medical Center
College of Pharmacy
University of Kentucky**
800 Rose St., C-117
Lexington, KY 40536-0084
Mon.-Fri. 8 AM-5 PM
Tel: 606-323-5320
Fax: 606-323-2049

LOUISIANA

MONROE

Drug Information Center
St. Francis Medical Center
309 Jackson St.
Monroe, LA 71210-1901
Tel: 318-327-4250
Fax: 318-327-4125

NEW ORLEANS

Xavier University Drug
Information Center
Tulane University
Hospital and Clinic
Box HC12
1415 Tulane Ave.
New Orleans, LA 70112
Mon.-Fri. 9 AM-5 PM
Tel: 504-588-5670
Fax: 504-588-5862

MARYLAND

ANDREWS AFB

Drug Information Services
89th Med Gp/SGQP
1050 W. Perimeter Rd.
Suite F1-121
Andrews AFB, MD 20331
Mon.-Fri. 7:30 AM-6 PM
Tel: 301-981-4209
Fax: 301-981-4544

ANNAPOLIS

Drug Information Services
The Anne Arundel
Medical Center
Franklin & Cathedral Streets
Annapolis, MD 21401
7 days/week, 24 hours
Tel: 410-267-1130
    410-267-1000
Fax: 410-267-1628

BALTIMORE

Drug Information Services
Franklin Square
Hospital Center
9000 Franklin Square Dr.
Baltimore, MD 21237
7 days/week, 24 hours
Tel: 410-682-7744
Fax: 410-682-8181

Drug Information Service
Johns Hopkins Hospital
600 N. Wolfe St., Halsted 503
Baltimore, MD 21287-6180
Mon.-Fri. 8:30 AM-5 PM
Tel: 410-955-6348
Fax: 410-955-8283

Drug Information Center
University of Maryland at
Baltimore School of
Pharmacy
506 W. Fayette, 3rd Floor
Baltimore, MD 21201
Mon.-Fri. 8:30 AM-5 PM
Tel: 410-706-7568
Fax: 410-706-0897

BETHESDA

Drug Information Service
National Institutes of Health
Building 10, Room 1S-259
10 Center Drive (MSC1196)
Bethesda, MD 20892-1196
Mon.-Fri. 8:30 AM-5 PM
Tel: 301-496-2407
Fax: 301-496-0210

EASTON

Drug Information Center
Memorial Hospital
219 S. Washington St.
Easton, MD 21601
7 days/week, 7 AM - Midnight
Tel: 410-822-1000
Fax: 410-820-9489

MASSACHUSETTS

BOSTON

Drug Information Services
Brigham and Women's
Hospital
75 Frances St.
Boston, MA 02115
Mon.-Fri. 7 AM-3:30 PM
Tel: 617-732-7166
Fax: 617-732-7497

Drug Information Service
New England Medical
Center Pharmacy
750 Washington St., Box 420
Boston, MA 02111
Mon.-Fri. 9 AM-5 PM
Tel: 617-636-8985
Fax: 617-636-5638

WORCESTER

Drug Information Center
U.M.M.C. Hospital
55 Lake Ave. North
Worcester, MA 01655
Mon.-Fri. 8:30 AM-5 PM
Tel: 508-856-3456
    508-856-2775
Fax: 508-856-1850

MICHIGAN

ANN ARBOR

Drug Information Service
University of Michigan
Medical Center
1500 East Medical Center Dr.
UHB2 D301 Box 0008
Ann Arbor, MI 48109
Mon.-Fri. 8 AM-5 PM
Tel: 734-936-8200
    734-936-8251
Fax: 734-923-7027

DETROIT

Drug Information Services
Harper Hospital
3990 John R. St.
Detroit, MI 48201
Mon.-Fri. 8 AM-5 PM
Tel: 313-745-2006
    313-745-8216
    (after hours)
Fax: 313-745-1628

LANSING

Drug Information Center
Sparrow Hospital
1215 E. Michigan Ave.
Lansing, MI 48912
Mon.-Fri. 8 AM-4:30 PM
Tel: 517-483-2444
Fax: 517-483-2088

PONTIAC

Drug Information Center
St. Joseph Mercy Hospital
900 Woodward
Pontiac, MI 48341
Mon.-Fri. 8 AM-4:30 PM
Tel: 248-858-3055
Fax: 248-858-3010

ROYAL OAK

Drug Information Services
William Beaumont Hospital
3601 West 13 Mile Road
Royal Oak, MI 48073-6769
Mon.-Fri. 8 AM-4:30 PM
Tel: 248-551-4077
Fax: 248-551-4046

SOUTHFIELD

Drug Information Service
Providence Hospital
16001 West 9 Mile Rd.
P.O. Box 2043
Southfield, MI 48075
Mon.-Fri. 8 AM-4 PM
Tel: 248-424-3125
Fax: 248-424-5364

MINNESOTA

ROCHESTER

Drug Information Service
Mayo Clinic
1216 2nd St., SW
Rochester, MN 55902
Mon.-Fri. 8 AM-5 PM
Tel: 507-255-5062
    507-255-5732
    (after hours)
Fax: 507-255-7556

MISSISSIPPI

JACKSON

Drug Information Center
University of Mississippi
Medical Center
2500 N. State St.
Jackson, MS 39216
Mon.-Fri. 8 AM-5 PM
Tel: 601-984-2060
    (on call 24 hours)
Fax: 601-984-2063

MISSOURI

SPRINGFIELD

Drug Information & Clinical
Research Services
1235 E. Cherokee
Springfield, MO 65804
Mon.-Fri. 7:30 AM-4:30 PM
Tel: 417-885-3488
Fax: 417-888-7788

ST. JOSEPH

Drug Information Service
Heartland Hospital West
801 Faraon St.
St. Joseph, MO 64501
Mon.-Sat. 8 AM-8 PM
Tel: 816-271-7582
Fax: 816-271-7590

NEBRASKA

OMAHA

Drug Information Service
School of Pharmacy
Creighton University
2500 California Plaza
Omaha, NE 68178
Mon.-Fri. 8:30 AM-4:30 PM
Tel: 402-280-5101
Fax: 402-280-5149

Drug Information Center
Pharmacy Department, NHS
981090 Nebraska
Medical Center
Omaha, NE 68198-1090
Mon.-Fri. 8 AM-4:30 PM
Tel: 402-559-7205
　　　402-559-6747
Fax: 402-559-5463

NEW MEXICO

ALBUQUERQUE
New Mexico Poison &
Drug Information Center
University of New Mexico
Albuquerque, NM 87131-1076
7 days/week, 24 hours
Tel: 505-272-2222
　　　800-432-6866 (NM)
Fax: 505-272-5892

NEW YORK

BROOKLYN
International Drug
Information Center
Long Island University
Arnold & Marie Schwartz
College of Pharmacy
1 University Plaza
RM-Z509
Brooklyn, NY 11201
Mon.-Fri. 9 AM-5 PM
Tel: 718-488-1064
Fax: 718-780-4056

COOPERSTOWN
Drug Information Center
The Mary Imogene
Bassett Hospital
1 Atwell Rd.
Cooperstown, NY 13326
Mon.-Fri. 8:30 AM-5 PM
Tel: 607-547-3686
Fax: 607-547-3629

JAMAICA
Drug Information Center
St. John's University College
of Pharmacy and Allied
Health Professions
8000 Utopia Parkway
Jamaica, NY 11439
Mon.-Fri. 8:30 AM-3:30 PM
Tel: 718-990-2149
Fax: 718-990-2151

NEW YORK CITY
Drug Information Center
Bellevue Hospital Center
462 1st Ave.
New York, NY 10016
Mon.-Fri. 9 AM-5 PM
Tel: 212-562-6504
Fax: 212-562-6503

Drug Information Center
Memorial Sloan-Kettering
Cancer Center
1275 York Ave.
RM S-702
New York, NY 10021
Mon.-Fri. 9 AM-5 PM
Tel: 212-639-7552
Fax: 212-639-2171

Drug Information Center
Mount Sinai Medical Center
1 Gustave Levy Place
New York, NY 10029
Mon.-Fri. 9 AM-5 PM
Tel: 212-241-6619
Fax: 212-348-7927

Drug Information Service
The New York Hospital
Cornell Medical Center
525 E. 68th St.
New York, NY 10021
Mon.-Fri. 9 AM-5 PM
Tel: 212-746-0741
Fax: 212-746-8506

ROCHESTER
Drug Information Service
Dept. of Pharmacy -
Poison Division
University of Rochester
601 Elmwood Ave.
Rochester, NY 14642
24 HRS. 7 Days Week
Tel: 716-275-3718
　　　716-275-2681
　　　(after hours)
Fax: 716-473-9842

STONY BROOK
Suffolk Drug
Information Center
University Hospital
S.U.N.Y. - Stony Brook
Room 3-559, Z7310
Stony Brook, NY 11794-7310
Mon.-Fri. 8 AM-3:00 PM
　No Holidays
Tel: 516-444-2672
　　　516-444-2680
　　　(after hours)
Fax: 516-444-7935

NORTH CAROLINA

BUIES CREEK
Drug Information Center
School of Pharmacy
Campbell University
P.O. Box 1090
Buies Creek, NC 27506
Mon.-Fri. 8:30 AM - 4:30 PM
Tel: 910-893-1478
　　　800-327-5467 (NC)
Fax: 910-893-1476

CHAPEL HILL
Drug Information Center
University of North
Carolina Hospitals
101 Manning Drive
Chapel Hill, NC 27514
Mon.-Fri. 8 AM-4:30 PM
Tel: 919-966-2373
Fax: 919-966-1791

GREENSBORO
Triad Poison Center
Moses H. Cone
Memorial Hospital
1200 N. Elm St.
Greensboro, NC 27401
7 days/week, 24 hours
Tel: 336-574-8105
Fax: 336-574-7198

GREENVILLE
Eastern Carolina Drug
Information Center
Pitt County
Memorial Hospital
Dept. of Pharmacy Service
2100 Stantonsburg Rd.
Greenville, NC 27835
Mon.-Fri. 8 AM- 5 PM
Tel: 919-816-4257
Fax: 919-816-7425

WINSTON-SALEM
Drug Information
Service Center
Wake-Forest University
Baptist Medical Center
Medical Center Blvd.
Winston-Salem, NC 27157
Mon.-Fri. 8 AM-5 PM
Tel: 336-716-2037
Fax: 336-716-2186

OHIO

ADA
Drug Information Center
Raabe College of Pharmacy
Ohio Northern University
Ada, OH 45810
Mon.-Fri. 9 AM - 5 PM
Tel: 419-772-2307
Fax: 419-772-2289

CLEVELAND
Drug Information Center
Cleveland Clinic Foundation
9500 Euclid Avenue
Cleveland, OH 44195
Mon.-Fri. 8 AM - 5 PM
Tel: 216-444-6456
Fax: 216-445-6221

COLUMBUS
Central Ohio Poison Center
700 Children's Drive
Columbus, OH 43205
24 HRS. 7 Days/Week
Tel: 614-228-1323
　　　800-682-7625 (OH)
Fax: 614-221-2672

Drug Information Center
Ohio State
University Hospital
Dept. of Pharmacy
Doan Hall 368
410 W. 10th Avenue
Columbus, OH 43210-1228
Mon.-Fri. 8 AM - 4 PM
Tel: 614-293-8679
Fax: 614-293-3264

Drug Information Center
Riverside Methodist Hospital
3535 Olantangy River Road
Columbus, OH 43214
8 AM - 5 PM
Tel: 614-566-5425
Fax: 614-566-5447

TOLEDO
Drug Information Services
St. Vincent
Mercy Medical Center
2213 Cherry Street
Toledo, Ohio 43608-2691
Mon.-Fri. 8 AM-4 PM
Tel: 419-251-4227
Fax: 419-251-3662

OKLAHOMA

OKLAHOMA CITY

Drug Information Center
Integris Health
3300 Northwest Expressway
Oklahoma City, OK 73112
Mon.-Fri. 8 AM-4:30 PM
Tel: 405-949-3660
Fax: 405-951-8274

Drug Information Center
Presbyterian Hospital
700 NE 13th St.
Oklahoma City, OK 73104
Mon.-Fri. 7:30 AM-3:30 PM
Tel: 405-271-6226
Fax: 405-271-6281

TULSA

Drug Information Service
St. Francis Hospital
6161 S. Yale Ave.
Tulsa, OK 74136
Mon.-Fri. 9 AM-5:30 PM
Tel: 918-494-6339
Fax: 918-494-1893

PENNSYLVANIA

PHILADELPHIA

Drug Information Center
Temple University Hospital
Dept. of Pharmacy
Broad and Ontario St.
Philadelphia, PA 19140
Mon.-Fri. 8 AM-4:30 PM
Tel: 215-707-4644
Fax: 215-707-3463

Drug Information Center
Thomas Jefferson
University Hospital
111 S. 11th
Philadelphia, PA 19107-5098
Mon.-Fri. 8 AM-5 PM
Tel: 215-955-8877
Fax: 215-923-3316

PITTSBURGH

The Pharmaceutical
Information Center
Mylan School of Pharmacy
Duquesne University
431 Mellon Hall
Pittsburgh, PA 15282
Mon.-Fri. 8 AM-4 PM
Tel: 412-396-4600
Fax: 412-396-4488

Drug Information and
Pharmacoepidemiology
Center
University of Pittsburgh
Medical Center
137 Victoria Hall
Pittsburgh, PA 15261
Mon.-Fri. 8:30 AM-4:30 PM
Tel: 412-624-3784
Fax: 412-624-6350

UPLAND

Drug Information Center
Crozer-Chester
Medical Center
Dept. of Pharmacy
1 Medical Center Blvd.
Upland, PA 19013
Mon.-Fri. 8 AM-4:30 PM
Tel: 610-447-2851
    610-447-2862
    (after hours)
Fax: 215-447-2820

WILLIAMSPORT

Drug Information Center
Susquehanna Health System
Rural Avenue Campus
Williamsport, PA 17701
Mon.-Fri. 8 AM-4 PM
Tel: 717-321-3289
Fax: 717-321-3230

PUERTO RICO

SAN JUAN

Centro Information
Medicamentos
Escuela de Farmacia RCM
P.O. Box 365067
San Juan, PR 00936-5067
Mon.-Fri. 8 AM-4:30 PM
Tel: 787-763-0196
Fax: 787-763-0196

RHODE ISLAND

PROVIDENCE

Drug Information Service
Dept. of Pharmacy
Rhode Island Hospital
593 Eddy Street
Providence, RI 02903
7 days/week, 24 hours
Tel: 401-444-5547
Fax: 401-444-8062

SOUTH CAROLINA

CHARLESTON

Drug Information Service
Medical University of
South Carolina
171 Ashley Ave.
Room 604-SFX
Charleston, SC 29425-0810
Mon.-Fri. 8 AM-5:30 PM
Tel: 803-792-3896
    800-922-5250
Fax: 803-792-5532

SPARTANBURG

Drug Information Center
Spartanburg Regional
Medical Center
101 E. Wood St.
Spartanburg, SC 29303
Mon.-Fri. 8 AM-5 PM
Tel: 864-560-6910
Fax: 864-560-6017

TENNESSEE

KNOXVILLE

Drug Information Center
University of Tennessee
Medical Center
1924 Alcoa Highway
Knoxville, TN 37920-6999
Mon.-Fri. 8 AM-4:30 PM
Tel: 423-544-9125

MEMPHIS

South East Regional Drug
Information Center
VA Medical Center
1030 Jefferson Ave.
Memphis, TN 38104
Mon.-Fri. 7:30 AM-4 PM
Tel: 901-523-8990

Drug Information Center
University of Tennessee
847 Monroe Avenue
Suite 238
Memphis, TN 38163
Mon.-Fri. 8:30 AM - 4:30 PM
Tel: 901-448-5555
Fax: 901-448-5419

TEXAS

GALVESTON

Drug Information Center
University of Texas
Medical Branch
301 University Blvd. - G01
Galveston, TX 77555-0701
Mon.-Fri. 8 AM-5 PM
Tel: 409-772-2734
Fax: 409-747-5222

HOUSTON

Drug Information Center
Ben Taub General Hospital
Texas Southern
University/HCHD
1504 Taub Loop
Houston, TX 77030
Mon.-Fri. 8 AM-5 PM
Tel: 713-793-2917
Fax: 713-793-2937

Drug Information Center
Methodist Hospital
6565 Fannin (MSDB109)
Houston, TX 77030
Mon.-Fri. 8 AM-5 PM
Tel: 713-790-4190
Fax: 713-793-1224

LACKLAND A.F.B.

Drug Information Center
Dept. of Pharmacy
Wilford Hall Medical Center
2200 Berquist Dr., Suite 1
Lackland A.F.B., TX 78236
Mon.-Fri. 7:30 AM-5 PM
Tel: 210-292-7100

LUBBOCK

Methodist Hospital
Drug Information and
Consultation Service
3615 19th St.
Lubbock, TX 79410
Mon.-Fri. 8 AM-5 PM
Tel: 806-793-4012
    (Attn: Pharmacy)
Fax: 806-784-5323

TEMPLE

Drug Information Center
Scott and White
Memorial Hospital
2401 S. 31st St.
Temple, TX 76508
Mon.-Fri. 8 AM-6 PM
Tel: 254-724-4636
Fax: 254-724-1731

UTAH

SALT LAKE CITY

Drug Information Center
University of Utah Hospital
Dept. of Pharmacy Services
Room A-050
50 N. Medical Dr.
Salt Lake City, UT 84132
Mon.-Fri. 8:30 AM-4:30 PM
Tel: 801-581-2073
Fax: 801-585-6688

WEST VIRGINIA

MORGANTOWN

West Virginia Drug
Information Center
WV University-Robert C. Byrd
Health Sciences Center
1124 HSN, P.O. Box 9550
Morgantown, WV 26506
Tel: 304-293-6640
        800-352-2501 (WV)
Fax: 304-293-7672

WISCONSIN

MADISON

University of Wisconsin
Hospital & Clinics
600 Highland Ave.
Madison, WI 53792
Voice mail/24 hrs. a day,
responses in 3 days
Tel: 608-262-1315
Fax: 608-263-9424

WYOMING

LARAMIE

Drug Information Center
University of Wyoming
P.O. Box 3375
Laramie, WY 82071
Mon.-Fri. 8 AM-5 PM
Tel: 307-766-6128
Fax: 307-766-2953

STATE BOARDS OF PHARMACY

Questions on local regulations governing prescription and over-the-counter drugs, controlled substances, and pharmacy licensure can often be answered by your local state board of pharmacy. For your convenience, a contact name, address, and phone number for each state board is listed in the directory that follows.

ALABAMA
Jerry Moore, R.Ph.
Executive Secretary
1 Perimeter Park S.
Ste. 425 S
Birmingham, AL 35243
205-967-0130
Fax: 205-967-1009

ALASKA
Debbie Stovern
Licensing Examiner
Department of
Commerce and Economic
Development
P.O. Box 110806
Juneau, AK 99811
907-465-2589
Fax: 907-465-2974

ARIZONA
L.A. Lloyd, R.Ph.
Executive Director
5060 N. 19th Ave.
Ste. 101
Phoenix, AZ 85015
602-255-5125
Fax: 602-255-5740

ARKANSAS
John T. Douglas, P.D.
Executive Director
101 E. Capitol Ave.
Ste. 218
Little Rock, AR 72201
501-682-0190
Fax: 501-682-0195
aspb@mac.state.ar.us

CALIFORNIA
Patricia Harris
Executive Officer
400 "R" St., Ste. 4070
Sacramento, CA 95814
916-445-5014
Fax: 916-327-6308
patricia_harris@dca.ca.gov

COLORADO
W. Kent Mount
Program Administrator
1560 Broadway
Ste. 1310
Denver, CO 80202
303-894-7750—ext. 313
Fax: 303-894-7764
kent.mount@state.co.us

CONNECTICUT
Margherita R.
  Giuliano, R.Ph.
Board Administrator
State Office Building
Rm. 110
165 Capitol Avenue
Hartford, CT 06106
860-566-3290
Fax: 860-566-7630

DELAWARE
David W. Dryden,
  R.Ph., Esq.
Executive Secretary
P.O. Box 637
Dover, DE 19903
302-739-4798
Fax: 302-739-3071

DISTRICT OF COLUMBIA
Barbara Hagans
Contact Representative
614 "H" St., NW,
Rm. 904
Washington, DC 20001
202-727-7468
Fax: 202-727-7662

FLORIDA
John D. Taylor, R.Ph.
Executive Director
Agency for Health
Care Administration
Board of Pharmacy
2020 Capital Cir. S.E.
Bin# C04
Tallahassee, FL 32399
850-488-0595
Fax: 850-413-6982

GEORGIA
Caluha L. Barnes
Executive Director
166 Pryor St. SW
Atlanta, GA 30303
404-656-3912
Fax: 404-657-4220

HAWAII
Ruth Gushiken
Executive Officer
P.O. Box 3469
Honolulu, HI 96801
808-586-2698
Fax: 808-586-2874

IDAHO
R.K. Markuson, R.Ph.
Director
P.O. Box 83720
Boise, ID 83720-0067
208-334-2356
Fax: 208-334-3536

ILLINOIS
Ed Duffy, R.Ph.
Executive Administrator
Drug Compliance
Illinois Department of
Professional Regulation
100 W. Randolph,
Ste. 9-300
Chicago, IL 60601
312-814-4573
Fax: 312-814-3145

INDIANA
Frances L. Kelly
Director
402 W. Washington St.
Rm. 041
Indianapolis, IN 46204
317-232-2960
Fax: 317-233-4236

IOWA
Lloyd K. Jessen,
  R.Ph., J.D.
Exec. Sec./Director
1209 East Court Ave.
Executive Hills West
Des Moines, IA 50319
515-281-5944
Fax: 515-281-4609

KANSAS
Larry Froelich
Director
900 Jackson St. S.W.,
Rm. 513
Topeka, KS 66612-1231
785-296-4056
Fax: 785-296-8420

KENTUCKY
Michael A. Moné,
  R.Ph., J.D.
Executive Director
1024 Capital Center Dr.
Ste. 210
Frankfort, KY 40601
502-573-1580
Fax: 502-573-1582

LOUISIANA
Fred H. Mills, Jr., R.Ph.
Executive Director
5615 Corporate Blvd., 8E
Baton Rouge, LA 70808
504-925-6496
Fax: 504-925-6499

MAINE
Susan Greenlaw
Board Clerk
Maine Board of Pharmacy
35 State House Station
Augusta, ME 04333
207-624-8603
Fax: 207-624-8637

MARYLAND
Norene Pease
Executive Director
4201 Patterson Ave.
Baltimore, MD 21215
410-764-4755
Fax: 410-358-6207

MASSACHUSETTS
Charles Young
Executive Director
100 Cambridge St.
Rm. 1514
Boston, MA 02202
617-727-0085
Fax: 617-727-2366

MICHIGAN
Sheldon Rich, R.Ph.
Chairman
611 W. Ottawa St.
P.O. Box 30018
Lansing, MI 48909
517-373-9102
Fax: 517-373-2179

MINNESOTA
David E. Holmstrom,
  R.Ph., J.D.
Executive Director
2829 University Ave. SE
Ste. 530
Minneapolis, MN 55414
612-617-2201
Fax: 612-617-2212
david.holmstrom@state.
mn.us

MISSISSIPPI
William L. Stevens
Executive Director
P.O. Box 24507
Jackson, MS 39225
601-354-6750
Fax: 601-354-6071
bstevens@its.state.ms.us

MISSOURI
Kevin E. Kinkade, R.Ph.
Executive Director
P.O. Box 625
Jefferson City, MO 65102
573-751-0093
Fax: 573-526-3464
kkinkade@mail.state.
mo.us

MONTANA
Warren R. Amole, R.Ph.
Executive Director
111 N. Jackson
P.O. Box 200513
Helena, MT 59620-0513
406-444-1698
Fax: 406-444-1667

NEBRASKA
Katherine A. Brown
Executive Secretary
Board of Examiners in
Pharmacy
P.O. Box 94986
Lincoln, NE 68509-4986
402-471-2118
Fax: 402-471-3577

NEVADA
Keith W. MacDonald,
R.Ph.
Executive Secretary
1201 Terminal Way
Ste. 212
Reno, NV 89502-3257
702-322-0691
Fax: 702-322-0895

NEW HAMPSHIRE
Paul G. Boisseau, R.Ph.
Executive Director
57 Regional Dr.
Concord, NH 03301
603-271-2350
Fax: 603-271-2856

NEW JERSEY
H. Lee Gladstein, R.Ph.
Executive Director
124 Halsey St., 6th Floor
Newark, NJ 07102
973-504-6450
Fax: 973-648-3355

NEW MEXICO
Jerry Montoya
Executive Director
1650 University Blvd. NE
Ste. 400-B
Albuquerque, NM 87102
505-841-9102
Fax: 505-841-9113
nmbop@nm-
us.campus.mci

NEW YORK
Lawrence H. Mokhiber,
R.Ph.
Executive Secretary
Cultural Education Center
Rm. 3035
Albany, NY 12230
518-474-3848
Fax: 518-473-6995

NORTH CAROLINA
David R. Work, R.Ph.
Executive Director
P.O. Box 459
Carrboro, NC 27510
919-942-4454
Fax: 919-967-5757

NORTH DAKOTA
Howard Anderson, R.Ph.
Executive Director
P.O. Box 1354
Bismarck, ND 58502
701-328-9535
Fax: 701-258-9312

OHIO
William T. Windsley
Executive Director
77 S. High St.,
17th Floor
Columbus, OH 43266
614-466-4143
Fax: 614-752-4836

OKLAHOMA
Bryan Potter, R.Ph.
Executive Director
4545 N. Lincoln Blvd.
Ste. 112
Oklahoma City,
OK 73105
405-521-3815
Fax: 405-521-3758

OREGON
Ruth Vandever, R.Ph.
Executive Director
State Office Bldg.
Ste. 425
800 NE Oregon St., #9
Portland, OR 97232
503-731-4032
Fax: 503-731-4067

PENNSYLVANIA
W. Richard Marshman,
R.Ph.
Penn. State Board of
Pharmacy
Executive Secretary
P.O. Box 2649
Harrisburg, PA 17105
717-783-7157
Fax: 717-787-7769

PUERTO RICO
Giselle Rivera, R.Ph.,
Pharm.D.
President
Call Box 10200
Santurce, PR 00908
787-725-8161
Fax: 787-725-7903

RHODE ISLAND
A. Jeffrey Newell
Chairman of the Board
Department of Health
Board of Pharmacy
Three Capitol Hill
Room 205
Providence, RI 02908
401-222-2837
Fax: 401-222-2158

SOUTH CAROLINA
Louis H. Hutto, Jr.
Chairman
P.O. Box 11927
Columbia, SC 29211
803-896-4700
Fax: 803-896-4596

SOUTH DAKOTA
Dennis M. Jones, R.Ph.
Executive Secretary
4305 S. Louise Ave.
Ste. 104
Sioux Falls, SD 57106
605-362-2737
Fax: 605-362-2738

TENNESSEE
Kendall M. Lynch
Director
500 James
Robertson Pkwy.
Nashville, TN 37243
615-741-2718
Fax: 615-741-2722

TEXAS
Gay Dodson, R.Ph.
Executive Director
333 Guadalupe
Ste. 3-600, Box 21
Austin, TX 78701-3942
512-305-8001
Fax: 512-305-8075

UTAH
J. Craig Jackson
Director
Utah Department of
Commerce
P.O. Box 146741
Salt Lake City,
UT 84114
801-530-6628
Fax: 801-530-6511

VERMONT
Carla Preston
Staff Assistant
109 State St.
Montpelier, VT 05609
802-828-2875
Fax: 802-828-2465
cpreston@sec.state.vt.us

VIRGINIA
Elizabeth Scott Russell,
R.Ph.
Executive Director
6606 W. Broad St.
4th Floor
Richmond, VA 23230
804-662-9911
Fax: 804-662-9313
www.dhp.state.va.us

WASHINGTON
Donald H. Williams, R.Ph.
Executive Director
P.O. Box 47863
Olympia, WA 98504
360-753-6834
Fax: 360-586-4359

WEST VIRGINIA
Sam Kapourales, R.Ph.
President
232 Capitol St.
Charleston, WV 25301
304-558-0558
Fax: 304-558-0572

WISCONSIN
Patrick D. Braatz
Administrator
P.O. Box 8935
Madison, WI 53708
608-266-2811
Fax: 608-267-0644

WYOMING
Jim Carder
Executive Director
1720 S. Poplar St.,
Ste. 4
Casper, WY 82601
307-234-0294
Fax: 307-234-7226

reported. Even when Wilson heard unexpectedly good tallies, he muted his feelings, simply saying, "That is encouraging."

After dinner, the family retired to Ellen's studio. Woodrow stood before the hearth, awaiting each bulletin. There were no surprises, just steadily positive updates. The Wilsons amused themselves with conversation for a while; and then, to fill a lull, Wilson grabbed a volume of Robert Browning and read aloud. Nobody paid much attention. Nell kept slipping out of the room, anxious to learn the latest. A little before ten, she was about to return to the reading when she heard the sound of a distant bell. Within a moment, it was clanging wildly; and that unmistakable peal from Nassau Hall drew Ellen to the front door. Tumulty burst from the crowd of newspapermen, calling out, "He's elected, Mrs. Wilson!"

Ellen returned to the studio and found her husband examining the latest tabulations. No words were required. She simply placed her hands on Woodrow's shoulders and raised her face toward his as he leaned forward and kissed her gently. Margaret, Jessie, and Nell approached, and he hugged each of them. And then others entered the room to congratulate him, while a crowd gathered outside. Messenger boys kept arriving with telegrams. "I cordially congratulate you on your election and extend to you my best wishes for a successful administration," read President Taft's from Cincinnati. Theodore Roosevelt had wired from Oyster Bay, New York, "The American people by a great plurality have conferred upon you the highest honor in their gift. I congratulate you thereon."

The final numbers would not be known for days, but that great plurality held through the night. With a four-way race making a majority virtually impossible, Wilson was racking up a decisive victory—50 percent more votes than his closest competitor. In the end, he would win 6,293,454 votes (41.9 percent) to Roosevelt's 4,119,538 (27.4 percent), Taft's 3,484,980 (23.2 percent), and Debs's 900,672 (6 percent). The electoral vote was much more lopsided, as Wilson carried all but eight states: California, Washington, South Dakota, Minnesota, Michigan, and Pennsylvania (88 electoral votes), which went to Roosevelt; and Utah and Vermont (8 electoral votes), which went to Taft. Wilson's 435 electors were more than the nation had ever bestowed upon a single candidate.

Amid the increasing excitement, Nellie Wilson had a chilling moment as she watched all the elation drain from her father's face. In the meantime,

the clamor outside demanded his presence. By the time Wilson reached the front door to confront the crowd, his countenance reflected only the gravity of the moment. He was able to suppress his emotions until he looked out and perceived a sea of undergraduates surging into Cleveland Lane, waving flags and singing "Old Nassau." The ancestral wail of a bag-pipe pierced the cool night air. At last, the old schoolmaster wept.

For a moment, vanity got the best of him. Mindful of the patch on his head, he wanted to stand above the crowd. Tumulty and Dudley Malone carried a rocking chair to the portal and held it fast, so that Wilson could stand on it. "Gentlemen," he said, "I am sincerely glad to see you. I have no feeling of triumph tonight, but a feeling of solemn responsibility. . . . You men must play a great part. I plead with you again to look constantly forward. I summon you for the rest of your lives to support the men who like myself want to carry the nation forward to its highest destiny and greatness."

After less than two years—only 658 days—of public service, Woodrow Wilson had been elected the twenty-eighth President of the United States. It had all happened so swiftly as to seem predestined, as though millennia of circumstances had paved the way to this moment . . . and all that lay ahead.

PART THREE

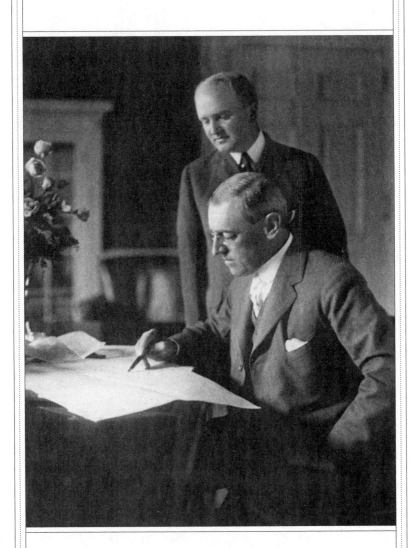

8

DISCIPLES

On the next day . . . they heard that Iesus was com-
ming to Hierusalem . . .
    And Iesus, when he had found a yong asse, sate
thereon, as it is written . . .

—IOHN, XII:12–14

The President-elect slept well.

The revelers on Cleveland Lane had dispersed
around midnight, leaving Woodrow Wilson to turn in by
one. He did not awaken until nine. When he faced the
waiting phalanx of reporters, he revealed, "It has not quite
dawned on me. I had been in an impersonal atmosphere for
the last three months, reading about myself, reading that I
was to be elected, and now I can hardly believe that it is
true."

Before requesting the details of his own historic
election—becoming the first Democrat elected to the
White House in twenty years and the first Southerner since
the Civil War—Wilson inquired about the Congressional
results. In an election with the lowest turnout (58.8 percent) in seventy-six years, he had coattails. Democrats fortified their majority in the House of Representatives by
picking up sixty-one new seats; and while most state legislatures still elected their United States Senators, Democrats
were poised to start the next session of Congress with a

seven-vote majority. The results, Wilson told the press, filled him with "the hope that the thoughtful Progressive forces of the Nation may now at last unite to give the country freedom of enterprise and a Government released from all selfish and private influences, devoted to justice and progress." When somebody pointed out that many in the press had already chosen his departmental secretaries, Wilson replied, "Well, then, you have to forbid me reading the newspapers for they might prejudice me." That afternoon, Wilson and his bodyguard walked to the far perimeter of the Princeton campus—greeting friends along the way and tramping around much of Lake Carnegie.

The next few days brought more than fifteen thousand letters and telegrams and what felt like as many visitors. Overnight, influence peddlers and office seekers pushed the well-wishers aside. Those who restrained themselves least met Wilson's resistance most. As the chairman of his successful campaign committee, William McCombs had every reason to make his way to Cleveland Lane, as he did late Election Night; but his erratic nature, periodic misjudgments, and blatant intentions troubled Wilson. "Before we proceed," the President-elect said upon greeting him, "I wish it clearly understood that I owe you nothing." As McCombs began to recount his contributions, Wilson interrupted to say, "God ordained that I should be the next president of the United States. Neither you nor any other mortal could have prevented that." And though McCombs lingered in Princeton for most of that week, Wilson allowed him no private audience as he confined his few political conversations to telephone calls with Colonel House, whose judgment he already prized above all others', as he would for most of his Presidency.

Colonel House left a remarkable record of his hundreds of encounters with Woodrow Wilson—three thousand typed pages, which he dictated almost daily. They provide telling glimpses of Woodrow Wilson, so long as one never forgets that House is their focal point and that diary can be the falsest art. House presents himself as the man who often suggested Wilson's best ideas and who had cautioned against the worst, an intimate who never overstepped or even misstepped. In truth, Wilson was phlegmatic on few topics. He appreciated new facts and entertained outside opinions; but from those closest to him, he preferred constancy over contention. He generally expected his advisers to react to his thoughts rather than supply him with new ones.

In that capacity, House complemented Wilson perfectly. Stockton Axson wondered how much House actually did see and how much "he, Polonius-like, merely confirmed what the President saw." He seemed "never to say anything rememberable" and was, in fact, "usually silent; and when he spoke, . . . deferentially in agreement with everything W. W. said." Axson granted that most of their serious discussions took place behind closed doors, but he was never aware of House's arguing with Wilson; and he noticed that House "had the tact to refrain from even mentioning public affairs at the luncheon or dinner table unless the President himself should shift the table talk from anecdote and limericks to something serious." No intellectual, House was a rapt listener, a challenging but undemanding conversationalist. He could keep a confidence.

House's greatest talent was in "playing" Wilson—tuning his temperament to Wilson's and seldom striking a discordant note. He was vain but devoid of venality, seeming to want "nothing for himself." That lack of greed kept him, in Wilson's eyes, "clear-sighted"—for he looked at both national and international questions without a personal agenda. Unlike legislators, who had to consider their home districts, and even Cabinet members, who were responsible to their departments, House had a constituency of one. He drew the blueprints of plans Wilson could only sketch; as Axson said, "He relished the personal details involved, which the President disliked." He was not afraid to speak his mind, but was careful never to cross the President. Wilson did not suffer fools; and he enjoyed listening to House—because, in large measure, that meant hearing himself. For his companionship as much as his counsel, House become an indispensable friend.

Over time, House evolved into a figure unique in American history—a full-time unpaid adviser with singular and total access to the President of the United States, and answerable only to him. So long as Woodrow Wilson was pleased, Colonel House operated of his own volition and on his own dime, always behind the scenes. No man in American history ever wielded so much power yet remained so unaccountable. "Take my word for it," said the blind Senator T. P. Gore of Oklahoma, "he can walk on dead leaves and make no more noise than a tiger."

"Clearly," William G. McAdoo wrote of House and Wilson, "he was the friend to whom he could turn and to whom he did turn" when it came to selecting the Cabinet. Moving "outside the periphery of official life," McAdoo noted, House was "better situated than the Governor to look into

golfed, napped, and even indulged in solitaire. He and Nell went several times to the small theater in town, where a stock company performed "excruciatingly bad" productions. ("I shall never grow up," he told her. "I would rather see poor acting than not go to a play when I have a chance.") He devoted part of every morning dictating to Swem, and over the next four weeks, they worked through the stack of vital correspondence, responding to seven hundred letters. Wilson even made time to review the proofs of a book called *The New Freedom*, a compilation of his campaign speeches about to be published. When a newspaper photographer snapped a picture of the President-elect behind the walls at Glencove, Wilson confronted him, declaring, "You're no gentleman, and I'll thrash you if you do that again." The photographer apologized profusely.

Beyond that, Wilson engaged in an activity Presidents seldom allow themselves—contemplation. His experiences as president of Princeton and Governor of New Jersey had taught him that the most opportune moment to institute change was at the beginning of one's tenure—with the wind of optimism at one's back and before the forces of resistance had a chance to gather. And so, Wilson began prioritizing his programs so that he might set them in motion upon his arrival at the White House. He turned directly to those decisions by which the public first judges its Chief Executive, the selection of a Cabinet—ten departmental heads. "In his usual methodical way," Nell observed, "he made a series of charts—a page for each man under consideration, listing the details of their careers, their qualifications, their friends, even the sort of wives they had." And then, in his own form of solitaire, Wilson shuffled the charts, discarding one name each time he considered another. His family grew so exasperated with the secrecy of his process, it began to lose interest. "I don't really care who you choose," Nellie blurted one day, "as long as you make McAdoo Secretary of the Treasury." That delighted her father. "Imagine!" he said to Ellen. "Nell wants me to appoint a man to the Cabinet just because she likes him."

With the President-elect sporting a tropical tan, the Wilsons returned on the *Bermudian* on December 16, 1912. Margaret Wilson and Joseph Tumulty met them at the pier. The four-week sojourn had been "an unmixed blessing," Wilson wrote Mary Hulbert, then Stateside, as those "healing days in Bermuda gave us a great store of peace and vitality upon which to live in the months to come." He would need it, as opposition forces were already plotting to reclaim New Jersey for themselves. Governor

Wilson insisted that he had not finished fighting there—that he had no intention of resigning immediately or even of changing his residence. "It is very important that the people should feel that I am still connected with New Jersey," he said, at least until "the progressive program is complete, even to the dot above the i." Within hours of disembarking, he was on a train to Trenton, where—with the recent Democratic victories—a new generation of would-be state bosses was dispensing patronage, a young Frank Hague of Jersey City among them.

A few weeks later, with his second annual message to the state legislature, Wilson hoped to turn the last year's accomplishments into the drumbeat of the Progressive march onward. For immediate consideration, the Governor raised such matters as the need to alter the state's corporation laws, regulation of investment companies, reform of the criminal justice system, an examination of tax assessment and collection, further empowerment of the Public Utility Commissioners, encouragement of the commission form of government, and conservation of natural resources, including forest preservation. He strongly urged approval of two amendments to the Constitution of the United States that awaited ratification—the Sixteenth, which would empower Congress to levy taxes on incomes, and the Seventeenth, which would establish the direct election of Senators by popular vote. While his ambitious program would face mixed results, Wilson saw the New Jersey legislature address all of it. The State Senate passed a woman suffrage resolution; and legislators agreed to enact a law that would remove jury selection from the hands of sheriffs. Before leaving office, Wilson would sign a set of anti-trust bills—called the "seven sisters"; and shortly thereafter, New Jersey would ratify the constitutional amendments.

Between mid-December and his inauguration, Wilson also delivered a handful of speeches outside the state, reiterating a few basic themes. On his second night after returning from Bermuda, he addressed the New York Southern Society at the Waldorf-Astoria, telling the roomful of transplants from Dixie that America was "not what it was when the Civil War was fought"—that while regional pride was to be appreciated, sectionalism was not, and that the Progressive principles for which he had been fighting in New Jersey should apply across the country. Weeks later, addressing the Commercial Club of Chicago, Wilson said he hoped to bring about an end to "the old feeling that the Southerner was not of the

same political breed and purpose as the rest of American citizens" and that he hoped to see the death of "many another prejudice, particularly of these prejudices which are getting such formidable root amongst us as between class and class, as between those who control the resources of the country and those who use the resources of the country."

"The business future of this country," Wilson asserted, "does not depend upon the government of the United States. It depends upon the business men of the United States. . . . only the temper and the thought and the purpose of business men in America is going to determine what the future of business shall be." Wilson indicated several fights he intended to pick—against the protectionist Payne-Aldrich tariff, the banking structure, and the constricting monopolies in America.

Between the New York and Chicago addresses, Wilson visited Virginia. His train stopped at five stations, each crowded with cheering throngs—especially in Charlottesville, where the student body had turned out en masse. In Staunton, most of the town greeted him, including a band playing "Home, Sweet Home." Wilson spent the night in the manse at the top of the hill, in the very bedroom in which he had been born. The next day, December 28, the celebration of his fifty-sixth birthday began with a rhapsodic introduction from his host, a successor to the Reverend Joseph Wilson. "He went out from us as a very little boy, laden with the prayers and benedictions of a small congregation of Christian people," said the Reverend A. M. Fraser of the honoree. "He comes back to us to-day, by the favour of an overruling Providence, a proven leader of men." Wilson visited an old aunt, whom he had not seen since childhood. She had grown extremely deaf and required a long black ear-trumpet, which made conversation no easier. At one point, she said, "Well, Tommy, what are you doing now?" And Wilson said, "I've been elected President, Aunt Janie."

"Well, well," said old Aunt Janie, "president of what?"

Wilson told the citizens of Staunton exactly the sort of President of the United States he intended to be. For a generation, a Protestant-based movement called "the Social Gospel" had infused American thought. With it came improvements in health and housing, and the establishment of salvation armies and Christian associations to help young men from the country adjust to life in the city. The notion that Christian acts might cure social ills was nothing new to Wilson; he approached his new bully pulpit fully aware of his power as evangel in chief. Moral forces were at work,

Wilson told his audience at a birthday banquet at the Staunton Military Academy. In another talk, on the steps of the Mary Baldwin Seminary, he said, "There must be heart in a government; there must be a heart in the policies of government. And men must look to it that they do unto others as they would have others do unto them." Wilson believed such thought strengthened—not softened—him. "This is not a rosewater affair," he said. "This is an office in which a man must put on his war paint. . . . And there must be some good hard fighting, not only in the next four years, but in the next generation, in order that we may achieve the things that we have set out to achieve."

Republican opposition was already insinuating that the Democratic Party was going to institute changes destructive to the economy. Wilson assured his audiences that only those trying to create such panic had reason to fear. To those attempting to game the system, Wilson promised "on behalf of my countrymen, a gibbet as high as Haman."

A member of the press had recently suggested to Wilson that this Christmas must be the happiest of his life. "My young friend," he replied, "evidently you have never been elected President of the United States. Can you see how a man can have a light heart looking forward to the responsibilities of that great office, particularly at this time?"

"The President is not all of the Executive," Professor Woodrow Wilson wrote in *Congressional Government*. "He cannot get along without the men whom he appoints . . . and they are really integral parts of that branch of the government which he titularly contains in his one single person. The characters and training of the Secretaries are of almost as much importance as his own gifts and antecedents." Through the winter of 1912–13, Colonel House discreetly interviewed numerous prospects, arranging with Tumulty for Wilson to meet the most promising contenders in either Trenton or Princeton. With so short a political career of his own, Wilson had few political debts to service; but, reluctantly, he accepted that he headed a century-old party with political machinery in place. With that in mind, Wilson began wading through both enthusiastic and contradictory advice, starting with his first appointment.

"What will be done with Bryan?" was the urgent question. Edith Gittings Reid, an epistolary friend of Wilson's since his days in Baltimore, said, "The East was uneasy and prophesied dire results if Bryan was given a leading position. The West vowed that dire results would

impression that by accepting this great honor I would be doing him a favor." Although House had occasionally suggested that he was being considered for the post, McAdoo regarded himself unfit and told Wilson as much—that he was a man of business, not banking. "I don't want a banker or a financier," Wilson exclaimed. "The Treasury is not a bank. Its activities are varied and extensive. What I need is a man of all-round ability who has had wide business experience." McAdoo also had personal reservations: a widower for less than a year, with six (mostly grown) children, he was not a man of means. The job paid $12,000 a year, which would not go far in meeting the social expenses generally associated with the position. Wilson appealed to McAdoo's sense of duty, explaining that he could not perform the great responsibilities of office alone. "If I can't have the assistance of those in whom I have confidence," he said, "what am I to do?" McAdoo discreetly withdrew from the Hudson & Manhattan Railroad Company.

To serve as the Postmaster General, the largest employer in the United States, Colonel House recommended Albert S. Burleson, an eight-term Congressman from Texas who had become an aggressive Wilson supporter during the Baltimore convention. He struck Wilson as too much of an old-time politician, but House believed his familiarity with the inner workings of Congress and the patronage system would benefit both the department and the President. A letter from Oscar Underwood, the House Majority Leader and chairman of the Ways and Means Committee, with whom Wilson had already taken up the subject of a tariff bill, persuaded the President that Burleson was exactly what this highly political position required, if only because it would please the Speaker of the House. The first Texan ever to serve in a Cabinet and the son of a Confederate officer, Burleson was a known segregationist—which, at that time, was not a political liability. Upon receiving the official offer from the President-elect, Burleson told Wilson, "I will be loyal to your administration and sympathetic with your policies. When I reach the point where I cannot give you my undivided loyalty, I will tender my resignation. When I talk to you, I will always tell you my candid views. I can't know what is in your mind, but I can tell you what is in mine." As the boss of more Negroes in America than any other man, Burleson would prove to have enormous influence on life in Washington and the rest of the nation. For his vow of intense fealty to his administration, Wilson remained equally loyal to him, allowing him to run his department as he saw fit.

Colonel House recommended another Texan he knew well, one whose curriculum vitae closely resembled Wilson's. David F. Houston was born in North Carolina and educated at South Carolina College in Columbia, where he had studied under Wilson's uncle Dr. James Woodrow. After earning a master's degree at Harvard, Houston taught government at the University of Texas, where he became the school's president, a position he would subsequently hold at Texas A&M University before becoming chancellor of Washington University in St. Louis. Many found him cold and incommunicative but also "a man of intellectual force and solid information." Wilson had met him several times over the years and, upon learning of House's confidence in him, offered him the Department of Agriculture. Like most of the men in the Wilson Cabinet, he too wondered how he could relocate and live on the modest salary.

Josephus Daniels was a North Carolinian and, like Wilson, a nonpracticing attorney. This alumnus of the law school at Chapel Hill became active in state and then national Democratic politics, using the press to advance himself and his causes. He ran the Raleigh *News and Observer* and married into the political Worth family. A true Progressive and a friend of William Jennings Bryan, Daniels had helped defuse the "cocked hat" incident and had proved himself valuable as publicity director of the Democratic National Committee. For these reasons—not any maritime experience, for he had none—Wilson chose him to be Secretary of the Navy. His not knowing the ropes bespoke the lack of importance Wilson ascribed to the position. On the heels of the appointment, Wilson remarked to his friend and adviser Walter Page, "You do not seem to think that Daniels is Cabinet timber." Page replied, "He is hardly a splinter." Daniels was also an avowed white supremacist.

Upon receiving the appointment, Daniels immediately found his Assistant Secretary—the ambitious, anti-Tammany Franklin Roosevelt, a genuine lover of the sea. As Daniels noted in his diary, "He had supported Wilson for the nomination, and taken an active part in the campaign, and I found him a singularly attractive and honorable and courageous young Democratic leader." Wilson thought it was a "capital" idea. Although thirty-year-old Roosevelt had served but one term in Albany, he already provoked strong reactions. As soon as his name was floated, New York Senator (and TR's Secretary of State) Elihu Root warned Daniels that "every person named Roosevelt wishes to run everything and would try to be

the Secretary." Daniels told him that any man who feared being supplanted by a subordinate was tacitly confessing his own inadequacy for the job. When Wilson heard that story, he was convinced he had both the right Secretary and Assistant. That young FDR was an ardent Democrat and a cousin of TR—and was even married to the former President's niece—gave Wilson and the party some unexpected bragging rights.

A sign of the rising power of the conjoined labor and Progressive movements could be seen in 1913, as a bill arrived on President Taft's desk that would bisect the existing Department of Commerce and Labor. A reluctant Taft signed it on his last day in office, knowing the incoming President would establish the new position if he did not. The first man nominated for Secretary of Labor carried all the credentials Wilson needed to trust him: born in Scotland, the Presbyterian William Beauchop Wilson (no relation to his new boss) had worked in the coal mines of Pennsylvania as a child and then rose in the ranks of the labor movement, becoming an officer of the United Mine Workers of America before getting elected to Congress. McAdoo called him "level-headed, able, and trustworthy."

Wilson had intended his Secretary of Commerce to be one of America's staunchest Progressives, his adviser Louis D. Brandeis. Earliest mentions of his name, however, incited considerable protest. Politicians, businessmen, and attorneys denounced him as a radical—a reckless meddler who would queer any possibilities of investment in a Democratic-led prosperity. Wrote one Boston Brahmin to Cleveland Dodge, knowing he had the President-elect's trust, "I have no hesitation in pronouncing Mr. Brandeis treacherous, and I sometimes doubt if he is sane." Wilson overlooked the specific criticisms and even the unveiled anti-Semitism. But not only did Adamses, Lowells, and Peabodys oppose Brandeis, so too did many Jews themselves, such as Jacob Schiff, the financier and philanthropist—those who had a foot in the establishment door and did not want Brandeis's extremist reputation to spoil opportunities for more accommodating Jews. But plumbing fixture heir and Wilson insider—and latent anti-Semite—Charles R. Crane paid Brandeis nothing but his highest praise, calling him "the only important Jew who is *first* American and then Jew," a tribute that revealed the primary accusation American Jews then faced. Wilson wrote Brandeis supporter Bryan that he felt "the people's lawyer" had been "grossly aspersed," but he simply could not ignore the widespread prejudice against him. Not until a week before the inauguration did he settle on William C.

Redfield of Brooklyn, who had spent his life in business, mining, manufacturing, banking, and insurance before getting elected to Congress,
where he earned a reputation as a tariff specialist.

Wilson considered Brandeis a more obvious choice to serve as Attorney
General, but giving him that even more sensitive position would have created an even greater outcry. Wilson hoped to enlist Pennsylvania Congressman A. Mitchell Palmer, who had been an ardent supporter at the
Baltimore convention. Further study, however, revealed that Palmer had
been involved with a few clients with tenuous ties to trusts. And so House
lobbied for James C. McReynolds, an attorney who carried Progressive
credentials. A Kentucky-born graduate of Vanderbilt University in Tennessee who had studied law in Charlottesville, McReynolds taught and
then became an Assistant Attorney General in the Taft Administration. In
that capacity, he prosecuted the government's cases against the tobacco
and the anthracite coal monopolies. House persisted, and Wilson relented,
as both embraced McReynolds's independent spirit. They did not yet realize that his outspokenness included a repugnant personality and name-
calling racism.

Still hoping to include Palmer in his Cabinet, Wilson offered him the
War Department. Palmer seriously considered the honor up until a week
before the inauguration, when he declined. As he explained in a letter to
Wilson: "I am a Quaker. Many generations of my people have borne strong
testimony against 'war and the preparations for war.' Of course, as a Representative in Congress, I vote for the great supply bills to maintain the
military establishment . . . but I do this in response to the sentiment and
opinion of a vast majority of the people whom I represent. . . . As a Quaker
War Secretary, I should consider myself a living illustration of a horrible
incongruity." The very thought of such an appointment revealed how little
Wilson considered possible international conflagration. Palmer stood by
his conscience and chose not to "sit down in cold blood in an executive
position and use such talents as I possess to the work of preparing for such
a conflict." With only days remaining before Wilson took office, Tumulty
urged him to name somebody from their home state. He suggested Lindley M. Garrison, who had been an attorney in Camden and Jersey City
before he became a Vice-Chancellor of New Jersey. Wilson summoned
him to Trenton the next day and on the spot offered Garrison the position,
which he accepted.

For six decades the Department of the Interior had been the grab bag of the executive branch, looking after Indian affairs, patents, and the District of Columbia jails, among many concerns. Theodore Roosevelt had elevated its stature and deepened its purpose with his drive to protect America's wealth of natural resources, as water, oil, coal, and lumber had become lucrative enterprises. Taft had alienated TR, in fact, when he replaced his friend Gifford Pinchot, who headed the Division of Forestry, with a man more inclined toward private development than public use. There was no question where Wilson stood on the matter: "The raw materials obtainable in this country for every kind of manufacture and industry must be at the disposal of everybody in the United States upon the same terms." Thus, he considered several top Progressives for the Cabinet post, including Franklin K. Lane, a California Democrat who was then chairman of the Interstate Commerce Commission, having been appointed by Roosevelt.

Lane thought himself unworthy of the position; and when Colonel House sounded him out, he recommended another man. Beyond the self-effacement of Lane's letter, Wilson was impressed with his understanding of the job requirements. When his first choice, Mayor Newton D. Baker of Cleveland—a former student of Wilson's at Johns Hopkins and currently a reform Mayor only one year into his position—declined the nomination, Wilson nominated Lane, just four days before the inauguration.

"I must have the best men in the nation," Wilson had written Walter Hines Page at the start of the appointment process, when he had imagined only the most qualified would answer his calls to service. But as McAdoo would later write, "The judging of men is difficult at its best. When it happens to be entangled in a web of extraneous political considerations, it becomes frequently a matter of luck." Page pronounced the Cabinet "distinctly mediocre." In the end, Colonel House said only, "I think, in all the circumstances, we have done well."

Unlike modern Presidential cabinets, which portray as many facets of America as possible, the Wilson Cabinet of 1913 was a ten-way mirror, each panel of which reflected a different aspect of the man at the center. This was mostly a team of Rebels—lawyers from the South who had pursued other professions and never shed their Confederate biases, Anglo-Saxon Protestants all, mostly newcomers to Washington, if not politics altogether. Within the Wilson Cabinet, there would be much discussion

but little debate. For the most part, the President would delegate power to his Secretaries (all younger than he) to run their own departments, as he seldom found reason to countermand any of them. Every decision from this administration, noted one close observer, would contain a moral component, inspired by "the breath of God."

For the position of secretary to the President himself—a combination of political adviser and chief of staff—Wilson considered nobody but Tumulty. Although his experience was limited and he had seen little of the world beyond New Jersey, he had ably and loyally served Governor Wilson, keeping the Trenton office running smoothly during the months of transition. Many Democrats challenged Tumulty's understanding of national politics; and hundreds tried to block him from office because of his Catholicism. One letter asked Wilson if he was willing to have "the secrets of the White House relayed to Rome." But Wilson discarded the letter, saying only, "Asinine." In truth, Wilson trusted nobody's understanding of hand-to-hand politics more than Tumulty's. As he always remained behind the scenes, not even Wilson himself knew all that Tumulty did for him in the way of public relations and political maneuvering.

Among these appointments, two men remained conspicuously absent. The first was Colonel House, whom Wilson invited to join his "official family." Beyond the compliment of the offer, House never considered it. "I very much prefer being a free lance, and to advise with him regarding matters in general," House told his diary. He had no inclination to hold office, preferring "to have a roving commission to serve wherever and whenever possible." House created a niche for himself, with as much influence and as little responsibility as he desired. "Had I gone into the Cabinet," he admitted, "I could not have lasted eight weeks." In no time, anyone seeking Woodrow Wilson's attention realized that Colonel House provided the most direct access.

The second missing person was the most covetous of all the office seekers. After months of consideration, campaign manager William McCombs remained on Wilson's mind but never on a list. Wilson praised McCombs's intelligence but felt "he is never satisfied unless he plays the stellar role." Where Lincoln thrived on a gadfly such as William Seward in his Cabinet, Wilson said he feared McCombs could not "work in harness with the other men and that I should never get any real team work from him." More to the point, Wilson simply did not like him and resented even having

to spend time with him. After McCombs had accompanied the Wilsons to Staunton, during which time the two men had been alone together for more than an hour, Woodrow told Ellen he felt as if he had been "sucked by a vampire and had been left weak and ill."

When McCombs realized that Wilson favored McAdoo over him for Secretary of the Treasury, he bid to become Attorney General. Wilson's displeasure with the man turned into distaste. He asked McCombs why he suddenly preferred that position, and McCombs said that since he was a lawyer, the appointment would help him enormously when his term of office expired. "What a surprising statement for any man to make!" Wilson exclaimed to his secretary. "Why, Tumulty, many of the scandals of previous administrations have come about in this way, Cabinet officers using their posts to advance their own personal fortunes. It must not be done in our administration. It would constitute a grave scandal to appoint such a man to so high an office."

Many would later denounce Wilson for failing to reward McCombs with any spoils of victory. Unfortunately, he became his own worst enemy. His petty jealousies and grand insecurities became rampant, as did his consumption of alcohol—a bottle of whiskey a day, said Tumulty. And Wilson did remain loyal, offering him the ambassadorship to France. McCombs considered the posting for several months, vacillating daily—even after refusing it. Money was the mitigating factor, as Ambassadors had long been expected to foot the entertainment bills for their embassies, which excluded all but the rich from serving as diplomats in the major capitals. Wilson kept the position open for another year, allowing McCombs to change his mind once more, but he never did.

In his last Annual Message, President George Washington had urged the Congress of 1796 to compensate governmental officers sufficiently, suggesting that "it would be repugnant to the vital principles of our government virtually to exclude from public trusts talents and virtue unless accompanied by wealth." Wilson's overseas appointments reflected the dilemma at hand. He felt uncomfortable turning these positions into political rewards, but because the United States was at peace with the rest of the world and because there were so many envoys to name, he succumbed to repaying several men who were "conspicuous for [their] money." He had hoped to send his friend and former colleague Henry Fine to Germany; but even with the promise of a private stipend from Cleveland Dodge, Fine

believed life in the foreign court would strain his financial means. Wilson settled on James W. Gerard, a New York State Justice and onetime Tammany candidate, in part because Gerard had wealth and powerful friends in his influential home state. William Graves Sharp, a Congressman from Ohio whom Wilson sent to France, was a man of more modest means, as was Walter Hines Page, his newspaper friend, whom he named as Ambassador to Great Britain (after two others refused). Another writer, Thomas Nelson Page (no relation), came from an old Virginia family and became famous for his romantic evocations of the antebellum South before Wilson posted him to Rome. Frederic Courtland Penfield, a Wilson supporter with time and money, would spend the next several years in Vienna, the capital of the Austro-Hungarian Empire; Henry van Dyke, from the Princeton faculty, agreed to serve in the Hague; and Henry Morgenthau accepted the ambassadorship to the Ottoman Empire, which then included the Holy Land, where Wilson thought a Jew might provide the necessary balance between the Muslim and Christian populations. While Wilson's diplomatic corps was a diversified group, it lacked the academic heft he had once envisioned; few were expert in their territories, though such proficiency hardly seemed a prerequisite for any of the jobs during that international lull.

While most of Wilson's supplicants pressed for jobs, some pressured for a cause. Samuel Gompers, the president of the American Federation of Labor, went to Trenton expecting a ten-minute conference. Wilson gave the Jewish former cigar maker an hour and a half, during which time Gompers called for more protection of labor in upcoming anti-trust legislation. The appointment of William B. Wilson, a "labor man," pleased him.

Then came advocates of the Negro cause. In the final moments of the campaign, Wilson had sent an open letter to civil rights leader Bishop Alexander Walters of the African Methodist Episcopal Zion Church, assuring "my colored fellow citizens of my earnest wish to see justice done them in every matter, and not mere grudging justice, but justice executed with liberality and cordial good feeling." He said, "They may count upon me for absolute fair dealing and for everything by which I could assist in advancing the interests of their race in the United States." Since the election, rumblings from the South especially suggested that what little progress Negroes had made would be rolled back. Hoping that was not the case, Walters reminded Wilson that the Negro vote numbered 750,000,

scattered among several large states; more important were the "moral, religious and industrial uplift of my people." Giles B. Jackson, an African
American lawyer who had organized the National Negro Wilson League,
hoped Wilson might even refer to the "Negro Question" in his forthcom-
ing inaugural address.

Wilson's pre-inaugural rhetoric suggested that he was grappling with
the issue and preparing to stand up to America's sectionalism. At the Mary
Baldwin Seminary he had spoken of Jefferson's efforts to "divest his mind
of the prejudices of race and locality and speak for those permanent issues
of human liberty which are the only things that render human life upon
this globe itself immoral." To the businessmen of Chicago, he made an odd
argument for fighting monopoly, saying, "We are of the same race, that
splendid mixed race into which has been drawn all the riches of a hundred
bloods. And now, as a united people we are going to redeem the ancient
pledges of America." When Mrs. Oscar Underwood invited the Wilsons to
attend the Southern Democratic League ball in early March, Wilson declined, explaining to the Speaker himself, "While I myself am deeply glad
to be a Southern man and to have the South feel a sense of possession in
me, we shall have to be careful not to make the impression that the South
is seeking to keep the front of the stage and take possession of the
administration."

New thoughts were bound to collide with old ideas. Wilson's major
campaign promises involved reforming the country's financial structure.
He was already communicating regularly with Congressman Carter
Glass—who represented Staunton, Virginia. Chairman of the House Committee on Banking and Currency, Glass was also a staunch proponent of
poll taxes and literacy tests for Negroes. They were also discussing a measure that would divide the country into financial zones, each of which
would have a federal bank that issued currency, instead of requiring credi-
tors to borrow from a single central bank. Even with "the full power of the
administration," Glass warned, enacting legislation in this area would be
difficult. Discussion of increased rights for African Americans could only
make it more so. As Wilson drafted his inaugural address, he would refer
to equality and justice in America, but as a matter of the economy, not
ethnicity.

Among all the radical changes that faced the nation, Wilson had to
uproot his family. For almost a quarter of a century, his home had been

Princeton—"where we have enjoyed and suffered so much." Frankly, he admitted to Mary Hulbert, "we dread the change,—not so much the new duties as the novel circumstances in which they must be performed." And yet, for all the anxiety, his neuritis and his headaches had quieted since he left academia for politics. His digestion remained delicate, but he was enjoying his longest stretch of good health in years.

At the start of 1913, Wilson wrote the sitting President about domestic matters at the White House, and Taft took the liberty of replying to Mrs. Wilson. He recommended retaining Mrs. Elizabeth Jaffray, a widow of great efficiency and initiative, in her position as housekeeper in the White House, and Arthur Brooks, the official custodian and valet. Taft called him "the most trustworthy colored man in the District of Columbia" and praised his efficiency in recording every delivery to the Executive Mansion and in preparing for trips and entertainments. Taft wrote Wilson himself that Congress would be willing to spend $5,000 to refurbish a number of bedrooms on the third floor to accommodate guests; and he offered to recommend to the Appropriations Committee a small provision so that the President could have a military aide at his disposal. Beyond that, he informed his successor, "Your laundry is looked after in the White House, both when you are here and when you are away. Altogether, you can calculate that your expenses are only those of furnishing food to a large boarding house of servants and to your family, and your own personal expenses of clothing, etc." With the Presidential salary of $75,000 per annum, and another $25,000 for traveling expenses, the Tafts had been able to save $100,000 during their four years.

To assist further, Ellen Wilson hired a social secretary—a "cave dweller," as the locals referred to the city's permanent residents—named Belle Hagner. Nell Wilson fretted because she was known to be a friend of the Roosevelts; and so Ellen invited their favorite cousin, Helen Bones, to live with them as well, to serve as a personal secretary.

While organizing her move, Ellen disappeared to New York one day on a mysterious errand. That night she handed each of her daughters an "inauguration present"—pearl necklaces for Jessie and Margaret and a bar pin set with small diamonds for Nell. They were the first pieces of jewelry any of them had ever owned. As it had not even occurred to Ellen to get something for herself, Woodrow presented her the next day with a diamond pendant. Ever after the family called it the "crown jewel." Because

of all the relocation expenses (on top of this small indulgence) before his new salary kicked in, Wilson secured a $5,000 bank loan, the most he had ever borrowed in his life. "He hated to do it," Nell remarked, "but we could not have made the move to Washington without it."

Bidding New Jersey farewell, the Governor attended a series of meetings and meals with the legislators who had been his allies in reforming the state, what he called the New Jersey "surprise." In an after-dinner talk to the Senators gathered in Atlantic City, he recalled the night he had led them in a cakewalk, which was the first time they had realized "that my long, solemn face was not a real index to my countenance, and that I was . . . a human being." On this occasion Wilson led the twenty-one Senators along the boardwalk for a two-mile midnight stroll in the brisk winter air. He resigned from office on March 1, 1913, and, upon handing the seal of office to his successor, he said, "The rarest thing in public life is courage, and the man who has courage is marked for distinction; the man who has not is marked for extinction, and deserves submersion."

That night the townspeople and students of Princeton said goodbye to Wilson, gathering on Nassau Street and marching with flares to Cleveland Lane, where the band played "Hail to the Chief," "My Country, 'Tis of Thee," and "Auld Lang Syne." The president of the First National Bank presented Wilson with a silver loving cup on behalf of "the Citizens of Princeton." An emotional Wilson addressed the crowd, unable to resist one anecdote of "mortification": he had recently entered a shop to buy an item from a man whose face he had known for years. When Wilson asked if the salesman might send the item to the house, the shopkeeper said, "What is your name, sir?" Now he told his well-wishers that the "real trials of life" were the connections one broke. "I have never been inside of the White House, and I shall feel very strange when I get inside of it," he said. "I shall think of this little house behind me and remember how much more familiar it is to me than that is, and how much more intimate a sense of possession there must be in the one case than in the other." Upon the conclusion of his remarks, the Princetonians in the crowd broke into "Old Nassau."

On Monday the third, Secret Service men, a large crowd, and a line of motorcars waited outside 25 Cleveland Lane. At 10:30, Woodrow and Ellen exited the house, choosing to walk to the train station instead of riding in one of the automobiles. They made a slight detour, strolling down

Library Place, past the house they had built years earlier. Friends and neighbors paid their respects along the way, though most of the towns-people waited for them at the train—a special car followed by a half dozen coaches filled with six hundred rollicksome undergraduates. The family stood on the back platform as the train pulled out of the campus depot at eleven, the First Couple smiling and waving and looking wistful as the spires and towers disappeared from view.

Passing flag-waving crowds all along the route, the train pulled into Washington's Union Station at 3:45. The students hastily detrained, in order to form a double line through which the Wilsons made their way from the Presidential car to the street, where a limousine took them through side streets to the Shoreham Hotel at 15th and H Streets. They completely bypassed the chaotic gathering of woman suffragists who were staging a "pageant" down Pennsylvania Avenue and commanding most of the attention that afternoon—5,000 women demanding their rights as they paraded in front of a crowd of 500,000. One of the guests of honor, the deaf and blind and militant Helen Keller, got waylaid in the con-gestion and never got to address the crowd; but she had her say in the next day's newspapers, assuring the public and the incoming President that the demonstration symbolized "the coming of the new, not the passing of the old" and that it would "not be long before a president shall ride down these broad avenues elected by the people of America, women and men."

The Wilsons encountered friendlier commotion at the Shoreham. Be-cause the hotel served as headquarters for Princeton alumni, hundreds donned orange and black as they secured badges that would admit them to a number of special events. During one encounter that day, a plump and dapper gentleman approached Wilson to introduce himself: it was Frank-lin Lane, the new Secretary of the Interior. By late afternoon, the stress of moving caught up to Ellen. The color left her face, and she repaired to her room to rest behind locked doors. After a while, Nell entered, to help her dress for a six-o'clock tea at the White House. Sitting before a mirror, ar-ranging her hair, Ellen put both hands over her face and burst into tears. But she managed to pull herself together before she had to join her husband.

Full of charm, the Tafts explained the White House to the new ten-ants, and conversation came easily. In the background that afternoon stood a short, handsome, dark-haired lieutenant in the naval medical corps,

thirty-five-year-old Cary Travers Grayson. Virginia-born and -educated, Grayson—an Episcopalian—radiated modest confidence. He was quiet and deferential by nature but a lively raconteur when called upon, and Washington hostesses considered him the ideal "extra man." Before the Wilsons departed, Taft jovially drew his successor under his arm and said, "Mr. Wilson, here is an excellent fellow that I hope you will get to know. I regret to say that he is a Democrat and a Virginian, but that's a matter that can't be helped!"

The Wilsons returned to their hotel, where Ellen, exhausted but undaunted, announced, "It's just a bigger Prospect—Sea Girt with no servant problem." A Wilson cousin hosted a dinner at the Shoreham for a few dozen intimates, including Fred Yates, the Wilsons' artist friend visiting from England's Lake District. After dinner the President-elect excused himself to appear at a "smoker"—a dinner of eight hundred Princeton alumni—on the tenth floor of the nearby New Willard Hotel, where he spoke briefly but emotionally about the "comradeship" he felt within the Princeton family, largely because of the university's great role in the nation's service.

Under gray skies, Woodrow Wilson left the hotel the next morning at ten o'clock in a two-horse open victoria. Some one thousand Princeton students—all wearing orange sashes—along with five hundred more from the University of Virginia, served as an honor guard, lining the carriage's route to the White House. Ellen and the girls remained at the hotel, giving themselves ample time to dress. The retinue of undergraduates was permitted to follow the carriage and then gather on the White House lawn, where, once again, they burst into song. A military band announced Wilson's arrival, but he waited on the front porch until the students had finished their medley, concluding, of course, with "Old Nassau"—at the end of which, a hatless Wilson bowed his head. Then he walked between the military aides in full dress uniforms to the Blue Room, where President Taft joined him, followed by the arrival of the new Cabinet and Vice President–elect Thomas R. Marshall. Taft took Wilson by the arm, leading him through the Red Room to the South Portico, where photographers had lined up cameras for official photographs. The incumbent was then tipping the scales at 340 pounds, twice Wilson's weight; and though he was born the year before the incoming President, his girth and big mustache—and, perhaps, his four years in office—made him look considerably older than his successor.

Taft and Wilson entered a large landau drawn by four horses. Great cheers greeted them all along Pennsylvania Avenue. In the meantime, White House chauffeurs drove the Wilson family in automobiles down side streets to the Capitol, where they took seats in the Senate Gallery to witness Marshall's being sworn into office. Senator Miles Poindexter took the floor to deliver a speech that droned on, standing as the only impediment between those inside the chamber and the largest audience that had ever assembled for an inauguration. Three times, as the minute hand of the chamber clock crept toward twelve, an attendant pushed it back. An indignant Nell Wilson wondered how a Senator could be so cavalier. Someone close by provided an explanation, which further described the political climate in Washington: "He's a Republican," said the voice, "—he's doing it on purpose." At last, Marshall took his oath, and everybody moved to seats on the portico of the Capitol. Back at the White House, the flag was lowered and a new one raised.

It was still overcast but a mild fifty-five degrees as the Presidential carriage pulled before the crowd, the incumbent appearing happier than the incoming President. With little pomp, Wilson took his place on the grandstand, which sat slightly above the heads of the 100,000 countrymen who stood there in anticipation. Wilson had asked to be sworn in with his hand on Ellen's small Bible, which Chief Justice Edward Douglass White opened and offered to a Deputy Clerk of the Court to hold. Upon completing the oath of office, Wilson followed the example of George Washington and stooped to kiss the pages of Scripture before him—the 119th Psalm: "So shall I keep thy Law continually: for ever and ever." In that moment, the sun broke through the clouds. The crowd started to push through the barriers to get closer to the platform, so they might better hear their new President. As the police began to force them back, Wilson said, "Let the people come forward."

He proceeded to deliver a stirring inaugural address. Equal parts lesson, sermon, and mission statement, his carefully chosen 1,800 words— composed over the last month—began with a simple proclamation of fact: "There has been a change of government." He described the Democratic takeover of both houses of Congress and the White House in the last two years; and then he asked what that meant. He spent ten paragraphs answering the question.

At first he inspired the audience, describing the bounty of America— "Our life contains every great thing, and contains it in rich abundance."

But he hastened to add that the riches had come at great human cost. He said the government had too often been used for private and selfish purposes, and those who used it had forgotten the people. The change in government, Wilson assured, meant new "vision." He said, "Our duty is to cleanse, to reconsider, to restore, to correct the vile without impairing the good, to purify and humanize every process of our common life without weakening or sentimentalizing it."

For the next few minutes he enumerated the specific Progressive ideas he intended to enact. Not least among them was "safeguarding the health of the nation," as the "first duty of law is to keep sound the society it serves." As he spoke of his ambitious program, many felt they were listening to the most glorious rhetoric from that podium in fifty-two years, when Lincoln summoned "the better angels of our nature" in his first inaugural address. Wilson proclaimed the "high enterprise of the new day: to lift everything that concerns our life as a nation to the light that shines from the hearthfire of every man's conscience and vision of the right. It is inconceivable that we should do this as partisans. . . . The feelings with which we face this new age . . . sweep across our heartstrings like some air out of God's own presence, where justice and mercy are reconciled and the judge and the brother are one."

"This is not a day of triumph," he concluded, "it is a day of dedication." With that in mind, he summoned "all honest men, all patriotic, all forward-looking men, to my side," assuring them that "God helping me, I will not fail them, if they will but counsel and sustain me!" He made no mention of foreign affairs. This speech was about restoring justice to a great but broken nation, a "government too often debauched and made an instrument of evil."

Speaking in his manner of heightened conversation rather than theatrical bombast, Wilson earned wave upon wave of applause at the end. Ellen Wilson quietly left her seat and unobtrusively descended the steps, to stand on a bench directly below her husband. She gazed up at him with a look of rapture.

The President and former President returned to the White House, while the Wilson women were chauffeured separately. Upon their arrival, Ellen and her daughters were taken to their second-floor quarters. Woodrow and Ellen's suite consisted of two bedrooms, a dressing room, and two baths. Bright and airy, with fires burning in the open grates, it overlooked

the Ellipse and the Washington Monument. When the girls checked on their mother, they found her at the window, looking down upon Mrs. Taft's formal garden with its graveled paths and geometrical flower beds. "Isn't it lovely, children?" she asked tentatively, already thinking of improvements. "It will be our rose garden with a high hedge around it."

They joined the Cabinet members and their wives and other distinguished guests—two hundred of them—who had gathered in the dining room for a stand-up buffet luncheon. Colonel and Mrs. House were there, though he had chosen not to attend the actual inauguration. "Functions of this sort do not appeal to me and I never go," he wrote in his diary. The former and new Presidents arrived and awkwardly stood together in the vestibule. Wilson invited Taft to remain for the lunch honoring the new administration, never expecting him to accept. But Taft stayed, only to find himself in the unfortunate position of standing alone as the new President received congratulatory handshakes. At last, Wilson returned to Taft, who said in parting, "Mr. President, I hope you'll be happy here." Wilson questioned the sentiment: "Happy?"

"Yes, I know," Taft replied. "I'm glad to be going—this is the loneliest place in the world."

Nellie Wilson overheard the comment and thought the strength of their family would keep that from happening. And then a minor mishap occurred, which, strangely, would ensure that Wilson would never be alone. The President's sister Annie Howe slipped on one of the marble staircases and gashed her scalp and forehead. Several Army and Navy aides were on hand, Dr. Grayson among them. Equipped for medical emergencies, he stitched her wound. This began what would become the most constant and intimate relationship the President had with a man for the rest of his life—a unique affiliation characterized by trust beyond that of any official, as Dr. Grayson would literally have his hand on the President's pulse and, thus, on the well-being of the world. "My official connection with Mr. Wilson was almost accidental," Grayson himself would later explain, "though, as I look back over the long stretch of years, I should like to call it providential."

A little after three, the Presidential party went outside to the reviewing stand in front of the house to watch the longest parade in inaugural history, forty thousand participants over the course of four hours. Young cadets from the service academies marched, including West Point "yearling"

Dwight D. Eisenhower. Woodrow Wilson stood throughout the procession, repeatedly doffing his tall silk hat, while Ellen smiled and waved her lace handkerchief. After the parade, fourteen of the innermost circle dressed for dinner in the State Dining Room. Profusions of roses filled the table, under the soft glow of the great silver candelabra. Everybody stared admiringly at the man sitting quietly at the head of the table. Afterward, a display of fireworks lit up the sky before the various family members set about finding their bedrooms, shrieks of excitement signaling each new discovery. For the first time since Franklin Pierce's inauguration in 1853, there would be no official ball. While other Presidents held to the festive tradition even in times of war and national hardship, Wilson chose to omit the occasion, considering it not just an unnecessary expense but also a source of "graft." Local vendors did not care for this curtailment of their quadrennial windfall, but they got a clear sense of the austerity of their new neighbors. Ellen Wilson appeared too weak to have danced that night anyway.

Wilson dropped into his office, to get a feel of the place and to meet briefly with Colonel House; but he soon rose from his desk to head to the Shoreham Hotel, where he arrived at the tail end of a dinner being held by the Class of 1879. After his strenuous day, the Princetonians had fully expected an announcement that he was too tired to appear; but Wilson beamed as he sat between reelected Congressman Charles Talcott—with whom he had once made a "solemn covenant" to devote themselves to the political arts—and Taft-appointed Justice of the Supreme Court Mahlon Pitney. The "Witherspoon Gang" was there in force.

The President stayed past midnight. Not long after he had returned to the White House and found his bedroom, he began pushing several of the mother-of-pearl buttons set in the wall, hoping to summon an attendant. A doorkeeper hastened to the second-floor residence, only to find Woodrow Wilson standing in his underwear. One of his trunks, which happened to hold his pajamas, never got delivered. It was immediately located at the train station, but it did not arrive at the White House until one o'clock, by which time the President of the United States was sound asleep.

9

BAPTISM

And Iesus, when hee was baptized, went vp straight-
way out of the water: and loe, the heauens were
opened vnto him, and he saw the Spirit of God de-
scending like a doue, and lighting vpon him.

—MATTHEW III:16

Article I, Section 8, of the Constitution of the United
States ordained the creation of a "District (not exceeding ten Miles square) as may . . . become the Seat of the
Government of the United States." It was christened Columbia, the elegiac term for America, and its "federal city"
was named for the first President. Congress held its first
session in the District of Columbia in 1800, even before the
completion of the Capitol. A National Mall extending from
this great hub to the Potomac River would gradually fill in
with monuments and buildings worthy of the Acropolis.
"Slowly," Henry Adams commented upon the end of the
nineteenth century, "a certain society had built itself up
about the Government; houses had been opened and there
was much dining; much calling; much leaving of cards."
Unlike most world capitals, Washington was neither its nation's chief commercial nor cultural center. Government
was its only industry, powered by the fact that every elected
official held a temporary job with limited time to achieve

his goals. In 1913, Washington, D.C., was a gracious Southern city of 350,000 people.

African Americans accounted for nearly a third of that population, the largest Negro congregation in the country. Most were invisible, unseen or overlooked in their subservient positions. Practically all the black women served as domestics, while the men worked as servants, waiters, and manual laborers. For the most part, Negroes knew their place. The city appeared to have no slums, because the overcrowded ghettos were on its periphery or made up of shacks tucked in the downtown alleys, where thousands subsisted in poverty. With the establishment of the Civil Service, a few Negroes began rising to the middle class, entering through the front doors of the Postal Service and the Treasury Department, where they could hold jobs similar to those of white people. A small upper middle class of blacks had risen in the capital; but, so far as Nell Wilson could tell, the "undisputed leaders of Washington colored society" were the dozens of footmen, doormen, maids, and butlers who staffed the Executive Mansion at 1600 Pennsylvania Avenue. They wore elegant uniforms; and, unlike the masters of the house, they held their jobs for life.

"The White House" became the official name for the sandstone Georgian mansion during TR's stay, referring to both the President's home and his workplace. Because his family had filled so many rooms at a time when the executive branch was expanding, TR had ordered construction of wings off the sides of the house to provide office space. His successor, Taft, created an elliptical room within the West Wing, which became the President's office.

Sunshine filled the White House on March 5, 1913, Woodrow Wilson's first full day at his new job. Arthur Brooks, his personal valet, had laid out his clothes. At precisely 8:30, Wilson sat at the mahogany table in the small family dining room on the north side of the house. Fred Yates joined him and his family, and they rehashed the prior day's events as the President ate his customary breakfast—two unbeaten raw eggs in orange juice, swallowed like oysters, a bowl of porridge, and coffee. The President left at nine for what was then called "the oval room in the Executive offices."

During his first official appointment—with friend and future diplomat Charles Crane—Wilson commented on the days of Washington and Jefferson, when "the President had time to think." His first policy decision revealed his determination to find the hours in which to free his mind. He

was going to rid himself of one of the "chief burdens" of his job, the meeting of candidates for appointment to public office. Wilson had telegraphed as much in his constitutional government lectures just a few years earlier, when he predicted that "as the multitude of the President's duties increases," holders of the great office should be "less and less executive officers and more and more . . . men of counsel and of the sort of action that makes for enlightenment."

At ten o'clock Wilson met informally in the Cabinet Room with his ten departmental Secretaries, who were mostly strangers to him and to one another. Thereafter, their semiweekly meetings would usually begin at eleven with Wilson relating an anecdote before presenting issues of immediate concern. Then he would call upon each Secretary in turn, practically simulating a Princeton preceptorial. Shortly after this first meeting, Wilson developed nicknames for all the Cabinet members, which doubled as ciphers during confidential telephone conversations and telegrams between him and Colonel House. Bryan became "Prime"; Secretary of War Garrison was "Mars"; and Secretary of the Navy Daniels became "Neptune." Wilson considered his Cabinet "executive counselors"; and from that day forward, observed Neptune, he gave them "free rein in the management of the affairs of their department. No President refrained so much from hampering them by naming their subordinates. Holding them responsible, he gave them liberty, confidence, and co-operation. More than that: he stood back of them when criticized and held up their hands." The West Wing functioned with a staff of six, including the stenographer Charles Swem, who had accompanied Wilson from New Jersey.

Ceremonial duties consumed most of Wilson's first day in office, as he greeted more than a thousand guests. There was a "Woodrow luncheon" for the two dozen relatives from his mother's side and a "Wilson dinner" for those from his father's. For almost an hour, he received well-wishers in the East Room, the "public audience chamber," which, at almost three thousand square feet and running the width of the house, was the largest in the mansion. Guests arrived by appointment, but many brought guests of their own: one Illinois Congressman arrived with 150 Chicago Democrats; an Atlanta editor ushered in 150 of his newsboys. And then the entire Democratic National Committee appeared. Not until after dinner did Wilson discover the most satisfying moment of the day—when he could

address the piles of letters and reports that awaited him next to his old familiar typewriter in the private book-lined study on the second floor.

Although Tumulty had announced that the government would not be conducting Presidential appointments as usual, Wilson immediately faced that disparity between aspiration and accommodation in the thousands of non-Cabinet appointments at his discretion. He believed no President had ever entered the White House so free of political debt, but he quickly learned that he owed more than he had thought. "I am not going to advise with reactionary or standpat senators or representatives in making these appointments," Wilson announced at the start of his administration, as he intended to place capability above party loyalty. "Mr. President," Postmaster Burleson, the savviest political mind in the Cabinet, replied, "if you pursue this policy, it means that your administration is going to be a failure. It means the defeat of the measures of reform that you have next to your heart. These little offices don't amount to anything. They are inconsequential. It doesn't amount to a damn who is postmaster at Paducah, Kentucky. But these little offices mean a great deal to the senators and representatives in Congress."

Burleson put a practical example before him—the nation's fifty-six thousand postmasterships. "The Cardinal," as Burleson was nicknamed, said he hoped he could apply Wilson's standards to all the appointees, but the Congressmen and Senators expected to have their say. "They are mostly good men," Burleson explained. "If they are turned down, they will hate you and will not vote for anything you want. It is human nature. On the other hand, if you work with them, and they recommend unsuitable men for the offices, I will keep on asking for other suggestions, until I get good ones." Wilson remained unconvinced until Burleson addressed the appointment atop a stack of papers—a recommendation from the Congressman in southeastern Tennessee. Wilson had received objections to the appointment and said he could not endorse it. Burleson proceeded to describe the little town near Chattanooga and the Representative's familiarity with the people there. Wilson sat in silence during the long descriptive discourse, finally saying, "Well, Burleson, I will appoint him." Seeing another 55,999 similar instances before him, Wilson relinquished control in the matter, simply asking Burleson where he should sign their commissions. Except for the ability to bring nonpolitical figures (especially academicians) into the government, Wilson found little pleasure in dispensing

patronage. Sometimes it actually pained him, as he rejected friends—even family members—who sought judgeships or other appointments.

With ten years between them, Woodrow had always been more of a father figure to Joseph Wilson, Jr., than a brother. While Josie had built his own modest career in the newspaper business in Tennessee, by his late forties, he had reached a dead end and sought a new career. He had been working for the Democratic Party, and McAdoo thought he might make a good candidate for the Senate. Short of that, the current junior Senator from Tennessee, Luke Lea, had another idea.

Since the founding of the Congress, a little-known position called Secretary of the Senate has existed. The Senators themselves elect this officer, who originally had served as their clerk, archivist, and quartermaster. By Wilson's day, the job included overseeing the Senate payroll, its pages, and the public records; it paid $6,500 per annum. After the election of 1912, Senator Lea believed putting Joseph Wilson in that position might give Lea some special access. Josie bought into the idea, and, for a moment, so did his brother—until the Senator from Oklahoma, T. P. Gore, reminded Wilson of, as he put it, "something called the separation of powers."

Even before the Senate elected somebody else, Josie cast his eye on another position, Postmaster of Nashville. Shortly after taking office, the President wrote his brother that it would be "a very serious mistake both for you and for me if I were to appoint you," despite his "struggle against affection and temptation." The brothers' relationship did not change after that—as, after all, they already wrote each other irregularly and saw each other infrequently.

Wilson demonstrated more fraternal feelings toward his advisers, three in particular. "Mr. House is my second personality," the President said, when asked of his silent partner in formulating policy. "He is my independent self," and "his thoughts and mine are one." The two men discussed House's relocating; but, House wrote in his diary, "we both realize that one soon becomes saturated with what might be termed the Washington viewpoint, and that everything is colored by that environment." They concluded it would be best for House to continue living in New York, Massachusetts, and Texas, and shuttling to Washington whenever beckoned, relying on the telephone and on letters in between. House visited the White House ten times that spring alone, as they charted administration policy.

Joseph Tumulty continued as Wilson's political adviser. More than

merely tending to the pesky details of office for which Wilson had no patience, Tumulty's Trenton-tested instincts allowed him to deal with the press, take the public's pulse, interact with the legislature, and serve as gatekeeper to the Oval Office—tasks that future Presidents would divide among a dozen men.

The third crucial member of the Wilson team was Cary T. Grayson, who was already becoming the most indispensable. After five days as President—during which he had received nine Justices, dozens of envoys, and hundreds of commissioners and other governmental functionaries—Wilson fell ill. He suffered from a severe headache and gastric disorder—which he referred to as "turmoil in Central America." Dr. Grayson, who had been monitoring Wilson's sister since her Inauguration Day accident, found the President in bed. "When you get to know me better," Wilson explained, "you will find that I am subject to disturbances in the equatorial regions." Grayson's first recommendation for Wilson to rest would become chronic advice.

Grayson did not yet know the extent of his new patient's hypertension, but he promptly saw that Wilson had been overmedicating his headaches with coal-tar analgesics—such as the new wonder drug aspirin—which upset his stomach. His medicine cabinet already held a quart-sized can of tablets and a stomach pump, which he used regularly in a procedure that involved inserting a rubber hose from his mouth to his stomach and funneling in enough saline solution to siphon out the gastric acid. Recognizing a pernicious cycle, Grayson took Wilson off the drugs. The patient accused the doctor of being a "therapeutic nihilist." Shortly thereafter, the President invited Dr. Grayson to lunch with Secretary of the Navy Daniels. "There is one part of the Navy that I want to appropriate," Wilson said. "There have been a good many applications for the position but Mrs. Wilson and I have already become acquainted with Doctor Grayson and we have decided that he is the man we should like to have assigned to the White House." He became the President's personal physician, and soon a lot more.

As such, he learned all he could about his new patient from various sources. Long associating Woodrow's prior history of "neuritis" and visual impairment with the strains of work, Ellen had privately consulted with Dr. Francis X. Dercum of Philadelphia (who treated her brother Stockton for his persistent breakdowns), to ask if he thought her husband could shoulder the Presidency. Dercum knew of Wilson's ruptured blood vessel

years earlier and saw no great danger; but another famous neurologist, Dr. S. Weir Mitchell, disagreed, prophesying that Woodrow Wilson would not live out his first term.

Dr. Grayson reminded Wilson that "he had four hard years ahead of him and that he owed it to himself and the American people to get into as fit condition as possible and to stay there." The regime, Grayson would later recollect, "included plenty of fresh air, a diet suited to his idiosyncrasies as I discovered them by close study, plenty of sleep, daily motor rides, occasional trips on the *Mayflower* [the Presidential yacht], and especially regular games of golf, together with treatment for a persistent case of neuritis from which he had long suffered." As a result of keeping the President engaged in leisure activities every day, Grayson became his regular companion, "drawn into close personal association with him."

Once out of bed, Wilson conscientiously attempted to maintain a balanced schedule. After breakfast, he would dictate correspondence from nine until ten and then receive visitors until one. He would lunch with family members and then work another hour or two. Every afternoon included an automobile ride; and except for some light paperwork, he worked at night only during crises. Sundays he slept in before attending services at the Central Presbyterian Church. He even made time for recreational reading, asking the Librarian of Congress to keep him supplied with detective novels. From the very start of his term, Wilson set his sights on its completion. "The day after I am released from this great job," he wrote, "I shall take a ship for Rydal!" Until then, Wilson had an ambitious legislative program he hoped to bequeath, but every President quickly discovers that he must first untangle the state of affairs he has inherited.

In the centuries since Columbus, Spain, Germany, France, and England had all plundered Central and South America. Mexico became their piñata, which they repeatedly bashed so that more of its treasures would fall at their feet. In the mid-1800s, the United States took some swings as well, annexing Texas and grabbing Mexican land as far north as Oregon. In his *History of the American People*, Wilson characterized the Mexican-American War as "inexcusable aggression and fine fighting." The American presence steadily increased south of the Rio Grande, as Mexico's abundance of oil became more precious than its metals.

Longtime dictator General Porfirio Díaz invited outside investment; and under America's Republican administrations at the start of the twentieth century, "dollar diplomacy"—the belief that the government should exploit all possible business opportunities in foreign countries—earned handsome dividends for Americans. With the rise of this private imperialism, Mexican resentment grew. In 1910 a reform-minded landowner, Francisco Madero, ran against Díaz in a "free election"—only to be imprisoned by his opponent. So began the Mexican Revolution, with Madero marshaling the forces of Emiliano Zapata, Pascual Orozco, and Francisco "Pancho" Villa—all of whom kept turning on one another. In the spring of 1911, Díaz fled the country, and Madero was named President. Not two years later, General Victoriano Huerta had him shot and on February 18, 1913, became President of Mexico.

Two weeks later, President Huerta sent congratulations to the newly inaugurated President Wilson. The gesture was barely reciprocated. Wilson wired a seven-word formal reply—carefully addressed to General—not President—Huerta, to avoid even suggesting diplomatic recognition of what Wilson considered an illegal regime. Days after the inauguration, the New York *World* implicated America's Ambassador, Henry Lane Wilson (no relation), in the overthrow of Madero. Tensions in Latin America were the subject of the first official Cabinet meeting on Friday, March 7; and when they reconvened the following Tuesday, the President read aloud a statement he had written on the subject, taking his first steps into a quagmire not of his creation.

These initial words about Mexico would become the cornerstone of his foreign policy for as long as he held office; and they further signaled his intention to serve largely as his own Secretary of State. "Cooperation is possible only when supported at every turn by the orderly processes of just government based upon law, not upon arbitrary or irregular force," he said. "We hold . . . that just government rests always upon the consent of the governed, and that there can be no freedom without order based upon law and upon the public conscience and approval. . . . We shall lend our influence of every kind to the realization of these principles in fact and practice. . . . We can have no sympathy with those who seek to seize the power of government to advance their own personal interests or ambition. . . . We shall prefer those who act in the interest of peace and honor, who protect private rights and respect the restraints of constitutional provision."

Some other Cabinet members commented that such a statement suggested the new administration was unnecessarily rushing into places where it did not belong. Wilson averred that "something had to be said, that the agitators in certain countries wanted revolutions and were inclined to try it on with the new Administration." As Agriculture Secretary David Houston recalled, "He intimated that he was not going to let them have one if he could prevent it." Secretary Bryan nodded and smiled.

However reluctantly, the United States was taking its first steps along a new path into international affairs, becoming a global overseer. Under Woodrow Wilson, American foreign policy would increasingly find itself clucking its disapproval, if not disdain, for the misbehavior of other nations. The situation in Mexico was just the beginning of a series of conundrums in which Wilson questioned himself as to whether his actions imposed sound public policy or just his own personal morality—all the while questing, of course, to do both.

While the change in Mexico's government had occurred in the prior administration, Taft had postponed taking a position, perhaps out of respect to the incoming President. A quick study of the situation reported that the conditions resulting from American nonrecognition of the Huerta government were already producing "serious inconvenience." Several matters between the two countries hung in abeyance, from water rights along the Colorado River to a border dispute in El Paso; loans from American banks were coming due and would go unpaid. The professor who wrote the report allowed that the circumstances by which Huerta rose to power were deplorable; but, he added, "We cannot become the censors of the morals or conduct of other nations and make our approval or disapproval of their methods the test of our recognition of their governments without intervening in their affairs." Others insisted that standing on the sidelines would threaten American lives, property, and profits.

"I will not recognize a government of butchers," said the President, digging in his heels. "While recognition of Huerta was the *wise* course, as practicality defines wisdom," an ardent supporter later wrote of his decision, "it was not the *right* course." With American land, mineral, and industrial investors pleading for Wilson to change his mind, Wilson told Tumulty, "I have to pause and remind myself that I am President of the United States and not of a small group of Americans with vested interest in Mexico."

Despite suspecting his motives and disapproving his actions, Wilson kept Taft's Ambassador Wilson on the job. If nothing else, he would protect current American business interests in Mexico. But President Wilson also dispatched an emissary of his own to gather intelligence, somebody who could quickly ascertain the Ambassador's role in the coup as well as the legitimacy of Huerta's government. This first secret intelligence agent in the Wilson Administration, William Bayard Hale, had no connection to Mexico and could not even speak Spanish; but, as an Episcopalian priest who had written a campaign biography of Wilson, he could be trusted.

Hale reported a shocking tale of cold-blooded treachery, in which Ambassador Wilson had conspired with Huerta and several other sympathetic foreign ministers to overthrow Madero. Furthermore, Hale noted, "Madero would never have been assassinated had the American Ambassador made it thoroughly understood that the plot must stop short of murder." Hale thought this tale of "treason, perfidy and assassination in an assault on constitutional government" was the most shocking ever to involve an American diplomatic officer. And though it had transpired on President Taft's watch, it was Wilson's problem now. What was worse, Hale concluded, "thousands of Mexicans believe that the Ambassador acted on instructions from Washington and look upon his retention under the new American President as a mark of approval and blame the United States Government for the chaos into which the country has fallen."

Within days, Wilson set in motion the recalling of the "unspeakable" Henry Lane Wilson; and within two months he had been replaced by John Lind, a former Minnesota Congressman and Governor whose knowledge of the territory was negligible. Lind arrived in Mexico with an invitation from Wilson to Huerta—to abandon his office. He suggested that the country hold a general election, in which Huerta would not run. Even Madero's Foreign Relations Secretary Manuel Calero would later write that Wilson's not choosing to recognize Huerta was well within his rights; to destroy him, however, was not. "Huerta was a usurper," Calero granted. "But did it belong to the President of the United States to drive him from the place usurped? This was a matter that concerned exclusively the people of Mexico."

Wilson's initial attempts to push Huerta out of office only strengthened the Mexican leader. As Calero observed, American nonrecognition

offered Huerta "the occasion of exhibiting himself as champion of the national dignity, as defender of the sovereignty of Mexico against the intrusion of a foreign government." Resorting to a policy Wilson called "watchful waiting," he and his new diplomatic team in Mexico appraised the alcoholic Huerta's regime one day at a time.

At the Cabinet meeting on March 12, 1913, Secretary Bryan brought up another country going through a revolution. After four thousand years of dynastic rule, Sun Yat-sen had recently declared a Republic of China and was encouraging foreign investment there. The Taft Administration had approved the participation of American banks in an international consortium that might lend $125 million. Wilson had been in office a week when representatives from J. P. Morgan & Company and Kuhn, Loeb & Company called upon Bryan, saying they would not close the deal without express authorization from the government. Wilson was sympathetic to the emerging nation—in part because of almost a century of Presbyterian missionary work in China. In May, the United States recognized China as a republic, one of the first nations to do so. Bryan called it "one of the pleasant duties of this administration." But Wilson strongly disapproved of this so-called Six Power Loan.

The next day, he composed his official response: "The conditions of the loan seem to us to touch very nearly the administrative independence of China itself; and this administration does not feel that it ought, even by implication, to be a party to those conditions." Wilson felt the problem lay in certain demands the loan placed upon the Chinese, who were pledging to secure the loan with burdensome taxes and supervision by foreign agents. His primary objection, however, was that "it gave the monopoly of this nation's interests in China's finances to a small group of American bankers to the exclusion of all other American financiers"—for the present and in the future. That representatives of J. P. Morgan & Company further expected the United States government "to utilize both its military and naval forces to protect the interest of the lenders" in the event of the Chinese defaulting was all Wilson needed to hear. Such responsibilities, he stated, were "obnoxious to the principles upon which the government of our people rests."

Wilson's statement assured the citizens of both the United States and China that he wanted to promote "the most extended and intimate trade relationship between this country and the Chinese republic," and that he

hoped to pursue opportunities through "the open door—a door of friendship and mutual advantage." But, he added, this loan overly entangled America in the affairs of China. Ever since the Spanish-American War, the United States had been navigating an imperialistic course, guided most recently by "dollar diplomacy." With Wilson's quashing the China deal, he semaphored a change in direction.

That meant immediate reconsideration of agreements the Roosevelt and Taft administrations had made with a number of other countries whose governments were in turmoil. Chief among them were the Philippines, an American territory, fought and paid for in 1898—a takeover the Republican administrations had justified by insisting the Filipinos were not prepared to govern themselves. Hostilities between the islands and the United States had existed ever since. Wilson considered whether the Philippines were, in fact, "prepared for independence"; and he decided they were not. Nor did he believe that the United States had made its best efforts to help them. To the dismay of many Americans, including a few of his own Cabinet members, Wilson announced that American policy there was no longer to be "for the advantage of the United States, but for the benefit of the people of the Philippine Islands." Toward that end, he announced that a majority of seats on the governing Philippine Commission, which the American President appointed, would be filled by Filipinos. Tensions dramatically abated, as the Philippines were, at last, on a track toward independence.

And then there was a political temblor in California that was felt as far as Tokyo and Washington, D.C., one that also called for moral adjudication. Americans had for the last decade invested in Asia, and now Asians wanted to own land in America. There had long been an overt prejudice against "Orientals" in California, which only intensified as Japanese immigrants especially prospered in agriculture. When enough started to buy land, the state legislature proposed a bill forbidding foreign ownership. Japan was deeply insulted. Foreign policy was suddenly conjoined to domestic policy, in a state whose leader, the great Progressive Governor Hiram Johnson, was also a racist. For the next several months, Wilson attempted to get California to temper the language of the law, but not only did he wish to avoid trespassing onto states' rights, he also needed all the Congressional support he could muster for his legislative agenda.

In Washington, he introduced another kind of "open door" policy, one

in which the executive branch of government was literally open to the public. By the second week of the Administration, the press and the public were startled to find that anybody was welcome to observe their officials at work. Nobody had ever seen a government so candid and accessible. War Secretary Garrison would swivel in his desk chair and answer questions from strangers who had entered his office; Josephus Daniels said he intended to become the first Secretary of the Navy who would actually visit the Navy yards across the country. Even in the White House, citizens could walk back to the executive offices.

At 12:45 on March 15, 1913, the Wilson Administration made history when it established what would become a convention of the Presidency. That Saturday afternoon, Tumulty ushered 125 members of the press corps into Wilson's office; and for the first time, a President held a White House press conference. Wilson was hardly the first President to talk to a journalist; indeed, Taft met occasionally with newspapermen after hours and granted them a few minutes of questions; and TR cherry-picked members of his "newspaper cabinet," allowing them to transcribe what he chose to dictate. To promote government transparency, Wilson announced that he intended to schedule regular conferences at which any journalist could ask whatever he wanted.

If nothing else, the exercise was a good publicity tool for Wilson. Few could speak off the cuff with such ease, and he sometimes simply chose not to answer a question. Most of his responses—terse and precise—revealed nothing more than necessary, but his witty interplay with the press set the tone for relations between the press and future Presidents. "As he went on talking, the big hit he was making with the crowd became evident," reported *The New York Times* after the first gathering. "There was something so unaffected and honest about his way of talking . . . that it won everybody, despite the fact that many of the men there had come prejudiced against him." Between March and December 1913 alone, Wilson appeared at sixty press conferences.

At the second conference—which moved to the much larger East Room—Wilson took the press into his confidence and asked for its help. "The only way I can succeed is by not having my mind live in Washington," he said. "My body has got to live there, but my mind has got to live in the United States, or else I will fail." Wilson hoped the newspapermen would bring him a sense of the nation beyond the city in which they

worked, considering themselves importers as much as exporters. And with that metaphor in mind, Wilson turned to what he believed would be his administration's defining piece of legislation, one that had eluded his predecessors for decades and that required a radical presentation.

In the northwest corner on the second floor of the United States Capitol—just off the Senate chamber—is an anomalous gilt-trimmed salon with a vaulted frescoed ceiling and a brilliantly colored tile floor. It is called the President's Room. George Washington had proposed such a room so that the Chief Executive and Senators might conduct their joint business; but not until the mid-nineteenth century, when the great legislative edifice was expanded and crowned with its iron dome, did it come into existence. In the interim, the Chief Executive almost never came to Capitol Hill. After John Adams left the Presidency in 1801, Presidents virtually discontinued their visits to the two legislative houses. Ostensibly to keep "the President's Annual Message to Congress" from becoming a throne speech—though possibly because he was not a good speaker—Thomas Jefferson messengered his texts to the legislature for a clerk to read, and that practice became standard. Because new Congressional sessions began on the fourth of March every other year, a President might visit his special room but twice a term, to sign any bills passed under the wire on the third. Beyond that, this jewel of a room remained a museum piece.

The Constitution states that the President shall from time to time not only give to the Congress information on the state of the Union but also "recommend to their Consideration such Measures as he shall judge necessary and expedient; he may, on extraordinary Occasions, convene both Houses, or either of them." The morning after his election, Woodrow Wilson had contemplated that clause, thanks to a journalist named Oliver P. Newman. In an off-the-record interview about executive style, Newman had suggested that Wilson might abandon the 112-year-old tradition and deliver important speeches in person. Wilson had stood at the window in his library on Cleveland Lane and stared out, as if into the future. "Newman," he said, "that would set them by the ears."

On second thought, Wilson did not want to antagonize Congress. But the idea kept growing. Thinking it would emphasize the cruciality of all that he wished to propose, Wilson asked the legislature to convene. Reaction from Capitol Hill was swift. Republicans, such as William O. Bradley of Kentucky, cautioned him to remember the separation of powers, saying,

"If Mr. Wilson comes to the Capitol to influence legislation, he will be more foolish than the donkey that swam the river to get a drink of water." Several Democrats, such as John Sharp Williams of Mississippi, denounced the notion as a reversion to royalty. "The practice instituted by Jefferson was more American than the old pomposities and cavalcadings between the White House and the Capitol," Williams said. On April 8, 1913—for the first time since November 22, 1800, when John Adams delivered his fourth annual message—a President of the United States rode the mile and a half from the White House to the Capitol for the purpose of addressing a joint session of Congress.

Wilson staged the appearance with predictable simplicity, arriving by automobile with only a Secret Service guard. He wore a black frock coat and light trousers, his cravat a gray four-in-hand. A small committee of Representatives greeted him, ushering him to Speaker Champ Clark's office for a moment while the Representatives took their places in the House chamber. Then the House doorkeeper stepped into the main aisle and announced, "The Vice President of the United States and members of the United States Senate." They filed in, the Senators sardining themselves on the benches in the first two rows, as Vice President Marshall went to a big armchair on the rostrum facing the crowd, to the Speaker's right. The gallery was packed with visitors who had requested tickets, the President's wife and three daughters, and members of the Cabinet, who were invited to attend informally on their own, so as not to give the appearance of a state occasion. Just before one o'clock, the President appeared in the chamber, escorted by members of each house; and everybody rose and applauded. Wilson shook hands with the Speaker and the Vice President before taking his stand at the Reading Clerk's desk. Speaker Clark formally introduced the President; and everybody applauded again. Wilson bowed.

The President began by stating his primary reason for delivering this message in person, which was his long-held belief in humanizing institutions. He said he wanted them to know that the President of the United States "is a person, not a mere department of the Government hailing Congress from some isolated island of jealous power, sending messages, not speaking naturally and with his own voice—that he is a human being trying to cooperate with other human beings in a common service." The audience applauded.

In a natural voice—stressing history over histrionics—Wilson explained that he had summoned the Congress to emphasize the essential need for tariff reform. This extraordinary session, he said, was a task laid upon him and his party that it had to perform promptly, "in order that the burden carried by the people under existing law may be lightened as soon as possible and in order, also, that the business interests of the country may not be kept too long in suspense as to what the fiscal changes are to be to which they will be required to adjust themselves." While industrial and commercial life had drastically changed in America, the tariff schedules had not; certain manufacturers were benefiting at the expense of consumers. The sooner rates were adjusted, Wilson said, "the sooner our men of business will be free to thrive by the law of nature (the nature of free business) instead of by the law of legislation and artificial arrangement."

"Consciously or unconsciously," Wilson told America's lawmakers, "we have built up a set of privileges and exemptions from competition behind which it was easy . . . to organize monopoly." He said it was necessary to "abolish everything that bears even the semblance of privilege or of any kind of artificial advantage, and put our business men and producers under the stimulation of a constant necessity to be efficient, economical, and enterprising, masters of competitive supremacy, better workers and merchants than any in the world." He insisted this was not only the best thing for American business in an increasingly global economy but also the right thing. His speech lasted nine minutes. Amid the applause, Wilson left the chamber.

In the car with his wife, on the way back to the White House, Wilson kept chuckling under his breath. When, at last, Ellen asked what he was laughing about, he said, "Wouldn't Teddy have been glad to think of that—I put one over on Teddy and am totally happy."

Doubtless, the speech got the better of Teddy Roosevelt, who never shook his contempt for Wilson. At a luncheon in Oyster Bay, during which TR made one snide remark after another about "Professor" Wilson, a New York newspaper editor took the former President to task, suggesting that Wilson also embraced progressive principles. "I am a little hard on Wilson," Roosevelt conceded. "What I object to about him is his mildness of method. I suppose, as a matter of fact," he said, thumping his chest, "Wilson is merely a less virile *me*."

Washington was agog over the precedents Wilson appeared to be

breaking every day, and the very next afternoon he returned to the lion's den. With the eleven Democratic members of the Senate Finance Committee, he sat for an hour and a half around the hand-carved table in the middle of the President's Room. In a cloud of cigar smoke, the men strategized passage of the tariff bill, despite political opposition and the power of special interests. Wilson had always been persuasive; now the Senate was realizing that he could also be relentless in getting what he wanted. There had not been a systemic reduction of rates since 1857; and after months of working with Representatives Clark, Underwood, Palmer, and Glass, Wilson was not about to see this bill turn back on itself as the Payne-Aldrich bill had under Taft.

The protective tariff had played an important role in the economy of America, protecting its young industries against foreign competition; but over time, as monopolies evolved, it became, in the words of Treasury Secretary McAdoo, "a general tax on the entire population for the benefit of private industry." If a few vendors of a particular product conspired to fix its price even one cent below the foreign import price, they could continue to monopolize the domestic market and share the wealth among themselves. Wilson believed the reduction, if not the removal, of these tariffs would drive a stake into the heart of the various trusts—whether they controlled the manufacture and sale of steel rails, leather gloves, or sugar. The aim of his administration was to allow high duties on luxury items but to lower those on raw materials and necessities, optimally to no tariff.

Sugar, for example, cost less to produce in Puerto Rico or Cuba than it did in the United States, and the Louisiana planters claimed they would be ruined without tariff protection. The President, the only elected official with a national constituency, had to convince each Representative to look beyond the borders of his district and to consider the nation at large. The "whole art of statesmanship is the art of bringing the several parts of government into effective cooperation for the accomplishment of particular common objects," he had noted back when he was just a political scientist. And in order to turn theory into practice, Wilson had told one Congressman, he intended to play the part of the President as though he were a Prime Minister—"as much concerned with the guidance of legislation as with the just and orderly execution of the law." Wilson's appearance in the Capitol two days in a row expressed not only his belief that the two

branches could more effectively run the government when harnessed together but also that he intended to return to the President's Room often.
Not ten weeks after Wilson had taken his oath, the tariff bill sailed
through the House, where the Democrats enjoyed a 291–134 majority. Of
the five Democrats who opposed the bill, four came from Louisiana.

The Senate would be another matter, what with its fifty-one Democrats to forty-four Republicans (and one Progressive). To secure passage,
Wilson realized he would need sticks and carrots. Furnifold McLendel
Simmons was the ranking Democrat on the Finance Committee, an outspoken white supremacist and the powerful third-term Senator from
North Carolina. He was the presumed chair apparent of the committee—
until President Wilson questioned his ability to push through the Underwood bill that would lower tariffs. Simmons represented the conservative
wing of their party and was long opposed to the Progressive. With his
power threatened, Simmons changed his position, assuring Wilson that he
would support the reforms.

Wilson lured with patronage those Senators who staunchly defended
their state's crops and industries. After he spoke to his new friends in the
press corps of the disturbing power of lobbyists—what he called the "invisible government"—editorials and news reports incited public outcry
across the country. He regularly invited Senators to the White House; and
during one of his visits to the President's Room, he held twenty-three separate conferences. He asked that a special telephone be installed, linking
the Senate and the White House. Because the American Woolen Company
had become the only significant purchaser of wool in the country, he called
upon Attorney General McReynolds to investigate the legality of their
operations, to see that anti-trust laws were not being violated. The "college
professor" had obviously learned the lessons of politics he had taught for so
many years.

Summer descended upon Washington as the Senate tariff debate heated
up, turning into a partisan fight. "The last thing I ever think of doing is
giving up," Wilson wrote Mary Hulbert on June 22, 1913. "But, among
other things, this business means that I am to have no vacation." The
President called upon Congress to remain in session and sweat through
the summer with him. During several months of testimony and debate,
the Underwood-Simmons bill whittled down the basic tariff rates in the
United States from 40 percent to 25 percent. Many items would

get reduced to 0. The 56 percent tariff on woolens would be shrunk to one-third that amount, and the tariff on raw wool would go from 44 percent to 0; the President granted that the sugar tariff should not be immediately eliminated but reduced to 1 percent for a period of three years, after which there would be "free sugar."

In the fiscal year ending on June 30, 1913, the United States Treasury would have received $318 million from customs duties. With the new rates, that would drop to $270 million. The Administration, having to compensate for that shortfall, turned to the recently ratified Sixteenth Amendment to the Constitution, which provided Congress the "power to lay and collect taxes on incomes, from whatever source derived . . ."

The income tax was not new to America. Lincoln first imposed it in order to pay the Union army. It was, in fact, a redistribution of wealth, with the rich paying more than the poor. Congress had repealed it after the Civil War, but the tax reappeared in 1894 to deal with the nation's financial crisis. It provided relief to the agrarian West and South, where incomes lagged behind those in the industrial Northeast, until the Supreme Court declared it unconstitutional because it was not apportioned according to the states' populations. The new amendment overrode that stipulation, thus allowing for a progressive tax structure—with the lowest earners paying no tax while the highest would pay as much as 7 percent. That would affect less than 1 percent of the population but would, in fact, yield $71 million in its first year, more than offsetting losses from the reduced tariffs. The implementation of this new income tax was bundled into the Underwood-Simmons Revenue Act.

So long as the lawmakers were a captive audience that summer, Wilson took advantage of his momentum. On June 23, he returned to address another joint session of Congress—because of what he considered "a clear and imperative duty." Despite the oppressive summer heat, he insisted that "there are occasions of public duty when . . . the work to be done is so pressing and so fraught with big consequence that we know that we are not at liberty to weigh against it any point of personal sacrifice." The need for a new banking and currency system, he said, presented such an occasion. "We must have a currency . . . elastically responsive to sound credit . . . the normal ebb and flow of personal and corporate dealings," he said. "Our banking laws must mobilize reserves; must not permit the concentration anywhere in a few hands of the monetary resources of the

country or their use for speculative purposes in such volume as to hinder or impede or stand in the way of other more legitimate, more fruitful uses." Wilson called for a national institution to keep those reserves of money flowing—an archipelago of Federal Reserve Banks.

Because of the inflexibility of the existing banking system, one in which banks across the country were beholden to the trust on Wall Street, the national economy had clogged five times since the Civil War, producing panics. Small rural banks and even the United States Treasury had found themselves at Wall Street's mercy, and a Congressional committee chaired by Representative Arsène Pujo was investigating the power of the bank trust. The Wilson Administration's philosophy was to decentralize the reserves by creating a government-supervised national bank for banks, with twelve branches scattered across the country.

Republicans especially fought this Federal Reserve legislation. As Secretary McAdoo recalled, "They said it was populistic, socialistic, half-baked, destructive, infantile, badly conceived, and unworkable." As the name-callers became educated to the intricacies of the bill, many realized the national economy would be strengthened because there would be more local control of credit and debt. As McAdoo analogized, "The country as a whole was like a town of wooden houses, where the only water for fighting fire was in barrels in back yards, except for one gigantic reservoir many miles away—too far away to be effective." Under the Wilson plan, there would be "twelve large and efficient reservoirs located at strategic points in the community itself," and there would be no need for the "ineffective water barrels in the back yards; the reservoirs are so near, and they are always full." Debate raged about the management of this bucket brigade.

In fact, a similar plan had been devised in 1910 at a secret meeting of the nation's most powerful bankers at the exclusive Jekyll Island Club, a Morgan playground off the coast of Georgia. These members of the trust had proposed a pre-emptive solution to the very problems Wilson now sought to fix—a central bank with regional branches, but one that was privately owned and under their control. John D. Rockefeller's son-in-law, Senator Nelson Aldrich, had presented the bill, and it faced crushing Democratic opposition. Now the President hoped to employ the solid structure of the concept but place it more under the authority of the people, by providing quasi-governmental oversight.

Wilson had discussed the problem for months with Treasury Secretary

McAdoo; Congressman Carter Glass, who was chairman of the House Committee on Banking and Currency; Dr. H. Parker Willis, a University of Chicago economist and adviser to that committee; and longtime advocate of reform Secretary Bryan. During one conversation, McAdoo ironed out a plan regarding interest on the money the government would advance to the Federal Reserve Banks: "What we ought to do," he suggested, "is to give the Federal Reserve Board the power to impose, from time to time, such rates of interest as in its judgment may be wise, or to charge no interest or circulation tax at all. This will make the arrangement flexible and responsive to the needs of the country." Wilson called upon his former Princeton colleague Professor Royal Meeker to poll the nation's leading economists on the state of banking.

After finding a mostly positive consensus, two bones of contention remained—one regarding the backing of the currency issued by the banks, the other regarding the composition of the central board of control. Wilson consulted Louis Brandeis. As he had done in helping forge the basics of the New Freedom, Brandeis articulated what he considered the basic principles of the plan, thus bolstering Wilson's proposals and confidence. First, he said, it was best to enact a "confidence-inspiring" currency bill at an early date, as a watered-down proposal would serve nobody. He said the "power to issue currency should be vested exclusively in Government officials," and that bankers needed government oversight. He told Wilson that whatever bill got passed would have little effect "unless we are able to curb the money trust, and to remove the uneasiness among business men due to its power." Finally, he said the "conflict between the policies of the Administration and the desires of the financiers and of big business, is an irreconcilable one. Concession to the big business interests must in the end prove futile." While the Administration had to consider carefully the recommendations of the banking trust, it was dangerous to heed its advice despite its technical proficiency. This bill was meant to win the public trust, not woo the banking trust. Two days after conferring with Brandeis, Wilson began drafting his speech to Congress, incorporating all the lawyer's ideas.

Brandeis's arguments boiled down to the need for federal supervision. Representative Carter Glass disagreed, believing the banks should have representation; Senator Robert L. Owen of Oklahoma, the chairman of the Committee on Banking and Finance and a longtime Bryan supporter, felt otherwise. McAdoo sought a compromise, but the President had made up

his mind. This chronic problem demanded a bold remedy of "public participation and direction"—government control.

When a number of liberal Midwestern bankers protested, their supporter Carter Glass could envision only one unlikely means of turning the President around. He arranged an audience for the financiers to sit directly across from Wilson at his desk. Each banker made his best argument regarding representation on the governing board of the Federal Reserve, after which Wilson turned toward the most vehement of them and quietly asked, "Will one of you gentlemen tell me in what civilized country of the earth there are important government boards of control on which private interests are represented?" The question hung there in silence until Wilson posed a second question: "Which of you gentlemen thinks the railroads should select members of the Interstate Commerce Commission?" The bankers were struck dumb. Carter Glass converted to Wilson's position before they had even exited the office.

One last obstruction threatened passage of the bill, with the Bryan liberals withholding their support unless this condition was met. It involved the Federal Reserve notes—the actual issuance of currency—as being the "obligations of the United States" instead of the regional reserve banks issuing them. Without the United States Treasury standing behind the currency, Bryan felt this bill should not even be presented to Congress, for fear that its omission might antagonize their own party members and even jeopardize the tariff bill. In a meeting with Wilson, the former standard-bearer of the party went even farther. "I called his attention to the fact that our party had been committed by Jefferson and Jackson and by recent platforms to the doctrine that the issue of money is a function of government and should not be surrendered to banks," Bryan recalled. Wilson considered all the opposition—including that of Carter Glass, who felt the government's issuing currency was an unnecessary obligation. The next time Bryan saw Wilson, he learned that "the two difficulties which had seemed insurmountable had been removed."

In the end, Wilson had confected this bill by melding idealism with pragmatism, and nobody questioned that its success or failure should redound upon him. Wilson himself only questioned the timing. "Shall we hasten to change the tariff laws and then be laggards about making it possible and easy for the country to take advantage of the change?" he asked the joint session of Congress. "There can be only one answer to that

question. We must act now, at whatever sacrifices to ourselves," he said, landing hard on the word "now" and clenching his jaw. "I should be recreant to my deepest convictions of public obligation did I not press it upon you with solemn and urgent insistence." Opposition sprang: House Minority Leader James Robert Mann criticized Wilson for showing no interest in reaching out for bipartisan support and, just as bad, for addressing the Congress as though he were "a schoolmaster telling fourth-grade school children to be good." A hard fight lay ahead.

After only four months in office, Wilson was already feeling the pressures. With the President's having set such an accelerated pace out of the gate, Colonel House cautioned him to conserve his strength. Wilson would not slacken, and he was already speaking of "the loneliness of his position" in a way that House found "saddening." Having worked behind the scenes on all the President's major initiatives, House deserted Washington for a long vacation. Wilson had no such luxury.

He had intended to spend the summer with his family in Cornish, New Hampshire, a charming village on the Connecticut River, with an active colony of artists for Ellen—chief among them sculptor Augustus Saint-Gaudens, painter Maxfield Parrish, and Impressionist Robert Vonnoh, whose work had greatly influenced hers. Based on little more than photographs, Wilson signed a two-summer lease on Harlakenden, a stately Georgian house that belonged to American writer Winston Churchill. Surrounded by two hundred acres, it offered spacious but simple living and a view of the river and Mount Ascutney. Work in Congress demanded Wilson's presence in Washington—"I can't be cool and comfortable at Cornish while Congress perspires here all summer at my request," he said. He would have to vacation around the legislators' schedule; but he insisted upon his family's leaving him behind—especially his wife, who had been drawn into a maelstrom from the moment she had arrived in Washington.

In addition to the endless succession of afternoon receptions for one hundred and evening banquets for fifty, over which she had to preside, Ellen Wilson imposed additional demands upon herself, the only way she could justify her new role. Unlike many of her predecessors, she had no interest in the frills of being First Lady. A true disciple of the Social Gospel, however, she became the first President's wife to embrace the

humanitarian potential of her position, the ability to draw attention to social injustices. "I wonder how anyone who reaches middle age can bear it," she once told a cousin, "if she cannot feel . . . that whatever mistakes she may have made, she has on the whole lived for others and not for herself." And so, Ellen Wilson promptly made it her mission to inspect government buildings, including the Post Office Department and the Government Printing Office, where she found working conditions for women substandard—unsanitary lavatories and insufficient light and fresh air. She also took it upon herself to visit the city's slums, leading members of Congress through squalid alleys right outside their office doors and then urging remedial legislation for the Negroes who lived there.

And Ellen made the White House a home for her husband. She catered to all his needs, still serving as his most discriminating editor and adviser, and encouraging the professorial evenings of old, during which he might study and write and then recite poetry or sing around the piano with his daughters. She maintained Sunday as his day of observance, filled only with family and a restorative ride by automobile or on horseback. In accordance with Dr. Grayson's advice, she kept his meals simple—plain fish and meat courses, a vegetable and potatoes, a salad, and ice cream—served at seven, he in black tie, as was the custom of the house. Never much of a wine drinker, he occasionally allowed himself a "wee dram"—a shot of Scotch whisky. Congress allotted almost $10,000 for the conversion of the third floor of the White House—formerly attic space—for family use, which she spent creating more guest rooms and baths. She took down from the second-floor walls the dark green burlap and animal heads of the Roosevelt era and substituted light pastels and "craft" fabrics. She decorated the master suite in Delft blue and white, its furniture in chintz. The adjoining sitting room housed the Lincoln Bed. Ellen was able to obtain a further appropriation from Congress to remodel the gardens flanking the South Portico. She asked Princeton's landscape architect Beatrix Farrand to design the East Garden—which would feature low hedges and a rectangular lily pond in the center. For the West Garden, she maintained her initial concept of long rows of rosebushes, which not only afforded a pleasant view from her bedroom window but also provided Woodrow with a more becoming "President's walk" from the residence to his office. It became a permanent feature of the White House.

Even though Ellen wanted to spend the summer by her husband's side,

Woodrow insisted his worry over her health in the Washington heat would distract him more than her absence. On the train to New Hampshire, Ellen went to her berth and cried. She was hardly gone before Woodrow wrote the first of that summer's many lachrymose letters to her, explaining his growing understanding of his life in the highest office in the land, where duty superseded all other considerations. "I cannot choose as an individual what I shall do," he wrote on June 29; "I must always choose as President, ready to guard at every turn and in every possible way the success of what I have to do for the people. Apparently the little things count quite as much as the big in this strange business of leading opinion and securing action." Indeed, he found, "The President is a superior kind of slave," and somebody was always watching his every move, analyzing his every gesture, resenting his ever enjoying a holiday.

Wilson at least hoped to have Independence Day off, especially as he had already declined an appearance at Gettysburg; but, he wired Ellen on June 28, "FIND SO LONG AS I AM PRESIDENT, I CAN BE NOTHING ELSE." The next day he wrote to explain that Pennsylvania Congressman A. Mitchell Palmer had informed him that that year's commemoration at the battlefield was to be "no ordinary celebration," as it would mark the semicentenary of the great turning point of the Civil War. "Both blue and grey are to be there," he explained to Ellen. "It is to celebrate the end of . . . all strife between the sections." The President's absence, he noted, would be publicly resented. "It would be suggested that he is a Southerner and out of sympathy with the occasion. In short, it would be more than a passing mistake; it would amount to a serious blunder."

Washington, D.C., became a ghost town, the houses on the best residential streets emptying of all who could escape the summer torpor, the furniture in the great rooms of the White House all covered in white sheets. Feeling "marooned," Wilson prevailed upon Tumulty and Dr. Grayson to move into the Executive Mansion, and he found them good company. The former was married with small children, whom he joined on weekends on the New Jersey Shore; Grayson remained the President's boon companion and constant medical consort. They spent practically all their free time together—dining, theatergoing twice a week, even attending church together. Dr. Grayson prescribed a daily dose of golf.

"An ineffectual attempt to put an elusive ball into an obscure hole with implements ill-adapted to the purpose" is how Wilson delighted in

describing the pastime. And perhaps because of the devotion, concentration, difficulty, and even prayer it required, golf became his second religion. He played every day that weather and work permitted. Wilson had supreme powers of concentration, and he loved impossible challenges; but he never became expert at the sport—in part because of his bad eye, which limited his peripheral vision. And so he played a methodical game that compensated for the ocular handicap—short, perfectly straight shots—though once he required twenty-six strokes on a single hole. Seldom did his score rise above 100, because upon reaching three digits, he was inclined to pack up his clubs and quit. One day at the Piping Rock Club in Locust Valley on Long Island, he shot 146, and even admitted as much to a reporter. He liked to play on the less exclusive courses around Washington—especially when they included a relaxing drive across the Potomac to Virginia. He was extremely selective about those in his party, as he forbade any talk of business and never played a second time with anybody who violated the rule. "Each stroke requires your whole attention and seems the most important thing in life," he wrote Edith Reid that summer. "I can by that means get perfect diversion of my thoughts for an hour or so at the same time that I am breathing the pure out-of-doors." His scorecard was not a barometer of his ability—which never changed—but of his mental state, the ease with which he could sink the ball into the hole suggesting how free from his responsibilities he had become. No President before or since played as much golf in the White House as Woodrow Wilson.

The President and his physician found slight relief from the heat on Capitol Hill by cruising down the Potomac and Chesapeake Bay on the Presidential yacht, the *Mayflower*. They spent a sweltering July 3 in Yorktown. Wilson and Grayson eluded the Secret Service agents by saying they were going ashore with the captain of the ship and several sailors. But once the small motor launch had reached the wharf, the two men lost the others and spent the day wandering the sleepy streets of the old town by themselves. They visited the local courthouse and the battlefield and continued up the York River to see the farm that had once been Washington's headquarters—crawling through brambles, shooing away bees, and encountering an angry bull along the way. The locals paid no attention to their visitors until a twelve-year-old girl saw them and said, "Excuse me, sir, but you certainly do remind me of the pictures of President Wilson."

He returned to Washington, only to leave by train early the next morning with Tumulty for Gettysburg, Pennsylvania. There, exactly fifty years prior, Union and Confederate soldiers had fought the costliest battle of the Civil War. The fifty-one thousand casualties (nearly eight thousand deaths) were almost equally divided; but, in retrospect, it proved to be the turning point of the war, as the Confederates steadily retreated over the next two years. In November of 1863, Lincoln delivered his deathless 272-word address, dedicating a portion of the battlefield as a final resting place for those who gave their lives there. In the half century since the battle, Gettysburg came to represent the reuniting of the nation. The symbol was so important that the Congress appropriated more than $2 million to mount a reunion, offering to transport any Civil War veteran from anywhere in the country and to feed and house him during this three-day "Peace Jubilee."

More than fifty thousand veterans flocked to the small town, proudly wearing uniforms and decorations and waving flags. Each man was provided with a cot and bedding in a 280-acre camp of eight-man tents. In the scorching heat, thousands gathered for speeches under a gigantic big top, walked the battlefield, and healed old wounds. The most compelling moment of the reunion came when two small teams of white-whiskered survivors of Pickett's Charge faced each other and shook hands, reaching across the same stone wall each side had once fought to overtake. Goodwill seemed restored, but so little had been resolved: slavery had been abolished, but regionalism and racism in America were as rampant as ever. The survivors looked to Wilson for inspiration.

The world would little note what he said there. The President's entrance into the great tent brought the crowd of ten thousand to its feet. In a black frock coat, he put his top hat down and stood without a podium before the assembly. Holding his text in his left hand, he delivered a peculiarly hollow speech—full of ethereal questions ("Who stands ready to act again and always in the spirit of this day of reunion and hope and patriotic fervor?") while offering few concrete answers. He called upon his countrymen to serve "the people themselves, the great and the small, without class or difference of kind or race or origin." That was as close as he got to the underlying themes of the terrible war that had torn the nation apart. Within a half hour of his arrival, Wilson had returned to his train. He left behind a stillness at Gettysburg—which, in some ways, was his intention.

The nation dedicated to the proposition that all men were created

equal was, in fact, built atop an active fault of discrimination. A deep fissure of intolerance remained. State laws, especially in the South, went a long way toward keeping the races apart; but even Northern states were enacting anti-intermarriage statutes. The purportedly color-blind Civil Service had long operated under the "rule of three," by which an employer was able to select from the trio of top applicants, allowing him to bypass Negro candidates. Many in the white majority were unable to accept the concept of all races being on equal footing; and where statutes proved inadequate, some took the law into their own hands. In parts of America, racial violence was so common, Negroes instinctively kept their distance from whites and held their tongues. Lynchings in America occurred weekly. As President, Wilson wished to promote racial progress—equal opportunities and peaceful coexistence—by shocking the social system as little as possible. With both impatient blacks and intolerant whites clamoring for action, there seemed only one solution that might avert upheaval and allow social evolution to take its course.

There were already two Americas. Negro activist James Weldon Johnson wrote of such commonplace practices as the refusal to tip one's hat to a colored woman or to address a Negro as "Mister" as more than trivialities; he added that "they connote the whole system of race prejudice, hatred, and injustice; their roots go to the very core of the whole matter." Such mere trifles, he said, declared that "there is no common ground on which we can stand." At the same time, Agriculture Secretary David Houston, a highly regarded educator and political scientist, was considering the problem of discrimination against the Japanese in California and how they rated more favorably than Negroes—who were as a rule, he would write years later, "of low mental capacity and lazy." So it hardly took anyone aback when Postmaster General Burleson had raised a prickly policy matter at one of the first Cabinet meetings back in the spring: Burleson wanted to segregate white and Negro employees not just in the Postal Service but in all departments of the government.

Many Negroes worked in the railway mail service, he explained, often in the same car with white men. In those instances, he suggested, it was presumed that the white men would outwork the black and resentments would grow. Furthermore, Burleson said, "It is very unpleasant for them to work in a car with negroes where it is almost impossible to have different drinking vessels and different towels, or places to wash."

More than any of Wilson's Cabinet members, Burleson understood the practice of politics; and he had done his due diligence. He had spoken with African American leaders, including organizer Bishop Alexander Walters of the African Methodist Episcopal Zion Church, who, he claimed, endorsed the idea of separating the races. Josephus Daniels wrote in his diary that Burleson said "he had the highest regard for the negro and wished to help him in every way possible, but that he believed segregation was best for the negro and best for the Service." Burleson went even farther that day, asking the President to reconsider even the appointment of Negroes to midlevel clerical offices—including the Register of the Treasury, which a black man had held for years.

Segregation was not new to Washington, having flourished since the Roosevelt Administration. TR may have invited Booker T. Washington to dine in the White House, but he was publicly chastised for it and decades would pass before another African American would find a place at the White House table. Under Taft the dining room for White House employees divided along a color line. So did the Census Bureau. In the few Washington departments that hired Negroes, many worked without question in areas apart from white workers. Some divisions simply became known as "Negro colonies." A Harvard- and Howard-educated attorney named Robert H. Terrell spent a few years in the Treasury Department before Taft appointed him to the Municipal Court of the District of Columbia, making him the nation's first Negro judge; government office lunchrooms refused to serve him or other equally distinguished black men. Negroes who sought equal treatment at lunch counters were only inviting violence.

Legalized segregation—"Jim Crow" laws—seemed a logical way to avoid friction, as it would keep blacks and whites literally from having to rub shoulders. Fifty years after Gettysburg, it seemed unimaginable to most Southerners that white men might have to serve under a black boss. Wilson was still inclined to let each Secretary run his department as he saw fit; and so, on the two racial issues before him, he rendered a split decision: he permitted Burleson and McAdoo to segregate their departments; and he proceeded to appoint a Negro, Adam E. Patterson, as the Treasury Register.

That settled nothing, as each announcement incited intense reaction. Although Wilson believed the purity and fidelity of the white women of the South were its very backbone, he did not subscribe to the primal

fear—mongering of many other Confederates. His Johns Hopkins colleague Thomas Dixon, the author of the Ku Klux Klan trilogy, wrote Wilson that he was "heartsick" over the appointment, that unless he withdrew Patterson's name, "the South can never forgive this. . . . The establishment of Negro men over white women employees of the Treasury Dept. has in the minds of many thoughtful men & women long been a serious offense against the cleanness of our social life." Dixon asked Wilson to "purge Washington of this iniquity" and withdraw the appointment.

"I do not think you know what is going on down here," an exasperated Wilson replied, trying to explain the shifting mores in a city where the black population could not be ignored. "We are handling the force of colored people who are now in the departments in just the way in which they ought to be handled." At Treasury, for example, the President was standing by his appointment, as that particular office was being reconfigured into an all-black unit, one of several such divisions there: "I am trying to handle these matters with the best judgment but in the spirit of the whole country," he wrote with some impatience, "though with entire comprehension of the considerations which certainly do not need to be pointed out to me." Wilson considered this plan of putting "certain bureaus and sections of the service in the charge of negroes" a thoughtful means of "rendering them more safe in their possession of office and less likely to be discriminated against."

As Burleson's proposals had portended, Southerners in Congress felt this was their moment to rise again. Senators James Vardaman of Mississippi, Benjamin Tillman of South Carolina, and Hoke Smith of Georgia all announced their refusal to support not only Patterson but any Negro who would be in a position to boss white women. A gracious Patterson requested that Wilson withdraw his name, which he did.

In the meantime, McAdoo and Burleson segregated their departments with all deliberate speed. They supervised the creation of separate but ostensibly equal work, lunch, and lavatory facilities. That summer, Robert N. Wood, president of the United Colored Democracy of the State of New York, wrote Wilson that his people deeply resented the segregation of clerks in the Civil Service throughout the federal government—

> . . . not at all because we are particularly anxious to eat in the same room or use the same soap and towels that white people use, but because we see in the separation . . . of the races in the matter of soup

and soap the beginning of a movement to deprive the colored man entirely of soup and soap, to eliminate him wholly from the Civil Service of the United States. For just as soon as there is a lunch-room or a work-room which the colored man may not enter in a government building, there will be separate tasks assigned the colored men and these will be, as the promoters of segregation have declared, the tasks which white men do not want.

Even Booker T. Washington—"the great accommodator," considered an "Uncle Tom" by uprising black leaders—wrote Oswald Garrison Villard of the NAACP that he had recently spent several days in Washington and that he had "never seen the colored people so discouraged and bitter as they are at the present time."

In a letter signed by Villard, Director of Publicity W. E. B. Du Bois, and President Moorfield Storey, the NAACP vigorously protested the new government policy. "Never before has the Federal Government discriminated against its civilian employees on the ground of color," they wrote. States drafting discriminatory laws were one thing; segregating federal buildings in the District of Columbia was quite another. "It has set the colored people apart as if mere contact with them were contamination," they wrote.

Wilson had not intended such a result, as he did not equate segregation with subjugation. Rather, he considered it a way for Negroes to elevate themselves, getting a foothold in American institutions so that they could start assimilating. He thought the new forces of black workers in the federal government first had to occupy the same buildings as whites before they could share the same rooms. Gradually, he believed, proximity would breed familiarity, and, in time, harmony. Powerful bigots saw segregation as a means to keep the black man down; but Wilson viewed it "with the idea that the friction, or rather the discontent and uneasiness, which had prevailed in many of the departments would thereby be removed. It is as far as possible from being a movement *against* the negroes. I sincerely believe it to be in their interest." While his Cabinet members had put the policy in motion, Wilson stood behind it and owned it. "My own feeling," he told Villard, "is by putting certain bureaus and sections of the service in the charge of negroes we are rendering them more safe in their possession of office and less likely to be discriminated against." Or so he had convinced himself.

"I hope that you will try to see the real situation down here," an exasperated Wilson tried to explain to Oswald Villard. He wished Villard understood the hatred that festered in the hearts of so many Southerners. Wilson suggested that left to his own devices, he would not have instituted these new measures; but finding what he considered a middle ground, he believed a period of tranquillity would open more doors of opportunity for the Negroes. "I believe that by the slow pressure of argument and persuasion the situation may be changed and a great many things done eventually which now seem impossible," Wilson said. "But they can not be done, either now or at any future time, if a bitter agitation is inaugurated and carried to its natural ends." He appealed to Villard and the NAACP to "aid in holding things at a just and cool equipoise until I can discover whether it is possible to work out anything or not." Wilson believed there was so much intolerance in the nation just then that it would take "one hundred years to eradicate this prejudice"; if they could all avoid stirring emotions with incendiary talk and rely on evolution, they might be able to avoid revolution.

For Wilson, segregation remained secondary to the advancement of his New Freedom, though both matters were bound together. "It would be hard to make any one understand the delicacy and difficulty of the situation I find existing here with regard to the colored people," the President of six months wrote Villard. In the matter of appointments, he explained, "I find myself absolutely blocked by the sentiment of Senators; not alone Senators from the South, by any means, but Senators from various parts of the country."

Villard sympathized with Wilson's position, but he did not empathize. "I believe that as with your most immediate predecessors," he wrote, "the time will come when you will find it necessary to go ahead and do what is right without considering their feelings." Villard believed the President was not a bigot, that he supported the advancement of the Negro; and that made it all the more frustrating to see him knuckling under to the Southern Senators. In a subsequent conversation with journalist John Palmer Gavit, Wilson said he had to deal with a Congress dominated by men of such fundamental beliefs; and Gavit understood that the President's opposition to such views "would certainly precipitate a conflict which would put a complete stop to any legislative program." In that moment, then, it seemed the only way to further the New Freedom was on the back of the Negro.

By the end of the year, the Post Office Department and the office of the Auditor for the Post Office were segregated; and soon the District's City Post Office would establish separate windows for Negro patrons as well as the personnel who manned them. At the office of the Auditor of the Navy, screens separated white workers from black, the latter group no longer finding their lavatory on the same floor but in the basement. The Bureau of Engraving and Printing followed suit. Secretary McAdoo proudly removed every white from the Register's Division, not realizing, as Villard wrote Wilson, "that this division will immediately be called the 'nigger division' and that the precedent thus established will be of the utmost danger to the colored people long after the motive has been forgotten and Mr. McAdoo has disappeared from public life." Civil Service positions now required photographs, which tempted some employers simply to overlook the "rule of three." The number of positions available to Negroes, along with the level of those jobs, went in the same direction as their lavatories.

Despite the opposition from the bloc of bigoted Southern Senators, Wilson did repeatedly nominate Negroes to refill positions that they had traditionally held—including the reappointment of Judge Robert H. Terrell to the Municipal Court. In tangling with a Senator or even Speaker Champ Clark, Wilson flatly explained the promise he had made to the black community and that he was honor-bound. He expected equality in all the facilities within the federal buildings.

In the early fall of 1913, the NAACP conducted an investigation of the segregation of colored employees within the government departments. Villard sent the results to Wilson, as he had requested. At the Bureau of Engraving and Printing, the investigator—NAACP Secretary May Childs Nerney—reported that colored women who had dined for nine years with white women had been relegated to a separate table. At the Post Office Department there was an attractive dining room for the white employees but none for the black, which some excused with the argument that there were no restaurants in Washington that would serve blacks and so neither should the government be expected to. Treasury boasted 270 colored employees; but May Nerney found many had been consigned to areas of the building that were poorly lighted and ventilated. Those segregated, she added, were regarded as "a people set apart, almost as lepers. Instead of allaying race prejudice . . . it has simply emphasized it." Because Negroes could now advance only so far, they seemed to have lost their competitive

drive. She felt many Negro workers would look for employment elsewhere.
Jim Crow, some feared, would next overtake public transportation. Wilson
wrote Villard that he intended to right the wrongs within the policy but
not to change the policy itself.

As McAdoo asserted in a letter to Villard, "There is no 'segregation issue' in the Treasury Department." He contended that white women had
long complained of having to sit at desks with colored men. His personal
feelings articulated the current administration's policy: "I shall not be a
party to the enforced and unwelcome juxtaposition of white and negro employees when it is unnecessary and avoidable without injustice to anybody,
and when such enforcement would serve only to engender race animosities
detrimental to the welfare of both races and injurious to the public service."
Protesters across the country were already organizing that summer, and an
anti-segregation petition with twenty thousand signatures would soon land
on the President's desk. In just a few months, Wilson had become entangled
in what journalist Gavit would call "the most difficult and embarrassing
and dangerous subject" before him—what was merely the culmination of
"the crimes and hypocrisies of three centuries."

Wilson managed to find relief in Cornish a few times that summer.
The family made time to take long drives together through the New
Hampshire countryside; and at night they sat on the terrace, under the
stars, as Woodrow regaled them with stories of life in "hectic" Washington. They often entertained neighboring artists; and one night actress Marie Dressler, who summered across the river in Windsor, Vermont, came to
perform an evening of songs and stories. But the Wilsons most appreciated
their time alone, especially as they announced Jessie's engagement to Frank
Sayre that July. Wilson heartily approved of his future son-in-law, especially as he had converted to the Democratic Party and—reminiscent of
her father—was giving up the practice of law for a career in academia,
starting as an assistant to President Harry Garfield of Williams College.

Harlakenden had an artist's studio, where Ellen painted every day, creating some of her most accomplished canvases to date. Her landscapes had
become slightly more Impressionistic, revealing looser brushwork and
genuine mastery of composition and color. Robert Vonnoh called Ellen "a
real artist" and declared that if she continued, her work would become
"really *very* distinguished." In fact, five of her paintings from the summer
would be part of an exhibition of the Association of Women Painters and

Sculptors in New York that fall. In reviewing her work, *The New York Times* would say, "Mrs. Wilson is a serious art student and she observed in nature aspects that appeal to the lover of outdoor life." Three of the pictures sold in the $100 range.

As in the earliest days of their courtship—and through thirty years of periodic separations—Woodrow and Ellen still corresponded copiously when they were apart. The duties of office restricted him from writing more than twice a week. Although his letters were largely about his work, his passion still permeated them. He wrote his wife of twenty-eight years that his "dearest indulgence" that summer was in occasionally daydreaming of her beauty and charm. "I adore you! No President but myself ever had *exactly* the right sort of wife! I am certainly the most fortunate man alive!" he declared.

Ellen's feelings ran just as deep, and she sublimated them by immersing herself in family and her artwork. She said she felt like "a soldier's wife," as she suffered through Woodrow's absences. "I *idolize* you," she wrote him, "—I love you till it *hurts*." Ellen passed much of the time without Woodrow by reading his letters from the White House to their three daughters. "And although she still skipped the 'sacred parts,'" remembered Nell, then twenty-three, "we knew by the tender pride in her face that after all the years together they remained the poetic messages of a lover."

Midsummer, Ellen could endure the separation no longer. Accompanied by Nell, she braved the steamy twenty-hour journey to Washington to pay a surprise visit. Woodrow's obvious elation alone made the entire journey worthwhile. He looked tired, strained as he was marshaling votes for his two sweeping economic bills; but he was rejuvenated having Ellen by his side again. They were both amused when Secretary McAdoo called on the President that night and, upon seeing Nell, invited her to play tennis with him the next day. Within a few days of Ellen's arrival, Dr. Grayson encouraged her return to Cornish because of the overwhelming heat and Woodrow's concern about her.

In September, New Jersey Democrats held a primary election, and Wilson took the train to Princeton so that he could vote. Away only six months, he already felt strangely detached from his home of so many years. With a few minutes to kill, he walked through Nassau Hall, only to learn that a crowd was gathering out front. Wishing to avoid a spectacle,

Wilson asked a young man whether a certain back door was unlocked, which would allow for an unobserved exit. Strangely, the man misinterpreted Wilson's inquiry as interest in seeing the president of the college, who was then at home. The fellow raced to inform him, and in a moment, Jack Hibben was on horseback, galloping to Nassau Hall. Flushed with anticipation, he found his former intimate, who had spurned him for years now. "I was told, Mr. President, that you were looking for me," he said. Offering a cold smile but not his hand, Wilson replied, "No, no, you are mistaken." And with that, he turned toward the station, adding, "Good afternoon, Sir." Before boarding the train, Wilson apologized to a member of his small party, explaining, "The man who stopped and spoke to me was my friend. I did more to make him than I did for any other person in the world. I unbosomed my very soul to him. And in the crucial moment of my life, he turned against me. I can never forgive him."

Washington had become Wilson's home now, legislative battles and all. "I of course find a real zest in it all," he wrote Edith Reid. "Hard as it is to nurse Congress along and stand ready to play a part of guidance in anything that turns up, great or small, it is all part of something infinitely great and worth while, and I am content to labour at it to the finish." In the late afternoon of September 9, 1913, the Senate passed his tariff bill, almost entirely along partisan lines. Louisiana's Senators—protecting sugar and cotton—were the only two Democrats to vote against it; and the two most Progressive Republicans (including Robert "Fighting Bob" La Follette of Wisconsin) voted for it. Looking back on the five months in which this bill had been kicked around the floor of the Capitol, opposition Senator Albert B. Cummins of Iowa said that the Congress had surrendered its primacy to "a single will." He told the press that he intended to read the writings of "the man who has more influence in the Congress of the United States than any man ever before had. I refer to Woodrow Wilson."

At nine o'clock on the night of October 3, 1913, fifty guests in evening clothes—including the Congressional leaders and most of the Cabinet—gathered around the President's desk in the Oval Office. A buoyant Wilson entered to applause and took his seat, the tariff measure printed on parchment awaiting his signature. He gilded the ceremony by introducing what would become a Presidential tradition for future historic signings: he autographed the bill with two different gold pens—one for his first name,

one for his last—which he presented to Congressman Underwood and Senator Simmons.

"I have had the accomplishment of something like this at heart ever since I was a boy," he told those assembled, "and I know men standing around me who can say the same thing—who have been waiting to see the things done which it was necessary to do in order that there might be justice in the United States." Referencing Shakespeare's *Henry V*, the President said, "If it be a sin to covet honour, then am I the most offending soul alive." He did not choreograph this occasion to pat the men on their backs so much as to push them forward. Their job was only half done. "We are now about to take the second step," he said, ". . . in setting the business of this country free." The House had already passed the currency bill, and now he urged its passage through the Senate.

"How profoundly I thank God for giving you the chance to win such victories," Ellen wrote from Cornish, "—to help the world so greatly;—for letting you work for Him on a *large* stage;—one worthy of the splendid combination of qualities with which He endowed you. . . . It has been the most remarkable life history I ever even *read* about,—and to think *I* have *lived* it with you. I wonder if I am dreaming, and will wake up and find myself married to—a bank clerk,—say!"

Into the fall of 1913, the subject of banks consumed most of Wilson's waking hours. And on September 18, his audacious currency bill—the Federal Reserve legislation, with its restructuring of the nation's banking system—passed the House by a vote of 287 to 85. Forty-eight Republicans supported the President while only three Democrats opposed him. Outside the Capitol, wealthy conservatives quickly weighed in. The president of the National City Bank suggested that Federal Reserve notes would hardly be worth the paper they were printed on; railroad tycoon James J. Hill pronounced the proposal "socialistic"; a Yale economist said American gold would seek investment in Europe and massive inflation would descend; Republican leader James Mann had already denounced the entire plan but now suggested it was a moot point, as none of the 7,500 national banks would even enter the Federal Reserve System.

Seven Democrats and five Republicans sat on the Senate Banking and Currency Committee, and it came as a great surprise when one of the majority, Gilbert M. Hitchcock of Nebraska, announced he had so many objections to the bill that he joined the opposition. A Democratic

colleague, James A. Reed of Missouri, followed. That gave the Republicans the edge in keeping the bill from ever leaving their committee. Then Democratic Senator James A. O'Gorman of New York, mindful of his constituents on Wall Street, joined forces. Former Senator Nelson Aldrich trotted out his old plan of a central bank. Thus began, said Vice President Thomas R. Marshall, "the most illuminating and exhaustive discussion of a public question ever held in the Senate of the United States."

Not forgetting the great debates of Clay, Calhoun, and Webster, Marshall said the next five months saw "a practical history of all the banking systems of the world; of all the debts, assets and incomes of all the races of the world; of their armies, their navies, their taxes." Through it all, Wilson maintained his equanimity, though he fumed in private. "Why *should* public men, senators of the United States, have to be led and stimulated to what all the country knows to be their duty!" he rhetorically asked Mary Hulbert. Wilson repeatedly convened with his party's dissenters, separately and together, as well as with Republican members of the committee, winning over one mind at a time. With the able support of Colonel House, McAdoo, and Bryan, he steadily plied his powers of persuasion, arguing that structural change was needed immediately. The off-year elections in early November signaled that Progressivism was still in the air; and one by one, Democrats wandered back into the party fold. Bankers—especially those outside New York—began to embrace the banking bill. Even the final Republican arguments in early December felt stale.

On December 19, 1913, the Senate passed the bill 54 to 34. Every Democrat present, along with six Republicans and one Progressive, voted aye. With a Christmas holiday beckoning, it took only three days of conferences to reconcile the bill with the House version. And on December 23, the President held another signing ceremony in his office, surrounded by his family as well as the officials who had contributed to the bill. For this occasion, he had purchased three gold pens, which he handed to Congressman Glass, Senator Owen, and Secretary McAdoo. He spoke for a few minutes, expressing his belief that, on the heels of the tariff bill, this act "furnishes the machinery for free and elastic and uncontrolled credits, put at the disposal of the merchants and manufacturers of this country for the first time in fifty years." Wilson could not find the words to express his "deep emotions of gratitude" at being part of something so beneficial to the business of America.

It was a profoundly emotional time for Wilson in other ways as well. Only weeks earlier, on Tuesday, November 25, 1913, Jessie Woodrow Wilson had married Francis Bowes Sayre in the East Room of the White House. The bride had hoped for a small and informal wedding; but with the President's soaring popularity in Washington, that became impossible. Four hundred guests—Cabinet members, Senators and Representatives, Supreme Court Justices, and diplomats, along with friends and family of the wedding couple, gathered in the great salon. Just before 4:30, Sayre and his groomsmen (one of whom was Charles Evans Hughes, Jr., son of an Associate Justice) descended the stairway and entered the East Room, where Dr. Sylvester Beach, the Wilsons' pastor in Princeton, and Sayre's brother, a minister, would perform a combined Episcopalian and Presbyterian ceremony.

The procession of attendants entered to the musical accompaniment of the Marine Band, resplendent in scarlet. When all were in place, a bugle heralded the entrance of the President, who was dressed in a dark gray cutaway. Her arm linked through his, the bride wore a white satin dress of her own design, with a long veil and a train three yards in length. To the traditional strains of *Lohengrin*, they walked to the raised platform that had been erected before the great east window. This makeshift chancel was flanked by two large blue vases, filled with gigantic clusters of white lilies. When Dr. Beach asked "who giveth this woman," the President stepped forward and placed his daughter's hand in that of the groom.

The wedding party received guests in the Blue Room, and refreshments were served in the dining room. As there was a $1,000 reward to any journalist who could report on the newlyweds' honeymoon plans, they had prearranged a getaway in Joseph Tumulty's car from the south entrance of the White House. Before they left, Jessie stood halfway up the main staircase and threw her bouquet, right into the hands of her sister Nell. When the festivities had wound down, Woodrow placed his arm across Ellen's shoulders and drew her close as they walked wistfully to the elevator. "I know; it was a wedding, not a funeral," Ellen said to some of the relatives who remained, "but you must forgive us—this is the first break in the family."

And then a second shoe dropped. Over the last few months, Secretary McAdoo, known to his friends as Mac, had become a familiar presence in the White House. The President increasingly relied upon him; and, in

time, the young widower frequently appeared during off-hours, calling on Miss Eleanor, as he referred to Nell, to join him for tennis or horseback riding. They enjoyed dancing together at social events; and he soon became a regular visitor in the evenings, hoping they might have a chance to sit alone in the Green Room. Often he would walk with Miss Eleanor to the Washington Monument, where they would sit and watch the sunset. Although she was the most frivolous of the Wilson daughters, McAdoo found her unusually well-informed and opinionated—as she would be, having sat at her father's dinner table for twenty-three years. "It was not long before I discovered that my interest in her was more than platonic," McAdoo later recalled. For a while, he kept his feelings to himself. He was twice her age, and he worked for her father. But the next time they waltzed, he decided to marry her.

At the same time, Dr. Grayson—McAdoo's closest friend and Washington's other most eligible bachelor—grew concerned about his two patients, the President and Mrs. Wilson. He convinced them that they desperately needed a vacation. With Jessie away on her honeymoon in London and Paris, Grayson urged Wilson to spend the Christmas holiday with the rest of his family in the Gulf country. Mississippi Senator John Sharp Williams recommended Pass Christian as an ideal winter resort. One evening just before the Wilsons' departure, knowing that she would be gone for weeks and that he was leaving on a tour of the nation to select sites for the Federal Reserve Banks, Mac revealed his intentions. They agreed to search their souls before committing to each other, or even telling her parents.

Pass Christian was everything Senator Williams had promised—balmy and restful. The Wilsons, Helen Bones, and Dr. Grayson stayed at Beaulieu, an antebellum mansion with tall white columns and garlands of moss hanging from the trees. They celebrated Christmas and Wilson's fifty-seventh birthday; and, inevitably, the President began to chart the next stage of his New Freedom. Returning from a round of golf with Grayson one day, Wilson noticed smoke curling from the roof of a house. They ran to the door to inform the residents, only to have the mistress of the house invite her guests into the parlor to sit down. "I haven't time to sit down," the President said, "—your house is on fire." They were able to get to the roof in time to extinguish it; and afterward, the local firefighters elected Wilson and Grayson members of their department. At that

moment, however, the President had much bigger fires to put out—across the Gulf.

Two months earlier, Woodrow Wilson had delivered an address on foreign affairs at a convention of the Southern Commercial Congress in Mobile, Alabama, which several ministers from Latin America attended. The Panama Canal was approaching completion, and the isthmus was about to become the new crossroads of the globe. Before the world rushed in, Wilson wanted to articulate a new policy for his nation. He had every desire to expand the economy but only "upon terms of equality and honor." For Wilson, that meant one principle: "the development of constitutional liberty in the world."

President Wilson hoped to change the course set by his predecessors, as the only American Empire he wished to create was one of ideas. "Human rights, national integrity, and opportunity as against material interest," he said, "is the issue which we now have to face." He seized this occasion to insist "that the United States will never again seek one additional foot of territory by conquest. She will devote herself to showing that she knows how to make honorable and fruitful use of the territory she has; and she must regard it as one of the duties of friendship to see that from no quarter are material interests made superior to human liberty and national opportunity." What distinguished America, he said, were the beliefs on which it was founded. "I would rather belong to a poor nation that was free," he said, "than to a rich nation that had ceased to be in love with liberty." For a century, the Monroe Doctrine had served to keep Europe from securing political control over the nations of the Western Hemisphere; and Wilson believed—as Colonel House realized one day while lunching with him— that it was "just as reprehensible to permit foreign states to secure financial control of these weak and unfortunate republics."

A storm was brewing the January night Wilson went out to a cruiser at sea to confer with John Lind, his special agent in Mexico. Lind reported on Mexico's recent elections, which had prompted General Huerta to nullify the results, dissolve the legislature, and remain as dictator. Regional opposition continued to mount, but the leaders remained too wary of one another to join forces. To defend himself against the insurrections of Venustiano Carranza in the north and Emiliano Zapata in the south,

Huerta mobilized a vast army of federal forces, literally kidnapping men off the streets.

When Wilson had addressed a joint session of Congress months earlier on the subject of Mexico, he had recommended neutrality, forbidding the United States to export munitions there. When this policy did nothing to weaken Huerta, Wilson changed tack, lifting the embargo in order to help arm General Francisco "Pancho" Villa, a popular leader from the north who also held Huerta in great contempt. When that showed little effect, Lind urged an aggressive attack against Huerta. Unfortunately, the Ambassador was neither knowledgeable nor sensitive enough to recognize that the Mexican people preferred Huerta to foreign imposition. Knowing he was not receiving enough reliable information, Wilson returned from his shipboard meeting badly shaken. He felt it was as essential as it was inevitable that the Huerta regime should fall, but he was committed to Mexico's determining its own government—no matter how badly he wanted to intervene.

The Wilsons returned to Washington, where Ellen's ongoing efforts for slum clearance resulted in a bill being introduced in Congress. Although this pleased her, she was always weary and often looked drawn and pale. One night in early March 1914, after shaking hands with three thousand people at a White House reception, she fainted, falling hard on the polished floor of her bedroom. There was no sign of any deep injury, but she was sore for weeks. Ellen insisted she was fine and, referring to her husband, said, "This goose keeps worrying about me for no reason at all!"

Not until April did Ellen show signs of her old self, at which time Woodrow took the entire family—along with Dr. Grayson and a nurse—to the Greenbrier in White Sulphur Springs. The West Virginia resort offered golf, tennis, riding, even a new indoor pool. After a few days, William McAdoo joined them, his engagement to Eleanor having just been announced. In asking for her hand, Mac had suggested to his boss that he would resign to spare the President any embarrassment. "I appreciate your generous and considerate attitude," Wilson said, "but I hope you will dismiss all thought of such a thing. You were appointed Secretary of the Treasury solely on your merit. No one imagined, at that time, that the present situation would arise." He then paused and said with a wink, "But I must admit . . . that, if you had married into my family before I became President, I could not have offered you a position in the Cabinet, no matter

how outstanding your record and qualifications might have been." It was a happy Easter for all of them, especially Woodrow and Ellen, who quietly rejoiced in each other's company during long rides in a buckboard, reminiscent of their courtship in Rome, Georgia, thirty years earlier.

On April 9, 1914—the day the Wilsons had left for the Greenbrier—a whaleboat attached to the American war vessel *Dolphin* docked at Tampico—then under Huerta's martial law—and a few sailors disembarked for a routine supply run. These bluejackets did not produce the permits that were required. Mexican soldiers boarded the whaleboat, which flew American flags at the bow and stern, and took the unarmed Paymaster and his crew into custody. When they were but a few blocks into town, an officer of higher authority ordered the Americans' return to the wharf until further instructions arrived. Within ninety minutes, Huerta's forces ordered their release and issued an apology, complete with "an expression of regret" from Huerta himself. The apology did not satisfy Admiral Henry T. Mayo, commander of the naval squadron, who unilaterally demanded a twenty-one-gun salute to the American flag.

The next morning, Secretary of State Bryan wired the President about the incident. Although everything Huerta said or did provoked him, Wilson was annoyed with Mayo, whose demand seemed unnecessary. Colonel House said Mayo should be admonished against making such decisions without authorization, but the Commander in Chief supported his Admiral: "Mayo could not have done otherwise," Wilson wired Bryan back. The Mexican commander in Tampico felt unqualified to order that salute, and the matter escalated to a diplomatic incident. Huerta informed the American Chargé d'Affaires that he would accede to the demand, provided an American ship responded in kind. Wilson agreed, and the confrontation could have ended with forty-two bullets being fired into the air. But then Huerta tried to reopen the negotiation, demanding that a protocol between the two governments be signed. Wilson knew that action could be construed as his recognition of the Huerta government, to which he would not accede. For the first time in his life, Wilson had difficulty sleeping.

Eleven days after the incident, Wilson opened his press conference assuring everybody that there was not about to be a war between the United States and Mexico; but when he took the matter to Congress that afternoon, jingoism filled the air. His welcome before the joint session in the House was disturbingly enthusiastic. "The incident cannot be regarded as

a trivial one," he told the legislators—especially as two of the men arrested had been removed from the boat itself, and thus seized from United States territory. Furthermore, the President asserted, this was not an isolated incident. A few days later, an orderly from the USS *Minnesota* was arrested in Veracruz while obtaining his ship's mail. Wilson reaffirmed that he had no intention of going to war, but he asked for Congress's approval to "use the armed forces of the United States in such ways and to such an extent as may be necessary to obtain from General Huerta and his adherents the fullest recognition of the rights and dignity of the United States, even amidst the distressing conditions now unhappily obtaining in Mexico."

Several Republicans saw this as an opportunity for America, once again, to carry a big stick. Alongside Henry Cabot Lodge, the most forthright speaker that day was Senator Elihu Root of New York, who said the insult to Old Glory was the least of the matter: behind that lay "years of violence and anarchy in Mexico" that warranted bold action to reinforce America's position of power in the world. "People seem to want war with Mexico," Wilson told his family after seeing the Congressional reaction, "but they shan't have it if I can prevent it." The Senate authorized the President to employ the armed forces to back his demands "for unequivocal amends for affronts and indignities." Thus empowered, Wilson would have to keep resisting the urge to remove the sword from its scabbard in Haiti and the Dominican Republic as well, nearby nations that had endured years of revolts and coups d'état and which had required American fiscal assistance as well as its occasional military presence to stabilize them and their economies.

Woodrow Wilson had no intention of becoming another TR, an imperialistic warrior who exerted his might because he could; but he did see himself as a Christian soldier, fighting for what was right. Blinded by his desire to remove Huerta, Wilson did not see the irony of demanding a salute from a government he did not even recognize. Between his speech to Congress and the Senate approval, the Administration learned that a ship had left Havana for Veracruz laden with 1,333 boxes of German guns intended for Huerta. Wilson discussed the matter with his Secretaries of State and the Navy. Daniels said, "The munitions should not be permitted to fall into Huerta's hands." The President hesitated to act pre-emptively, but his advisers maintained that if the arms did reach the usurper, it would increase the loss of Mexican lives and the guns might later be

turned upon Americans. "There is no alternative but to land," said Wilson. Daniels immediately cabled Admiral Frank F. Fletcher, commander of the Atlantic Fleet, "Seize custom house. Do not permit war supplies to be delivered to Huerta government or to any other party."

On the morning of April 21, 1914, Fletcher's fleet steamed to Veracruz, and eight hundred Marines and Navy bluejackets filled their whaleboats and sailed to the waterfront. By nightfall they had captured the customs house as well as the post and telegraph offices and the railroad station; the next day they overtook the rest of the town. Nineteen Americans lost their lives, and another seventy were wounded; more than a hundred Mexicans died.

On May 11, Wilson went to New York to take part in a memorial for the American sailors killed at Veracruz. Past huge silent crowds, his carriage followed the slow procession of horse-drawn caissons up Broadway from the Battery to City Hall, and then across the Manhattan Bridge to the parade ground of the Brooklyn Navy Yard. Speaking there, he rambled slightly as he attempted to define not only the justification for the action at Veracruz but also the precepts of his nascent foreign policy.

Wilson remained conflicted. Just three weeks earlier, he had told Congress, "The people of Mexico are entitled to settle their own domestic affairs in their own way"; then he resorted to embargoes, invasion, and occupation of Veracruz—punishing Mexico's misbehavior. On this occasion, after a few paragraphs extolling the selfless duty and service of the fallen nineteen, he reached the undefined core of his remarks: "We have gone down to Mexico to serve mankind if we can find out the way. We do not want to fight the Mexicans. We want to serve the Mexicans if we can, because we know how we would like to be free, and . . . a war of service is a thing in which it is a proud thing to die." He would later admit that he could not dismiss the thought of the young men killed in Mexico. "It was right to send them there," he said, "but that does not mitigate the sorrow for their deaths—and *I* am responsible for their being there."

Other news contributed to Wilson's distress that day. The Secret Service had just foiled a plot against his life, and new threats appeared. Officials urged him to review the parade from a stand, which offered some protection. Mayor John P. Mitchel concurred, saying, "The country cannot afford to have its President killed." More important, Wilson replied, "the country cannot afford to have a coward for President."

Just when the Mexican crisis weighed heaviest on Wilson, three men from South America arrived to ease the burden. Ambassadors from Argentina, Brazil, and Chile—the A. B. C. Powers—offered to mediate a settlement between Mexico and the United States. Both parties eagerly accepted, though Wilson made it clear his interest was not in resolving the incident at Tampico but in the "settlement by general pacification of Mexico." Ridding Mexico of its dictator, of course, had been the subtext of Wilson's actions all along, but he hoped this entire matter might establish a policy the United States could pursue going forward. At a time when American mining interests, English oil interests, German commercial interests, and French banking interests were all exploiting Mexico, Wilson told a journalist that he wanted the United States to be more than a good neighbor. The "business, prosperity, and contentment of Mexico mean more, much more, to us than merely an enlarged field for our commerce and enterprise." House's metaphor for the President's foreign policy cheered him: "If a man's house was on fire he should be glad to have his neighbors come in and help put it out, provided they did not take his property, and it should be the same with nations."

William Jennings Bryan had already done a lot of the spadework for America's new foreign policy. As of mid-1914, more than thirty nations—representing four-fifths of the world's population, including most of Europe except Germany—had signed his treaties. These accords provided for the submission of international disputes to a permanent tribunal and the agreement that there would be no hostilities for a year, during which time complaints would be investigated. The notion reminded Wilson of a rule a headmaster at a Southern school had imposed under which any student with a grievance might fight another provided he came first to the headmaster and agreed to fight under his supervision according to the Queensberry rules; it stopped fighting on campus altogether. Wilson decided to put America's new code of ethics to the test.

In 1901, Secretary of State John Hay and British Ambassador Sir Julian Pauncefote had signed an agreement permitting the United States to construct and maintain a canal in Central America; Article III of the Hay-Pauncefote Treaty dictated that the Panama Canal "shall be free and open" to vessels "of all Nations . . . on terms of entire equality." Furthermore, it stipulated, "such conditions and charges of traffic shall be just and equitable." During Taft's last year in office, as the great pathway approached

completion, Congress passed an act exempting U.S. vessels engaged in noninternational trade from paying tolls. After all, the lawmakers reasoned, the United States had underwritten the canal's construction, and this exemption applied only to American ships going from coast to coast, not competing against the ships of other nations conducting international commerce. Most Republicans—especially the vocal ex-President Roosevelt—considered the exemption an entitlement; even Democrats endorsed it. Great Britain believed the exemption violated the spirit, if not the letter, of the Treaty.

So did Wilson. The exemption had been on his mind from the start of his term, but he felt he needed a few important legislative notches on his belt before he could persuade even his own party members to defy public sentiment as well as basic accounting. On March 5, 1914, the President returned to Congress with his briefest message ever, urging the repeal of the exemption provision of the Panama Canal Act. He asked the legislators to think beyond themselves. "We ought to reverse our action," he said, ". . . and so once more deserve our reputation for generosity and the redemption of every obligation without quibble or hesitation."

Wilson's position was sound, not only morally but also politically. "When everything else about this administration is forgotten," the President once told his brother-in-law, "its attitude in the Panama Canal Tolls will be remembered as putting the conduct of nations on the same basis as that which prevails among honorable individuals, where a promise is a promise and is kept regardless of personal advantage." He thought the Hay-Pauncefote Treaty was foolish in many ways; but, he said, "We gave Great Britain our word and that word must be respected by us."

As he did whenever he needed to gather legislative support, Wilson dispatched McAdoo and Burleson—his "wet nurses," he called them behind their backs—to the Senate floor, where they threatened and cajoled. The repeal became law by a vote of 50 to 35 in the Senate, and 247 to 162 in the House. Sir Edward Grey, the British Foreign Secretary, thereafter became a great friend of Colonel House and the United States government. The recently retired British Ambassador James Viscount Bryce told friends he considered Wilson's words and deeds in the Panama matter "the finest, most dignified, most courageous thing done in the United States for many years: perhaps, indeed, since Lincoln's second inaugural." Bryce wrote the President himself that his behavior reminded him of the one British

statesman "in whom the sense of moral obligation always found expression in the simplest and noblest words"—John Bright. Bryce could have heaped no greater praise.

In his annual message to Congress in December 1913, Wilson had spoken of the need to protect the business communities of America by letting the Sherman Anti-Trust Act of 1890 stand unaltered, even with its large gray areas that allowed some leeway for monopolies. Six weeks later, carried by the strong current of his legislative successes, he returned to Congress to sharpen the definitions—if not the teeth—within that law. Rather than create a new political conflict, he approached the task by encouraging cooperation between two traditionally hostile adversaries. "The Government and businessmen are ready to meet each other half way in a common effort to square business methods with both public opinion and the law," he said. Having turned once again to Louis Brandeis for advice, Wilson proposed several means to correct the nation's unfair business practices.

The core of the problem remained the elite club of tycoons who sat on boards of the nation's major banks and railroads, as well as its industrial, commercial, and public service entities. Those who borrowed and those who lent, those who bought and those who sold, were one and the same—a group with the power to stifle competition. And so Wilson recommended a prohibition of "interlockings of the *personnel* of the directorates of great corporations." Such a prohibition, Wilson contended, "will bring new men, new energies, a new spirit of initiative, new blood, into the management of our great business enterprise," thereby enriching the nation's business activities. Second, he hoped to see the Interstate Commerce Commission superintending the financial operations of the nation's railroads; "the prosperity of the railroads and the prosperity of the country are inseparably connected," he said, and without greater oversight, the interests of the transportation systems were subordinated to their financiers.

Wilson also believed there were enough ambiguities in existing laws to discourage America's entrepreneurs. "Nothing hampers business like uncertainty," Wilson said; and nothing daunted business more than "the risk of falling under the condemnation of the law before it can make sure just what the law is." He believed there should be an interstate trade commission—not another watchdog agency but a bureau that would serve

"only as an indispensable instrument of information and publicity, as a clearinghouse for the facts by which both the public mind and the managers of great business undertakings should be guided." As he had asserted when he had run for Governor of New Jersey, Wilson did not believe there were bad corporations, only individuals who did bad things under the corporate guise. "It should be one of the main objects of our legislation to divest such persons of their corporate cloak and deal with them as with those who do not represent their corporation," he said, "but merely by deliberate intention break the law." In other words, malfeasants should be held individually responsible, "and the punishment should fall upon them, not upon the business organization of which they make illegal use." Wilson listed other injustices, insisting that "conscientious businessmen the country over" would be unsatisfied until they had rewritten the "constitution of peace, the peace that is honor and freedom and prosperity."

Congressman Henry D. Clayton of Alabama, who headed the House Judiciary Committee, sponsored a comprehensive anti-trust bill that would bear his name and which contained most of the remedies Wilson had requested and included language that protected labor organizations from being considered illegal combinations themselves in restraint of trade. It passed in both houses with overwhelming majorities. With the cooperation of Senator Francis G. Newlands of Nevada and Commerce Secretary William C. Redfield, Congress also created the Federal Trade Commission just as the nation was entering a period of vast international commerce. The Commission, said Agriculture Secretary Houston, would "give legitimate and honest business advice and guidance and protect it from the unfair competition and practices of dishonest enterprises."

Meanwhile, Wilson did not neglect rural America. Houston estimated that little more than half the country's arable land was under cultivation, and of that, but an eighth was yielding its potential. From the start, the Administration set several programs into motion to stimulate the agricultural economy. More innovative were the plans to unite the scientific and agricultural communities. Houston created an Office of Information to disseminate in readable English the latest discoveries in soil improvement, plant and animal breeding, and the eradication of farm diseases. And then two Southerners—Senator Hoke Smith of Georgia and Congressman A. F. Lever of South Carolina—sponsored a bill that yoked land-grant colleges

across the country to farms that would put the latest agricultural methods into practice.

The Smith-Lever Act also promoted greater cooperation between federal and state governments. It hitched most of the nation's three thousand rural counties together to make the United States the world's most productive supplier of food. In 1913, Secretary Houston observed, the rural roads between Richmond, Virginia, and Washington, D.C., were too muddy to allow an automobile to make the journey. Soon the Federal Aid Road Act was put in motion so that the federal and state governments could work together to create highways, linking the modernizing nation's backcountry with its metropolises.

After just a few of Wilson's legislative triumphs, the *New York Evening Post* had asserted that he had "more powerfully shaped more important legislation than any Executive of our time." Wilson maintained his mantra of "cooperation" well into the spring of 1914, transcending the usual political bickering so often that he had produced the greatest spate of legislation the Republic had seen since its founding. Colonel Harvey had recently written that no President, save Lincoln, had been inaugurated with a larger number of perplexing problems before him. And, he added, "no President of the United States has demonstrated greater capacity for true leadership." Reform-minded journalist Ray Stannard Baker wrote in his diary, "The government seems really to have become a popular government. Progress is really being made." The very soul of the District of Columbia seemed revived.

The social event of that season began at six o'clock on May 7, 1914—a Thursday evening—when Eleanor Randolph Wilson married William Gibbs McAdoo in the White House. Largely in deference to Ellen Wilson, whose health remained fragile, the event was as modest as Jessie's wedding had been grand. Beyond McAdoo's fellow Cabinet members and their wives, the attendees were almost entirely old friends and family members. The groom arrived with his six children—half of whom were older than the bride, the youngest of whom served as flower girl. Nell wore a long-trained gown of heavy ivory-colored satin. For the second time in six months, the President walked one of his daughters down the aisle, this time in the Blue Room, which was adorned with lilies and white apple blossoms. The Washington Monument and the blue hills of Virginia stood witness in the background. Once again the Reverend Beach performed the

ceremony. The wedding couple stepped into the Red Room, fragrant with American Beauty roses, and received their guests beneath the Gilbert Stuart portrait of Washington. Refreshments followed in the State Dining Room, where Nell cut the wedding cake with one of the military aides' swords. Woodrow and Ellen—she in a creamy lace dress, wearing amethysts he had given her—stood at the front door, holding hands, as their youngest daughter kissed them goodbye. The newlyweds managed to evade the press as they boarded a train for their two-week honeymoon at Harlakenden.

The difference in age between the bride and groom concerned Wilson, though he believed Mac was a "noble man" who would make Nell happy. But selfishly, the marriage left him despondent. Daughter Margaret would never marry and would always remain his favorite intellectual challenger; he and Jessie would be bound forever by their deep faith. But Nell was her father's "chum," the sprite who could release the boyishness that few got to see. "Ah! How desperately my heart aches that she is gone," he wrote Mary Hulbert three days after the wedding. "She was simply part of me, the only delightful part; and I feel the loneliness more than I dare admit even to myself." Nell was torn as well, though she knew her father was not suffering from "the desolate sense of being only half alive" that overwhelmed him whenever he and her mother were separated.

The contraction of the family circle drew Woodrow and Ellen even closer. For months he had been "dreadfully worried" about the health of his wife of twenty-nine years; but at Nell's wedding, Ellen's brother Stockton asked if he was still apprehensive. "No, not now," he said. "She is coming out of the woods. . . ."

10

ECCLESIASTES

To euery thing there is a season, and a time to euery purpose vnder the heauen.

A time to be borne, and a time to die . . .

A time to weepe, and a time to laugh: a time to mourne, and a time to dance. . . .

A time to loue, and a time to hate: a time of warre, and a time of peace.

—ECCLESIASTES, III:1–8

Five hundred people waited on the steps of Blair Arch that Saturday—June 13, 1914—as the little shuttle train pulled up to the back door of the Princeton campus. Two Secret Service men jumped out, followed by Dr. Grayson, Joseph Tumulty, the newlywed McAdoos, and a beaming Wilson. Wearing a snappy blue jacket, white trousers, white shoes, and a straw boater, he fit right in among his classmates who were there to welcome him. They mingled among hundreds of men of all ages in bright-colored baseball uniforms, sailor suits, and kilts; there was even a cohort in Arab garb leading a camel and another group dressed as buccaneers, with three mules pulling their pirate ship. The merrymakers were all Princeton alumni, indulging in their annual rite of spring—Reunions, the highlight of which would be that afternoon's "P-rade," a procession of all the returning graduates through the campus by class, from oldest to youngest. A class member offered Wilson a

'79 hatband and an automobile ride to the class headquarters in Seventy-nine Hall, his former office building. The President of the United States said he preferred to walk.

Other than an official handshake with university president Hibben, the only special distinction accorded Wilson that day was the unusually raucous "locomotive" cheers when the men of 1879 "P-raded" before the alumni sections of other years. Later, at dinner, he spoke briefly, saying, in an obvious reference to his successor, "I hope never again to be fool enough to make believe that a man is my friend who I know to be my enemy."

Only those closest to the President knew that pressures in his current position had recently induced nightmares, in which—curiously—his old Princeton enemies recurred. "Those terrible days," Colonel House noted in his diary, "have sunk deep into his soul and he will carry their marks to his grave."

Meanwhile, severe problems mounted at the White House. Even as Argentina, Brazil, and Chile were at Niagara Falls mediating the role America should play in the stabilization of Mexico, revolutionary leaders Carranza, Villa, Pablo González, and Álvaro Obregón were terrorizing each other. And the labor movement in America was reeling from a massacre in the Colorado town of Ludlow, where coal miners had been on strike for more than six months. The Colorado National Guard attacked their tent city of 1,200, killing a score of people—including women and children. The United Mine Workers of America—who counted more than half the nation's colliers among its members—tried to organize the strikers in the region by arming them and exhorting them to take action against the owners and their guards. The ensuing violence resulted in the deaths of dozens more. Not until Wilson dispatched federal troops was order restored. The strike would persist through the end of the year, when the UMWA would run out of money; mine owner John D. Rockefeller, Jr., would ultimately offer acceptable reforms, but Ludlow's mines would be abandoned, becoming a silent monument to the bloodiest struggle in American labor history. During all this time, the nation slogged through a recession that had begun under Taft, waiting for Wilson's bold fiscal reforms to jump-start the economy.

Wilson's most distressing problem, however, was his wife, who continued to weaken. "There is nothing at all the matter with her organically," a distraught Woodrow wrote Mary Hulbert. Mindful of the Axson family's

psychological history, he feared the possibility of a nervous breakdown. Characteristically, Ellen kept insisting that Dr. Grayson maintain her husband's regimen of golf, automobile rides, and regular visits to the theater. But for weeks, Woodrow could not help awakening at three o'clock in the morning so that he could sit at Ellen's bedside and monitor her sleep. Nell McAdoo visited daily and observed her father's gait slowing and the lines in his face deepening.

Then, on June 28, 1914, there was a new wrinkle: a teenaged Bosnian Serb shot Archduke Franz Ferdinand in Sarajevo, killing the heir apparent to the Austro-Hungarian Empire. The assassin was a member of a revolutionary group committed to liberating the Slavs from Habsburg rule. Over the next month, his bullet would ricochet around the globe, piquing animosities everywhere. One empire seemed to have been spoiling for just such an international brawl.

After the Franco-Prussian War of 1870–71, dozens of small Germanic states had unified under Chancellor Otto von Bismarck, who spun a web of strategic alliances to assure Germany's domination of Europe without further conquest. Kaiser Wilhelm II, however, had ideas of his own—"to increase this heritage for which one day I shall be called upon to give an account." Every major power was soon poised to tackle age-old enemies.

In July, this bad situation worsened. Diplomatic efforts to avert war came up against unresolved disputes and petulant personalities, especially the crowned heads of Europe. Upon learning from Ambassador Frederic C. Penfield in Vienna of the Archduke's assassination, Wilson sent his shocked condolences to Emperor Franz Joseph. Because the German military felt equipped to take on all its neighbors, a cautious Ambassador James W. Gerard in Berlin wrote Chancellor Theobald von Bethmann Hollweg, asking, "Is there nothing that my country can do . . . towards stopping this dreadful war? I am sure that the President would approve any act of mine looking towards peace." He received no reply.

Upstairs at the White House, Wilson told himself that his wife's strength was returning, until a sudden decline impelled Dr. Grayson to bring in three additional physicians. They concurred that Ellen was suffering from Bright's disease, a fatal inflammation of the kidneys. Dr. Grayson went to the President's office to deliver the dreadful news. Wilson listened in pained silence. "Let's get out of here," he said; and the two men ambled around the South Lawn of the White House, saying little. At last, Wilson

exclaimed, "What am I to do!" In a moment, he answered his own question, saying, "We must be brave for Ellen's sake." He rose and marched directly to her room, where he sat by the side of her bed—as he would in the days that followed, whenever the duties of his office permitted. Discussion of her illness was confined to the second floor of the White House.

At a press conference on July 27, a reporter asked the President to comment on America's plans to maintain peace in Europe. Wilson limited his answer, saying only, "The United States has never attempted to interfere in European affairs." The next day—exactly one month after the Archduke's assassination—Austria declared war on Serbia. Lunching with the McAdoos, Wilson merely said, "It's incredible—incredible." Then he added, "Don't tell your mother anything about it." Nell asked her father if the declaration would implicate the rest of the world. Wilson only stared and then covered his eyes with his hand, saying, "I can think of nothing—nothing, when my dear one is suffering."

Nor could he have done anything. By then a war in Europe was inevitable, with more at stake than vengeance for a slain prince. Because of pre-existing treaties, Russia mobilized in defense of Serbia and called upon France to honor the provisions of their Triple Entente with Great Britain. On August 1, Germany declared war on Russia and, two days later, announced war with France, which meant trampling over Belgium, which was neutral. When Germany did not heed a British warning to withdraw from the tiny nation, Great Britain declared war on Germany. Because of an old alliance with Britain, Japan was forced to declare war on Germany as well. In less than a week, seventeen million men were engaged in a fight among at least eight nations.

On August 4, Woodrow sat at Ellen's bedside as she slept. One of his hands held hers while the other wrote a message to the Emperors of Germany and Austria-Hungary, the President of France, the King of England, and the Czar of Russia offering to "act in the interest of European peace, either now or at any other time that might be thought more suitable." At that moment, one of the doctors told the First Family that Ellen was dying. For the first time in their lives, Wilson's daughters saw their father weep.

By Thursday, August 6, Ellen sensed her demise, and she kept asking about the status of her slum clearance bill on Capitol Hill. At the President's urging, Congress instantly passed the Alley Dwelling Act. Learning of the legislation brought a smile to her face. She felt that her business on

earth was done—except for making one wish, which she expressed privately to Cary Grayson. She drew him near and whispered, "Please take good care of Woodrow, Doctor."

Grayson summoned the family, and Wilson held her hand as their daughters sat vigil with him. At five o'clock that afternoon, Ellen drew her last breath. She was fifty-four. Tenderly, Woodrow folded her hands across her breast and wandered to the window, where he broke down and cried.

"It is pathetic to see the President," Frank Sayre wrote his mother that weekend; "he hardly knows where to turn." Fortunately, the White House was prepared to make all the arrangements on behalf of a traumatized President. A heavy band of black crepe was hung on the bell-knob at the front door of the White House, and the flag above was lowered to half-mast. A funeral was held at two o'clock on Monday the tenth in the East Room, where America's three assassinated Presidents and President Benjamin Harrison's deceased wife had all lain in state. The service could not have been simpler, with as few people beyond family as protocol required— Cabinet members and their wives, Supreme Court Justices, a Senate delegation headed by Vice President Marshall, and a Representative from each of the forty-eight states. After a few words of Scripture and a prayer, Wilson and his family left the room and then the officials took their leave. An hour later, six policemen who had served in the White House bore the coffin from the East Room to the horse-drawn hearse in front of the mansion. The family, staff, and Secret Service followed in motorcars to Union Station, where the cortege boarded a special train to take Ellen home.

They arrived in Rome, Georgia, at 2:30 the next afternoon, the sleepless President having sat by the casket almost the entire journey. Thousands of people flocked to the station to pay their respects. Every store in town closed that day; and all the church bells tolled as the funeral procession wended through the streets. Eight hundred mourners sat inside the First Presbyterian Church, where Ellen had first heard her father preach; thousands more—including schoolgirls dressed in white, each holding a myrtle branch—stood on the road as the procession moved from the service to the Myrtle Hill Cemetery. A light rain turned torrential as the Wilsons and Axsons stood under a tent for the final prayers before Ellen's coffin was lowered into the ground next to her mother and father. While those around him quietly wept, the President made no effort to conceal his grief. His body shook, and he sobbed openly.

. . .

"The days . . . that followed were heartbreaking," recalled Dr. Grayson, committed to honoring Ellen Wilson's deathbed wish. This was no simple task, for he knew his patient's history of prostration when under pressure. As Wilson himself had written Mary Hulbert the day after his wife died, "God has stricken me almost beyond what I can bear."

But not beyond. A few weeks later, the President reported, "In God's gracious arrangement of things I have little time or chance to think about myself." With the destruction of his universe, he found strength in the collapse of the world. And like most Americans, he thanked God for the isolation the Atlantic Ocean provided.

Germany activated a modified version of its two-front Schlieffen Plan—which had been sitting in a drawer for a decade—invading France by overwhelming Belgium and Luxembourg and attacking Russia through East Prussia, while Austria-Hungary attacked Serbia. "My own attitude towards the conflict was . . . simple and clear," one young German volunteer would later write in his book *Mein Kampf.* "I believed that it was not a case of Austria fighting to get satisfaction from Serbia but rather a case of Germany fighting for her own existence. . . . And if this struggle should bring us victory our people will again rank foremost among the great nations. Only then could the German Empire assert itself as the mighty champion of peace." He spoke for millions of his countrymen.

The opening salvos had created the gravest international situation in history. During the five-day Battle of Tannenberg on the Eastern Front, the Russians suffered 30,000 casualties; the three-day Battle of Cer in Serbia resulted in 18,500 Austro-Hungarian victims; and in ten days in August, France endured 150,000 casualties—half the numbers of the year-long Franco-Prussian War. And more than lives were lost. In late August, German troops pulverized the Belgian city of Louvain, for five centuries the intellectual capital of the Low Countries, firebombing its church of St. Pierre, the markets, the university, and its famous library.

The President of the United States had issued a formal proclamation of neutrality on August 4. It forbade any American citizen from accepting and exercising a commission in service of any of the belligerents, and it proclaimed that American waters and ports would not provide a haven for any of the belligerents' ships of war. Two weeks later—while acknowledging

hundreds of condolence letters—Wilson reminded the people of the United States that they were "drawn from many nations, and chiefly from the nations now at war." It was, therefore, natural that each American would want to choose sides. But such division within the nation, he cautioned, "might seriously stand in the way of the proper performance of our duty as the one great nation at peace." And then he suggested the seemingly impossible: "We must be impartial in thought as well as in action, must put a curb upon our sentiments as well as upon every transaction that might be construed as a preference of one party to the struggle before another."

Ambassador Page in London adhered to Wilson's policy but could not disguise his own feelings. "A government can be neutral," Page wrote his brother, "but no *man* can be." And Charles W. Eliot, former president of Harvard, confidentially urged Wilson to combine the British Empire, France, Japan, Italy, Russia, and the United States in both "offensive and defensive alliance to rebuke and punish Austria-Hungary and Germany for the outrages they are now committing, by enforcing against those two countries non-intercourse with the rest of the world by land and sea." Even Woodrow Wilson—the man who worshipped Bagehot, Bright, and Wordsworth—was not above personal predilection. While his public statements remained neutral, his private conversation revealed contempt for the German people and their leaders. He said that "German philosophy was essentially selfish and lacking in spirituality." The destruction of Louvain moved him deeply; and he condemned the Kaiser for the rise of militarism. But Wilson sustained his public position, writing Eliot that he favored neither an alliance nor entrance into the war; and, he suggested, public opinion would not support such actions. Even the bellicose Teddy Roosevelt backed the President—for a while. But the Republican leader Henry Cabot Lodge took issue with Wilson from the start, agreeing that American neutrality should be "rigidly honest and fair" but complaining that the demand was "a perfectly unsound as well as utterly impractical position to take."

Sinking into a depression, Wilson tried to maintain the routine of his married life as much as possible. He insisted that his family take advantage of Harlakenden by spending at least the last weeks of summer there, and he would steal as many days in Cornish as he could. But back in the White House, Wilson was wracked by loneliness and guilt. "I sometimes feel that the Presidency has had to be paid for with Ellen's life," he confessed to Dr. Grayson; "that she would be living today if we had continued

in the old simple life at Princeton." Stockton Axson did not disagree, but insisted that "she would rather have died when and where she died than have lived at the cost of any diminution of the career in which her husband realized to the fullest his talents and his powers."

"I never understood before what a broken heart meant, and did for a man," Wilson wrote Mary Hulbert in late August. "It just means that he lives by the compulsion of necessity and duty only." Although he was operating on willpower alone, Wilson accepted Dr. Grayson's recommendation that he spend the occasional morning in bed. When Grayson went in to check his condition one day that month, he found the President lying there, tears streaming down his face. "It was a heart-breaking scene," the doctor later recounted to a friend.

At the end of the month, doctor and patient traveled to Cornish, where Harlakenden exuded none of the mirth of previous visits. Colonel House—recently back from an extended European tour, where he had met mostly with diplomats in London and Berlin, and with the Kaiser as well—joined Wilson for two days. One of House's goals had been to discuss disarmament with the Germans, but he encountered mostly contempt and distrust. German Undersecretary for Foreign Affairs Arthur Zimmermann had claimed that the Kaiser's "strong and sincere efforts to conserve peace" had collapsed because Russia had mobilized, destroying any possibility of an understanding.

Wilson hung on House's every word. For the first time he was considering geopolitics tactically, not historically. This war was already challenging the idealistic hopes he had for the future, as he feared a German victory would force the United States into becoming "a military nation." Whoever won, he predicted the war would "throw the world back three or four centuries" and that the future would hold two superpowers—Russia dominating Europe and part of Asia and the United States dominating the Western world. House agreed but added a third superpower: China, he suggested, would dominate Asia.

The two men discussed every policy under the sun, foreign and domestic—including a new vacancy on the Supreme Court. Upon the death of one of Taft's six appointees, Wilson reflexively appointed his Attorney General, James McReynolds, who still carried trust-busting credentials. An unpredictable malcontent who never blended with the rest of the Cabinet, McReynolds quickly revealed himself to be one of the most

disagreeable Justices in the Court's history, a cantankerous bigot whose prejudices led him to take archconservative positions utterly at odds with Wilson's belief that constitutions "are not mere legal documents: they are the skeleton frame of a living organism." To take his place in the Cabinet, Wilson promoted Thomas W. Gregory, another Southern Presbyterian, an Austin attorney who had served as a special assistant to McReynolds and was part of House's Texas posse. But however the conversations between Wilson and House began, they always ended by remembering Ellen.

Except for the steady presence of Dr. Grayson and cousin Helen Bones, who served as his hostess when Margaret was not in town, Wilson returned from his brief vacation to a big empty house. His spirits steadily declined that autumn, though he maintained a "steady front" for the world. "My loss has made me humble," Wilson wrote Mary Hulbert in September. "I know that there is nothing *for me* in what I am doing. And I hope that that will make me more serviceable." Into October he performed his required duties but little more, descending into deep lassitude on Sundays—sleeping all morning, and dozing during his motor rides around the city in the afternoon. "I want to run away," he wrote his friend Nancy Saunders Toy, an academician's wife in Boston, that November. "All the elasticity has gone out of me," he added in December. "I have not yet learned how to throw off the incubus of my grief and live as I used to live, in thought and spirit, in spite of it. Even books have grown meaningless to me. I read detective stories to forget, as a man would get drunk!"

With Dr. Grayson enforcing a strict physical regimen, the President at least looked healthy. Tan, clear-eyed, and weighing a lean 176 pounds, Wilson dictated letters to Swem in the house after breakfast, received visitors in the Oval Office from ten until one, allowed a few formal visits after lunch, and then changed into his golfing togs for afternoons on the links. He would find himself with but a few minutes to dress for dinner, after which he might permit a few consultations before secluding himself for the solitary state business of reading and writing. Washington felt like a penitentiary to him. "There is no human intercourse in it," he said, "—at any rate for the President."

One night Wilson restlessly jumped the prison wall, traveling by train with Margaret and Dr. Grayson to New York City. They breakfasted with Colonel House in his apartment at 115 East Fifty-third Street. After a round of golf with the Colonel's son-in-law, Gordon Auchincloss, at Piping

Rock Club, Wilson spent the late afternoon alone with House discussing an American relief effort for Belgium. At nine o'clock they walked from House's apartment just east of Park Avenue to Seventh Avenue, and then down Seventh to Broadway. Periodically they would stop, but once discovered they quickened their pace. By the time they had reached Herald Square, a throng had formed in their wake. They dashed into the Thirty-fourth Street door of the old Waldorf-Astoria, went up in the elevator, crossed to the Thirty-third Street side, and continued their quiet walk down Fifth Avenue to Twenty-sixth Street . . . where they boarded a motor bus back to Fifty-third Street. For the first time in a long time, Wilson seemed to breathe more easily; but when they returned to the apartment, House recalled, the President said "he could not help wishing when we were out tonight that someone would kill him."

The President was not suicidal. But House clearly understood him to say "he had himself so disciplined that he knew perfectly well that unless someone killed him, he would go on to the end doing the best he could." Wilson never doubted his faith. "There are people who *believe* only so far as they *understand*," he said, "—that seems to me presumptuous." The power of religion, he insisted, made *his* life "worth living."

Autumn 1914 brought the first test of the nation's faith in Woodrow Wilson's Presidency—the midterm elections. "The successful leader ought not to keep too far in advance of the mass he is seeking to lead, for he will soon lose contact with them," Wilson had once said by way of dismissing TR as a President who had promised Heaven without delivering it. Because Wilson considered the tariff and the currency at the heart of the movement for enduring reform in America, he thought the Democrats could successfully run more on their program than on their promises. When Frank Doremus, chairman of the Democratic Congressional Campaign Committee, invited the President to take an active role in the campaign, Wilson replied that his administration had been "more fruitful in important legislation of permanent usefulness to the country" than any within memory. With the world in crisis, Wilson felt he could not "turn away from his official work even for a little while" in order to campaign.

Nobody knew how the war abroad would affect the economy at home, but there were already early signs that neutrality would not necessarily

protect American commodities. The Governors of the New York Stock Exchange had met just before the war was declared to discuss the possibility of closing the Exchange. Before the meeting, J. P. Morgan himself called Secretary McAdoo for his advice. Whether it was simply a preemptive action to avert a panic or because he did not want to disrupt the establishment of the Federal Reserve System, which was meant to protect banks from such panics, McAdoo recommended shutting down. The Exchange did—for the next four and a half months, the longest closure in the history of the market.

Entering the twentieth month of its recession, the United States confronted a new reality in international commerce: America transported virtually none of the nation's product. Now, with all the major countries of Europe pressing most of their ships into military service, America's stream of maritime commerce dried up. Eight million bales of cotton, to name but one significant export, sat on its wharves and in its warehouses. The excess glutting the market, cotton's price plummeted from 13.5¢ per pound to 6¢, while the cost of shipping what cotton could be stuffed into a cargo ship soared.

The laws of capitalism should have suggested that private enterprise would find a way to profit from the great demand abroad. But, as Treasury Secretary McAdoo observed, "Private initiative becomes extremely timid in times of peril and uncertainty." With a faraway war of indefinite length, American business withdrew from risky investments. McAdoo opposed government ownership of business enterprises—except, he said, "in extraordinary circumstances where the intervention of the government is urgently demanded in the interest of the public welfare."

Lying in bed early one morning, pondering these extraordinary circumstances, McAdoo had an idea. He grabbed a pad and pencil and dashed off a "ship purchase" bill before breakfast—a radical concept of "a shipping corporation of which the American government would own all, or a major part, of the capital stock." Later that day, he presented the idea to Wilson. The President liked it but wanted to sleep on it, as no matter how desperate the need for merchant ships, such a bill was sure to arouse the hostility of every reactionary in the country and the opposition of every powerful business interest. He said they would dismiss the idea as "socialistic."

A short time later, Wilson handed the proposal back to McAdoo and said, "We'll have to fight for it, won't we?" McAdoo said yes. And the

President replied, "Well, then, let's fight." Neither could have predicted the invective of the ensuing partisan battle. "Anyone who did not know the political motives behind our opponent's words would have thought that we had set out deliberately . . . to destroy legitimate commerce, and that our shipping plan was the first step on the road to national ruin." The bill sailed through the House; but the Senate fought against it for almost two years. Much of the resistance came from its fear of Wilson's advancing too far ahead of the public. That September, Congress passed the War Risk Insurance Bill, a measure the Administration backed when the marine insurance companies refused to indemnify against such new perils as mines and torpedoes. That bill seemed just as socialistic but encountered less opposition, McAdoo believed, because businesses calculated that there was no money for them to make in such a venture; it seemed best to allow the government to suffer the loss.

Although the struggle over the ship purchase bill had hardly begun by the time of the midterm elections, the people got the strong sense of the President's passion for it. Republicans used the bill to reunite and challenge the Administration. Even after seven Democratic Senators defected, it appeared that the bill still had enough votes. That prompted the Republicans to resort to one of their most obstructive weapons—the filibuster, the right of one or a series of Senators to hold the floor as long as he could stand and speak. Cots were rolled into the Senate cloakrooms as tag-team speeches—including Ohio's Senator Theodore Burton holding forth for thirteen hours—evolved into the longest continuous session in the history of Congress: fifty-four hours and eleven minutes. It effectively prevented passage of the bill for almost two years, at which point a version of it was voted through. McAdoo reckoned that the Senate delay cost a billion dollars, as the cost of ships rose dramatically while the war persisted. The war risk insurance during that time returned better than a 35 percent profit.

Meanwhile all that cotton sat on the docks as the next crop was being picked. Everybody suspected the war would create a greater need for the bales, though many feared it might be declared contraband, which would reduce further demand. Money in the South—where cotton was the foundation of the financial infrastructure—tightened, threatening an already stressed economy. Once again the Administration stepped in, issuing currency to Southern banks for loans to the farmers, to finance storage of the

new crop and to invest for the following year. Once again, the New Freedom was creating elasticity, allowing supply and demand to find their
equilibrium. Within weeks, cotton had bounced to 8.5¢ per pound; and
Wilson's success at jump-starting a disabled but essential American industry would provide precedent for future Presidents.

The President consulted with J. P. Morgan, Jr., who was concerned that
the war and the restrictions imposed by the New Freedom legislation
would hurt the American economy. The value of securities was his immediate concern; but Morgan, who was powerful enough to bail out whole
countries, was thinking worldwide. The curtailment of international trade,
Morgan suggested, should be "a tremendous opportunity for America, but
the country is not in a position to take advantage of that opportunity if it
does not feel that its own capital invested in its own country is safely and
remuneratively placed." In fact, France had just retained the House of Morgan in hopes of securing $100 million.

J. P. Morgan & Company asked the Department of State if there were
any objections to such a loan. Robert Lansing, an expert in international
law and an adviser to the Department, could offer no legal grounds, but
Secretary Bryan suggested several reasons to oppose the transaction—all
rooted in the President's stated position. "Money is the worst of all contra-
bands because it commands everything else," Bryan wrote Wilson on August 10, 1914. "I know of nothing that would do more to prevent war than
an international agreement that neutral nations would not loan to belligerents." Bryan contended that a loan to France would sanction future loans
to Great Britain or Germany or Russia or Austria, which would tend to
factionalize American citizens. Lending institutions would find themselves exerting pressure on the media to support the governments they
were financing. All that, Bryan announced, was terribly "inconsistent with
the true spirit of neutrality." Wilson agreed, at first.

One of the President's strengths was in remaining as flexible as his nation's currency. Wilson appeared before another joint session of Congress
to urge the raising of $100 million in internal taxes to compensate for the
loss of revenues from customs. When he saw that the nation's railroads
needed financial relief, he expressed as much to the Interstate Commerce
Commission. And two months after Bryan spoke against the Morgan loan
to France, Wilson reversed himself, as the funding involved was not to be
considered loans so much as "credits" for American goods—including

guns as well as grains, machinery, meat, and cotton. The nation emerged from its recession.

Without straying from Ellen's rose garden, Wilson limited his midterm campaigning to a few statements, primarily a long letter to House Majority Leader Oscar Underwood—written for publication. In it the President catalogued the Sixty-third Congress's accomplishments and announced the agenda for the Sixty-fourth. (That included a conservation program protecting natural resources and developing water power, in the name of economy as much as ecology.) Without "a Congress in close sympathy with the administration," Wilson wrote, "a whole scheme of peace and honor and disinterested service to the world of which they have approved cannot be brought to its full realization."

The Republican Party remained divided, its Progressive insurgents still unsettled, while the Democrats were uncharacteristically unified. *The New York Times* credited this "reversal of ancient tradition" to the personality of the President himself, saying, "He has inspired the nation with confidence in him as a leader; he has inspired the world with confidence in him as a statesman; it is not strange that he has inspired his party with confidence in him as its chief." In the weeks before the midterm elections, Wilson even extended his hand to Tammany Hall candidates in New York, a machine boss in Illinois, and the old Smith-Nugent machine in New Jersey, where he still voted. In truth, Wilson admitted to Tumulty after two years in office, he had developed new respect for some of the old party warhorses, even a few of the hacks, who loyally stood by his side "without hitching."

Under the newly ratified Seventeenth Amendment, the midterm elections of 1914 marked the first time the people—not the state legislatures— directly elected its Senators. The vote skewed Democratic, with Wilson's party attracting Progressive voters and picking up four seats. The House of Representatives, on the other hand, revealed a growing desire to slow, if not stop, all the radical changes, and the Democrats lost sixty votes there. They maintained a lead of thirty-four votes, but the results distressed the President. He said it did not seem worthwhile to work as hard as he had in the past two years only "to have it scantily appreciated." Colonel House tried to console the President, reminding him that he was not on the ballot; but Wilson said, "People . . . know that to vote against a democratic ticket is to vote indirectly against me." While the Republicans had found

votes in the industrial Midwest, Tumulty took heart in the Democrats' successfully planting their flag in the West—where he believed the 1916 election would be won. The President himself took to touting that his party, which had been called "sectional," was becoming "unmistakably national." The biggest loser in the election proved to be the Progressive Party, which ran almost 150 candidates for Congress in 1914 and saw only a handful elected. Insurgents from each of the two major parties drifted back to their respective folds.

After that, Wilson sagged into a diagnosable "acute depression"—the thirteenth such "breakdown" in his adult life. He continued to perform his duties, but he slumped with fatigue at the end of each day. Colonel House shuttled from New York to Washington almost weekly and spent several nights at a time at the White House. His companionship proved to be as valuable as his counsel; when the Colonel could not engage the President after dinner with talk of politics, he would ask him to read aloud. Wordsworth or Thomas Gray's "Elegy Written in a Country Church Yard" always revived him. But Wilson's melancholia persisted. He said that Ellen's death had broken his spirit and that he simply "was not fit to be President because he did not think straight any longer, and had no heart in the things he was doing." On November 12, 1914, his nerves were so frayed that he lost his temper for the first time in the White House.

William Monroe Trotter, a Negro activist and a Wilson supporter in the 1912 election, had already presented the President with a national petition signed by African Americans in thirty-eight states protesting the Administration's segregation of the Departments of Treasury and the Post Office. At that time, Wilson had assured the suppliants that he would personally investigate their complaints. A year later, Trotter appeared in the West Wing of the White House with representatives of the National Independence Equal Rights League to inform Wilson that the conditions for the Negro had only worsened. Negroes felt so betrayed that they had just registered their protest to Wilson's policies at the polls. Discovering their strength as a bloc, they voted against every Democratic candidate except those who opposed segregation.

"In the first place," the President said, bridling at Trotter's remarks, "let's leave politics out of it." Wilson insisted this was "a human problem, not a political problem," and that if "the colored people made a mistake in voting for me, they ought to correct it and vote against me if they think

so." As a whole, he said, the American people wished to support the advancement of the Negro race; but Wilson acknowledged that friction still existed and that prejudice in America ran deep. "It takes the world generations to outlive all its prejudices," Wilson said, insisting this was not "a question of intrinsic equality, because we all have human souls." It was a current question of "economic equality—whether the Negro can do the same things with equal efficiency." Once he had proved it, he said, "a lot of things are going to solve themselves."

Trotter had no use for such talk. "Only two years ago you were heralded as perhaps the second Lincoln," he said, "and now the Afro-American leaders who supported you are hounded as false leaders and traitors to the race. What a change segregation has wrought!" Trotter did not stop there. "You said that your 'Colored fellow citizens could depend upon you for everything which would assist in advancing the interest of their race in the United States.'" And then he asked if there was a "new freedom" for white Americans and a "new slavery for your 'Afro-American fellow citizens.'"

That did it. "Your tone, sir," Wilson announced, "offends me." The President said that he had enjoyed the exchange of ideas expressed by this delegation, but Trotter's last personalization had crossed a line. "You are an American citizen, as fully an American citizen as I am, but you are the only American citizen that has ever come into this office who has talked to me with a tone . . . of passion that was evident. Now, I want to say that if this association comes again, it must have another spokesman." Trotter did not back down, insisting he was "from a part of the people" who waited to hear that the President was without prejudice, and then implied that they would defect from the Democratic Party. Trying to dismiss the delegation, Wilson told Trotter, "You have spoiled the whole cause for which you came."

Trotter said he was sorry to hear that, especially—he added, now baiting the President—in an America that professed to be Christian. A fuming Wilson snapped, "I expect those who profess to be Christians to come to me in a Christian spirit." For several more minutes, Trotter held the floor of the Oval Office, expounding upon each of his arguments, insisting that Wilson's policy brought more dangers than advantages. At last, Trotter led his colleagues to the street, where he announced to the press a protest meeting the following Sunday. He intended to take this movement to the churches.

The confrontation galvanized the black community. James Weldon

Johnson—then editing *The New York Age*, the city's oldest African American newspaper—addressed the President in an editorial, saying, "Mr. Wilson, the men who waited upon you did not go to ask any favors; neither did they go . . . to be patted on the head and told to be 'good little niggers and run home.'" No, Johnson said, they were simply citizens asking their "Chief Magistrate" to right a wrong. The President had preached the New Freedom and sent his Army and Navy "in the interest of the landless peons of Mexico," he said, "but not one word has he uttered for fair play to the ten million Negroes in this country." For Johnson, the episode revealed a basic truth about Woodrow Wilson: he "bears the discreditable distinction of being the first President of the United States, since Emancipation, who openly condoned and vindicated prejudice against the Negro."

The white liberal press took Wilson to task as well. Oswald Garrison Villard sent copies of newspaper editorials to the President, lamenting that "an Administration so noble in its feeling for the under-dog . . . cannot do simple justice when it comes to the color line." The *New York Evening Post* suggested that Trotter's "bad manners" aside, the Wilson Administration had drawn a color line where it had not existed. Blacks and whites had worked side by side for half a century, and this administration "went out of its way to create the issue it now deplores."

Wilson regretted the encounter with Trotter, but not for any substantive reason. "Daniels," he later remarked to his Secretary of the Navy, "never raise an incident into an issue. When the negro delegate threatened me, I was damn fool enough to lose my temper and to point them to the door." In retrospect, he believed he should have listened quietly and said he would consider their petition, allowing the matter to pass. "But I lost my temper," Wilson said, "and played the fool." A few months later, Wilson got sucker punched again—but this time from the other side.

In 1914, David Wark Griffith—a former actor from Kentucky who became the predominant filmmaker of his time, transforming motion pictures from a nickel-and-dime novelty into a storytelling art—adapted a bestselling novel called *The Clansman*, by Thomas Dixon, Jr., into a film. Part of a trilogy, the book was inspired by *Uncle Tom's Cabin*. But where Harriet Beecher Stowe's classic novel exposed the evils of slavery, Dixon's rabble-rousing work meant to portray the injustices of Reconstruction. Subtitled *An Historical Romance of the Ku Klux Klan*, it picked the scabs off the nation's Civil War wounds, hoping to incite a reaction to what

he considered a growing acceptance of racial equality. A proud white supremacist—who deplored miscegenation and the government in the postwar Confederacy—Dixon depicted Reconstruction from the losing side, suggesting that Negroes had once happily worked in the cotton fields before the war had freed them to run amok. He preyed upon the reader's sentiments by presenting the most blatant racial stereotypes: one character—a former slave—lusts after an innocent white girl; when she plummets to her death from a cliff, to evade his touch, the righteous Klan gallops forth to mete out the ultimate justice, a lynching.

The result was an epic film—the most expensive ($112,000) and the longest (190 minutes) that had ever been produced. Rich in detail and wondrous in scope, *The Clansman* reenacted visceral battle sequences, sentimental love scenes, and even the assassination of Abraham Lincoln. (White actors in blackface assumed the important Negro roles.) Less than a week before its premiere, Dixon arranged a meeting at the White House with the President, his friend and colleague from Johns Hopkins—whose early writings were quoted in the movie's title cards.

A born self-promoter, Dixon could think of no better means of publicizing his work than a Presidential endorsement. He appealed to Wilson, as one historian to another, describing how the camera could record and disseminate history. "Of course," Dixon later wrote Tumulty, "I didn't dare allow the President to know the *real big purpose back of my film—which was to revolutionize Northern sentiments by a presentation of history that would transform every man in my audience into a good Democrat!*" What he did tell the President was "that I would show him the birth of a new art—the launching of the mightiest engine for moulding public opinion in the history of the world." Wilson was still in mourning and said he could not attend a theater, but he was not averse to a small unpublicized viewing.

On February 8, 1915, *The Clansman* premiered at Clune's Auditorium in Los Angeles and became an overnight sensation. Nobody in the new industry had ever witnessed such spectacular storytelling. The Los Angeles chapter of the NAACP sought an injunction against exhibiting the film, claiming it was a threat to public safety because of the violence it would incite. The show went on, but word about the incendiary nature of the film spread. Then, on February 18, Wilson and his daughters and his Cabinet gathered in the East Room for the first running of a motion picture in the White House.

"It is like writing history with lightning. And my only regret is that it is all so terribly true," Woodrow Wilson purportedly said when the lights came up. In fact, Wilson almost certainly never said it. The encomium does not even appear in the unpublished memoirs of the self-serving Thomas Dixon. The only firsthand record of Wilson's feelings about the film appear in a letter three years later, in which he wrote, "I have always felt that this was a very unfortunate production and I wish most sincerely that its production might be avoided, particularly in communities where there are so many colored people." There is no record of his sentiments beyond that, though he surely would have been troubled by the political implications of publicly supporting a movie mired in controversy. Another member of the audience that night reported that the President seemed lost in thought during the film and exited the East Room upon its completion without saying a word to anybody.

The first sentence of the famous "review" definitely captures the voice of a lyrical historian; the second, however, sounds more like Chief Justice Edward White, whom Dixon invited to another screening and who admitted to having shouldered a rifle as a Klansman in New Orleans. Whether the remark was a conflation of the two men's thoughts or a complete fabrication, the comment did not appear in print for more than two decades. In any case, word of a White House screening circulated, and that was tantamount to a Presidential endorsement. By the time the film opened in New York City on March 3, Dixon had urged Griffith to drop the title in favor of the subtitle—*The Birth of a Nation*. Not only did it carry more weight, but it also took the klieg lights off the worst of the controversy.

Before the New York premiere, the NAACP appealed to the courts and the National Board of Censorship to block the film. Its racism disturbed some of the liberal members of the board, but art trumped politics; and the courts followed suit, taking no action. The NAACP picketed the Liberty Theatre, but the protesters went virtually unnoticed by the people in the endless queues. Small riots and protests broke out in Northern cities; William Monroe Trotter led a protest rally in Boston's Faneuil Hall. City councils, editorial pages, and cocktail party guests debated the right to screen the film wherever it played. A former Massachusetts Congressman sought confirmation that the President had viewed the film and had voiced no objection. Wilson turned the controversy over to Tumulty, instructing him to write that the President had seen the film but "was entirely

unaware of the character of the play before it was presented and has at no time expressed his approbation of it. Its exhibition at the White House was a courtesy extended to an old acquaintance."

The Birth of a Nation became a national phenomenon. In less than a year, almost a million people saw it at the Liberty Theatre alone. But the stink of racism clung to the movie, and intensified as time rendered society more tolerant. In parts of the South, however, it played like a recruiting film, sparking a revival of the moribund Ku Klux Klan, which now added Catholics, Jews, and immigrants to its list of enemies.

"It seems, indeed," Wilson wrote Mary Hulbert the Sunday before Thanksgiving 1914, "as if my *individual* life . . . consisted only of news upon which action must be taken."

Within a matter of weeks, a man whose worldview hardly extended beyond England's Lake District faced issues on virtually every continent. The Senate was delaying a treaty Bryan had signed with Nicaragua to stabilize the government. Politics forced the President to refuse to grant financial assistance to a desperate Liberia. Exiled in Tokyo, Sun Yat-sen appealed to Wilson to prevent J. P. Morgan & Company from making a loan to Yüan Shih-k'ai, the despotic self-proclaimed Emperor of China. From England, Ambassador Page wrote of how American commerce was tied to Britain's naval operations and how the Germans had carpeted the North Sea with so many mines that at least one ship a day was blown up. Page further declared that he could no longer personally finance his required entertaining in the Embassy. Luckily, one letter from Wilson to Cleveland Dodge elicited the necessary $25,000 to keep him as Ambassador; the money was quietly transferred through Colonel House and Page's son.

On December 1, the conscientious Secretary Bryan presented a memorandum urging American mediation in Europe. It was early enough in the conflict that Bryan felt "these Christian nations" might get past the pride that started the war and kept it from ending. Now, "when all must confess failure to accomplish what they expected," Bryan said, ". . . when new horrors are being added daily, it would seem to be this nation's duty, as the leading exponent of Christianity and as the foremost advocate of worldwide peace," to bring everybody to the table. For all its good intentions, Bryan's memorandum made the President wonder if his Secretary of State was suited to his current office. Foreign policy was no longer a simple

matter of signing treaties. It required a more sophisticated view of a world in which every country had become enmeshed with every other and whose political workings had become Byzantine. When Wilson asked Bryan to compose a note to the English government protesting their detention of American ships bound for neutral ports, the President found the draft undiplomatic and unliterary. Wilson rewrote much of it, hoping Bryan would improve upon it further. Three days later he found that Bryan had not changed it at all. The President increasingly turned to Colonel House—whose intellect he respected and whose intuition he trusted. Above all, House enjoyed the diplomatic arts—for which Wilson had limited patience.

Based on his own private conferences, House felt Bryan's plan showed little understanding of the world. House said that the Allies would consider mediation "an unfriendly act" at that moment, that the United States should not be talking peace with Germany until she had reason to change her aggressive military policy, that even though Austria-Hungary had privately indicated a willingness to negotiate, Germany had already declined to do so. The President believed that House could "do more to initiate peace unofficially than anyone could do in an official capacity."

And yet, Wilson did not dismiss Bryan's memorandum out of hand. Its general concepts reinforced his own evolving thoughts, especially the notion of arriving at some enduring international concord without any nation having to achieve victory. For all his lack of experience, Wilson was hardly blind to America's potential role in the world. As early as the second week of August 1914, he had told Stockton Axson that he feared Germany's maritime policies would jeopardize American neutrality.

Wilson began to sketch his own permanent structure for peace. He believed the days of seizing land to build empires had past; great powers had long exploited small states, but even those nations were entitled to democratic ideas and equal opportunities. Private manufacturers of armaments should not be allowed to urge war, for they stood to profit. The world had become a single neighborhood of nations, wherein it would never again be possible for any country to regard a quarrel between two nations as a private quarrel, and "an attack in any quarter was an attack on the equilibrium of the world." Wilson then articulated what he believed were four fundamental principles: there "must never again be a foot of ground acquired by conquest"; it "must be recognized in fact that the

small nations are on an equality of rights with the great nations"; ammunition "must be manufactured by governments and not by private individuals"; and there "must be some sort of an association of nations wherein all shall guarantee the territorial integrity of each." Others had considered some of these elements in the past; but nobody had drawn such a bold blueprint.

The holidays proved to be a time to grieve and a time to rejoice. Wilson traveled to Williamstown, Massachusetts, for Thanksgiving with the Sayres, and the family reunited at the White House for Christmas. Wilson's profound loneliness pervaded both occasions. When his friend Nancy Saunders Toy visited in early January, she found the President's sadness at the dining table as palpable as ever. Jessie, eight months pregnant, remained in Washington, while Frank returned to Massachusetts—only to be summoned weeks later, on the seventeenth of January. By the time he arrived, his son had been born—the President's first grandchild and the first baby born in the White House since Grover Cleveland's daughter twenty-one years prior. Wilson was elated but also, as he wrote Mary Hulbert, full of pity "that the sweet, sweet mother could not have been here to share her daughter's joy!" Wilson would not consent to the seven-pound, twelve-ounce boy being named for him; and so, his parents chose Francis Bowes Sayre, Jr., instead.

On December 8, 1914, Wilson appeared before Congress to deliver his Annual Message, the primary topic of which was national defense. To recent outcries that America was not "prepared for war," Wilson granted that the United States was not ready to put a trained military force into the field. What was more, that was how he intended to keep things. "We are at peace with all the world," he said with pride. Toward maintaining that position, he assured the nation, "We never have had, and while we retain our present principles and ideals we never shall have, a large standing army." Wilson hoped to hold America to its tradition of relying upon volunteer soldiers. He supported strengthening the National Guard but also feared the maintenance of a large military machine would only encourage its use.

In January 1915, Wilson began venturing from home, delivering the annual Jackson Day speech at Tomlinson Hall in Indianapolis. Much of his speech was partisan horseplay—calling the Republican Party nothing more than "a refuge for those who . . . want to consult their grandfathers about everything." But he also reiterated his message of neutrality.

Standing before a crowd in Middle America reminded Wilson of an often forgotten truism. The United States is actually an electorate composed of a majority of independent voters sandwiched between two minority parties. "You have got us in the palm of your hand," Wilson told that silent majority. "I do not happen to be one of your number, but I recognize your supremacy because I read the election returns." Wilson believed the way to attract that voter was not by bowing to him but by standing up taller for his beliefs—for he felt his party offered not only "good society" but also "great emotions." Wilson himself admitted to Mary Hulbert that the trip got him out of his rut and that it was "good to get my blood moving in a speech again."

Wilson saw the war in Europe as an opportunity to expand the crusade he had begun in Mexico—liberating "people everywhere from the aggressions of autocratic forces." At a time when TR was attacking him for not assuming a more aggressive posture in the matters of Mexico and Belgium—accusing him of "poltroonery"—the President sent Colonel House back to Europe "to ascertain what our opportunities as neutrals and as disinterested friends of the nations at war are in detail with respect to the assistance that we can render, and how those opportunities can best be made use of." House met with Secretary Bryan to tell him of his mission. "He was distinctly disappointed when he heard I was to go to Europe as the peace emissary," House noted in his journal. "He said he had planned to do this himself."

In a goodbye letter, the President said he hoped the mission might "prove the means of opening a way to peace." He had no delusions regarding its success, and he was unambiguous in defining House's role: "You are to act only as my private friend and spokesman, without official standing or authority. . . . Your conferences will not represent the effort of any government to urge action upon another government." Although Colonel House had never accepted a dime from either a state or the national government for any of his political work, the nature of this trip suggested extraordinary demands at a price beyond his means, and he agreed to a travel and social allowance of $4,000. "Of course you know," the President wired, "my heart goes with you."

On January 30, 1915, Colonel and Mrs. House boarded the largest, fastest, and poshest ship afloat—the Cunard Line's RMS *Lusitania*. The voyage launched a new phase in American foreign policy, that of an unofficial

American diplomat operating with carte blanche. Then, on February 4, while House was still at sea, Germany declared the waters surrounding the British Isles a war zone and warned civilian travelers that they crossed the ocean on belligerent nations' passenger ships at their own risk. The next day, as the *Lusitania* approached the Irish coast, the captain raised the flag of the United States, feigning neutrality.

Upon his arrival in London, House was granted an hour-long audience at Buckingham Palace with King George V, whose contempt for his first cousin the Kaiser prevented any talk of peacemaking. Meetings with British diplomats ensued, including numerous conversations with Sir Edward Grey, an Oxford-educated Liberal Member of Parliament and longtime Foreign Secretary. After a month, House crossed the Channel to France—passing a floating mine along the way—and then proceeded to Berlin, where he met Undersecretary Arthur Zimmermann. All parties showed indifference toward settling the war.

Only months earlier, Ambassador Morgenthau in Constantinople had written that the Ambassadors of England, Russia, and Germany all looked to Wilson to step in as "Peacemaker," that they recognized the folly of this war. But now, each nation was convinced it was winning. Britain's and France's lists of contraband deeply troubled the United States. Britain further declared the North Sea a war zone and began taking into custody ships trading with Germany. This blockade—even of necessities from neutral nations—spurred Germany to expand the war zone to include all waters surrounding the British Isles and to declare that all enemy merchant ships in those waters would be destroyed. On February 10, Bryan notified Germany that he expected assurances that American citizens and vessels would not be in danger even if their ships traversed the war zone; and he said the United States government would hold Germany accountable for inflicting damage upon American citizens or vessels. The British government was warned against deceptive use of the American flag.

In January 1915, Germans destroyed the *William P. Frye*, an American ship transporting wheat from Seattle to England; in March, they torpedoed the British ship *Falaba*, taking the life of an American passenger; in April a German airplane attacked the American steamship *Cushing*; and on May 1, a German submarine torpedoed the American tanker *Gulflight*. Wilson wanted to call the German government to account for its repeated attacks. Bryan felt the President should warn the American people before

taking on the Germans, saying that while under international law Americans had a technical right to go where they pleased, there was "a moral duty which they owe to their government to keep out of danger . . . and thereby relieve their government from responsibility for their safety." It was not difficult to depict the Germans as the devils in this struggle, but the British were no angels. Germans wondered why there was so much outrage over the loss of a few innocent American lives when a blockade was starving an entire nation.

"I go to bed every night absolutely exhausted, trying not to think about anything," Wilson wrote Mary Hulbert. He found time to maintain his few correspondences with his women friends; but the President had to resign himself to the fact that there was little hope for a widower of his age to have another stab at romance, especially while he was incarcerated in the White House. There was "a void in his heart," Dr. Grayson recalled. He knew that "however bravely he smiled upon the world he was lonely." As Wilson himself put it in a letter to his daughter Jessie at the end of winter, "My heart has somehow been stricken dumb."

In the spring, Cary Grayson fell in love, and he hoped his feelings might be contagious. He had become smitten with a beautiful young heiress in Washington named Alice Gertrude Gordon, whose friends called her Altrude. Before his death, Altrude's father—a wealthy mining engineer—had prevailed upon a longtime friend, Edith Galt, to "look out for" his motherless teenaged daughter. Mrs. Galt knew her only slightly; but, recently widowed, she agreed to serve as an unofficial guardian. A five-month trip to Europe together bonded the two lonely women; and, as it happened, Mrs. Galt was also friendly with Cary Grayson. One day, while he and the President were motoring through town, they passed her on the street and Grayson bowed in salutation. "Who," the President asked, "is that beautiful woman?"

The question startled Grayson, for it was one of the President's few spontaneous comments in months and his first romantic flutter since Ellen's death. He wondered how he might arrange a meeting. He called upon Mrs. Galt and cleverly asked for her help in dealing with a sick friend—Helen Bones. The President's sometime hostess and longtime houseguest was just then recovering from a serious illness, he said; and, with the

White House still devoid of any social life, Helen Bones desperately needed companionship and exercise. "My dear Doctor," Mrs. Galt said by way of refusing, "as you know I am not a society person. I have never had any contracts with official Washington, and don't desire any. I am, therefore, the last person in the world able to help you."

Trying another approach, Dr. Grayson telephoned Mrs. Galt one morning, asking if he might call upon her. He arrived in a White House car, along with Nell McAdoo and Helen Bones. As it was a beautiful day, Mrs. Galt agreed to join them for a drive. The women delighted in each other's company and arranged to see each other again; and they quickly became friends, exactly as Grayson had hoped. Mrs. Galt—famously the first woman in Washington to drive her own automobile—would take Helen in her electric car out to Rock Creek Park, where they walked along the bridle paths before returning to her house for tea.

She was born Edith Bolling on October 15, 1872, in Wytheville, Virginia—150 miles southwest of Staunton—the seventh of eleven children of William Holcombe Bolling and the former Sallie White. Her ancestors were among the first families of Virginia—predating them, in fact, as she was a direct descendant of the Indian princess Pocahontas. The Bollings lived on a plantation in eastern Virginia until the Civil War destroyed their life of "slaves and abundance." A graduate of the University of Virginia Law School, William Bolling moved to Wytheville, where he established a practice and became a Circuit Court Judge.

His big brick house in the center of town was filled with several generations of the family, plus an old freed slave who had insisted on remaining with them. With so many mouths to feed, they lived modestly. Edith was thirteen before she got past the town limits of Wytheville; and she spent most of her time tending to her father's mother, a sharp-tongued semi-invalid who seldom left the house, her condition the result of a riding accident in her youth. Always dressed in black, Grandmother Bolling taught Edith how to read and write, and then she added French, Bible studies, and all the needle arts. Although tough-skinned, Edith was tender toward those in need. She adored her father, who read the great books aloud at night and the Good Book on Sundays as the lay reader at the Episcopalian Church.

Edith received a boarding school education for a few years, until the limited family funds had to be spent on her younger brothers. By that

time, she had shot up to her adult height, a striking five feet nine inches. While hardly well educated, she was a capable young woman—exuberant and domestic. She developed a shapely figure and carried herself with regal bearing.

Edith's oldest sister, Gertrude, had married a man named Alexander Hunter Galt and moved with him to Washington. The winter after her schooling ended, Edith stayed with them for four months and was introduced to a world of culture. Returning one night from a concert to the house on G Street, she found the Galts dining with Alexander's cousin Norman. A decade older than Edith, the lonely bachelor lived with his father in a gloomy brownstone and worked in the family business—"Galt & Bro., Jewellers," established in 1801, the city's leading emporium for silver, timepieces, and fine stationery. Edith Bolling made an immediate impression upon him.

Norman sent her flowers and candy, visited her in Wytheville, and was often at his cousin's house when Edith returned to Washington the following winter. He became so much a part of the family that it never crossed her mind that he would want to marry, especially as she luxuriated in her independence. But at twenty-four, with no plans for a career, she accepted his proposal.

It was a union without passion, but not unhappy. Edith moved into her father-in-law's house until she and Norman could afford a small place of their own. Within a few years, Norman's father, brother, and brother-in-law died, as did Edith's father. In 1903, at age thirty, she gave birth to a son, but complications quickly developed: she would not be able to conceive again; and the infant died after three days. Edith and Norman drifted apart. He became the sole owner of the family business, providing positions for Edith's brothers. Yearning for gaiety, she traveled to New York, attended theater, and shopped for fashionable clothes. In 1908, two years after the couple moved into a larger house at 1308 Twentieth Street NW just off Dupont Circle, Norman died.

"I was left with an active business either to maintain or to liquidate, upon which all my income was dependent," Edith later recounted. She had no business experience, and the estate still owed money to the Galt relatives Norman had bought out. Edith felt further indebted to the employees who had served the firm for decades and to her own three brothers who worked there, supporting their mother and unmarried sister. Edith, at

age thirty-five, decided to run the company. She drew the smallest possible salary for herself until her debts were paid. Afterward, she could indulge in an annual grand tour of Europe but always returned to an empty house. By forty, she was settling into a comfortable but lonely widowhood.

Edith had both the time and inclination to enjoy her new friendship with Helen Bones. She delighted in hearing stories about Helen's cousin Woodrow, because they contrasted so sharply with his public image. Edith had previously considered the President "a human machine, devoid of emotion." Now she felt only sympathy for the "lonely man . . . uncomplainingly bearing the burden of a great sorrow and keeping his eye single to the responsibilities of a great task."

One afternoon in March 1915, instead of riding in Edith's electric car, Helen insisted on changing their routine by having a White House limousine take them to the park. After a long walk along muddy paths, Edith suggested returning to her house, where she would have Helen's boots cleaned. "We are not going to your house," Helen said. "I have ordered tea at the White House this afternoon, and you are to go back with me." Edith insisted she could not for fear of being seen with such muddy shoes; but Helen explained that there was nobody home. Cousin Woodrow was playing golf with Dr. Grayson, and they could take the White House elevator directly to the private quarters. "Cousin Woodrow asked me the other day why I never brought my friends back there," she explained. "He really wishes I would have some one in that lonely old house."

But exiting the elevator, Edith was surprised to see the President and his physician, just returned from golf, their shoes as muddy as those of the women. Helen explained that they were about to have tea, and she invited the gentlemen to join them. After the men had changed and everybody's shoes had been cleaned, they gathered for an hour in the oval sitting room on the second floor, where Edith displayed her vivacity and tart sense of humor. Wilson was struck by his guest, with her wide smile and buxom figure. Dr. Grayson had clearly arranged the "chance encounter." Wilson and Helen invited Edith to remain for dinner, but she chose not to overstay her welcome.

The two women continued their walks together, and Edith redeemed her rain check on Tuesday, March 23. The White House sent a car for her, and they picked up Dr. Grayson along the way. Grayson left dinner early

to make a house call at the McAdoos', leaving the President alone to entertain Helen and Edith. He charmed them with stories and, upon Helen's request, the reading of several poems. Edith reported to her sister-in-law that night that as a reader, "he is unequalled."

Two weeks later, Helen invited Edith for a drive. The big White House open touring car picked her up, and returned to get Helen, only to find the President ready to join them as well. He sat up front with the chauffeur, while the Secret Service agent took a seat in the back with Helen and Edith. Wilson and Helen begged Edith to dine with them, explaining that they would otherwise be alone. After dinner, the three of them sat by the fire, where the President felt so much at ease that he shared stories of his youth and of his father. Edith did the same, animatedly talking in her Virginian accent about the heartache of Reconstruction. The whole evening passed quickly for Edith; and she was touched by Wilson's "warm personality" and "boylike simplicity."

The following Wednesday, Wilson invited Edith to join his party at Griffith Stadium, where he tossed out the first ball at the opening game of the baseball season. They got to watch the Washington Senators shut out the New York Yankees, 7 to 0. Edith's walks with Helen continued, and soon Nell and Margaret joined them. With the arrival of warm weather, Woodrow and Edith and Helen took rides in the afternoon and the evenings in the comfortable open-air car. Mrs. Galt became a regular dinner guest at the White House, and the staff began to talk amongst themselves. "She's a looker," the doorkeeper told Colonel Edmund W. Starling, the newest member of the White House Secret Service detail and Wilson's personal bodyguard. "He's a goner," confirmed Arthur Brooks, the President's valet. One evening Edith outshone herself, wearing a smartly tailored black charmeuse dress designed especially for her by Worth, the leading Paris designer, and a pair of gold slippers—all meant to match the corsage of golden roses that had arrived earlier that day with the President's card. The evening ended early only because the President was leaving the next morning for his grandson's baptism in Williamstown.

Wilson returned a few days later, on May 3, and invited Mrs. Galt to dine the next night. Margaret and Helen and Dr. Grayson were there, as were Wilson's sister Annie Howe and her daughter. It was a prematurely warm evening; and after dinner, Wilson suggested having coffee on the South Portico, with its privileged vista of the city. Dr. Grayson left right

after the meal, and suddenly—as if on cue—all the other guests decided
to walk around the South Lawn, leaving Edith alone with the President. In
that moment, he pulled his chair closer to hers. "I asked Margaret and
Helen to give me an opportunity to tell you something tonight that I have
already told them," he said. And then, he declared his love for her.

Without thinking, Edith blurted, "Oh, you can't love me, for you don't
really know me, and it is less than a year since your wife died."

"Yes," he said, "I know you feel that; but, little girl, in this place time
is not measured by weeks, or months, or years, but by deep human experiences; and since her death I have lived a lifetime of loneliness and heartache. I was afraid, knowing you, I would shock you; but I would be less
than a gentleman if I continued to make opportunities to see you without
telling you what I have told my daughters and Helen: that I want you to
be my wife."

Before she could speak again, the President addressed the unique obstacles of his proposal, those even greater than his having known her for
only two months. With a spotlight always directed upon the White House,
he explained, all who enter were observed; and no matter how hard he
worked to protect her, gossip would inevitably begin.

After Woodrow and Edith had talked for more than an hour, she told
him if he required an answer that night, it was no. Never having given
herself wholly to any man—certainly not to one of Wilson's passions—she
had to consider whether she wanted to sacrifice her independence at this
stage of her life. She had to ask herself not just how she felt about Woodrow Wilson but also about becoming a wife again—and a public figure at
that. At ten o'clock, he and Helen escorted Edith home in silence.

Edith could not sleep that night. She sat in the big chair by her window and stared into the darkness, thinking how he had made her "whole
being . . . vibrant!" In the morning hours, she calmed herself by committing her thoughts to paper. Edith considered it "an unspeakable pleasure
and privilege" to share the President's "tense, terrible days of responsibility" but felt inadequate, unable to offer any gift so great. "I am a woman,"
she wrote Woodrow, trying to get used to the very "thought that you have
need of me."

Hours later, Helen arrived for their walk through Rock Creek Park.
She said nothing of the night before until they sat on some stones in the
middle of the woods. "Cousin Woodrow looks really ill this morning," she

said. Then she burst into tears and added, "Just as I thought some happiness was coming into his life! And now you are breaking his heart." Edith tried to explain how unprepared she had been for the suddenness of Woodrow's announcement—that up until then she had not allowed herself to think of him as anything but the President and a delightful new friend. At the same time, she knew she was right in asking for time to sift through her feelings.

She was in a quandary—"more and more torn by the will to love and help him, and yet unconvinced that I could." Edith handed her late-night letter to Helen, who became the lovers' go-between. She nicknamed her cousin "Tiger"—not, as some have suspected, for his animal desires nor even because of his Princeton connection but because Helen found him "so pathetic caged there in the White House . . . that he reminded her of a splendid Bengal tiger she had once seen—never still, moving, restless, resentful of his bars that shut out the larger life God had made him for."

So began the most ardent chase of Wilson's life. His hundreds of letters to the former Ellen Axson had expressed every romantic sentiment he could conjure, but they were callow sentiments alongside the torrent of words that would now engulf Edith—billets-doux employing every manner of entreaty. There was urgency in the Tiger's pursuit, fueled by the gratitude that he had been granted one final stab at love. The same held true for Edith, except she realized that this was her first.

The last twenty-four hours had left Wilson spent, but Edith's letter replenished him. And that night, he shamelessly stripped his emotions bare. "Here stands your friend, a longing man, in the midst of a world's affairs," he wrote, "—a world that knows nothing of the heart he has shown you . . . but which he cannot face with his full strength or with the full zest of keen endeavor unless you come into this heart and take possession."

Meetings and briefings, of course, came between his morning letters and evening dinners with Edith. He learned of a new conflict between China and Japan and once again offered the protection of the Monroe Doctrine to a new President of Haiti. He was even more troubled by Colonel House's informing him that Allied diplomats were suggesting that the President was pro-German, just as England—with more than two million men in its military ranks—expected to get through the Dardanelles and help Russia, which was already running out of munitions. But until Edith

accepted his proposal, Wilson felt as if his world stood still. And then came news that put everything out of mind, not just for America but for most of the world.

On May 7, 1915, the President had just finished lunch and was preparing to play golf when he learned that a submarine had sunk the *Lusitania*. That first bulletin reported no loss of life, but the President canceled his game nonetheless, opting for a drive instead. News dribbled in through the night, giving him time to write Edith, "My happiness absolutely depends upon your giving me your entire love." He feared that she was overthinking the situation, second-guessing what was best for him— "when the only thing that is best for me is your love."

The President was beside himself that night. Possessed, he stepped right past his Secret Service guards and out the front door of the White House onto Pennsylvania Avenue, into a light shower, as though he were headed to Edith's house. Then, instead of veering left toward Dupont Circle, he felt duty pulling him home. By ten o'clock, more details of the day's events were available. It seemed that, without any warning, the German submarine *U-20* had fired two torpedoes into the belly of the *Lusitania*— seven days out of New York and in the Irish Sea. The great liner sank in eighteen minutes, taking 1,198 souls with it—413 crewmembers and 785 passengers, 128 of whom were American citizens.

"The country was horrified, and at that moment the popular feeling was such that if the President, after demanding immediate reparation and apology to be promptly given, had boldly declared that . . . it was our duty to go to war, he would have had behind him the enthusiastic support of the whole American people," recalled Senator Henry Cabot Lodge. Although the sinking of the ship was not a targeted attack on the United States, the *Lusitania* became a battle cry for a growing number of jingoes. Nobody sounded the charge more loudly than Theodore Roosevelt. Even before all the facts were known, he bellowed to the media that the incident was "an act of piracy." He said, "We earn as a nation measureless scorn and contempt if we follow the lead of those who exact peace above righteousness." Roosevelt told his son Archibald, "Every soft creature, every coward and weakling, every man who can't look more than six inches ahead, every man whose god is money, or pleasure, or ease, and every man who has not

got in him both the sterner virtues and the power of seeking after an ideal, is enthusiastically in favor of Wilson."

There was, of course, an opposing view, which Secretary Bryan voiced in the Cabinet Room. He felt Americans had to take responsibility for their actions. One week before the *Lusitania*'s crossing, the Imperial German Embassy in Washington had posted admonitory advertisements in fifty American newspapers in a box beneath the Cunard Line's schedule. It reminded travelers that a state of war existed between Germany and her allies and Great Britain and her allies and that travelers sailing in the war zone on British or Allied ships did so at their own risk.

When Bryan heard the news, he immediately wondered if the ship carried "munitions of war." If she did, he said, "it puts a different phase on the whole matter!" Assistant Secretary Lansing reported that an examination of the clearance papers revealed that there had been ammunition on board. International law permitted ships to carry small quantities of ammunition; but upon learning the actual numbers, Bryan said the 4,200 cases of rifle cartridges and 1,250 cases of shrapnel, along with cases of fuses, shell castings, and high explosives meant the United States should rebuke not only Germany for destroying the *Lusitania* but also England for interference in international shipping, particularly for "using our citizens to protect her ammunition." From London, Colonel House cabled that an "immediate demand should be made upon Germany for assurance that this shall not occur again." More than that, the United States must consider the inevitability of going to war. America, he added, "must determine whether she stands for civilized or uncivilized warfare. Think we can no longer remain neutral spectators. Our action in this crisis will determine the part we will play when peace is made, and how far we may influence the settlement for the lasting good of humanity." Ordinary citizens were even more outspoken. One wired the White House, "In the name of God and humanity, declare war on Germany." To that, Wilson took offense, telling his secretary, Charles Swem, "War isn't declared in the name of God; it is a human affair entirely." *The Washington Post* editorialized that it had faith in the "courage, patience and wisdom of President Wilson," and it waited to see how he intended to "uphold the honor and interests of the United States."

In truth, Wilson was not thinking straight—laboring, as he was, over two, even three love letters a day, some requiring more than one draft as

he felt Edith was coming around at last. "You ask why *you* have been chosen to help me! Ah, dear love," he wrote on May 9, "there *is* a mystery
about it . . . but there is no mistake and there is no doubt!"

On May 10, 1915, Woodrow and Edith saw each other in the afternoon
and professed their mutual love. "The most delightful thing in the world,"
he told her, was "that I am permitted to *love you*." With that, the Chief of
State entrained to Philadelphia, where he addressed fifteen thousand people at Convention Hall—including four thousand recently naturalized
citizens. Speaking from his shorthand outline, he spun some romantic ideals before settling down to the issue of American neutrality in the face of
that week's disaster. "The example of America must be a special example,"
he said, ". . . not merely of peace because it will not fight, but of peace
because peace is the healing and elevating influence of the world, and
strife is not." Full of humanity that evening, he blurted, "There is such a
thing as a man being too proud to fight. There is such a thing as a nation
being so right that it does not need to convince others by force that it is
right."

"Too proud to fight," became the next day's headline and an easy target
for the political opposition. "This was probably the most unfortunate
phrase that he ever coined," said Henry Cabot Lodge, the Republican
leader, who always resented Wilson's rhetorical gifts and who intended to
make political hay out of the comment. With 128 Americans at the bottom of the Irish Sea, it struck many as tone-deaf. "It was not the moment
for fine words or false idealism," said Lodge; and this turning the other
cheek gave Wilson's opponents—especially those disavowing neutrality—
the chance to strike again. "The phrase 'too proud to fight,' uttered at such
a moment, shocked me, as it did many others," Lodge said, "and I never
again recovered confidence in Mr. Wilson's ability to deal with the most
perilous situation which had ever confronted the United States in its relations with the other nations of the earth."

The four-word phrase was, in fact, a re-articulation of his attitude
about American neutrality as a badge of "splendid courage of reserve moral
force." But even Wilson himself admitted he was not sure what he had
said in Philadelphia, since Edith remained foremost in his mind. "If I said
what was worth saying to that great audience last night," he wrote her the
next day, "it must have been because love had complete possession of me."

At a press conference the next morning, the President backpedaled,

insisting he had not been dictating any policy in Philadelphia, merely speaking for himself. The significance of the *Lusitania* was not lost on him. He told Tumulty that he could not bring himself to ponder the details of the tragedy because, if he did, he was afraid that "when I am called upon to act . . . I could not be just to any one." He vowed not to "indulge my own passionate feelings."

"I could go to Congress to-morrow and advocate war with Germany," Wilson said, "and I feel certain that Congress would support me, but what would the country say when war . . . finally came, and we were witnessing all of its horrors and bloody aftermath." He knew that once the people began poring over the casualty lists, they would wonder why Wilson had not tried to settle the matter with Germany peaceably. "When we move against Germany," he said, suggesting that day would come, "we must be certain that the whole country not only moves with us but is willing to go forward to the end with enthusiasm. I know that we shall be condemned for waiting, but in the last analysis I am the trustee of this nation, and the cost of it all must be considered in the reckoning before we go forward." Wilson insisted he was not afraid to fight; but the deaths of 128 Americans who had been warned against sailing on a belligerent's ship into a war zone did not demand a declaration of war. The next day, the President received unexpected support from his predecessor and former rival: William Howard Taft urged Wilson to stick to his guns. He believed it was the duty of every patriotic citizen to resist the "impulse of deep indignation which the circumstances naturally arouse" and not to second-guess the President.

In the quiet of his study, Wilson typed his nation's response to the loss of American lives at German hands. He reminded the Imperial German government that its current policy was infringing upon the "sacred freedom of the seas." He said its delineation of a war zone touched upon the coasts of many neutral nations (which, in fact, was not true, as the Netherlands was the only neutral country in the war zone) and further infringed upon the rights of noncombatants bound on lawful errands. Submarines, Wilson wrote, "cannot be used against merchantmen without an inevitable violation of many sacred principles of justice and humanity." Wilson called upon the German government to disavow its recent unjust acts, to make reparations, and to take immediate steps to prevent the recurrence of further subversion of the principles of warfare. American citizens were

within their rights to travel on the high seas, he insisted, especially as the United States and Germany were bound by "special ties of friendship."

Wilson sent the draft to Bryan for his and Lansing's suggestions—in diction, not direction. Bryan still thought the American government should condemn Allied violations and urge arbitration; Lansing, on the other hand, urged a tougher position. The President followed his instincts and instructed the Secretary of State to transmit his message. Bryan did so, but—he made clear to his boss—"with a heavy heart." Without doubting Wilson's "patriotic purpose," Bryan disagreed with his approach. He believed in "playing the part of a friend to both sides in the role of peace maker," and he feared this note would upset the balance. Bryan did not convey that he felt further compromised by Wilson's increased reliance on Colonel House. Indeed, House was digging back channels, trying to get Britain to lift its embargo if Germany would curb its use of submarines and lethal gases.

At the Cabinet meeting on Tuesday, May 11, the President shared House's latest dispatch from London, which questioned American neutrality. Bryan was hurt that the President had not shared the cable with him before discussing it with the Cabinet as a whole. He became visibly perturbed as the meeting progressed, until he heatedly accused some members of the Cabinet of no longer being neutral. With that, the President turned his steely gaze on the Secretary of State and fixed his jaw. "Mr. Bryan," he said, "you are not warranted in making such an assertion. We all doubtless have our opinions in this matter, but there are none of us who can justly be accused of being unfair." Bryan apologized.

The President and several family members escaped that weekend to the *Mayflower*, which was sailing to New York for the President to review the Atlantic Fleet. "The night was clear and the Potomac River like silver," Edith recalled; and after dinner she and Wilson drifted off alone into the moonlight. He did not speak of romance that night; instead, he leaned on the rail and discussed something she sensed had been troubling him. "I am very much distressed over a letter I had late today from the Secretary of State," he allowed, "saying he cannot go on in the Department as he is a pacifist and cannot follow me in wishing to warn our own country and Germany that we may be forced to take up arms; therefore he feels it is his duty to resign." Edith was no student of politics, but Woodrow was surely testing her instincts. "Good," she said, without a moment of hesitation;

"for I hope you can replace him with someone who . . . would in himself command respect for the office both at home and abroad."

When Wilson said he was thinking of appointing Robert Lansing in his place, she replied, "But he is only a clerk in the State Department, isn't he?" In truth, Lansing was more than that—indeed, a counselor to the Department and a son-in-law of John W. Foster, a former Secretary of State who, Wilson thought, might provide some guidance to the less experienced Lansing. Edith realized she had much to learn if she was to become First Lady; Woodrow realized Edith was full of knee-jerk opinions—all of which would always be what she considered were in his best interests.

At the end of the month, Wilson received a reply from the Germans. They expressed deep regret to the neutral nations that lost lives in the sinking of the *Lusitania* but asked the United States to examine further the details of the event: the *Lusitania* had been constructed with government funds as an auxiliary cruiser in the British navy; and the ship had been transporting ammunition and arms, including guns "which were mounted under decks and masked." In addition, the ship had been known to sail under neutral flags and, in this instance, had been transporting Canadian troops. The German government said it had acted in "just self-defense," that it was protecting the lives of its soldiers by destroying ammunition destined for its enemy. The note suggested that the British had been using Americans as human shields, violating American law, which prohibited the carrying of passengers on ships with explosives on board. Wilson found those paragraphs "wholly unsatisfactory."

But the nation sighed in relief, as the rest of the German note assured the United States of its intentions to renew its instructions to avoid attacking neutral vessels. Wilson and Bryan continued to disagree on the tone with which they should proceed. The President's excruciating headaches returned, but he continued to draft a second note to the Germans. He challenged their assertion that the *Lusitania* was transporting troops and masked guns, and argued that the sinking of a passenger ship involved principles of humanity—"a great steamer, primarily and chiefly a conveyance for passengers . . . was sent to the bottom without so much as a challenge or a warning and that men, women, and children were sent to their death in circumstances unparalleled in modern warfare."

Bryan disapproved. The note omitted any mention of his preference for mediation; there was to be no simultaneous protest sent to England; and it

did not bar Americans from traveling on ships carrying ammunition. Worst of all, Bryan felt it offered Germany "no chance to do anything but refuse to discontinue her submarine warfare." Refusing to sign the document, Bryan preferred to resign from office.

After a few sleepless nights, he met with the President for an hour. "Mr. Wilson would not yield a point, nor would Mr. Bryan," recalled Mrs. Bryan. At last her husband said, "Colonel House has been Secretary of State, not I, and I have never had your full confidence." Wilson could not deny the charge. He accepted the Secretary's resignation that night, though they waited a day to make it public. Strangely, after all his doubts about Bryan, the severance hurt Wilson. "It is always painful to feel that any thinking man of disinterested motive, who has been your comrade and confidant, has turned away from you," Wilson told Edith, ". . . and it is hard to be fair and not think that the motive is something sinister. But . . . I have been deserted before. The wound does not heal, with me, but neither does it cripple." In a touching note of valediction that would be published, Wilson wrote Bryan, "Even now we are not separated in the object we seek but only in the method by which we seek it. . . . We shall continue to work for the same causes even when we do not work in the same way."

"Hurrah! old Bryan is out!" Edith wrote Woodrow the morning of June 9. "I know it is going to be the greatest possible relief to you to be rid of him. Your letter is *much* too nice, and I see why *I* was not allowed to see it before publication." Jubilantly she told him "that at last the world will *know* just what he is." William Jennings Bryan had been, in fact, an earnest and principled public servant, making the most of a position in which he was never fully empowered. But Edith called him "that awful Deserter." Wilson realized he would not have to carry grudges so long as he had Edith by his side. "I will be glad when he expires from an overdose of peace or grape juice," she wrote ten days after Bryan's resignation, "and I never hear of him again." With a loving but objective eye, Woodrow wrote Edith, "You are, oh, so *fit* for a strong man! . . . What a dear partisan you are!" He loved her for that—"and how you can *hate*, too. Whew! . . . In my secret heart (which is never secret from you) . . . he *is* a traitor, though I can say so, as yet, only to you."

The second *Lusitania* note went to Germany signed by Robert Lansing, the interim Secretary, who would soon officially assume the post. The German response, sent through Ambassador Gerard in Berlin, showed a

willingness to cooperate but asked for the same. Foreign Minister Gottlieb von Jagow said submarine warfare was his nation's only chance of breaking the Allies' blockade. While Germany would not consider the mere presence of Americans on a ship enough to spare it, he did promise protection for American vessels and Americans on neutral vessels—so long as they were not transporting contraband. The seas were calm well into the summer.

Then on August 19, 1915, a German U-boat torpedoed the White Star Liner *Arabic* off the coast of Ireland. Submarines carried orders not to sink passenger ships without warning, but the commander of *U-24* said he interpreted the *Arabic's* zigzag route as an indication that it was about to ram his boat. Two Americans died. A stern rebuke from Lansing elicited several demotions within the Kaiser's navy and a renewed pledge from the German government not to attack unarmed liners without warning. Less than three months later, *U-38* torpedoed the Italian passenger liner *Ancona* off the coast of Tunisia, taking two hundred lives, nine Americans among them; but in dealing with Germany, America continued to rely on epistolary diplomacy.

Never had so many parts of the world demanded a President's attention. In Mexico, the Carranza forces appeared strong enough to overpower Zapata and Villa and warrant American recognition, vindicating Wilson's policy of "watchful waiting." But Wilson felt obligated to tell the factional leaders that "if they cannot accommodate their differences and unite for this great purpose within a very short time, this Government will be constrained to decide what means should be employed by the United States in order to help Mexico save herself and serve her people." Cotton remained a political football. Great Britain vacillated on its status as contraband, expecting the right to buy American munitions, but then confiscated shipments of America's great export staple intended for even neutral countries. Secretary Garrison continued discussing a regular Army of 300,000 men at the astronomical cost of $1 billion, though Wilson still believed too strong an Army created the compulsion to unleash it. At the same time, delegations of women petitioned the President to support their right to vote; the NAACP pressured the President to demonstrate sympathy for the Negro's cause; while in the Ottoman Empire, the party of "Young Turks" was now helping massacre Armenians; in Denmark, the government negotiated for the American purchase of its territories in the West Indies; and in America, citizens anxiously anticipated the next submarine attack. And through

it all, the President wrote Edith Galt, "love has set me free from all real distress." Until May 27.

Woodrow and Edith went for a ride after dinner that night for almost two hours. The driver and Helen Bones sat up front, offering the couple privacy in the back. Only they knew what transpired behind the drawn curtains; but their letters to one another the next morning suggest that Woodrow made advances, which an unready Edith rebuffed. "For God's sake try to find out whether you really love me or not," Woodrow wrote in frustration. "You owe it to yourself and you owe it to the great love I have given you. . . . Remember that I need strength and certainty for the daily task and that I cannot walk upon quicksand." Edith wished she could ease his pain. The young widow was not prudish so much as inexperienced, and in insisting that she loved him, she promised to get past her own barriers. "But *you*," she said, "must conquer!"

The President launched a relentless campaign. "You have invited me to make myself the master of your life and heart," he wrote, coaxing her to trust her instincts. "The rest is now as certain as that God made us . . . and *I shall win*, by a power not my own, a power which has never been defeated, against which no doors can be locked, least of all the doors of the heart." He added, "We will take hands now and walk together without fear withersoever our infallible guide may lead us."

At this ticklish moment in their courtship, an unfortunate guest arrived in Washington—Mary Hulbert. On May 31, Helen Bones was dispatched to meet Mary's early morning train; and Mrs. Jaffray gave her a private tour of the White House. The President made time to take a long drive with her—with Helen Bones chaperoning. It turned out that Mary had not come for romance but for money. Her hard-luck son had suffered a streak of bad health, and he needed cash to close a deal on some land in California's San Fernando Valley, where he intended to grow avocados.

For $7,500 the President assumed the mortgages on two properties the Hulberts held in the Bronx. And he supplemented that by recommending Mary's writing to a few publishers. She left the East Coast for several hapless years in Los Angeles, where neither her literary efforts nor the avocados ripened into sustainable careers. Wilson wrote Mary that he would miss her, but bade her farewell with polite "sympathy and hope," closing that chapter of their lives. From then on, she cobbled together a life of shabby gentility—publishing a cookbook, calling upon the friends she

had once stylishly entertained, even picking up work as an extra in motion pictures—one of which, *The Great Love*, was directed by D. W. Griffith.

The day after seeing Mary Hulbert, Woodrow presented Edith with a ring. It was not an engagement ring, for he knew not to force the issue; but he knew enough to keep pressing. "There is no one else in the world for me now," he wrote her on June 1. Edith was accustomed to removing her rings each night, but this one, she said, would remain, as it gave her "the most exquisite pleasure." In addition to his inundation of love letters—which now spoke of "gentle caresses" and "precious kisses"—Woodrow filled Edith's house with roses and orchids. She became a more frequent visitor to the White House, arriving for tea with Helen but stealing moments with Woodrow. She made herself comfortable in Wilson's study among all his books.

In June, Wilson intensified his campaign by arranging a vacation with Edith in Cornish. Helen Bones and Margaret Wilson invited her to be their guest, and the women left by automobile on the first day of summer, stopping in Princeton, where Helen gave Edith a tour of the campus. As they arrived at Harlakenden, Wilson set out from Washington with Dr. Grayson, stopping in Roslyn, New York, to spend the day with Colonel House.

They spoke of international matters for a while, until Wilson leaned in, saying he had "an intimate personal matter" to discuss. "What would you think of my getting married again?" he asked. Wilson explained that he had met "a delightful woman" and was thinking of asking for her hand. "Do you believe I would lessen my influence with the American people by taking such a step? And when do you think I could do it? I have led such a lonely life that I feel it is necessary for me to have companionship of that sort, and my dear dead wife would be the first to approve." Although House did not let on to the President, Dr. Grayson and Attorney General Gregory had both intimated that such rumors had been swirling within the White House.

House himself approved—if only because the President's health demanded it and because he believed "Woodrow Wilson today is the greatest asset the world has." House confessed to his diary, "If he should die or become incapacitated, it is doubtful whether a right solution of the problems involved in this terrible conflict and its aftermath would be possible." But he cautiously urged postponement until the following spring.

House's advice made sense; but once Woodrow and Edith were reunited

in Cornish, all logic went out the window. For the first time, the middle-aged lovers could spend extended periods alone, sometimes even away from the eyes of the Secret Service. "He was like a boy home from school," Edith recalled of those Arcadian days that summer, whenever the President was able to leave Washington. After breakfast they would sit on the terrace together and fish through the pouch of official mail, examining the catch together. When finished, they walked along the banks of the Connecticut River; in the afternoons, they invited the rest of their party to join them on long motor rides through the countryside, after which Dr. Grayson and the family took turns reading aloud from Wilson's *History of the American People*. Edith's favorite time came after a late dinner, when just the two of them sat before a fire in a room where the curtains had been drawn to shut out the cold night air. Together they would read the latest dispatches from around the world. "The President would clarify each problem for me," Edith recalled, "and outline the way he planned to meet it."

"Those days in Cornish had brought the banishment of any doubt of my love for Woodrow Wilson," she later recorded, "but had not overcome my reluctance to marry him while he was in the White House." She was, at heart, a provincial girl unready for a public international life. "I told him if he were defeated for re-election I would marry him, but if not I felt still uncertain." Then on June 29, 1915, she consented, in a note she composed on the West Porch of Harlakenden, while he was close at hand.

Wilson returned to an empty White House on July 19, 1915; and though the walls had been stripped for the summer and the furniture was dressed "in white pajamas," he did not feel lonely. "*You* were not actually here," he wrote Edith, "but your thought and love were here to greet me." For the rest of the summer, he scrawled long letters, sometimes a dozen pages or more, to Edith—interspersing accounts of the day's events with passionate expressions of his preoccupation: "You are everything to me," he wrote the following afternoon.

For the next several months, the President intensified what surely became the most romantic correspondence ever to emanate from the White House—250 letters between them, most of them expressing the desperate fervency of a world leader in crisis. In the middle of the night, precisely one year after Ellen died, he suddenly awakened. He did not know why exactly, but he recounted that in his dream Edith had disappeared and he found

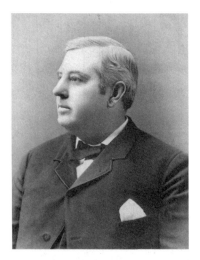

"Sugar Jim"—New Jersey Democratic Party boss James Smith, Jr., who offered Wilson the opportunity to run for Governor, expecting the academician to serve as his puppet. Instead, Wilson promptly dismantled the party machine.

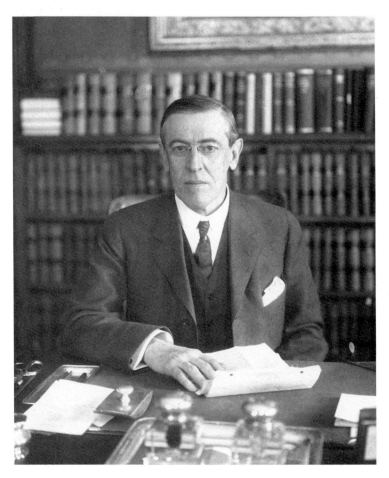

Governor Wilson in his office in the New Jersey State House in Trenton, 1911.

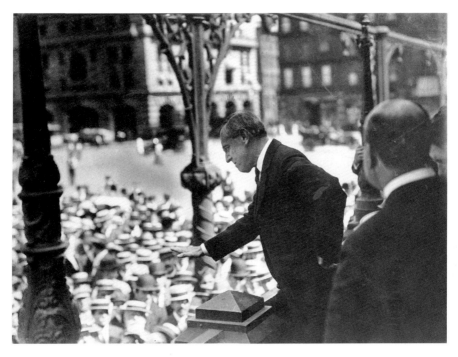

Wilson proved to be an effective campaigner for his political agenda,
executing the most progressive slate of laws in the nation.

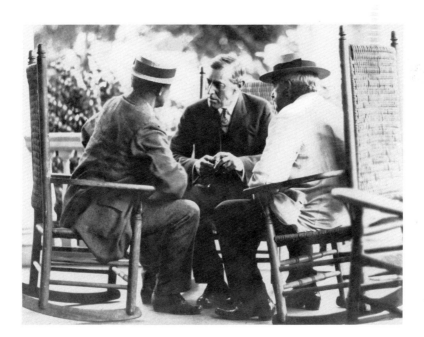

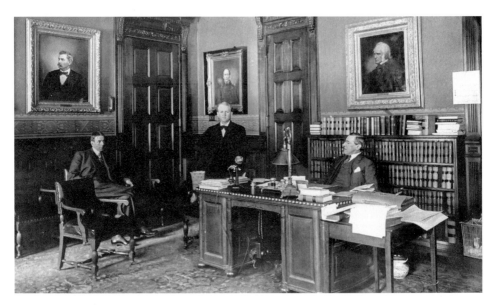

After less than a year of public service, Wilson allowed others to promote his candidacy for President. He had no supporters more loyal than newspaperman William Bayard Hale and former state legislator Joseph Patrick Tumulty, who became Wilson's private secretary and political adviser.

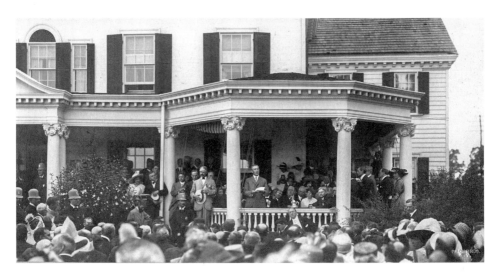

After a weeklong convention in Baltimore, the Democrats nominated Wilson as their candidate. On August 7, 1912, at the Governor's summer cottage in Sea Girt, New Jersey, Wilson accepted the nomination.

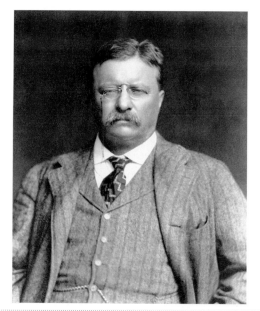

The election of 1912 pitted Wilson against an incumbent President, William Howard Taft, and a former President, Theodore Roosevelt (seen here), who ran as the candidate for the Bull Moose Party, and Socialist Eugene V. Debs.

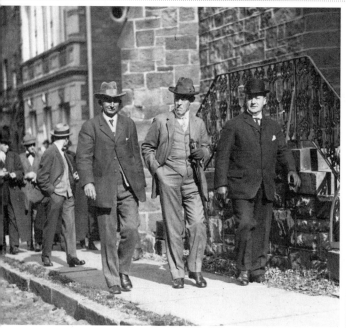

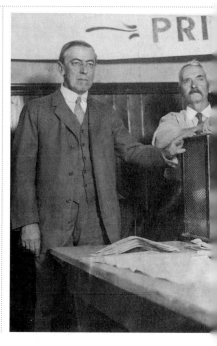

On November 5, 1912, Governor Wilson walked to his Princeton polling place and cast his vote. He was elected the twenty-eighth President of the United States in a landslide.

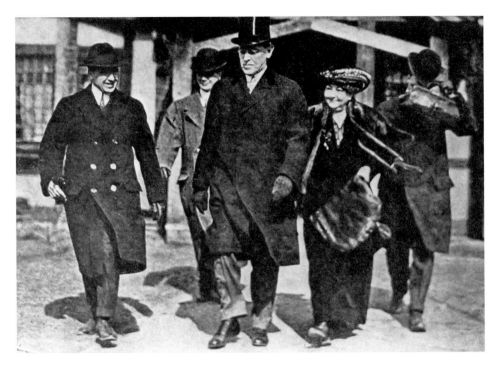

March 3, 1913—the President-elect and Mrs. Wilson walked to the Princeton depot and then departed to Washington, D. C.

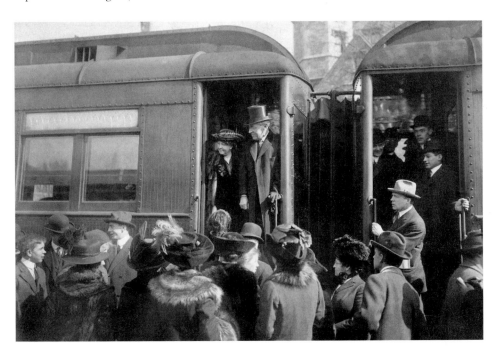

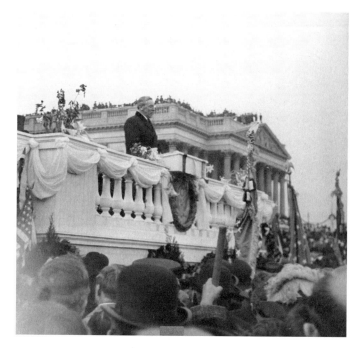

"There has been a change of government,"
Wilson proclaimed in his inaugural address on March 4, 1913.

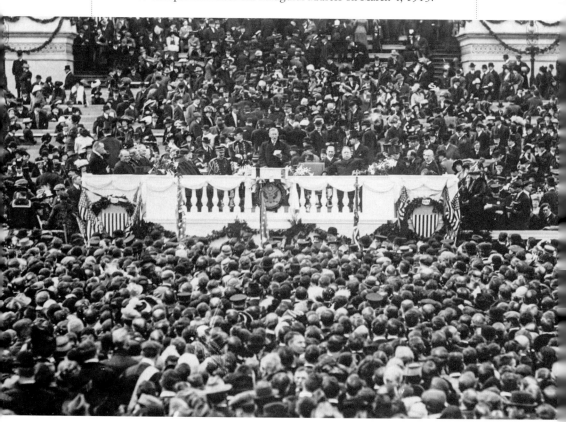

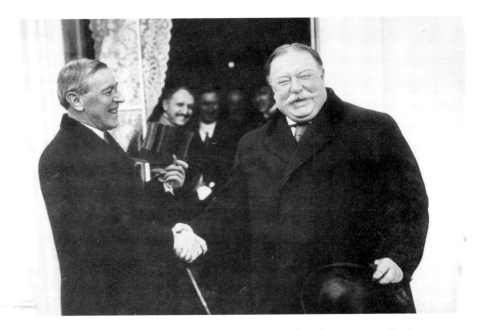

"I'm glad to be going," President William Howard Taft told Wilson upon leaving the White House, "—this is the loneliest place in the world."

The First Lady used her social position to lobby for improved housing in Washington's slums.

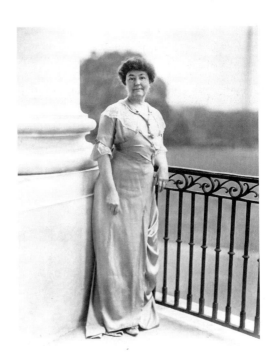

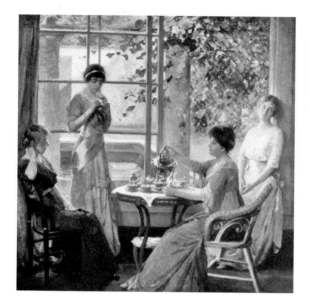

Ellen Wilson pouring tea, with her daughters Jessie, Eleanor, and Margaret—as painted by American Impressionist Robert Vonnoh, one of Ellen's teachers when she studied at the Lyme Art Colony in Connecticut.

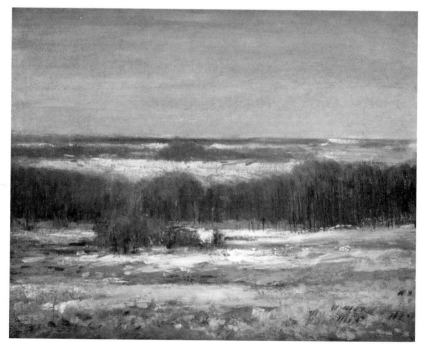

An accomplished artist, Ellen created a makeshift studio on the third floor of the White House, and exhibited her work in New York and Philadelphia. This oil on canvas—*Winter Landscape*—was painted probably in late 1911–early 1912.

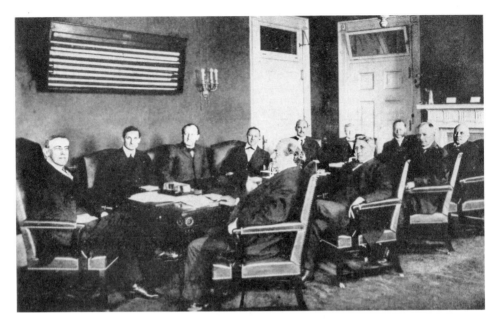

A team of Rebels: the Wilson Cabinet—mostly Southerners who never shed their Confederate biases. Clockwise from the left: Wilson, W. G. McAdoo, J. C. McReynolds, J. Daniels, D. F. Houston, W. B. Wilson, W. C. Redfield, F. K. Lane, A. S. Burleson, L. M. Garrison, W. J. Bryan.

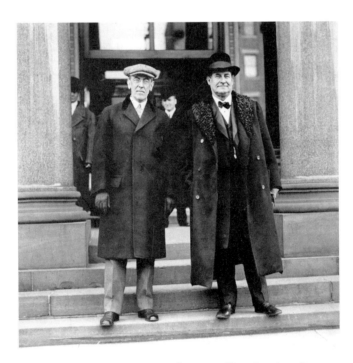

The President and his Secretary of State, William Jennings Bryan— the longtime standard-bearer of the Democratic Party, who had lent his support to Wilson's nomination. Disagreeing with his handling of the sinking of the *Lusitania* in 1915, Bryan resigned.

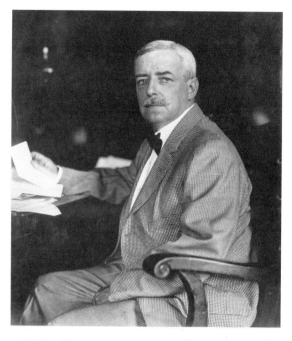

Robert Lansing—the son-in-law of one Secretary of State and uncle of another, John Foster Dulles—succeeded Bryan at the State Department.

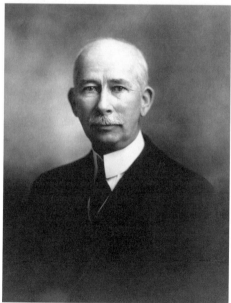

"My second personality," Wilson called Colonel Edward Mandell House. Unpaid and answerable to nobody but the President, he became Wilson's most trusted roving diplomat and adviser—for a while.

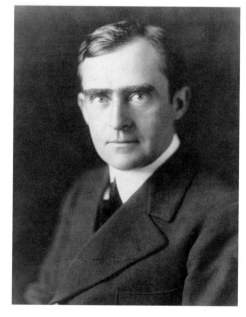

Wilson met Cary Travers Grayson, M.D., a lieutenant in the naval medical corps, at the start of his administration. Over the next eight years, he became Wilson's personal physician and most loyal friend.

Louis D. Brandeis was the leading architect of Wilson's "New Freedom," a program of progressive legislation that included establishing the Federal Reserve System and anti-trust regulation. After a bitter confirmation hearing, he became the first Jew to sit on the Supreme Court.

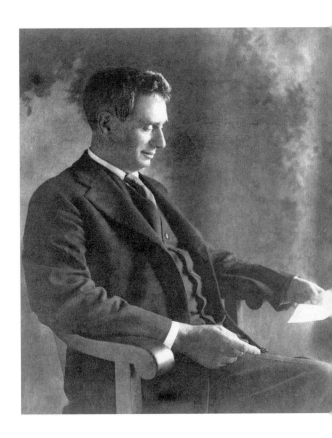

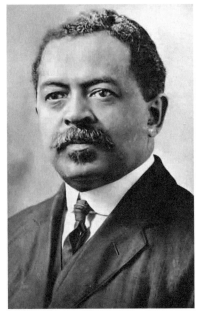

Wilson was at his most regressive in his civil rights policies, permitting segregation in federal workplaces. He always kept his door open to African American petitioners until activist-journalist William Monroe Trotter arrived with his grievances. "Your tone, sir, offends me," Wilson said, banning him from the White House for the duration of his term in office.

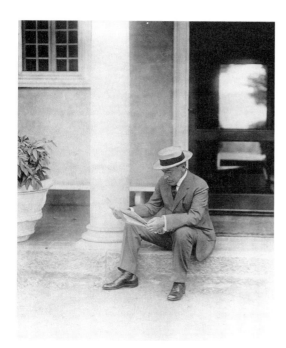

At Dr. Grayson's urging, Wilson sought recreation whenever possible. In the summers, he joined his vacationing family in Cornish, New Hampshire, where he could read a newspaper at his leisure.

Wilson played more golf than any President in White House history—an estimated twelve hundred rounds while in office.

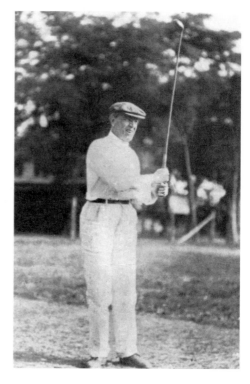

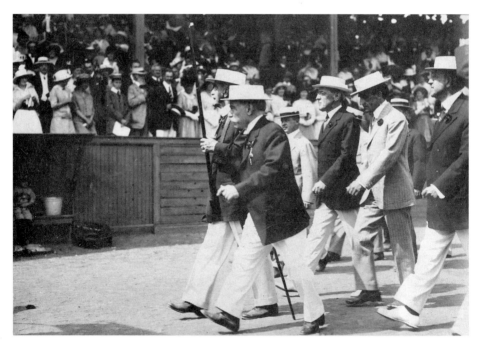

In June 1914, he "P-raded" with his Class of 1879 at their 35th Princeton Reunion.

Tragedy struck in the summer of 1914 when war broke out across Europe and Ellen Wilson unexpectedly died of Bright's disease. Severely depressed, the President relied more than ever on the company of his inner circle— Tumulty, Dr. Grayson, and, as seen here, Colonel House.

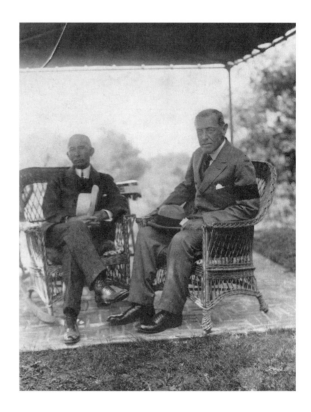

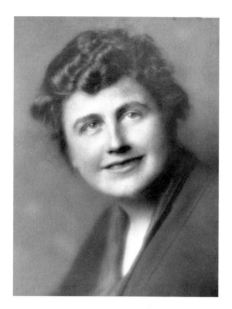

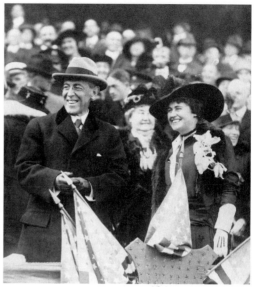

In March 1915, Dr. Grayson introduced Wilson to a young Washington widow, Edith Bolling Galt, whom he quietly courted.

That October, they appeared together at a World Series game in Philadelphia; and that December, they married.

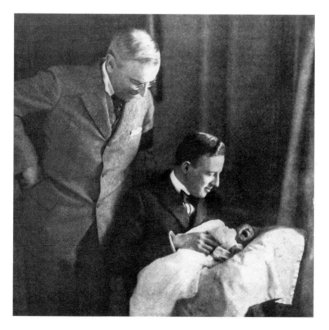

Wilson's other great joy that year was the birth of his first grandchild, seen here in the arms of his father. Francis Bowes Sayre, Jr., the last child to be born in the White House, would become the dean of the National Cathedral.

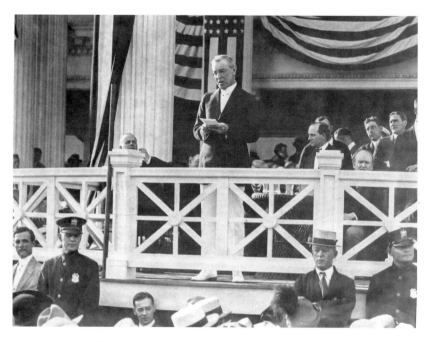

Wilson received official notification of his re-nomination for President on September 2, 1916, at Shadow Lawn in Long Branch, New Jersey. Standing below him (far left), in a light suit, is Assistant Secretary of the Navy Franklin D. Roosevelt.

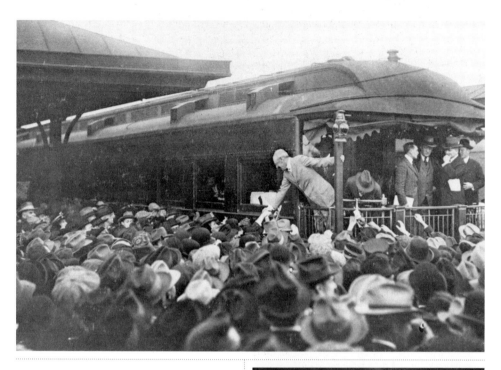

Despite a nasty campaign, Wilson was always happy on the hustings. Running against Charles Evans Hughes, a former New York Governor and former Associate Justice of the Supreme Court, Wilson won on the slogan "He kept us out of war."

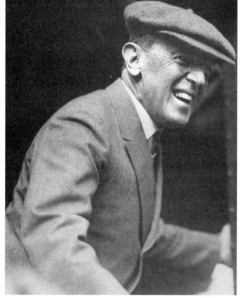

himself exclaiming, "Edith, my Darling, *where are you?*" Even though they gave themselves that month away from each other—in part to quell any gossip—Woodrow was revived.

Edith Bolling Galt was engaged in the first full-blown love affair of her life—and a Cinderella story at that. As she explained in a letter to Woodrow, "*I*—an unknown person—one who had lived a sheltered inconspicuous existence, now having all the threads in the tangled fabric of the world's history laid in her hands for a few minutes, while the strong hand, that quicks the shuttle, stops long enough in its work, to press my fingers in token of the great love and trust with which you crown and bless my life." Edith felt new purpose in her life and began training for it with gusto. She boned up on foreign affairs and United States history; she took golf lessons; she adopted Woodrow's quirky use of "okeh"—a Choctaw word meaning "it is so"—which he insisted was the proper form of "O.K." And she offered ferocious support for his decisions and fearless assessments of those who surrounded him, even his innermost circle: Dr. Grayson was above reproach, and the President was already in the process of promoting him; Tumulty she considered "common"; and Colonel House, she dared say, was "not a very strong character." She knew what a "comfort and staff" he was to Wilson, but she considered him "a weak vessel." Woodrow explained that House possessed a strong character and was noble, loyal, devoted, prudent, farseeing, and wise; but, he admitted, "His mind is not of the first class. He is a counsellor, not a statesman." Woodrow suggested that Edith would come to love House—"if only because he loves me and would give, I believe, his life for me." In preparing to become Mrs. Woodrow Wilson, Edith even found herself trying to match his eloquence. "Do you feel my arms 'round your neck and my lips on yours while I whisper— goodnight?" she wrote him mid-August.

When Edith returned to Washington at the start of September, she saw how world events had turned his eyes into "pools of tragic suffering." During their traditional drive, Wilson spoke of the increasing struggle to avoid entrance into the war, to say nothing of all the complications closer to home. "And so, little girl," he said, "I have no right to ask you to help me by sharing this load that is almost breaking my back, for I know your nature and you might do it out of sheer pity." And in that moment—despite the presence of the chauffeur, the Secret Service, and Helen Bones—Edith threw her arms around Woodrow's neck and said, "Well, if you won't ask me, I

will volunteer." She agreed to marry him as soon as he was ready. She presumed he would suggest the American public would need a year to get used to the idea of the President taking a second wife.

Wilson divulged his intentions to his daughters, and each responded with enthusiasm. Margaret spoke for her sisters when she wrote Edith late that summer, "I'm so glad that he has your love to help him and support him in these terrible times! . . . I love you dear Edith, and I love to be with you." Edith revealed her secret to her mother and siblings, allowing Woodrow to reach out to them. He made them feel welcome at the White House, and he wrote Edith's mother that he hoped "that you will love me and accept me as your own son." The couple prepared to go public.

But then they encountered the first naysayers—right in the West Wing of the White House. Grayson, the matchmaker, knew how therapeutic it had been for the President to be in love again, but the rest of Wilson's advisers worried about the politics of the situation. Rumors of a love affair would not play as well with the electorate as the suffering of a grieving widower—especially in the quarter of the states (mostly in the Progressive West) that permitted women to vote. With Ellen dead only a year and the Presidential election only twelve months away, the Cabinet decided somebody had to advise the President to wait. They selected the President's son-in-law.

McAdoo—evidently in concert with Colonel House—devised a strangely devilish ploy. Over lunch on September 18, he told the President that he had received an anonymous letter asserting that rumors of his engagement had spread and that the desperate Mrs. Hulbert had been shopping his letters. Whatever her motive, McAdoo suggested, the letters were sure to create a scandal, possibly one that would portray their latest exchange as a $7,500 payoff. Wilson was aghast that Mary Hulbert could ever do such a thing. He knew the innocence of the correspondence, but he could also imagine how desperate Mary had become and how the political opposition in Washington would respond.

Shaken to the core, he dispatched a note to Edith, informing her that there was "something, personal to myself, that I feel I must tell you about at once." He took the liberty of asking if he might defy propriety and call upon her at home. "Of course, you can come to me," a distressed Edith replied, though she asked him to bring Dr. Grayson along, to provide the necessary cover.

Woodrow bared his soul. He told Edith—as he would later record in a letter to her—all about his relationship with "Mrs. Peck" and what he called "a passage of folly and gross impertinence in my life." For that, he was "deeply ashamed and repentant," and also tormented and confused. He could not understand what would possess anybody to publish such letters, knowing the humiliation they would bring. Wilson was contrite—not because Mrs. Peck was unworthy of the sentiments expressed in the letters but because Wilson felt he did not have "the moral right to offer the ardent affection which they express." In fact, the whole cache of mail seems to corroborate that the "affair" with Mrs. Peck did not trespass into the physical. Wilson said his "utter allegiance to my incomparable wife [had not been] in any way by the least jot abated."

None of that lessened either the shame Wilson suffered or the grief "that I should have so erred and forgotten the standards of honorable behavior by which I should have been bound." Now that indiscretion implicated Edith Galt. "Stand by me," he pled. "Don't desert me."

Edith hesitated, and Woodrow left her to sort out her feelings. Each endured a restless night. He lamented the pain he had brought to her. "When it was the deepest, most passionate desire of my heart to bring you happiness," he wrote her the next morning, ". . . I have brought you, instead, mortification and thrown a new shadow about you." After spending the night in her big chair by the window, she wrote Woodrow to apologize for having faltered.

"This is my pledge, Dearest One," she wrote. "I will stand by you—not for duty, not for pity, not for honor—but for love—trusting, protecting, comprehending Love. And no matter whether the wine be bitter or sweet we will share it together and find happiness in the comradeship." Woodrow was overjoyed.

House told the President he did not believe the issue of "the Peck letters" would ever amount to anything. The Colonel never mentioned that he knew that the entire incident had been trumped up. Instead, he graciously accepted the responsibility for planning the impending wedding, which the two men agreed could take place before the end of the year. House conceded that the salutary benefits of Wilson's remarrying far outweighed any political fallout.

A private telephone wire was installed between the White House and Edith's, avoiding any switchboards; letters passed between them several

times a day, as did a pouchful of memoranda, with the President's comments and notations, so that Edith could brief herself on his activities. He continued to send flowers every day—orchids if they were dining out or attending the theater, a corsage that she would wear high on her left shoulder. He also changed the routine of his regular automobile ride by making time to stroll with Edith through Rock Creek Park; it was Agent Starling's task to follow them. He wanted to look away, to afford the lovers some privacy, but his job did not permit it. "He was an ardent lover," Starling recalled. "He talked, gesticulated, laughed, boldly held her hand. It was hard to believe he was fifty-eight years old."

The White House announced their engagement on Wednesday, October 6, 1915. In an accompanying statement, the President declared his intention to vote for woman suffrage in New Jersey the following month. He added that he would be voting as neither the leader of the nation nor of his party, only as a citizen of New Jersey. Although there was a strong movement for an equal rights amendment to the Constitution—which his daughter Margaret strongly advocated—Wilson believed this was a matter for each state to settle. The press credited Edith with turning Wilson into a suffragist; but, as Cary Grayson wrote Altrude Gordon, "The joke is that she's against it: but she's too good a diplomat to say anything on the subject these days."

Woodrow and Edith went to New York that Friday, to spend time with Colonel House and his wife. The President bunked at their apartment, while Edith and her mother stayed at the St. Regis Hotel. Before they went to dinner and the theater, Wilson received a jeweler, who arrived at the apartment with thirteen diamond rings, one of which Edith selected. Saturday the couple went to Philadelphia, where Wilson became the first President to attend a World Series game—as the Boston Red Sox beat the Philadelphia Phillies, 2 to 1. Thanksgiving weekend, the President showed off his bride-to-be at the annual Army and Navy football game at the Polo Grounds in New York. They sat in a box on the Army side of the gridiron until halftime, when the Admirals of the Navy came to escort their Commander in Chief across the field to the enthusiastic cheers of the entire stadium. "Every one," Edith observed, "seemed to be our friend." Even though the couple chose to send announcement cards in lieu of wedding invitations, gifts from all over the world began to arrive. Many came from manufacturers, hoping for a White House endorsement, while foreign

delegations sent glassware, silverware, jewelry, and furniture. The only gift the President officially accepted was a nugget of California gold, which the state hoped they might hammer into a wedding ring.

Ironically, once the President and Mrs. Galt had made their relationship public, they could spend more time together in private. As they were engaged to be married, there was no need for furtiveness. On Sundays, after attending church, the couple would seclude themselves all day. Almost every night, a Secret Service agent accompanied Wilson to Twentieth Street and sat vigil outside Edith's house, usually until midnight. Often Wilson wanted to walk home along the late-night deserted streets; and Agent Starling could not but notice that the President would unconsciously jig a few steps whenever he had to wait for an occasional milk truck to pass. He also realized that when Wilson got lost in his own thoughts, he often whistled—softly, through his teeth—invariably the same tune, one he undoubtedly had heard in one of his visits to the theater: "Oh, you beautiful doll! You great big beautiful doll! Let me put my arms around you, I could never live without you."

The White House came alive again. The President smiled for most of his photographs. There were frequent small celebrations among intimate friends and family. On November 30, seventy-five members of the Class of 1879 went to the White House for a mini-reunion; the members of the old Witherspoon Gang spent the night in the guest rooms upstairs. "Dinner went off delightfully," Woodrow wired Edith, who had gone to shop in New York. ". . . You were unanimously elected an honorary member of the class amidst loud cheers."

Wilson delivered his State of the Union address on December 7, 1915. While it covered a variety of subjects, they encompassed one overall theme: "national efficiency and security." With war spreading across the globe, Wilson stood confidently behind his firewall, remaining "studiously neutral." While the British push through the Dardanelles had resulted in a bloodbath costing 100,000 lives, Wilson maintained that America's task was domestic—making "a common cause of national independence and of political liberty in America." He said the United States would "aid and befriend Mexico, but we will not coerce her. . . . We seek no political suzerainty or selfish control." He endorsed Pan-Americanism, the notion that the states of the Americas "are not hostile rivals but cooperating friends" and that there was "none of the spirit of empire in it." He

would be welcome at the ceremony. Edith read the Bishop's letter twice and handwrote her reply, thanking him for his explanation of the embarrassing situation . . . and then relieving him from his duty of performing the ceremony.

Before sealing her note, she rang the President and read the Bishop's letter and her reply. Woodrow agreed that the Bishop had overstepped but suggested that his position demanded some respect. "No," Edith told Woodrow, "this letter goes to him right now. I will postpone our wedding rather than be bludgeoned into a thing of this kind."

"Yes," replied the President, "I was afraid of that. But, after all, the poor fellow has enough to stand with a wife like that." Edith called upon the rector of her local church to replace the Bishop.

Two days later, on December 18, 1915, White House usher Ike Hoover took charge of Edith's house. He emptied the lower floor of all furniture and moved in a team of decorators and caterers. In the recess of the window in the front room, florists created a semicircular bower filled with maidenhair ferns and a canopy lined in Scotch heather, a tribute to the President's roots. There were many sprays of purple orchids, Edith's favorites, in the room; and the rest of the space was decorated with palms and American Beauty roses. The prie-dieu that had served in several White House weddings was covered in white satin and adorned with more orchids. Back at the White House, the President worked with his stenographer in the morning and hosted the wedding guests for lunch. Late in the afternoon, he and Edith went for a drive, returning to the White House at six. He presented her with a brooch of white diamonds.

With only his Secret Service escort, Wilson arrived at Edith's house at eight o'clock and went upstairs to her sitting room. He waited alone for a half hour, until Hoover tapped on the door. The nearly fifty-nine-year-old groom, in a cutaway coat, white waistcoat, and gray striped trousers, looked upon his forty-three-year-old bride, wearing a black velvet gown and matching hat and her brooch. They descended the stairs together as a small string section from the Marine Band played the wedding march from *Lohengrin*. Downstairs waited their families and a handful of friends, including Tumulty, a few Bolling retainers, Edith's doctor, her "ward" Altrude Gordon, and, of course, Cary Grayson. There were no attendants; and when the minister asked, "Who giveth this woman to be married to

this man?" Edith's mother stepped forward and placed her daughter's hand in that of the President of the United States.

A buffet supper followed—oyster patties, boned capon, Virginia ham, chicken salad, caramel ice cream, and a three-tiered wedding cake. While the party was in full swing, Woodrow and Edith slipped upstairs to prepare for their departure. The guests cheered as they left, as did a crowd outside, thrilled to catch a glimpse of the couple as they ducked into the waiting limousine, its Presidential crests covered with pieces of carbon paper. Only the driver and the Secret Service car behind them knew their immediate destination; and they were ultimately able to shake the fleet of newspapermen and the police cars that were in hot pursuit. Several minutes later, they arrived in Alexandria, Virginia. Agent Starling stood at the siding at the edge of the freight yard, where the baggage coach of their special train had already been loaded with luggage and two automobiles, one for the President and one for the Secret Service. As both the White House limousine and the train from Washington pulled up, Starling blinked his flashlight three times and escorted the newlyweds onto their special car virtually unnoticed.

Only then, around midnight, did the engineer receive orders from the officials of the Chesapeake and Ohio directing him to his destination—Hot Springs, Virginia, halfway between Edith's and Woodrow's respective birthplaces. About seven o'clock the next morning, the train pulled into the siding of the station in the small resort town. As it came to a stop, Agent Starling went back to the private car, quietly walking the corridor between the bedrooms. Approaching the sitting room, he heard a familiar tune—as there before him stood a man in a top hat, tailcoat, and morning trousers, his hands in his pockets. He was dancing a jig. Unaware that he was being watched, he suddenly clicked his heels in the air. And then Starling heard the President sing, "Oh, you beautiful doll! You great big beautiful doll. . . ."

complete and strong for whatever may betide. I am indeed blessed beyond my (or any other man's) deserts."

On December 30, 1915, a German U-boat fired a torpedo into the British cruiser *Persia* off the coast of Crete. The 500 passengers aboard the merchant ship should have been permitted to disembark; but no warning shot had been fired, and 350 passengers died. Days later came reports of two more vessels torpedoed in the Mediterranean, also without warning. "Personally," Secretary of State Lansing telegraphed the President, "I am very much alarmed over the seriousness of the situation." Woodrow and Edith reluctantly ended their honeymoon.

The President returned to the White House—and the start of an election year, a phenomenon that exaggerates even the pettiest issues. Remaining focused on but one objective—keeping his country from war—Wilson was in for some of the angriest discord ever to come a President's way. Isolationists and pacifists felt he had been too aggressive in response to the German attacks, and the jingoes felt he had been too passive. Even though all the facts regarding the *Persia* were still not known, Tumulty argued for "vigorous action." When he reported that a growing constituency in the country suggested a lack of leadership, Wilson stiffened in his chair. "Tumulty," he said, "you may as well understand my position right now. If my re-election as President depends upon my getting into war, I don't want to be President.

> . . . I have made up my mind that I am more interested in the opinion that the country will have of me ten years from now than the opinion it may be willing to express today. Of course, I understand that the country wants action . . . but I will not be rushed into war, no matter if every damned congressman and senator stands up on his hind legs and proclaims me a coward.

This renewal of German attacks, in clear violation of naval law and international treaties, demanded an escalated response. The United States could not keep sending admonitory notes, protesting one naval incident while coming to terms on another. Severance of diplomatic relations, which Wilson considered the "forerunner" of war, would be the next logical step. Ambassador Page in England wrote Wilson that the British thought the United States was being "hoodwinked" by the Germans and that

America's response was laughable. He said Londoners were referring to Americans as "Too-prouds" and that they hissed when an American image appeared on their moving-picture screens. Colonel House conferred with the new Minister of Munitions, David Lloyd George, and several other Cabinet members, the consensus being that only Wilson's intervention could stop the war. Toward that end, House echoed Lloyd George's feelings that it would enormously strengthen Wilson's hand if he would start building an impressively large Army and Navy.

Such comments meant little to Wilson. He did not work for Great Britain, he reminded Tumulty. "I believe that the sober-minded people of this country will applaud any efforts I may make without the loss of our honor to keep this country out of war." Constantly weighing his military options against the diplomatic, Wilson believed it was time for both—readying America for battle, all the while grasping at solutions to resist it.

After conferring with several leaders on the Continent, House returned to England, where he dined on Valentine's Day 1916, with past, present, and future Prime Ministers Arthur James Balfour, H. H. Asquith, and Lloyd George, along with Foreign Secretary Lord Grey. Although their constituents were far from ready to lay down arms to negotiate, the statesmen all agreed to discuss the matter; and, a week later, House confided in Lord Grey the possible terms for a sweetheart deal, which the latter recorded in what became known as the House-Grey Memorandum. House had said that Wilson was ready to propose a conference that would summon the Allies and the Germans together; and he noted, "Should the Allies accept this proposal and should Germany refuse it, the United States would probably enter the war against Germany." Furthermore, the memorandum said, "if such a Conference were held, it would secure peace on terms not unfavourable to the Allies; and, if it failed to secure peace, the United States would leave the Conference as a belligerent on the side of the Allies, if Germany was unreasonable." Among its terms would be the restoration of Belgium, the transfer of Alsace and Lorraine to France, and the acquisition by Russia of an outlet to the sea in the south.

Wilson approved this peculiar document, which had little value. He did not support secret covenants, and its vagueness suggested that it was little more than an exercise in mediation. House, of course, was not empowered to speak for the United States; and, indeed, the President

1916, "I love peace." And the price for that peace, Wilson said, required "a great plan for national defense of which we will all be proud and which will lead us to forget partisan differences in one great enthusiasm for the United States of America."

Wilson's speech in Cleveland marked a turning point in his campaign for preparedness. David Lawrence, who was part of the touring press corps, discerned a shift in the President's rhetoric—as the long poetic sentences yielded to a punchier delivery. "The President talked," Lawrence observed, ". . . like a man who had really convinced himself." And in so doing, he recovered the unvarnished sincerity that had uplifted people when he first ran for office.

In vast auditoriums and from caboose platforms, Wilson addressed citizens in five Midwestern states, scaffolding the argument that he would later build for America's increasing involvement in the world. In Chicago on January 31, he said it was "a very terrible thing . . . to have the honor of the United States entrusted to your keeping," especially with the great task that had been assigned to his nation—"to assert the principles of law in a world in which the principles of law have broken down." The war, he said, "was brought on by rulers, not by peoples, and I thank God that there is no man in America who has the authority to bring war on without the consent of the people."

Three American Presidents had been assassinated in Wilson's lifetime, as had been a dozen international leaders. Although the incident was kept from the public and even from the President himself, a man tried to take Wilson's life during his preparedness tour. After his speech in Chicago, Wilson had retired to his suite at the Blackstone Hotel for the night. Dr. Grayson went to a supper party, and, upon returning to the Blackstone, discovered the entourage of Secret Service detail in a state of high excitement. "A man had tried to get to the President threatening to kill him," Grayson wrote his fiancée late that night. He turned out to be an unstable "crank," who had written a note saying that he was going to sneak into the President's room and stab him to death with a pair of scissors. The would-be assassin never got closer than a few floors above the Presidential suite before jumping to his death. Wilson slept through the entire incident, until Dr. Grayson entered his room on another pretense, so that he could lock the window, ensuring that everybody else might sleep as soundly as Wilson. Security for the President was subsequently beefed up to prevent any

such event from recurring. On February 3, in St. Louis, the President insisted that America was at peace with all the world "because she entertains a friendship for all the nations of the world."

In speech after speech, he turned the argument of national safety into one of "national dignity" and, ultimately, one of forging a new national identity. The trip left Wilson inspired, reminding him of the importance of getting out of Washington, to hear the real voices of America. Upon returning to the White House, however, Wilson found himself listening to just one.

No President and First Lady spent as much of their time together as the Wilsons did, as neither wished to revisit the loneliness each had experienced. Even the possessive Wilson daughters delighted in their stepmother, seeing in her, observed Dr. Grayson, "the deliverer of their father from sadness into joy, and she, in turn, always showed the utmost consideration and affection for them."

The President now took to rising at six o'clock in the morning, at which time he would have a small sandwich and a cup of coffee from a plate and thermos that had been set on a small table outside his bedroom. Then he and Edith (and a Secret Service agent) would go to a course for at least an hour of golf. They would be home in time to breakfast together at eight o'clock sharp and then go to his study together to check "the Drawer," the bin in his desk in which all documents demanding immediate attention had been placed. Edith would sort the papers, placing those requiring his signature before him and blotting each as she set down the next item. Time permitting, he discussed each document with her. By nine o'clock, stenographer Charles Swem would arrive; and Edith would sit close by, listening to Woodrow dictate replies to his mail, marveling at "the lucid answers that came with apparently no effort from a mind so well-stored."

Edith would then leave to tend to housekeeping and social matters along with her own mail, which she dictated to her secretary, Edith Benham. From the big window seat at the end of the west hall, she could see her husband signal to her, as he left the study, to accompany him to the West Wing. If possible, they would stroll through the garden; if not, they would grab the few minutes together walking directly to the Oval Office. Edith tried to schedule her appointments to coincide with his so that they could reconvene for lunch, which they generally reserved for each other.

They did not discuss business over meals. The President spent two afternoons a week in Cabinet meetings; the other days were filled with individual Secretaries or legislators. Whenever possible, Edith and Woodrow
would cram in a round of golf or a motor ride before dinner; afterward
Wilson tended to his most serious work, assessing problems and addressing them on paper—confidential correspondence, speeches, or policy papers, which he would type himself. Edith would sit up with him, decoding
top secret memoranda. They often worked past midnight, until he might
say, "You don't know how much easier it makes all this to have you here
by me. Are you too tired to hear what I have written?" Beyond their personal bliss, the rest of the world steadily darkened.

Trouble had been mounting within the War Department for months,
as its disgruntled Secretary, Lindley M. Garrison, increasingly found himself at odds with his boss. Garrison's views about preparedness and international intervention had long been more aggressive than the President's:
Garrison favored a large and permanent conscripted Army, while Wilson
preferred a smaller armed force with a large, trained reserve of volunteer
citizens at the ready. In truth, the conflict ran deeper than that, as Garrison believed Wilson had "little or no interest in the Army and had rather
a disparaging attitude toward it." Within less than a week of Wilson's return from the Midwest, Garrison resigned.

Wilson wasted no time in wiring Newton D. Baker—the former Mayor
of Cleveland who had, in fact, refused Wilson's prior offer to serve as Secretary of the Interior. In proffering this post, the President told him, "It would
greatly strengthen my hand." The men had met when Baker was an undergraduate at Johns Hopkins and Wilson was lecturing there. He accepted his
former professor's offer and appeared in Washington three days later. After
Baker—an Episcopalian with pacifistic leanings—had recited a litany of
reasons why he should not be named Secretary of War, Wilson asked, "Are
you ready to take the oath?" There was good reason for Wilson's urgency.

Wilson realized his Army was so small that he lacked sufficient manpower even to prevent bandits from crossing the long Mexican border. And
a few hours before dawn on March 9, 1916—Secretary Baker's first day in
office—Pancho Villa and an army of 1,500 descended upon the town of
Columbus, New Mexico, three miles across the border. While most of the
town slept, the Villistas burned buildings, looted stores, and shot at will,
killing seventeen Americans, half of whom were soldiers. Two hundred

fifty troopers of the 13th United States Cavalry fought back and chased the marauders five miles into Mexican territory, killing seventy-five.

In fact, the bandits were primitive political operatives, retaliating against Wilson for his recent acceptance of Carranza's de facto government, which Villa hoped to topple by embarrassing both leaders. Until then, such raids as these allowed him to feed and arm his troops, refueling his own dreams of national leadership. Any account of the fearless peasant challenging the Goliath to the north only enhanced his legend. As he fled back to safety, Villa dropped a stash of personal papers, including what appeared to be his final orders just before the Columbus attack, which revealed his true mission: "Kill all the Gringos."

From Fort Sam Houston, Texas, General Frederick Funston wired Secretary Baker that "unless Villa is relentlessly pursued and his forces scattered, he will continue raids." Even before consulting the Carranza government, Wilson authorized a punitive expedition whose sole objective was the capture of Pancho Villa, dead or alive. He ordered Brigadier General John J. Pershing, a Missouri-born graduate of West Point who had distinguished himself in Cuba and the Philippines, to command this force and secure the United States–Mexico border.

Wilson never viewed Pershing's expedition as "an invasion of that Republic nor an infringement of its Sovereignty." Indeed, its whole idea was "to cooperate with the forces of General Carranza in removing a cause of irritation to both Governments and to retire from Mexico so soon as this object is accomplished." In an effort to avoid a war with the United States, Carranza agreed to work with the Americans with mutual permission for American and Mexican forces to cross into each other's territory in pursuit of bandits. While Pershing prepared for his mission, one of Carranza's Colonels declared that should American troops cross the border, he would immediately attack. Caught in a pickle, Wilson told Tumulty and Secretary Baker that should that case arise, he would not send troops into Mexico—because that would amount to waging an interventionist war against Mexico.

Many accused the President of timidity, of failing to seize a political opportunity—nationally and internationally. Tumulty argued that if Wilson did not send troops after Villa, he might "just as well not contemplate running for the Presidency, since he would not get a single electoral vote." When Tumulty found Wilson intractable, he sought out Secretaries

Burleson and Houston; and with their input, Tumulty wrote an urgent letter, restating his case—insisting that biding any more time "would be not only disastrous to our party and humiliating to the country, but would be destructive of our influence in international affairs and make it forever impossible to deal in any effective way with Mexican affairs." Colonel House supported Tumulty, at least in the pages of his diary, saying Wilson's failure to act would destroy his influence in Europe as well.

In the meantime, Villa and his men withdrew deeper into the Mexican wilderness, hiding out in the mountainous country. Even though Carranza now considered Villa his rival, it was awkward allying with American soldiers to pursue a lone Mexican. On March 15, General Pershing led almost five thousand men across the border; Secretary Baker even encouraged the use of Curtiss "Jenny" airplanes based in Texas to conduct aerial reconnaissance. By the end of the month, Pershing was hot on Villa's trail.

Ambivalence filled the Cabinet Room. By early April, Secretaries Baker and Lansing favored withdrawal of the troops from Mexico; the former thought the mission had been accomplished, that the Villistas had been dispersed to the point of ineffectiveness. Secretary Houston argued that if the troops were withdrawn, Villa would rebound into action. After listening to all their arguments, Wilson believed America must remain in Mexico until Carranza could assume the responsibility for bringing Villa to his knees.

That would not be any time soon, as Mexicans were calling Carranza a traitor for consenting to the occupation of his country by a foreign army. Although diplomats from both countries had been negotiating for weeks, he would not commit to an agreement because the United States refused to set a withdrawal date for its troops. And then, on June 20, Pershing's forces encountered resistance in the town of Carrizal—seventy-five miles into Mexico—when a local commandant announced that he would defy the Americans if they sought entry. An hour of battle left nine Americans dead and twenty-five taken prisoner. "The break seems to have come in Mexico," Wilson wrote House; "and all my patience seems to have gone for nothing. I am infinitely sad about it. I fear I should have drawn Pershing and his command northward just after it became evident that Villa had slipped through his fingers; but except for that error of judgment (if it was an error) I cannot, in looking back, see where I could have done differently, holding sacred the convictions I hold in this matter."

Again, Tumulty insisted upon the President's taking stronger action. He told Wilson that he should send a message to Carranza saying, "Release those American soldiers or take the consequences." That, said Tumulty, "would ring around the world." Wilson sent instead for his private secretary, to whom he delivered a long monologue, trying to explain foreign affairs from his chair in the Oval Office.

"Tumulty," he said, "you are Irish, and, therefore, full of fight." And while Wilson appreciated the depth of Tumulty's feelings on the Mexican situation, he—not Tumulty and not the Cabinet—had to bear the responsibility for every action to be taken. "I have to sleep with my conscience in these matters," the President said, "and I shall be held responsible for every drop of blood that may be spent in the enterprise of intervention." He knew declaring war would be politically advantageous, but Wilson insisted, "*There won't be any war with Mexico if I can prevent it*, no matter how loud the gentlemen on the hill yell for it and demand it."

"I came from the South and I know what war is," Wilson reminded Tumulty, "for I have seen its wreckage and terrible ruin." To those who had never seen such devastation, the President suggested, declarations of war came easily. Wilson could only think of a poor farmer's boy or the son of a poor widow in a modest town who would have to fight and die. Some American Presidents have seized the first possible opportunity to pull the trigger; speaking of Mexico, but just as surely meaning anywhere in the world, Wilson said, "I will not resort to war . . . until I have exhausted every means to keep out of this mess."

Wilson's lips quivered as he insisted that he would be just as ashamed to be rash as to be a coward. "Valor," he said, "withholds itself from all small implications and entanglements and waits for the great opportunity when the sword will flash as if it carried the light of heaven upon its blade." Someday, Wilson said, "the people of America will know why I hesitated to intervene."

And then the President revealed an unspoken intricacy of the Mexican situation. Eager for war between Mexico and the United States, Germany had planted propagandists in Mexico to encourage hostilities with its North American neighbor. "She wishes an uninterrupted opportunity to carry on her submarine warfare," said Wilson, "and thus believes that war with Mexico will keep our hands off her and thus give her liberty of action to do as she pleases on the high seas." With war appearing "inevitable," the

Stronger disagreements raged in Congress, cutting across party lines and creating strange alliances. Leading Republican and interventionist Henry Cabot Lodge sided with Wilson in his stance against Democrats Gore and McLemore; and isolationist Midwestern Republicans, such as Wisconsin's Robert La Follette, allied with powerful Southern Democrats, such as William Stone and Mississippi's James K. Vardaman. On April 19, 1916, the President walked through the political minefield of the Capitol to address a joint session of Congress. Without abandoning his position of peace and neutrality, he delivered a solemn sixteen-minute speech devoid of rhetorical flourishes and moved the nation one step closer to war.

After summarizing the Imperial German government's maritime practices and policies of the prior fourteen months, Wilson insisted his own government had been "very patient." At the same time, Wilson said, it had accepted in good faith Germany's repeated explanations and assurances, despite its continued commitment to "the use of submarines for the destruction of an enemy's commerce." Wilson felt the United States was compelled to issue an official warning: "that unless the Imperial German Government should now immediately declare and effect an abandonment of its present methods of warfare against passenger and freight-carrying vessels this government can have no choice but to sever diplomatic relations with the government of the German Empire altogether."

America realized the seriousness of the situation—*The New York Times* dedicated its entire front page to the speech—and so did Germany. On May 4, 1916, the German government responded at last to the American note in a manner designed to save face for both nations. Germany said it was "prepared to do its utmost to confine the operations of war for the rest of its duration to the fighting forces of the belligerents, thereby also insuring the freedom of the seas." But so long as Great Britain maintained its illegal blockade, Germany said, neutrals could not expect them to restrict the usage of their most formidable weapon. The United States had evidently won this diplomatic battle, as Wilson, once again, averted entry into the war. Colonel House warned Count von Bernstorff that "the least infraction would entail an immediate severance of diplomatic relations," and Bernstorff said he did not believe any further transgressions would occur. In a world of aggressors, Wilson now insisted that "the peace of society is obtained by force." Across America his people began arguing such issues as militarism, compulsory military service, and an armament race.

On the night of May 30, the Wilsons took a small party to Baltimore, where the Friars Club of New York performed an out-of-town "Frolic." Songwriter and performer George M. Cohan was the headliner that night, but a lanky young Oklahoman—part cowboy, part Cherokee—just starting out in vaudeville stole the show by spinning political commentary and a rope at the same time. Will Rogers would later look back on that night as the most nervous performance of his life. With the President right in front of him, he told jokes about the attempted capture of Pancho Villa, saying, "There is some talk of getting a Machine Gun if we can borrow one. The one we have now they are using to train our Army with in Plattsburgh. If we go to war we will just about have to go to the trouble of getting another Gun." Wilson led the entire audience in laughter. After more jokes about Mexico, Rogers turned his attention to Europe, stopping the show when he said, "President Wilson is getting along fine now to what he was a few months ago. Do you realize, People, that at one time in our negotiations with Germany that he was 5 Notes behind?" The President guffawed.

The Presidential election sparked most of the punch lines and rhetoric that year. While Woodrow Wilson still enjoyed the luxury of comfortable Democratic majorities in both houses of Congress, the Republicans were gathering forces to end his progressive program, which had hardly slowed. He encouraged citizens to become as active as his administration. In June 1916, Wilson addressed an open-air convention behind Independence Hall in Philadelphia, to whom he said that Americans needed more than a simple understanding of their ideals. He summoned each citizen to ask not what his country could do for him but "to think first, not of himself or of any interest which he may be called upon to sacrifice, but of the country which we serve." He offered a new motto: "America First."

Not to be confused with a noninterventionist policy that would adopt the same moniker a generation later, "America First" meant "the duty of every American to exalt the national consciousness by purifying his own motives and exhibiting his own devotion." When Wilson said this meant putting the country first in their thoughts—being "ready . . . to vindicate . . . the principles of liberty, of justice, and of humanity"—the crowd cheered. "You cheer the sentiment," Wilson said, looking up from his outline, "but do you realize what it means?" He explained that it carried the responsibility not only of being just "to your fellow men, but that, as a nation, you have got to be just to other nations."

In a "fighting mood," Wilson then said he wanted to take a number of domestic actions, each of which was sure to antagonize large segments of the population, mostly the business community. These issues had all been among his original campaign promises. The President had long favored legislation to prevent the waste or control of the country's natural resources by special interests. While a few of Wilson's predecessors had reserved more than a dozen national parks—comprising millions of acres of natural wonderland—no President had established a proper bureau to preserve that land. Interests clashed: Wilson had signed a bill in 1913 damming the Hetch Hetchy Valley within Yosemite National Park in order to provide more water to San Francisco, and conservationist John Muir went to his death the next year damning the action, which altered the ecology of many square miles of territory. Strict preservationists supported the great parks for the public's benefit, but their interests often conflicted with those of groups promoting tourism—the railroads and land developers who might allow more people to enjoy the parks. Following Taft's example, Wilson approved a third naval oil reserve in the West—Teapot Dome— but his Secretary of the Interior, Franklin Lane, found himself repeatedly blocked in his efforts to get Wilson to sign leases allowing private businesses to tap into those reserves. And so in the summer of 1916, President Wilson signed the National Park Service Act, which not only regulated the existing parkland but allowed for the regulation and expansion of a vast network of hundreds of parks, monuments, and recreation areas. His administration's negotiations with Great Britain (on behalf of Canada) resulted in the Migratory Bird Treaty Act, which protected hundreds of species at a moment when commercial interests threatened to destroy them. In environmental matters, Wilson's guiding principle was to preserve as much as possible while serving as many as possible.

With close to ten million foreigners coming to America in the preceding decade—many from nations with growing hostility toward the United States—xenophobia descended upon this "nation of immigrants" with its 100 million people. After a year of work, Congress passed a bill requiring a literacy test of prospective citizens. Wilson vetoed it. As President, he was loath to exercise this power of one man opposing the majority of two houses of Congress, but he felt this bill violated the spirit of the nation, as it excluded those "to whom the opportunities of elementary education have been denied, without regard to their character, their purposes, or

their natural capacity." When the bill appeared before him a second time, he vetoed it again, condemning it as "a penalty for lack of opportunity." But this time the Congress prevailed, planting the first of many hedges against foreign invaders, as the United States inched closer to war.

Wilson had run for President on the proposal of shortening the standard ten-hour workday to eight. At the start of 1916, the railroad workers agitated for that concession from the railway executives. They threatened to strike, which would affect the lives of every American. Henry Ford wired the President that the moment such a strike should occur, the Ford Motor Company—then manufacturing 2,200 cars a day and dependent upon the railroads to transport its product—would shut its factory and all its assembly plants across the country, taking more than forty-nine thousand workers off the payroll. The President reasoned with the railroad brotherhoods to table the rest of their demands while convincing management, in essence, to put America first. Many accused the President of cozying up to labor; but Wilson issued a statement of his own composition stating: "I have recommended the concession of the eight-hour day . . . because I believed the concession right."

Wilson did not leave the capital that summer, so that he could put this legislation—which would become the Adamson Act—on a fast legislative track. After addressing Congress as a whole, he spent the next several days and even nights on the Hill stoking support. The bill's passage averted the strike and marked the beginnings of controversial government intervention into the private enterprise system, bold Presidential action Wilson believed national necessity demanded.

During this time he kept appearing unannounced in the President's Room in the Capitol to lobby Democratic leaders. He also wanted to see the immediate passage of the Keating-Owen child labor bill, which would prohibit the sale in interstate commerce of goods manufactured by children, and the Kern-McGillicuddy bill, a workmen's compensation bill that would protect federal employees in the event of injury or death, thus establishing guidelines for disability insurance. All three pieces of labor legislation quickly passed and received Wilson's signature, establishing guidelines throughout the nation's businesses and industries.

Seldom if ever in American history had a President made good on as many campaign promises as Woodrow Wilson. They were bold pledges, and to help safeguard them, he sent to Congress his most audacious

request yet. In January 1916, a vacancy occurred on the Supreme Court when Joseph Rucker Lamar, Wilson's boyhood friend from Georgia, died. A week later, the President asked McAdoo whom he might suggest to take Lamar's place, and without hesitation McAdoo recommended "the people's lawyer," Louis Brandeis. Nobody embodied the principles of the New Freedom more than this essential member of candidate Wilson's first brain trust; and nobody engendered more of Wilson's admiration than this profound liberal thinker, social activist, and spokesman for the voiceless. But Wilson asked McAdoo if he thought Brandeis could be confirmed. "Yes . . . if you appoint him," McAdoo said, "but it will be a stiff fight." Nobody could have known how rigid that opposition would be.

For all his admirers, Brandeis had enemies everywhere. Because he was a trust-buster, Wall Street regarded him as a radical, or worse; because he was "a militant crusader for social justice," as future Justice William O. Douglas would write, the establishment considered him a troublemaker; because he was an attorney who relied on sociological and psychological data, strict constructionists considered him dangerous, a casuist who would use the Court to activate social change. No less an eminence than former President Taft himself (who had long cast a sheep's eye on the high court) privately called the nomination "one of the deepest wounds that I have ever had as an American and a lover of the Constitution and a believer in progressive conservatism."

Largely unspoken, at least in public, was that Brandeis was a Jew—not only the first to be nominated for a position on the Supreme Court, but an active Zionist at that. To Woodrow Wilson—who had appointed the first Jewish professor at Princeton and the first Jewish Justice to the New Jersey Supreme Court—Brandeis's religion meant nothing, except in its controversial correction of a longtime oversight. If nothing else, Brandeis's presence on the Court would neutralize the biggest mistake Wilson felt he had made as President; it would be the only possible antidote to the conservative anti-Semite James C. McReynolds, whom he had named two years prior.

Since George Washington had begun filling the bench, twenty-one nominees had got tangled in the process of Senate confirmation. Some sensed rejection and withdrew, while eight actually failed to obtain the necessary votes. Historically, the process had been a routine vote, aye or nay—generally the same day the nomination was presented. Opposition to

Brandeis was as rabid as it was rapid. Overnight the establishment press proved especially virulent, attacking his character more than his qualifications. Harvard's President A. Lawrence Lowell—who was about to urge a Jewish quota and segregated dormitories on his liberal campus—mustered more than fifty signatories to a petition denouncing the nomination; six former members of the American Bar Association—Taft and Elihu Root among them—formally objected to the appointment. The Senate Committee on the Judiciary announced an investigation of the many charges already leveled against Brandeis; and McAdoo shrewdly urged Brandeis to ask the committee to hold their hearings in public, as he figured most of the objections would fade in the light of day. The nominee stuck to his work and avoided the press, though he did quietly marshal supporters to hold a brief for him in Congress, where he had no intention of appearing.

On February 9, 1916, a Senate subcommittee considering a high court nominee held a public hearing for the first time. Three Democratic and two Republican Senators listened to testimony before a standing-room-only crowd. More than forty witnesses—largely Boston Brahmins or other establishment figures from the losing side of cases that Brandeis had prosecuted—paraded before the tribunal, cloaking their personal criticisms in rhetoric about dishonorable and unprofessional conduct. More compelling advocates countered every charge, while Felix Frankfurter and Walter Lippmann defended Brandeis in the press and former Harvard President Charles W. Eliot sent the committee a ringing endorsement, as did nine of Harvard Law School's eleven law professors. The arguments came down to a partisan vote. To help seal the nomination, chairman Charles Culberson of Texas asked Wilson to expound upon his reasons for nominating Brandeis.

The President happily obliged. As the committee had already put to rest any personal accusations and aspersions, Wilson cited former Chief Justice Melville Fuller, who had called Brandeis "the ablest man who ever appeared before the Supreme Court of the United States." Speaking for himself, Wilson wrote:

> I cannot speak too highly of his impartial, impersonal, orderly, and constructive mind, his rare analytical powers, his deep human sympathy, his profound acquaintance with the historical roots of our

institutions and insight into their spirit, or of the many evidences he
has given of being imbued to the very heart with our American ideals
of economic conditions and of the way they bear upon the masses of
the people.

Culberson made the letter public; and Brandeis supporters arranged a few
private social encounters between wavering Senators and the nominee
himself. The four-month confirmation process was as brutal as any the
Court, if not the country, had ever seen—a "low-tech lynching." It opened
the doors for future examination of judicial nominees, who were soon required to defend themselves in person.

After partisan committee votes, the full Senate confirmed Brandeis on
June 1 as the sixty-seventh Supreme Court Justice by a vote of 47 to 22.
One Democrat and three progressive Republicans crossed the aisle. "I
never signed any commission with such satisfaction as I sign his," Wilson
told Henry Morgenthau in concluding another highly successful Congressional inning, with no action more far-reaching than that appointment: if
a Jew could ascend to the country's highest court, there was no stopping
other minorities from shattering other glass ceilings, even though it would
take generations to slough off age-old prejudices. Whenever Brandeis
spoke in judicial conference, for example, Wilson's first appointee, Justice
McReynolds, was known simply to rise and leave the room. He went so far
as to avoid official Court pictures because he did not want to be photo-
graphed with a Jew. And when Brandeis retired in 1939—leaving a distinguished legacy of liberal decisions behind him—he received the customary
panegyric letter, signed by his colleagues . . . all except one.

"That summer of 1916 was crowded with every sort of thing," Edith
Wilson would recall. "First on the list was the ever-encroaching menace of
the War in Europe. Then came the Presidential campaign." Nationalism
had become a global epidemic, and it had at last infected the United
States. The First Lady was still trying to process how she had awakened
from her uncomplicated quiet life into a world in which every public
moment was fraught with significance. Woodrow encouraged her to learn
all the verses of "The Star-Spangled Banner," for she would surely need to
know them. Indeed, it had become a season of endless flag-waving, a

coming of age for the nation, its first reunion since the country had divided a half century earlier.

June 14—the day in 1777 on which Congress had adopted the Stars and Stripes as the emblem of the Union—had been sporadically observed ever since the start of the Civil War; but in the spring of 1916, Wilson officially proclaimed it a day for "special patriotic exercises" on which Americans might "rededicate ourselves to the nation, 'one and inseparable,' from which every thought that is not worthy of our fathers' first views of independence, liberty, and right shall be excluded." It had an electrifying effect.

The entire month was filled with one parade after another. The message was the same everywhere: "Americanism" and preparedness. Chicago staged the largest parade in its history, in which more than 130,000 people—each carrying a flag—marched for more than eleven hours. There were neither floats nor costumes, just people from all walks of life— telephone operators, bankers, judges, firemen, Spanish-American War veterans, and druggists—marching to the cheers of one million onlookers. Even militant feminist Alice Paul leading a troop of fifty suffragists down Michigan Avenue, against the flow, drew cheers from the crowd as fellow marchers diverted themselves to the curb so that the ladies might pass. On Long Island, 2,500 "Pilgrims" marched through Oyster Bay to the Roosevelt home at Sagamore Hill—each carrying a flag—to appeal to the Colonel to lead the nation once again. In Hollywood, German-born Carl Laemmle had his Universal Film Manufacturing Company release a forty-reel serial called *Liberty*, and his studio staged a preparedness parade.

Nobody exhibited more patriotism that season than the President himself. At Arlington National Cemetery on Memorial Day, he raised George Washington's time-honored argument against "entangling alliances"; but, by way of national preparation, Wilson suggested, "I would gladly assent to . . . an alliance which would disentangle the peoples of the world from those combinations in which they seek their own separate and private interests and unite the people of the world to preserve the peace of the world upon a basis of common right and justice." On Flag Day, he led a parade of sixty-six thousand down Pennsylvania Avenue, from the Capitol to the White House, and spoke of the flag's importance as it united a people whose citizenship was derived from every nation in the world. "Americanism" became the shibboleth of the day, as Wilson urged citizens

to pledge their allegiance to the flag of the United States of America instead of honoring the hyphen that linked every American to the country of his ancestry. Wilson insisted the time had come for "hyphenated" citizenship to end.

That same week, Wilson addressed the graduating class of the United States Military Academy, where he seemed to allude to Teddy Roosevelt as he asserted, "I am an American, but I do not believe that any of us loves a blustering nationality—a nationality with a chip on its shoulder, a nationality with its elbows out and its swagger on. We love that quiet, self-respecting, unconquerable spirit which doesn't strike until it is necessary to strike, and then strikes to conquer." A decade later, Vice President Marshall would reflect on those "long and weary" months of 1916, remembering that Wilson was "busy with the hope of finding some loophole through which he might enter as the great pacifier of the conflict in Europe."

Amid this patriotic fervor, the Republican Party opened its National Convention in the Chicago Coliseum on June 7, 1916. The delegates hoped to select from among a half dozen candidates the one most likely to beat Wilson, but their own house was still in disarray. They had not resolved the differences that had riven the Grand Old Party in 1912 and driven it to defeat. The Republicans remained so divided that the Progressive Party, their offshoot, opened its own convention a mile away, in the Auditorium. The Bull Moosers were eager to rejoin their old herd, should the Republicans be of the same mind. They nominated Theodore Roosevelt, hoping that would incite the Republicans to do the same so they could all join forces.

But the Republicans were not ready to reembrace the man they believed had put personality and even principles before party. As the convention opened, the delegates seemed predisposed to an undeclared candidate who said he would accept the nomination—the former Governor of New York and current Associate Justice of the Supreme Court Charles Evans Hughes. Eager to be drafted, he received as many votes on the first ballot as the next two contenders combined, while former President Roosevelt ran a distant sixth. Hughes obtained the nomination on the third ballot. Running with TR's former Vice President, Charles W. Fairbanks of Indiana, he remained pro-business and eager to enter the war.

As Hughes became the only Supreme Court Justice ever to leave the bench in order to run for President, Wilson promptly elevated the

progressive John Hessin Clarke, whom he had appointed as a District Court Judge. Clarke would become a reliable vote within the liberal bloc, though he would remain on the Court only six years. Insiders knew that animosity between him and Justice McReynolds contributed to his early departure; and, indeed, the retirement letter from his brethren—like Brandeis's—would fall one signature short.

Wilson spent the early weeks of June drafting the national Democratic platform. The document expanded upon the programs of the New Freedom; and it made particular mention of extending the franchise to the women of the country, though he maintained that the most effective means of achieving such equality was through state-by-state ratification.

The following week, Democrats gathered at the St. Louis Coliseum for their convention, which was more of a coronation. Although the incumbent did not appear for the ceremonies, he controlled the convention from the White House. The three days of ballyhoo played according to the script, with the exception of one speech. Former New York Governor Martin H. Glynn, at Wilson's behest, delivered the keynote address. Seeing one issue overshadowing all the rest, Glynn provided a brief review of moments in history when Presidents of all parties could have drawn the nation into international hostilities but refrained. As Glynn cited example after example, from Washington to Benjamin Harrison, he recited a simple chorus—"But we didn't go to war." Adams, Jefferson, Van Buren, Pierce, and Grant all "settled our troubles by negotiation just as the President of the United States is trying to do today." The applause at the end of the speech raised the Coliseum's rafters and resonated across the country. While there were plenty of issues on which to run, the Democrats chose to peg their campaign to one irrefutable theme: "He kept us out of war."

The office of the Vice President of the United States was still something between a figurehead and a fool; and in each capacity, Thomas R. Marshall excelled. A few Vice Presidents served as liaisons between the White House and the Senate; but because Wilson made regular Congressional visits, Marshall was redundant even in that role. The President invited him to attend Cabinet meetings but showed so little interest in his opinions, Marshall saw no reason to appear. Like many of his predecessors who served as President of the United States Senate, Marshall considered the Executive Mansion out of bounds. In his four-hundred-page memoirs, Marshall would mention Woodrow Wilson's name only a handful of times.

Even so, he remained a popular figure in Washington. TR's acerbic daughter Alice Roosevelt Longworth especially enjoyed poking fun at him, claiming that his business card read "Vice President of the United States and Toastmaster." Indeed, Marshall was a delightful speaker and always had an amusing quip on the tip of his tongue. During one session when a Senator was holding the floor too long, yammering about all the things "this country needs," Marshall leaned in toward a clerk and said in a stage whisper, "What this country needs is a really good five-cent cigar." The quotation stands as Marshall's most durable legacy, coupled, perhaps, with his anecdote of a mother who had two sons, one of whom became Vice President while the other was lost at sea . . . "and nothing has been heard from either of them since." But while Wilson and Marshall had private policy disagreements, the Vice President never displayed anything but loyalty toward the President. There was no reason to break up a winning ticket. Besides, Indiana—with its admixture of rural and industrial populations—was sure to be a close race in the national election; and the Republican nominee, Charles Fairbanks, had been a popular Hoosier Senator, a political figure once so promising that he even had a town in Alaska named after him.

The railroad crisis and insufferable heat that summer exacerbated Wilson's gastric distress, severe headaches, and extreme fatigue. "I get desperately tired somedays," he wrote his daughter Jessie, "and am glad to get to bed every day." Colonel House was especially mindful of how tired he had looked at Dr. Grayson's recent wedding.

The Wilsons were not able to leave Washington until the first of September for their summer vacation at a large estate called Shadow Lawn, in Long Branch, New Jersey, near Asbury Park. The big white house—complete with a semicircular portico—suggested a seaside version of the Wilsons' home in Washington. Edith said it felt like a hotel and referred to the entry as "the lobby." Woodrow said it reminded him of a gambling hall. But the expansive grounds could accommodate crowds for campaign speeches, and the gates in front provided privacy. Hoping to avoid the scourge of infantile paralysis that plagued the East Coast, the McAdoos, with their two young children, joined the President at the Jersey Shore. The Wilsons and the rest of their extended "family"—which included her brother Randolph, Helen Bones, the Graysons, and Tumulty—quickly settled into Shadow Lawn until the election, in part to reassert Wilson's

right to vote in New Jersey. The other reason they abandoned the Executive Mansion for several months, according to Edith, was "my husband declined to use the White House, the Nation's property, for a political purpose."

Because custom prevented Presidential nominees (even sitting Presidents) from attending their nominating conventions, the conventions came to them. On September 2, the Notification Committee of the Democratic Party arrived at Shadow Lawn, with the Vice President, the Cabinet, Congressmen, and party leaders in tow, and twenty thousand partisans in their wake. A speaker's platform had been erected for Wilson. After thanking the party for renewing its trust in him, he catalogued the formidable record the Administration had amassed—from the revision of the tariffs to its most far-reaching piece of legislation, that very week's Revenue Act of 1916. This statute incorporated several items dating back to the Populist movement a quarter century earlier, including a graduated tax rate based on ability to pay. The bill raised the tax from 1 to 2 percent on net annual incomes above $4,000 and included a surtax as high as 13 percent on incomes above $2 million; it also imposed an estate tax as high as 10 percent on $5 million legacies, and, foreseeing a windfall for one particular industry, a steep tax on the manufacture of munitions. Critics gasped at this redistribution of wealth; Wilson considered it "equitable."

His speech—with its recital of 1912 campaign promises delivered— ran justifiably long; but it emphasized America's commitment to the future. "We are to play a leading part in the world drama whether we wish it or not," he said. "We shall lend, not borrow; act for ourselves, not imitate or follow." Far from his 1914 insistence upon neutrality, Wilson now insisted that no nation "can any longer remain neutral as against any wilful disturbance of the peace of the world. The effects of war can no longer be confined to the areas of battle. No nation stands wholly apart in interest when the life and interest of all nations are thrown into confusion and peril. . . . The nations of the world must unite in joint guarantees that whatever is done to disturb the whole world's life must first be tested in the court of the whole world's opinion before it is attempted."

He left New Jersey to make several speeches—including one at Lincoln's birthplace in Kentucky—before bringing his "non-campaign" to a halt when he learned that his sister Annie, ill in New London, Connecticut, had taken a turn for the worse. Woodrow and Edith immediately

went north to visit and remained there for several days. Because of the obvious strain on the President, and because nobody could predict how much longer Annie Wilson Howe might live, her physician urged him to return to Shadow Lawn. Two days later, Annie died. They accompanied her coffin to her funeral in South Carolina, where Woodrow walked his wife through his childhood house. He would assume his sister's debts.

Upon returning to New Jersey, the President undertook the double duty of running the country and campaigning for the privilege of continuing to do so. Every Saturday he delivered a political address from the front porch at Shadow Lawn; and any given day brought Cabinet members, Colonel House, Ambassador Page from England, or Vance C. McCormick, a former Mayor of Harrisburg, Pennsylvania, whom Wilson had anointed the new chairman of the Democratic National Committee. Henry Ford, who admired Wilson's strength in maintaining American neutrality and in keeping the trains running, offered nominal (though not monetary) support. He told the President that based on their conferences, he had taken the unusual step of providing pay equality for his women employees. Ignacy Paderewski, the brilliant Polish pianist and political activist, paid a visit, asking the President to remember the Poles caught in the crossfire between Russia and Germany. Edith could not help kneeling on the landing above the two men, watching Paderewski's moving expression as he pled so earnestly for his people.

Wilson did take to the hustings in a few of the many toss-up states. Half the electoral college map was already accounted for: Republican New England plus New York, Pennsylvania, and Michigan would deliver the same number of electors as the solid Democratic South. Thus, the battleground became the Midwest and the less populous but more Populist states of the far West. Except for California, the stakes were so low in each of the farthermost Western states that they hardly merited a nominee's time. Wilson traveled only as far as Ohio, Indiana, Illinois, and Nebraska.

Political campaigns had grown savvier in analyzing demographics; and the Democrats targeted specific constituencies, sending the most appropriate surrogates to address them. In multicultural New York, Jewish, Polish, and Italian leaders mobilized their neighborhoods. William Jennings Bryan campaigned aggressively for Wilson in the West. And, because he was the most consistent vote for peace and progressivism, the National Democratic Speakers' Committee sent the popular blind Senator

T. P. Gore to speak up and down the California coast. Gore disagreed with the President on several issues, but he effectively argued that Wilson had kept America out of war and showed the most promise to continue doing so.

W. E. B. Du Bois wrote the President of his disappointment in his tenure and called upon him to account for the dismissal of colored public officials and for segregation in the Civil Service. As a member of that underclass, he asked what progress Negroes had seen, even when it came to lynching. Wilson replied through Tumulty that he had tried to live up to his original assurances, "though in some cases my endeavors have been defeated." He had, in fact, issued a strong statement condemning lynching—hardly conscience-challenging, one would have thought, though it did mark the first time a President had gone on record doing as much. Although some Negro organizations continued to trust Wilson enough "to do the just thing at the proper time," Du Bois urged his followers to vote Socialist.

Wilson was still the most inspiring orator on the stump. His refusal to talk down to audiences continued to elevate them; and the inevitable patriotic punch line with which he closed every speech went straight from his heart to that of his audience. He was so eloquent the day he addressed the National American Woman Suffrage Association in Atlantic City—maintaining his position of state-by-state enfranchisement—even outgoing NAWSA president Dr. Anna Howard Shaw could not resist him. The very fact that he did not pander for votes by coming out in favor of the federal amendment as so many wanted him to do, she said, "showed such respect for our intelligence" and a "sincerity of purpose when he said he would fight with us."

Wilson could also play rough. An Irish agitator named Jeremiah O'Leary was president of the American Truth Society, an ostensibly nonpartisan—but fanatically anti-English—organization. With their support, O'Leary released an unusually vitriolic letter to Wilson, condemning his "dictatorship over Congress" and his "truckling to the British Empire." Wilson called a press conference, at which he read the wire he had sent in reply: "Your telegram received. I would feel deeply mortified to have you or anybody like you vote for me. Since you have access to many disloyal Americans and I have not, I will ask you to convey this message to them."

And he could be funny. The President instinctively knew how to warm up audiences, invariably opening with a light remark. One of his favorites

was about a magazine correspondent researching the life of Mark Twain. The writer had gone to Hannibal, Missouri, where he encountered the only local who actually remembered Samuel Clemens as a child. He was, unfortunately, somewhat feebleminded; and so the interviewer had to keep jogging recollections out of him. He tried prompting the old fellow with the names of famous Twain characters—such as Tom Sawyer and Huckleberry Finn. But upon hearing each name, the old Missourian just blankly scratched his head. In a final attempt, the interviewer asked if he had ever heard of Pudd'nhead Wilson. "Oh, yes," said the old man, looking up and beaming, "I voted for him last year."

Although Wilson appeared younger than his opponent, Charles Evans Hughes—with his sculpted beard and mustache—was, in fact, six years the President's junior. But the two men were in many ways alike. The son of a (Baptist) minister, Hughes was a skilled debater, a lawyer, and a scholar (who had taught Greek and mathematics and, later, law at Cornell); and he too was a compelling orator. But his campaign never expressed either a consistent vision or a positive message. The Republicans' pro-business platform criticized Wilson's positions against tariffs and trusts, but the recession he had inherited had dissipated within two years and citizens felt the Democrats were looking after their interests. Wilson announced to a group of businessmen in Detroit that the United States had just become a creditor nation. It currently held more of the surplus gold in the world than ever before, and "our business hereafter is to . . . lend and to help and to promote the great peaceful enterprises of the world." Finding little traction, the Republicans offered derogatory generalizations or carped over tax tables.

The Republicans denounced Wilson's halting foreign policy, but they had to keep from sounding bloodthirsty. Hughes was nowhere near as vituperative as TR, or even Henry Cabot Lodge, who summarized Wilson's foreign policy after the German sinking of the *Sussex* as little more than "brave words. More notes. More conversation." Because Hughes often restrained his feelings, some Republicans called him "Wilson with whiskers." His tendency to make one set of arguments for pro-German audiences and another for the pro-British earned him the nickname "Charles Evasive Hughes." In the words of Vice President Marshall, the Allies revealed themselves to be the "less corrupter" of the two sides in the Great War; but still, "war was abhorrent to the great mass of Americans, and the

campaign of 1916 . . . [was] based largely on the fact that the president had kept us out."

The Republican Party never united behind its candidate. "It had no constructive policy," recalled Secretary McAdoo. "The Republicans carried on a campaign of criticism. Professional critics are seldom elevated to positions where creative talent is the chief quality required." Roosevelt's contempt for Wilson grew satanic—enough for him to set aside his own reservations about Hughes and campaign in a few strategic states for him. "Instead of speaking softly and carrying a big stick," said TR in Louisville, "President Wilson spoke bombastically and carried a dishrag."

TR never stopped attacking the President for reducing the country to an "elocutionary ostrich." Roosevelt derided Wilson's "He kept us out of war" slogan as nothing more than "ignoble shirking of responsibility . . . clothed in an utterly misleading phrase, the phrase of a coward." In reality, Colonel Roosevelt explained, "war has been creeping nearer and nearer, until it stares at us from just beyond our three-mile limit, and we face it without policy, plan, purpose or preparation." Because Roosevelt endorsed Hughes, the Bull Moose Party disbanded. TR hoped to lead his Progressives home to the Republican Party. The more chauvinistic patriots among them followed, but many found greater kinship among the Democrats.

Unlike Wilson, Hughes barnstormed the country. While campaigning in California, he checked into the Virginia Hotel in Long Beach, where Governor Hiram Johnson happened to be staying while running for the Senate. This popular figure rather expected to receive at least a message if not a courtesy call from his party's leader, but none came; and Johnson resumed his campaign running for himself and not his party. Hughes's widely reported snub did nothing to stanch the flow of Progressives to the Democrats, and the Republicans turned even more mean-spirited. Secretary Daniels believed "that no campaign in the history of the country has been quite so marked by viciousness, bitterness and invective. All the elements of hate and misrepresentation were brought into play." As the election neared, Wilson felt his opposition had sunk to unspeakable depths, so low, he told a reporter, that he had "an utter contempt for Mr. Hughes."

Indeed, Hughes shouted for months about the Adamson Act and the intrusion of government into the lives of Americans. He cried that he was not "too proud to fight"; some Republicans whispered about "Mrs. Peck" and the spurious affair while the first Mrs. Wilson was alive, and a party

representative offered Mary Hulbert several hundred thousand dollars for Wilson's letters, an offer she refused; other Republicans shrieked that the Revenue Act was nothing less than Socialism. As for the Socialists themselves, their leader, Eugene Debs, forwent a fifth consecutive run for the White House in favor of a more pragmatic path to power. He ran for Congress from his home district in Indiana, railing against the President. "Mr. Wilson, who had all his life been opposed to militarism, has now become the avowed champion of plutocratic preparedness," he argued, "and today he stands before the country pleading in the name of Wall Street and its interests for the largest standing army and the most powerful navy in the world." But after months of campaign cacophony—and with German U-boats cruising the waters off Connecticut and Rhode Island—one phrase continued to resonate: "He kept us out of war."

Social reformers Jane Addams and Lillian D. Wald rallied behind Wilson, as did leftist intellectuals Max Eastman, John Reed, Herbert Croly, a cofounder of *The New Republic,* and one of his first staff members, Walter Lippmann. The latter became Wilson's strongest advocate through articles in his influential magazine of Progressive thought. Where he had once been a strong TR supporter and Wilson critic, Lippmann had now come to appreciate that the President was a man of vision. He argued to his colleagues, "What we're electing is a war President—not the man who kept us out of war. And we've got to make up our minds whether we want to go through the war with Hughes or with Wilson." Lippmann appreciated that truly thoughtful people could—and inevitably should—have the power to change their minds, as he did in the pages of *The New Republic* just before the election. "I shall not vote for the Wilson who has uttered a few too many noble sentiments," he wrote, "but for the Wilson who is evolving under experience and is remaking his philosophy in the light of it."

"If I understand myself," Wilson told Ida Tarbell in an interview in *Collier's* that ran the week before the election, "I am sincere when I say that I have no personal desire for reelection." Indeed, he admitted that he regretted not having been able to read a serious book in years. "It would be an unspeakable relief to be excused, but I am caught in the midst of a process." He reminded the voters that his progressive program was a work in progress; and he asked, "Is it wise that the country should change now, leaving so much at loose ends?" Tarbell could not help thinking of Lincoln in

August 1864, when he felt he might not be reelected and made a secret compact with himself to cooperate as much as possible with the President-elect, to save the Union in the period between the election and the inauguration. For weeks Wilson had been developing a secret compact of his own.

Since 1886, the law had stipulated that in the event of vacancies in the offices of both the President and the Vice President, the line of succession ran through the Cabinet, starting with the Secretary of State. In light of the seriousness of the world situation and the speed with which crises required handling, Wilson devised an exit strategy should Hughes win. He would ask Marshall and Lansing to resign from their positions so that he could appoint Hughes Secretary of State; then Wilson would resign, allowing Hughes to take office immediately instead of having to wait until the following March.

On Sunday, November 5, 1916, the President of the United States sat in his office at Shadow Lawn and typed a strictly confidential letter to the Secretary of State, one unique in Presidential archives. He outlined the plan, not overlooking the "consent and cooperation" of the Vice President and Secretary Lansing himself. Wilson thought his argument compelling enough for both men to accept: "No such critical circumstances in regard to our foreign policy have ever before existed. It would be my duty to step aside so that there would be no doubt in any quarter how that policy was to be directed. . . . I would have no right to risk the peace of the nation by remaining in office after I had lost my authority." He sent the letter and fully intended to act upon it, if necessary—"just as soon as the result of the election was definitely known."

Only that morning, Edith had spoken to her husband about losing the election, which she expected. Such a result was difficult for Wilson to imagine, having just faced tens of thousands in cheering throngs at Madison Square Garden and Cooper Union in New York City. But the candidate's wife had endured sleepless nights, tossing and turning over the opposition to Wilson's Mexican policy, the daily news from Europe, and, most of all, the massive amounts of money the Republicans had spent to smear him. Without knowing of Woodrow's plan, she told him how happy they would be living their own lives. Upon hearing her, Woodrow stood and said, "What a delightful pessimist you are! One must never court defeat. If it comes, accept it like a soldier; but don't anticipate it, for that destroys your fighting spirit." They took a long ride along the Jersey Shore.

Tuesday morning the Wilsons drove to Princeton, arriving a little before nine. Crowds of students and photographers watched the President
vote in the firehouse. He spent the rest of the day back at Shadow Lawn
working, making lists of states with the number of electors from each. The
telegraph company offered to run a special wire into the house so he could
receive the election results as they were transmitted, but Wilson said he
would rather learn the news by telephone from his campaign directors.
Early indications from Colorado and Kansas suggested that Wilson would
do better there than he had in 1912. After a quiet dinner, the family
passed the time playing Twenty Questions. Then at ten o'clock the telephone rang. A friend of Margaret's in New York was calling with condolences. Margaret could barely speak, spluttering that it was too early to
know any results, that the polls were still open in the West. The caller
explained that *The New York Times* had announced that it would indicate
the winner with a colored light atop its building—white for Wilson, red
for Hughes—and there was no mistaking the flash of crimson.

Dr. Grayson arrived from the executive offices in Asbury Park with the
news that the New York *World* had also predicted a Hughes victory; and
when the President phoned Tumulty, the normally cheery Irishman delivered the same verdict. In spite of that, Tumulty issued a statement that
Wilson would win, once the results from the West arrived. Wilson laughed
over the phone and said, "Well, Tumulty, it begins to look as if we have
been badly licked." Tumulty heard no sadness in his boss's voice and offered more positive signs from the West. "Tumulty, you are an optimist,"
Wilson replied. "It begins to look as if the defeat might be overwhelming.
The only thing I am sorry for, and that cuts me to the quick, is that the
people apparently misunderstood us. But I have no regrets. We have tried
to do our duty."

Shadow Lawn darkened. At last, Wilson said, "Well, I will not send
Mr. Hughes a telegram of congratulation tonight, for things are not settled." And then his face turned grave as he acknowledged the inevitability
of Hughes's bringing the country into the war. Hughes himself remained
properly silent that night, but Theodore Roosevelt could not help himself from issuing a statement at ten o'clock, saying, "I am doubly thank-
ful as an American for the election of Mr. Hughes. It is a vindication of
our national honor." At Shadow Lawn, the butler brought a tray of sandwiches and beverages to the family. At 10:30, Wilson grabbed a glass of

milk, said his goodnights, and added, "I might stay longer but you are all so blue."

Edith joined him a few minutes later. "Well, little girl," he said, "you were right in expecting we should lose the election. Frankly I did not, but we can now do some of the things we want to do." She sat on his bed, holding his hand, ready to discuss the future. In an instant he fell into a deep sleep, as though a great burden had been lifted.

Edith was less fortunate. Feeling her husband's pain, she was wide awake at 4 a.m., when someone knocked on her door. Margaret had just spoken to Vance McCormick at Democratic headquarters in New York and learned that the West was reporting unexpectedly favorable results. Margaret asked if they should awaken her father, and Edith said, "Oh no, do let him sleep."

At daybreak, the results remained in doubt. Some newspapers reported the Hughes victory, while the more cautious press only hinted as much— what with New York, Pennsylvania, and Illinois having gone Republican by hundreds of thousands of votes. New Jersey went solidly for Hughes, as did Iowa. But the electoral race remained neck and neck all day. New Hampshire and Delaware were each tipping Republican by only 1,000 votes, and Minnesota by 392 votes. And then Ohio surprisingly swung Democratic. Idaho followed; and so did New Hampshire by 56 votes. A reporter was said to have called Hughes in New York that morning hoping to get his comments on this possible Democratic trend. "The President can't be disturbed," the aide said. "Well," replied the reporter, "when he wakes up tell him he's no longer president."

That comment was premature as well. The race had come down to the one state that had yet to report its results—California, with 13 electoral votes. Poll watchers there guarded every ballot box amid allegations of voter fraud. Each ballot was painstakingly tallied. Into the morning after the election, the race remained a dead heat. A significant reason for the delay was that Sierra County, one hundred miles northeast of Sacramento and high in the Sierra Nevada, had not been heard from. An early snow had fallen upon sixteen rural precincts there. Voters had turned out, but now an entire nation had to wait for horse-drawn wagons carrying the ballot boxes to traverse the snowy crude roads so that the votes of this tiny county could be counted and certified.

Margaret Wilson knocked on her father's bathroom door while he was

shaving that morning to tell him that *The New York Times* had printed an "Extra" edition of the paper that day suggesting that the election was still in doubt but leaning Wilson's way. "Tell that to the Marines," Wilson said, running the razor across his face. Incertitude persisted through the day and into the next. On Thursday the ninth, Woodrow and Edith went to Spring Lake to play golf, and while they were at the eighth tee, Dr. Grayson arrived with news from headquarters about California, which was favorable but not definitive. Throughout the ordeal, the President maintained his calm, though Edith discerned his tension. On November 10, California officially went for Wilson by 3,806 votes and the election was over.

Pundits suggested that Hughes's snub of Hiram Johnson cost him the Presidency. A sounder explanation for the traditionally Republican state's turning Democratic that year was that in the final stretch of the campaign, Senator Gore of Oklahoma kept driving the same point to the crowds he drew in the West: "A vote for Hughes is a vote for war. A vote for Wilson is a vote for peace." A decade later, Gore himself concluded, "The women voters in the west elected Wilson on the peace issue." Indeed, twelve states in the Union then allowed women to vote in the Presidential election, eleven of which were in the West, ten of which went for Wilson. Despite their small numbers, women had become an electoral constituency in the United States.

The final electoral vote count was 277 to 254, which fairly reflected the popular vote: 9,126,868 for Wilson and 8,548,728 for Hughes—49.2 percent to 46.1 percent. The Socialist candidate captured 3 percent of the vote, and a few minor candidates less than that. Wilson became the first Democratic President elected to a second consecutive term since Andrew Jackson in 1832. He was also the first man since James K. Polk in 1844 to get elected without carrying his home state. There were other signs of erosion of public support: in Congressional races, the Democrats lost two seats in the Senate, leaving them with a comfortable but decreasing margin of 54 to 42; and they suffered another bad hit in the House of Representatives, dropping to 214 members against 215 Republicans. Because three Progressives chose to caucus with the Democrats, the President's party could cobble together a coalition and maintain control of both houses. The South remained Wilson's igneous base, where he carried some states with more than 90 percent of the vote.

Wilson's dearest friend from Charlottesville, Heath Dabney, pointed out that the President had received more votes than any candidate had ever received for any office on earth—three million votes more than he had received in 1912—and his tallies in the individual states were almost always larger than those of Democratic candidates for Congress or governorships. Woodrow and Edith left directly for Williamstown, Massachusetts, for the baptism of Frank and Jessie Sayre's daughter, named Eleanor Axson; and then the President and his wife returned to the White House, after months away, to begin his second term. Charles Evans Hughes did not concede by telegram until November 22, 1916, claiming he had waited for the official count in California to end. Wilson replied graciously, though he commented to his brother, Josie, that Hughes's wire "was a little moth-eaten when it got here but quite legible."

"My husband . . . was weary and unwell," Edith would recall, "—reaction from the strain of the campaign." Other factors, of course, weighed heavily upon him. Thousands of miles away, the war continued to rage, as the British persisted in blockading and the Germans in torpedoing. The Continent became a charnel house—1916 seeing more slaughter than any year in history, with three of the bloodiest battles ever fought. The months-long Battle of Verdun produced 800,000 casualties; twice that number were wounded or killed in the second half of the year in the Battle of the Somme (where the prescient American poet Alan Seeger had his "rendezvous with Death"); another 1,600,000 people fell that summer in the Brusilov offensive, in which Russia defeated the Central Powers on the Eastern Front; and lesser battles in 1916 saw another 600,000 killed or wounded.

While the seas had remained quiet since the *Sussex* note of the spring had demanded that the Germans stop attacking ships with American passengers, turbulence returned. In less than three weeks, U-boats sank four ships conducting trade between Britain and the United States, taking several American lives. The Germans insisted they were playing by the rules, and notes continued to be exchanged as Germany offered reasonable enough excuses to warrant months of investigation. "Foreseeing an inevitable crisis with Germany over the frequent sinking of our ships," Tumulty recorded, Wilson believed that he could not "draw the whole country with

him in aggressive action if before he took the step leading to war he had not tried out every means of peace." His enemies decried his "meekness and apparent subservience to German diplomacy." In truth, the British did not make Wilson's life any easier.

That summer England had imposed a "black list," which forbade Britons from dealing with eighty-five American companies the government perceived as conducting business for the benefit of their enemies. Congress considered retaliation in the form of an embargo on loans and supplies, but the President argued otherwise. He recalled a similar vengeful action in 1807 in which "the states themselves suffered from the act more than the nations whose trade they struck at."

To complicate matters, neither side in Europe was ready to throw in the towel. "Never before in the world's history," observed Wilson, "have two great armies been in effect so equally matched; never before have the losses and the slaughter been so great with as little gain in military advantage. Both sides have grown weary of the apparently hopeless task of bringing the conflict to an end by the force of arms; inevitably they are being forced to the realization that it can only be brought about by the attrition of human suffering, in which the victor suffers hardly less than the vanquished." The brutal fighting had lasted so long, each side was punch-drunk, convinced that the next blow would provide the knockout.

By December, a chink had appeared in the German armor. Wilson received intelligence revealing that "Germany as a whole"—its most militaristic factions aside—appeared "ready to welcome steps toward peace as the food situation, while by no means critical, is becoming more and more difficult and as there is a general weariness of war." Chancellor von Bethmann Hollweg and new Foreign Secretary Arthur Zimmermann showed signs of budging. In London, Colonel House met with a colleague of David Lloyd George's and said that England had become "the only obstacle to peace." Wilson was eager as ever to mediate a settlement, one he felt could include everything England had been fighting for. Even though House had said that the United States had been "quite unneutral in its friendliness to England," both sides complained that America had been partial toward the other. Each wanted commercial advantages from America—in the way of food and munitions—without offering anything in return, not even a willingness to negotiate peace.

On November 25, Wilson sat at his desk and considered the uniqueness

of his position. "Perhaps I am the only person in high authority amongst all the peoples of the world who is at liberty to speak and hold nothing back," he wrote. He could speak "as an individual" and "as the responsible head of a great government." As such he felt compelled to speak not only for the people of the United States but "for friends of humanity in every nation." He hoped to produce a series of terms that would deliver "an enduring peace." Unlike prior conflicts, Wilson believed this war—"with its unprecedented human waste and suffering and its drain of material resource"—presented "an unparalleled opportunity for the statesmen of the world to make such a peace possible." Toward that end, Wilson drafted what came to be called a "peace note" to all the powers at war. He told Edith it "may prove the greatest piece of work of my life."

Wilson called upon leaders on both sides to clarify their respective war aims and to consider their progress in the last two years. "The conflict moves very sluggishly," he suggested; and a prolonged war could only lead to "irreparable damage to civilization." Wilson proposed a conference of representatives of the belligerent governments and of the governments whose interests were directly involved. He was not butting in either to mediate or even to propose peace. He was merely calling for "a concrete definition of the guarantees which the belligerents on the one side and the other deem it their duty to demand as a practical satisfaction of the objects they are aiming at in this contest of force." The answers to these questions, he said, would be nonbinding, merely suggestions to help neutral nations determine their future courses of action. "The United States," he said, "feels that it can no longer delay to determine its own."

The next night, Colonel House arrived at the White House, and the President read to him what he had drafted thus far. House thought it was "a wonderfully well written document" but that Wilson's suggestion that "the causes and objects of the war are obscure" would enrage the Allies. House explained that such a remark suggested no understanding of the Allies' viewpoint, which held "that Germany started the war for conquest; that she broke all international obligations and laws of humanity in pursuit of it." The British claimed to be fighting "to make such another war impossible, and to so break Prussian militarism that a permanent peace may be established."

Over the next two weeks, Wilson edited his "peace note." In calling upon the leaders to articulate their objectives, Wilson believed he might

get the antagonists to realize that "peace is nearer than we know; that the terms which the belligerents . . . would deem it necessary to insist upon are not so irreconcilable as some have feared." On Friday, December 15, he read his revised version to his Cabinet. McAdoo and Houston strongly opposed sending it, as it "might be regarded as an act of friendship toward Germany and possibly as a threat." After a lengthy discussion, the President said, "I will send this note or nothing." And at 9:30 p.m. on December 18, he sent it. House revealed to his diary, "I find the President has nearly destroyed all the work I have done in Europe. He knows how I feel about this and how the Allies feel about it, and yet the refrain always appears in some form or other." Although he kept his feelings private, he remained angry at the President for weeks—though not as angry as the President became with Secretary Lansing for a highly indiscreet blunder.

Feeling that the "peace note" gave the appearance of complicity with the Germans' recent overtures, the Secretary of State issued his own statement, in which he indicated that the note had sprung from America's increasing involvement with the belligerents. "I mean by that," he added, digging a shallow grave for himself, "that we are drawing nearer the verge of war ourselves, and therefore we are entitled to know exactly what each belligerent seeks, in order that we may regulate our conduct in the future." Wilson was furious. The note not only second-guessed him but provided what he considered an unnecessary addendum, one that would only further cloud the murky waters of diplomacy. Worse, it revealed that Lansing was not in sympathy with Wilson's desire to stay out of this war. The stock market plummeted, as war jitters triggered the most precipitous one-day drop in fifteen years.

The President all but called for Lansing's resignation. Instead, he dictated a follow-up statement for the Secretary to release—which offered both his correction and his contrition. Wall Street bounced back the next day. The "peace note" episode reminded the American foreign policy team that it was essentially a one-man band.

Twenty-two relatives gathered at the White House to celebrate Christmas 1916 and Wilson's sixtieth birthday. "We thank God for all you mean to the World, and trust that your life and strength may be spared for many years," wrote Cleveland Dodge, "to solve the great problems which you, better than anyone else, can solve." Wilson believed as much himself. With the belligerents failing to reply with the terms he had requested, Wilson decided to state his own. He formulated a general resolution to the great

conflict and something more—"making the keystone of the settlement arch the future security of the world against wars, and letting territorial adjustments be subordinate to the main purpose." On January 3, 1917, he and Colonel House conferred, laying cornerstones of the foundation. The main tenet was "the right of nations to determine under what government they should continue to live." Beyond that, Wilson thought Poland should be free and independent, Belgium and Serbia should be restored, and the vast Turkish Empire should be dismantled. House urged granting Russia maritime access to the south—"a warm seaport"—without which, he feared, they would surely go to war again. Wilson set to work on a speech that would outline not only an end of the war but also the start of a new age of peace.

For two weeks he toiled, and at one o'clock on January 22, 1917, he appeared before the Senate. While the nation's legislators had grown accustomed to the President's addressing them to explain any number of audacious programs, this visit was singular, for it came with little advance notice and no explanation of its purpose.

Wilson spoke of the duty of the American government in building a new structure of peace in the world. "It is inconceivable that the people of the United States should play no part in that great enterprise," he said. He added that the country owed it to itself and the other nations of the world to "add their authority and their power to the authority and force of other nations to guarantee peace and justice throughout the world." He wanted the American government to originate a "League for Peace." In ending this war, he sought treaties and agreements "which will create a peace that is worth guaranteeing and preserving, a peace that will win the approval of mankind, not merely a peace that will serve the several interests and immediate aims of the nations engaged."

Such a "covenant of cooperative peace," Wilson said, must include the people of the New World if it was meant to "keep the future safe against war." In reassembling a shattered world, Wilson said, there must be "not a balance of power, but a community of power; not organized rivalries, but an organized common peace." That, Wilson said in a statement that would resonate for generations, would require "a peace without victory."

Victory would mean peace forced upon the loser, a victor's terms imposed upon the vanquished. It would be accepted in humiliation, under duress, at an intolerable sacrifice, and would leave a sting, a

resentment, a bitter memory upon which terms of peace would rest, not permanently, but only as upon quicksand.

"Only a peace between equals can last," he said.

Wilson was formulating a number of specific points—regarding Poland, armaments, and "freedom of the seas." Above all, he proposed the ideas of "government by the consent of the governed" and that "no right anywhere exists to hand peoples about from sovereignty to sovereignty as if they were property." Wilson concluded by insisting, "These are American principles, American policies. We could stand for no others. And they are also the principles and policies of forward looking men and women everywhere. . . . They are the principles of mankind and must prevail."

Having sat through the speech in rapt silence, the audience in the gallery and the Senators on the floor broke into sharp applause, led by Republican Robert La Follette, who afterward commented, "We have just passed through a very important hour in the life of the world." Senator "Pitchfork Ben" Tillman said it was "the most startling and noblest utterance that has fallen from human lips since the Declaration of Independence." Other members of Congress suggested this expression of a new world vision was the most important pronouncement of an American President since the Monroe Doctrine. (Wilson had even suggested in his text that the rest of the world should adopt Monroe's doctrine—that "no nation should seek to extend its polity over any other nation or people, but that every people should be left free to determine its own polity." *The New York Times* wrote that the speech offered more than a contract for peace; it was "a moral transformation."

But, as expected, Republican critics pounced. Senator Francis E. Warren of Wyoming gibed that "the President thinks he is the President of the world." Others suggested that Wilson was abandoning the Monroe Doctrine, inviting non-Americans to tamper with the workings of the Western Hemisphere. Alice Roosevelt Longworth took wicked delight in the way Wilson had converted the Capitol into his own personal theater and turned each Presidential message into a "show." On this occasion, she thought he had outdone himself. "Peace without victory," she said, "amounted to nothing more than a continuation of cowardly temporizing."

A sanguine Wilson told the press, "I have said what everybody has thought impossible. Now it appears to be possible." He did not expect the

Senate to take specific action as a result of his remarks. This was simply a rare moment in the nation's history in which a President asked the people and its representatives to embrace a philosophy.

Foreign reaction was mixed. Ambassador Page in London said the British admired the idealism of the speech but felt the defeat of Germany was essential for any long-term tranquillity, a peace *with* victory. Privately, some Allied Ambassadors in the United States questioned the President's right to propose terms of a peace to a war in which he was not engaged. The most positive foreign reaction came from the Germans. Ambassador von Bernstorff was still pushing his government to respond to Wilson's earlier request for peace, and he remained in quiet contact with Colonel House.

But on January 31, 1917, Germany announced a new policy, an offensive of unrestricted submarine warfare whereby all ships, belligerent or neutral, in the war zone surrounding Great Britain, France, and Italy, or in the eastern Mediterranean Sea, would be sunk. A specified route would be provided to permit a limited number of well-marked American ships to enter this zone. Bernstorff wrote Colonel House that Berlin had instructed him to inform Wilson that Germany had been prepared to meet virtually all the Allies' peace terms back in December, but no longer. They now believed their new submarine policy would bring the war to its swiftest conclusion. As soon as Tumulty had the German bulletin in hand, he brought it to the President and watched as he read and reread it. Wilson turned gray, his lips tightened, and his jaw locked. Placing the paper back in Tumulty's hand, Wilson quietly said, "This means war. The break that we have tried so hard to prevent now seems inevitable."

Still, Wilson resisted. Despite resenting Germany for misleading him for so many months, he believed "it was for the good of the world for the United States to keep out of the war in the present circumstances." He insisted that he would not allow this turn of events to incite military action "if it could possibly be avoided." He was willing to bear the criticism and contempt that would come from all sides. On February 2, Secretary Lansing, voicing the sentiments of most of the Cabinet, wrote Wilson, "The situation can no longer be tolerated. The time for patience has passed."

The next day, the President returned to Congress. After reviewing Germany's provocative behavior, Wilson announced that he had directed the Secretary of State to inform His Excellency the German Ambassador "that all diplomatic relations between the United States and the German

Empire are severed and that the American Ambassador at Berlin will immediately be withdrawn." Should German naval commanders violate the
laws of the sea and humanity, Wilson said, he would "take the liberty of
coming again before the Congress, to ask that authority be given me to use
any means that may be necessary for the protection of our seamen and our
people in the prosecution of their peaceful and legitimate errands on the
high seas." Even at this late date, Wilson kept the diplomatic doors open.
"We shall not believe that they are hostile to us unless and until we are
obliged to believe it."

At two o'clock that afternoon—as Wilson walked before both houses
of Congress, an Assistant Solicitor for the State Department appeared at
the German Embassy in Washington and handed Count von Bernstorff
his passport. "I am not surprised," Bernstorff said, wistfully granting that
there was "nothing else left for the United States to do." After eight years
in Washington, he told the press that he was finished with politics and
expected to retire to his farm to grow potatoes.

Colonel House recorded that Wilson was still of a mind that "it would
be a crime for this Government to involve itself in the war to such an extent as to make it impossible to save Europe afterward." The President
maintained that his recent declaration was intended to lay "the bases of
peace, not war." Wilson spent much of the next week engaged in the same
practice that he had as a young boy organizing his baseball team: he
drafted a constitution. In this instance it was for that League of Peace to
which he had referred, an organization of neutral nations that would be
committed to a number of basic precepts—mutual guarantees of political
independence, territorial integrity, arms limitation, and a refusal to take
part "in any joint economic action by two or more nations which would in
effect constitute an effort to throttle the industrial life of any nation or
shut it off from fair and equal opportunities of trade." Roosevelt wrote
Lodge that he now doubted whether Wilson would go to war under any
circumstances. "He is evidently trying his old tactics," he said; "he is en-
deavoring to sneak out of going to war under any conditions. . . . He is
yellow all through in the presence of danger. . . . Of course it costs him
nothing, if the insult or injury is to the country, because I don't believe he
is capable of understanding what the words 'pride of country' mean. . . ."

On February 28, Wilson granted an audience to a delegation of peace
advocates—church leaders, a Socialist labor organizer, a historian, and

Jane Addams among them. Their mission was to impress upon the President his own comments in his "peace without victory" speech and to offer historical examples and moral imperatives for why America should stay out of the war. When Professor William Isaac Hull, one of his former students, urged Wilson to send an appeal to the German people, circumventing the militaristic hierarchy, the President brought the conversation to a close. "Dr. Hull," he said, "if you knew what I know at the present moment, and what you will see reported in tomorrow morning's newspapers, you would not ask me to attempt further peaceful dealings with the Germans."

"GERMANY SEEKS AN ALLIANCE AGAINST US; ASKS JAPAN AND MEXICO TO JOIN HER; FULL TEXT OF HER PROPOSAL MADE PUBLIC," blared the *New York Times* headline the next day. This exposed plot had come in the form of a coded telegram from Foreign Minister Zimmermann to the German Ambassador in Mexico, who was to encourage President Carranza to ally with Germany and to invite Japan to do the same. In return, Mexico would not only receive financial reward but could also reclaim Texas, New Mexico, and Arizona.

In truth, the British had intercepted Zimmermann's note in mid-January but had not relayed it to Wilson, via Ambassador Page, until February 25. The following afternoon, the President appeared before a joint session of Congress. With just days until the arrival of the new legislature, he called upon the Sixty-fourth Congress to take one more bold position. "Since it has unhappily proved impossible to safeguard our neutral rights by diplomatic means," he said, ". . . there may be no recourse but to *armed* neutrality." Without proposing war, Wilson requested certain tools with which to fight German weapons—most especially the authority to supply American merchant ships with defensive arms. That day, a German U-Boat sank the *Laconia*, a former British ocean liner converted to an armed merchant cruiser, as it approached Ireland. Twelve people from among the 75 passengers and crew of 217 died, including a mother and daughter from Chicago.

The House immediately passed an armed ship bill by a vote of 403 to 13, but the Senate balked. Several Senators believed arming merchantmen left the nation only one incident away from war. Midwesterners such as La Follette, along with O'Gorman from New York and Vardaman from Mississippi, decided to dramatize their opposition with a filibuster. In this

case, they had only to delay for the two days before the Sixty-fourth Congress would terminate—at noon on March 4. Although seventy-six Senators said they would approve the bill, eleven men held the government hostage.

Because March 4 fell on a Sunday, the formal inauguration of the President was scheduled for the next day. But, as required, Chief Justice White swore Woodrow Wilson in for the second time, in a quiet ceremony. Wilson had been in the President's Room since 10:30 that rainy morning, attending to business and monitoring the filibuster down the hall. The Cabinet gathered over the next hour, along with Tumulty, Colonel House, and Dr. Grayson. No more than thirty people witnessed Wilson take the oath. Edith, the only woman present, stood behind him. Afterward, Wilson kissed the Bible, which was opened to the Forty-sixth Psalm: "God *is* our refuge and strength: a very present help in trouble."

There were no festivities that day, only complaints about the filibuster. With the bill killed, a seething President returned to the White House, where he went to his desk. That night he released a long statement to the press, taking the Senate to task. "In the immediate presence of a crisis fraught with more subtle and far-reaching possibilities of national danger than any other the Government has known within the whole history of its international relations," the President raged, "the Congress has been unable to act either to safeguard the country or to vindicate the elementary rights of its citizens." He felt the United States, especially in times of crisis, could not proceed in this manner. "A little group of willful men, representing no opinion but their own," he said, "have rendered the great Government of the United States helpless and contemptible," making it "the only legislative body in the world which cannot act when its majority is ready for action." The President saw a single remedy—a change in the rules. Within days, Wilson would call upon the newly seated Sixty-fifth Congress to institute an essential of Senatorial procedure—the rule of "cloture," by which a (then) two-thirds majority of the Senate could end a filibuster.

A cold wind blew across the East Portico of the Capitol that Monday, March 5, as the sun tried to burn through the clouds that remained from a recent storm. "The inauguration was not a festival," one onlooker observed; "it was a momentary interlude in a grave business, and it must be got over with as briefly and as simply as possible." Because of new threats

against Wilson's life, security was reinforced, with twenty Secret Service agents surrounding him. Only fifty thousand people gathered for the ceremonies; the inaugural parade was half the length of the first; and, again, there would be no Inaugural Ball. For the first time, a First Lady accompanied her husband to and from the Capitol and stood by his side while he delivered a brief speech of 1,500 words.

This address was as unlike his first inaugural as was the spirit infusing the occasion. In 1913 he had spoken not a word about foreign affairs, only of his optimistic domestic agenda. Now he talked almost entirely of the "tragical events of the thirty months of vital turmoil through which we have just passed," which had made "us citizens of the world." There could be no turning back, he said. "The shadows that now lie dark upon our path will soon be dispelled and we shall walk with the light all about us if we be but true to ourselves." Without quite defining the mission, he said, "United alike in the conception of our duty and in the high resolve to perform it in the face of all men, let us dedicate ourselves to the great task to which we must now set our hand."

With that, Woodrow Wilson commenced his second term, delivering the nation to a place it could not even have imagined four years ago. While the United States was far from prepared militarily, its President had conscientiously made it ready mentally and morally to address the inevitable ordeal ahead. To clarify that task, Wilson reminded his countrymen, "We are provincials no longer."

12

ARMAGEDDON

*And the nations were angry, and thy wrath is
come . . .*

—REVELATION, XI:18

With the events of the inauguration behind them,
Woodrow and Edith went home, where the family
had gathered upstairs in the oval sitting room of the White
House to watch the fireworks. Curtained off by themselves
in his study, a weary First Couple invited Colonel House to
sit with them. He found the President holding Edith's hand
and pressing his cheek against hers.

After reviewing the highlights of the day, a revived
President suggested that they take to the streets, where they
could enjoy the new system of lights that illuminated much
of Washington. Wilson had a chauffeur drive them without a Secret Service agent, despite that day's bomb threats.
A car with guards followed closely, as much of Washington
turned out to admire the public buildings along Pennsylvania Avenue, all the way up to the Capitol, with its glow-
ing dome. Within minutes, crowds on the street recognized
the President and cheered. He and his wife retreated to the
White House, where they talked with Colonel House until
eleven.

Two days later, Wilson was suffering from a terrible
cold and exhaustion. Dr. Grayson ordered him to bed,

where he remained for the better part of the next two weeks. Edith had already taken note of the conditions that tended to incite his minor collapses, "when every nerve was tense with anxiety . . . and the burdens resting on his shoulders [were] enough to crush the vitality of a giant."

A slight but discernible change in White House procedure occurred during his convalescence. The filibuster having defeated the armed ship bill, Wilson asked Attorney General Gregory whether he could arm merchant ships without Congressional authorization. When Gregory said yes, the White House asked Secretaries Lansing and Daniels to prepare for the new policy. Curiously, however, communications with the Secretaries passed via Mrs. Wilson. The President was learning that he could use his wife as an operative—"a blind" is how she described herself, blocking unwanted visitors and relaying essential messages in both directions. Edith sat by her husband's bed and read the long memoranda detailing the plans for arming merchant ships. "Mr. Lansing, especially," observed Mrs. Wilson, "saw no hope for peace and urged that we proceed on the theory that we should soon be at war with Germany."

Adding further confusion to a world spun out of control, the people of Russia revolted. After years of steady decimation in the war under an unheeding monarchy, the Imperial Guard mutinied, the Duma formed a provisional government, and—hopelessly fighting his "Cousin Willy," the Kaiser—Czar Nicholas II abdicated his throne, bringing three hundred years of Romanov rule to an end. While the future of that empire remained unclear, the certain death of the dynasty lent greater credence to Wilson's conception of "war against autocracy." It now clearly defined this war as one between Democracy and Absolutism. March 18 brought word of three torpedoed American merchant vessels, with the loss of more than a dozen lives.

Wilson appeared at the 2:30 Cabinet meeting on Tuesday, March 20, his old genial self. Almost immediately he sought advice regarding America's relations with Germany. With the nation in a growing state of agitation, the Cabinet found the President's calmness sobering and reassuring. "Excitement," Robert Lansing noted, "would seem very much out of place at the Cabinet table with Woodrow Wilson presiding." The President gravely posed two questions: Should he summon Congress to meet before April 16, for which he had already issued a call? And what should he say?

McAdoo answered first. He said the war seemed a "certainty," and he

could see no reason for delaying American participation. If we did not respond at once, he said, "the American people would compel action and we would be in the position of being pushed forward instead of leading, which would be humiliating and unwise." More than supplying men, which he doubted the country could do at that time, he felt the United States could underwrite the Allies' loans. Houston picked up the ball and said that Germany was already at war with America and that the country should not hesitate to fight back. "The quickest way to hit Germany," he said, "is to help the Allies." Until the United States had amassed a large Army, it could speed up the production of submarines and destroyers, build multitudes of fast ships for freight, and extend liberal credits to Germany's enemies. War Secretary Baker said the current state of affairs demanded drastic action without delay—"that the Germans did not intend to modify in the least degree their policy of inhumanity and lawlessness," and that such acts meant war. He advocated preparing an Army at once. Lansing said it behooved the President to appear before Congress to declare that a state of war already existed between Germany and the United States and to "enact the laws necessary to meet the exigencies of the case." With the Russian Revolution, Lansing added, the time was ideal for entering the war, to fight for a League of Peace with no powerful autocracies among its members. With increasing excitement, he added that public sentiment was strong enough at that moment to sway Congress.

The President asked Lansing to lower his voice. He did not want people in the corridor overhearing their discussion. He remained unsure how to introduce the Russian situation into this American decision. Lansing said those were not causes to go to war; but he believed the character of the autocratic German government—"as manifested by its deeds of inhumanity, by its broken promises, and by its plots and conspiracies against this country"—pertained. Wilson absorbed all of Lansing's words, saying only, "Possibly."

Lansing argued that the sinking of a few American ships, even with the loss of American lives, did not provide a sound enough basis to declare war. The "duty of this and every other democratic nation to suppress an autocratic government like the German . . . because it was a menace to the national safety of this country and of all other countries with liberal systems of government," however, did.

"We have not yet heard from Burleson and Daniels," said the President

in a professorial tone. With reluctance, the Postmaster General expressed regrets about having to abandon neutrality but agreed that if the President did not take action, the people would force it. "I do not care for popular demand," Wilson said. "I want to do right, whether popular or not." And so Burleson urged an immediate declaration of war—and, he added, "I want it to be understood that we are in the war to the end, that we will do everything we can to aid the Allies and weaken Germany with money, munitions, ships and men, so that those Prussians will realize that, when they made war on this country they woke up a giant which will surely defeat them." He recommended the issuance of $5 billion in bonds. Wilson turned to the other side of the table and said, "Well, Daniels?"

The eyes of the Secretary of the Navy filled with tears. The most pacifistic of the Cabinet members and a friend of Bryan's, he took his colleagues aback when he announced that he too favored war. "Having tried patience," he said, there was "no course open to us except to protect our rights on the seas." The President's faced dropped.

Once everyone had spoken his piece—all starting from different positions but ending with the same conclusion—the President said, "Well, gentlemen. I think that there is no doubt as to what your advice is. I thank you." As the Secretaries adjourned, Wilson asked Burleson and Lansing to remain, so that he could inquire when he might ask Congress to convene should he decide to do so. Two Mondays hence would be the earliest possible date, they explained. "Thus ended a Cabinet meeting the influence of which may change the course of history," Lansing wrote in a memorandum to himself. "The ten councilors of the President had spoken as one," he said, "and he— well, no one could be sure that he would echo the same opinion and act accordingly." Fifty newsmen waited in the outer executive offices for word about the meeting; but the Secretaries could not say much because they honestly did not know how Wilson would act. They revealed only that he would probably call Congress into extra session within the next two weeks. The President attended the vaudeville show at Keith's Theatre that night.

Over the next several days, the President got outside of the White House as much as possible—not fleeing his responsibilities so much as freeing himself so that he could think. He played golf and took long automobile rides. When he had business to conduct with Cabinet members, he went to their offices—on foot. Wilson was not completely alone, of course: the Secret Service accompanied him. And so did Edith. Observed

Thomas Brahany, the chief clerk of the White House staff, "I think this is the first time in American history that a President's wife has accompanied the President in a purely business call on a Cabinet Officer."

On Friday, March 30, Woodrow Wilson was ready to prepare his remarks to Congress. He knew his next public utterance would alter the world. For this momentous address, he summoned the country's most successful speechwriter, one of its foremost historians, one of its first political scientists, one of its most elegant wordsmiths, a spiritual thinker to provide moral grounding, and, finally, his most trusted stenographer to get it all down on paper. There in the second-story study, Woodrow Wilson sat alone.

Actually, Edith was in the room with him, decoding cipher messages for her husband. They closed the office door with orders that nobody was to disturb him. He started with an outline, graduated to a shorthand draft, which he corrected in shorthand and longhand, and then put his fingers to the keys of his Hammond typewriter. The Wilsons lunched alone, after which Edith took him for an hour's ride in the park. And then it was back to the desk for ten hours over the course of the weekend, finishing after church on Sunday.

Upon the completion of the speech, Edith recalled, Wilson summoned a newspaper friend, Frank I. Cobb, editor of the New York *World*. "I'd never seen him so worn down," the journalist said. "He looked as if he hadn't slept, and he said he hadn't." Indeed, Wilson had wrestled with the situation over several nights. "He tapped some sheets before him," added Cobb, "and said that he had written a message and expected to go before Congress with it as it stood. He said he couldn't see any alternative, that he had tried every way he knew to avoid war." And then the boy who had grown up in the battle-ravaged South added, "I think I know what war means. . . . Is there anything else I can do?" Cobb said Germany had forced his hand.

After breakfast the next morning, Wilson passed to the Public Printer a sealed envelope containing the draft of his self-typed address, and he asked Tumulty to notify Congress that he was prepared to appear as soon as the two houses could organize. He spent the rest of the morning playing golf with Edith. In the afternoon, he walked across the West Executive Avenue from the White House to the State, War, and Navy Building (a grand monstrosity of an edifice, later called the Executive Office Building)

to brief Secretaries Lansing and Daniels. Later that day, American Ambassador Sharp further justified the Administration's course of action when he notified Washington that a U-boat had torpedoed the freighter *Aztec*, the first armed American merchantman, taking a dozen lives.

Tension spread. Sensing what lay ahead, seven pacifists from Boston confronted their senior Senator, Henry Cabot Lodge, as he was leaving a committee room. Their spokesman approached Lodge and said his constituents opposed entering the war. Lodge disagreed, replying, "National degeneracy and cowardice are worse than war." The young man said that anyone who wanted to go to war was a coward; and with that, the sixty-seven-year-old Senator called the man a liar and threw a punch, sending him to the floor. Similar arguments broke out across the nation. In the White House, Wilson gave his speech a dry run, reading it to Colonel House. The Colonel admired it immensely, not least of all because he felt it contained concepts he had been urging upon the President since the war began—differentiating between the German government and the German people, demanding the same codes of honor and morals for nations as for individuals, stating that the United States should not join a league of nations of which an autocracy was a member. But the speech, regardless of House's or anyone else's contribution, was pure Woodrow Wilson. Whether or not he was the first to utter them, the ideas and ideals were his. At 6:30, the two joined Wilson's family for a small dinner, during which the war was not discussed.

At 8:10 the household left the Executive Mansion, followed ten minutes later by the President and Mrs. Wilson, accompanied by Tumulty and Dr. Grayson. Despite a light spring rain, cheering crowds lined the streets all the way to the Capitol, where searchlights illuminated the massive flag atop the bright dome. Two troops of United States cavalry in dress uniform with sabers drawn greeted the President at the entrance to the House of Representatives. The members had been in session all day; and now, after an hour's respite, they returned to the great chamber. In a semicircle directly before the Speaker's desk sat the entire Supreme Court—Chief Justice White front and center—without robes. The Cabinet flanked them in the front row to the Speaker's left; the diplomatic corps—including the Ambassador of newly elected President Carranza of Mexico—in evening dress, filled the seats behind. It was the first time the foreign envoys as a cohort had been invited to the great hall. Led by Vice President Marshall,

the Senate entered, almost every man carrying or wearing a small American flag. The press and special invited guests packed the gallery, 1,500 people all together. Edith sat with her mother and Margaret Wilson in the front row of the balcony. At 8:32 the Speaker's voice announced the President of the United States. The Justices were the first to rise and cheer, leading a two-minute ovation—the greatest welcome Wilson had received in all his visits to the chamber. The audience settled into silence so deep, Edith said one could hear only the sound of people breathing.

The President appeared nervous at first. He looked pale; his voice quavered, and his fingers trembled. In plain terms, Wilson explained the reason for this extraordinary session: "There are serious, very serious, choices of policy to be made, and made immediately, which it was neither right nor constitutionally permissible that I should assume the responsibility of making." For several minutes, the audience was silent, as Wilson calmly recited a list of recent German atrocities. He pointed out that some of the unarmed ships that had been sunk were carrying relief to stricken Belgians, that there had been not only violations of international law but a disregard for human life, and that property "can be paid for; the lives of peaceful and innocent people cannot be." The "present German submarine warfare against commerce," he insisted, was nothing less than "a war against all nations" and a "challenge to all mankind."

Each nation, Wilson said, must decide for itself how to meet that challenge. "Our motive," he asserted, "will not be revenge or the victorious assertion of the physical might of the nation, but only the vindication of right, of human right, of which we are only a single champion." Armed neutrality, he declared, was no longer an option. "There is one choice we cannot make, we are incapable of making," he said to the utterly still audience: "We will not choose the path of submission—"

The chamber erupted in cheers. Chief Justice White dropped the big soft hat he had been holding so that he could raise his hands in the air and clap. The applause spread from the floor to the galleries. At last the President, having found his voice, continued from the point at which he had been interrupted:

> —and suffer the most sacred rights of our nation and our people to be ignored or violated. The wrongs against which we now array ourselves are no common wrongs; they cut to the very roots of human life.

With a profound sense of the solemn and even tragical character of
the step I am taking and of the grave responsibilities which it involves,
but in unhesitating obedience to what I deem my constitutional duty,
I advise that the Congress declare the recent course of the Imperial
German government to be in fact nothing less than war against the
government and people of the United States; that it formally accept
the status of belligerent which has thus been thrust upon it; and that
it take immediate steps not only to put the country in a more thorough state of defense but also to exert all its power and employ all its
resources to bring the Government of the German Empire to terms
and end the war.

Justice White sprang to his feet, triggering an even greater ovation. He
fought back tears.

The President was in full command as he cogently articulated how
this had become a war of necessity for America. "Neutrality is no longer
feasible or desirable where the peace of the world is involved and the freedom of its peoples," he said, "and the menace to that peace and freedom lies
in the existence of autocratic government backed by organized force which
is controlled wholly by their will, not by the will of their people."

"We have no quarrel with the German people," Wilson emphasized,
because this "was a war determined upon as wars used to be determined
upon in the old, unhappy days when people were nowhere consulted by
their rulers and wars were provoked and waged in the interest of dynasties
or of little groups of ambitious men who were accustomed to use their fellow men as pawns and tools." But the actions of the German leadership
demanded a global response, which included an affiliation of democratic
nations. "It must be a league of honour," he said, "a partnership of opinion." Wilson rejoiced at the recent events in Russia and pronounced that
emerging nation a "fit partner" for that league now that it had shaken off
the "autocracy that crowned the summit of her political structure."

The United States was going to have to pay the price of going to war;
and some of those costs were immediate. They included: extending "the
most liberal financial credits" to those countries already fighting Germany; "the organization and mobilization of all the material resources of
the country to supply the materials of war and serve the incidental needs
of the nation in the most abundant and yet the most economical and

efficient way possible"; the immediate equipping of the existing Navy to deal with the enemy's submarines; and the immediate addition to the armed forces of at least 500,000 men. Toward that end, Wilson believed not in a volunteer Army but the "principle of universal liability to service," along with authorization for additional men as soon as they were needed and could be trained. Wilson said he did not wish to borrow money to pay for all these efforts; he believed it was "our duty . . . to protect our people" through equitable taxation.

In short, Wilson said, Germany had become an international menace, and the United States was "about to accept gauge of battle with this natural foe to liberty and shall, if necessary, spend the whole force of the nation to check and nullify its pretensions and its power." That meant America would fight for nothing less than "the ultimate peace of the world and for the liberation of its people, the German peoples included: for the rights of nations great and small and the privilege of men everywhere to choose their way of life and of obedience." And then Woodrow Wilson justified going to war—with a declaration that would long resonate:

"The world must be made safe for democracy."

The sentence elicited no response at first. Then Senator John Sharp Williams of Mississippi stopped the speech with his applause. Everybody present rapidly comprehended the importance of those eight words, and the acclamation steadily mounted. When it finally subsided, Wilson completed his thought, which was meant to define further America's role in the conflict and to characterize the nation's place in the world for at least the next century. The world's peace, he continued,

must be planted upon the tested foundations of political liberty. We have no selfish ends to serve. We desire no conquest, no dominion. We seek no indemnities for ourselves, no material compensation for the sacrifices we shall freely make. We are but one of the champions of the rights of mankind. We shall be satisfied when those rights have been made as secure as the faith and the freedom of nations can make them.

With Lincolnesque charity, Wilson reminded his audience that for all of America's arguments with Germany's allies, the Imperial and Royal Government of Austria-Hungary had not actually engaged in warfare

against citizens of the United States. Furthermore, Wilson reminded his fellow Americans, "We are . . . sincere friends of the German people," including those living amongst them—unless and until they displayed any disloyalty to the United States.

After thirty-six minutes, Wilson concluded, adapting the words of no less a reformer than Martin Luther himself. "God helping her," Wilson said of America's new crusade, "she can do no other."

All members of the three branches of government stood as one. The Senators waved their small flags wildly, all except Senator La Follette, who conspicuously stood in silence, chewing gum, with his arms folded. As the President hastily departed, Senator Lodge strode toward him, extended his hand, and said, "Mr. President, you have expressed in the loftiest manner possible, the sentiments of the American people."

Wilson waited for Edith to descend from the gallery, and they rode with Tumulty back to the White House. Applause accompanied them all the way home; but inside the car, they remained silent. Before the President joined his family, he and Tumulty sat for a few minutes in the Cabinet Room. "Think of what it was they were applauding," said Wilson, utterly drained. "My message to-day was a message of death for our young men. How strange it seems to applaud that."

And then in a startling soul-baring moment, the President told Tumulty that maintaining his impartiality during the last thousand days of war had been a terrible ordeal. "From the beginning I saw the utter futility of neutrality, the disappointment and heartaches that would flow from its announcement," he confessed, "but we had to stand by our traditional policy of steering clear of European embroilments." While he had appeared indifferent to criticism, Wilson said few had sympathized with his situation. One person who had recognized those pressures bearing down on the President was the editor of the *Republican* in Springfield, Massachusetts, who had recently sent an empathic note. Wilson read its few paragraphs to Tumulty, after which he pulled out a handkerchief and mopped his eyes. And then, Tumulty recalled, the President lay his head on the Cabinet table and sobbed "as if he had been a child."

Reviews of the speech were reverential, its historical significance lost on nobody. Walter Lippmann, whose admiration for Wilson had been ascending, sent the President a sample of what he had just written for *The New Republic*: "Any mediocre politician might have gone to war futilely for

rights that in themselves cannot be defended by war," he said. "Only a statesman who will be called great could have made America's intervention mean so much to the generous forces of the world, could have lifted the inevitable horror of war into a deed so full of meaning." From London, Ambassador Page cabled that the pronouncement was "comparable to only two other events in our history—the achievement of our independence and the preservation of the Union." James Gerard, America's recently disinvited Ambassador to Germany, commented that the speech contained "a lofty idealism about it which puts this war on the plane of a crusade. No more momentous document has ever been written in the history of the world." A nearly eighty-year-old director of the United States Chamber of Commerce called the President's office simply to say that he had heard Lincoln speak his immortal words at the Pennsylvania battlefield. "Mr. Wilson's address on Monday," the director said, "will rank with the Gettysburg speech of Lincoln."

The outcome of the ensuing Congressional debate was never in doubt. The Senate began the discussion early on April 4 and voted that night— 82 to 6 in favor of war. The House debate opened the following morning and dragged into the early morning hours of April 6, with some 150 members having their say. Although corralling every vote was hardly a necessity, this particular issue had the rare distinction of seeing virtually every member in his seat. During the first roll call, however, one voice in the back row failed to make itself heard—that of Jeannette Rankin of Montana, the first woman elected to the House of Representatives, in her first month in office. She had endured a long, excruciating day: the National American Woman Suffrage Association had lobbied hard for her to vote for war, to demonstrate that women could be as hawkish as men; and the Congressional Union, representing another faction of suffragists, urged her to show that women were doves. She seemed to vacillate until former Speaker "Uncle Joe" Cannon walked over to the Democratic Representative and said, "Little woman, you cannot afford not to vote. You represent the womanhood of the country in the American Congress. I shall not advise you how to vote, but you should vote one way or the other—as your conscience dictates." When the roll was called for the second time, the Clerk of the House went to Rankin's side to record her choice. "I want to stand by my country," she said, "but I cannot vote for war." It was close to 4 a.m. when all the votes were tallied—373 to 50.

At lunch the next day, Good Friday, the President was informed that a printed copy of the War Resolution—signed by Vice President Marshall and Speaker Clark—was on its way from the Congress. Wilson rushed through his meal and exited the State Dining Room just as the messenger arrived at Ike Hoover's office. The staff discussed moving to the President's study, but Wilson said he would sign it right there, at the usher's desk. "Stand by me, Edith," he said as she handed him a gold pen he had given her. His jaw clenched as he affixed his bold signature to the parchment. He rose from his chair, returned the pen to Edith, and excused himself. Executive clerk Rudolph Forster informed the reporters waiting in the executive offices; and a naval officer in the West Wing went outside and wigwagged to another officer in the window of the Navy Department building that the President had signed the resolution. In an instant, wireless operators were transmitting the news to the world. For only the fourth time, the United States of America had declared war on a foreign nation; and Woodrow Wilson was commanding unprepared forces—just 300,000 men, fewer than 10,000 of whom were officers. The German General Staff ranked the United States militarily "somewhere between Belgium and Portugal."

Weeks later, Wilson drafted his five-sentence last will and testament. The President left all his property to "my beloved wife Edith for her lifetime," with the request that she distribute Ellen's personal articles—such as clothing, jewelry, and art—to his daughters, and an additional stipulation that Margaret Wilson receive $2,500 annually so long as she remained unmarried. Upon Edith's death, the estate was to benefit his children equally.

The day after war was declared, the President wrote a memorandum for himself, a list of measures he hoped Congress would pass in order to "put the country in a thorough state of defense and preparation for action." They included not only fortifying the existing military bills but also amending policies related to shipping, the Federal Reserve, the railroads, and interstate commerce. He believed the nation needed to unify behind a single set of principles, and a single leader. "My mother did not raise her boy to be a War President," Wilson said after a Cabinet meeting, "—but it is a liberal education!"

The naval forces of the United States mobilized immediately, putting

every government ship—the commissioned fleet, reserve warships, Coast Guard and Lighthouse Service boats—into active service. In a related action, the United States government seized ninety-one German-owned vessels—twenty-seven in New York harbor, including the *George Washington*. It was a merchant fleet with an estimated value of $100 million and the capacity to transport forty thousand troops—tonnage that would have required a year to manufacture. Most of the ships were not immediately seaworthy. In anticipation of the war declaration, the German crews inflicted wounds on their own vessels, sawing off bolt heads, which would require weeks to replace. By nightfall, more than one thousand Germans—including ship captains and cooks and musicians—were peaceably interned on Ellis Island, where they awaited deportation.

The President issued a proclamation to the American people, which the nation's newspapers carried on their front pages. Because, as he put it, the "entrance of our own beloved country into the grim and terrible war for democracy and human rights" created "so many problems of national life and action," he immediately presented an anxious nation "earnest counsel." This remarkable appeal outlined for the people not only the immediate problems before them but also the many types of "service and self-sacrifice" in which every one of his fellow countrymen could engage.

Besides fighting, the most basic task was to supply food—for Americans at home as well as fighting men abroad, along with the starving people of the nations "with whom we have now made common cause." Once adequately fed, America could consider the rest of the operations of the war—manpower, materiel, machinery, even mules. Wilson said all American industries must be made "more prolific and more efficient than ever," that the industrial forces of the country would become "a great international . . . army . . . engaged in the service of the nation and the world, the efficient friends and saviors of free men everywhere."

In the face of worldwide industrialization, Wilson urged a recultivation of America's agricultural roots. The supreme need of the nation just then was "an abundance of supplies, and especially of foodstuffs." Wilson urged America to "correct her unpardonable fault of wastefulness" and to increase her harvests. Almost overnight, male high school students were released from class, allowed to earn diplomas by manning the family farms. In the cities and suburbs, "Victory Gardens" cropped up almost overnight, as the people began planting vegetables in their backyards and on their

rooftops. In Washington, the government offered its unoccupied property to anyone who would farm it; along the Potomac Drive, where cherry blossoms would later bloom, society ladies tended edible gardens. Every housewife was further exhorted to practice strict economy in all her spending, even beyond household purchases, for that would put her "in the ranks of those who serve the nation." Curbing excess, Wilson decreed, was a public duty—"a dictate of patriotism which no one can now expect ever to be excused or forgiven for ignoring."

That applied especially to businesses. Wilson cautioned America's middlemen—whether they were handling foodstuffs or factory goods— that the "eyes of the country will be especially upon you." The country, he said, expected its businessmen to "forego unusual profits, to organize and expedite shipments of supplies of every kind." To the American merchant, he suggested a simple motto: "Small profits and quick services." He begged all editors to publish this appeal; he urged advertising agencies to resound its message; he hoped clergymen would consider these themes worthy of homilies. From his own bully pulpit, Wilson said, "The supreme test of the nation has come. We must all speak, act, and serve together!"

Unity became the driving force behind all Wilson's actions in making the nation ready to fight. The President was determined to centralize as many of the agencies and industries as possible under a single command. That meant training a nation of rugged individuals to come together as one, in working for their common cause. He appointed men of all political persuasions to scores of new positions, based solely on ability, regardless of their political histories. An air of nonpartisanship in the capital would allow the Congress to enact two dozen major pieces of legislation in the next year—each of which helped put the nation on war footing, changing the very character of the country.

Loyalty was the standard by which Wilson measured every one of his countrymen, starting with those in his administration. Despite Edith's dislike for Tumulty's commonness, Wilson could not deny his decade of unimpeachable devotion. Although Colonel House scarcely veiled his pretensions to power, he had never refused the President, and he possessed expertise in foreign affairs that nobody else in the Administration did. And though Dr. Grayson had made an "indelicate and objectionable" request for an admiralship, Wilson promoted him over many who had served longer, largely because he could never dismiss his personal allegiance to

the man who had introduced him to his wife. Edith confidentially divulged her dislike for the President's son-in-law—finding him ambitious and "thoroughly selfish"; but Secretary McAdoo had consistently proved himself the ablest member of the Cabinet, proactive and persuasive. Now Wilson called upon him to serve as the controller of European war loans and as Chairman of the Federal Farm Loan Bureau, General Manager of the Liberty Loans, and Chairman of the War Finance Corporation.

Transportation provides the lifeblood of a nation, and as 1917 wore on, Wilson came to grips with the fact that the United States simply had no continental railway system. It also lacked a sufficient number of railcars and the capital to build more. The Anti-Trust Act of 1890 prohibited the major companies from merging competing lines or making rate agreements among themselves. "Federal control of the railroads was, in fact, inevitable," McAdoo later wrote of the situation; but neither Wilson nor anybody else in the Administration wanted to put his hand on the throttle. By year's end Wilson felt compelled to say "that it is our duty as the representatives of the nation to do everything that is necessary to do to secure the complete mobilization of the whole resources of America by as rapid and effective means as possible." He seized the railroads with nothing more than a proclamation.

The Army Appropriations Act of the prior year had not only earmarked money to augment America's fighting force but had also authorized the President to exercise federal control whenever emergency war measures were required. Opposition immediately voiced the fear that this marked the first step of government ownership of the railroads. The Administration readily pointed out that in England, where private corporations owned the railways, the government had taken control the day His Majesty had declared war on the Kaiser; France, Italy, and Germany also exerted the same control. Wilson explained to the nation, "Only under government administration can an absolutely unrestricted and unembarrassed common use be made of all tracks, terminals, terminal facilities and equipment of every kind."

Based on his earlier experience building the Manhattan tunnels, McAdoo recommended several railroad executives, any of whom might run this new Railroad Administration. After discussing the list, Wilson asked McAdoo himself to direct the operation. "I don't want to urge it," Wilson said. "I am merely asking if you think you could undertake it?" Upon

reflection, McAdoo said that he could, and that the problems were more than questions of transportation. "It is a matter of finance as well as of operation," he said. With one hand running the trains and the other holding the Treasury's money, McAdoo was inclined to think it would be less of a burden for him to be in charge himself than working with somebody else. Two million railroad workers were suddenly in his employ, as McAdoo became the first man to consider the nation's 240,000 miles of railway lines as a whole. By consolidating services, McAdoo eliminated a superfluous one-sixth of the nation's passenger-train miles, enhancing efficiency and saving more than $100 million; the railway-car shortage of 1917 would become a surplus a year later; a coal famine was averted through greater efficiency; and McAdoo increased the pay for practically every railroad worker to a "decent living wage." Nobody objected until the war was over, when the railroads were returned to private hands and political opponents accused him of throwing money around so that the workers would elect him President of the United States.

The Army Appropriations Act had also established the Council of National Defense, a committee of a half dozen Cabinet Secretaries (War, Interior, Navy, Commerce, Agriculture, and Labor) who worked in concert with a seven-member commission, boasting the likes of labor leader Samuel Gompers and a half dozen business tycoons, including Julius Rosenwald, the president of Sears, Roebuck and Co. The committee's most significant personage from the private sector was an almost mythical figure named Bernard Baruch, who was identified in a press release as a banker.

"I am not a banker, and never have been," Baruch himself would later state; ". . . I regarded myself as a speculator." The son of a German Jewish doctor and a mother whose Sephardic ancestors settled in colonial New York, Baruch grew up in South Carolina and then New York, where he graduated from its City College. A self-made millionaire by thirty, mostly through shrewd investing, he continued to amass a fortune, along with a reputation for being a scrupulous financial wizard. As the war approached, Baruch had been so concerned that the nation was not prepared for all eventualities that he had written friends within the Administration. The President invited him to the White House for an exchange of ideas, and—shortly after that—to join the Council of National Defense. "Next to my father," Baruch would recall, "Wilson had the greatest influence on my

life. He took me out of Wall Street and gave me my first opportunity for public service."

The Advisory Commission of the Council of National Defense was created to advance "the coordination of industries and resources for the national security and welfare." That meant managing the logistics as well as the economics of mustering, lodging, training, equipping, and transporting millions of men. As his Cabinet showed, Wilson believed in tapping leaders from outside the government to serve inside his administration. Baruch admired how each of his colleagues naturally assumed the lead in his field of expertise. The president of the Baltimore and Ohio Railroad headed the committee on transportation, the director general of the American College of Surgeons oversaw medicine and sanitation, Rosenwald supervised dry goods, clothing, and supplies, and Baruch looked after raw materials and minerals. "From the time the problem of industrial mobilization first gripped my interest," Baruch recalled, ". . . I had recognized that victory in modern war depended upon the speed and efficiency with which the nation could convert its economy from peace and employ its resources for war."

He created a template for all the major industries in America by enlisting national leaders in each industry—from aluminum to zinc. When a demand for copper, for example, suddenly surged along with its price, Baruch called on Daniel Guggenheim and other magnates and reasoned with them to meet the government's needs at a fair price. Not only did this price-fixing save the government $9 million but it led industry to put patriotism before profits, enabling cooperation between people instead of corporations. When French Ambassador Jean-Jules Jusserand complained that gasoline shipments to France were being stalled, Baruch got to the heart of the problem with one telephone call to a colleague on the oil committee. Through these powerful appointments and cooperative committees, Wilson was able to cut through endless red tape.

Baruch urged the President to create "a centralized purchasing agency with authority over prices and the closing of defense contracts." Wilson could not go that far, but he did establish a War Industries Board, in which military leaders sat with industrial bosses and could at least coordinate the purchase of war supplies. Products were simplified and standardized, allowing for mass production, which was more efficient and economical. The WIB's power was minimal; but once Baruch was named its

chairman, he realized he could regulate where he could not negotiate. His committee assumed influence by becoming the nation's "priority machine"—directing, restraining, and stimulating war production as situations demanded, allocating materials where required, and ending unhealthy competition. Practicalities often determined policies. Should a locomotive, for example, be sent overseas to transport soldiers to the front or sent to South America to haul nitrates for bullets? Taking the stays out of women's corsets supplied enough metal for two warships.

Like Wilson, Baruch found it abhorrent that they should have to discuss prices and profits when "blood will flow so freely and suffering will become so great"; but the American entrance into the war was about to create the greatest burst of production in the nation's history. With it would come torrents of money. From the start of his work, Baruch sought to "reduce prices to the point we believe proper, yet keep wages up, preserve our financial strength, keep production of these absolutely vital materials at full blast and increase our resolution and determination to conduct the war to a successful conclusion." Instead of fixing prices, Baruch preferred flexibility; and he thought a strong centralized purchasing power could do much to control the economy, through the contracts it dispensed and "moral suasion."

President Wilson created an alphabet soup of boards and agencies to supervise the various aspects of the war effort, all of which he coordinated. While the President never saw the value in a "coalition cabinet" that consciously teamed rivals, he observed a policy of inclusion. His administration benefited from literally dozens of Republicans, many from the worlds of banking and business: three Republican Assistant Secretaries of War served Newton Baker, alongside Morgan banker E. R. Stettinius, who was put in charge of supplies; five of the eight members of the War Trade Board were prominent Republicans, as was the Red Cross chief, H. P. Davison, another Morgan banker; Republicans Frank Vanderlip of National City Bank ran the War Savings Stamps Campaign, and Russell C. Leffingwell (later a Morgan partner) became an Assistant Secretary of the Treasury. Former President Taft headed the National War Labor Board; and Harvard Law Professor Felix Frankfurter, a former Bull Mooser, left Cambridge to become an assistant to Secretary Baker, to act as Judge Advocate General and to chair the War Labor Policies Board, on which Navy Undersecretary Franklin Roosevelt would serve. Wilson also created a special

War Cabinet—which met on Wednesdays in his study. Its core included: the Secretaries of the Treasury, War, and Navy Departments as well as Baruch; Williams College President (and son of a Republican President) Harry Garfield, whom Wilson named to oversee the Federal Fuel Administration; Edward N. Hurley, a tool industry tycoon who had chaired the Federal Trade Commission and was reassigned to the United States Shipping Board; Democratic Party chairman Vance McCormick, head of the War Trade Board; and the man who distinguished himself more in the war years than any other Wilson appointee, a mild-mannered Quaker named Herbert Clark Hoover.

Orphaned at nine, Hoover was raised by an uncle in Oregon before entering the inaugural class at Stanford University, from which he graduated with a degree in geology. Starting his career as a mining engineer, he traveled to Australia and China, where he devised a process for extracting zinc. He became both a respected scholar in his field and a wealthy consultant. By the time the war began, Hoover had become a financier living in London. With over 100,000 Americans—mostly tourists—desperate to get home, he organized a committee to engineer their return. So effective was he, Ambassador Page called upon him to consider applying that same sort of American know-how to the feeding of Belgians in need. Hoover excelled at the task, performing feats of diplomatic and commercial magic in getting millions of tons of food distributed to ten million starving men and women. Shuttling across Europe, Hoover saw German deprivation as well, the result of the British food blockade. At Wilson's behest, he returned to Washington, where the President asked him to organize American food activities. He agreed, so long as he could continue to head the Belgian relief as well. He imposed one other condition: that he would receive no payment for his services and that the whole of the force under him, exclusive of clerical assistance, would do the same.

Unsentimental and brusque, Hoover expressed alarm and pessimism after assessing the current food situation, and with good reason. America's prior year's production of cereals—including wheat, corn, oats, barley, rice, and rye—was four-fifths of the six billion bushels it had been the year before; and adverse weather already assured that the coming year would yield even less. To make matters worse, adequate national rail service was not yet up and running to accommodate the crops on hand.

At age forty-two, he embarked upon what one scholar called "the

greatest experiment in economic organization the world had seen"—a nationwide exercise in extra production and economy. The President strong-armed Congress into passing a Food and Fuel Control Bill that granted power to the Administration to fix prices and exert other controls over the production and distribution of living essentials. The Lever Act—named for its South Carolinian sponsor—became an omnibus bill overloaded with excess baggage, riders from Representatives who bartered for inclusion of their pet causes in exchange for their votes. In this instance, the growing movement of Prohibitionists had their say, attaching a rider that banned the production of distilled spirits from any produce that might be used for food.

The entire nation rolled up its sleeves and tightened its belt so that as much food could be sent to Europe as possible. The Administration called upon the nation to go "meatless" at least one meal a day and one day a week, commonly Monday; it sent a similar request to go "wheatless," at least once a day and all day Monday and Wednesday. In time, at least one "sweetless" day of the week was encouraged, usually Saturday. Billboards and newspapers featured appeals to save food. Housewives enrolled as "members of the Food Administration"; their numbers included Edith Wilson, who signed a pledge endorsing "food conservation," for which she received a red, white, and blue card featuring spears of wheat, which she displayed in a White House window, like an ordinary housewife. Herbert Hoover's moon face became the symbol of economizing, if not deprivation, as mothers withheld spoonfuls of sugar from their children's cereal in his name; and the verb "Hooverize" entered the lexicon—"to be sparing or economical."

Hoover delivered phenomenal results. At the start of the war, the United States could pledge to export 20 million bushels of wheat; it sent 141 million. In just one quarter of a year, the country restricted its consumption of sweets enough to send 500,000 tons of sugar abroad. In addition to beef, the nation increased its pork production by a million tons. American restaurants reported having saved thousands of tons of meat, flour, and sugar in a single two-month period. Dumps nationwide noticed discernible decreases in garbage. Its first year in the war, America sent Europe twice as much food as it had the year before.

Americans conserved fuel as well. Because the industrial and military need for coal and oil became insatiable, management rewarded workers

with wages and the basic standard of living increases that unions had been demanding for years; union membership soared. Energy czar Garfield closely monitored the national fuel supply; and when shortages appeared, he ordered non–war related factories to shut down for days at a time or one day a week. Citizens and businesses protested the clumsy manner in which the Administration dropped such actions upon them; and, in fact, the government never adequately explained that the closures were more about allowing a day for the transportation system to meet war demands. Political opponents grumbled persistently about the Administration's lack of readiness, harshly criticizing Wilson's inadequacy as a leader; but all good citizens bundled up nonetheless as they endured "heatless" Mondays. Even the Wilsons observed "gasless Sundays," substituting a ride in a horse-drawn carriage for their weekend limousine drives. The switch was thrown on electric advertisements, streetlights dimmed, and "lightless" nights were eventually ordered, twice a week, even on Broadway. Wilson introduced Daylight Saving Time to America, which created an extra hour of farm work every day and which saved an hour of artificial light, reducing the use of electric and coal power.

Within weeks of America's entry into the war, Edith Wilson was tending eight sheep her husband had brought to graze on the White House lawn. The flock trimmed the grass, thus saving manpower; and at shearing time, they provided ninety-eight pounds of "White House Wool"—two pounds of which were sent to each state and the Philippines—which raised at auction close to $100,000 for the Red Cross. Edith also pulled out her old sewing machine and sat for hours, making pajamas for the sick and injured. (Whenever their fingers were free, all the Wilson women observed the Red Cross motto of "Knit Your Bit," by producing socks and sweaters. Margaret contributed to the war effort by embarking on two long concert tours, which earned some $10,000 for the cause.) Whenever the President saw a Food Administration or Red Cross card in somebody's window, his eyes filled. "I wish I could stop and know the people who live here," he would say, "for it is from them that I draw inspiration and strength."

The President hoped the rest of the country might share his feelings. Toward that end—and to carry the "Gospel of Americanism" to every corner of the globe—the President established the most controversial board of all, the Committee on Public Information. While other government boards dealt primarily with the nuts and bolts of winning the war,

the CPI dealt with the ephemeral business of public perception—what Secretary Baker called "mobilizing the mind of the world so far as American participation in the war was concerned." Where the knee-jerk reaction for most countries going to war, he said, was to impose strict censorship, the CPI intended to expose information. Or so it would have people believe.

Because the United States had entered the Great War for neither territory nor treasure but for intangible ideals, the President felt the need to capture the public's hearts and minds. He hired a journalist named George Creel—a muckraker out of Denver who had been a Wilson loyalist in the last two elections—to head the CPI. The Great War differed most essentially from previous conflicts in its recognition of public opinion as a major force, Creel wrote in his memoir *How We Advertised America*. "The trial of strength was not only between massed bodies of armed men, but between opposed ideals, and moral verdicts took on all the value of military decision."

Ever since the incursions in Mexico, there had been a delicate balance between the White House and the newspapers regarding coverage of military operations. Although the number of press conferences had sharply declined from weekly events to only two in all of 1916, Wilson's administration still offered plenty of access and transparency. "Starting with the initial conviction that the war was not the war of an administration, but the war of one hundred million people," Creel would write, "we opened up the activities of government to the inspection of the citizenship. A voluntary censorship agreement safeguarded military information of obvious value to the enemy, but in all else the rights of the press were recognized and furthered." But "information" was a product manufactured by people's minds; and as such, it could not be measured like wheat, meat, and sugar. And though the CPI maintained that no other belligerent nation allowed "such absolute frankness with respect to every detail of the national war endeavor," the fine line between fact and opinion—between morale-building and manipulation—all but disappeared. With $100 million to spend at its own discretion, the CPI would issue all the war news it considered fit to print. The department did not overtly censor information, but it covertly shaped it.

Secretary Baker said the war "was to be won by the pen as well as by the sword." Tellingly, Creel enlisted teams of not just historians but also

publicists to write pamphlets outlining "America's reasons for entering the war, the meaning of America, the nature of our free institutions, our war aims" and stacking them alongside the "misrepresentations and barbarities" of the German government. A few dozen of these booklets went into production, each extolling a different aspect of the American vision. An army of volunteers blanketed the country with seventy-five million copies; millions more were spread around the world. Another team issued an official daily newspaper, reporting on the activities of each government department. And Creel conscripted some of the most respected writers in America—including Owen Wister, Booth Tarkington, William Dean Howells, and Edna Ferber as well as journalists Ida Tarbell, Ray Stannard Baker, and William Allen White—to write about the American way of life in "letters," which were translated and delivered to any foreign press that would publish them.

To help fight years of German propaganda and to recraft what the Administration considered an unfair image of the United States, Creel hired several bright young men, including one who would not only distinguish himself immediately but would also emerge later as one of the most important propagandists of the century, a pioneer in the field of public relations. Edward Bernays, a nephew of Sigmund Freud, headed the CPI's export service. Born in Vienna and raised in New York, where he became a press agent shortly after graduating from Cornell, Bernays appreciated his uncle's work in exploring unconscious desires; and, perhaps better than anybody else at the CPI, he recognized the importance of tapping less into what the masses thought than into what they felt.

The CPI created a speakers division, which organized meetings across the country—forty-five "war conferences," providing information about America's evolving status in all the battles. It oversaw an organization called the Four Minute Men—seventy-five thousand speakers who volunteered in more than five thousand communities, where they generally appeared in motion picture theaters during the four minutes it took for the projectionists to change the reels. More than 750,000 speeches, on topics ranging from food conservation to "Maintaining Morals and Morale," were delivered to an estimated eleven million audience members—every one, Creel said, "having the carry of shrapnel."

Another division of the CPI produced motion pictures, which were initially documentary in nature. As the war continued, the film industry

produced feature films centering on the war that grew increasingly brutal in their portrayal of the enemy. Lon Chaney starred in *The Kaiser, the Beast of Berlin*. In *The Heart of Humanity*, Erich von Stroheim played a brutal "Hun" who attempts to rape a nurse before throwing a baby out a window. D. W. Griffith himself produced another wartime epic, about young lovers in France torn apart by the war and reunited by killing a sadistic German rapist. If that were not enough to rouse any American, the CPI distributed posters and window cards—based on almost 1,500 original drawings contributed by the artists themselves. At the beginning of the war, the artwork represented mostly romantic evocations of the glories of the great cause. Howard Chandler Christy and James Montgomery Flagg painted flag-clad beauties urging Americans to "Sow the Seeds of Victory" by considering "every garden a munitions plant." Flagg would also create one of the most enduring American images, a recruiting poster showing a white-haired Uncle Sam wearing a star-spangled top hat and declaring, "I WANT *YOU* FOR U.S. ARMY." A year later, the American posters turned ugly, depicting Germans as slobbering apes carrying off Lady Liberty. War exhibits traveled the state-fair circuit, not only spreading the American message but also generating income in the millions of dollars.

Beyond America, the CPI spread its word to the Allies, the neutral nations, and the enemy. Creating a daily news service to publicize stories by both wire and the wireless, America opened small offices in all the major capitals of the world, except those of the Central Powers. Stories about American education, finance, labor, medicine, and agriculture were sent everywhere, as were the speeches of Woodrow Wilson, marking the first time in history that the speeches of a head of state received universal distribution. "Every conceivable means was used to reach the foreign mind with America's message," Creel said; that included the novel idea of inviting leading foreign correspondents—particularly those from neutral nations—to come to America. Upon America's entrance into the war, the CPI had received $5.6 million from the President's discretionary fund and a Congressional appropriation of $1.25 million; in the end, it earned some $3 million from its films and expositions, thus costing the government less than $5 million. Creel called this a bargain for waging a "world-fight for the verdict of mankind." But there were hidden costs in trying to win that verdict.

On June 15, 1917, the Sixty-fifth Congress passed the Espionage Act—

one of the most provocative pieces of legislation in American history. It represented the greatest possible expression of patriotism and the suppression of free speech. In 1798, when the young nation had almost gone to war with France, President Adams had propounded the Sedition Act, which made the publication of "false, scandalous, and malicious writing" against the government or its representatives a crime. Adams's opposition— chiefly Jefferson and Madison—considered the act a violation of the First Amendment. Sixty-five years later, when the states were at war with one another, Lincoln suspended the writ of habeas corpus on several occasions and imposed martial law based on the Constitution's allowance whenever rebellion or invasion threatened "the public Safety." Furthermore, he stifled free speech in punishing critics of his policies.

At least as far back as the sinking of the *Lusitania*, Wilson had been concerned about Germany's covert activities. He had addressed the subject head-on in his 1915 State of the Union Address when he spoke of naturalized United States citizens "who have poured the poison of disloyalty into the very arteries of our national life." The President had asked Congress for legislation to help combat this problem. "Such creatures of passion, disloyalty, and anarchy must be crushed out," he said. On April 2, 1917, the President appealed for the authority Adams and Lincoln had been given, with enough power to make good on his vow to deal with any disloyalty in the nation "with a firm hand of stern repression."

Congress had introduced several new bills, including one from Representative Edwin Webb of North Carolina and Senator Charles Culberson of Texas targeting espionage and treason. They included all the powers the President might need, including a provision to monitor information of, from, and about the government—essentially making it illegal for a person to publish information that the President declared "useful to the enemy" in time of war. It amounted to nothing less than censorship.

While the bulk of the bill dealt with spies and saboteurs, a few sections wandered into gray areas, particularly in empowering the executive branch. One section, for example, declared it illegal even to "attempt to cause disaffection in the military," while another allowed the Postmaster General to determine which writings were of a "treasonable or anarchistic" nature and, as such, subject to the ban.

Democratic liberals, to say nothing of the journalists Wilson had courted for four years, could hardly believe that he could condone such

legislation. Progressive Republicans, such as Senators William E. Borah and Hiram Johnson, and the predictable chorus of right-wing Republicans, such as Henry Cabot Lodge, opposed him as well. Hearst editor Arthur Brisbane called upon the President to comment on the importance of "the absolute freedom of the press." Wilson replied that he could "imagine no greater disservice to the country than to establish a system of censorship that would deny to the people of a free republic . . . their indisputable right to criticize their own public officials." He insisted that he would regret the loss of "patriotic and intelligent criticism" during the trying times and said, "So far as I am personally concerned, I shall not expect or permit any part of this law to apply to me or any of my official acts, or in any way to be used as a shield against criticism."

Even with that assurance, the bill struck at the very heart of a free society. It asserted that the chosen leaders of a nation should have the right in times of war to suspend the normal freedom of the press. Opponents contended there was never good reason to withhold or doctor information, while supporters maintained that absolute transparency in a time of war might threaten national security.

Congressman Webb opened the House debate by condemning the press for conveying the impression that his bill trampled upon the First Amendment. At a time when men were offering their lives to win the war, he thought newspapers should be willing to sacrifice the right to publish stories the President thought injurious. The nation had given Wilson its trust to command its Army; so too should he be entitled to control its information. Representative Dick Thompson Morgan of Oklahoma, a Republican, said: "In time of great national peril, it is necessary sometimes that individual citizens shall be willing to surrender some of the privileges which they have for the sake of the greater good."

Morgan's own Senator could not have disagreed more. "I am opposed to any censorship of the press at this time," said Democrat T. P. Gore, "because censorship goes hand in hand with despotism." A strong disciple of the freedom of speech, he said that censorship strikes at the very foundation of a free democracy. Hiram Johnson called the amendment "vicious" and "un-American." Lucien Price, an astute political pundit, editorialized in *The Boston Daily Globe* that May, "The American people could not long endure the necessary war-time conscription of men and property, if the truth were also conscripted." He called his fellow citizens "the greatest

reading public in the world," one that could not tolerate "a shutdown of news just as they enter the war themselves."

Tumulty sent Wilson an excerpt from a biography of John Adams, which claimed that the greatest blunders of the Federalist Party were the infamous Alien and Sedition Acts and that "no one has ever been able heartily or successfully to defend these foolish outbursts of ill-considered legislation which have to be abandoned, by tacit general consent, to condemnation."

When a canvass of votes in the House suggested that censorship as included in the Webb bill would not prevail, the President stepped up to reaffirm his position that censorship was "absolutely necessary to the public safety." He sent Representative Webb a letter—to be released to *The New York Times*—expressing his confidence that the great majority of the American press would observe "a patriotic reticence about everything whose publication could be of injury"; but he still insisted that there were in every country "some persons . . . whose interests or desires will lead to actions on their part highly dangerous to the nation in the midst of a war."

The censorship section was cut from the bill, and that compromise allowed the overwhelming nonpartisan passage of the Espionage Act. What remained left a watchdog government with enough authority to intimidate. Much of what had been excised was inserted in a later piece of legislation, the Sedition Act of 1918, which prohibited "disloyal, profane, scurrilous, or abusive language about the form of government of the United States," or its military or naval forces or the uniforms or the flag thereof; and it prohibited any language intended to cast upon them "contempt, scorn, contumely, or disrepute."

For all his experience raking muck, Creel proved himself remarkably adept at sanitizing. While the recent debate had raged, he composed a detailed memorandum to help organize the CPI. Topic number one was "censorship," a word, he said, that was "to be avoided." Creel suggested nothing nefarious; indeed, he insisted the entire spirit of his agency must be "one of absolute co-operation. It must go upon the assumption that the press is eager and willing to do the handsome thing, and its attitude must be one of frankness, friendship and entire openness." He and the President were on the same page; and, for the most part, the White House and the press remained mutually respectful throughout the war.

Wilson seldom abused the arsenal of powers the Congress had granted

him. "From the war's beginning," David Lawrence observed, "Mr. Wilson made frequent visits . . . to the different war bureaus. He developed the habit of dropping in when least expected." Lawrence suggested these visits were part of his exercise and relaxation regimen—a chance to stretch his legs—but he was also exerting the common touch, keeping the rapidly expanding government bureaucracy a place where even the President might drop in on any given day.

With Wilson's "ability to delegate work, his loyalties to subordinates, and his speed in evaluating problems," Herbert Hoover would recollect forty years later, "he proved a great administrator." Hoover added that Wilson's "religious and moral upbringing expressed itself in a zeal for financial integrity which characterized the conduct of a war practically without corruption."

To the stirring drumbeat of the CPI, the people of the nation compensated for their deprivations with a spirit that had not united them since the country's founding. Everybody pitched in. Just as the British Royal Family shook all German nomenclature from its family tree—Battenbergs becoming Mountbattens, and the House of Saxe-Coburg and Gotha adopting the family name Windsor—so too did Americans expunge all things Teutonic. Across the country, hamburgers were rechristened "liberty steaks," and sauerkraut became "liberty cabbage." German shepherds were called Alsatians; Berlin, Iowa, turned into Lincoln, Iowa; and Brooklyn's Hamburg Avenue was renamed after Wilson. Some school boards discontinued teaching the German language. Otto Kahn, a German-born partner in the New York banking firm of Kuhn, Loeb & Company as well as the chairman of the Metropolitan Opera Company, wrote the President to ask whether he felt opera in German sung by German artists should continue in his opera house. Wilson hated to see the loss of German opera, but he left the decision to Kahn and his board—which chose to bar German works. With all the changes, German Americans unavoidably became victims of hysteria, discrimination, and, in one instance, lynching. Aware of the bigotry, Wilson urged tolerance, speaking repeatedly and reassuringly of his "confidence in the entire integrity and loyalty of the great body of our fellow-citizens of German blood." Considering the general spirit of the nation, he would later reflect "that America was never so beautiful as in the spring, summer and autumn of 1917 when people were

stirred by a passion in common, forgot themselves and political differences in an urge to put all they had, all they were, to use in a great purpose."

Despite Woodrow Wilson's having no military experience, he proved to be a highly effective Commander in Chief—decisive and delegative. His battle plan had two fundamentals: first, that the nation would submit to a national draft; second, that the United States would not send those fighting men abroad as "replacement troops" for the Allies but as United States soldiers fighting under the American flag.

Among Congress's first pieces of business after its declaration of war was a Selective Service bill. Recognizing the inadequacy of mustering a volunteer Army (only thirty thousand men had signed up by the end of April 1917), Congress debated the need for conscription, America's first mandated military service since the Civil War. While such an act struck many as the very sort of autocracy the soldiers would be sent to fight against, Wilson asserted that the heart of the selective draft was the idea that "there is a universal obligation to serve and that a public authority should choose those upon whom the obligation of military service shall rest." It provided for a system that was both fair and functional, giving control to local draft boards in their creation of a national Army, determining not only who but how each man in the pool might serve. A local board might determine that a fellow volunteering to fight in France could better serve by remaining in his wheat field or coal mine. Wilson believed such a bill would create the greatest impression of "universal service in the Army and out of it, and if properly administered will be a great source of stimulation." A section of the Selective Service bill stated that, unlike in the Civil War draft, nobody could purchase or otherwise furnish a substitute for himself.

One fifty-eight-year-old Rough Rider could hardly contain himself. Itching to be back in uniform and in the spotlight, Theodore Roosevelt had quietly assembled his own division, communicating for months with men all over the country who wanted to serve with him. Only three days after the declaration of war, he went to Washington, determined to see Wilson. He had no formal appointment; but he told those around him, "I'll take chances on his trying to snub me. He can't do it! I'd like to see him try it!"

Late the next morning, Tumulty telephoned to say that the President would see the former President at noon. They met in the Green Room and

promptly got past the awkwardness of their previous vicious rivalry. In truth, Wilson had invited TR to the White House three years earlier for a delightful half hour of nonpolitical conversation over glasses of lemonade; but on this spring day, the Colonel came on a very specific mission. He commended Wilson on his war message and on his bill for selective conscription and then proposed the division he hoped to lead. Roosevelt found Wilson slightly awkward, sounding defensive about his policy of the last three years over which they had crossed swords. "Mr. President," Roosevelt interjected, "what I have said and thought, and what others have said and thought, is all dust in a windy street, if now we can make your message good. Of course, it amounts to nothing, if we cannot make it good. But, if we can translate it into fact, then it will rank as a great state paper, with the great state papers of Washington and Lincoln. Now, all that I ask is that I be allowed to . . . help get the nation to act, so as to justify and live up to the speech, and the declaration of war that followed." After half an hour, the two men were bantering and laughing together.

Before leaving the White House, TR asked if he might call upon Tumulty in the executive office. Wilson summoned his secretary to the Red Room, where there were handshakes and backslaps. Roosevelt heartily greeted several of his former household staff and said to Tumulty, "You get me across and I will put you on my staff, and you may tell Mrs. Tumulty that I will not allow them to place you at any point of danger." Back on the street, he told the crowd of newsmen, "The President received me with the utmost courtesy and consideration," and said that the President would rule on his request "in his own good time." Wilson asked Tumulty what he thought of the Colonel, and he replied that the man's enthusiasm was overwhelming. "Yes," said Wilson, "he is a great big boy. I was, as formerly, charmed by his personality. There is a sweetness about him that is very compelling. You can't resist the man. I can easily understand why his followers are so fond of him." Not aware that TR still felt little more than contempt for Wilson, the President seriously considered the Colonel's proposition.

Roosevelt lingered in the capital, where he granted audiences and courted old friends from Congress, hoping they might include a provision in the Selective Service bill that would allow volunteer forces to go directly to the front while America trained her conscripted Army. "We owe this to humanity," he wrote the Democratic chairman of the Senate Committee on Military Affairs. The Selective Service Act passed on May 18, 1917, and

included this Roosevelt exception, to be executed at the President's discretion. Wilson announced that day that he would not avail himself of any volunteer divisions, that to do so "would seriously interfere with . . . the prompt creation and early use of an effective army." He determined that such divisions would contribute little to the effective strength of the armies currently engaged against Germany.

No matter what good theater it might make to send TR to the Western Front, Wilson could see no strategic reason to do so. He wired Roosevelt that his conclusions were based "entirely upon imperative considerations of public policy and not upon personal or private choice," but the Roosevelt camp had its doubts. "It seemed to us that the President's refusal was undoubtedly influenced by political considerations," wrote TR's daughter Alice Roosevelt Longworth, who suggested that there simply was not room for another star on the world stage—one President behind a desk, another leading a charge. Said Alice, "It was the bitterest sort of blow for Father."

Ten million American men between the ages of twenty-one and thirty, on the other hand, registered for the draft on June 5, 1917. Although there had been threats of resistance, the day passed without incident. Over the next year and a half, almost five thousand local boards would register nearly twenty-five million men, assigning each a number between 1 and 10,500. Then, a little before ten o'clock in the morning of July 20, 1917, in a room in the Senate Office Building, Secretary of War Baker stood before a crowd of government officials. Wearing a blindfold, he dipped his hand into a large glass jar and fished out a capsule, inside of which was the number 258. It was announced and written on a chalkboard, and newsreel cameras recorded the event. Over the next sixteen and a half hours, other officials and eventually local college students pulled the 10,499 remaining capsules, thus completing the first and largest such lottery in history. Shortly thereafter, more than 10 percent of those registered would be called up and then selected according to five categories of eligibility—factoring marital, medical, and occupational status along with the number of dependents one supported. Not everybody answered the call: 350,000 men—including a discernible number of German Americans, Socialists, and pacifists—simply resisted. Over the course of America's involvement in the war, the age limits would stretch to include all men between eighteen and forty-five. Over 150,000 lads under military age joined the Students' Army Training Corps, getting a jump on their preparation for

service, usually on a college campus; and 80,000 men—mostly young businessmen—earned commissions after three months of twelve-hour days at officers' training camp. A Presbyterian minister wondered whether he could serve his country best by going to the front or staying in his parish; Wilson said that "it is the duty of these gentlemen to stand by their flocks, unless it is very evident that they can be dispensed with."

Suddenly the United States government was responsible for feeding, housing, clothing, and training millions of men. In just three months, thirty-two encampments requiring hospitals, power stations, sewage systems, theaters, libraries, and, often, railroad tracks and stations were built, a marvel of administration and construction. At a cost of roughly $10 million each, half these "cantonments" provided wooden barracks for the national Army; the other half provided tent camps, with wooden floors, for the National Guard. Stretching from Camp Devens in Massachusetts to Camp Kearney in California—all named for military heroes and most clustered in the South—each cantonment accommodated 40,000 soldiers. According to Secretary Daniels's final reckoning, 4,272,521 men served in the wartime Army.

Manpower proved easier to supply than firepower. By the time enlisted men appeared in camp, only a small fraction of the standard-issue Springfield rifles were on hand. By the end of the war, Springfield could supply only half the American Expeditionary Force's needs, forcing the government to purchase weapons from other companies. Because time was of the essence, Secretary Baker could not afford to gather competitive bids on every item the government needed. The War Department placed orders at once with Colt, Lewis, and Vickers for machine guns, anything to get weapons into soldiers' hands as quickly as possible. For months, American soldiers used European equipment. Indeed, not until late in the war would an American squadron fly American planes. As Charles G. Dawes—a Midwestern banker who became a Brigadier General in charge of supply procurement—quickly learned, it was essential to acquire any weaponry on hand and pay the going rate. The result was a fighting force that was never completely standardized but one that could improvise when necessary.

The Commander in Chief encouraged as much in what Josephus Daniels called the "most remarkable address of the war." It seemed to Wilson that the greatest obstacle in this "unprecedented war" was the German

submarine, which the legendary British Admiralty had been unable to overcome—largely because of its timorous approach to the problem. (They repeatedly rejected America's idea of including convoys to accompany their ships across the Channel, for example.) On Saturday, August 11, 1917 as the core of the United States Navy was preparing to transport men and materiel overseas—the Wilsons cruised down the Potomac on the *Mayflower* for their regular summer weekend jaunt. Then, without any public announcement, they sailed into the York River, where the massive dreadnoughts that constituted the Atlantic Fleet were at anchor. Unceremoniously, Wilson boarded the flagship *Pennsylvania*, where he found all the officers of the fleet gathered on the quarterdeck. With no press even aware of his presence, Wilson addressed the men "in confidence," delivering a personal inspirational message.

Wilson asked the sailors before him—from Ensigns to Admirals—to strategize beyond the lessons in their manuals, to

> please leave out of your vocabulary altogether the word "prudent." . . . Do the thing that is audacious to the utmost point of risk and daring, because that is exactly the thing that the other side does not understand. And you will win by the audacity of method when you cannot win by circumspection and prudence.

Wilson believed "the most extraordinary circumstance of modern history is the way in which the German people have been subordinated to the German system of authority, and how they have accepted their thinking." The purpose of this war, he told those about to fight, was "to see to it that no other people suffers a like limitation and subordination. . . . We are in some peculiar sense the trustees of liberty." Edith saw that her husband had inspired the men profoundly. He shook hands with every officer.

Thus began the most colossal conveyance of fighting men the world had ever known. The United States Navy swelled from 65,000 to 500,000; and, by the end of 1917, it had transported 145,918 men across the Atlantic Ocean. The next year it carried two million more. In all the months of mass passage, only 768 American soldiers and sailors were lost at sea.

In truth, Wilson had not anticipated building so sizeable a war machine. He read every night from a khaki-covered pocket edition of the

Bible that a soldier had sent him, and he prayed for the hostilities to end. The threat of the American invasion might encourage the Germans to withdraw to the peace table; and there was always the hope that the Allies might just win the war on their own before the Yanks arrived.

In August 1917, Pope Benedict XV appealed to the leaders of all the belligerent governments, asking them to stop turning the civilized world into "a field of death" and forcing Europe to take "a hand in its own suicide." He insisted that there should be a simultaneous and reciprocal reduction of armaments and that arbitration should begin right away. Secretary Lansing presumed this appeal emanated from Austria-Hungary—with its heavily Catholic population and strong support of the Vatican. He questioned the Pope's motives and suggested that he had become an unwitting "agent of Germany," eager to restore peace to Catholic Belgium and Poland but making no mention of Slavic Serbia and Montenegro. Wilson felt the Pontiff offered nothing more than a return to the status quo before the war, without removing any of the elements that provided the pretext for the war. "It is none of our business how the German people got under the control of such a government or were kept under the domination of its power and its purposes," he wrote in shorthand in preparing his reply, "but it is our business to see to it that the history of the world is no longer left to their handling." Wilson expressed doubt that such a peace could be based upon a restitution of the German government's power or upon "any word of honor it could pledge in a treaty of settlement and accommodation." He would not take the word of the present German rulers as "a guarantee of anything that is to endure, unless explicitly supported by such conclusive evidence of the will and purpose of the German people themselves as the other peoples of the world would be justified in accepting." The President looked forward to the possibility of a "covenanted peace."

On December 4, 1917, the President delivered his State of the Union Address and spoke almost entirely about the war, clarifying America's objectives. "We shall regard the war as won only when the German people say to us . . . that they are ready to agree to a settlement based upon justice and the reparation of the wrongs their rulers have done," he said. Observing that Austria-Hungary had become nothing more than "the vassal of the German Government," he now recommended a declaration of war against that empire. Three days later, Congress complied—by a

unanimous vote in the Senate (La Follette was absent) and by all but one vote in the House.

The declaration cemented the bond between the United States and the Allies, signaling that all Germany's friends were now America's enemies. That only induced new talk that Austria-Hungary wished to arrive at a separate peace and extract itself from the war, which would, in turn, weaken Germany. In fact, Britain would soon enter secret talks with Austria on that very subject, as it desperately waited for the Americans to train and unleash the full force of their Army. When Vice Admiral William Sowden Sims—who was appointed Commander, United States Naval Forces Operating in European Waters—arrived in London, he learned a shocking truth that the British government had withheld from its people and the rest of the world. It was underreporting the tonnage of ships it had been losing each month. It was in the millions.

Some bumptious Englishmen—including Winston Churchill—would later claim that "America should have minded her own business and stayed out of the World War," that the Allies were on the verge of making peace with Germany in the spring of 1917. But few of Churchill's countrymen agreed. Most were undyingly grateful for American participation. Admiral John Jellicoe, head of the Royal Navy, privately told Admiral Sims upon his arrival, "They will win, unless we can stop these losses—and stop them soon." King George summoned Ambassador Page to Windsor Castle to tell him how much his nation appreciated the help of the Americans and to confess how badly they needed it. In September 1917, new Prime Minister David Lloyd George sent Wilson some hard facts, specifically that "in spite of the efforts of the Allies to raise and equip armies and to manufacture munitions, in spite of their superiority in men and material and the perfection to which they have brought their offensive arrangements, the Germans . . . find themselves in possession of more and not less Allied territory." As the American convoy plan met immediate and long-term success, the hopes of the King, like those of every citizen of the Allied nations, rested on American leadership.

General Frederick Funston was the presumptive leader of the American forces until his sudden death just weeks before the declaration of war. Many supposed that General Leonard Wood, leading spokesman for America's Preparedness Movement, might fill his boots, though his close relationship to TR did not endear him to Wilson. Ironically, Wilson had

distrusted Wood since a meeting in early 1913, at which the General had done nothing but badmouth Roosevelt, in an obvious attempt to curry favor with Wilson. That only made the President doubt Wood's discretion and loyalty. And so, Secretary Baker and Wilson turned to General John J. Pershing, then fifty-seven years old. Tall, stiff-backed, and square-jawed, with a manicured mustache and a commanding voice that he used as little as possible, Pershing consistently had displayed leadership as he had risen through the ranks: with the 6th Cavalry, fighting Apaches and Sioux; commanding the 10th Cavalry—a regiment of the African American "buffalo soldiers," which earned him the nickname "Black Jack"; teaching at West Point; fighting in Cuba and the Philippines; and serving in diplomatic postings in Japan and the Balkans before leading the 8th Calvary in the punitive expedition along the Mexican border. He had said little during the preparedness quarrels.

After one meeting at the White House on May 24, Wilson immediately sent Pershing to Europe, with several thousand troops, to establish his command and demonstrate support for the Allies. Those Americans fortified morale more than they did the front lines. Despite constant pressure to fill in with "doughboys" wherever the French "poilus" and British "Tommies" had suffered great losses, Wilson reiterated that "we will leave to General Pershing the disposition of our troops, but it must be an American Army, officered and directed by Americans, ready to throw their strength where it will tell most." Like Wilson's Cabinet officers, Pershing was given virtually free rein of his personnel, creating a centralization of his forces and avoiding internecine warfare by having the absolute approval and obedience of his Generals. Pershing did not want his troops to lose their national identity by becoming absorbed in the Allied armies. Wilson felt the same about all his country's war efforts: when he saw a poster from the Food Administration referring to "Our Allies," he asked Herbert Hoover to substitute the words "Our Associates in the War," explaining, "I have been very careful about this myself because we have no allies and I think I am right in believing that the people of the country are very jealous of any intimation that there are formal alliances."

Pushing the United States into the international arena, Wilson relied heavily on Colonel House's secret intelligence-gathering project—"the Inquiry"—which Secretary Lansing helped define in a memorandum he wrote in optimistic preparation for the peace talks. Because it would be

impossible to find any negotiators who possessed full knowledge of the myriad of issues involved, Lansing had recommended assembling a team of experts whose knowledge cut across different countries and different disciplines, each of whom would prepare a pamphlet that could assist in deciding the United States' role in the determination of boundaries and the redistribution of colonial possessions. He had further recommended that House supervise the entire effort.

Working out of unimposing offices, the Inquiry quietly went about its work, as House assigned Sidney Edward Mezes to administer this think tank. Mezes happened to be Mrs. House's brother-in-law; and House insisted that he was not only trustworthy but also supremely qualified. A lifelong academician and philosopher, Dr. Mezes was then president of the City College of New York and was "well grounded in both political and economic history," had a progressive outlook, and was conversant in French, German, Italian, and Spanish. To serve as his secretary, House recommended Walter Lippmann, whose abilities were so impressive, the anti-Semitic House surmounted his objections—because "unlike other Jews he is a silent one." The mission of the Inquiry was not simply to gather information but also to apply it in rebuilding the world after the current apocalypse.

At the end of 1917, its secret work grew complicated when a newspaper revealed its existence. Then a series of secret agreements among the Allies, predetermining how the Central empires would be dismantled and divided after the war, came to light. Great Britain, France, Russia, Japan, and—perhaps most problematic—Italy (which had joined the Allies) had all privately agreed to new covenants, creating a system of alliances as labyrinthine as those that had kindled the war. They imagined whole new countries drawn from territory between Germany and the Middle East. Affixing such territorial purposes to the war contradicted Wilson's ideals. One cannot determine precisely what the President knew and when he knew it, because he proceeded to act as though these pacts did not exist. He believed he would be able to bring everybody around to his way of thinking—regardless of secret treaties—in due time. As the President wrote Colonel House: "When the war is over we can force them to our way of thinking, because by that time they will, among other things, be financially in our hands." By year's end, however, it looked as though the Allies might not have a chance at any spoils.

During the first four weeks of autumn, the Austro-Hungarian and German armies overwhelmed the Italians at Caporetto. Starting with a surprise attack, from which the Italians never recovered, the battle effectively knocked its army out of commission; the retreat felt like a turning point in the war, as in addition to some 30,000 Italian casualties, 250,000 of their men were taken prisoner. Morale sank, and soldiers deserted. The retreat broke more than the back of the Italian armed forces; it fractured the spirit of the entire Allied cause. One young Red Cross ambulance driver from Oak Park, Illinois—Ernest Hemingway—would later capture that moment, saying, "Abstract words such as glory, honor, courage, or hallow were obscene." In the meantime, in Russia the Bolshevik government was hoping to draft a separate peace with the Germans. Such a treaty would hurt the Allies, allowing the Germans to remove their armies from the Eastern Front so they could fight on the Western. And in the far reaches of the Ottoman Empire, one small plot of sand proved to have far-reaching implications.

Commander of Britain's Egyptian Expeditionary Force since June 1917, British General E. H. H. "Bloody Bull" Allenby had steadily pushed his campaign east across the Sinai desert. How Palestine might figure into an Allied victory in the war had not been determined; Zionists had long prayed it might become a permanent homeland for the millions of Jews dispersed around the world. On November 2, 1917, after consideration by the British War Cabinet, Foreign Minister Balfour wrote Lionel, the 2d Baron Rothschild, a representative of the Zionists, a short letter, the core of which read:

> His Majesty's Government view with favour the establishment in Palestine of a national home for the Jewish people, and will use their best endeavours to facilitate the achievement of this object, it being clearly understood that nothing shall be done which may prejudice the civil and religious rights of existing non-Jewish communities in Palestine, or the rights and political status enjoyed by Jews in any other country.

By December 9, Allenby's troops had captured Jerusalem; and at noon on the eleventh, the Bloody Bull and his officers dismounted so that they

could enter the Holy City on foot. They were the first Christian army to seize the city from the Turks since 1099. The Balfour Declaration was not a legal document, merely a statement of intention; but it became the groundwork for the Jewish state that would remain a bone of contention over the next century. Secretary Lansing suggested to the President that he refrain from taking any position on Zionism—as the United States was not at war with Turkey, the Jews were far from united in their own feelings about a Jewish state, and there were many Christians who would "undoubtedly resent turning the Holy Land over to the absolute control of the race credited with the death of Christ." But Wilson told Lansing that he had already assented to the Balfour Declaration, recognition that would prove to be fundamental to the region.

The President dispatched House to Europe, to sit at the Inter-Allied War Council meeting in Paris, where they discussed means of coordinating all their war efforts. With the Allies stumbling on the European fronts, Wilson saw the opportunity for his man to "take the whip hand" in directing the global agenda, for the United States not only to "accede to the plan for a unified conduct of the war but insist upon it." General Pershing apprised Baker that he hoped to have America's fighting forces in active service by the summer of 1918. "Winning the war is vital to our future," he said, "and if humanly possible it ought to be done in 1918. There is no telling what might happen if we defer our utmost exertion until 1919."

"A supreme moment of history has come," Wilson said in concluding his State of the Union Address that December. "The eyes of the people have been opened and they see. The hand of God is laid upon the nations. He will show them favour, I devoutly believe, only if they rise to the clear heights of His own justice and mercy." To assist in this ascent, the President asked Colonel House for a memorandum from the Inquiry that would pose the different questions a peace conference must consider and propose achievable answers. Mezes, attorney David Hunter Miller, and Walter Lippmann generated a comprehensive but highly readable document—*The Present Situation: The War Aims and Peace Terms It Suggests*. It delineated America's political and military objectives from Berlin to Baghdad— paying particular attention to the Poles, Czechs, South Slavs, and Bulgarians. It enumerated America's assets, laying out especially how money, if

skillfully handled, could be wielded like a weapon, used both to threaten enemies and to lure friends; and it assessed its liabilities—the military impotence of Russia, the "strategic impossibility" of any military operation that could cut to the heart of Middle Europe, the "costs and dangers" of a war of attrition on the Western Front, the possibility that the Germans might agree to a settlement over Alsace-Lorraine without changing the basic balance of power in Western Europe, and the instability of Italy, where social revolution loomed. The proposal offered a program for a "diplomatic offensive," the best possible scenarios for each of the players in the world drama—including ways of creating discord between Austria-Hungary and Germany and harmony among the Allies. Finally, and most incisive, the Inquiry memorandum offered a statement of peace terms—ten items, territory by territory.

Colonel House delivered the report on December 23. It evidently went unread through the holidays, during which time representatives of the newly established Bolshevik regime under Vladimir Lenin officially opened talks with the Central Powers in Brest-Litovsk (which would become Brest, Belarus) to discuss a settlement.

At the first plenary session of the Brest-Litovsk Peace Conference, Russia presented a manifesto—six principles that centered on a theme of liberation. They included banning "forceable annexation of territory seized during the war," restoring independence where it had been seized, protecting minorities in multinational territories with "special laws," safeguarding weaker nations against such bullying tactics as boycotts and blockades, and, most important, allowing national groups to determine their own political futures through referendums. British Ambassador Cecil Spring-Rice had a private audience with Wilson shortly after those terms were made public; and from Washington, he promptly confided to Foreign Minister Balfour, "Situation here is such that the President must in self-defence make some answer to the Bolshevists' appeal."

That very day—Friday, January 4, 1918—Colonel House handed the President an expanded version of the Inquiry's statement of peace terms. Over the next twenty-four hours, Wilson could not help incorporating at least the sentiments of Lenin's principles, if not a few specifics, into his own thinking, especially where Russia was concerned. At half past ten on Saturday morning, he and his right-hand man outlined general provisos and then proceeded to specific territorial adjustments. Working directly

from the Inquiry's memorandum, they considered each proposition from both the Allied and Central Powers vantage points. House generally served as the anvil against which Wilson hammered his ideas. The President defined most of the basic stipulations in shorthand and then refined them at his typewriter. Two hours later—having "finished remaking the map of the world," as House put it—Wilson asked the Colonel to number his short typed statement. They agreed upon the sequence, with one exception—the creation of a peace association, which Wilson thought should come at the very end, as a way of rounding out the message. That became his fourteenth point.

Also that day, Prime Minister Lloyd George delivered a long speech to the Trade Union Conference in London in which he articulated his nation's position. The basis of any territorial settlement in the war, he said, was the principle of "government by consent of the governed"—what he now called "self-determination." When the text reached Washington, Wilson's spirits sank; he thought the address made many of his very same points. House argued that Lloyd George's remarks simply laid a foundation for Wilson's speech and that Wilson "would once more become the spokesman for the Entente, and, indeed, the spokesman for the liberals of the world."

On Sunday, Wilson secluded himself in his study and incorporated his fourteen points into a speech. He toiled until day's end, at which time he read his address to Colonel House. A single theme ran through the text— what Wilson would describe as "the principle of justice to all peoples and nationalities, and their right to live on equal terms of liberty and safety with one another, whether they be strong or weak." House called the address "a declaration of human liberty and a declaration of the terms which should be written into the peace conference." More than that, he diarized, "I felt that it was the most important document that he had ever penned." The next day Wilson read the speech to Secretary Lansing.

Two days later, the President appeared before both houses of Congress at noon and got right down to business. "We entered this war," he said, "because violations of right had occurred which touched us to the quick and made the life of our own people impossible unless they were corrected and the world secured once for all against their recurrence. What we demand . . . is that the world be made fit and safe to live in." All the peoples of the world, Wilson added, were partners in this interest; and with that,

he stood before the Congress and the world to present his Mosaic "programme of the world's peace . . . the only possible programme."

Wilson's first five points were edicts for all the nations to obey: "open
covenants of peace, openly arrived at" (thus, no secret treaties); "absolute
freedom of navigation upon the seas"; "the removal, so far as possible, of all
economic barriers" and an equality of trade conditions among all the nations consenting to the peace; a reduction of national armaments "to the
lowest point consistent with domestic safety"; and "a free, open-minded,
and absolutely impartial adjustment of all colonial claims."

The next eight points eradicated the old imperial borders of specific
territories and entreated the rest of the world to honor the new boundaries.
Several of the stipulations carried their own Wilsonian homilies. Point VI
called for the German evacuation of all Russian territory and the allowance for "the independent determination of her own political development
and national policy," so that she might join the community of free nations
under institutions of her own choosing; more than that, Wilson said, the
"treatment accorded Russia by her sister nations in the months to come
will be the acid test of their good will, of their comprehension of her needs
as distinguished from their own interests, and of their intelligent and unselfish sympathy." Point VII insisted upon the evacuation and restoration
of Belgium—as no other single act would so much serve "to restore confidence among the nations in the laws which they have themselves set and
determined for the government of their relations with one another. Without this healing act the whole structure and validity of international law
is forever impaired." Point VIII demanded the release of all French territory and the restoration of its invaded portions—particularly "the wrong
done to France by Prussia in 1871 in the matter of Alsace-Lorraine, which
has unsettled the peace of the world for nearly fifty years." Point IX sought
a readjustment of Italy's frontiers "along clearly recognizable lines of nationality." Point X said the peoples of Austria-Hungary "should be accorded the freest opportunity of autonomous development." Point XI
addressed the Balkan states, granting "political and economic independence and territorial integrity," especially in according Serbia "free and
secure access to the sea." Point XII disassembled the Ottoman Empire,
assuring the Turkish portion a secure sovereignty and the other nationalities the right to develop autonomously, and mandating that the Dardanelles should be permanently opened as a free passage to ships of all

nations. And Point XIII urged the creation of an independent Polish state, complete with free and secure access to the sea.

Three and a half years earlier, when the fighting in Europe broke out, H. G. Wells published a series of articles that were compiled into a book entitled *The War That Will End War*. As the fighting persisted, so did that phrase, which modulated into "the war to end all wars." As Woodrow Wilson became the principal voice of the era—and because that sentiment encapsulated his outlook—the slogan was attributed to him. And nothing addressed that concept—thus permanently affixing it in the public's mind—more than his Fourteenth Point: "A general association of nations must be formed under specific covenants for the purpose of affording mutual guarantees of political independence and territorial integrity to great and small states alike."

President Wilson said the United States would fight until those fourteen "arrangements and covenants" were achieved. As he had suggested in the past, America carried no vendetta against Germany, no jealousy of German greatness, no desire to block her legitimate influence or power. "We wish her only to accept a place of equality among the peoples of the world—the new world in which we now live,—instead of a place of mastery," he said. "The moral climax of this the culminating and final war for human liberty has come," he concluded on behalf of the people of the United States, "and they are ready to put their own strength, their own highest purpose, their own integrity and devotion to the test."

"God was satisfied with Ten Commandments. Wilson gives us fourteen," France's Premier Georges Clemenceau would gibe; the British wondered how Point II might affect their ruling the waves; and the German press took Wilson to task for employing "all his demagogic artifices . . . to prevent Russia from closing a separate peace with the Central Powers." But most of the rest of the world heartily embraced Wilson's speech. The "extreme radicals, even the socialists, approve it," House triumphantly noted in his diary, "and so do the conservatives and reactionaries." Paderewski of Poland sent grateful salutations; speaking in Edinburgh, Balfour referred to the speech as a "magnificent pronouncement"; muckraker Lincoln Steffens and peace activist Jane Addams both conferred their praise; and the French press, cabled General Pershing, offered "unqualified approval." Even Colonel Roosevelt told *The New York Times* that he was "much pleased" with it. Thanks to George Creel, when the Germans advanced into Russia in early

1918, they found the walls of the towns placarded with the Fourteen Points—not just in Russian but also translated into German; 300,000 handbills were distributed in five days in Petrograd alone. The CPI printed and disseminated more than four million copies of Wilson's speech.

The Germans were just as eager as the Allies to end the war, but Chancellor Georg von Hertling showed no signs of embracing the Fourteen Points. Factions within the Reichstag were prepared to compromise but—as the ongoing talks at Brest-Litovsk indicated—only on their terms and to their advantage. Strikes broke out in Berlin and Vienna, and revolution was in the air. House delighted at the schisms the Fourteen Points had created among the German politicians; and Wilson capitalized on the divisiveness by returning to Congress on February 11 to reaffirm his points, offering four principles for their enactment.

Each part of the final settlement must "be based upon the essential justice of that particular case," especially in its striving for a permanent peace; the peoples and provinces were not to be bartered "as if they were mere chattels and pawns in a game, even the great game, now forever discredited, of the balance of power"; every territorial settlement must be in the interest of the populations concerned and not as a part of an adjustment against rival states; and all "well defined national aspirations" must be considered in light of their effect on "perpetuating old elements" that might break the peace of Europe and beyond. Wilson said he offered no threats, insisting that the power of the United States "will never be used in aggression or for the aggrandizement of any selfish interest of our own"—only to serve freedom. The subtext of Wilson's speech was clear: he welcomed peace efforts but intended to fight until Germany forsook its militaristic ways.

"What is at stake now is the peace of the world," Wilson continued. "What we are striving for is a new international order based upon broad and universal principles of right and justice,—no mere peace of shreds and patches." The President explained that in raising his Fourteen Points he had meant only "that those problems each and all affect the whole world" and that "unless they are dealt with in a spirit of unselfish and unbiased justice, with a view to the wishes, the natural connections, the racial aspirations, the security, and the peace of mind of the peoples involved, no permanent peace will have been attained." When Germany suggested it would determine the futures of Russian territory and a place for an

independent Poland, Wilson became even more outspoken. "People are not to be handed about from one sovereignty to another by an international conference of an understanding between rivals and antagonists," he said. "National aspirations must be respected; peoples may now be dominated and governed only by their own consent." And then he added, " 'Self-determination' is not a mere phrase. It is an imperative principle of action, which statesmen will henceforth ignore at their peril." Two weeks later— after losing two million soldiers—Russia would surrender a third of its population and farmland and half its industrial centers.

Germany realized it had only a few months before American troops would arrive in Europe. And so, beginning on March 21, it committed all possible resources to a spring offensive. This involved four major attacks, the goals of which were to break through the Allied lines, outflank the British forces, which extended to the English Channel, and close in on the French. Under the direction of Generalquartiermeister Erich Ludendorff, the Germans forced the British 5th Army to retreat thirty miles and lose 100,000 men. They continued to inflict serious damage to the French as they drove them back, coming within striking distance of Paris. Severely compromised, the Allies closed ranks behind a single leader, naming Marshal Ferdinand Foch Supreme Commander of the Allied Armies. While the Germans gained significant ground and suffered fewer losses than the Allied armies, Foch was able to keep the enemy from inflicting the coup de grâce. After four years of horrific warfare, victory on neither side was in sight: German casualties in the spring offensive practically equaled those of the British and French combined. There were more than 1.5 million casualties all together.

That was the same number of doughboys who reached France by June 1918—all fresh and inspired by one of Wilson's most stirring speeches. Before fifteen thousand people at a rally in Baltimore on April 6—the anniversary of "our acceptance of Germany's challenge to fight for our right to live and be free, and for the sacred rights of free men everywhere"— Wilson had delivered not just a call to arms but an announcement of America's new military strength. With all the passion of one of his heroes, Shakespeare's Henry V, Wilson cried, "Force, Force to the utmost, Force without stint or limit, the righteous and triumphant Force which shall make Right the law of the world, and cast every selfish dominion down in the dust." America's former prince of peace had become a full-fledged war-

rior king, dispatching millions of young men unto the breach of the greatest carnage the modern world had ever seen.

"In Flanders fields the poppies grow," began the most popular poem of the era, an elegy that laced propaganda with pastoral imagery. But the casualties on those fields mounted so high they opiated the mind, keeping people from processing all the horror. With its profusion of noble sentiments and heartwarming songs, the Great War still presented itself as a romantic conflict; but it would be for the last time, as new technology mechanized war, turning from conventional weaponry to more diabolic tools of devastation. Sophisticated automatic rifles and machine guns took more lives in more efficient and gruesome new ways. In the century since shrapnel was introduced, it had developed to the point that each cylinder shot into the air could now release dozens of exploding lead marbles, damaging their human targets not only immediately but also later through the infections the lead balls induced. The Germans developed a highly effective flamethrower. And by 1915, both sides in the war employed poison gas—starting with tear gas and chlorine and progressing to mustard gas. The latter had the ability to corrode the skin and erode the lungs, leading to blindness if not death. Submarines, tanks, and airplanes contributed to the ever-increasing slaughter as armies spent months at a time living and fighting in trenches, behind barbed wire, sometimes losing hundreds of thousands of lives while gaining only a few feet of muddy ground.

With sanitation facilities crude at best, the soldiers were subjected to every imaginable disease, from nephritis to pneumonia along with trench fever (a form of rickets) and trench foot (similar to frostbite). Rats were rampant, dangerous for the parasites and diseases they carried; lice bred beyond control. "Shell shock" became a familiar auditory and psychological affliction; and corpses tangled in barbed wire became a common sight. Poetry now reflected a discernible shift in tone, as much of the early idealism succumbed to grotesque reality.

And then appeared the Fourth Horseman of the Apocalypse— Pestilence. During the unusually cold winter of 1918, a lethal influenza spread, evidently from Camp Funston, Kansas. With some fifty thousand men in close quarters, most of them shipping out overseas and scattering across Europe, only to share crowded unsanitary foxholes, the war created a global Petri dish for a pandemic. Within a year, the Spanish flu—as it came to be called because Spain's King Alfonso XIII became its most

publicized survivor—would be responsible for half the deaths of American soldiers. Lasting four centuries, the Black Death had killed 75 million people. This outbreak of influenza would infect a billion people, killing 100 million of them.

War inflates peacetime numbers, particularly economic statistics. A military workforce in the millions, supported by thousands of new bureaucracies—from draft boards to the National Screw Thread Commission—had to be funded. "I now had to face the prodigious problem of war financing," recalled Treasury Secretary McAdoo. "With each fresh calculation the sum had grown larger, and the figures were appalling. There were so many uncertain factors in the problem that a definite conclusion was not possible." But McAdoo realized that he had to generate several billion dollars within a few months. His predecessor during the Civil War, Salmon P. Chase, had been afraid to appeal to the people for money, and so he relied heavily on private bankers and agents to sell bonds; McAdoo considered this a fundamental error. "Any great war must necessarily be a popular movement," he believed. "It is a kind of crusade; and, like all crusades, it sweeps along on a powerful stream of romanticism."

The day after the war was declared, McAdoo went to Congress to confer with members of the House Ways and Means Committee and the Senate Finance Committee. He submitted a draft of a bill seeking authorization to issue $7 billion worth of bonds. "The request for such an enormous amount of money startled Congress and the country," McAdoo recalled. But he explained that he did not intend to offer the entire batch of bonds at once. He also detailed the importance of sending $3 billion as loans to the Allies—"substitutes for American soldiers" until they had actually arrived. North Carolinian Claude Kitchin, Majority Leader and chairman of the House committee, noted that the bill contained "the largest authorization of bond issues ever contained in any bill presented to any legislative body in the history of the world." With near unanimous support, it passed both houses of Congress within two weeks.

Selling bonds became one of the great morale builders during the war. Business was good enough that anybody with money could earn a higher rate of interest from other financial instruments; but the Administration literally capitalized, as McAdoo said, on "the profound impulse called patriotism." They took the campaign to the people—farmers and factory workers and millionaires alike—giving every citizen an opportunity to

serve the country by investing in it. After consulting with several business titans, particularly two of the nation's leading financiers—J. P. Morgan and Paul M. Warburg—McAdoo settled on $2 billion at a 3.5 percent rate of interest, high enough to maximize widespread participation but low enough to minimize the government's burden. Calling them "Liberty Loans," he embarked on a four-week speaking tour to drum up subscribers. With the support of the major banks, the Four Minute Men, women's clubs, and politicians of all persuasions (with the notable exception of Ohio's Republican Senator Warren G. Harding), and with newspapers and billboard owners and advertising agencies offering free services, the First Liberty Loan drive ended after one month, oversubscribed by more than $1 billion. Four million citizens had invested, 99 percent of them paying from $50 to $10,000. On May 31, 1917, the President invested $10,000. In order to give the Treasury greater flexibility by not requiring approval each time it needed to float a bond—and to empower Congress with control over the amount of moneys the nation could borrow—in September 1917, Congress created a limit it called a "debt ceiling," this first one set at $11.5 billion.

Three more drives followed over the next fifteen months. McAdoo had been so unsure about the first bond issue that Congress had exempted the income the bonds produced from all but inheritance taxes. Now he returned to Congress to suggest that surtaxes be applied in certain instances. To ensure the success of these subsequent campaigns, Washington called upon the nation's most powerful new sales force—movie stars. In the last five years, a Los Angeles community of orange groves and pepper trees had blossomed into Hollywood, the home of one of the most lucrative industries in the nation; and its famous players did whatever they could to boost the war effort—appearing at benefits, drawing publicity, and raising spirits as well as money. After Wilson received Charlie Chaplin, Mary Pickford, and Douglas Fairbanks at the White House, they accompanied McAdoo on his bond tours and turned throngs of fans into subscribers wherever they went. Sometimes the crowds grew too vast to hear the stars talk, and the actors resorted to their pantomime skills in encouraging the public to invest in the nation. On one tour, stone-faced cowboy William S. Hart crammed rallies in nineteen cities into ten days and sold $2 million worth of bonds. The four Liberty Loan campaigns raised $17 billion. By

then the Victory Liberty Bond Act had raised the debt limit to $43 billion, far above the $25.5 billion in total federal debt.

McAdoo had never intended for bonds to finance the entire war; he believed the "soundness and stability" of America's financial structure depended on raising not less than one-third of its expenditures through taxation. The Revenue Act of 1916 sought to raise $200 million, more than half derived from the income tax; the basic rate inched from 1 percent to 2 on annual incomes over $3,000, and there was a surtax of 6 percent on incomes over $500,000 that slid upward to 13 percent on incomes over $2 million. The next year, the United States experienced the sharpest spike in its tax history. A 2 percent tax was imposed on incomes of $1,000, with graduated surtaxes amounting to as much as 67 percent in the cases of multimillion-dollar incomes; this not only generated more revenue but enrolled more taxpayers. Congress introduced excess-profits taxes—8 percent on businesses and individuals earning more than $6,000 annually. In the years just before the war, hundreds of employees of the Bureau of Internal Revenue had collected $280 million annually. After America entered the war, ten thousand workers collected $2.8 billion.

On May 23, 1918, McAdoo urged a higher tax on profits generated by war industries, an increase in the income tax on unearned incomes, and a heavy tax on luxuries. The only reasons to challenge the legislation, said McAdoo, were political. Congressional elections were less than half a year away, and he noted that many members had told him they were worried that such taxation would result in the Republicans seizing the House of Representatives. McAdoo said he felt the fear was "ill-founded." He believed the electorate would have more respect for those representatives who were willing to announce their positions than those who dodged the issue. Either way, he asked the President, "how can we allow any political consideration to stand in the way of our doing the things which are manifestly demanded to save the life of the Nation?" The question launched what would become a perennial debate between people who insisted that businesses—the very people who invested in the growth of America— were being treated unfairly and those who contended that the redistribution of wealth was not only equitable but stimulative to the economy. Between 1917 and 1918, the nation's gross domestic product grew from $60 billion to $75 billion; and the federal deficit—that is, the amount by

which government expenditures exceeded revenues—shot from $1.1 billion to $9 billion.

On May 27, Wilson appeared briefly before another joint session of Congress and presented the facts as McAdoo had laid them out. Winning the war was paramount; hundreds of thousands of America's men—"carrying our hearts with them and our fortunes"—were hastening to Europe; there could be "no pause or intermission" in their crusade; and that required raising additional moneys. "Only fair, equitably distributed taxation . . . drawing chiefly from the sources which would be likely to demoralize credit by their very abundance," he said, "can prevent inflation and keep our industrial system free of speculation and waste."

"No new taxes" would later become an evergreen American political slogan; but Wilson proposed the exact opposite. He insisted it was the government's duty in that moment to introduce new taxes and raise the old ones. While no elected official ever wanted to take such a position, the President exhorted Congress to embrace the challenge. That required a major concession on all their parts, which he audaciously presented in a slogan of his own: "Politics is adjourned."

Both houses of the Sixty-fifth Congress had cooperated with the executive branch in enacting Wilson's vigorous wartime agenda, and so he reluctantly asked them to extend themselves further by abrogating the very essence of their existence—the playing of politics. So long as they were waging war, the President of the United States blandished, "the elections will go to those . . . who go to the constituencies without explanations or excuses, with a plain record of duty faithfully and disinterestedly performed." Whether one agreed with the President or not, his rousing speech offered a profile in courage.

Debate extended for several months, though it would prove nearly impossible to resist a Commander in Chief who spoke with such unabashed patriotism. "Have you not felt the spirit of the nation rise and its thought become a single and common thought since these eventful days came in which we have been sending our boys to the other side?" he asked that May. He believed Americans were so united in their resoluteness to win the war, they would undergo any sacrifice toward that end. "We need not be afraid to tax them," Wilson added, "if we lay taxes justly."

The great variable in the equation, of course, was in the definition of the word "justly." McAdoo favored taxing "war profits," as the chemical

and the steel industries, for example, were benefiting hugely from the conflict. He pointed out that the Allies borrowed about $9.5 billion from America during the war years, but they spent close to $12 billion there in that period. Most of that money went to munitions-makers, who were notorious profiteers. McAdoo estimated that gains from war profiteering amounted to close to $3 billion. In the meantime, progressive Representative Kitchin targeted "excess profits." He noted that that such companies as Ford, Standard Oil, and American Tobacco had been earning excessive profits before and during the war and deserved to be taxed accordingly after the war. Henry Cabot Lodge cautioned that so much taxation would curb future investment, thus generating less in income taxes and keeping average Americans from buying Liberty Bonds. Such debates would last months as well, but Wilson still had no compunction asking for these new revenues. After all, he said in his speech on May 27, 1918, "Just as I was leaving the White House I was told that the expected drive on the western front had apparently begun."

From the moment he landed in London, it had been General Pershing's plan to hang fire until he had mustered a substantial enough force to win the war. Before late May 1918, American troops had barely muddied their boots, obtaining only occasional battle experience. Because of the exigencies of the spring offensive, Pershing temporarily allowed Marshal Foch to intersperse some of his troops among the combined British and French forces. Then, on May 28, 1918, some 3,500 soldiers of the 28th Infantry Regiment of the U.S. 1st Division took offensive action in a small battle at Cantigny, seventy-five miles north of Paris. Assisted by French airplanes above and tanks on the ground, the Americans overtook the town and advanced into German-held territory in a matter of hours. Beyond the military victory was the psychological boost. This small band proved that Americans knew how to fight, and it offered a preview of what millions of robust doughboys could do. The Battle of Belleau Wood lasted almost the entire month of June and ended in an American victory. The Yanks won again in July at Château-Thierry. By August, Foch decided to take advantage of the shift in momentum and commence his own offensive, one that would last the next hundred days. The Allied armies fought in the Battle of Amiens (the first day of which Ludendorff called "the Black Day

of the German Army," as a massive arrival of British tanks allowed the soldiers to emerge from the trenches to fight), the Battles of the Somme, the Battle of the Argonne Forest, and at St. Mihiel, where the Americans won another decisive battle.

Even Winston Churchill, chary in praising outsiders, could not help acknowledging the vitality the Americans brought to the bloody battle-fields. He would later cite a Frenchman's account of country roads sud-denly filled with that "inexhaustible flood of gleaming youth in its first maturity of health and vigour." Backhanded though the compliment may have been, he added, "Half trained, half organized with only their courage and their numbers and their magnificent youth behind their weapons, they were to buy their experience at a bitter price. But this they were quite ready to do." According to one military historian, the American Expedi-tionary Force "seized 485,000 square miles of enemy-held territory and captured 63,000 prisoners, 1,300 artillery pieces, and 10,000 mortars and machine guns."

In the words of Woodrow Wilson, "Our men went in force into the line of battle just at the critical moment when the whole fate of the world seemed to hang in the balance and threw their fresh strength into the ranks of freedom in time to turn the whole tide . . . so that henceforth it was back, back, back, for their enemies, always back, never again for-ward!" In short order, "the commanders of the Central Empires knew themselves beaten." But Churchill was right about the bitter cost. While the decisive streak of American military victories was not exactly Pyrrhic, it was pricey. In 150 days of combat, the AEF suffered the loss of 116,516 soldiers and sailors, almost half of whom died in combat, while most of the rest succumbed to influenza; another 204,002 were wounded; and 3,350 men were reported missing.

Half those losses came in the first six weeks of the fall of 1918 in the Argonne Forest, a dense wood next to the Meuse River, where the United States fought the largest battle in its history, before or since, with 1.2 million soldiers. It would result in the deaths of 26,277 Americans, more than had ever died in a single battle. There Alvin York, a sergeant born in a log cabin in Tennessee, led an attack on a machine gun nest, which resulted in the killing of 28 Germans and the capture of 132 more, rendering him a symbol of American heroism. Captain Harry Truman of Independence, Missouri, led a battery that supported the tank brigade of George S. Patton, without

losing a single man. He would return Stateside and become a haberdasher. And overhead, an Indianapolis 500 racecar driver from Ohio named Edward Rickenbacker was becoming one of the war's flying aces. American, French, and German casualties totaled 300,000 in the Meuse-Argonne offensive.

The war fomented great social change, as it imbued the nation with moral force and generated economic growth. On foreign battlefields, soldiers with roots in more than fifty different nations came together, as bankers shared foxholes with bums. Historian and future Yale President Charles Seymour observed that "the youthful plutocrat saw life from a new angle, the wild mountaineer learned to read, the alien immigrant to speak English." Materially speaking, the gross domestic product of the United States had doubled since 1914—to $75.8 billion—with half that rise coming since America's entrance into the war; and the gross public debt had almost trebled, to $14.6 billion. More than the steel and explosives industries benefited. Gillette, to name but one company, signed a deal with the government to produce 3.5 million razors, to be shipped to all enlisted men. With the muscle of the American workforce—its young males—largely in uniform, unemployment reached record lows, halving to 3 percent in 1918, some months dipping below 2. More women worked outside the home than ever before. Typewriters and telephones created a demand for clerical workers and operators, jobs deemed appropriate for them. The need for workers in the industrial North—notably Chicago, Cleveland, and Detroit—caused a migration of African Americans from sharecropping farms in the South. Even "colored girls" were able to find nondomestic work. But racial hatred and segregation persisted.

Less than a week after Congress had declared war, the President heard from the black pastor of Shiloh Baptist Church in Washington, D.C. He reminded Wilson that "the Colored people" accounted for one-tenth of the American population and that the time had come for their President to assure them that he and his administration desired their "hearty, united and enthusiastic support in carrying on the War" and that "no discrimination or injustice will be practiced by the Government." Days later, Wilson received a more stringent document from the Boston branch of the National Equal Rights League, signed by William Monroe Trotter, his former adversary, who suggested that the war allowed for some progressive social reordering. "There is need no longer of subjection of Americans to the race prejudices of fellow Americans," insisted the long proclamation.

"In the presence of a common danger and a common obligation, with a war devastating Europe caused by racial clannishness and racial hatred . . . let the United States of America and the people thereof give up race proscription and persecution at home." In short, they entreated Wilson to give the same encouragement for volunteering or enlisting to all Americans "by vouchsafing the same free chance to enlist, to rise by merit, and on return home, the same right to civil service, and to civil rights without bar or segregation."

Wilson saw no signs that the country was ready for that. Localized racial violence had become commonplace in the South, and now disturbances moved north, as blacks were taking jobs held formerly by whites. The old bugaboos of black men preying upon white women and black women seducing white men played into people's fears. Such had been the talk for months in East St. Louis, Illinois. After a few isolated incidents of brutality, the city conflagrated into what came to be called a "race riot." In truth, it was a pogrom.

On July 2, 1917, a phalanx of whites marched down a thoroughfare of the city and waited at a main intersection. As black people appeared, the mob attacked, pointlessly and relentlessly shooting, clubbing, stoning, and stomping people to death; they set fire to two hundred homes in the African American neighborhood; they dumped bodies into the Cahokia Creek. State troopers and the Illinois National Guard came to quell the melee, but witnesses saw men in uniform turn on the black victims as well. During two days of chaos, thousands of blacks took flight; and though officials tallied thirty-nine deaths, anti-lynching activist and journalist Ida B. Wells figured 150 people died. Governor Arthur Capper of Kansas wrote President Wilson not only to convey his outrage at the savagery but also to condemn the "damning effects of liquor," which had evidently fueled the massacre.

William English Walling—a wealthy, Harvard-educated grandson of Kentucky slave-owners, who cofounded the NAACP—wrote the White House, declaring the "unchecked savagery" in East St. Louis the worst since the Civil War. "There is no oversupply of labor anywhere in America today," Walling wired, "massacre clearly due to effort of the anti-Negro element of the South to check exodus of colored labor which promised to force south to suspend the reign of terror which has ruled there for half a century and to give negroes better pay and to treat them like human beings." Walling added, "There should be an immediate Presidential pro-

clamation that in the present military exigency the full military power of the nation will be used in defense of the lives and liberty of our colored fellow citizens."

Wilson called upon Attorney General Gregory to get to the bottom of "these disgraceful outrages." But, as Wilson soon wrote the Republican Congressman in St. Louis, Missouri, the federal attorneys and agents investigating the case required violations of federal statutes in order to act. "Up to this time," he admitted sadly, "I am bound in candor to say that no facts have been presented to us which would justify federal action." The President seemed as surprised as he was appalled that such a "tragical matter" should have been possible. As protesters across the country took to the streets and petitions seeking action arrived at the White House, Wilson offered little more than assurances that this local matter was being investigated. Of greater concern was the global war and the national conscription of an Army which he believed was clearly not ready for integration.

Secretary of War Baker wrote the President in August "that this is not the time to raise the race issue," for it was now his intention "to preserve the custom of the Army, which has been to organize colored people into separate organizations." Necessity would dictate that some colored men would train in Southern camps with white soldiers. Racist South Carolina Governor Coleman Livingston Blease insisted that he did not wish Negro troops to be stationed in his state; Congressman Lever feared the worst should such integration be forced upon his district—as did the President. Late that July, the 3rd Battalion of the 24th Infantry Regiment—654 black enlisted men serving under eight white officers—was sent to Houston; from the moment of their arrival, the black soldiers had clashed with white civilians. On August 23, some black troops mutinied, breaking into the arsenal and procuring guns, which they used indiscriminately as they rampaged through town. Fifteen people were killed and twelve others assaulted. Congressman Joe Eagle telegraphed the President to say that this behavior "conclusively proves tragic blunder committed in ordering negro troops to Southern camps. Besides this tragedy the presence of negro troops here has largely demoralized local negro feeling and conduct. Unless all these negro troops are sent away quickly my opinion that last night's tragedy is but a prelude to a tragedy upon enormous scale." Race riots flared from Philadelphia to Chicago. In Estill Springs, Tennessee, a Negro charged with murder was tortured with red-hot irons, then doused

in oil and burned to death before a crowd of men, women, and children. Lynchings across the South became epidemic, and the sight of black bodies swinging from trees was common.

In February 1918, civil rights activist James Weldon Johnson led a small delegation of ministers from the New York branch of the NAACP to the White House for an audience with the President. It was one of the few important congregations of black leaders to visit the White House since Wilson's dismissal of William Monroe Trotter in 1914. Johnson's mission on this day was specific, though it carried a broad message. In the immediate aftermath of the Houston race riot, a court-martial had sentenced thirteen men to death; and the condemned were hanged in pre-dawn darkness, without review. A subsequent court-martial sentenced another sixteen soldiers to death, but that verdict came just days after a new policy from the War Department declared a suspension of military death sentences without Presidential review. And so the NAACP delegation arrived with a petition with 1,200 signatures requesting clemency for those Negro soldiers facing the gallows. Johnson stood as he read the document, which spoke, he claimed, for the "great mass of the Negro population of the United States," the twelve million patriotic Negroes, many of whom wanted nothing more than to express their loyalty through military service. It detailed the "long series of humiliating and harassing incidents" that had sparked the riots, all part of an ingrained anti-Negro culture that was becoming increasingly institutionalized inside the American military as it had long been in Southern communities.

The presentation moved Wilson deeply. He asked for more facts about the immolation at Estill Springs—about which he had heard nothing— and he expressed dismay "that such a thing could have taken place in the United States." The delegation pressed him to offer a public utterance against mob violence and lynching, but Wilson said that he did not think word from him would have any "special effect." When the gentlemen from Harlem disagreed—stressing that "his word would have greater effect than the word of any other man in the world"—Wilson promised to "seek an opportunity" to say something.

For more than half an hour, the President sat with the delegation. Johnson had seen Wilson before from a distance and found him an austere figure. Now, sitting only a few feet away, the President struck him as "very human. His head, no longer inclined forward, rested back easily, and the

sternness of his face relaxed and, occasionally in a smile, became completely lost." He asked questions about the Negro in America and even offered a few reminiscences of his boyhood in the South. After the meeting, Johnson confessed that he could not rid himself of "the conviction that at bottom there was something hypocritical about him." But, he noted, "I came out . . . with my hostility toward Mr. Wilson greatly shaken."

The President made good on his word on July 26, 1918, when he found his "opportunity" and released a thoughtful statement, which he tied to the war effort. "I allude to the mob spirit," he said, without pointing to a particular individual or region. "There have been many lynchings," he added, "and every one of them has been a blow at the heart of ordered law and humane justice." He declared such actions nothing less than un-American. "We are at this very moment fighting lawless passion," Wilson stated, and lynchers only emulated Germany's disgraceful example by disregarding the sacred obligations of the law. He said, unequivocally, "Every American who takes part in the action of a mob or gives it any sort of countenance is no true son of this great Democracy, but its betrayer, and does more to discredit her by that single disloyalty to her standards of law and of right than the words of her statesmen or the sacrifices of her heroic boys in the trenches can do to make suffering peoples believe her to be their savior." He implored every Governor, law officer, and citizen to cooperate, "not passively merely, but actively and watchfully—to make an end of this disgraceful evil."

One month later, Wilson issued another race-related statement, this one based upon his review of the Houston riot cases, particularly those of the sixteen men facing the death penalty. He upheld six of the sentences—"because the persons involved were found guilty by plain evidence of having deliberately, under circumstances of shocking brutality, murdered designated and peaceably disposed civilians." The rest he commuted to life imprisonment because the men were not shown to have caused any deaths, despite their engagement in riotous and mutinous behavior. Wilson did not stop there. He said, "I desire the clemency here ordered to be a recognition of the splendid loyalty of the race to which these soldiers belong and an inspiration to the people of that race to further zeal and service to the country of which they are citizens and for the liberties of which so many of them are now bravely bearing arms at the very front of great fields of battle."

Not even James Weldon Johnson had made a case for the innocence of the six men who would be hanged. He acknowledged that President Wilson maintained his policy of reviewing death sentences from the courts-martial, and he praised his anti-lynching statement. In the autobiography he wrote fifteen years later, Johnson granted that his earlier "estimate of Mr. Wilson was actually colored and twisted by prejudice."

Four hundred thousand black American soldiers served during the war—in segregated units. Some camps were integrated, but the black soldiers trained separately. Most of the black regiments sent overseas were service units, digging trenches and burying bodies—the "nasty side of army life"; but forty thousand engaged in actual combat. To ease racial tensions, the War Department created a Negro officer training camp, so that black soldiers could take orders from men their own color. Whenever Negro soldiers stepped beyond the boundaries of segregation, they faced indignities; but the numbers in which they enlisted suggested that they were eager to prove their worthiness as first-class citizens. As the Texas Grand Master of the separate-but-equal Prince Hall Freemasonry said, "We believe that our second emancipation will be the outcome of this war. If the world is to be made 'safe for democracy,' that will mean us also." Even at a death rate more than twice that of the white American dough-boy, the black soldier was willing to stake his life on the promise that noble service would free him from segregation and mob violence.

Each pace forward incited efforts to push the Negro back. The war created enough circumstances in which the two races proved that they could coexist. But as 1918 drew the races into their closest contact ever, it also created the greatest repulsion. More lynchings than the nation had seen in a decade and a revitalized nationwide Ku Klux Klan lay just ahead. In addressing delegates from the National Race Congress at the White House on October 1, 1918, Wilson reminded the Negroes, "We all have to be patient with one another. Human nature doesn't make giant strides in a single generation. . . . I have a very modest estimate of my own power to hasten the process, but you may be sure that everything that I can do will be accomplished."

It both encouraged and disheartened African Americans to see the President's power at work when it came to challenging discrimination for another group—women, whose movement for suffrage began back in 1848 at a convention in Seneca Falls, New York. Even in the front lines of

this surge for equality, division existed between those who supported the evolution of their cause by working within the system and the revolutionaries, who sought immediate change and were prepared to defy the law if it would help achieve it. Arguments over class and race within each division had impeded progress for two generations. For a few decades, the National American Woman Suffrage Association, headed by medical doctor Anna Howard Shaw and a former teacher, Carrie Chapman Catt, had made considerable headway. It was not enough for Alice Paul, a highly educated activist from Pennsylvania with legal training, who joined the more militant Congressional Union for Woman Suffrage, which she transformed into the National Woman's Party in 1916. Decades younger than the NAWSA leadership, she felt it was time to revolt.

For years Wilson had endorsed women's suffrage and received its proponents in the White House, even when they disagreed with his approach. He admired Dr. Shaw and Mrs. Catt, but as this inveterate drafter of constitutions told a delegation seeking his support for an equal suffrage amendment in January 1915, "I . . . am tied to a conviction, which I have had all my life, that changes of this sort ought to be brought about state by state."

To many, Wilson was hiding behind states' rights. A year later, he tried convincing another suffrage delegation otherwise, as he remained committed to pushing New Jersey to adopt a state amendment. "It may move like a glacier," Wilson told two hundred members of the Congressional Union at the Waldorf-Astoria, "but when it does move, its effects are permanent." After Wilson had spoken, an emboldened Mary Ritter Beard, wife of Columbia University historian Charles A. Beard, asked the President whether the Clayton Anti-Trust Act had been enacted state by state. "I do not care to discuss that," an annoyed President said, and the meeting came to an end, with visible disappointment. Even his unmarried daughter, Margaret, who could always appeal to his sense of reason, steadily urged him to back a federal amendment, and she pressured Colonel House as well.

The battle lines in the matter of women's suffrage were drawn more between generations than genders, as the issue was not yet of imperative concern to the American public. Not even Progressives and, more important, women themselves were of one mind on the subject. The issue was not just about voting, or even keeping women in their place; many enlightened people considered it the beginning of a breakdown in traditional

family values. Theodore Roosevelt wrote, "Women do not really need the suffrage," though he did not think "they would do any harm with it." His two sisters opposed it; his younger wife supported it, mildly. Wilson was still unable to envisage a world in which women might play a strong political role. "Suffrage for women," he said one morning when his old friend Nancy Saunders Toy was staying at the White House, "will make absolutely no change in politics—it is the home that will be disastrously affected. Somebody has to make the home and who is going to do it if the women don't?" But, valuing people of intelligence exercising their democratic rights, Wilson strongly favored their enfranchisement; and, as he had promised, he applied personal and party pressure on each state legislature as it considered this question.

Growing numbers of disgruntled women continued to coerce the White House. For several months before Wilson's second inauguration, Alice Paul's National Woman's Party protested outside the Executive Mansion—several hundred "silent sentinels" every day, standing at the north gates, carrying banners. "Mr. President, how long must women wait for liberty?" was a favorite slogan; "Kaiser Wilson" was another. They reported at ten o'clock and remained until 4:30. Sometimes they chained themselves to the White House fence. Believing the angry protesters would thrive on opposition, the Administration instructed the police to take no action against them, thus limiting their press coverage.

On the first extremely cold day of their protests, the President sent Ike Hoover outside with a message for the dissidents. Just as they expected to be shooed from the vicinity, Hoover invited them all inside to the lower corridor of the White House, where the President specifically asked that they be served hot tea or coffee. "Excuse me, Mr. President," Hoover reported a moment later, "but they indignantly refused." Wilson asked that a servant carry hot bricks to the White House gates to provide warmth, a courtesy they accepted through the winter.

Although the passion of the suffragists moved him, in May 1917, Wilson wrote Mrs. Catt that he felt the time was inopportune for women to press their claim, as the Congress was consumed with the conduct of the war. The President continued his own efforts—lobbying state legislatures and urging the formation of a House committee to promote a Nineteenth Amendment to the Constitution, which had been defeated in that chamber three years earlier. When a mission of Russian diplomats arrived at the

White House in June, a boldly stenciled ten-foot-wide banner greeted them, declaring: "We, the women of America, tell you that America is not a democracy. Twenty million American women are denied the right to vote. President Wilson is the chief opponent of their national enfranchisement." Many women in the crowd expressed outrage that the protesters unfairly chose to speak for them; some cried "Treason!" Several men ripped the banner to pieces. Upon the President's orders, neither the police nor the Secret Service took any action other than maintaining order. Dr. Shaw of NAWSA said this sort of agitation only injured the suffrage cause; even sympathizers in Congress condemned the action. Alice Paul announced to the press, "We have ordered another banner with the same wording, and we intend to show it in the same place." The President wrote of the fracas to his daughter Jessie, "They certainly seem bent upon making their cause as obnoxious as possible."

On Bastille Day, Alice Paul's National Woman's Party took a different approach. It assembled sixteen socially prominent women—including the daughters and wives of distinguished Americans—to march quietly to the front gates of the White House. Carrying banners exclaiming "LIBERTY, EQUALITY, FRATERNITY," they refused to move on and waited to be arrested. It was an entirely peaceful demonstration, as courteous as a cotillion. An officer approached each woman, removed his hat, bowed, and advised her of the law she was breaking, before placing each of them under arrest. Even the crowd of thousands who turned out regularly to menace the protesters, watched in silence except for their quiet applause. Three days later a judge found the suffragists guilty of unlawful assembly and sentenced each to a twenty-five-dollar fine or sixty days in the District of Columbia workhouse in Occoquan, Virginia. They chose Occoquan.

No sooner were they incarcerated than the President summoned the District Commissioner in charge of the police. "Mr. Wilson was highly indignant," recalled Commissioner Louis Brownlow. "He told me that we had made a fearful blunder, that we never ought to have indulged these women in their desire for arrest and martyrdom, and that he had pardoned them and wanted that to end it." Brownlow then had the painful duty of informing the President that the women had refused his pardon. In the meantime, the incident provoked exactly what Wilson had feared—unwanted publicity. Newspapers ran accounts of the daughter of a former Secretary of State and the sister-in-law of a former Secretary of War being

required to rise at 6:30, wear loose gray dresses, and eat hominy, cabbage, and vegetable soup. Most "unnecessarily humiliating" of all, reported *The New York Times*, was that the suffragists had been quartered with Negro women.

Wilson was further humiliated when Dudley Field Malone, the Collector of the Port of New York, decided to represent the women. The President met with his old friend for more than half an hour. Malone insisted that Wilson could enact national suffrage almost immediately if he sincerely believed in it. At that point, with the nation mounting its war effort, Wilson said he did not feel he could go to Congress with such a demand. Malone asked why Wilson considered it right to demand of Congress all the important legislation he had pushed through and not this measure.

"I know of nothing that has gone more to the quick with me or that has seemed to me more tragical than Dudley's conduct," Wilson wrote Colonel House, "—which came upon me like a bolt out of the blue. I was stricken by it as I have been by few things in my life." Rather than accept that he had inadequately justified his position, he dismissed Malone's new role in the women's rights movement as an overreaction. "Here is one more item of tragedy added to this time of madness. We must not let the madness touch us," he wrote House, replaying in his mind what Kipling had said about keeping his head when all about were losing theirs.

During the 1916 election, Malone had campaigned hard for Wilson, notably in the woman suffrage states; California, of course, had delivered the President his cliffhanging victory. Malone had promised the women there that if they reelected Wilson, he would devote himself to the passage of the federal suffrage amendment. Now Malone felt hypocritical working for an administration that would not allow him to honor that commitment. As England and Russia in the midst of the Great War had promised women national enfranchisement, he could not reconcile the President's position. Unless the government took a step in that direction, Malone asked, how could it "ask millions of American women in our homes, or toiling for economic independence in every line of industry, to give up by conscription their men and happiness to a war for Democracy in Europe, while these women citizens are denied the right to vote on the policies of the Government which demands of them such sacrifice?" He told the President, "It is high time that men in this generation . . . stood up to battle

for the national enfranchisement of American women." On September 7, 1917, he tendered his resignation, which the President reluctantly accepted.

Wilson steadily continued his work on behalf of the movement at the state level. In the November 1917 elections, another five states embraced woman suffrage—most notably New York. Wilson had advanced the cause there by addressing a large delegation of its Woman Suffrage Party at the White House shortly before the election and then releasing his remarks to the press. Women had played a significant role in the war effort—not least of all the women of NAWSA, who sold a million dollars' worth of bonds. Praising their "ardor and efficiency," Wilson had insisted then that "this is the time for the states of this Union to take this action." In a post-election White House meeting, the woman leaders praised the President for his support; but even Mrs. Catt said "the time had come to grant the Federal amendment." This time, Wilson agreed.

Until she saw some actions to back the President's words, Alice Paul and her followers escalated their war for equality. They continued to write quotations on their banners that they thought would embarrass the President, such as the one that read "WE SHALL FIGHT FOR THE THINGS WHICH WE HAVE ALWAYS HELD NEAREST OUR HEARTS—FOR DEMOCRACY, FOR THE RIGHT OF THOSE WHO SUBMIT TO AUTHORITY TO HAVE A VOICE IN THEIR OWN GOVERNMENTS." They were, of course, quoting Wilson himself and were consequently immune from charges of sedition. When Alice Paul was hauled into court for obstructing traffic, she claimed she was exempt from the court's jurisdiction on the grounds that she and her sisterhood had no part in making the laws that brought her there. Paul was released, only to find herself back in court a few weeks later, at which time she was sentenced to Occoquan. There she demanded to be considered a "political prisoner" and began a hunger strike.

Wilson called for both a physician and a Commissioner of the District of Columbia to examine the prisoner's conditions. On November 9, 1917, Commissioner W. Gwynn Gardiner filed a detailed report, with the surprising observation that Miss Paul had volunteered that "she recognized the fact that President Wilson was a friend to the suffragists, but that they had determined upon picketing as a means of bringing the cause before the people of the country and keeping it before them." She stated further that she had decided upon this hunger strike as a means of "compelling those in authority to accede to her demands." Because she was

physically frail and refused to eat, the workhouse insisted on force-feeding her through a tube that would be inserted down her throat. Gardiner consulted with Dr. William Alanson White, a renowned psychiatrist and superintendent of St. Elizabeth's Hospital, the government hospital for the insane. White explained that this was "an every-day occurrence" at his institution, that for twenty years he had been feeding patients in this manner with no ill effect, and he recommended it for Miss Paul. Her room, Gardiner reported, was "well-lighted, well-ventilated, and perfectly clean." On the night of November 14, however, Occoquan became Bedlam. After Paul had undergone her forced feeding, many of her fellow soldiers protested what they considered inappropriate indignities—including the wearing of prison stripes. Their obstinacy ignited what became known as the "Night of Terror," complete with threats and physical abuse.

By the first week of 1918, another vote on the women's suffrage amendment was advancing in the House of Representatives. Elizabeth Bass, who headed the Women's Bureau of the Democratic National Committee, sent the President a short letter wondering "if you know how a word or two from you today . . . would enthrone you forever in the hearts of the women of the United States as the second Great Emancipator." Of greater significance was Bass's observation that they were living in fast-changing times—"when all foundations are shifting," and even the most extreme advocates of states' rights had just abandoned their position and passed a Prohibition amendment, of which Wilson did not approve. On January 9, Wilson advised the Democratic members of the House Suffrage Committee to vote for the federal amendment "as an act of right and justice to the women of the country and of the world." The next day the House voted 274 to 136 in favor of the Nineteenth Amendment to the Constitution, without a single vote to spare in attaining the requisite two-thirds majority. Republicans supported the measure four to one, while Democrats, mostly from the South, split down the middle. A far more difficult fight lay ahead in the upper house.

All that year Wilson and the suffragist leaders lobbied Senators. The vote was set for September 30, and according to every straw poll, the amendment would be two votes shy of passage. On the twenty-eighth, women from NAWSA called on Secretary McAdoo to discuss eleventh-hour strategy. They handed him a list of Senators they believed might still be talked into voting for their cause. McAdoo looked it over and said he

had already talked himself hoarse pleading the case. But the next morning, Sunday, he had an idea. The only possible means of winning was to have the President address the Senate. There were, unfortunately, two significant obstacles: Wilson did not discuss public questions on the Sabbath; and there was no precedent for a Chief Executive to address a chamber of Congress in order to influence a vote on pending legislation.

McAdoo called his father-in-law at ten o'clock that morning and stated his case. He said he did not believe anything at this point would change two votes; but, knowing how to appeal to the President's penchant for lost causes, he said, "I felt that since no President of the United States had ever spoken in favor of woman's suffrage, and that since we were fighting a war for democracy, it seemed to me that we could not consistently persist in refusing to admit women to the benefits of democracy on an equality with men." McAdoo argued that even if the speech fell on deaf ears within the legislature, the public, just weeks away from electing a new Congress, would hear his message. Wilson said that not only was there no precedent for such a speech but it would provoke resentment. At five o'clock that afternoon, Edith called McAdoo on the telephone to say that her husband was writing his speech.

At one o'clock the next day, Wilson appeared at the Capitol. The chamber quickly filled with Senators, their umbrage apparent. Through the "frigid atmosphere," he spoke for fifteen minutes, hoping that the "unusual circumstances of a world war in which we stand" justified his presence. He said, "I regard the concurrence of the Senate in the constitutional amendment proposing the extension of the suffrage to women as vitally essential to the successful prosecution of the great war of humanity in which we are engaged."

Wilson reminded his audience that the entire world was looking "to the great, powerful, famous Democracy of the West to lead them to the new day . . . and they think, in their logical simplicity, that democracy means that women shall play their part in affairs alongside men and upon an equal footing with them." In the past, some anti-suffragists had maintained that men's defense of the nation with bullets entitled them to ballots; for the first time, a Commander in Chief argued that the nation had made partners of the women in this war: "Shall we admit them only to partnership of suffering and sacrifice and toil," he asked, "and not to a partnership of privilege and right? This war could not have been fought,

either by the other nations engaged or by America, if it had not been for the services of the women." He went further, saying, "This measure which I urged upon you is vital to the winning of the war." Just as women had helped in the war effort, so too would they help in drafting the peace: "We shall need their moral sense to preserve what is right and fine and worthy in our system of life as well as to discover just what it is that ought to be purified and reformed. Without their counsellings we shall be only half wise." The President asked the Senate to lighten his task by placing in his hands the "spiritual instruments" he needed to close the war.

He swung no votes that day. With victory still out of reach, the two factions of the suffrage movement joined forces, each side having learned from the other. Alice Paul softened her approach to President Wilson while Carrie Chapman Catt got tougher. Moving their armies to the Capitol, the two suffrage leaders privately assured Southern legislators that giving women the vote was not meant to diminish states' rights or augment Negroes' powers; it was simply about lifting the "sex restriction." Publicly, they targeted anti-suffrage legislators from both houses in the upcoming elections. A number of longtime Senators saw reason to worry. "The women have earned it," Wilson told Stockton Axson. "I am sorry it had to come in this way"—through the agitations of war—"but they must have what they have justly won."

With the young men of the American Expeditionary Force at last in the line of fire, Wilson considered virtually every act of Congress a measure of patriotism. That meant not only giving full voting rights to women but also seizing certain rights from other Americans. To ensure that the soldiers had the complete support of the Americans at home, Congress passed the Sedition Act on May 16, 1918. With the strong encouragement of Attorney General Gregory, this amendment to the Espionage Act of 1917 conferred certain policing powers upon the Postmaster General and further curbed citizens in expressing political opinions. Protest against this new law was vehement, but it found little backing in any branch of government.

When still teaching at Princeton, Wilson had written that the Sedition Act of 1798 had "cut perilously near the root of freedom of speech and of the press. There was no telling where such exercises of power would stop. Their only limitations and safeguards lay in the temper and good sense of the President and the Attorney General." Now as President, with Americans dying for their country, Wilson would brook no speech that

even suggested sedition. He left the actual pursuit of violations to his hard-line Postmaster General and Attorney General. Both men were leery of the Socialist Party and the Industrial Workers of the World because both organizations had opposed American entry into the war, which they considered a capitalist struggle at the expense of the workers. Questions arose as to whether vocal opposition to the war qualified as seditious.

Paranoia permeated the nation. Local watchdog organizations formed to ferret out enemies within America's borders. The largest and best-organized group of this nature banded under the Justice Department's Bureau of Investigation. Calling itself the American Protective League, by 1918 it claimed over six hundred branches with 250,000 card-carrying members whose only real power was intimidation. Gregory boasted to McAdoo that after almost a year of operation, there had been only three instances of "objectionable" APL conduct.

The American Union Against Militarism—which became the American Civil Liberties Union—begged to differ. In August 1917, this left-leaning pacifist organization sent the President a list of recent cases they thought would convince him that civil liberty in America was being "seriously threatened under pressure of the war." The authors of the letter—including Lillian D. Wald and Roger Baldwin—provided evidence that constitutional rights were being overlooked. They cited unlawful arrests of people exercising their rights of free speech and peaceable assembly—meetings and parades that had been disrupted by the military, orders from overzealous District Attorneys, and arbitrary actions by Post Office officials who declared certain publications "unnmailable" because of their content. Wilson assigned the Attorney General to investigate the charges because he personally esteemed the people who had signed the letter. When the Postmaster General clamped down on eighteen periodicals, the President immediately received a letter from Max Eastman, Amos Pinchot, and John Reed, who asked, "Can it be necessary, even in war time, for the majority of a republic to throttle the voice of a sincere minority?" Again, Wilson intervened, writing Albert Burleson, "These are very sincere men and I should like to please them." The Postmaster General insisted that their opposition to the war, especially the conscription law, went so far as to "obstruct the Government in its conduct of the war." The matter quickly moved through the courts, until the Supreme Court ruled in favor of the government.

On June 16, 1918, Eugene Debs campaigned for the Socialist Party in Canton, Ohio, where he had just visited three comrades who were serving time in a workhouse for having encouraged young men to refuse induction into the Army. Debs kidded with his audience about the care he had to take in selecting his words, and then he proceeded to inform his 1,200 listeners that the government had been trying to suppress the Socialist message, that the master class had always taught and trained the workers "to believe it to be your patriotic duty to go to war to have yourselves slaughtered at their command." He urged his listeners "to know that you are fit for something better than slavery and cannon fodder," and he harangued the government for prosecuting those who resisted what the ruling class called "patriotic duty." Two weeks later, Debs was arrested and charged with ten counts of sedition.

At his trial in September, Debs's attorneys presented no witnesses, only the defendant himself, who spoke for two hours. The court found him guilty. Upon receiving a ten-year prison sentence, he spoke once more, telling the judge: "Your Honor, years ago I recognized my kinship with all living beings, and I made up my mind that I was not one bit better than the meanest on earth. I said then, and I say now, that while there is a lower class, I am in it, and while there is a criminal element I am of it, and while there is a soul in prison, I am not free." The words would echo for decades; but Woodrow Wilson still considered Debs a traitor.

Within months his case came before the Supreme Court. The Espionage Act of 1917 criminalized the conveyance of "information with intent to interfere with the operation or success of the armed forces of the United States or to promote the success of its enemies"; and, for all of Debs's elocutionary caution, the Justices considered his Canton speech an obstruction of military recruitment. In considering whether the defendant's conviction violated his First Amendment right to the freedom of speech, the Justices referred to a nearly identical case decided the preceding week, *Schenck v. United States*. The Court had ruled that an individual distributing leaflets urging opposition to the draft was not safeguarded. Justice Oliver Wendell Holmes, Jr., had written the unanimous opinion for the Court, which famously asserted that "the character of every act" depended upon its context.

The most stringent protection of free speech would not protect a man in falsely shouting fire in a theatre and causing a panic. . . .

The question in every case is whether the words used are used in such circumstances and are of such a nature as to create clear and present danger that they will bring about the substantive evils that Congress has a right to prevent. . . . When a nation is at war many things that might be said in time of peace are such a hindrance to its effort that their utterance will not be endured so long as men fight and that no Court could regard them as protected by any constitutional right.

Holmes wrote the opinion in the Debs case as well, which was also unanimous.

Woodrow Wilson felt Debs had violated every tenet of unity and loyalty that he held dear. The President was quick to note that Debs had every right to exercise his freedom of speech before the war. But, Wilson maintained, "once the Congress of the United States declared war, silence on his part would have been the proper course to pursue." It galled Wilson that while "the flower of American youth was pouring out its blood to vindicate the cause of civilization, this man, Debs, stood behind the lines, sniping, attacking, and denouncing them."

America entered a period of repression as egregious as any in American history. Members of the Cabinet manipulated the offensive laws, but Woodrow Wilson's fingerprints were all over them. "The new espionage act," wrote H. L. Mencken, "gives the Postmaster General almost absolute power to censor American magazines. He may deny the mails to any one that he doesn't like, for any reason or no reason. No crime is defined; no hearing is allowed; no notice is necessary; there is no appeal." Wilson periodically asked Postmaster Burleson to show leniency toward some potential scofflaws, especially left-wingers he knew to be intellectually sincere; but the government arrested 1,500 citizens in 1918 for little more than criticizing it; and close to 2,500 "enemy aliens" were interned during the war.

Worse than the actual suppression of written material was the atmosphere of suspicion the Administration created, one so noxious that it coerced most "law-abiding" citizens into censoring themselves, inhibiting one of the very freedoms for which America was fighting overseas. Only later did Mencken write, "Between Wilson and his brigades of informers, spies, volunteer detectives, perjurers and complaisant judges, and the Prohibitionists and their messianic delusion, the liberty of the citizen has

pretty well vanished in America. In two or three years, if the thing goes on, every third American will be a spy upon his fellow citizens."

Wilson was not blind to the injustices his administration had imposed. But at a moment when many American soldiers were marching off to their deaths, he considered temporary restraints on civil liberties minor infringements. He conceded his own uncertainty about finding the right balance in his policies but not about erring on the side of precaution. As he wrote liberal activist Max Eastman: "I think that a time of war must be regarded as wholly exceptional and that it is legitimate to regard things which would in ordinary circumstances be innocent as very dangerous to the public welfare, but the line is manifestly exceedingly hard to draw and I cannot say that I have any confidence that I know how to draw it. I can only say that a line must be drawn and that we are trying, it may be clumsily but genuinely, to draw it without fear or favor or prejudice."

In the beastly hot summer of 1918, Wilson could no longer avoid another problem that had long troubled him. "I have been sweating blood over the question what it is right and feasible (*possible*) to do in Russia," he wrote Colonel House on July 8, months after that empire had collapsed and surrendered, leaving its problems for the Allies to solve. France and Britain abhorred the thought of Bolshevism spreading to their countries; and they realized that the German armies at the Eastern Front would now be reassigned to the Western Front, increasing their threat. Allied supplies were stockpiled in the northwesternmost cities of Murmansk and Archangel, which Russia could no longer defend. For months, the Allies relentlessly pressured the United States to join them in an invasion.

Wilson wanted no part of the plans. His recent forays into Mexico (where he had been ensnared his entire first term) and the Dominican Republic and Haiti (where American troops would remain mired until 1924 and 1934, respectively) had proved certain limitations of foreign policy: not even boundless military might offered a guarantee of stabilizing a foreign government. Although averse to Bolshevism, Wilson was not adverse. He believed armed resistance could easily backfire and that trying to stop a revolutionary movement with ordinary armies was "like using a broom to sweep back a great sea." Wilson continued to resist the Allies' pleas.

Lord Reading—a justice rendering temporary ambassadorial service in Washington—gathered that the President feared that once American

troops were in Russia, some action by the French or British would interfere with Russian domestic affairs and suck America in even deeper. Reading reported to Prime Minister David Lloyd George that "the President is apprehensive lest any intervention should be converted into an anti-Soviet movement and an interference with the right of Russians to choose their own form of government." In their efforts to enlist American support, the French went so far as to send Henri Bergson to Washington, but the renowned philosopher failed in his efforts. Wilson had just read a report from an explorer named George Kennan—well versed in Russia (and a cousin of a teenager of the same name, who would later become an influential diplomat in the same region). He wrote the Administration of the need to eschew the Bolshevik government—as they were "usurpers," criminals, and enemies of the Allies, with nothing to offer them, not even the ability to restore order across Russia's vast geography. A massive Siberian intervention—involving as many as a million men—was then being staged to help White Russian forces overtake the Reds.

In the extreme opposite corner of Russia, seventy thousand interned Czech freedom fighters found themselves stranded in Vladivostok. They had been plotting to return to the front by journeying across the Pacific, where they would go by ship to America and on to France; but the Bolsheviks detained them. The Allies could only benefit from the addition to their ranks; and the Czechs' freedom-loving spirit appealed greatly to America. Philosopher and politician Tomáš Masaryk met with Wilson in Washington, and the President proved susceptible to the cause. On August 5, 1918, he agreed to commit military aid in the Siberian expedition— five thousand American troops to help protect the Allied stockpiles in the northwest and seven thousand more to help the Czech legions in the southeast. If nothing else, an American presence in Russia could keep a closer eye on imperialistic Japan, which saw an opportunity to harpoon Russian territory for itself. Masaryk thanked Wilson for his action. "Your name," he wrote him, ". . . is openly cheered in the streets of Prague,—our nation will forever be grateful to you and to the people of the United States."

Unfortunately, by the time American and Allied troops reached the northern military stores, winter had put any defensive operations on ice, and the war on the Eastern Front had shut down. The United States asked Japan to match its troops, but they sent twelve thousand men instead.

Within months, seventy thousand Japanese troops had arrived, with more on the way; and they had seized the Chinese Eastern Railway. "The presence of our troops in Siberia is being used by the Japanese as a cloak for their own presence and operations there," Secretary Baker wrote the President, "and the Czecho-Slovak people are quite lost sight of in any of the operations now taking place." Baker suggested that the longer America stayed, the more Japanese would arrive; but it seemed just as dangerous to leave the Japanese unchecked as they increased their presence. The United States would remain for several more years, seeing once again that military interventions—like the memories of invaded nations—are never short. While the American Expeditionary Force Siberia was not the actual start of the subsequent Cold War, it planted the seeds of distrust that Russians would recall decades later.

As the war in Europe expanded, the President's life contracted. He continued to delegate the running of specific operations to his Generals, Cabinet Secretaries, and Commissioners, leaving him to focus on the panoramic vision of the war's aims. While others sorted out details, he treasured his time alone with Edith, and socialized with few people beyond his family. He obeyed Dr. Grayson's advice to the letter, allowing for as much daily exercise and leisure as possible. He played golf every morning—at least nine holes, knowing he could play eighteen on weekends. In the winter, the White House staff painted his golf balls red, so that he could spot them more easily on the snow-covered links. Nothing eased his worries more than visits to the theater. He especially enjoyed the vaudeville offerings at B. F. Keith's Theatre just across Fifteenth Street from the White House grounds. He tended to enjoy these shows more than dramatic plays, because even a bad variety act was sure to be followed by something amusing. The family delighted in hearing him laugh.

Beyond the diversion, an evening at Keith's offered the President a microcosm of America, a mixture of ethnicities presenting all-American entertainment. Any given night featured a variety of animal acts, circus acrobatics, classical and popular music, and comedy. A Hungarian-born Jew named Erik Weisz performed feats of magic and "escapology" as Harry Houdini; and English-born Vernon Castle and his wife, Irene, introduced American audiences to the tango and fox-trot. Countless Italian-, Irish-, and Jewish-American comedians became headliners, as lacing their

monologues with hearty ethnic humor, and laughing at themselves before others could, proved an effective means of integrating their people into white, Protestant America. Negro storytelling was a popular feature as well—usually mocking the colored man's laziness or ignorance. The sketches were good-natured, no more derogatory in content than those of any other ethnicity; the only difference, of course, was that white people in black makeup delivered the anecdotes. These "darkey stories" and minstrel songs carried Wilson back to his childhood in Dixie. He was a devoted fan of George Primrose, a tap-dancing fireball in blackface; and in the privacy of the Oval Room upstairs at the White House, Woodrow would frequently slip a record on the Victrola and break into a spirited jig solely for Edith's entertainment. She marveled at how light on his feet he was, and he often said he envied Primrose and "wished he could exchange jobs" with him.

Nobody dominated the current stage more than George M. Cohan, who came from a family of Irish Catholic vaudevillians and wrote dozens of plays and revues and hundreds of songs. During the war they turned unusually patriotic, and his song "Over There" became America's wartime anthem. It was a rousing call to arms whose lyrics announced that "the Yanks are coming." Wilson could not get the number out of his head; and at a time when he anguished over dead and wounded soldiers, he often sang it to himself. Stockton Axson noticed that his voice invariably broke whenever he reached the last line—"And we won't come back till it's over over there."

Remarkable for someone whose health had been so fragile all his life, the President maintained his strength through the war. Apart from the occasional cold that kept him in bed, he did suffer two medical incidents, neither neurological. On April 19, 1918, while taking part in a campaign to promote Liberty Bonds, Wilson dismounted from a British tank and set his left hand down upon a red-hot exhaust pipe. He suffered serious burns, which required dressing his hand for months. "Now I am going about like a hotel waiter with a white glove over the bandages," Wilson wrote his daughter Jessie, ". . . feeling as if I ought to be handing something to somebody!" (The President's insurance company refused to pay indemnity on the grounds that he was ambidextrous and, therefore, not incapacitated.) And in the early fall, Wilson's nasal passages became so congested that he went weeks without breathing properly or sleeping well. Dr.

Grayson discovered polyps and determined that they should be removed. Wilson agreed to a polypectomy but insisted the procedure be kept secret. Without telling anybody but their respective wives, Wilson and Grayson sneaked out of the White House on September 7 and went to a local doctor, who removed the growths. The operation proved to be more complicated than anybody had anticipated, but neither the press nor the public ever had an inkling their President had been ill. It would not be the last time Dr. Grayson and the Wilsons would keep a medical matter from not only the public but even the innermost circles of the White House. For the moment, Grayson believed the President could live another ten years, even endure a third term—"if nothing untoward happened."

From the moment America entered the war, Woodrow Wilson proved to be a formidable Commander in Chief, directing the conversion of a peacetime nation into the globe's mightiest military-industrial complex, one in which every citizen played a role. He ruled mostly with his rhetoric, which remained as sharp as a bayonet. On September 27, he kicked off the Fourth Liberty Loan drive saying, "The common will of mankind has been substituted for the particular purposes of individual states." While the doughboys continued to lead the Allies to one victory after another, the nations of Europe—the Allied and Central Powers alike—could already envision the future. "Individual statesmen may have started the conflict," Wilson said that night, "but neither they nor their opponents can stop it as they please. It has become a peoples' war, and peoples of all sorts and races, of every degree of power and variety of fortune, are involved in its sweeping processes of change and settlement."

Wilson presented truths he now considered axiomatic: a nation's military power should not determine the fortunes of its people; strong nations should not be free to wrong weak nations; people should be ruled by their own will and choice, not by arbitrary and irresponsible force; there should be certain common standards of right and privilege; and the assertion of right should not be haphazard but the result of "common concert to oblige the observance of common rights." The audience stood and cheered, and the government raised $7 billion with this bond.

Two days later, Bulgaria became the first of the Central Powers to surrender; and independence spread across the region. Within eight days, Poland declared itself an independent state; the following week a provisional government of Czechoslovakia formed; and eleven days later a

council established itself in Budapest preparing to create a Hungarian nation separate from Austria. The Germans, recognizing the inevitable, realized that their best hope for rational terms of surrender was with the opponent they had fought for the shortest time. On October 6, 1918, Prince Max von Baden, the German Imperial Chancellor, formally requested the President of the United States "to take steps for the restoration of peace, to notify all belligerents of this request, and to invite them to delegate Plenipotentiaries for the purpose of taking up negotiations." Prince Max accepted as a basis of those negotiations Wilson's Fourteen Points and his pronouncements in his address of September 27.

Wilson requested explication. He presumed Max's letter meant that Germany accepted his terms, that further discussion was warranted only to sort out the practical details, and that German withdrawal of all her armies to German territory was implicit in this acceptance. Another volley of notes discussed the American demand that the process of evacuation and the conditions of an armistice all be matters left to the judgment of the American and Allied governments and that no arrangement could be accepted by the United States "which does not provide absolutely satisfactory safeguards and guarantees of the maintenance of the present military supremacy of the armies of the United States and of the Allies in the field." On October 12, the Germans accepted Wilson's demands, but their army kept fighting. Days later, Germany agreed to cease submarine warfare; and by the end of the month, the Allied commanders met to discuss means of rendering Germany militarily impotent. While the Kaiser went into seclusion in Belgium, refusing to abdicate, Sultan Mehmed VI of the Ottoman Empire requested terms of capitulation, as did the Emperor of Austria. At the end of the first week of November, Prince Max sent a delegation of diplomats to France to negotiate specifics of his nation's surrender and then announced his resignation.

Before Wilson could claim victory in the Great War, he had to engage in one last battle—the midterm Congressional elections of 1918. Although politicians had to some degree abided since January by Wilson's decree of adjourning politics, each party longed to blame the other for the nation's woes and to claim its successes. The Republicans were powerless so long as they remained mute, as the successful culmination of the war put the Democrats at an advantage. By the end of that summer, the Republicans realized they could bite their tongues no longer. Republican National

Committee chairman Will Hays toured the country repudiating the Administration's policies; in August, Senator Lodge spoke out against the Fourteen Points; in September, Republican Congressmen urged the election of a Republican Congress; on October 24, Colonel Roosevelt wired three influential Republican Senators, encouraging them to reject the Fourteen Points. While Germany had already consented to those terms, Roosevelt said, "such a peace would represent not the unconditional surrender of Germany but the conditional surrender of the United States."

Wilson intended to refrain from campaigning, and he instructed his Cabinet not to embark on political tours. Roosevelt's comments, however, warranted a Presidential response. In stressing the critical nature of the times, he boiled his argument down to a peculiarly political point:

> If you have approved of my leadership and wish me to continue to be your unembarrassed spokesman in affairs at home and abroad, I earnestly beg that you will express yourself unmistakably to that effect by returning a Democratic majority to both the Senate and the House of Representatives. I am your servant and will accept your judgment without cavil, but my power to administer the great trust assigned me by the Constitution would be seriously impaired should your judgment be adverse, and I must frankly tell you so because so many critical issues depend upon your verdict.

He emphasized the need for "unified leadership" in the nation, which a Republican Congress would divide. Adding to this strangely inappropriate statement, Wilson said, "The return of a Republican majority to either House of the Congress would, moreover, certainly be interpreted on the other side of the water as a repudiation of my leadership." In ordinary times, he said, he would not feel at liberty to make such a public appeal. "But these are not ordinary times."

"Criticism and ridicule," to use Tumulty's terms, were hurled at Wilson, justifiably. In politicizing the war, he had committed a serious gaffe. He had not only "lowered himself," as Secretary Lane noted privately, but he had also diminished his constituents. Outside the capital, Republicans had joined the war effort as much as Democrats; and the President's message seemed to ignore their contributions, to say nothing of the Republican support he had received within the Capitol. Democrats offered

numerous examples of Presidents from Washington to TR who had made similar electoral appeals. Even Lincoln midwar had campaigned by cautioning the electorate against "swapping horses in midstream." By Election Day, however, some simply made Wilson the whipping boy for the staggering confusion in the world.

Western Civilization lay prostrate from the most convulsive four years it had ever known. Four dynasties that had long dominated much of the world had fallen; and the combat itself produced stunning statistics: 885,000 British soldiers died, as had 1,400,000 French (more than 4 percent of their population) and 1,811,000 Russians; the Central Powers lost over 4,000,000 soldiers. All together, close to 10,000,000 soldiers died in the Great War, and more than 21,000,000 were wounded; counting civilian deaths, as the result of disease, famine, massacres, and collateral damage, somewhere between 16,500,000 and 65,000,000 people died—1.75 percent of the population of the participating nations. Wilson could already sense that the men in the trenches on both sides were undergoing an emotional change, that they would "return to their homes with a new view and an impatience of all mere political phrases, and will demand real thinking and sincere action." With American soldiers still in harm's way, Wilson resented that the Republicans—especially Roosevelt and Lodge—used the final weeks of the campaign to clamor for "the undesirable and impossible," namely "a vengeful peace." Wilson would not engage in that argument. "So far as my being destroyed is concerned," he wrote Senator Henry F. Ashurst, "I am willing if I can serve the country to go into a cellar and read poetry the remainder of my life. I am thinking now only of putting the US into a position of strength and justice. I am now playing for 100 years hence."

The United States had undergone profound changes of its own, arguably more in the last two years than at any other time in its history. Such paroxysms offered voters countless reasons to ignore Wilson's appeal for a Democratic Congress. Conscription and governmental restrictions—especially of gasoline and coal—persisted; tax rates remained at unprecedented highs; race relations dipped to historic lows; and hatred of foreigners and contention over labor prevailed.

Despite the impending victory in Europe, America was suffering. Naïveté and idealism had soured into skepticism and disillusionment; and influenza spiked in the United States that fall, killing in a single week

almost five thousand people in Philadelphia, to name but one city. The disease sent more than a quarter of the nation to bed, killing more than a half million Americans. Many public events and venues—including political rallies and even Keith's Theatre in Washington—shut down. Many voters were either too ill or too afraid of getting ill to go to the polls. Those who took their chances found many of their fellow citizens wearing face masks.

While Republican candidates vociferously challenged the President's request for political support, Wilson fell silent, right up to Election Day. On November 5, turnout was light, but the message was emphatic. Republicans took control of both chambers of Congress. In the House, they picked up twenty-five seats, which marked more than a one-hundred-seat gain since Wilson had entered the White House, giving them the majority and the speakership that went with it. In the Senate, Republicans gained seven seats—reclaiming, at last, their pre-Wilson majority. Despite his joy that the war was ending, Wilson privately revealed that he was "of course disturbed by the result of Tuesday's elections, because they create obstacles to the settlement of the many difficult questions which throng so on every side."

No longer the peacetime nation that long disavowed foreign entanglements, America had become a mighty fortress, the first industrial superpower of the twentieth century. The country boasted a towering infrastructure for a massive system of defense, replete with the machinery for further expansion. Its heavy industries had demonstrated their ability to work in concert with the government and one another, becoming proficient if not expert in mass production. Because of its vast natural resources, the United States could feed not only itself but the rest of the world as well.

America had become an extroverted nation, a force of morality for all humanity. It was prepared to unleash its power whenever necessary—to protect its citizens and their globalizing interests and to stand vigil over the rest of mankind. Colonel House believed the war had given Wilson "a commanding opportunity for unselfish service." He told the President that the great figures in history—from Alexander to Napoleon—"had used their power for personal and national aggrandizement"; but Wilson now had the rare opportunity to "use it for the general good of mankind."

While it was Woodrow Wilson's intention to lead his nation into a millennium, he now faced a hostile incoming Congress. Notwithstanding, he remained confident that "by one means or another the great thing we have to do will work itself out." After all, he reminded one junior member of the Administration, "I have an implicit faith in Divine providence. . . ."

PART FOUR

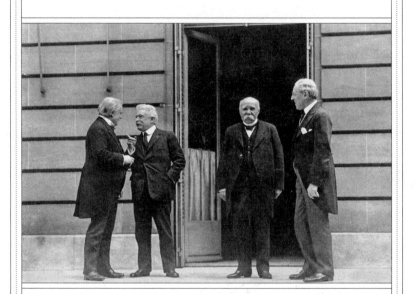

13

ISAIAH

*The Spirit of the Lord God is vpon me, because the
Lord hath anointed me, to preach good tidings vnto
the meek, hee hath sent me to binde vp the broken
hearted, to proclaime libertie to the captiues . . .*

—ISAIAH, LXI:1

At noon on Thursday, November 7, 1918, the United
Press Association's office in Paris cabled its headquarters in New York that Germany and the Allies had signed
the Armistice. Within three minutes, the national censors
had approved its dissemination; and within half an hour,
word had spread nationwide.

By one o'clock, all of New York City's bells and sirens
had sounded, and similar demonstrations across the country followed. People in Manhattan poured into the streets—
in what *The New York Times* called "a delirious carnival of
joy which was beyond comparison with anything ever seen
in the history of New York." Factories in Boston closed,
and parades spontaneously erupted through the town. Chicago's stores, offices, munitions plants, and City Hall shut
down, while its opera company interrupted rehearsal and
broke into "The Star-Spangled Banner." In Columbus,
Ohio, the massive crowds surrounding the State House demanded remarks from Governor James M. Cox. And in
Washington, D.C., people gravitated to the South Lawn of

the White House, where the euphoric crowd, dancing and tossing their hats in the air, waited for the President to appear. Nell McAdoo was leaving the Treasury Building, only to have a total stranger throw his arms around her and kiss her. Edith Wilson bustled to her husband's study, urging him to the portico, where he might address the gathering below, but he refused. He was one of the few men in the world who knew for a fact that this national hysteria was based on a false report.

Correspondents in Europe soon got their stories straight, and the next day the New York *Globe* characterized the misinformation as "the greatest and most cruel hoax in the history of journalism." The source of the falsehood was never discovered, but many suspected a German agent had perpetrated the deception "to create popular desire and demand among the Allied people for the German-sought armistice." Wrote Arthur Hornblow, Jr., a young intelligence officer, "From a psychological point of view the best possible way of making the public *want* an armistice would be to tell them that there *was* an armistice, and let them taste of the joy that would naturally await upon the news." That very day, in fact, German delegates were on their way to surrender at a secret site.

Marshal Foch spent the night on the outskirts of the village of Rethondes in the forest of Compiègne. At dawn, a train carried him, his staff, and British officers to an obscured railroad siding. Around seven, another train—including a carriage still marked with Napoleon III's coat of arms—shuttled the German plenipotentiaries to another siding in the woods. At nine, the German representatives walked the heavily guarded hundred yards that separated the trains and entered the Wagon Lits Company car 2419D. After formal salutations, the teams sat across from each other at a long wooden table. Foch told his interpreter to ask the Germans what they wanted. Matthias Erzberger, the civilian head of the German delegation, said, "We have come to receive the Allied Powers' proposals for an armistice." An offended Foch interrupted to say, "Tell these gentlemen that I have no proposals to make to them." The Frenchman made motions to leave, when another member of the German team interceded, asking Foch to put semantics aside. Count Alfred von Oberndorff said they had come—after receiving a note from President Wilson—to accept Foch's terms.

The parley proceeded, but not without hiccups. For more than a week, Germany had been in the middle of a revolution. Sailors had mutinied; Bolsheviks were seizing power across the country; and Kaiser Wilhelm

clung to his throne. And so, while Foch had given his enemies seventy-two hours in which to sign the terms of surrender, Erzberger questioned his legal ability to do so. The Kaiser did not abdicate until November 9— when he retreated to Holland, where he would spend the rest of his days in what he considered temporary exile. As the clock was running out, a second team of German diplomats arrived, announcing that a Republic had been proclaimed under a Socialist Chancellor. Several hours later, they received the requisite authorization.

Wilson spent the morning of Sunday the tenth with Edith at services in the Presbyterian Church. They lunched alone and took a long drive in the afternoon. Several Bollings joined them for an anxious dinner, after which Edith's mother said to her son-in-law, "I do wish you would go right to bed; you look so tired." Woodrow said he wished he could—"but I fear The Drawer; it always circumvents me; wait just a moment until I look." He returned with four or five long encrypted cables, which he handed to Edith. Her brother Randolph stayed until one o'clock, helping her decode the important messages, though none contained the news the world awaited. Back in the train car outside Rethondes, the delegates ironed out minor wrinkles; and shortly after five o'clock in the morning Paris time, they signed the documents. It was agreed that the Armistice would officially begin on the eleventh hour of that eleventh day of the eleventh month. Around three o'clock Washington time, word reached the White House in a series of telegrams from Colonel House, who was in France. Together Edith and Woodrow decoded his cable: "Autocracy is dead. [Long live] democracy and its immortal leader. In this great hour my heart goes out to you in pride, admiration and love." Edith would later recount that stunning moment in which they simply stood mute, "unable to grasp the full significance of the words."

The President caught a few hours of sleep before he issued a simple announcement that the Armistice had been signed and that work was suspended that day for all government employees. "A supreme moment of history has come," he handwrote. "The hand of God is laid upon the nations. He will show them favour, I devoutly believe, only if they rise to the clear heights of His own justice and mercy." Pandemonium broke out once again across the country and in the major capitals of the world. Wilson spent the rest of the morning in his study writing the speech he would deliver at one o'clock that afternoon.

Wearing a black tailcoat and light gray pants, he strode before the Congress. A standing ovation welcomed him, the audience's cheers extending to the gallery as the presiding officers permitted the spectators to join in the demonstration. Wilson quieted the chamber and launched into defining the terms to which the Germans had agreed in "these anxious times of rapid and stupendous change." Eleven military clauses pertained to the Western Front, from the cessation of operations to the immediate evacuation of invaded countries; five clauses dictated Germany's actions on the eastern frontier, including its abandonment of territory that had belonged to Russia, Romania, or Turkey before August 1, 1914. Germany had one month in which to capitulate unconditionally in East Africa; and similar terms applied to all hostilities at sea, including the surrender of submarines and surface warships, as well as the Allied freedom of access to and from the Baltic and Black Seas and the evacuation of seized Russian war vessels. The existing Allied blockade would continue. Repatriation of all civilians from the Allied or Associated nations must occur within a month. Applause interrupted several of these points, its intensity commensurate with the severity of the terms against the Germans. The mention of the return of Alsace-Lorraine to France, for example, brought the spectators to their feet. Any suggestions of leniency toward the enemy met silence. After modestly reciting all thirty-five terms of the Armistice, the President of the United States declaimed one last sentence. "The war," he said, "thus comes to an end."

America had won a decisive victory. Even Senator La Follette, who had sat silent until then, broke into applause. Arizona Senator Henry F. Ashurst dined with French Ambassador Jusserand in the Senate restaurant, only to see the diplomat burst into tears of joy. Cheering throngs lined the streets as Wilson returned to the White House, and for weeks praise was heaped upon him wherever he went. King George V sent a "message of congratulation and deep thanks in my own name and that of the people of this empire." The next day, *The New York Times* lauded the nation and, even more, Woodrow Wilson, whose "clear vision of the moral objects for which the nations took up arms against Germany . . . won for him very early acknowledged pre-eminence as the spokesman of the allied cause." As most of the world agreed, "He has been a great leader."

Washington celebrated all day, sweeping even Wilson into the festivities. November 11 happened to be the birthday of the King of Italy, and

the Italian Ambassador was celebrating the occasion that night with a ball. A little before eleven o'clock, the President proposed to Edith that they crash the party. The Ambassador was only too happy to welcome a giddy Wilson, who toasted the King and lingered for another hour. Back at the White House, Woodrow and Edith sat on a couch by her bedroom fireplace, where he read a chapter from the Bible before retiring.

The next morning the President felt the first undertow of politics amid the waves of congratulation. The mere possibility that Wilson himself would attend the Peace Conference caused considerable controversy, at home and abroad, as its location and leadership could alter the outcome. Two neutral nations, Switzerland and the Netherlands, offered to host the meeting, which meant Wilson might preside; but the great blood-soaked battleground, France, felt entitled to hold the event. Colonel House reported from Paris that the French thought Wilson should not even appear for the negotiations. A ceremonial visit would be welcome, but even Americans in France, he said, "are practically unanimous in the belief that it would be unwise for you to sit in," for fear "that it would involve a loss of dignity and your commanding position." It would certainly overshadow House's own presumed position there. Premier Clemenceau got word to Wilson that "he hoped you will not sit in the Congress because no head of a State should sit there. The same feeling prevails in England."

Wilson understood the situation but considered his presence nonnegotiable. He maintained that he played the same role in the United States that Prime Ministers played in their countries. "The fact that I am head of the state," he wrote House, "is of no practical consequence." As journalist David Lawrence observed, "To have stayed in America and sent a member of his Cabinet as head of the delegation would have permitted the Prime Minister of Great Britain and the Premiers of the other countries to outrank the chairman of the American delegation." The President would never accept such an arrangement, as it would belittle both the role of the United States in the peace talks and the influence America had exerted in defining the aims of the war. Wilson already inferred that the French and English leaders wished to exclude him for fear he might lead the weaker nations against them. Beyond that, the more Wilson saw of the Allies' postwar posturing, the more convinced he became that they would insist upon "a peace of force and vengeance." The President, on the other hand, contended that only on "a peace of justice could a stabilized Europe be rebuilt."

More than ever, Wilson believed his League of Nations was essential to the new world order. An organization in which every sovereign member state had pledged to discuss disputes before going to war, he insisted, was the only way to prevent future local disagreements from turning global. Wilson also believed this league had to be an integral part of the Peace Treaty, not an afterthought. "Such was his faith," observed Dr. Grayson, "and he was fully aware that he himself must be the chief apostle of that faith . . . in the face of many who called themselves 'realists' and would demand that the business of the day be dealt with rather than future contingencies." Wilson's decision to head the American Peace Commission was less a matter of convention than of conscience. In the words of Cary Grayson, "He *must* go."

Not everybody shared Wilson's vision, of either America or the world. Less than two weeks after the Armistice, Theodore Roosevelt was building opposition to Wilson's plans and support for his own possible Presidential run in 1920. In a letter to fellow imperialist Rudyard Kipling, he called the League of Nations a "product of men who want everyone to float to heaven on a sloppy sea of universal mush." Even though he had recently been bedridden with lumbago, arthritis, and the symptoms of what would prove to be an embolism of the lung, TR continued to write world leaders and dictate newspaper editorials denouncing Wilson and his Fourteen Points. Meanwhile, Wilson quickly assembled his team of four Peace Commissioners.

The President sought associates less to help craft his peace plan than to execute it. He presumed Colonel House's participation, though a few of House's recent comments had made him look twice at the man he had once called his "second personality." He found Secretary of State Lansing unimaginative but dutiful, and his absence would have presented an overt diplomatic breach. He thought Secretary McAdoo, who had literally made the American trains run on time during the war, while also heading the Treasury Department and overseeing domestic and international war loans, would be enormously useful applying his expertise to prostrated Europe; but, after years of public service, McAdoo was exhausted and so were his financial assets. Three days after the Armistice, he tendered his resignation to his father-in-law. He and Nell would leave for a three-month holiday in Santa Barbara before settling in New York, where he would launch a lucrative law practice and contemplate a run for the Presidency. It

would be an ambition Wilson would never fully support. He believed McAdoo was a man of action and that the next President would inherit a world that required a man of reflection. Wilson replaced his son-in-law at the Treasury with Congressman Carter Glass.

Although Secretary Baker was inexpert in military matters, his proficiency during the war would have made him a worthy counselor at the talks. But with Lansing absent, McAdoo departing, and the sudden announcement by Attorney General Gregory that he would be tendering his resignation for "pecuniary" reasons, everybody thought it best to keep Baker in the Cabinet Room, where he could keep a steady hand on the rudder. He recommended General Tasker Bliss, who had served as the Army's chief of staff and on the Supreme War Council in France.

The final chair became somewhat controversial, as Wilson hoped to provide at least the suggestion of nonpartisanship. Because the Senate had to approve all treaties, several prominent Republicans in the upper house were mentioned, Henry Cabot Lodge chief among them. He was not only the leading Republican Senator, but he also chaired the Senate Foreign Relations Committee. His well-known enmity toward the President kept anybody from seriously considering the idea, though pundits ever since have suggested that if chosen, he would have ensured passage of the Treaty.

Recognizing that he would have enough foreign adversaries to contend with at the conference table, Wilson chose not to borrow trouble by commissioning his bitterest foe. Beyond that, he believed the Constitution prohibited appointing Lodge, or any other legislator, because of the stipulation that "no Senator or Representative shall, during the time for which he was elected, be appointed to any civil office under the authority of the United States, which shall have been created."

Wilson's opponents would further question the President's right even to negotiate a treaty, but as he had stated as a college professor, a President "may guide every step of diplomacy and to guide diplomacy is to determine what treaties must be made." The Senate possessed the power to disapprove of a treaty, but the executive branch of the American government could dictate its terms.

Tumulty recommended Elihu Root—TR's Secretary of State, a former United States Senator, and a Nobel Peace Prize laureate. But Wilson worried about Root's conservatism and his aggressive opposition to the Administration's early policy of neutrality. William Howard Taft was also

considered, but the idea of a former President serving as an aide to a sitting President seemed awkward for both parties.

Eventually, Wilson settled on a seasoned diplomat, Henry White— who had served in Roosevelt's administration as the First Secretary in London under Ambassador Hay and subsequently as TR's Ambassador to Italy and then to France. Roosevelt called him the "most useful man in the entire diplomatic service." Republicans—Lodge among them—immediately denounced the appointment as cosmetic, dismissing White as a Republican in name only. With the delegation filled, Woodrow Wilson prepared for Paris. A page from one of his own books reminded him that "the initiative in foreign affairs, which the President possesses without any restriction whatever, is virtually the power to control them absolutely." The Senate—even Democrats—already felt Wilson was freezing them out.

In the course of a long conversation about postwar hopes, Wilson received advice from Stockton Axson, who recommended that he gather at the White House all the leaders in the American war effort, Democrats and Republicans alike. He hoped Wilson might imbue them with a sense of his personal gratitude and then say "that the worst and hardest was yet to come . . . in the readjustment of the world," and "that their cooperation, their loyalty to the country, and to the great cause, will be even more needed then, than it was during the war." Edith looked up from her knitting and concurred. Axson insisted that Wilson could have the leaders from both sides of the aisle eating out of his hand. Wilson acknowledged the wisdom of the notion but said there was no place large enough to hold that many people. Axson recommended the East Room. The President nodded and even conceded that it "would be a step that would help to suppress party opposition." But he never acted upon the idea, and antagonism festered.

By the time Wilson tried to rally the Congress behind him in his sixth Annual Message on the State of the Union, the lawmakers felt marginalized. He entered the overflowing chamber on December 2, 1918, to what one onlooker called an "ominous silence." Even delivering a patriotic speech did little to thaw his audience. Starting with an evaluation of the nation's war effort, Wilson attributed most of its success to "the mettle and quality of the officers and men we sent over and of the sailors who kept the seas, and the spirit of the nation that stood behind them." He singled out various bureaus and constituencies that had contributed to the nation's

success—especially America's women. He spoke of the specific challenges ahead as the country returned to a peacetime economy. Still, little received applause, even when his supporters tried to incite an ovation. Secretary Daniels found the Congressional reserve nothing short of "churlish." But one diplomat's wife, who viewed the proceedings through her opera glasses, wrote in her diary that "the President's *complete* disregard of the Senate following on top of his very tactless appeal to the country to return a Democratic Congress, has made him just about as thoroughly and completely unpopular in his own country as any president has been or could be."

Wilson concluded his speech by announcing his intention to leave for Paris. He reminded the Congress that the Central empires had accepted the bases of peace that he had outlined to the Congress the prior January and that they were ideals for which American soldiers had fought. Now, he explained, "I owe it to them to see to it, so far as in me lies, that no false or mistaken interpretation is put upon them, and no possible effort omitted to realize them." Wilson said it was his duty to "play my full part in making good what they offered their life's blood to obtain."

Toward that end, Wilson said in parting, "May I not hope . . . that in the delicate tasks I shall have to perform on the other side of the sea . . . I may have the encouragement and the added strength of your united support?" Emphasizing the magnitude of his undertaking, he assured the lawmakers, "I am the servant of the nation. I can have no private thought or purpose of my own in performing such an errand." He said he would make his absence as brief as possible, hoping to return having translated into action "the great ideals for which America has striven."

Even before Wilson had exited the Capitol, it was clear that both the House and Senate were divided. His valedictory wishes felt labored, and the response was the "ice bath" the Republicans had promised. One Washington Brahmin, Caroline Astor Drayton Phillips, kept her eye on Edith Wilson as she departed, and it was the first time the woman had seen the First Lady look "pale and stern and terribly sad." The next day, Republicans in both houses did what they could to constrain the President. Senator Knox of Pennsylvania offered a resolution that would limit America's role at the Peace Conference to those matters germane to America's entry into the war, which would postpone discussions involving laws of the sea and a League of Nations. Senator Sherman of Illinois denounced the

President for leaving the country and asked his colleagues to declare his absence "an inability to discharge the powers and duties" of his office. More than that, he accused Wilson of "an act of legislative and executive sabotage against the government" so long as Congress was in session and domestic conditions were unstable.

Amid such hostility, the President still possessed the ability to exude what some considered a spiritual glow. No fan of Wilson, Mrs. Phillips, for one, had felt "a sensation of light and warmth" when the President had spoken. "My heart and mind became filled with confidence in the President, with faith in his ideals," she wrote in her diary. As Woodrow Wilson boarded his midnight train for Hoboken, Mrs. Phillips foresaw for him a "hard and bitter fight at the Peace Congress." She felt "that he was sacrificing all personal ambition to obtain what he believes to be a paramount necessity for the world." She believed "that he will reveal the . . . subconscious ideal, which lies in the souls of men all over the world, for something far better than we have ever known."

And so the *George Washington* set sail on December 4 and landed in France on the thirteenth. Woodrow Wilson had jettisoned any doubts the dissidents might have instilled about the world's readiness for his ideals. The unprecedented sendoff in New York harbor made him feel that failure to achieve his goals was not an option. He proceeded to the historic receptions in Brest and Paris and London, which only boosted his confidence. On New Year's Eve, the President and First Lady rode the Royal Train to Dover and crossed the Channel; and then the President of France's train took them from Calais to Paris. The next morning he played his first game of golf on French soil at St. Cloud; and in the afternoon he called a conference of the members of the American Mission at the Hôtel de Crillon, where they were quartered. With a few weeks before the official meetings got under way, Wilson consented to one more state visit.

Italy hoped to show its appreciation of the United States and, in so doing, curry favor with the man who would soon determine many of its new borders. At the government's insistence, the Wilsons rode from Paris in the King of Italy's train—with its china and glassware bearing Italian arms and its servants in royal scarlet livery. Crowds lined the tracks across Italy; and when it stopped at one small town, the Mayor compared the President's visit to "the second coming of Christ."

The Royal Train reached the Eternal City at 9:30 on the morning of

January 3, 1919. "The reception in Rome," recalled Secret Service agent Edmund Starling, "exceeded anything I have ever seen in all my years of witnessing public demonstrations. The people literally hailed the President as a god—'The God of Peace.'" The people of Rome filled the cobble-stone streets with flowers, and a blizzard of white roses fell from the windows above as Wilson rode through hysterical mobs who were shouting, singing, and weeping. Wilson addressed the Italian Parliament, the nation's press, King Victor Emmanuel III and Queen Elena, and their guests at a state dinner at the Quirinal Palace. The Mayor of Rome honored Wilson with citizenship of his city. Ike Hoover had witnessed the French and English receptions for the President; but the Italians, he observed, seemed "to consider him as another Savior come to earth."

The next day, Wilson and his entourage faced more hysteria at the only venue that then seemed worthy of his presence—the Vatican. The major-domo escorted him through dozens of chambers, past colorfully costumed Swiss Guards and courtiers, until he arrived at a small throne room. At the tinkling of a bell, the diminutive Pontiff, dressed all in white except for his red sandals, entered. Accompanied only by a pair of interpreters, Benedict XV took the President by the hand into the Papal study for a brief private conversation—the first meeting between an American President and a Pope. Strangely, by the time the President had left the Vatican, the crowd had vanished. The officials later told Wilson that the police had dispersed the multitudes because of a potential threat of a riot. But later, Wilson explained to Edith that the government had broken up the demonstration for fear that the President might try to enlist the people's support for his Fourteen Points—to which Italy had agreed as the basis of the Armistice but to which it did not necessarily intend to adhere.

The First Couple left Rome the next morning, stopping in Genoa and Turin (where a thousand mayors from Piedmont gathered to greet the President) and Milan (where the Wilsons attended a performance of *Aida* at La Scala). Of all the places they had visited, Milan provided the apotheosis. Beyond the overwhelming crowds, observed Grayson, "there was a reverence everywhere that touched the President deeply." People lit votive candles before his picture. "There is bound to be a reaction to this sort of thing," Wilson told his doctor. "I am now at the apex of my glory in the hearts of these people, but they are thinking of me only as one who has come to save Italy, and I have got to pool the interests of Italy with the

interests of all the world, and when I do that I am afraid they are going to be disappointed and turn about and hiss me."

Wilson recognized that once the international conference began, it would be every world leader for himself, advancing his own country's agenda. Upon his arrival in Paris, Wilson returned to his supreme priority. He pulled out his draft of a Covenant for the League of Nations, to which he now added finishing touches.

Theodore Roosevelt—who that very week had complained to a newspaper editor about Wilson's being a "silly doctrinaire at times and an utterly selfish and cold-blooded politician always"—would have had plenty to say in the impending debate. But on January 6, 1919, he fell silent, dying in his sleep. The State Department drafted a proclamation for the President to sign, but Wilson felt it was inadequate. He enhanced the tribute to his longtime rival, praising the Colonel's war record and his awakening the nation "to the dangers of private control which lurked in our financial and industrial systems." The President ordered suitable military honors at his funeral and the display of flags at half-staff at the White House and departmental buildings. In addition to the Vice President's temporary new duties of running the Cabinet meetings, Wilson asked Marshall to represent him at both TR's private and state memorial services.

The absence of Wilson's most persistent critic did not lessen opposition to the President's policies. In fact, Henry Cabot Lodge doubled his own efforts. Two weeks before Roosevelt died, Lodge had sat with him, discussing the proposed league. Neither man subscribed to such a global plan. Opposed to Wilson's direction, Roosevelt had said just before his death, "Let each nation reserve to itself and for its own decision, and . . . make it perfectly clear that we do not intend to take a position of an international Meddlesome Mattie. The American people do not wish to go into an overseas war unless for a very great cause, and where the issue is absolutely plain."

To anybody abroad, such talk seemed petty. The Armistice was in effect, but the devastation was part of every European's life. The great victory for Democracy had left millions of lives in disarray, with many of its cities wanting reconstruction amid the rubble of the fallen autocratic empires. Parts of two continents would have to be built from scratch: revolutions had created seventeen new constitutional republics; and ten new nations had declared their independence and were struggling to find their

footing in constitutional governments. People rejoiced at being rid of their dictators, but they yearned for stability. Communists said they could offer as much to the Russians, and the Germans continued to consider that alternative for themselves.

Since his arrival in Europe, Woodrow Wilson had delivered seven formal speeches, each full of high-minded ideals and inspiration. When adviser Herbert Hoover suggested that Wilson must not ignore "the shapes of evil inherent in the Old World system," the President replied that a new spirit infused all of humanity. Hoover agreed. He did not hyperbolize when he stated, "Woodrow Wilson had reached the zenith of intellectual and spiritual leadership of the whole world, never hitherto known in history."

Across the Seine from the Place de la Concorde stood a two-story edifice of the Second Empire, the Ministry of Foreign Affairs, known simply by its location—the Quai d'Orsay. Its ground floor contained a succession of heavily gilded reception rooms with high ceilings and tall windows, each salon more splendid than the last. This would become the theater for the great diplomatic drama about to unfold.

While more than two dozen nations would make up the Peace Conference, the principals realized the need for a smaller leadership group if they were to accomplish anything. The heads of government and the foreign ministers of France, Great Britain, Italy, the United States, and Japan formed the Council of Ten. On Sunday, January 12, 1919, the leading players engaged in two full dress rehearsals at the Quai d'Orsay: at 2:30 the Supreme War Council met to discuss an extension of the Armistice; and at 4 p.m. the Council of Ten convened to discuss the ground rules for the upcoming plenary sessions, at which all the invited nations would be seated. The afternoon allowed everybody to get a feel for the room and one another. It was quickly recognized that the crucial arguments concerned a quartet of nations and that their leaders could best resolve those matters in private conversations, in an aptly named Council of Four.

The most towering personality in this foursome belonged to the diminutive Georges Clemenceau. Seventy-seven and sporting a bristling white walrus mustache, the French Prime Minister was a lifelong Radical Republican who had become a physician, a writer-publisher, and a political prisoner all before turning twenty-four. To evade further harassment, he

had sailed for America, where he learned English, started a medical practice in New York City, sent articles to Paris newspapers, and taught French
and horseback riding at a girls' school in Stamford, Connecticut, only to
marry one of his students. He returned to Paris and politics, as both a
public official and a newspaper publisher, who was derided and later redeemed for printing "J'Accuse," Émile Zola's historic defense of the falsely
persecuted Captain Alfred Dreyfus. In 1906, he became the seventy-
second Prime Minister of France for three years and was reinstated as the
eighty-fifth eight years later. Because of a skin condition, he almost always
wore gloves. John Maynard Keynes, then a young economist advising the
British delegation, later noted that Clemenceau—a friend of Claude
Monet—"felt about France what Pericles felt of Athens—unique value in
her, nothing else mattering." He maintained that Clemenceau was "a foremost believer in the view of German psychology which thinks that the
German understands and can understand nothing but intimidation, that
he is without generosity or remorse in negotiation"—that one must never
conciliate, only dictate to a German. The Gallic leader sought security and
revenge; and for his longtime ferocity as his nation's advocate, France nicknamed him "the Tiger."

An even more cunning political animal was David Lloyd George, at
fifty-six the youngest of the Big Four. Born in 1863, and losing his father
the following year, he put himself on a fast track of law and politics and
never deviated, becoming a Member of Parliament at twenty-seven and
rising steadily in the government. In 1916 he became the first and only
Welsh Prime Minister of England. With an outsider's eagerness to
please, he proved unusually adroit in speaking and writing his second
language, English; and few men could read a room as insightfully as Lloyd
George. He held the unfortunate position of head of a coalition government, forced to juggle the wishes of all sides in matters of colonies and
concessions. In a sketch he wrote but withheld for years, Keynes said,
"Lloyd George is rooted in nothing; he is void and without content." And
yet, he granted, the Prime Minister had highly sensitive political instincts.
"To see the British Prime Minister watching the company, with six or
seven senses not available to ordinary men, judging character, motive, and
subconscious impulse, perceiving what each was thinking and even what
each was going to say next, and compounding with telepathic instinct the
argument or appeal best suited to the vanity, weakness, or self-interest of

his immediate auditor," he wrote, "was to realize that the poor President would be playing blind man's buff in that party." Lloyd George traveled to Paris with a personal secretary, who was also his mistress and whom he addressed in their private correspondence as "My dear Pussy." Dr. Grayson thought Lloyd George was "as slippery as an eel."

The commedia dell'arte featured a favorite stock character—the Capitano—a braggart and coward who carried a sword he never used and who burst into emotional fits when challenged. Vittorio Orlando—who was Italy's third Prime Minister during its four years of war—filled that role whenever he appeared. Clemenceau would soon call this stumpy Sicilian-born lawyer with Mafia ties "the Weeper." Italy wanted a place at the table, like the other victors of the war, and expected its spoils as spelled out in a secret pact, the Treaty of London.

Then there was the President of the United States—tall, trim, with fine-cut features—hailed not only as a victor but also a prophet. "In addition to this moral influence the realities of power were in his hands," young Keynes perceived.

> The American armies were at the height of their numbers, discipline, and equipment. Europe was in complete dependence on the food supplies of the United States; and financially she was even more absolutely at their mercy. Europe not only already owed the United States more than she could pay; but only a large measure of further assistance could save her from starvation and bankruptcy. Never had a philosopher held such weapons wherewith to bind the princes of this world.

These four men and their associates gathered on the garden side of the Quai d'Orsay, in the Bureau du Ministre, the office of Stéphen Pichon. It was a large salon lined with eighteenth-century Gobelins tapestries and high bow windows and double-doors that opened onto a magnificent rose garden. Clemenceau sat before its great fireplace, facing all the others, who sat classroom style in chairs before him.

They began by considering the many matters of representation, providing a small sample of the conundrums that lay ahead. Montenegro, for example, was in the process of formation; the United States recognized the government of its king, and Wilson urged its accreditation. There were questions about the British Empire—whether Australia, for example,

deserved greater representation than, say, New Zealand. While Wilson's "heart bled" for Belgium and Serbia, he wanted to limit their participation because neither had "made a voluntary sacrifice" in the war. Japan had been invited to bring five delegates to the Conference, even though, Clemenceau said, she "had not done very much in the War, and what she had done had been mainly in her own interests." Russia, in the midst of its civil war, would not be represented at all. Then, just as the leaders were making genuine headway, uniformed servants appeared to serve afternoon tea. Wilson had to restrain himself from voicing his surprise that with the weighty affairs of the world's future under discussion, the Conference should be interrupted by such triviality. But he honored the custom, even as he realized it was a political ploy, a way for the host to stage-manage every detail of the proceedings.

When these preliminary talks resumed, Grayson opened one of the windows, and Lloyd George remarked that it was the room's first breath of fresh air since the reign of Louis XIV. Clemenceau and his team immediately waved their hands in disapproval. They were embroiled in a heated argument with Italy's Foreign Minister, Sidney Sonnino, and Grayson had hoped the breeze might cool their tempers. But complaints from the French resulted in their closing the window. The repeated French objections to the open window, it appeared, were less about ventilation than about controlling the atmospherics of the peace talks. At the end of that first session, Wilson realized the Conference would be operating at a pace considerably slower than he had anticipated. That evening, he commented to his wife's social secretary, Edith Benham, that the first day reminded him "of an old ladies' tea party."

At the Council of Ten meeting on January 13, the leaders began to prepare the agenda for the Conference by proposing the topics they would consider. They included: new states; frontiers and territorial changes; and colonies—most especially the outposts of the German Empire, over which Japan, Great Britain, and Italy were already slavering. Because Wilson believed the dispensation of those colonies should fall under the jurisdiction of the League of Nations, he urged the establishment of that body as their primary order of business.

Every group encounter revealed more of each nation's desires. At the same day's meeting of the Supreme War Council, British Foreign Minister Balfour expressed his wish to seize Germany's navy; he suggested telling

the vanquished, "If you want food you must hand over your ships." French Minister of Industrial Reconstruction Louis Loucheur announced that the French had no interest in Germany's reparations being paid in kind, and they expected the return of all stolen goods. Wilson consistently argued that "so long as hunger continued to gnaw, the foundations of government would continue to crumble," and that food, therefore, should be distributed promptly to friends and enemies, if only to ward off Bolshevism. On January 15, the great powers debated which should be the official language of the Conference. The hosts naturally argued for their native tongue; Lloyd George thought French and English should be considered equally official, and Wilson concurred. Without denying the precision of French in diplomatic matters, he argued that English was the diplomatic language of the Pacific and was comprehended by more people—including Clemenceau—than any other language represented at the Conference. Orlando indicated that he spoke no English. It was late afternoon before they agreed that the Conference would be trilingual. It promised to be a very long conference.

Five days before the commencement of the full summit, Wilson raised the problem he believed would be the ultimate fly in the ointment—Italy. While mindful of treating Orlando as an equal in the Council of Ten (if not as one of the Big Four), the President pre-emptively pointed out that the secret "Treaty of London"—under which Italy was to receive territory for joining the Allies—could not be considered binding. Wilson said the anticipated boundaries in that agreement had been laid down to protect Italy from the Austro-Hungarian Empire, and that empire no longer existed. Furthermore, the empire had been broken up into a number of states no one of which would be strong enough to menace Italy. Thus, both the basis and the purpose of that treaty no longer existed. Before facing the Conference at large, Wilson wanted to assure Orlando that Italy's frontiers with its new neighbors would be fair, and he invited Orlando to step up as the representative of a great power in the new world order by sacrificing petty national interests for greater global principles. In this reasonable and direct manner, Wilson steadily asserted his authority. Herbert Bayard Swope, ace reporter for the New York *World*, suggested that the Conference was beginning with Wilson as "the central figure in the room, the others paying him marked deference." Those who had thought him cold at first now "thawed under his influence."

Hundreds of petitioners who had come to Paris in hopes of a moment on the world stage had requests for the President. The provisional government of Lithuania, to name one, sent Wilson a plea—not for a seat at the table but only for "standing room back against the wall—where we have stood so long—waiting to be heard when the question of our fate is to be determined." Zionist leader Chaim Weizmann wrote Wilson that the "Jewries of nearly every country" had assembled just across the Channel and were "united in favour of a Jewish Commonwealth in Palestine and that a large majority of them have already definitely pronounced themselves in favour of a British Trusteeship of Palestine." And Wilson was asked to address a congress of women workers at the Trocadéro Palace— which made Clemenceau object to any further demonstrations honoring him. That included any events that might glorify America's part in the war or endorse the League of Nations.

That did not stop anyone from trying to capture Wilson's attention. W. E. B. Du Bois had organized a Pan-African Congress with fifty-seven "representatives of the Negro race" and hoped to be heard. Samuel Gompers met with the President to discuss the international labor situation, particularly "to what extent it would be possible for the League of Nations to devise and control a labor plan that would prevent worldwide economic unrest and trade disturbances." Wilson informed the head of a delegation from Armenia that it was difficult to "assign representatives to political units which have not yet been received into the family of nations." And Nguyen Tat Thanh, a twenty-nine-year-old from Indochina, who eked out a living cooking, teaching Chinese, and colorizing photographs when he was not converting to Marxism, received no response to his asking Wilson to recognize his homeland. He would soon adopt the pseudonym Ho Chi Minh—which meant "He Who Enlightens"—and then spend the rest of his life seeking proper acknowledgment of Vietnam. "Paris is now filling up with all sorts of people from all the little corners of the earth, leaders of ambitious new nations, awaiting the coming peace conference," Ray Stannard Baker jotted in his notebook. "About every second man of this type one meets, fishes out of his pocket a copy of a cablegram that he or his committee has just sent to President Wilson. It is marvellous indeed how all the world is turning to the President! The people believe he means what he says, and that he is a just man, set upon securing a sound peace."

The opening weekend of the Conference began with torrential rains, and the President awakened that Saturday morning—January 18, 1919— with a cold that kept him in bed until noon. At 2:30, limousines began to arrive at the Quai d'Orsay, bearing small flags of their nations on their hoods or bunting in Allied colors across the tops of their windshields. Two thousand people lining the Quai cheered as Wilson's car pulled up at 2:50, its passenger sufficiently reenergized. Ten minutes later the ruffle of drums and blare of trumpets announced the arrival of President Poincaré, who joined the plenary session. The signature element in the small palace's gorgeous white and gold hall—with frescoed cupids dancing on high—was an imposing fireplace and its mantelpiece. A beautiful round clock set within the mantel gave the room its official name, the Salon de l'Horloge. Above the clock, in a large niche, stood a marble statue of France holding the torch of civilization. Four magnificent chandeliers, reflected in large mirrors, illuminated the chamber. Although the French renamed the grand hall the Salle de la Paix for the duration of the talks, Clemenceau had seen to it that they officially began on the forty-eighth anniversary of Bismarck's achieving national unification, which had set Franco-Prussian relations on the path to war.

The lesser powers believed they would be treated the same as the mighty but promptly realized that the table in the Salle de la Paix was not round. Each of the delegates found his designated crimson leather–covered chair at a great three-sided arrangement—a head table with two long arms, all covered in green baize. Seating indicated a country's standing. Clemenceau sat at top center, Lloyd George and his delegation and the other Commonwealth nations on his left, Wilson and the Americans on his right. Around that bend, as far from the center of power as Czechoslovakia and Serbia but not as far down as Belgium or Brazil, sat Premier Orlando, one of seventy representatives from thirty countries. Secretariats lined the four walls. Everyone rose for Poincaré and remained standing for his brief welcoming remarks, in French—which were translated—after which he withdrew.

Clemenceau asked for nominations of a permanent chairman of the Conference, and Wilson proposed Clemenceau. The President generously offered that this was no mere tribute to their host nation but was because "we have learnt to admire him and those of us who have been associated with him have acquired a genuine affection for him." Lloyd George and

Sonnino seconded the motion, which was adopted unanimously. Although this small ceremony was the only business of the day, Clemenceau used his acceptance speech as an opportunity to stake some ground.

"President Wilson has special authority for saying that this is the first occasion on which a delegation of all civilised peoples of the world has been seen assembled," he said. And then he laid his objectives on the table:

> The greater the bloody catastrophe which has devastated and ruined one of the richest parts of France, the ampler and more complete should be the reparation . . . so that the peoples may be able at last to escape from this fatal embrace, which, piling up ruin and grief, terrorises populations, and prevents them from devoting themselves freely to their work for fear of enemies who may arise against them at any moment.

While baring his hatred for the enemy, Clemenceau spoke repeatedly of the amicable relationships among those assembled, suggesting that "success is only possible if we all remain firmly united." He said, "We have come here as friends; we must leave this room as brothers." Toward that end, he did not let this first session close without an offering to Wilson.

"Everything must yield to the necessity of a closer and closer union among the peoples who have taken part in this great war," Clemenceau said. "The League of Nations is here. It is in yourselves; it is for you to make it live; and for that it must be in our hearts. As I have said to President Wilson, there must be no sacrifice which we are not ready to accept." After his remarks, Clemenceau invited the delegates to submit memoranda detailing the crimes and punishments to be assigned to "the authors of the war."

Every posture of these talks would be fraught with the politics of leadership, every gesture a play for power. In observing just a few perfunctory motions, young British diplomat Harold Nicolson already sensed Clemenceau's high-handedness, especially with the smaller powers. Whenever asking if there were any objections, he merely said with machine-gun rapidity, "Non? . . . Adopté." Two days later, Nicolson dined with Balfour, who told him that Clemenceau had worn a bowler to the opening session.

Balfour apologized to the "old Tiger" for his own top hat, saying, "I was told . . . that it was obligatory to wear one." Replied Clemenceau, "So was I."

From the moment of Wilson's arrival in Paris, Poincaré and Clemenceau and almost every other Frenchman urged the President to visit the war sites so that he could see the devastation the enemy had inflicted. It was a bald attempt to win his sympathies and influence his judgments as to the compensation France deserved. In truth, the repeated suggestion offended him, just as his refusals perturbed his hosts. One night after weeks of the entreaties, an American friend having nothing to do with the Conference casually asked the President when he intended to visit the devastated regions. "Et tu, Brute?" he said, only half joking. "I don't want to see the de*vast*ated regions," he replied, using a quirky archaic pronunciation of the word and offering an explanation:

> As a boy, I saw the country through which Sherman marched to the sea. The pathway lay right through my people's properties. I know what happened, and I know the bitterness and hatreds which were engendered. I don't want to get mad over here because I think there ought to be *one* person at that peace table who isn't mad. I'm afraid if I visited the de*vast*ated areas I would get mad, too, and I'm not going to permit myself to do so.

Steadily, the French convinced themselves that Wilson had grown unsympathetic to their cause; and, noted Edith Wilson's private secretary, Edith Benham, "they are fearful he may give too good terms to Germany if he doesn't see the horror of the war and is prejudiced in their favor." Dr. Grayson, who virtually shadowed the President, could see that the French simply did not understand Wilson's equanimity. "They did not realize that he as much as any of them hated Germany and all her ways," he observed, "but that he was holding himself in hand because he knew that peace terms drawn up in furious rage would defeat their own ends, that to destroy Germany economically would make just reparations impossible." Wilson continued to draw a distinction between the former German Imperial government and the German people. The people had done evil, but it was done under wrong leadership. He felt that "to keep cool" was the first essential to the making of "a peace of justice," that whipping himself

into "a passion of rage" would render him unfit for the present task. Germany must be punished, he asserted, "but in justice, not in frenzy."

"As a matter of fact," Wilson said, "if I had my way I'd adjourn the Peace Conference for one year, and let all these people go home and get the bile out of their systems." But he knew, of course, that a world of starvation and instability demanded immediate attention. Bolshevism fed off such conditions, and there was no time to lose. That very week, police in Lausanne arrested several German and Russian Bolsheviks carrying false passports on their way to Paris, where they had plotted to assassinate Clemenceau, Lloyd George, and Wilson. Rumors implicated the People's Commissar of War, Leon Trotsky, in this criminal cell. Communism was becoming not just a contagious sociopolitical movement with which democratic leaders disagreed; it was turning into an international terrorist threat.

At the next meeting of the Council of Ten, on January 21, Wilson read a proclamation he had prepared in an effort at least to acknowledge the Conference's greatest deficiency—namely, the absence of Russia. "The Associated Powers are now engaged in the solemn and responsible work of establishing the peace of Europe and of the world," he said, "and they are keenly alive to the fact that Europe and the world cannot be at peace if Russia is not." Recognizing the "absolute right of the Russian people to direct their own affairs without dictation or direction of any kind from outside" and not wishing to exploit the country in any way, Wilson proposed that all the political factions in Russia declare a truce and send delegates to a conference on the Princes Island—Prinkipo—in the Turkish Sea of Marmara, where representatives of the Associated Powers would help them sort out their differences enough to seat them at the table in Paris.

It was not a well-laid scheme, and it quickly went awry. Anti-Bolshevik forces refused to attend, and there was dissension among the Bolsheviks themselves. Furthermore, the invitation spurred Latvians, Letts, and Estonians to request audiences, in order to establish their own states, separate from whatever government might end up ruling Russia. In the meantime, the Allied Powers themselves disagreed on the merits of such a conference. British troops were still fighting alongside the White armies of Russia, and Lloyd George could not ignore the vociferous anti-Bolshevik rhetoric at home. "A poisoned Russia, an infected Russia, a plague-bearing

Russia; a Russia of armed hordes . . . preceded by swarms of typhus-bearing vermin which slew the bodies of men, and political doctrines which destroyed the health and even the souls of nations," was how Bolshevik Russia had recently been described by the new War Secretary, Winston Churchill. In a few weeks Churchill would add, "Of all tyrannies in history the Bolshevist tyranny is the worst, the most destructive, and the most degrading. It is sheer humbug to pretend that it is not far worse than German militarism." French diplomat Paul Cambon thought the idea of summoning a horde of Russian dissidents to an island in the Sea of Marmara was little more than the "idealistic promptings of President Wilson's mind."

At their second plenary session, on January 25, 1919, the delegates considered the creation of a League of Nations. Wilson took the floor. "We have assembled for two purposes," he explained, "—to make the present settlements which have been rendered necessary by this war, and also to secure the peace of the world." The League of Nations, he said, "seems to me to be necessary for both of these purposes." With his longtime penchant for humanizing institutions, Wilson asked his audience to remember that "we are not representatives of government, but representatives of peoples." He reminded the others present that the United States had not engaged in the war out of fear of enemy attack or with thoughts of "intervening in the politics . . . of any part of the world" and that the maintenance of future harmony required "the continuous superintendence of the peace of the world by the associated nations of the world." The League of Nations must be established not as some occasional organization "called into life to meet an exigency" but as one "always functioning in watchful attendance . . . that it should be the eye of the nations to keep watch upon the common interest, an eye that does not slumber, an eye that is everywhere watchful and attentive." Without that League, he said, "no arrangement that you can make would either set up or steady the peace of the world."

Ever since that day in Paris, many have considered Woodrow Wilson's idée fixe an idealistic pipe dream. For him, it was anything but. He did not consider the League part of a peace settlement so much as its very foundation—the chassis on which the framework of the peace could sit and the future of international cooperation could advance. To act otherwise meant perpetuating the ancient feuds over the same patches of territory.

Wilson still sought no gains for his country—other than the desire not to return to war. That, he said, required the creation of a League of Nations, for he regarded it "as the keystone of the whole programme which expressed our purpose and our ideal in this war and which the Associated Nations have accepted as the basis of the settlement." He insisted it was the mandate of his people, the reason for America's soldiers having shed blood; and his return to the United States without having made every effort to realize that program would only invite "the merited scorn of our fellow-citizens." Wilson spoke of the American doughboys he saw every day on the streets of Paris. "Those men came into the war after we had uttered our purposes," he said. "They came as crusaders, not merely to win the war, but to win a cause; and I am responsible to them, for it fell to me to formulate the purposes for which I asked them to fight." Wilson's oration played well. Colonel House said it was "the very best speech" the President had ever delivered. The delegates voted for the Commission to frame the League's constitution.

The rest of the plenary session was devoted to forming committees dealing with "the personal guilt and responsibility of the authors of the war," the internationalization of waterways, and reparation and damages, as well as one on the League of Nations. Wilson had no way of knowing that, just two days prior, England's Lord Curzon had written Lord Derby that the League of Nations held no more interest to him than writing rules about the freedom of the seas—that the League had "nothing whatever to do either with the war or with the immediate task of concluding peace." French diplomat Paul Cambon granted that Wilson possessed certain rhetorical gifts but said privately that he was "out of touch with the world, giving his confidence to no one, unversed in European politics, and devoted to the pursuit of theories which had little relation to the emergencies of the hour." The longer-serving combatants in the war held a shorter view of the world than Wilson's. "The business of the Peace Conference," said Cambon, is "to bring to a close the war with Germany, to settle the frontiers of Germany, to decide upon the terms which should be exacted from her, and as soon as possible to conclude a just peace."

Feeling one step closer to his goal, Wilson awakened early the next morning to visit some of the "devastated" areas between Paris and Rheims. It was not meant to be an in-depth tour, just a chance to add a dimension to names that had already become part of military history. A caravan of

eight motorcars stopped fifty miles northeast of Paris on the highway over-looking Belleau Wood. As a military aide explained the battle there, the President exited his car, climbed the hill, and visited a trench that Marines had occupied before advancing on the enemy. To the right, Wilson saw his first American graveyard since his arrival in France. He uncovered his head and gazed upon the lines of crosses. Then they proceeded to Château-Thierry. As it began to snow, Wilson and his party stopped for lunch in a special train that had followed them. Afterward, the party drove through one destroyed town after another. They stopped at Rheims, which the Germans had systematically bombarded, block by block, until its population of 250,000 had scattered, leaving just 3,000 people burrowing in cellars. Snow blanketing the city, the Presidential party boarded the train back to Paris at five o'clock. When asked, the President uttered, "No one can put into words the impressions received amid such scenes of desolation and ruin." Speaking later to a delegation from the Federation of Protestant Churches of France, he said, "Happily, I believe in God's providence. Simple human intelligence is incapable of taking in all the immense problems before it at one time throughout the whole world. At such a juncture if I did not believe in God I should *feel utterly at a loss.*"

The leaders of the Conference realized that President Wilson had to return to America in time for the closing of Congress on March 4 and that he would need something to show his people. After his stirring performance on January 25, they recognized the value in pacifying him with his League just so they might proceed to their own territorial wish lists. In allocating pieces of the German and Ottoman Empires, the only arrangement Wilson could countenance was the concept of "mandates," which South African General Jan Smuts had suggested. Under this arrangement, pieces of the fallen Central empires would be placed in the trust of the entire family of nations, the League. Wilson was most concerned that these mandates not be treated as colonies. In explaining to one journalist America's natural aversion to acquiring "outlying" new territory, he referenced the Philippines and how "impatient" the United States was until "we could give them autonomy." By the end of January, the Council of Ten had delineated three classes of mandates: those of countries whose populations were civilized but not yet organized, such as Arabia; distant tropical colonies, such as New Guinea, that were not an integral part of any mandatory country; and countries that formed "almost a part of the

organization of an adjoining power." One after the other, each country lodged its complaints and staked its ground.

Baron Makino of Japan reminded the Council that at the outbreak of the war, the German military and naval base at Kiaochow in China constituted a serious threat to international trade and shipping, to say nothing of the peace in that corner of the world. The Japanese government, in concert with the British, had given notice to the Germans to surrender that territory to China, and when it failed to reply, Japan had fought with the British and succeeded in taking hold of the region as well as its significant railway lines. He now justified his government's claims to the unconditional cession of territory in Shantung Province (including its railways) as well as all the German-owned islands in the North Pacific.

China saw things differently. Wellington Koo, the Columbia University–educated Chinese Minister to the United States, delivered an impassioned speech, insisting that Japanese domination of the railroad lines would give them "absolute control over all of China's natural resources." He demanded that they be returned to China with compensation. On most issues of "dividing the swag," Wilson found himself in the minority, insisting that captured colonies should be controlled by the League of Nations and administered under the mandatory system, whereby the nations best fitted to do so would control the territories, which could, in turn, always appeal directly to the League to remedy any injustice. The Japanese had already grabbed some of China's "most sacred soil," including the Tomb of Confucius. Wilson sided with the Chinese.

The principles of the League of Nations aside, Lloyd George questioned whether Wilson had thought through its practicalities. Developing colonies, he said, was less about dividing spoils than multiplying debt. "Great Britain had no Colony from which a contribution towards the national expenditure was obtained," he said; and he thought the same situation would apply to Mesopotamia, Syria, and other parts of the Ottoman Empire should the mandatory system be applied there. "Whoever took Mesopotamia would have to spend enormous sums of money for works which would only be of profit to future generations," he said; and he wondered who was to bear the costs in the present. "Was the League of Nations to pay?" he asked. "How would it be possible to raise sufficient money to carry out all the necessary works for the development of these countries from which no returns could be expected for many decades?" He asked if

the League would be levied to make good on the annual deficit of any nations under a mandate. Wilson granted that certain expenses—such as defense—would be borne by the League.

Sensing the sentiments in the room, Wilson added that the world would not accept many of the actions being discussed—such as "the parcelling out among the Great Powers of the helpless countries conquered from Germany." Such actions, he said, would make the League of Nations "a laughing stock." Orlando asked if Wilson intended all questions relating to the disposal of conquered territories to be referred to the League. If so, he suggested the world would think "that this Conference had done nothing, and a confession of impotence would be even more serious than disagreement amongst the delegates."

By the end of the month, the Allies were turning on one another. Premier William Morris Hughes of Australia "bitterly opposed" any agreement that did not transfer New Guinea to his nation—a position that galled Wilson, for Hughes appeared to hold the world hostage for his country's personal gain. "Australia and New Zealand with 6,000,000 people between them," he said, "could not hold up a conference in which, including China, some twelve hundred million people were represented." And that was just one dispute that had to be settled. On January 30, 1919, alone, the Council of Ten also heard positions regarding the disposition of Samoa, Smyrna, Adalia, the north of Anatolia, Armenia, Syria, Mesopotamia, Palestine, Arabia, Uganda, Nigeria, Algeria, Morocco, Kurdistan, the Caucasus, Baku, Lebanon, Odessa, Persia, the Czechoslovak Republic, the Congo, the Cameroons, Romania, and Serbia. Delegates began to realize the necessity of abandoning singular national desires in favor of a worldview.

Through patient and eloquent reasoning, Wilson was able to sway Lloyd George and then Japan and Italy to his side, resulting in the approval of the mandatory system for African and Pacific territories. He granted that many of these mandates were more duty than privilege; and while he was disinclined to see the United States reap any advantage from the war, he was equally against letting his nation shirk any duty. But any demand for America to share in that burden, he said, would require a postponement until he could explain the matter to his people, most particularly the Senate. Charles Seymour of the American Peace Commission found it discouraging to see the Council of Ten wasting so much time on

details of technical disputes that should be left to subordinates; and with Wilson's departure impending, Colonel House thought the President should devote his time to the League. "I urged him," House wrote in his diary on January 31, 1919, "to . . . make it his main effort during the Conference. I thought he had a great opportunity to make himself the champion of peace and to change the order of things throughout the world."

On the afternoon of February 3, Wilson opened the first meeting of the Commission on the League of Nations at the Hôtel de Crillon. Although he was the first world leader to support such an organization, Wilson readily acknowledged it was the work of many heads and many hands. A few academicians and Liberal politicians in England had actually devised just such an international society in the middle of the war; and a few American associations—including the League to Enforce Peace, which former President Taft had led—organized simultaneously. Wilson had authorized David Hunter Miller, a law partner of House's son-in-law, Gordon Auchincloss, to work with British adviser Cecil Hurst in putting together a draft of a constitution that would incorporate suggestions from General Smuts and Great Britain's Lord Robert Cecil. Being the last and foremost proponent of the document, Wilson would forever be acknowledged as its "author," despite his earnest efforts to correct the record.

From February 3 to 13, the Commission—representing fourteen nations—met ten times, parsing every word of the document and perfecting its fine points. At almost every turn, the French attempted to interject their need to scold Germany. The Covenant had thirteen articles of governance and organization and ten Supplementary Agreements, which defined the structure of mandates, called for "humane conditions of labor," promised "to accord to all racial or national minorities . . . exactly the same treatment and security" accorded the majorities, and insisted upon "no law prohibiting or interfering with the free exercise of religion." The document contained several more utopian elements: Article IV, for example, required "the reduction of national armaments to the lowest point consistent with domestic safety"; Article V maintained that disputes among the "Contracting Powers" would be subjected to arbitration before armed force would be considered.

The backbone of the League Covenant came in Article X with its establishment of collective security. It asserted that hostile actions by a non-signatory party against any of the League members would result in a

united effort of members to blockade the infractor—"closing the frontiers of that Power to all commerce or intercourse with any part of the world, and to employ jointly any force which may be agreed upon to accomplish that object." The member nations would agree to unite in coming to the aid of their colleagues "against which hostile action has been taken, and to combine their armed forces in its behalf."

The French were paranoid about a rearmed Germany; and at the February 11 meeting of the Commission, they questioned whether they should enter into the League if it lacked an international army. Wilson explained that the only method by which the organization could achieve its ends was through a "cordial agreement" and goodwill. "All that we can promise, and we do promise it," he said, "is to maintain our military forces in such a condition that the world will feel itself in safety. When danger comes, we too will come, and we will help you, but you must trust us. We must all depend on our mutual faith." After the meeting, Lord Cecil privately warned one of the French diplomats that the League of Nations was "their only means of getting the assistance of America and England, and if they destroyed it they would be left without an ally in the world." At another formal gathering of diplomats, Cecil had spoken to the French off the record, saying that "America had nothing to gain from the League of Nations"—that she could ignore European affairs and look after her own—and that "the offer . . . for support was practically a present to France." The Commission spent the entire next day reading each of what had become twenty-seven Articles of the Covenant as reported back from the Drafting Committee.

With his departure drawing near, Wilson conferred with Colonel House about his role during this absence. House said he had four objectives—reducing Germany's military forces to their peacetime footing, delineating Germany's boundaries, reckoning Germany's reparation bill, and determining how Germany should be treated economically. He told the President he thought he could "button up everything" during the four weeks the President would be away. Wilson looked startled, even alarmed, knowing how long drafting the Covenant had taken—and those talks had begun with a general consensus. Wilson now perceived a change within House, an increasing sense of empowerment over the last few weeks, one that seemed to grow as Wilson's embarkation approached. House hastily added that he did not intend to settle all these matters, merely to "have

them ready" for Wilson's return. House asked the President to bear in mind that "it was sometimes necessary to compromise in order to get things through. Not a compromise of principle, but a compromise of detail." He reminded Wilson of his own compromises since their meetings began. "I did not wish him to leave expecting the impossible in all things," House wrote in his diary. In fact, Wilson never expected House to broker any deals in his absence, nor did he desire it.

Turning to domestic politics, House suggested that the President sail not to New York or even Virginia, as planned, but to Boston. He thought it would prove beneficial if the Europeans could see Wilson receive an enthusiastic homecoming after his two months away and that he could expect that from New England, which he had seldom visited. With legislators already preparing for battle, it would also allow him to plant his flag in the home state of his archrival, Senator Henry Cabot Lodge. House further proposed a dinner at the White House for the Senate and House Foreign Relations Committees as soon as was practicable. Wilson thought an address to Congress would provide an adequate platform from which to describe his peace efforts. But House convinced him that it would deprive the essential legislators of a chance for "discussion, consultation, or explanation." Wilson agreed.

As this meeting in Paris was the biggest story of the century, the press questioned its access to the proceedings, always expecting more from the man who demanded open covenants of peace, openly arrived at. Wilson believed in the transparency of their business, but he also understood the fragility of the situation—dozens of nations, often with conflicting desires. The fate of the League of Nations was too delicate to leave to journalists to misrepresent. More than impractical, allowing newspapermen to sit in on intimate discussions among the Council of Ten or the Big Four seemed impertinent. Befriending the press might have helped his cause, especially in having to proselytize to a skeptical Senate and an agnostic public; but Wilson never believed journalistic access could guarantee greater support. He wanted to offer the public a fully realized plan rather than some half-baked ideas. He fretted over leaks in the press and European portrayals of him as a dreamer with little practical sense.

Within days of Wilson's arrival in Paris, George Creel had recommended a daily press conference, a concept to which Wilson subscribed. Immediate demands, however, made it clear that the President would

rarely have time for such an exercise, and the constantly changing situation would make it impossible to talk "with any degree of certainty" until things were in writing and approved. And so, even before formal talks had begun, Wilson had invited Ray Stannard Baker to join the Peace Commission as its press representative, an intermediary between the Commission and the other journalists. Ironically, this lack of direct access to the President forced the newspapermen to rely on less reliable outsiders—representatives of smaller countries or low-level diplomats who did not know the entire picture. Major players realized they could control stories through the very leaks Wilson feared.

"It is highly important that the right news be given out," Wilson had said, at a time when the volatility of the talks fueled rumors on a daily basis. He had asked Baker to visit him every night at seven o'clock, at which time he would recap that day's events, suggesting that any completed business be furnished to the press but that pending matters be omitted. Edith Wilson said that she could set her watch to the nightly arrival of Baker, who never missed an appointment, though he sometimes had to wait more than an hour if the President was detained. She sat in on the briefings so that she could be fully apprised of the work of the Conference without her husband's having to repeat himself.

On February 14, 1919, the President awakened to what would be the most momentous day of the Conference thus far. As he would be leaving for home that night, he made a point of providing an hour-long interview with almost twenty American correspondents, his first press conference since arriving in Europe. As House observed, he addressed them "in the pleasantest and frankest way." He expressed his regret that he had not been able to converse with them daily, adding, with a laugh, that "every one else had had his ear." And though his own schedule in the last few weeks had been filled with League activity, he gravely emphasized that "the most tremendous issue in the world to-day concerns the economic situation." Everything else, he said, could wait until the wheels of industry were again in motion. "You can't talk government with a hungry people," held the President. That said, he diplomatically added that all the participating nations wanted to reassure France that "what she has just gone through never will occur again." While the weeks of talks had been full of tension, Wilson confessed that he learned how to take advantage of long speeches by stealing catnaps, knowing he could awaken in time to hear the

translations. Colonel House marveled at Wilson's performance before the press. "It is to be remembered that he did not want to see them," House told his diary, "and yet when he got to talking, he was so enthused with what he had to say that it looked as if he would never stop."

As much as anybody, Edith Wilson knew that Colonel House had been of "inestimable help" to her husband, and she liked him personally; but she could not help voicing a long-held suspicion that spoke to the root of his character: House almost never disagreed with her husband. "It seems to me that it is impossible for two persons *always* to think alike," she told Woodrow. "I find him absolutely colourless and a 'yes, yes' man." As in the past, Wilson defended him; but it was not the first time Edith had cast a baleful eye on her husband's most trusted adviser.

Even though she knew the meetings in Paris permitted participants only, Edith had set her heart on attending that Valentine's Day session of the Conference at which her husband was to submit the report of the League of Nations Commission. It was nothing less than the Covenant for the League, for which he had garnered the unanimous approval of the fourteen nations on his committee. Knowing that her husband reflexively resisted asking for favors, Edith disclosed her desire to Dr. Grayson, who hoped to attend the session as well. He thought of approaching Clemenceau, who, he believed, would permit their attendance. Edith presented this plan to Woodrow, who said, "In the circumstances it is hardly a request, it is more a command, for he could not very well refuse you." That suited Edith. "Wilful woman," he said, "your sins be on your own head if the Tiger shows his claws." And Edith replied, "Oh, he can't, you know; they are always done up in grey cotton."

Clemenceau did consent to Edith's eavesdropping on the session—with conditions. At the far end of the grand salon, opposite the great clock, heavy red brocade curtains concealed a narrow alcove, which had space for two chairs. If she and Grayson agreed to remain concealed—so that the wives of other delegates would not pester him in the future—they could take their places before the diplomats arrived and remain until the last of them had exited. By peeking through the curtains, they could witness this moment of history.

At 3:30 that afternoon, Edith and Dr. Grayson were in their places, able to see President Wilson open the third plenary session. "I had arranged most of the program," House wrote in his diary; but Woodrow

Wilson had prepared all his life for this day. With only a few expository detours, Wilson read out loud the Covenant for a new world order, while delegates followed along with their reading copies. The most eye-popping article remained the defensive alliance to which the United States and all the other signatories would be committed. This article allowed that certain cases might require the Executive Council "to recommend what effective military or naval force the members of the League shall severally contribute to the armed forces to be used to protect the covenants of the League." The members would further pledge to "support one another in the financial and economic measures which are taken under this Article." He insisted that this armed force would be used only as a last resort, "because this is intended as a constitution of peace, not as a league of war."

"Your speech was as great as the occasion. I am very happy," Colonel House jotted on a slip of paper, which he passed to the President. "Bless your heart," Wilson replied. "Thank you from the bottom of my heart." House would note the exchange in his journal entry for the day, writing that the President was unfailingly interesting when he spoke. But the Colonel, about to exercise his new authority with the delegation, could not help himself from adding, "The President . . . talks entirely too much."

A number of speeches in approval of the Covenant filled the rest of the plenary session, after which Wilson ducked into a second press conference. The Covenant presentation behind him, Wilson relaxed and turned anecdotal. He told of one private conversation between him and Clemenceau, in which the old Tiger accused the President of having "a heart of steel." Wilson disagreed, saying, "I have not the heart to steal." Wilson prophesied that the difficult portion of the Conference lay ahead—upon his return from America—when they would approach the great territorial questions, many of which were snarled by secret treaties. For now, Wilson rejoiced that the concept of the League that had been adopted at the plenary session of January 25 had on this day received near unanimous approbation. The first phase of the Peace Conference had produced the tangible results the President had sought. Observed one junior member of the American Commission in his diary, "It seems impossible now that what Wilson has started out to do will not be done. . . . Today will be perhaps the greatest date in the history of the world. The birth of the brotherhood of man."

Wilson attended one more conference on February 14, at the Quai

d'Orsay. Under Lloyd George's aegis, Britain's new War Secretary, Winston Churchill, hoped to address the leaders on the subject of Russia before the President sailed for home. Clemenceau said the subject seemed too important for such a brief and unexpected meeting; but Wilson politely allowed that Churchill had made the effort to anticipate his departure, and so they should at least hear his concerns. Wilson insisted that they were all in need of more intelligence on the subject, which was why he had hoped the conference at Prinkipo might have come to fruition. "What we were seeking was not a *rapprochement* with the Bolsheviks," Wilson said, "but clear information." And if the Bolsheviks would not come to Prinkipo, Wilson was now thinking that emissaries should go to them.

In fact, he and House had discussed just such a plan raised by William Bullitt, a brilliant Yale-educated Philadelphian. Only twenty-eight years old, this member of the American delegation proposed his own mission to Moscow to meet with the Lenin government—not to negotiate but to investigate. As Wilson strongly felt "there should be no interference with internal affairs of Russia, but that the Allies would do everything possible . . . to help the Russian people from the outside," he approved the plan. At best it might buy some time in which some of the diverse Russian factions might consolidate; at worst it could yield facts about the cryptic Lenin government. Accompanied by legendary muckraker Lincoln Steffens, who had turned Marxist, Bullitt left on this sub rosa operation.

Fearing that the Allies might cozy up to Lenin, Churchill had crossed the Channel to warn the Supreme War Council that a complete withdrawal of Allied troops from Russia would mean the destruction of all non-Bolshevik armies there. Without further military resistance to the Red Army, he insisted, an "interminable vista of violence and misery was all that remained for the whole of Russia." Wilson said the existing forces of the Allies were not enough to stop the Bolsheviks, and the United States, for one, was not prepared to reinforce its troops. It was "certainly a cruel dilemma," he added. The removal of Allied soldiers would result in Russian deaths; but, Wilson said, "they could not be maintained there forever and the consequence to the Russians would only be deferred." With the *George Washington* awaiting his arrival in Brest, Wilson cast his lot with the group's decision. With no intention of acceding to Churchill's suggestions, Wilson did not understand why Lloyd George had even allowed him to appear in the first place.

That long day over at last, Edith Wilson blended into the crowd of diplomats and well-wishers among the fleet of motorcars, each with a flag flapping in the cool night breeze. She found her husband in the blue limousine with the Presidential seal. As she entered the car, he removed his top hat and leaned back. "Are you so weary?" she asked.

"Yes, I suppose I am," he said, "but how little one man means when such vital things are at stake." He elaborated, articulating the very essence of his mission. "This is our first real step forward, for I now realize, more than ever before, that once established the League can arbitrate and correct mistakes which are inevitable in the Treaty we are trying to make at this time," he said. "The resentments and injustices caused by the War are still too poignant, and the wounds too fresh. They must have time to heal, and when they have done so, one by one the mistakes can be brought to the League for readjustment, and the League will act as a permanent clearinghouse where every nation can come, the small as well as the great." He smiled at his wife and added, "It will be sweet to go home, even for a few days, with the feeling that I have kept the faith with the people, particularly with these boys, God bless them." Edith let Woodrow savor the moment in silence the rest of the way to their residence, where soldiers stood at salute as they entered.

Colonel House accompanied them to the train station. Despite a heavy rain, a long crimson carpet lined with palms extended from the curb to where President Poincaré, Clemenceau and his entire cabinet, and numerous diplomats were waiting. Wilson bade House adieu, placing an arm around his shoulders and all his faith in House's hands. In Wilson's absence, Lansing would be the titular head of the American Commission, but House was entrusted to speak on the President's behalf. Wilson knew that France, especially, would be eager to exploit his absence by rushing into place certain terms about the geographical boundaries of Germany and the inclusion of war costs in the reparations demands. Wilson said he was unwilling to allow anything beyond mechanical basics to be determined while he was gone. With so many matters involving "the fortunes and interests of many other people," he said, "we should not be hurried into a solution arrived at solely from the French point of view." As he plainly expressed to House, "I beg that you will hold things steady with regard to everything but the strictly naval and military terms until I return."

At 10:30 the next morning, the Presidential train pulled up to the pier in Brest, where American soldiers and local French officials awaited. Wilson thanked the people of France and their government for treating him as a friend. At 11:15 the ship set sail, carrying a number of hitchhikers, including Assistant Secretary of the Navy Franklin D. Roosevelt and his wife, Eleanor. The majority of the passengers were sick and wounded soldiers. The President himself was visibly fatigued from his two-month ordeal in Europe. Still, he brimmed with optimism, his spirits soaring as high as the dove bringing the olive leaf to Noah.

Stateside, Joseph Tumulty had kept the White House functioning and the President fully briefed. He also planned Wilson's arrival in Boston and his Foreign Relations Committee dinner at the White House, as the nation and its legislators were already taking sides. "Plain people throughout America for you," he radiogrammed the President. "You have but to ask their support and all opposition will melt away." Despite the rough crossing and another cold, the President used much of the voyage for rest and recreation—exercise in the sun by day and movies after dinner. While aboard ship, he received joyous word from his son-in-law Frank Sayre, whose message simply said: "Woodrow Wilson Sayre and Jessie send love." The namesake was the President's fourth grandchild.

On the morning of February 19, while Wilson was mid-Atlantic, a French anarchist shot five times at Clemenceau while he was en route to the Quai d'Orsay. One of the five bullets passed through his neck, miraculously missing any major arteries, and lodged in his shoulder. By day's end, the old Tiger had returned to his residence and was making light of the matter. But it served as a grim reminder that this was still an age of anarchy. Three days later, Clemenceau summoned House and urged a speedy settlement with Germany.

The Wilsons threw a small shipboard luncheon in honor of Washington's birthday on the twenty-second. They invited the Franklin Roosevelts, whom they found charming company. Conversation turned naturally to the League, which Ambassador to Russia David R. Francis said he believed the people of the United States would support. "The failure of the United States to back it," Wilson said, "would break the heart of the world,

for the world considers the United States as the only nation represented in this great conference whose motives are entirely unselfish."

The *George Washington* arrived in Boston Harbor in a fog, but Woodrow Wilson had never been so clear. Even though he had been absent from his desk longer than any President in history, he knew the political realities that awaited. He asked Tumulty to explain to the local authorities that his immediate duty was "to get to Washington and take hold of my work there." He had hoped to minimize all formalities and, if possible, even eliminate having to speak, for fear of giving his visit a political taint. Tumulty trimmed the schedule to a reception at the pier, a private luncheon, and a short public address; to do any less, he suggested, would not only embarrass the local officials but would also disappoint the many thousands who would assemble to greet Wilson. "Your arrival awaited in Boston with splendid and entirely non-partisan enthusiasm," he explained.

Boston declared Monday the twenty-fourth a local holiday in honor of the President's return. An estimated 200,000 Bostonians cheered him and the fifty-car procession along most of the three-mile route from the pier to the Copley Plaza Hotel. For security reasons, some of the streets were roped off and emptied, with a sharpshooter standing atop every block of buildings along the way. After lunch, Wilson went to Mechanics Hall, not having imagined the throngs that were waiting. By the time Republican Governor Calvin Coolidge had introduced him to the crowd of seven thousand, with a surprising pledge to support the President in his plans if it meant an end to war, Wilson's adrenaline was pumping.

He delivered an especially deft speech, masking its politics in patriotism and addressing any concerns about his long absence. "I have been very lonely . . . without your comradeship and counsel," he told the enthusiastic crowd. He said the proudest fact he could report was "that this great country of ours is trusted throughout the world"; and he said the Conference was moving slowly due to "the complexity of the task which is undertaken." The Europe he left was full of hope, he said, "because they believe that we are at the eve of a new age of the world, when nations will understand one another. . . . If America were at this juncture to fail the world, what would come of it?"

Anticipating the donnybrook ahead, Wilson explained that he had not gone to Europe merely to spout idealism. "We set this nation up to make

men free," he said, "and we did not confine our conception and purpose to America, and now we will make men free. If we did not do that, all the fame of America would be gone, and all her power would be dissipated." Throwing off the gloves, he said, "I have fighting blood in me, and it is sometimes a delight to let it have scope."

To sustained applause, Wilson exited the hall for South Station. After brief whistle-stop speeches in Providence, Rhode Island, and New London and New Haven, Connecticut, Wilson went to sleep, awakening in Washington. He went directly to the White House, where he signed the large number of documents that had piled up in his absence. That afternoon, he presided over a Cabinet meeting, at which he detailed the chicanery with which he had to deal in Paris. Although his detractors suggested that the Europeans were duping him at the Peace Conference, Wilson was, in fact, wise to their subterfuge from the start. He knew that the French were constantly trying to weaken his position by coercing the press to emphasize the power of Republican opinion in the United States or by exaggerating fears of a renewed German offensive. At the same time, he was parrying not only the Allies' insistence upon extensive German reparations but also their entreaties to forgive their own respective debts. And though the spreading threat of Bolshevism had been enough for him to authorize the Bullitt mission, Wilson felt that much of the reported chaos in Russia was exaggerated.

On February 26, his second night back in the White House, Wilson hosted the dinner Colonel House had recommended, that of members of Congress on their respective foreign affairs committees. For the first time in two years, the White House was illuminated as though for a state dinner. But the lights did little to brighten the mood of half the guests. Promptly at eight, thirty-four legislators were directed to the State Dining Room. After the meal, Henry Cabot Lodge escorted Edith Wilson, the only woman present, to the East Room, where chairs were set up in an elongated circle. As the President took his place at the top of the oval, his wife took her leave. He opened the discussion with an informal statement, explaining that the other world leaders had "agreed upon the need and the importance of forming a League of Nations, of doing something practical to bind the nations together"—to prevent any flare-ups of the past war and the ignition of any future wars. With that, he said, "Ask anything you want to know, gentlemen, and ask it as freely as you wish." They did—until midnight.

Wilson fielded questions about disarmament, the Monroe Doctrine, and what some considered a surrender of American sovereignty. Wilson explained that the Executive Council of the proposed League could issue no order without unanimity and that any such orders must be submitted to each of the governments represented on the council. With every country overseeing every other, any arms race would be limited and transparent. He suggested that the sanctity of the Monroe Doctrine must be maintained, that the century-old policy was the bedrock of the Covenant. Wilson asserted that any attempts to eliminate war would require some sacrifice, each nation yielding something for the greater good of the whole world. And while he showed great respect for the power of the Senate Foreign Relations Committee to withhold its approval of a treaty, he expressed the hope that the present draft of the Covenant would not face radical changes from the committee, as it had been framed to mutual satisfaction by fourteen nations. Wilson imposed no limits on what his guests might say to the press. But everyone in the East Room recognized the political importance of this issue. While winning the war may have occurred on the Democrats' watch, the Republicans were not about to let them co-opt the peace.

Republican Senator Frank Brandegee of Connecticut assured reporters that nothing Wilson said that night changed his opinion about the League of Nations. "I am against it," he told *The New York Times*, "as I was before." An indifferent Henry Cabot Lodge thought the dinner was perfectly pleasant; but, he noted in his diary, "We went away as wise as we came." And while Lodge had chosen not to confront Wilson in his own house, he noted that "the President's performance under Brandegee's very keen and able cross-examination was anything but good."

Two days later, Lodge delivered a long speech in the Senate, shredding the Covenant article by article. "My effort," Lodge later recounted, ". . . was to try, by showing the objections to the League proposed, to make it apparent that the thing to do was to make peace and deal with the League later when we could take our time in doing so, and thereby to demonstrate the League should not be yoked with the treaty of peace and thus create the risk of dragging them both down together." Lodge asked his colleagues, "What is it that delays the peace with Germany?" And then he answered his own question: "Discussions over the League of Nations; nothing else. Let us have peace now, in this year of grace 1919. That is the first step to

the future peace of the world. The next step will be to make sure if we can that the world shall have peace in the year 1950 or 2000."

While the President was still in residence and the Sixty-fifth Congress still in session, Lodge took aggressive action. With no time to launch a full-scale resolution against the League, he circulated among Republican Senators and Senators-elect (not yet eligible to vote) a round-robin letter pledging opposition to the League. He gathered thirty-seven signatures. While not a binding document, it publicly demonstrated that the President faced serious opposition. Adding insult to that injury, the Republicans invoked a filibuster in the Congress's final hours, allowing certain appropriations simply to wither without approval. The only reason Wilson had even sailed home from France was to sign eleventh-hour bills. Bringing the body to a screeching halt served only to humiliate him. The Republicans signified that Wilson's resumed absence from Washington would only rile an even unfriendlier Sixty-sixth Congress. More irritated than chagrined, Wilson left the Capitol and proclaimed: "A group of men in the Senate have deliberately chosen to embarrass the administration of the Government. . . . It is plainly my present duty to attend the Peace Conference in Paris. It is also my duty to be in close contact with the public business during a session of the Congress. I must make my choice between these two duties, and I confidently hope that the people of the country will think that I am making the right choice."

In his time home, Wilson had been able to complete just one significant piece of business—the appointment of a new Attorney General. From the moment Thomas Gregory had announced his intention to step down from the office, Tumulty had recommended former Congressman A. Mitchell Palmer, a strong supporter of the Administration—a man of intelligence and integrity. For over a year, he had acted as the nation's Alien Property Custodian, seizing and sometimes selling "enemy property." Gregory advised against appointing him Attorney General, as had House, who found the glad-handing Palmer overbearing. In this politically challenging moment, Wilson listened more to his two savviest Cabinet members, Burleson and Daniels, as well as party chairman Vance McCormick, all of whom strongly endorsed Palmer as progressive, fearless, and "effective on the stump." This Swarthmore-educated Pennsylvania Quaker, who used "thee" and "thou," seemed a welcome addition to a heavily Southern Cabinet. He was also levelheaded, especially when it came to the incendiary

issues of sedition. While he had been aggressive in his seizure of German-owned property during the war, he also sought to release ten thousand German aliens in government custody; and he had opposed the local raids of the American Protective League as America was entering the war, publicly pronouncing the organization "a grave menace." Within days of his return to the White House, Wilson had announced his selection of Palmer, but in its session-end filibuster, the Senate took one more dig at the President by failing to approve him.

The Department of Justice required particularly strong leadership in that moment. With the war over, the Administration faced a number of vital issues, including the matter of clemency toward America's "political prisoners." In his final days in office, the hard-nosed Gregory had received a number of communications referring to the Espionage Act. He maintained that not one person had been convicted for *"mere expression of opinion"* but that all had been convicted at trials by jury of willful violations of the law whose aim was to prevent "deliberate obstruction to the prosecution of the war." Since the end of the war, Gregory had reconsidered all those convicted and found several no longer deserved their sentences. He asked Wilson to review individual cases, if not the entire policy; and the President hoped to put a new Attorney General immediately in place to do the same. Wilson recommended to Postmaster General Burleson that it was also time to reconsider their position in combating sedition. "I cannot believe that it would be wise to do any more suppressing."

Congress closed on March 4, and Wilson boarded a train at Union Station that day at two o'clock, returning to the *George Washington* in Hoboken. He made two stops along the way. The first was in Philadelphia, where he went to Jefferson Hospital to visit his daughter Jessie and his newborn grandson. The President delighted in the plump infant, who was yawning as his eyes remained closed. "With his mouth open and his eyes shut," Wilson said, "I predict that he will make a Senator when he grows up." The Presidential entourage continued its journey, reaching New York City, where he addressed a capacity crowd at the Metropolitan Opera House, sharing the great stage with none other than former President Taft, who spoke in favor of the League. When it was Wilson's turn to speak, a band struck up George M. Cohan's signature tune, and Wilson told the enthusiastic crowd, "I will not come back 'till it's over, over there.'"

He explained how the last war could have been avoided if Germany

had stopped to consider that Great Britain would ally with France and Russia. He said that the League of Nations was meant to serve as a signpost, "as a notice to all outlaw nations that not only Great Britain, but the United States and the rest of the world, will go in to stop enterprises of that sort."

After the speech, the Wilsons were ferried across the river to the Hoboken wharves, where they boarded their ship. The President was exhausted from having driven himself harder in the last three months than at any other time in his life. But he remained awake until past midnight, at which time he derived great satisfaction in commissioning A. Mitchell Palmer as his Attorney General through the power of a recess appointment.

Somebody observed that it had been exactly thirteen weeks since Wilson had first boarded the *George Washington,* a good omen that was not lost on Dr. Grayson. Except for another shipboard cold and fever during the eight-day crossing, Wilson had remained remarkably healthy in all that time. After examining him that week, Grayson found all his vital signs "unusually good" for a man of sixty-two. Even Ray Stannard Baker marveled not only at Wilson's strength—especially upon learning of the gastric and neurological conditions that had plagued him for years—but also his ability to disconnect from strife. Some days the President watched five hours of moving pictures. Confining himself to his cabin, where he slept or played a variation of solitaire called canfield, the President self-diagnosed his current bouts of neuralgia and an attack on his "equatorial zone" as nothing more than "a retention of gases generated by the Republican Senators," which he said were "enough to poison any man." Ray Baker further observed that Wilson was "a good hater—& how he does hate those obstructive Senators." He realized the President was now inclined to "stand by the Covenant word for word as drawn, accepting no amendment, so that the 37 of the round-robin will be utterly vanquished."

Wilson faced an even greater threat to his blood pressure. Colonel House's communiqués from Paris had become worrisome, to say the least. In one report, House had suggested that the issue of the League was still in play; in another he wrote of Clemenceau's requesting certain restraints against the republics on the west bank of the Rhine. Another noted that everything in Wilson's absence had "been speeded up." All together, the

wireless dispatches from the Continent suggested that House had overstepped in his role just as the French had overreached. Wilson urged withholding even provisional consent to policy decisions until his arrival.

The *George Washington* could not deliver him to France fast enough. For several more days, Wilson remained at sea, anxiously playing solitaire.

14

GETHSEMANE

Then commeth Iesus with them vnto a place called
Gethsemane . . .

—MATTHEW, XXVI:36

And being in an agonie, he prayed more earnestly,
and his sweat was as it were great drops of blood
falling downe to the ground.

—LUKE, XXII:44

The *George Washington* reached Brest at 7:45 in the evening of March 13, 1919. For reasons of security—and
the French government's desire to withhold any further
accolades for the American President—the reception was
reduced to a diplomatic minimum. The welcoming committee included only a few dignitaries, including Colonel
House. With little fanfare, the Wilsons boarded the special
train and were on their way to Paris by 10:30. Wilson and
House huddled privately in his stateroom while Edith retired to hers. The President listened to his most trusted
adviser report the latest French attempts to detach the
League Covenant from the Peace Treaty and to create a
Rhenish Republic, a buffer state between France and Germany. Before his return to America, Wilson had told
House he would not tolerate the latter, which would

"absolutely denude Germany of everything she had and allow Bolshevism
to spread throughout that country."

A little after midnight, Edith heard the Colonel leave. She opened the
connecting door to Woodrow's compartment. "The change in his appearance shocked me," she recalled later. "He seemed to have aged ten years, and
his jaw was set in that way it had when he was making superhuman effort
to control himself." Without saying a word, he held out his hand, which she
grasped. "What is the matter?" she asked. "What has happened?"

"House," he said, smiling sardonically, "has given away everything I
had won before we left Paris. He has compromised on every side, and so I
have to start all over again and this time it will be harder, as he has given
the impression that my delegates are not in sympathy with me." In Wilson's absence, the Colonel had apparently had his first taste of power.
House explained that upon learning the American press opposed linking
the League to the Treaty, he had made executive decisions relinquishing
certain points, for fear that the Conference would withdraw its approval.
"So," Woodrow told Edith, "he has yielded until there is nothing left."

She stood there, holding her husband's hand, dumbfounded—if only
because she believed the majority of the American press supported the
League. At last, Woodrow threw back his head, and Edith saw a steely
glint in his eyes. "Well," he said, "thank God I can still fight, and I'll win
them back or never look these boys I sent over there in the face again. They
lost battles—but won the War, bless them. So don't be too dismayed." The
Wilsons sat and talked for several hours, as the train rushed through
the night toward Paris.

Wilson conferred again with House in the morning. Although the
Colonel's diary reflects little of the President's displeasure, Wilson was
clearly distraught. "Your dinner to the Senate Foreign Relations Committee was a failure as far as getting together was concerned," he told House.
He spoke with "considerable bitterness" of his treatment that night at the
hands of Senator Lodge, who had refused to ask any questions or even "to
act in the spirit in which the dinner was given." House maintained that
the dinner had at least spiked criticism that Wilson was acting unilaterally, failing to consult the Senate about foreign affairs. House expressed no
culpability in his diary, only that "the President comes back very militant
and determined to put the League of Nations into the Peace Treaty."

Dr. Grayson immediately felt the chill in the air and realized that the

President was relying on him for more than medical advice. Grayson and Tumulty had periodically used each other to relay information to the President; and just that week Grayson intuitively asked Tumulty to "communicate freely with me, giving me any pointers and suggestions that you may see fit." The doctor monitored the President's every move and watched Clemenceau and Poincaré as they welcomed Wilson's train at the Gare des Invalides. The President told the old Tiger that he hoped he was not feeling any ill effects from the recent shooting. "On the contrary," said Clemenceau, "I think it did me good."

The Wilsons settled into a new "White House" at 11 Place des États-Unis, on a quiet block between the Étoile and the Seine. Although it came lavishly furnished—with pictures by Rembrandt, Delacroix, and Goya—it felt "more homey" than the Murat Palace. Its only drawback was that the bedrooms were on the ground floor. The President's, in the back, along with a study, faced a garden, while Edith's was streetside, facing a park with a Bartholdi statue of Lafayette and George Washington. As if to compensate for its exposure to the street, it came with a gold-fixtured bathroom so lavish it made her giddy. A grand hall and staircase led to a second floor of public salons; the third floor had five bedrooms and plenty of secretarial space; and quarters on the fourth floor could accommodate twelve servants. The President would have preferred to pay for his lodging, but Clemenceau insisted upon the Republic's hosting its distinguished guests. "This house," Edith recalled, "was suddenly transformed into a workshop as the President, without an hour's delay, laid about him to win back what had been surrendered by Colonel House."

Wilson assessed the damage, first by spending an hour with his neighbor Lloyd George, who spoke not only of the daily trials at the conference table but also the tribulations he faced at home—railway workers were threatening to paralyze all of England, while miners were urging government seizure of their industry. After lunch, Wilson visited the American Commissioners, who were bivouacked at the Hôtel de Crillon, and dressed them down for failing to protect the League and the Germans' basic territorial rights. The French had already announced the creation of a Rhenish Republic, which Wilson described as nothing less than a personal "embarrassment." From three to five in the afternoon, he met with Clemenceau and Lloyd George in Colonel House's room. And after dinner at his residence, Wilson conferred with Premier Orlando, who described his

private war with his cabinet ministers, many of whom were insisting on claims along the Adriatic coast, where Jugoslavs were already agitating.

The next morning, Wilson met again with Clemenceau and Lloyd George and asserted that any thought of a preliminary treaty without inclusion of the League was simply unacceptable. It contradicted the initial plenary session, at which the delegates agreed that the League was integral to the peace settlement—indeed, "the initial compelling paragraph of any peace treaty." Wilson insisted that "there were so many collateral questions which must be referred to the League of Nations . . . that its creation must be the first object, and that no treaty could be agreed upon that would deal only with military, naval and financial matters." The Premiers got the message. By day's end, Ray Baker had disseminated a statement denying all reports of a separate treaty with Germany that excluded the League. "It will cause a fluttering in the dove-cotes," Baker wrote in his diary, noting further: "Here is a man who *acts*: and has *audacity*."

Colonel House rendered a different picture of Wilson. Having occupied the seat of power for several weeks, he resented being put back in his place. His quiet petulance slowly surfaced. The next day, House and Lord Cecil met with Wilson to discuss how the Covenant might be amended, clarifications the Colonel thought would "make the Covenant a better instrument" and remove the Senate's objections. "The President, with his usual stubbornness in such matters, desires to leave it as it is, saying that any change will be hailed in the United States as yielding to the Senate," House wrote, "and he believes it will lessen rather than increase the chances of ratification." Again, House assured Cecil that the President would make "considerable concessions." Still inebriated with power, House wrote, "My main drive now is for peace with Germany . . . and I am determined that it shall come soon if it is within my power to force action." Days later, he soberly lamented, "I have no authority to decide questions on my own initiative as I did while the President was away."

"All to do over again," Woodrow grumbled to Edith. Through the month of March, six days a week, Wilson sat in one meeting after another, caroming from the Quai d'Orsay, where the Supreme War Council, the Council of Ten, and the League of Nations Commission met, to the Hôtel de Crillon, and then back to his private study, where the Council of Four convened, often twice a day. There, answers to all questions were always

close at hand from experts who could run down the stairs from the great ballroom, which had been converted into a vast office. Typewriters clattered day and night.

On the surface, the conferees in Paris were united in their initial task of reindustrializing and revitalizing the world. Toward that end, the United States had sent an American Commission that included more than one hundred of the nation's most distinguished men, current and future leaders among them: Samuel Gompers advised the labor panel; Bernard Baruch worked on economics and commerce; Herbert Hoover oversaw food and provisions, Thomas Lamont of J. P. Morgan & Company and Secretary of State Lansing's nephew John Foster Dulles assisted the banking and finance committee. The latter's brother, Allen, served as a technical adviser. Among the younger men were Ulysses S. Grant's grandson, Colonel House's son-in-law, Gordon Auchincloss, and Christian Herter. The specialists who had been part of the initial Inquiry—historians, geographers, and experts on Western Europe, the Orient, Italy, the Balkans, Russia, and Poland— continued to report to House's brother-in-law, Sidney Mezes. The delegations from other nations were just as prodigious—what with John Maynard Keynes advising the British delegation and Jean Monnet the French. A thirty-year-old protégé of French Minister of Commerce Étienne Clémentel, Monnet was already espousing an expansion of inter-Allied economic councils with which he had worked, creating the nucleus of what he called "the Economic Union of Free Peoples." The other participants were dealing with too many immediate problems to consider such an enormous proposal, but Monnet believed the notion of a European Economic Community would have its day. Wilson's constant challenge remained getting his peers to put long-term global needs ahead of immediate national interests.

His conscience was his guide, especially when it came to reparations. But there were countless factors to debate, mostly the Allies' unconscionable demands. The British wanted to bill the Germans for damage to civilian life and property and also wanted compensation for "improper treatment of interned civilians." The French sought compensation for the loot of food, raw materials, livestock, machinery household effects, and timber. In addition, they wanted compensation to French nationals who had been deported and forced into labor camps. Panels had to determine to what extent Germany's co-belligerents—Austria-Hungary, Bulgaria,

and Turkey—were liable. Then all those bills had to be stacked alongside the Central Powers' ability to pay.

A Sub-Committee of the Commission on Reparation of Damage was created to crunch the numbers. During the spring of 1919, this panel met thirty-two times, analyzing scores of reports on the assets of two continents— determining how much of the enemies' money was in cash, securities, or receivables in foreign countries and deciding how much might be paid in raw materials "of which each of the Allied States had most need and which the enemy might be required to deliver in part payment." The degree of detail approached ridiculousness. The fourth meeting of this subcommittee, for example, was devoted to the resources of Bulgaria. Investigators counted its grains in hundreds of millions of tons and its livestock and poultry into the billions—all 9.5 billion chickens, 405 million geese, 210 million tur- keys, and 162 million ducks. The statisticians determined how many hect- ares were owned by peasants, schools, monasteries, and farmers' banks. Because rose-growing was a specialty of Eastern Roumelia—the flowers' extract being a valuable commodity—the subcommittee counted the num- ber of petals that particular Bulgarian province yielded. The ninth meeting of the subcommittee examined the foreign securities owned by Germany. Copious tables listing the number of canal boats sunk during the war, the Portuguese worker's daily consumption of "albuminous substances," and the appraisal of artworks were all summarized in dizzying specifics, though sometimes the assessors pulled numbers from the sky. The subcommittee noted that enemy vessels destroyed 2,479 British mercantile vessels, the re- placement costs of which could be figured at $150 per gross ton; but when it came to evaluating the loss of cargoes, Keynes said, it was "almost entirely a matter of guesswork." Adding the costs of soldiers' pensions and allow- ances, the total assessment against Germany came in around $40 billion, though the French claimed it was really twice that much and that Germany could afford $100 billion, if not twice that sum.

With so many vying interests at the Peace Conference, no problem had a perfect solution. Every financial formula contained an X factor of human complications. Much of Germany's wealth, for example, lay in its natural resources—particularly in coal, the mines of which sat in territories that could not simply be annexed to other countries. The Saar Valley, on the west bank of the Rhine, was German in every trait; but the French wanted its coal for their iron fields in Lorraine. Upper Silesia had a mixed population

of Germans, Czechoslovakians, and Poles, all of whom also wanted its coal and iron ore. Keynes noted, however, that economically it was "intensely German," and that those resources fired the industries of eastern Germany. Their loss would flatten the economic structure of the German state, inhibiting Germany's ability to pay the very restitution the Allies sought. Where prior peace congresses allowed victors to grab their spoils, Wilson pled with the Big Four to settle their differences rationally, considering the historical, geographic, ethnological, and economic implications.

While restitution was an essential component of the peace talks, reconstitution of the fallen empires held equal importance. On March 20, 1919, the Council of Four (minus Orlando) met in Lloyd George's flat, where they opened the century's biggest can of worms—the Arab portions of the old Ottoman Empire that stretched from the Mediterranean and the Red Sea to the Persian Gulf. The region held the resource that would fuel the next century—oil. The opening discussion about the area just coming to be called "the Middle East" had two primary goals: creating an Arab Confederation of States detached from Turkey; and arbitrating the claims of Great Britain and France to that territory. Both issues were complicated by an early agreement the Arabs had struck with the British, parts of which conflicted with yet another of those well-kept secret treaties.

During the war, French diplomat François Georges-Picot and English adviser Sir Mark Sykes had sought to strengthen the bond between their two nations by anticipating victory and dividing the Ottoman Empire among themselves and Russia (before that nation's surrender) into spheres of influence. Essentially, the French would control Syria and Lebanon and the northern regions of modern Iraq; Great Britain would control Mesopotamia and Palestine, including what would become Jordan; and the Russians would obtain Armenia and Kurdistan. The remaining desert would be surrendered to the Arab empire as zones under British or French influence. The agreement was signed in May 1916. All but ignored in the agreement, of course, were the Arabs themselves, who had recently found a dynamic champion in a diminutive British army officer named Thomas Edward Lawrence. Transfixed by the region, Lawrence hoped to transform it, as he helped organize the Arab armies behind Faisal—a charismatic son of the Grand Sharif of Mecca—in their revolt against the Ottomans. At the same time, he led a diplomatic charge against his own country in promoting Arab independence. Even though England, France, and the Arabs had been

joined in opposing the Turks, the Sykes-Picot Agreement, which Lawrence learned about only after it was signed, was an affront to the Arabs. And the following year, the Balfour Declaration complicated matters further by acknowledging Britain's support for establishing an independent Jewish state.

The concerned parties descended upon Paris in 1919, with "Lawrence of Arabia" escorting Faisal, in full desert garb, into the salons of the Allied diplomats. Lawrence himself often appeared similarly robed, drawing attention to his cause. Wilson joked that Sykes-Picot sounded like a blend of tea, but the problems it created were no laughing matter. Lloyd George told the Council of Four that if Damascus, for example, fell under French administration, the British would have "broken faith with the Arabs." General Allenby topped that, suggesting that French imposition upon an unwilling Syria would surely lead to war. Wilson argued that France and Great Britain's positions were moot since they had accepted his Fourteen Points, which superseded all prior agreements.

In a further complication, shortly before the peace talks, Faisal had signed an agreement with Dr. Chaim Weizmann, president of the World Zionist Organization. It honored the Balfour Declaration and encouraged development of a Jewish homeland in Palestine. It suggested both parties— scions of the same Semitic family tree—felt like outsiders and needed each other in order to sustain harmony in their mutual quest for independence. Wilson had long believed compromise could prevail when even ancient enemies sat together at the same table. He hoped to establish Faisal's place in the Conference and argued further that because one of the parties to the Sykes-Picot Agreement—Russia—was no longer a participant, that agreement was nullified. Believing in "the consent of the governed," the President said establishing Middle East mandates would depend on the Syrians accepting French oversight and the Mesopotamians accepting that of Great Britain. Similar conundrums appeared daily, and the revelation of one secret treaty after another only contributed to what Harold Nicolson called "an atmosphere of discord and disorder."

"An undeniable tone of pessimism prevails here," Ray Baker wrote in his diary the day that Syria was first discussed. And the problems in the Middle East were the least of it. He worried about the instability in Germany and the industrial situation in England, to say nothing of the mounting attacks on Wilson and the League at home. But the problem in Paris was more fundamental than all that.

Each day, Wilson realized to a greater degree that he and the other world leaders approached the world with differing visions. Taking a macro viewpoint, Wilson looked at the entire forest; his fellow peacemakers examined the micro situations for their own countries, seeing only the trees. The President believed in doing everything possible to see that self-determination might prevail in the new nations but increasingly saw that he would have to keep placating the great powers in order to protect the lesser ones. It was a delicate balance, for at any given moment a world leader could simply walk out on the entire proceedings. And France increasingly revealed less interest in self-determination than in the simple castration of Germany.

The American Commission remained especially mindful of Poland, which it considered a keystone to a reconstructed Europe. Its land had been seized and partitioned for years; its people were struggling to establish themselves as a democratic state; and it provided a crucial buffer between Germany and Russia, a firewall between Communism and Western Europe. Secretary Lansing and his colleagues advised Wilson to appoint an Ambassador to the wobbly republic as soon as possible, which he did. In the meantime, Hungary underwent a series of revolutions, one of them organized by Communist Béla Kun. He promptly declared himself dictator, launching a Red Terror, confiscating property, and murdering thousands of his own people. Communism also seeped into the Baltic states of Latvia, Lithuania, and Estonia. In Riga, a Latvian Soviet Republic took hold, releasing thousands of prisoners who, with the Communists, looted stores, homes, and banks. They used machine guns to mow down innocent citizens, those deaths matched by starvation and disease. American food supplies seemed the best antidote to the raging ills and instability.

Twelve days after Wilson returned to Paris, William Bullitt came back from his Russian expedition. He had met Lenin himself, who charmed the young diplomat. "The Soviet government is firmly established, and the Communist Party is strong politically and morally," Bullitt reported. His fellow traveler Lincoln Steffens would later remark to Bernard Baruch, "I have seen the future, and it works!" Bullitt promptly submitted a white paper urging recognition of the Red regime. On March 28, the altruistic but pragmatic Herbert Hoover, while acknowledging the massive number of deaths due to hunger in Russia, insisted, "We cannot even remotely

recognize this murderous tyranny without stimulating actionist radicalism in every country in Europe and without transgressing on every National ideal of our own." Furthermore, he asserted, "I feel strongly the time has arrived for you again to reassert your spiritual leadership of democracy in the world as opposed to tyrannies of all kinds." He suggested an examination of Bolshevism from its political, economic, humane, and criminal points of view. Having more sway with the President than Bullitt, he urged Wilson to understand the movement's "utter foolishness as a basis of economic development." Hoover had no doubt that real democracy was the straighter road to "social betterment."

Increasingly, Wilson realized the Conference was becoming less about such humanitarian issues as feeding hungry peoples than it was about politics. That was mostly because of the French, with their endless political ploys. Clemenceau, who constantly reverted to positions he had already surrendered, became Wilson's bête noire. Repeatedly the President explained that much of the world's sympathy toward France was the result of their believing she had been wronged by Germany. "Now if the policies are to be carried out which you are advocating, and which wrong the German people," he tried reasoning with the French Premier, "the world must naturally turn against you and France, and through sympathy alone it may be likely to forget Germany's crimes." In talking about the Rhenish buffer state the French sought, Wilson finally convinced Clemenceau. But, as he confided to Lord Cecil after dinner on March 18, talking to the French was like pressing a finger into an India rubber ball: "You tried to make an impression," Wilson said, "but as soon as you moved your finger the ball was as round as ever." Wilson said that he would never consent to dividing the country on the west bank of the Rhine from Germany, but he was prepared to agree to something "in the nature of an alliance between England and America and France to protect her against sudden aggression, in addition to the protection which she would already have by the League of Nations." That appealed to the European leaders in the abstract, but one could never overestimate Clemenceau's insatiable desire for security and revenge.

Stalling had become Georges Clemenceau's greatest stratagem. He had the luxury of time, while the other world leaders had nations awaiting their returns. Wilson, especially, had fierce opposition mounting in his absence. And each day of dithering in Paris meant further starvation and destabilization in the world. By the end of his first week back at the

conference table, Wilson was reaching the end of his tether. That Saturday, after hours filled with discussion of Polish borders, thirty-seven amendments to the League Covenant, and a plea from the Japanese about racial equality, an exhausted President blurted to his wife and physician, "It is hard to keep one's temper when the world is on fire and we find delegates, such as those of the French, blocking all of the proceedings in a most stubborn manner simply by talking and without producing a single constructive idea designed to help remedy the serious situation existing." He complained that the French now considered the League just another hedge against Germany. "They talk and talk and talk and desire constantly to reiterate points that have been already thoroughly thrashed out and completely disposed of. . . . They simply talk."

The next morning at eight—accompanied only by Dr. Grayson and Miss Benham and as few guards as the Secret Service would permit—the Wilsons inspected some battle sites. Without French supervision, they revisited Rheims and Vaux and Château-Thierry before proceeding to Noyon, Lassigny, and Montdidier. The Germans had left the legendary medieval château in Coucy in ruins, prompting Wilson to shake his head and decry, "What a pity that a place like this should be destroyed when there was no military or other advantage to be gained—only wantonness." In Soissons he saw the remains of a town that had endured almost daily bombardment, forcing its inhabitants to live in cellars for months at a time. Townspeople swarmed around the local inn, where Wilson and his party took their lunch. There a French officer passed a message along that "the soldiers wanted the President to know that they were back of him and his plans of peace, and they did not want him to allow France to get a kind of peace that Clemenceau . . . [was] desirous of having made." Upon his return to Paris that night at eight, Wilson said that the day had been instructive but "exceedingly painful." He allowed that it had enabled him "to have a fuller conception than ever of the extraordinary sufferings and hardships of the people of France in the baptism of cruel fire through which they have passed."

At the Council of Four the next day, Wilson spoke of his trip, though he did not dwell on the horrors of the past. "At this moment," he said, "there is a veritable race between peace and anarchy, and the public is beginning to show its impatience." He told of a woman who had approached him amid the rubble of Soissons, asking, "When will you give us

peace?" Seeking an answer, Wilson said they had to address the most urgent questions—reparations, the protection of France against aggression, and the Italian frontier along the Adriatic coast—without delay. He told visiting Secretary Daniels, "The only exercise I get is to my vocabulary." Clemenceau muttered that Wilson "thought himself another Jesus Christ come upon the earth to reform men."

Because there was little time for recreation, Dr. Grayson urged the President to make his rounds from the "new White House" on foot, whenever possible. Wilson asked his wife to buy a map of Paris, so that he could chart different routes for himself; but within days, it fell into disuse. Grayson repeatedly implored him at least to slow the pace of his workday, but the President said, "We are running a race with Bolshevism and the world is on fire. Let us wind up this work here and then we will go home and find time for a little rest and play and take up our health routine again." Wilson's left cheek twitched. He was in a constant state of fatigue, his patience wearing thin.

Wilson harped on the same refrain, that crushing Germany would only result in another war. Prefacing his remarks with sympathy from having just seen the devastation of the countryside, Wilson argued that it was his duty to bring about permanent peace conditions that would benefit the entire world. "Don't you see," he asked Clemenceau on March 25, 1919, "that the very program that you propose to impose, carrying with it an excessive burden of taxation for generations, would be the greatest encouragement that could be held out to the German people to go over to Bolshevism?" On March 26, he added, "We owe it to the peace of the world" to present a treaty "founded on justice." On the twenty-seventh he said, "Our greatest error would be to give [Germany] powerful reasons for one day wishing to take revenge. Excessive demands would most certainly sow the seeds of war." At the end of that morning's session, Dr. Grayson asked Wilson how he was feeling. "I feel terribly disappointed," he said. "After arguing with Clemenceau for two hours . . . he practically agreed to everything, and just as he was leaving he swung back to where we had begun." Wilson, Lloyd George, and Orlando considered drawing up their own peace terms and departing, leaving Clemenceau's government to live with the consequences.

After a week of no progress in discussing reparations, the Council of Four turned again to the Saar Valley. Clemenceau insisted that its cession to France and the control of its mines had been among his country's

primary war aims and that he would not sign the Treaty without it. Wilson said that stipulation had never been disclosed. Tensions between the two leaders escalated until the Tiger growled that Wilson had become "the friend of Germany." To the man who had mobilized a nation and sent two million men to fight by France's side, at the cost of 100,000 American lives, this was more than Wilson could bear. His jaw tightening and his eyes burning, Wilson accused the Frenchman of deliberately stating untruths. In light of Clemenceau's persistent refusal to cooperate, Wilson asked, "In that event, do you wish me to return home?" Looking just as furious, Clemenceau humphed that he did not wish the President to leave . . . that he would instead. With that, he turned on his heel and exited.

The afternoon session resumed as though the morning exchange had never occurred. "Knowing the President as I do," however, Robert Lansing wrote, "I am sure that he will not forgive, much less forget, this affair. From now on he will look upon Clemenceau as an antagonist. He will suspect his every suggestion and doubt his honesty. The President is a wonderful hater." Clemenceau, who coughed profoundly throughout the proceedings, showed contrition only in saying that he would never forget "that our American friends . . . came here to assist us in a moment of supreme danger." But he expressed his conviction that Wilson was naïve in seeking justice for the Germans. "Do not believe that they will ever forgive us," he said; "they only seek the opportunity for revenge. Nothing will destroy the rage of those who wanted to establish their domination over the world and who believed themselves so close to succeeding."

The exchange that day summed up the peace talks in a nutshell. Where Wilson had idealistically maintained that "there is throughout the entire world a passion for justice," Clemenceau argued the realpolitik of the world based on experience. "The history of the United States is a glorious history," he said, "but short. A century for you is a very long period; for us it is a little thing. I have known men who saw Napoleon with their own eyes." The discussion turned to the historic tug-of-war over Alsace, which, Lloyd George reminded, dated as far back as 1648. Upon hearing that, Orlando spoke up at last, insisting they must exclude such historical arguments; "otherwise," he said, "Italy could, if she wished, claim all the former territories of the Roman Empire." Wilson laughed; Clemenceau did not.

On Monday the Big Four returned to the coal mines. They discussed a

promising proposal of France's owning the mines and administering the territory under a League mandate with a plebiscite in fifteen years to determine the nationality of the region. And then they agreed upon some Polish borders. But soon Clemenceau had backslid to his "interminable arguments." Dr. Grayson watched Wilson as he attempted to keep the conversation on point, but it was "very plain that the constant strain of trying to make men work, who had no desire to work, along the lines necessary was having its effect on the President." He was turning peevish. "I think the President is becoming unreasonable, which does not make for solutions," Colonel House imparted to his diary.

After another day bogged down in verbiage, Wilson spoke to House on the telephone for close to an hour, complaining about Clemenceau's stubbornness. House sensed that Wilson was feeling isolated, that having given him his League of Nations, everyone was prepared to hang him out to dry. In passing, the President said that he did not think Paul Mantoux, the recording secretary and interpreter, liked him; and then in a completely unguarded moment, he said, "Indeed, I am not sure that anybody does."

On Thursday, April 3, 1919—after an early afternoon visit from King Albert of Belgium—the President excused himself from the Council of Four meeting and staggered to his room. His doctor found him suffering from intense pains in his back and head, severe coughing spells, considerable upset in his "equatorial zone," and a fever of 103 degrees. Because he did not want anybody to interpret his absence as a sign of quitting, Wilson advised Grayson to announce that he had taken to his bed. At first, Grayson announced only that the President was suffering from a severe cold. Although he would subsequently diagnose this baffling illness as the onset of influenza, doctors have studied Wilson's symptoms over the decades and come to various conclusions. Some suggest that the President suffered from some other viral infection, as there had been no cases of Spanish influenza reported in Paris that spring, and most of his symptoms subsided within days. On the other hand, several doctors noted that influenza viruses attack not only pulmonary organs but also the heart and brain; and, along with his difficulty breathing, Wilson also endured an infection of the prostate and bladder. Strangely, despite a lethargy that lingered for weeks, he displayed a contradictory impulse to carry on without a "care in the world"—signs of anosognosia, a mental condition in which the disabled is unaware of his disability. That led some doctors to consider a case

of encephalitis, which was known to cause changes in personality and periodic spurts of heightened energy. Wilson's history of cerebral vascular disease also suggests a small stroke. One other possible label has been assigned to Wilson's condition, one as mysterious as it is unsettling.

Dementia is seldom diagnosed in its earliest stages because its manifestations are almost imperceptible at the onset. In retrospect, however, one can often trace its development. Early signs of the condition include apathy toward former enthusiasms, increased impatience, self-absorption to the point of insensitivity toward others, and a creeping sense of compulsive as well as suspicious behavior. Most of those symptoms were, in fact, chronic attributes of Woodrow Wilson, and the rest could be credited to a man with little leisure time, a President anxious to return to the Oval Office, from which he had been absent for close to half a year. But Wilson's current and future symptoms justify its consideration.

Theories have abounded for a century—none of which can be certified, though this much can be asserted: Woodrow Wilson had suffered for more than twenty years from hypertension and progressive cerebral vascular disease, which had resulted in small strokes; he had increasingly become aware of his own absentmindedness—enough to ask that memoranda of important conversations be written—a state he referred to as his "leaky" brain. And that metaphor might just have pinpointed the true nature of his neurological condition, that he had long been suffering from "lacunar infarctions"—a trickling of blood in the brain from lesser blood vessels— rather than an occlusion of a major vein or artery. Whatever the case, in April 1919, at a moment of physical and nervous exhaustion, Woodrow Wilson was struck by a viral infection that had neurological ramifications.

The President had long been a hero to his valet, and his sudden display of behavioral changes troubled Ike Hoover. Generally predictable in his actions, Wilson began blurting unexpected orders, often reversing his own household policies. Because his secretaries and innermost staff worked unusually long hours, Wilson had placed use of the automobiles at their disposal, urging them to see Paris whenever possible; suddenly, after that first weekend in bed, he issued orders that the cars were thereafter off-limits except for official use. Ike Hoover said Wilson also became "obsessed with the idea that every French employee about the place was a spy for the French Government." He sometimes stopped speaking when the help was present because he had convinced himself that all the domestics

understood English and were reporting his conversations to Clemenceau, even though the Secret Service found only one servant who spoke any English. Twice he created a scene over pieces of furniture that had suddenly disappeared, which nobody else in the household had observed. He began to require a Secret Service agent to guard his office when he was not present; and he now placed papers from his desk into a strongbox. Recalling the President's puzzling behavior, Ike Hoover said, "We could but surmise that something queer was happening in his mind" and that "he was never the same after this little spell of sickness."

Seeing no reason for the Conference to recess, Wilson designated House to take his place, even though the Colonel no longer held his complete confidence. With the meetings held downstairs from his bedroom, Wilson could not imagine House's allowing the conversations to drift too far from his principles. But the next day, Wilson insisted the meeting be moved upstairs to the sitting room off his bedroom, in and out of which House would pop like a character in a French farce. The Colonel boasted more than once that he could move the proceedings along with much greater dispatch than the President himself, and Ray Baker saw why: "The Colonel sides with the group which desires a swift peace on any terms," while "the President struggles almost alone to secure some constructive & idealistic result out of the general ruin."

With Wilson temporarily out of commission, Clemenceau and Lloyd George tried to chip away at his position on reparations. The British Prime Minister turned House's head with flattery, suggesting that it was better for him to conclude this particular round of the peace talks than the President. Sensing after three days that the talks were straying from his righteous path, Wilson asked that the Conference be held right in his bedroom. "To lie in bed and think of problems that you cannot pitch into and dispose of naturally make the mind more active and prevents sleeping," the convalescent explained to his doctor. "When you can handle them in person it is easy enough to dismiss them after you go to bed. To know that I am responsible for them and cannot take part in the proceedings makes me restless." He claimed that a little overexertion made him feel better. Having a number of issues he wanted to sort out, he asked Grayson to summon Bernard Baruch. And to make the arrangements for gathering his advisers one afternoon, he turned to his wife. "Can't I tell Colonel House to do it?" Edith asked. And Woodrow emphatically replied, "No."

Practically everything about House now irritated the President. By Monday, April 7, Wilson's temperature was normal, and with a clear head, he asked Grayson, "Do you see any change in House[?] . . . He does not show the same free and easy spirit; he seems to act distant with me as if he has something on his conscience." Grayson was loath to agree, but he did not hesitate to speak his mind regarding House's son-in-law, Gordon Auchincloss, who had come to be considered something of a joke because of his exalted opinion of himself. Even the President had heard that Auchincloss made constant digs behind his back and had commented that "little Woody's" fortunes at the bargaining table were because of his fa-ther-in-law. Wilson told Edith and Dr. Grayson that he no longer wished Auchincloss to conduct any business in his name.

The problem had deeper implications. Not only was Auchincloss feed-ing stories to the press that exaggerated Colonel House's importance at the peace talks, but House began to believe them. One afternoon Edith Wil-son read an article in an American paper that described House as "the brains of the Commission." At that moment, the Colonel arrived for a conference with the President, who was not available. After some friendly conversation, Edith asked House if he had been aware of any of the "awful attacks on Woodrow," such as the one before her. After she read several paragraphs aloud, House blushed and asked if her husband had seen the article. When Edith said he had not, the Colonel suddenly said that he had to leave, taking the newspaper with him. Later she related the story to Dr. Grayson, who suggested not only that Auchincloss was stirring up the stories but also that House himself was feeding self-serving tips to the press. "I don't believe it, Dr. Grayson," said Edith, who had always ques-tioned House's loyalty, "for if it were true Colonel House would be a trai-tor." Grayson told her that he had caught House talking to a journalist and posing on the roof of the Crillon for a photographer. The moment House saw Grayson, he hastily departed. Edith told Woodrow about her encoun-ter with the Colonel, omitting the information Grayson had given her. "Oh, if Colonel House had only stood firm while you were away none of this would have to be done over," she lamented. "I think he is a perfect jellyfish." Wilson replied, "Well, God made jellyfish, so, as Shakespeare said about a man, therefore let him pass, and don't be too hard on House. It takes a pretty stiff spinal column to stand against the elements centred here."

That defense aside, the President began considering House in the same terms Ray Baker had written in his diary:

> More & more he impresses me as the dilettante—the lover of the game—the eager secretary without profound responsibility. He stands in the midst of great events, to lose nothing. He gains experiences to put in his diary . . .

Meanwhile, Wilson trusted House less and less. The Colonel, without explanation, stopped visiting the Wilsons' residence except for business meetings. He now peppered his diary with criticism of the President's actions; and he liked one negative quip enough to preserve it in his journal: "Wilson talks like Jesus Christ and acts like Lloyd George." Before the spring was over, House wrote in his diary, "I seldom or never have a chance to talk with him seriously and, for the moment, he is practically out from under my influence."

Although still febrile, Wilson experienced a surge of emotional energy. Husbanding his strength, he showed an intolerance for wasted time and an inclination toward snap decisions, some in impetuous variance to positions he had long held. If definitive progress was not to be made in a timely manner, Wilson told Grayson, he would simply go home. On Sunday, April 6, Wilson asked him to ascertain the location of the *George Washington* and to order its immediate retrieval to Brest. "When I decide, doctor . . . to carry this thing through," he told Grayson, "I do not want to say that I am going as soon as I can get a boat; I want the boat to be here."

News of deploying the ship from dry dock in America was, according to Ray Baker, "the greatest sensation of the entire Peace Conference." Tumulty—minding the store in Washington—informed the President through Admiral Grayson that the action seemed politically ill-advised, that Washington viewed it "as an act of impatience and petulance on the President's part," if not an act of "desertion." And then Clemenceau and his Finance Minister, Louis Lucien Klotz, "talked away another day," producing nothing more than what Wilson called a "mass of tergiversations." After the meeting he complained to Grayson of having "Klotz on the brain." He knew he had made the right decision in beckoning his ship.

The American advisers in Paris considered Wilson's action a turning

point in the talks. Henry White thought the time had come for an end to private proceedings—that the Councils of Ten and Four were being used to discredit the President, that he should announce that all future decisions would be arrived at during plenary sessions, and that "not one American soldier, dollar or pound of supplies for military purposes will be furnished until Peace is made." Herbert Hoover was of a similar mind, believing the Allies were bound in the end to accept the League for fear of losing American financial support. "It grows upon me daily that the United States is the one great moral reserve in the world today," he wrote the President, and that "if the Allies cannot be brought to adopt peace on the basis of the Fourteen Points, we should retire from Europe lock, stock and barrel." Unfortunately, the Allies had the United States over a barrel, one the President had rolled out himself. Knowing Wilson's deathless adherence to the League, the other leaders believed he would yield ground on thirteen of the points in order to preserve his precious fourteenth, and they held it hostage.

Whether it was his stubbornness about the League or some euphoric manifestation of one of his medical conditions, Wilson emerged from his sickbed the second week of April in what one doctor later characterized as a "hypomanic state." The Big Four quickly came, at last, to several agreements, in which the President conceded points that differed from his prior positions. He agreed, for example, to a clause (written by John Foster Dulles of the Commission on Responsibilities) assigning Allies' damage to German aggression. Having once renounced such a policy, he now accepted a British proposal to try the Kaiser (living in exile in Holland) for war crimes. He relented on the matter of the Rhenish Republic, allowing French occupation with a future plebiscite. While many within his own delegation questioned his judgment, none of these positions, in truth, was vital enough for him to kill the peace process, especially as the French were showing a willingness to budge from some of their original positions. Wilson characterized all these agreements as diplomatic victories, and in one fundamental way, they were: they allowed him to preserve the League as part of the Treaty.

His recent behavior suggested a susceptibility to suppliants of all sorts and the possibility of further concessions. At a meeting of the League of Nations Committee on April 10, Wilson received a delegation representing the International Council of Women and the Suffragist Conference of

the Allied countries and the United States, which petitioned for universal suffrage and against sexual and slave trafficking in women and children. The next day, before his round of Council meetings, he received two Galician goatherds—who arrived in native mountain costume and reeking of goat—representing two small colonies that hoped the new Poland would include them. Only hours later, the President was hosting a lunch for the most glamorous visitor to Paris that season, Marie, the Queen of Romania, whom he had met the day before and who promptly invited herself to his residence. The scandalous blonde—who had boasted of a "love child"— did not endear herself to the President by arriving twenty minutes late and with extra guests. She obviously hoped to lobby for a favorable drawing of Romania's borders, though secretary Edith Benham could see from the tightening of Wilson's jaw that a sliver of Romania was being sliced off for each minute she was tardy. The President suggested starting the meal without her, but his wife persuaded him not to breach the rules of etiquette merely because she had.

Once she had arrived, the Queen proved to be a sparkling conversationalist, intelligent and fast-talking and outspoken, especially in hailing the virtues of monarchies for being "less liable to breed Bolshevism than were democracies." But her charms were utterly wasted on the President, who politely evaded all her blunt questions about the personalities at the Conference. He brought the luncheon to a close so that he could appear on time at the Quai d'Orsay for the three o'clock plenary session devoted solely to a presentation by the Commission on International Labor Legislation. The delegates adopted clauses establishing a forty-eight-hour workweek, banning child labor under the age of fourteen, and ensuring equal pay for women and men "for work of equal value in quantity and quality."

The following Thursday, Wilson endured his busiest day yet—eighteen appointments, mostly with spokesmen for minor nations and principalities. It began with a committee of Irish American politicians hoping to engage the President in influencing the establishment of an Irish Republic, a political hot potato for Great Britain. Since it struck Wilson as both imprudent and inappropriate to engage in Britain's internal politics, he kept future contact on an unofficial basis. The day's procession also included representatives from China, an Assyrian-Chaldean delegation seeking representation in what would become Iraq, and a Dalmatian delegation

wishing to be free of Italy, Albania, Romania, Armenia, and Serbia as well as the Orthodox Eastern Churches. "After all this ocean of talk has rolled over me," he told War Secretary Baker, who was visiting, "I feel that I would like to return to America and go back into some great forest, amid the silence, and not hear any argument or speeches for a month." But the most strident discussions had yet to begin.

After months of holding back—as Wilson knew he would—Vittorio Orlando held forth. In return for joining the Triple Entente, Italy cited the secret Treaty of London and claimed the South Tyrol up to the Brenner Pass. Rumors suggested the massive display of Italian affection for Wilson during his New Year's visit accounted for his inexplicably allowing close to a quarter of a million German-speaking Tyrolese to fall under Italian rule. Wilson himself would later admit that he conceded the territory based on "insufficient study" and that he came to regret this "ignorant" decision. The Treaty of London also guaranteed Italy portions of Dalmatia along the Adriatic, and some of the islands therein. Wilson was prepared to challenge these claims, but he knew that Britain and France would stand by the Treaty. Then came Italy's biggest challenge.

Nestled in an inlet of the Adriatic Sea—not forty miles from Trieste, where the coastline turned from Italy to Croatia—sat Fiume, a port that had long served Austria-Hungary. In the generation preceding the war, Fiume saw great economic growth, in large measure because Hungary (with its own Catholic persuasion) had encouraged Italian immigration there. Within the last decade, the population of the city itself had become home to more Italians than Croatians, though counting all the suburbs gave Fiume a Croatian majority. In signing the Treaty of London, Italy had not included the city among its demands. Now it did. On April 17, 1919, Ambassador Page in Rome wrote Colonel House that Italians had come to feel as passionate about Fiume as the French did about Alsace and Lorraine. Despite the recent spike in the Italian population there, Wilson insisted that Fiume—historically, culturally, geographically, and economically—was a Croatian port, one that properly belonged to the Jugoslavian nation that was taking form, whose people called it Rijeka.

Wilson believed he had conceded enough to Italy, and he considered the Dalmatian coast essentially Slavic. On April 18, he met privately with Lloyd George and Clemenceau, in hopes of creating a united front in

blocking Orlando, who was hinting that he would walk out of the Conference if his demands were not met. Wilson asked Ray Baker if he thought Orlando was bluffing, and Baker thought not. The other members of the Big Four had received enough bounty to present to their constituents—including an acknowledgment of the Monroe Doctrine, which Wilson could show naysayers back home. And now Orlando wanted his trophy.

On the morning of the nineteenth, Orlando presented his claims to the Council of Four, and Wilson flatly refused him. He disliked having to disappoint the Italian Premier, for whom he had developed a fondness, but he said it was impossible to accept conditions that so contradicted the very principles that Italy had accepted at the time of the Armistice. Wilson acknowledged Orlando's strongest argument—that natural borders must be strongly considered. "The slope of the mountains not only threw the rivers in a certain direction but tended to throw the life of the people in the same direction," Wilson observed; and that largely accounted for his assenting to the claims in the Tyrol, even in Trieste and most of the Istrian Peninsula. "Outside of these, however," recorded Sir Maurice Hankey, who kept the minutes of the meeting that morning, "further to the South all the arguments seemed to him to lead the other way. A different watershed was reached. Different racial units were encountered. There were natural associations between the peoples." Wilson maintained that something more than mountains and the flow of streams defined a nation. Despite Orlando's arguments that Jugoslavia had ports beyond the Italian-populated Fiume on which to rely, Wilson said the essential point was that "Fiume served the commerce of Czecho-Slovakia, Hungary, Roumania as well as Jugo-Slavia." Hence, it was necessary to establish its free use as an international port.

The inconstant Lloyd George announced that Great Britain would stand by the Treaty. Wilson argued that such a solution would draw the United States into an unfair, even impossible, situation. His country had entered the war in the name of certain principles that were at cross-purposes with the Treaty of London. Italy's Baron Sonnino unexpectedly reminded the President that in May of 1918, he had spoken publicly of America's interest in "the present and future security of Italy." Wilson insisted that "Dalmatia was not essential to the security of Italy." The foursome agreed to table the matter until the next day. That night Wilson attended the theater for the first time in a month—a divertissement that

worried members of the President's party as some of the girls onstage began to remove some of their garments. The President did not look away.

The next day—Easter Sunday—Wilson resurrected the question of Fiume. Orlando argued that a failure to grant the port to his people would result in a "reaction of protest and of hatred." When Wilson had heard enough, he read two of the Fourteen Points that applied to the frontiers of Italy and Serbia's right to access to the sea, and then he read Orlando the riot act. He reminded his fellow leaders that "the material and financial assistance of the United States of America had been essential to the successful conclusion of the War" and that the United States had declared its principles upon entry into that war, principles acclaimed by those present that morning. Wilson said it was "incredible" to him that Italy was turning its current position into an ultimatum, but he was clear that the United States would not sign a treaty that surrendered all that Italy demanded, even if that meant Orlando's walking out before signing. After the President's remarks, Orlando rose from his chair, walked to the window, and burst into tears. He did not appear at the meeting of the Council of Four the next day or the day after that.

"You will surely admit," Wilson said to Clemenceau and Lloyd George, "that it is I who caused America to enter the war, who instructed and formed American opinion little by little. I did it while standing by principles which you know. Baron Sonnino led the Italian people into war to conquer territories. I did it while involving a principle of justice; I believe my claim takes precedence over his." Wilson instructed financial adviser Norman Davis to sit on a $50 million loan Italy had requested—"until the air clears—if it does."

With Orlando showing no signs of rejoining the group, Wilson resorted to a tactic that had served him well ever since his days as an embattled college president. He would take his case to the people—in this instance by publishing a friendly and levelheaded statement outlining his position regarding Italy's territorial claims. It did not play well. Orlando responded with his own long statement to the press, in which he took the President to task. "The practice of addressing nations directly constitutes surely an innovation in international relations," he said sarcastically. "I do not wish to complain, but I wish to record it as a precedent, so that at my own time I may follow it, inasmuch as this new custom doubtless constitutes the granting to nations of larger participation in international

questions." Protesters marched in Rome; the crowds that had beatified Wilson months prior now burned him in effigy. The Italian press derided "Wilsonian peace," and Orlando announced that he was withdrawing from the Peace Conference.

On the heels of this Italian retreat from signing the Treaty or joining the League, the President faced an even more crucial ordeal. In late April, after sitting in silence, the Japanese wished to be heard. In fact, Japan had spoken up in February when it suggested amending the clause providing for "religious equality" by adding racial equality as well. Equating the yellow race with the white would not play well across the British Empire—nor in the United States, where anti-Asian laws persisted. The further implication that the black man might stand alongside the white man there was also still anathema. Harold Nicolson knew "no American Senate would ever dream of ratifying any Covenant which enshrined so dangerous a principle."

Nor would Woodrow Wilson. Only recently, the President had read an article on the strikes in Germany, and it rekindled his fear of Bolshevism. He had serious concerns about Communism creeping into America. The most likely vessel for that occurrence, he confided to Dr. Grayson, was "the American negro returning from abroad." He related an anecdote of a lady friend who wanted to employ a black laundress and offered to pay the standard wage, but she demanded that she be given more because that money "is as much mine as it is yours." In the millions of pages documenting Wilson's administration, the President rarely expressed a belief in inequality among the races; even his discussions of segregation expressed a policy meant for the good of both peoples. But on this incautious occasion, he revealed his true unreconstituted nature, what could only be perceived as genteel racism. He pointed out to Grayson that during the war, the French had placed their Negro soldiers shoulder to shoulder with the whites. That concept, Wilson said, "has gone to their heads." For all his talk of evenhandedness, Wilson did not consider the races fundamentally equal, and he had no intention of equalizing them under the law.

The topic of racial equality had been tabled in Paris for several months, but the Japanese now raised it once again, though they were prepared to sacrifice it in order to leverage a greater reward: Shantung Province—in the middle of China's east coast, on the Yellow Sea—the birthplace of

Confucius, a sacred region for Taoists and Buddhists, and a center of the Boxer Rebellion. Since the final days of the nineteenth century, much of the province had fallen under the German sphere of influence. In 1917, Great Britain, needing ships, appealed to Japan, which secretly agreed to supply them in return for all the Pacific islands that Germany held north of the equator plus the Chinese province of Shantung, including its prosperous ports, especially Kiaochow. Britain would receive the German islands south of the equator. This was practically the first Wilson had heard of this secret treaty. Now Baron Makino informed a plenary session that he would not press the "racial equality" clause he had sought earlier, but when it came to Shantung, his delegation was prepared to walk if it did not get its way. Losing two members of the Big Five would render the Conference a debacle.

According to every Wilsonian standard, Shantung should remain Chinese, but Japan's strategic advantage of already occupying Kiaochow bolstered her treaty-guaranteed right to the rest of the province. After dinner on April 25, Wilson tried to unknot this latest secret entanglement by talking to Dr. Grayson, rather the way he used to converse with Colonel House. "England's secret treaty with Japan would mean that when it came to a showdown England would side with Japan," he reasoned. That meant not only that Japan might not stand by the Fourteen Points and would withdraw from the Conference but that England might follow as well. "If I only had men of principle to stand by me," he lamented. By adhering to his principles without compromise, Wilson figured Japan, Italy, and England would not sign the Peace Treaty—and he would have to "shoulder the blame for obstructing the peace of the world." He wished the Japanese might see some way of saving face but yield in their demands and that the League of Nations might settle the matter later. Most of Wilson's experts advised his standing by the principles that had brought them this far. House admitted that his sympathies were "about evenly divided, with a feeling that it would be a mistake to take such action against Japan as might lead to her withdrawal from the Conference." Tumulty cabled from Washington that "the selfish designs of Japan are as indefensible as are those of Italy." But, Wilson noted, "they do not seem to realize what the results might be at this crucial time in the world's history."

He wrestled with what would become of the League of Nations if Italy

refused to return and Japan departed. Having watched the President sweat blood, Ray Baker wrote in his diary that night: "He is at Gethsemane."

Secretary of State Lansing wrote himself a memorandum, calling this submission to the Japanese a "surrender of the principle of self-determination, a transfer of millions of Chinese from one foreign master to another." He thought it better to exclude Japan from the League than to abandon China. Speaking on behalf of Henry White, Herbert Hoover, and himself, General Tasker Bliss went further, sending the President a long letter in which he concluded: "If it be right for Japan to annex the territory of an Ally [China], then it cannot be wrong for Italy to retain Fiume taken from the enemy." If the United States abandoned the democracy of China to the domination of the "Prussianized militarism of Japan," he said, "we shall be sowing dragons' teeth"—a reference to a mythical prince who planted such teeth, from which sprang armed warriors.

For one of the few times in his life, Wilson suffered from insomnia; and after lunch on April 30, Dr. Grayson urged the haggard President to ride with his wife through the Bois de Boulogne before that afternoon's meeting. Wilson consented, knowing that he was sure to fall asleep once inside the car. "My mind was so full of the Japanese-Chinese controversy," he told Grayson. "But it was settled this morning, and while it is not to me a satisfactory settlement, I suppose it could be called an 'even break.' It is the best that could be accomplished out of a 'dirty past' "—one that got even grimier when he learned that France had also signed a secret treaty with Japan.

The next morning, Wilson bowed to the Japanese demands, leaving the American delegation "mortified and angry." His loyal supporters tended to blame Colonel House, who was, in fact, the only supporter of the deal. Charles Seymour thought the decision revealed that Wilson was "more the practical politician than has sometimes been supposed." Instead of risking the dissolution of the Conference and the destruction of the Covenant, he based his decision not on the future conditional or the past imperfect but on the present indicative.

The Japanese promised to restore Chinese sovereignty to Shantung, though they intended to retain all the economic rights that formerly belonged to the Germans—specifically railways and the mines associated with them. Wilson maintained that had he not fallen on this sword, the Japanese would have departed from the Conference, which, he believed, would have led to an old-fashioned military alliance with Russia and

Germany, a perpetuation of the same thinking that had led to this war. With the acceptance of these terms, the Treaty was virtually settled—with the League of Nations still intact.

That same afternoon, May Day, had started quietly enough but ended with a number of bloody confrontations in the streets between labor and the cavalry. For Wilson, it seemed one stress more than he could bear. In addition to surrendering to the Japanese terms, he officially approved of arraigning the Kaiser and possibly trying him for war crimes. And then, after several more hours of intense discussion, he suddenly announced to Edith and Dr. Grayson after lunch, "I don't like the way the colors of this furniture fight each other.

> The greens and the reds are all mixed up here and there is no harmony. Here is a big purple, high-backed covered chair, which is like the Purple Cow, strayed off to itself, and it is placed where the light shines on it too brightly. If you will give me a lift, we will move this next to the wall where the light from the window will give it a subdued effect. And here are two chairs, one green and the other red. This will never do. Let's put the greens all together and the reds together.

Wilson's bizarre comments did not end there. He described the Council of Four meetings, how each delegation walked like schoolchildren each day to its respective corner. Now, with the furniture regrouped, he said each country would sit according to color—with the reds in the American corner, the greens in the British corner, and the rest in the center for the French.

Sensing it was a manifestation of stress, Grayson made little of the aberrant behavior, prescribing only an automobile ride. "Mr. President," he said lightheartedly, "I think if you ever want a job after leaving the Presidency you would make a great success as an interior decorator." Wilson smiled and said, "I don't mean to throw bouquets at myself but I do think that I have made a success of the arrangement of this furniture."

In retrospect, Wilson's behavior that day might have been "ludic"—activity somewhere between playful and delusional, and which sometimes accompanies improvement after brain injuries. Or perhaps it was nothing more than an attempt to impose order on circumstances beyond his control.

His thoughts about moving the furniture quickly passed, but Wilson's rearrangement in Asia did not. News of the settlement reached Peking on May 3, 1919, churning up a tsunami of shame and outrage. Students in Shanghai proclaimed that they had turned to Woodrow Wilson looking for the deliverance he had prophesied; "but no sun rose for China," they wrote. "Even the cradle of the nation was stolen." The next day, three thousand of them protested at Tiananmen Square before pouring into the streets, leaving angry petitions at the embassies of the Big Four and burning the house of one of China's envoys. This "May Fourth Incident" provided the tinderbox for pro-national and anti-imperialist sentiment, which ignited a political and cultural awakening, starting with a massive boycott of all things Japanese. For many it signaled the closing of the door the West had opened twenty years earlier. In Hunan it turned a young college graduate, Mao Tse-tung, into a radical newspaper publisher. "We are awakened!" read one of his editorials that summer. "The world is ours, the state is ours, society is ours!"

Centuries earlier Confucius had said, "To go beyond is as wrong as to fall short." That philosophy dominated Wilson's actions as the German delegation was about to arrive in Paris to receive the Peace Treaty. Wilson had heard that Germany still believed he was the one man who would see that "she would get justice at his hands." But he predicted to Grayson that he would become the object of their animosity once they got their hands on the document. "The terms of the treaty are particularly severe," Wilson granted, "but I have striven my level best to make them fair, and at the same time compel Germany to pay a just penalty. However, I fully realize that I will be the one on whom the blame will be placed. In their hearts the Germans dislike me because if I had kept America from entering the war Germany would have defeated the Allies. So I know that they blame me for their defeat."

The Allied leaders had grown contemptuous as well. Down to crafting the final paragraphs of the Treaty with Germany, they stopped at nothing in achieving their individual goals, each still thinking nationalistically. England and now even France forgot how they had beseeched the United States to join in their fight. Their lack of loyalty to President Wilson matched their growing lack of gratitude. Wilson complained about the

French, who had recently shown only "a lack of appreciation" as they assumed the attitude that "France did it all." The British behavior was even worse. Winston Churchill was already speechifying that the war had "proved the soundness of the British race at every point" and that "in every country, it is to the British way of doing things that they are looking now." It was only a matter of time before he would tell a New York newspaper editor that "America should have minded her own business and stayed out of the World War.

> If you hadn't entered the war the Allies would have made peace with Germany in the Spring of 1917. Had we made peace then there would have been no collapse in Russia followed by Communism, no breakdown in Italy followed by Fascism, and Germany would not have . . . enthroned Nazism.

Wilson—once "the prophet of the world"—found himself rolling in the political mud, preserving as much of his grand plan as possible. Said Ray Baker: "He must bargain and bluff, give way here, stand firm there. Miserable business—but *wise*."

And after four months of talks, the time had arrived to see how the Fourteen Points had translated into the Treaty of Versailles. While the printer was setting it in type, a member of the American Commission and Sir Maurice Hankey arrived at the temporary White House to point out two insertions that Clemenceau had made in the Treaty, unilaterally, presumably expecting them to slip by unnoticed. One was a liberty he had taken, which House called "a perversion of the entire mandatory system." Wilson simply ordered their excision. Over the next several days, John Foster Dulles combed the eighty-five-thousand-word text and discovered even more tampering. Bernard Baruch did the same. "The French seem to be always up to some skullduggery," Wilson commented; "the word 'honorable' doesn't seem to mean anything to them."

On the morning of Wednesday, May 7, 1919, while the Big Three were tying up a few loose ends before that day's official presentation of the documents to the German delegates, Premier Orlando entered the room and took his chair, as if he had never walked out. He did not want to miss that afternoon's pageant, which would be short on ceremony, though long on symbolism.

King Louis XIV had built the magnificent Château de Versailles, ten miles west of Paris, to stand as his monument "to all the glories of France"; and when Bismarck had dictated his harsh peace in 1871, he had added ignominy to the French defeat by selecting Versailles for the occasion. Now, on the perimeter of the château gardens, resplendent with lilacs and chestnut blossoms, world leaders gathered once again at the Trianon Palace Hotel, this time allowing the French to reclaim not only their land but also some of their glory. Tables and chairs were configured in the hotel dining room to replicate the Salle de la Paix at the Quai d'Orsay; and by three o'clock, all the Allied plenipotentiaries were seated (except for the habitually late Paderewski, who was evidently used to audiences being in their seats before he walked onto the stages of concert halls). In fact, the German delegation of six had been waiting in Versailles for a week—some of them believing the talks had slowed intentionally in order for this day to coincide with the fourth anniversary of the sinking of the *Lusitania*.

As soon as everybody was seated, Clemenceau, wearing yellow gloves, stood and announced that this was neither the time nor the place for "superfluous" words. "The time has come when we must settle our accounts," he said. "You have asked for peace. We are ready to give you peace." He offered to explain any terms the Germans might require, but he said there would be no oral discussion—only observations submitted in writing within the next fifteen days. With copies of the 413-page books (in French on the left-hand pages, English on the right, and illustrated with large folding maps) before them, Clemenceau added that "this Second Treaty of Versailles has cost us too much not to take on our side all the necessary precautions and guarantees that that peace shall be a lasting one."

Ulrich, Count von Brockdorff-Rantzau, the German Foreign Minister, did not stand, which delegates interpreted as insolence. "We cherish no illusions as to the extent of our defeat—the degree of our impotence," he said without repentance, ". . . and we have heard the passionate demand that the victors should both make us pay as vanquished and punish us as guilty." But he said they were required to admit that they alone were "war-guilty" and that "such an admission on my lips would be a lie." While he did not seek to exonerate Germany from all responsibility, he refuted the idea that Germany—"whose people were convinced that they were waging a defensive war"—should solely be "laden with the guilt," as the last half century of imperialism of all European states had "chronically poisoned

the international situation." He reminded the Conference that the blockade against Germany persisted to that day, taking the lives of hundreds of thousands of noncombatants since the Armistice. He made no attempt to delay the restoration of territory in Belgium and northern France that Germany had occupied. In order to do that, he said, they needed the technical and financial participation of the victors. "It must be the desire of impoverished Europe that reconstruction should be carried out as successfully and economically as possible," he said. Before even reading the Treaty, he endorsed the League of Nations. And he reminded the victors, "A Peace which cannot be defended in the name of justice before the whole world would continually call forth fresh resistance." Several people had observed that the Count was trembling violently when he entered the room, had fumbled with his chair in trying to sit down, and could not suppress the shaking of his hands and knees—all of which probably explained why he had not stood in the first place. Wilson dismissed the speech as "stupid," finding it "not frank & peculiarly Prussian!"

The Treaty of Versailles contained 440 articles, divided into fifteen sections. The first was the League Covenant. The second and third sections redrew Germany's borders, and much of the rest of Europe's. Germany would cede 5,600 square miles of Alsace-Lorraine to France, 382 square miles to Luxembourg and Holland, and almost 22,000 square miles, including West Prussia, to Poland. Dantzig would become a "free city," an internationalized zone under the guarantee of the League of Nations; and a separated East Prussia would hold a plebiscite to determine its nationality. Furthermore, Germany was to recognize the total independence of German Austria and Czechoslovakia, and to respect the independence of all territories that had been part of the former Russian Empire. Section IV itemized the German renunciation of all her overseas possessions—from Liberia, Morocco, and Egypt to Siam and Shantung, including whatever claims she had in Turkey and Bulgaria.

The next few sections were more onerous, as they compelled Germany to dismantle its military infrastructure. Its massive army of millions would be reduced to 100,000 soldiers, the once ominous navy to no more than 15,000 sailors manning three dozen vessels of war, including six small battleships and no submarines. Conscription was to be abolished, as were the manufacture, storage, and design of arms and munitions of war; no dirigibles could be kept, and only a limited number of unarmed

necessity for making it evident once for all that such things can lead only to the most severe punishment."

Over the next several weeks, the Council of Four pored over every territorial dispute. Tempers wore thin, reducing their efforts to playground politics that often required a referee. One morning session collapsed into an argument over Asia Minor, as Clemenceau accused Lloyd George of misrepresenting the terms of the secret treaties. The Welshman resented being called a liar and insisted upon an apology. The Frenchman said, "That's not my style of doing business." Wilson stepped in, and at the end of the meeting said, "You have been two bad boys, and so it would be well for you to shake hands and make up." They moved toward each other, but several seconds passed before Lloyd George held out his hand, which Clemenceau grasped. Turning toward a smiling Wilson, they both burst into laughter. The same day the Italians announced their intention to seize several Greek islands (under the pretense that they had been ceded by the Treaty of London), Wilson learned that Italy had just changed the name of a road from Via Wilson to Via Fiume. The President laughed at the news and called them "a big lot of babies." In one candid moment, Orlando unwittingly admitted that Fiume was only of sentimental value to Italy, but he had behaved so mulishly about it because his people made him. The Big Four often worked from a map in the President's room, one too large for any table to accommodate. Whenever it was needed, they spread it on the floor. One morning Dr. Grayson entered the salon, only to find the four most powerful men in the world on their hands and knees, studying the chart. "It had every appearance," noted Grayson, "of four boys playing some kind of a game."

In the spring of 1919, that quadrumvirate on the floor erased more boundaries and created more new nations than had ever been drawn at a single time. And whenever Clemenceau and Lloyd George fell into another argument, scrapping over patches of Asia Minor, Wilson reminded them that they were engaged in the "bargaining away of peoples." He vigilantly protected the Jews, wherever they settled, from Poland to Palestine. More than once did Wilson recall having reassured Rabbi Stephen Wise and the American Jewish Congress that he and the Allied nations fully agreed "that in Palestine shall be laid the foundations of a Jewish commonwealth."

While the United States had no direct interest in most of the territorial settlements, Wilson continued to involve himself as the others tore at the

Habsburg Empire. Austria and Hungary (then in the midst of a series of revolutions) would be divided into two separate landlocked countries, neither of which would ever be powerful enough to rise to any significant stature. The Treaty sanctioned a union of Czechs and Slovaks into a sovereign independent state. Similarly, the Independent Kingdoms of Serbia and Montenegro joined with the State of Slovenes, Croats, and Serbs as well as much of Dalmatia, and Bosnia and Herzegovina to form Yugoslavia. Parts of the Habsburg Empire—Bessarabia, Bukovina, and Transylvania—joined the Kingdom of Romania.

The Ottoman Empire offered a map with more blank space on which to draw. Out of the secret treaties and mandates and assurances to Arab leaders, new nations would be built in the sand. They proved problematic because they too bundled diversified populations, often with ancient ethnic and religious differences. Tensions naturally rose in the area as each of these disparate peoples sought self-government and independence while they were in conflict among themselves as well as with their mandatories. Adding to the friction was the steadily increasing demand for the oil beneath their feet. They agreed that the Allies would occupy for several years the nucleus of the empire—Constantinople, which bridged two continents—before the Republic of Turkey would be formed. To the south as far as Acre and to the east as far as the Tigris River, France collected on its claims from the Sykes-Picot Agreement, exercising its "tutelage" over the mandates of Syria and Lebanon. Great Britain assumed responsibility for Palestine, which divided in order to create Jordan on the East Bank of the eponymous river, and then beyond to Mesopotamia. In the end, this modern state of Iraq seemed destined to remain a delicate imbalance of incompatible, even warring, factions—Shi'ites, Sunnis, and Kurds— bound together by man-made borders when they might more naturally have divided into three separate countries.

The most unsettled and unsettling problem at the Peace Conference remained Russia, which had left more bodies on the battlefield than any of the belligerents. With neither a vote nor a voice at the Conference, it was consigned to watching the Allies grab all the bounty. Much of the problem was Russia itself, then more consumed with the revolution inside its borders than the political evolution on the outside. Ray Baker suggested that "Wilson's mind was never quite clear on the question of dealing with Bolshevist Russia." He seemed unable to comprehend the idea of building

a nation around an economic precept; and most of what he understood of the country's state of affairs, said Baker, "was repugnant to him."

William Bullitt tried to convince Wilson otherwise, as he advocated American recognition of the Bolshevik regime. He returned from his meeting with Lenin with an understanding that the Communist leader was prepared not only to make an armistice on all fronts but also recognize anti-Communist governments throughout most of the former Russian Empire—including what would become Baltic nations. Soviet expert George Kennan would later assert that the terms Bullitt conveyed did offer an opportunity for the Western powers to extract themselves from "the profitless involvements of the military intervention in Russia" and might have allowed for the "creation of an acceptable relationship to the Soviet regime." But Wilson put no faith in them because he believed the Bolsheviks were "the most consummate sneaks in the world." Kennan also suggested the unseasoned and "impatient" Bullitt was not the most effective advocate for his pro-Bolshevik position. And Bullitt did not realize that he had submitted his report the very moment that the President had become ill, which explained why the junior diplomat got no reply to his request for even a fifteen-minute meeting. He took further umbrage at Lloyd George's speaking dismissively in the House of Commons of "some American" who had investigated the proposal of recognizing the Bolshevik government in Moscow but who had evidently not turned up enough to warrant it. The Wilson Administration left him in the cold, claiming no interest in the mission. And Bullitt quit.

Further upset by the decisions Wilson made regarding Shantung, the Tyrol, Dantzig, and the Saar Valley, Bullitt fired off a scathing letter to the President of the United States explaining his resignation. Bullitt said he was one of the millions who had believed in Wilson's promises of "unselfish and unbiased justice," but "our government has consented now to deliver the suffering peoples of the world to new oppressions, subjections and dismemberments—a new century of war." In a final flurry of bitter disappointment, Bullitt added, "I am sorry that you did not fight our fight to the finish and that you had so little faith in the millions of men, like myself, in every nation who had faith in you." Lansing accepted Bullitt's resignation without comment. Wilson found it "insulting." He continued to believe, as he had told the Democratic National Committee when he had been Stateside in February, that the Conference might end before the vast Russian

territories had been recomposed, "but if we go home with a League of Nations, there will be some power to solve this most perplexing problem."

Lansing—who had been relegated to the role of errand boy for months—also thought the Treaty was "bad," insufficient to uphold the League; but he continued to perform his job, no matter how menial it became. Herbert Hoover believed the economic terms would ruin Germany and wreak Bolshevism there; but he continued in his unceasing efforts to supervise the feeding of Europe, where the ongoing blockade continued to starve masses of people. Wilson, of course, knew that opposition was building at home and granted that it was "a terrible compromise"; but he believed it would pass in the Senate—League and all—not because it was just, noted Baker, "but because the American people don't know, don't care, and are still dominated by the desire to 'punish the Hun.'" Several other members of the American Commission—including historian Samuel Eliot Morison and future FDR "brain-truster" Adolf Berle—left their posts before the Treaty was done. "The consequences of Wilson's refusal to turn his mind to the question of Russia were considerable," wrote Bullitt, presumably referring to the next several decades, in which relations between the Soviets and the Western powers would freeze over. "It is not impossible that Wilson's refusal to burden his 'one track mind' with Russia may well, in the end, turn out to be the most important single decision that he made in Paris."

Bullitt's animus toward Wilson swelled over the next several years, until he unburdened himself to his psychotherapist and subsequent friend, Sigmund Freud. Harboring his own resentment of the pious American president, the Austrian doctor agreed to analyze Woodrow Wilson in absentia, through the details of his life as Bullitt presented them. The result was a spiteful book that scorned practically everything about Wilson, with repeated references to his oversized ears and much more about what was between them—what Freud characterized as a Christ complex. The leitmotiv of the coauthored study was the subject's abnormal adoration of his father, the Reverend Wilson, and his lifelong wavering between self-identification with the Son of God and his need to assert himself as nothing less than God. "Tommy"'s repressed rage toward the Reverend Wilson, said Freud and Bullitt, manifested itself in a life of hypocrisy and self-contradiction. When *Thomas Woodrow Wilson: A Psychological Study* was published in the 1960s, critics suggested the book debunked Freud more than Wilson.

Valid or not, the analysis did capture some of the flaws of its subject,

and Bullitt was not the only man in Paris to perceive them. "The President, it must be remembered, was the descendant of Covenanters, the inheritor of a more immediate presbyterian tradition," wrote Harold Nicolson. "That spiritual arrogance which seems inseparable from the harder form of religion had eaten deep into his soul." Like Bullitt and Freud, Nicolson also wrote of Wilson's "one-track mind," saying,

> This intellectual disability rendered him blindly impervious, not merely to human character, but also shades of difference. He possessed no gift for differentiation, no capacity for adjustment to circumstances. It was his spiritual and mental rigidity which proved his undoing. It rendered him as incapable of withstanding criticism as of absorbing advice. It rendered him blind to all realities which did not accord with his preconceived theory, even to the realities of his own decisions.

He was like a brave knight-errant, John Maynard Keynes observed. "But this blind and deaf Don Quixote was entering a cavern where the swift and glittering blade was in the hands of the adversary."

Whether the European leaders had outfoxed Wilson or not, Keynes thought the problems with the Treaty were not the fault of one man. He found the Big Four themselves guilty of dwelling on the subject of reparation at the expense of rehabilitation. For all the redrawing of Europe, he felt nobody had thought enough to rebuild the defeated Central empires or to reclaim Russia or restore the "disordered finances" of France and Italy, or even to stabilize the new nations. "It is an extraordinary fact that the fundamental economic problems of a Europe starving and disintegrating before their eyes, was the one question in which it was impossible to arouse the interest of the Four. Reparation was their main excursion into the economic fields," Keynes wrote of Wilson, Clemenceau, Lloyd George, and Orlando, "and they settled it as a problem of theology, of politics, of electoral chicane, from every point of view except that of the economic futures of the States whose destiny they were handling." Like Bullitt, Nicolson and Keynes exited the Conference as disgruntled underlings, confident that they had more facts than their leaders, certainly more than Wilson. But political leaders view the world through different prisms from those of junior diplomats and with different perspectives. With his League in place, Wilson considered the Treaty a victory for mankind.

After the morning session of the Big Four on May 30, 1919, the Wilsons and Dr. Grayson rode to Suresnes, four miles west of Paris. There, on a gentle slope surrounded by acacia groves, the French government had offered a few acres to recognize the ultimate sacrifice of many Americans. The President was dedicating the cemetery that hot, sunny Decoration Day, consecrating a final resting place for 1,500 doughboys who were buried in a precisely measured grid, row after row of white crosses. Local women had decorated each grave with a wreath and a small American flag, a gesture that brought a lump to Wilson's throat as he entered the ground he was meant to hallow. Thousands of veterans in khaki filled the hillside, boys all looking older than their years, many with visible scars and empty sleeves.

Wilson stood on a small platform in the middle of the burial ground and removed his top hat. Edith could not help observing that in just the last few months, her husband's hair had turned white. Extemporizing from notes, he delivered one of the most poignant speeches of his life. The notes proved to be an essential crutch, for the pathos of the occasion almost broke the President's self-control. "No one with a heart in his breast, no American, no lover of humanity," he began, "can stand in the presence of these graves without the most profound emotion. These men who lie here are men of unique breed. Their like has not been seen since the far days of the Crusades. Never before have men crossed the seas to a foreign land to fight for a cause which they did not pretend was peculiarly their own, but knew was the cause of humanity and of mankind."

His mind filled with details of the final push to complete the Peace Treaty, Wilson extolled the spirit of the American soldiers as he reminded the world that "these men did not come across the sea merely to defeat Germany and her associated powers in the war. They came to defeat forever the things for which the Central Powers stood, the sort of power they meant to assert in the world, the arrogant, selfish dominance which they meant to establish; and they came, moreover, to see to it that there should never be a war like this again." It was left to civilians, such as himself, the President said, to "use our proper weapons of counsel and agreement to see to it that there never is such a war again." Of all the matters that had been thrashed out in the last six months, he said, only the concept of the League had met "unity of counsel" and unanimity of acceptance.

"I beg you to realize the compulsion that I myself feel that I am under," Wilson said in closing, striking a startling personal note. "By the Consti-

tution of our great country I was the Commander in Chief of these men. I advised the Congress to declare that a state of war had existed." And then, owning all that had befallen his troops, Wilson squarely confronted the most grievous task of any head of state. "I sent these lads over here to die," he said. "Shall I—can I—ever speak a word of counsel which is inconsistent with the assurances I gave them when they came over?" Wilson paused for a moment before saying that there was "something better . . . that a man can give than his life, and that is his living spirit to a service that is not easy, to resist counsels that are hard to resist, to stand against purposes that are difficult to stand against." And in that moment, he appeared to take a vow before the crowd, giving his countrymen at home and all the world a preview of what was to come: "Here stand I," he said, "consecrated in spirit to the men who were once my comrades and who are now gone, and who have left me under eternal bonds of fidelity."

Few bothered to fight back their tears. After renditions of Chopin's "Funeral March," the American and French national anthems, and a lone bugler sounding "Taps," the crowd was undone. The Wilsons drove back into town in silence, except for the President's own torrent of emotion.

"As lonely as God—a slave he is!" noted Ray Baker. "Yet he is the only great, serious responsible statesman here: when all is said, a great man: a Titan struggling with forces too great even for him."

But at home a drumbeat of anti-Wilson rhetoric continued. His critics kept hammering that Wilson's mission to France was purely political—that this entire expedition had been personal exploitation, building his base for a third term. Just as Wilson made it clear to his supporters that they must pour all their energies into the adoption of the League, the Republicans decided to channel all their powers into its defeat. If they could win that one issue, they might reclaim their authority in American politics.

Obviously, Wilson could not return in time to open the Republican-controlled Sixty-sixth Congress, but he sent a long message explaining why he had assembled the legislators and why he would not be present. Washington had to approve certain appropriations in order to keep the government running; and Paris was in the middle of negotiations. While the President hesitated to press any legislative suggestions in his absence, he sent close to three thousand words of recommendations. He revisited his early Progressive themes as he hoped the country would return to a

peacetime economy. He called for improvement in workers' conditions through "the genuine democratization of industry"; he addressed inequities in the tax system—calling for a reduction in sales taxes but an increase in excess profits taxes and estate taxes. With the demobilization of the military forces, he thought it safe to remove the wartime ban upon the manufacture and sale of wine and beer. And he asked Congress to endorse the cause he had been urging upon reluctant Senators that spring: suffrage for women. In a few weeks, the House would overwhelmingly pass the suffrage amendment; and two weeks after that, the Senate would deliver the two-thirds majority by two votes. The amendment moved to the states, where three-quarters of their legislatures were required for ratification. Alice Paul predicted that women would be voting for the next President.

With the opening of this Republican Congress, Wilson knew that passing any of his legislation would be an uphill battle. Ignoring the abuse already being hurled, Wilson hoped to continue leading the United States from its inherent provincialism to a more worldly vision. Off the record, he had derided his rivals for having "horizons that do not go beyond their parish" and said they were "going to have the most conspicuously contemptible names in history." He found himself thinking of March 5, 1921, for on that day he intended to return to a private scholarly life, and of having "the privilege of writing about these gentlemen without any restraints of propriety." Until then, however, he had to face not only the American Congress and the warring Allies as they completed the Treaty but also the one adversary that could reduce the last six months of work to naught.

"Will the Germans sign?" were the words on everybody's lips in Paris. Although the Armistice had been accepted, Allied armies prepared to resume battle and prolong the blockade. Germany was technically boxed into accepting the peace terms as handed to them. But the enemy stuck to its initial response that the "exactions of this Treaty are more than the German people can bear." The loss of treasury and the territory that might replenish it, and rendering Germany unable to assert itself in a modern world, all but ensured that this peace treaty would become a declaration of the next war. The Social Democratic government of Chancellor Philipp Scheidemann in Germany was against his country's signing.

So, strangely enough, were many leaders in Great Britain. In addition to fears of revenge, Liberal and Labour factions there questioned the

efficacy of creating a fiscal vacuum in the middle of Europe, one certain to suck the financial systems of the Continent down the drain with it. When Lloyd George returned to Paris from London in early June, he spoke of moderating the terms of the Treaty. At the Council of Four meeting on June 2, 1919, he discussed reducing reparations, redrawing borders, reexamining the need for more plebiscites, and removing multitudes of "pinpricks" whose cumulative effect was lacerating. Later, at a meeting of the American delegation, Wilson announced, "I have no desire to soften the treaty, but I have a very sincere desire to alter those portions of it that are shown to be unjust, or which are shown to be contrary to the principles which we ourselves have laid down." Clemenceau, of course, remained "absolutely rigid" about leaving all the terms as agreed upon.

In a moment of growing desperation, Lloyd George asked Bernard Baruch if he might arrange a private meeting between him and the President. In doing the Prime Minister's bidding, Baruch suggested that Lloyd George had been struggling between his campaign promises of toughness toward the Germans and "the dictates of his conscience." But his dilemma was greater than that. Once he and Wilson came face-to-face, Lloyd George told him that unless they altered the terms of the Treaty, neither the British army nor fleet would compel Germany to sign. The President sat in silence, his jaw clenched, while the Prime Minister reiterated the changes in the Treaty that he required. At last, Wilson had heard quite enough. "Mr. Prime Minister," he said, "you make me sick! For months we have been struggling to make the terms of the Treaty exactly along the lines you now speak of, and never got the support of the English. Now, after we have finally come to agreement, and when we have to face the Germans and we need unanimity, you want to rewrite the Treaty."

For months Colonel House had said Lloyd George "changes his mind like a weather-vane," and Wilson knew the political winds had not stopped blowing. While he maintained that the current terms were strict but fair, he said he would agree to the British proposals—if the French agreed. But in every delegation there were rivalries within rivalries, and even though Wilson knew that Marshal Foch, among others, feared Clemenceau's harsh insistences as well, he knew nobody in France was strong enough to defy him. Wilson could offer little more than his allowing the Prime Ministers to duke out their differences, telling them that he "did not desire a lenient

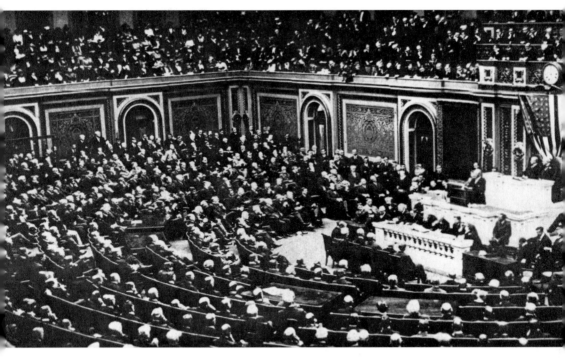

On April 2, 1917, less than a month after his second inauguration, President Wilson stood before Congress and delivered a war message, insisting, "The world must be made safe for democracy."

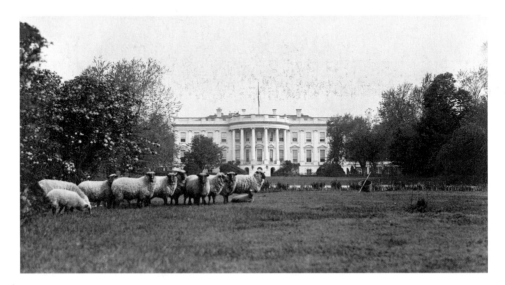

The Great War had been ravaging Europe since 1914, but the United States did not declare war until April 1917. The isolationist country, with an Army of a few hundred thousand, mobilized—shipping two million men to the front. At home, citizens poured all their resources into the war effort—including the Wilsons, who kept a flock of sheep at the White House, to trim the lawn and to grow wool for the Red Cross.

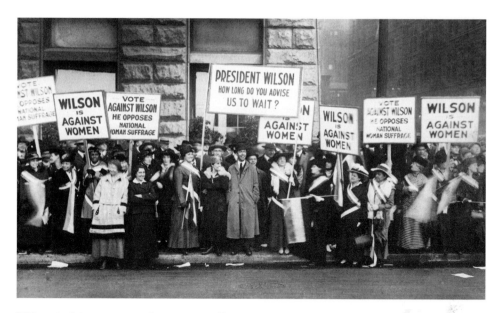

Wilson had long supported women's suffrage, but only through state-by-state adoption; with American women contributing to the war effort, he became the most persuasive advocate for the Nineteenth Amendment.

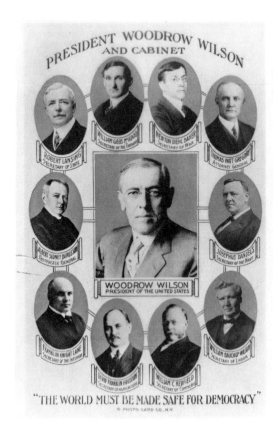

The Wartime Cabinet

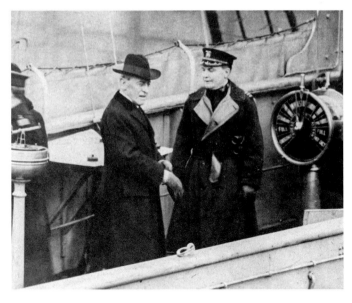

The war fought and won, President Wilson sailed to France on the *George Washington* in December 1918 to settle the peace. He would spend the next six months in Europe.

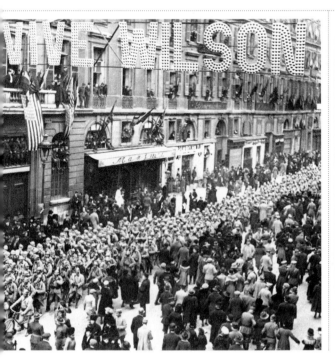

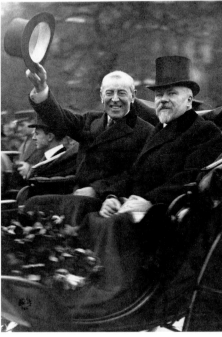

Paris welcomes its hero; on the right with French President Raymond Poincaré.

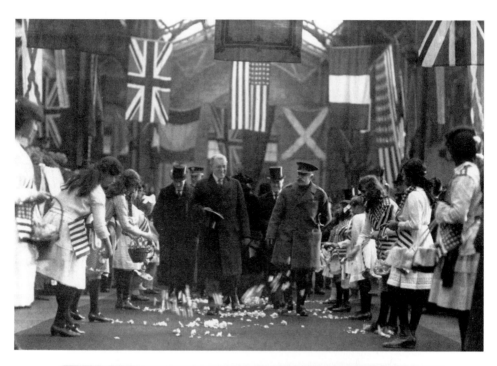

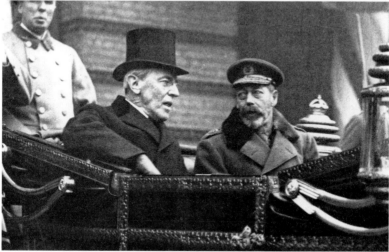

Wilson received further acclaim in England.
After his arrival in Dover, he was the guest of King George V.

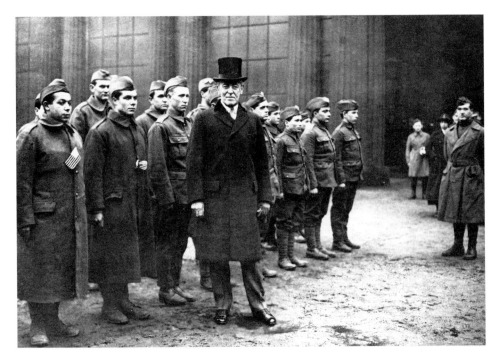

In the courtyard of Buckingham Palace, the President met American soldiers released from German prison camps.

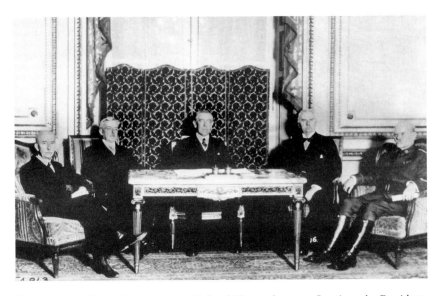

The American Peace Commissioners: Colonel House, Secretary Lansing, the President, Ambassador Henry White, General Tasker H. Bliss.

France's Premier Georges Clemenceau—
"the Tiger"—who sought revenge against
the Germans at every turn.

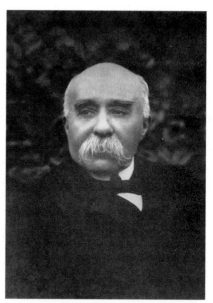

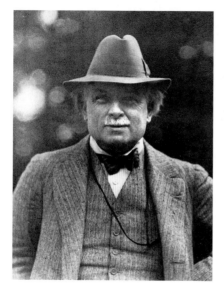

Great Britain's Prime Minister David
Lloyd George, whom one American
adviser said was "slippery as an eel."

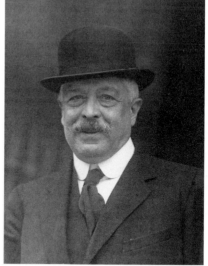

Italy's Prime Minister Vittorio Emanuele
Orlando, whom Clemenceau dubbed
"the Weeper," because he burst into tears
whenever his demands were not met.

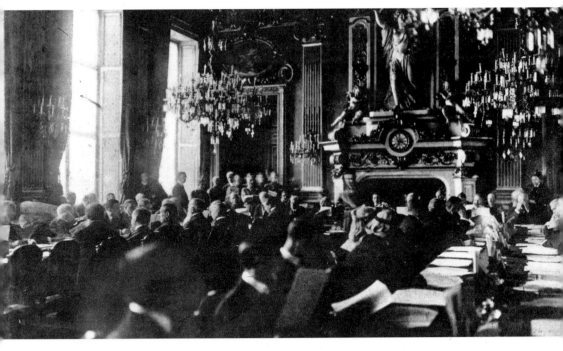

January 18, 1919—the opening of the Paris Peace Conference
in the Salle de la Paix in the Quai d'Orsay.

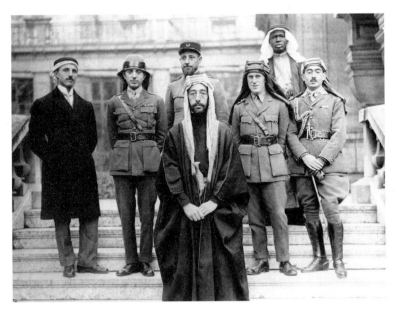

Representatives of nearly every population in the world flocked to Paris in the
first six months of 1919. Among them were Emir Faisal (center), who would
become the King of Greater Syria and the King of Iraq, and an Englishman
named T. E. Lawrence (third from right), known as "Lawrence of Arabia."

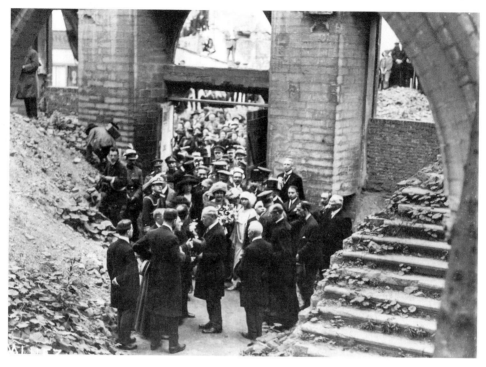

Wilson inspected the ruins of the library of Belgium's University of Louvain.

Official war painter Sir William Orpen captured the world-weariness of President Wilson in Paris, where he fought for an equitable peace based on his Fourteen Points.

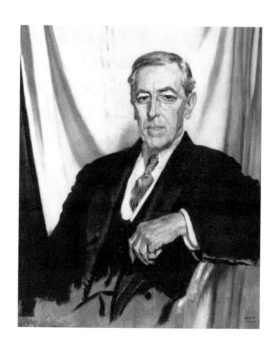

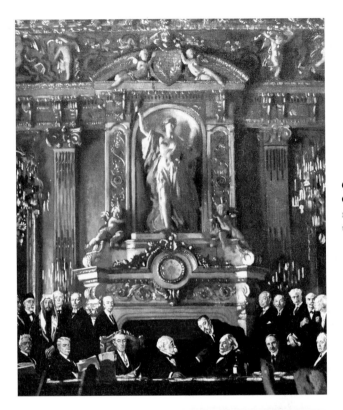

Orpen's rendition of the Council of Ten, which reshaped the world, at the Quai d'Orsay.

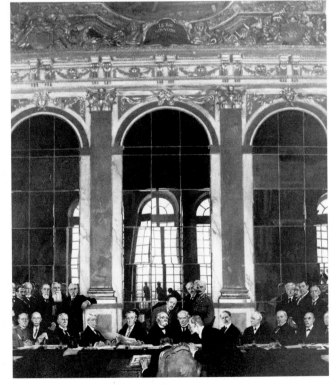

The Hall of Mirrors at the Palace of Versailles during the signing of the Treaty, the centerpiece of which was Wilson's League of Nations.

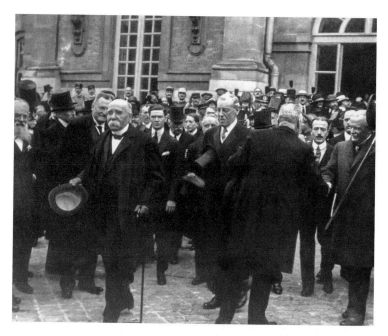

Clemenceau, Wilson, and Lloyd George (far right) exit the Palace of Versailles on June 28, 1919, after the signing. Their faces reveal exhaustion more than joy.

The United States Senate had to approve the Treaty, and Republicans had planned its obstruction even before the terms had been agreed upon. Wilson's nemesis was the senior Senator from Massachusetts, Henry Cabot Lodge.

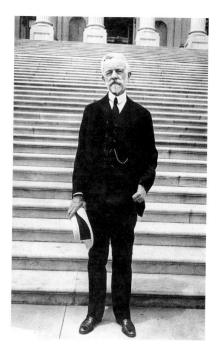

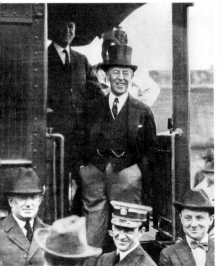
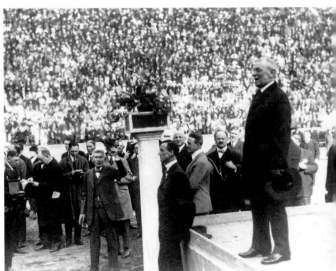
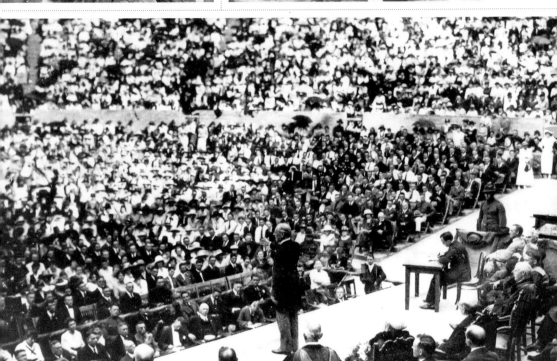

When Wilson found Senate resistance too great, he took his cause to the people. Despite excruciating headaches, he embarked upon a cross-country tour in September 1919. In St. Paul, Minnesota, at the Tacoma Stadium (upper right), and at the Greek Theatre at Berkeley (bottom) —Wilson rallied audiences in favor of the Treaty and the League of Nations.

After a speech in Pueblo, Colorado, Wilson broke down and returned to Washington, looking like a ghost of the man he had been three weeks prior. Days later, he suffered a stroke, which was kept from the public for the rest of his Presidency.

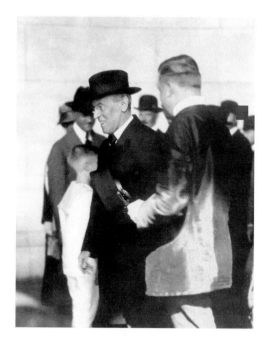

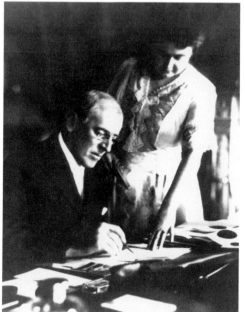

Wilson did not lose his powers to think or speak, but his left side was immobilized. For the next eighteen months, a conspiracy of Edith Wilson, Dr. Grayson, and Tumulty essentially ran the country. Some consider this "woman behind the man" (in a touched-up photograph) America's first female President.

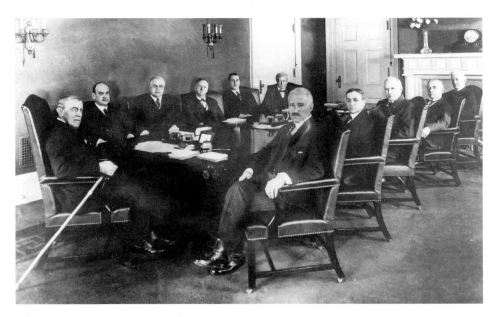

For more than six months, the President held no Cabinet meetings. By the time he was able to conduct minimal government business, he faced several new Secretaries (clockwise, after Wilson on the far left): D. F. Houston; A. Mitchell Palmer (who had authorized notorious raids during the President's illness, in hopes of ridding the country of seditious terrorists); Josephus Daniels, E. T. Meredith; W. B. Wilson; J. W. Alexander; J. B. Payne; A. S. Burleson; N. D. Baker; and Bainbridge Colby, who replaced a disgruntled Robert Lansing as Secretary of State.

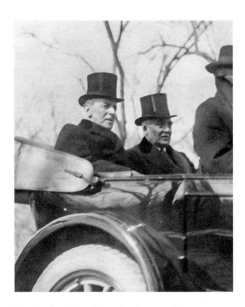

March 4, 1921. After the Senate did not pass the Treaty of Versailles, Wilson faced further humiliation: his successor, Warren G. Harding, reversed as many of Wilson's policies as possible.

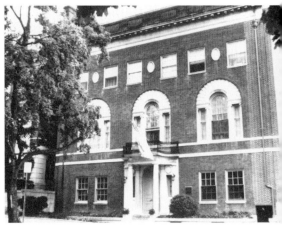

The Wilsons remained in Washington, retiring to an elegant house at 2340 S Street NW.

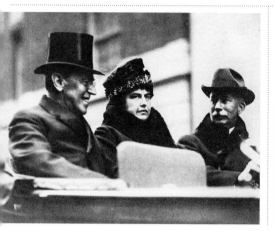
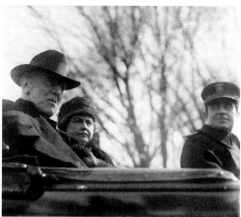

For years, Colonel House had enjoyed the honored position as Wilson's most trusted confidant. But during the Peace Conference in Paris, the President felt his adviser had overstepped. Upon his return to America, Wilson never spoke to him again. Only Dr. Grayson remained in Wilson's good graces to the end.

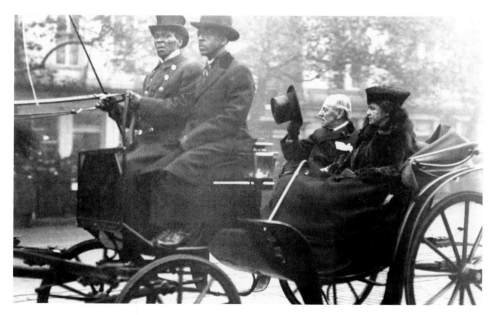

As Wilson's health declined, his post-Presidential popularity rose. Crowds greeted him whenever he appeared in public, as on Armistice Day 1921.

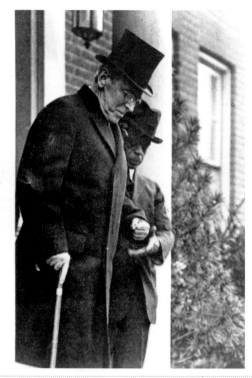

On Wilson's sixty-fifth birthday, servant Isaac Scott helped the hemiplegic ex-President.

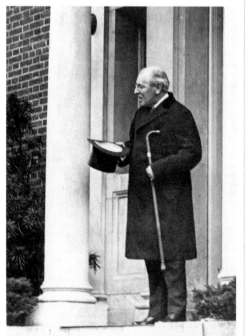

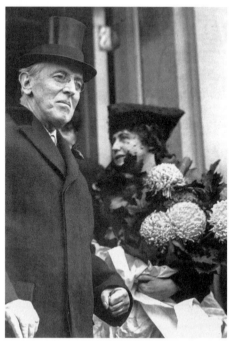

On special occasions, Wilson offered a few words from his doorstep—greeting women from the Pan-American Conference in April 1922; and again (with Edith at his side) on Armistice Day, seven months later.

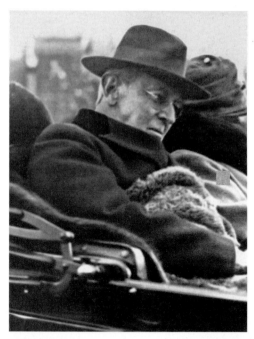

At age sixty-seven, on
December 28, 1923.

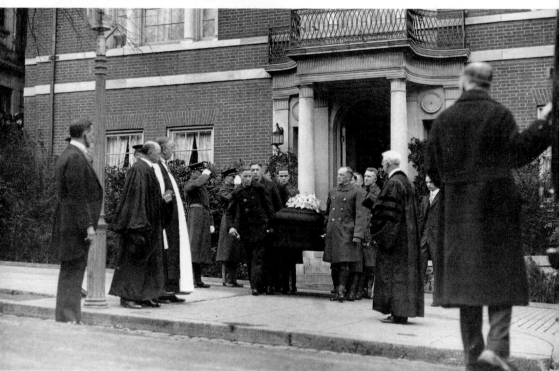

"I am a broken piece of machinery," Wilson uttered shortly before dying on February 3, 1924.
His casket was taken from S Street to the National Cathedral, where he remains buried.

treaty, but a just one." In the meantime, the Scheidemann government in Weimar stood firm, as the peacemaking appeared to be doomed.

While Lloyd George and Clemenceau found enough modifications between them to save face, the Wilsons accepted an invitation from the King and Queen of the Belgians to visit their country. For two days they toured by motorcar and train, sandwiching royal receptions between visits to Belgium's important sites. Beginning in the northwest corner of the country, between Nieuport and Ypres, they sometimes drove as fast as fifty miles per hour over dusty roads through territory where armies had fought and leveled whole towns. Skeletons of dead horses littered the woods, and clusters of graves dotted the landscape. Except for part of a tower, the old cathedral in Ypres was a heap of bricks; the once magnificent Cloth Hall, from the thirteenth century, was in ruins. As he walked the entire length of its seawall, Wilson listened to the wartime history of Zeebrugge, from which Germany had launched the terror of its submarine attacks. In Louvain, the university conferred a degree upon the President in its historic library, which had been reduced to a roofless shell with charred walls. Wilson delivered heartfelt talks throughout his visit and a proper address to the Belgian Parliament, in which he spoke with new understanding of this "valley of suffering." Now, more than any country in the world, it illustrated the need for a League. Minor adjustments were being made to the Treaty, but it still appeared that only divine intervention could impose German approval.

And then, the very day the Wilsons returned to Paris, the Scheidemann government collapsed under the strain of his refusal to ratify the Treaty. With the selection of a new coalition under Chancellor Gustav Bauer came the announcement from Weimar that the government of the German Republic was prepared to sign the Treaty of Versailles. The acceptance included a last-ditch effort to remove the "war-guilt clause," but the victors would yield no more.

The citizens of Paris danced in the streets. In Rome, Premier Orlando finally had something serious to cry about, as his government was overthrown. And before the Allies could appropriate the Kaiser's seventy-five ships that were interned in Scapa Flow, a bay in the Orkney Islands, the German navy ordered their immediate destruction. While burning French flags, the Germans scuttled most of their vessels. The action made Wilson think they were "savage enough to start war again." In Washington,

Republican leaders discussed how best to detach the League component from the Treaty and defeat it. They went so far as to consider a proposal to have Congress unconditionally declare a state of peace between Germany and the United States—for no better reason than to invalidate the last six months of Wilson's work. Official war painter Sir William Orpen put the finishing touches on his portrait of Wilson, showing a world-weary President with the creases and jowls and heavy lids over sunken eyes that the last six months had produced.

After the Council of Three session on Tuesday, June 24, Wilson, Clemenceau, and Balfour adjourned to Versailles to inspect the arrangements for the signing. Their host had selected the centerpiece of the palace—the Galerie des Glaces, the Hall of Mirrors—for the occasion, not only because it was one of the most spectacular rooms ever constructed but also because there the Germans had concluded the last war on a note of humiliation. This *grande galerie* was 240 feet long and 35 feet wide. Opposite its signature feature—a series of seventeen arches, each composed of twenty-one mirrors—matching windows opened onto extensive gardens. Upon seeing the space available to them, Wilson said he would like to include his wife and daughter at the proceedings. Clemenceau agreed that a few ladies should be present. Back at the Paris White House that night, the family circle found champagne glasses on the table. Miss Benham attempted to toast the President's health, but Wilson pre-empted her by raising his glass: "To the Peace, an enduring Peace, a Peace under the League of Nations."

The final settlement was not what Wilson had envisioned upon his arrival in Paris, as his critics never forgot. Maynard Keynes repeatedly called it a "Carthaginian peace," one so brutal that it would pulverize Germany into a wasteland. And Harold Nicolson enumerated his many grievances: the covenants of peace were not openly arrived at, as much of the Conference's work had been conducted in private; the freedom of the seas was not secured; the German colonies were distributed in a manner that was "neither free, nor open-minded, nor impartial"; several frontiers were drawn in contradiction to the nationalities as well as the desires of their populations.

On the other hand, the Treaty embodied the essence of the Fourteen Points and more. Belgium was restored; Alsace-Lorraine was returned; Poland was recognized; and Austria-Hungary was redrawn as a collection of

smaller, more discrete free and independent states. When public forums had proved unworkable for the volume of questions that required negotiation, discussions had gone private; but the final covenants were "open," with no secret treaties. Reductions of armaments and the removal of economic barriers were addressed in a global forum and seriously considered by experts of many countries. Wilson had indubitably tempered the revenge Clemenceau had sought; and he believed the League of Nations could correct what mistakes existed in the Treaty. For the first time, mankind had a blueprint for peace that was practicable, universal, and, theoretically, permanent. President Woodrow Wilson had left his country for more than six months, solely to promote the concepts of global responsibility, self-determination, collective security, and moral imperatives, establishing them as fundamentals of United States foreign policy.

Over the next several months, experts did the basic arithmetic, tallying the final costs of the war and how much Germany should pay. Even without reckoning such future expenditures as pensions and such losses as loans that would never be repaid, Lloyd George told Wilson that the war had cost the United Kingdom £8.5 billion. The sums from all the belligerents totaled $125 billion, a fifth of which the United States had run up. It would be another two years before the final bill for reparations would be sent to the Germans—£6.6 billion ($33 billion). Even at that figure, numerous concessions were made so as not to break the German bank. Over the next decade, the Germans would make good on £1.1 billion. On the eve of the Treaty signing, Lloyd George wrote Wilson that he hoped the United States would consider finding "some way of really assisting the financial needs of the world" by stepping up as its leading creditor.

After an early breakfast on Saturday, June 28, 1919, Wilson crossed the street to Lloyd George's flat, where Clemenceau also awaited. The German delegation had arrived in Paris early that morning, and now the Council of Three examined the credentials of Dr. Hermann Müller, the new Foreign Minister, and Herr Johannes Bell, the Minister of Communications. Finding everything in order, they sent word that the signing would occur at Versailles at three o'clock that afternoon.

At two o'clock the President and Mrs. Wilson and Dr. Grayson drove to the Élysée Palace, where they bade adieu to President and Madame Poincaré and then proceeded under cloudy skies to Versailles, the road to

which was lined with guards. As they approached the palace, the sun broke through.

The Hall of Mirrors shimmered. Again, the placement at the three-sided table approximated that at the Quai d'Orsay, with Clemenceau in the center, Wilson and the American delegation on his right, Lloyd George and his colleagues on his left. The remaining delegates assumed their familiar positions. Distinguished guests—such as Edith and Margaret Wilson—filled one end of the room, while the international press corps filled the other. Because the French had distributed more tickets to the event than there were seats and benches, several minutes of commotion ensued, as people scrambled to find standing room in the hall. It was five years to the day since a teenaged Bosnian Serb had shot Archduke Franz Ferdinand in Sarajevo.

At 3:10, Premier Clemenceau called the session to order. A small table had been set up directly before him on which sat the Treaty and several accompanying documents. To expedite the formalities, each of the signers had pre-impressed his personal seal. Wilson had used his signet wedding ring, which had been fashioned from the chunk of gold the State of California had presented him upon his marriage and which bore his name in stenographic ciphers. Once the Allies and Associated delegates were seated, a marshal ushered the German delegation into the room. Wilson had suggested that they be the first to sign the great document, so as not to give them any time to change their minds. Without flourishes and within three minutes, Ministers Müller and Bell approached the small table and affixed their signatures.

A beaming Wilson was next to sign the Japanese vellum document, rendering an unusually cramped signature. Lansing, White, House, and Bliss followed. Back at their seats, the President whispered to Lansing, "I did not know I was excited until I found my hand trembling when I wrote my name." The rest of the delegations quietly proceeded to the table—including the Italians, without the recently deposed Orlando. By 3:50, Clemenceau closed the proceedings with four words: *"La séance est levée."*

Only two incidents marred the occasion. When its request to sign the Treaty with a reservation regarding the Shantung settlement was denied, the Chinese delegation chose not to appear. And though he signed the Treaty because it meant ending the war, General Smuts filed a document declaring the peace unsatisfactory. For everybody else, it seemed a day of

glory—a historic moment marked, ironically, by a barrage of cannonfire from a battery in the southern part of the majestic gardens.

Afterward, Wilson, Clemenceau, and Lloyd George descended to the terrace at the rear of the palace, where thousands stood and cheered and, ultimately, pushed past the security so that they might get closer to the three leaders. The President's guards closed in to protect him; but as Dr. Grayson observed, "Women cried out that they just wanted to touch him." Planes circled overhead, and guns were fired into the air. After the Big Three and Barons Sonnino and Makino toasted the peace over glasses of wine, the Wilsons returned to Paris. The route was crowded with people waving flags and shouting, *"Vive Wilson."*

While Paris rejoiced, the Wilsons enjoyed a quiet last supper in France. Lloyd George stopped in to say goodbye and to explain that he was simply too fatigued to be part of the impending farewell ceremonies at the train station. Although they had quarreled often during the last six months, Lloyd George said, "You have done more than any one man to bring about further cordial and friendly relations between England and the United States. You have brought the two countries closer together than any other individual in history." The Wilsons left for the Gare des Invalides, where gendarmes held back a massive crowd. Inside, the principals of the Conference stood on the platform, along with practically every member of the French government and the American delegation. Clemenceau said he felt as though he were "saying good-bye to my best friend."

The man who had until recently claimed the distinction of being Wilson's best friend faced a decidedly different parting. After weeks of decreasing contact with the President, Colonel Edward Mandell House was little more than a face in the crowd on the train platform that night. His last conversation with Wilson, in fact, had left House unsettled. The Colonel had urged Wilson to return to the Senate in a conciliatory spirit, one of "consideration" instead of confrontation. "House," the President replied, "I have found one can never get anything in this life that is worthwhile without fighting for it." House disagreed, extolling the virtues of compromise and contending "that a fight was the last thing to be brought about, and then only when it could not be avoided." Those would be the last sentences the two would ever exchange in person, as the President chose never to see him again.

At 9:45 that night, the train left the station for Brest. Woodrow and Edith stood pensively at the window, relieved that they were, at last, on their way home. As the City of Light receded into the darkness, he broke the silence. "Well, little girl, it is finished, and, as no one is satisfied, it makes me hope we have made a just peace," he said, looking into her eyes; "but it is all on the lap of the gods."

15

PASSION

*And they spit vpon him, and tooke the reed, and
smote him on the head.*

*   *And after that they had mocked him, they tooke
the robe off from him, and put his owne raiment on
him, and led him away to crucifie him.*

—MATTHEW, XXVII:30–31

For more than six months, Dr. Grayson had prescribed
as much rest as possible, but not until the *George Washington* transported the President away from the unceasing
pressures did a weary and homesick Woodrow Wilson
comply. With more than a week of fair skies and calm seas,
he slept regularly into the late morning, walked and sun-
bathed on deck in the afternoon, and dined with guests,
watched movies, and joined the sing-alongs at night. He
could not abandon himself completely, however, for he
knew of the turbulence ahead.

Article II, Section 2, of the Constitution defined the
President's predicament: "He shall have Power, by and with
the Advice and Consent of the Senate, to make Treaties, provided two thirds of the Senators present concur." Wilson
spent hours on the Atlantic trying to compose the speech
with which he would present the Treaty of Versailles to
Congress. Anxious to measure the opposition that would
greet him, he asked Tumulty for a list of Senators inclined

to fight the Treaty and of any "particularly virulent" powers in the media. Tumulty named conservative publishing magnates William Randolph Hearst and Colonel Robert McCormick in Chicago, as well as liberals Oswald Villard of *The Nation*, former member of the Inquiry and Wilson supporter Walter Lippmann of *The New Republic*, and Wilson's earliest patron, George Harvey. Sailing into such formidable resistance from the press— and apparently two votes short of the sixty-four he would need in the Senate—Wilson had difficulty finding the right words.

For the first time since Grayson had met him, the President expressed complete dissatisfaction with his work on a speech. He blamed the "false start" on his disdain for his awaiting audience, insisting that if he had greater respect for Congress and its ability to reason, he could do a better job. Grayson wondered if that was all that ailed him. Wilson could collect his thoughts but had trouble organizing them; and his right hand was cramping so badly again that he had to write with his left.

On Tuesday, July 8, 1919, the ship docked in New Jersey. The Presidential party crossed the river to Manhattan. The largest crowd that had ever greeted Wilson in the city filled the sidewalks from the Twenty-third Street ferry to Carnegie Hall. There he delivered a brief address to an enthusiastic crowd—"a few words from the heart."

"Why, Jerseyman though I am," he said, "this is the first time I ever thought that Hoboken was beautiful." Speaking of America's new stature, Wilson said, "It is a wonderful thing for this nation, hitherto isolated from the large affairs of the world, to win not only the universal confidence of the people of the world, but their universal affection." He referred to the fight ahead only obliquely, talking about America's having done "the large thing and the right thing" in spreading freedom around the world. "I am afraid some people," he added, ". . . do not understand that vision. They do not see it. . . . [But] I have never had a moment's doubt as to where the heart and purpose of this people lay."

The Wilsons boarded their train at Pennsylvania Station. Although he had anticipated his return for months, he knew that Washington was about to engage in its most bitter debate since the Civil War. When his train pulled in at midnight, he was happily surprised to discover more than ten thousand people had gathered at Union Station to welcome him home. "It is very touching," he told Edith and Dr. Grayson. Thousands more waited for him outside the Executive Mansion, including one former

resident and ill-wisher—Alice Roosevelt Longworth, who stood in the crowd, crossing her fingers in the sign of the "evil eye" and crying, "A murrain on him!" Even though Wilson had come to regard his current home more as a prison than a palace, he heard only cheers that night. "This house," he said, "never looked so beautiful."

By morning, Wilson had made plain his desire to put the Treaty on a fast legislative track. He wanted to keep it as simple as possible—an up or down vote on the Treaty itself, without any Senate tinkering. He intended to make himself immediately available to the Foreign Relations Committee and to postpone presenting the side agreement to defend France. He held in reserve a plan to campaign for the League across the country should the Treaty's passage ever appear to be in jeopardy. At a press conference that morning, he insisted that Article X of the League Covenant—about collective security—was its very spine; if deleted, the League was "only a debating society."

The Republicans were in no rush. They believed every delay would contribute to the Treaty's derailment, which would allow them to fix the peace. They intended to deconstruct every clause of the President's handiwork, dissecting each word. While the Foreign Relations Committee indicated that it would honor a Presidential request to appear before it, the Republicans chose to postpone his testimony until a time that would serve them better. They suggested that the President had completed his duties in regard to the Treaty in Paris. One Kansas Congressman introduced a bill that day that would make it unlawful for a President to absent himself from the territorial jurisdiction of the United States during his term of office or to perform his duties beyond the District of Columbia. Tumulty's intelligence notwithstanding, anti-League forces were claiming forty-nine votes in the Senate, which included a few Democrats.

Although Woodrow Wilson's trips down Pennsylvania Avenue had become routine during the last six and a half years, his visits to the Capitol continued to make history. Not even torrential rains could keep crowds away that Thursday, July 10, 1919. The Senate chamber began filling two hours before he was expected. The President arrived minutes before noon and walked the familiar path to the President's Room on the second floor. A welcoming committee—which included Vice President Marshall and Henry Cabot Lodge, then the nation's most senior Senator—escorted him to the chamber. "Mr. President," Lodge asked, seeing the

twenty-by-fourteen-by-six-inch package under Wilson's arm, "can I carry the Treaty for you?" Wilson smiled and replied, "Not on your life." Democratic Senator John Sharp Williams from Mississippi said, "Don't trust him with it, Mr. President." And everybody laughed about the document . . . for the very last time.

The first President of the United States ever to enter the Senate and physically deliver a treaty, Wilson received a standing ovation, and even a few Rebel yells. But the Republicans withheld their applause. When the room had quieted, the President proceeded to discuss the Treaty, which he said constituted "nothing less than a world settlement." Reading from typewritten cards, he delivered an unexpectedly lackluster speech, largely an insipid lesson in history and politics, occasionally enlivened by rhetorical flourishes. Wilson explained that it was impossible to accommodate the varied interests of so many nations without what he called "many minor compromises." As such, he said, the Treaty "is not exactly what we would have written. It is probably not what any one of the national delegations would have written. But results were worked out which on the whole bear test." He refrained from detailing the compromises, letting the final document speak for itself.

Wilson had never liked reading from prepared texts and did so only when the solemnity of the occasion demanded. In the course of his nearly forty minutes that afternoon, he stumbled several times, going back to reread the sentences he had misread. Steadily he improved, especially as he approached the apex of his speech: "That there should be a league of nations to steady the counsels and maintain the peaceful understanding of the world," he explained, ". . . had been one of the agreements accepted from the first as the basis of peace with the central powers." It had "become the first substantive part of the treaty to be worked out and agreed upon." Now, twenty-one years after the Spanish-American War had thrust the United States into the world arena, the nation had "reached her majority as a world power." As such, he said, "a new role and a new responsibility have come to this great nation that we honour and which we would all wish to lift to yet higher levels of service and achievement." Wilson gathered his strength as he spoke of the "united power of free nations" that "must put a stop to aggression." The only hope for such peace, he insisted, was the League. "Shall we or any other free people hesitate to accept this

great duty?" he asked the Senate in Wilsonian fashion. "Dare we reject it and break the heart of the world?"

Only in these final seconds did the speech take flight. At last, the President looked up from his manuscript and faced the unresponsive bloc of Republicans and spoke from the heart:

> The stage is set, the destiny disclosed. It has come about by no plan of our conceiving, but by the hand of God, who led us into this way. We cannot turn back. We can only go forward, with lifted eyes and freshened spirit, to follow the vision. It was of this that we dreamed at our birth. America shall in truth show the way. The light streams upon the path ahead, and nowhere else.

Arizona Democrat Henry Ashurst wrote in his diary that day, "I was petrified with surprise."

Everybody on either side of the aisle had expected a masterpiece, an "accounting of the most momentous cause ever entrusted to an individual." If nothing else, the Senate would have liked to have been part of the treaty-making, if not as it was happening then at least in hearing about it now. But, the gentleman from Arizona noted, "his audience wanted raw meat, he fed them cold turnips." Republicans winked at one another. With that, Wilson set the bulky Treaty upon the Vice President's rostrum and left the chamber, unaware of his failure to deliver.

Ashurst, on the other hand, proved to be unusually observant that day. He seemed to be the only one to have noticed a pronounced "contraction" of the back of the President's neck during the speech. And—as if prompted by Wilson's speaking of a war in which masses had been "bled white"—he also detected a strange blanching of his ears. Ashurst lamented that his findings suggested "a man whose vitality is gone." But in fact, something more serious had apparently transpired, as the tightening in Wilson's neck surely suggested pain and the pallor an insufficiency of blood flowing to the head. Both, indeed, may very well have been harbingers of a cerebral episode, if not a minor incident itself.

In the President's Room, Wilson received thirty visitors, all Democrats but one. He issued talking points to get them over the Treaty's imperfections. He opposed reservations to the Treaty because they would only

delay if not destroy the fragile peace. The Monroe Doctrine, which was nothing more than a declaration of a nineteenth-century President, never had any legal standing, but the peacemakers in Paris had agreed to protect its position. Wilson had felt that the Treaty could take no action in the matter of Irish independence because the document disposed of territory taken from the enemy, not possessed by the Allies.

Republicans dismissed the speech as a string of glittering generalities. "Soap bubbles of oratory and souffle of praises," mocked Brandegee of Connecticut. Senator Borah of Idaho observed that the President had returned from six months in search of peace with little of substance beyond a sidecar arrangement with France that defined a new alliance for war. At a Sinn Féin rally of seventeen thousand Irish Americans at Madison Square Garden that night, the mention of Wilson's name prompted three minutes of booing.

Wilson continued to believe that popular sentiment supported the League; but he failed to realize that for six months, the most dynamic force within the Democratic Party had been an ocean away, allowing public opinion to drift. Secretary of Agriculture Houston, who was traveling in the West when the President returned, had grown increasingly aware of opposition efforts to denigrate the Treaty, especially the League Covenant. "I had the impression," he wrote, "that certain Republican leaders were determined, not so much to bring about the rejection of the Treaty, as to destroy the President's prestige, to pull him down, and to make such modifications of the Treaty, whether necessary or not, as would enable them to say that the final outcome was their accomplishment, and that they had saved the nation from the ills which the Treaty would have brought upon it." Houston urged Wilson to simplify his rhetoric. But Wilson did not see fit to listen, and in that moment, he began to lose his grip on the national argument.

Houston ascribed Wilson's hesitancy to overconfidence—less in himself than in his constituents. Wilson, he said, "is a firm believer in the doctrine that truth is mighty and will prevail. Seeing an issue very clearly himself, he trusts the masses of the people too implicitly also to see it clearly and to see it as he does, in the short run as well as in the long run." But Wilson did not realize that along with isolationist reactionaries, he lacked the support of many disenchanted liberals, several of whom had been with him in Paris. John Maynard Keynes was completing *The Economic Consequences of the Peace*, a devastating book that upbraided each of the Big Four, not least of all Wilson. Its three-part serialization in

The New Republic that year—at the urging of its New York editor, Walter Lippmann—would make an international name for the young economist as well as big problems for Wilson.

But neither Houston nor almost anybody else in Washington knew the full extent of the opposition Wilson was up against. The President himself did not know that the Republicans had been plotting the demise of his treaty for months before it even existed. Only years later did Franklin D. Roosevelt divulge a secret he had kept to himself about Henry Cabot Lodge and a small coven of Republicans, which included party chairman Will Hays. In late January 1919, as the Peace Conference was opening, this handful of Republicans held a clandestine meeting in Washington to discuss means of dismantling whatever accord Wilson brought home. As Roosevelt later imparted only as an unnamed source, "Hays, Lodge and others made up their mind before they knew anything about the Treaty or the League of Nations that they were going to wreck it whether their consciences demanded it or not."

Having been gone from home for so long, Wilson could not appreciate the tectonic shifts across the national landscape. Just as ramping up for war had rocked the nation, so too did demobilization. While Germany was the epicenter of massive economic inflation, prices in America had practically doubled between 1913 and 1919; in July 1919 alone, they spiked by 4 percent. The press referred so often to this inflation as the "high cost of living," it earned its own acronym. By the end of the month, the railroad brotherhood unions advised the President that unless they saw some severe action toward reducing the HCL, two million railroad workers would demand wage increases, which would amount to close to a billion dollars. Management, of course, attributed the inflation to such increases and linked these demands to the unions, many of which had foreign-born leaders, some of whom chanted the same slogans that were shouted in Bolshevik Russia.

James Weldon Johnson, field secretary for the NAACP, dubbed those hot months of 1919 the "Red Summer"—though for a different reason that had even graver consequences. Three dozen race riots erupted in America that season, half of them in July, producing the bloodiest rash of interracial violence in American history. Hundreds were killed, and tens of thousands were left homeless. At least five dozen black men died at the end of a rope. Many Negroes—especially those who had fought in the war—had viewed 1919 as the year in which they might advance in the mainstream

of American society. The very thought of such gains only threatened whites who wished to restrain them, and not just in the South. No less an authority than Mississippi's Governor Theodore Bilbo asserted that very month, "This is a white man's country, with a white man's civilization, and any dream on the part of the Negro race to share social and political equality will be shattered in the end."

Between Bisbee, Arizona, on July 3 and Syracuse, New York, on the thirty-first, whites ignited racial tensions in black communities, which spontaneously combusted into arson, looting, and gunfire in several Northern cities, including Philadelphia and Baltimore. The mayhem in Chicago lasted a week. After several days in which the local police could not quell the murderous riots in Washington, D.C., Secretary of War Baker called in two thousand federal troops, including three hundred Marines. But the fighting force that distinguished the bloodbath in the national capital was the Negro community itself, choosing, as Johnson wrote, "not to run, but to fight—fight in defense of their lives and their homes." Lamentable though these riots were, Johnson believed the Red Summer, especially those pogroms in Washington and Chicago, marked "the turning point in the psychology of the whole nation regarding the Negro problem," informing the white population as it empowered the black. The President expressed concern over the conflagrations, but considered them local problems at a time when he was concentrating almost exclusively on global issues.

Nationally, the most pressing domestic problem lay in the readjustment of the labor force, as American doughboys flooded the job market. Unemployment at the end of the war was less than 2 percent; two years later, it would be greater than 5 percent; a year after that, it would reach 12 percent. Not all the changes were as easily measured. Millions of Americans yearned for the peaceful normality of old, when the United States had flourished in wholesome isolation; millions more presumed the psyches of America's returning soldiers must have altered. The catchiest song of the day asked, "How ya gonna keep 'em down on the farm, after they've seen Paree?" The steady migration from rural communities to urban centers increased, marking the first moment that a majority of Americans lived in cities. The war had ended just before Second Lieutenant F. Scott Fitzgerald was supposed to ship overseas. In July 1919, he went home to Minnesota to rewrite his first novel, in which he proclaimed, "Here was a new generation . . . dedicated more than the last to the fear of poverty

and the worship of success; grown up to find all Gods dead, all wars fought, all faiths in man shaken."

A postwar recession accompanied the postwar disillusionment, and the Dow Jones industrial average instilled fears of continued stagnation at best—closing at the end of the year a little over 100, barely five points higher than when the decade began. But through the third and fourth quarters of 1919, the economy remained healthy enough for Wilson to focus almost exclusively on what he considered his legacy—the passage of the Treaty, complete with its Covenant. Unfortunately, that meant his having to face his most formidable enemy, an "HCL" of another sort.

Henry Cabot Lodge was the only son of a Bostonian widow whose ancestors had arrived in Massachusetts in 1700. Subsequent generations of Cabots amassed a fortune, mostly in shipping. "Boston incarnate," wrote Henry Adams, referring not only to Lodge's pedigree but also to his education, which revolved completely around Harvard College. He earned a bachelor's degree, a law degree, and the school's first doctorate in political science before teaching there for several years. As patronizing as he was patrician, Lodge suffered from what Adams called "Bostonitis," symptoms of which included "chronic irritability" and the quality of "thinking too much of himself." At the same time, Adams described his Harvard protégé as an "excellent talker, a voracious reader, a ready wit, an accomplished orator, with a clear mind and a powerful memory." About to launch his political career in the state legislature in 1879, Lodge also served as a junior editor of a New England journal called the *International Review*. In that capacity, he had accepted and published that first major literary effort of Princeton senior Thomas W. Wilson, six years his junior.

Barely in his twenties, Wilson had been strangely prescient. His treatise had challenged the very structure of American government, questioning a President's ability to lead in a system in which the legislature outweighed the executive branch and conducted most of its business in closed-door committee rooms. While young Wilson had not recommended demolishing the Congress in favor of a Parliament, in which its leader spoke for the majority; he had boldly recommended a cabinet that could sit among the representatives as a link between the two branches. Over the years, especially during TR's administration, Wilson saw how a vibrant personality could galvanize a Presidency. But the basic system still troubled him, as it fostered antagonism between the branches, especially

if different parties controlled them. Strong personalities on either side all but guaranteed hostile stalemates.

Lodge, the Republican leader in the Congress, considered Woodrow Wilson able, ambitious, and "by no means a commonplace man." He went so far as to praise him as a "master of the rhetorical use of idealism." In his posthumously published account of the League, he went to great lengths to insist that he never harbored any "personal hostility to Mr. Wilson"—a point he made five times on page 23 alone. But after six years of disagreeing with the President on practically every major position—and perhaps because Wilson had dethroned him as the nation's "scholar in politics"—Lodge's enmity toward Wilson had steadily escalated.

This petty academic rivalry in Lodge's mind should not be underestimated. His account of the League fight reminded his readers that, despite what newspapers said about Woodrow Wilson, "he was not a scholar in the true sense at all." Even his vaunted speeches, Lodge added, were practically devoid of classical allusion or literary quotation; and for all his education, Lodge said, he was "not a widely-read man." One Senator commented, "If only President Wilson had not been a college prof and didn't know how to write so well this issue would come out all right." Wilson tacitly bore his own grudge, one reminiscent of the fight over the graduate school at Princeton, when he battled the privileged, who had been handed everything for which he had to work. Before the end of the President's first term, Lodge had imparted to his dearest friend, TR, "I never expected to hate anyone in politics with the hatred I feel toward Wilson."

Seldom has the American body politic been so fractious as it was in 1919. Despite two victories at the polls, the President had not won either of his elections with a majority; and his strong, unyielding views further polarized his constituents. The Republicans held a majority in both houses, though only narrowly in the Senate. Each of the parties was further fractured by strong opposing factions within, especially when it came to the Treaty. Wilson was counting on all forty-six Democratic Senators, though two had already expressed their disapproval of the Treaty.

The Republicans were more divided. Lodge counted fifteen Republican Senators completely unwilling to vote for the Treaty under any circumstances. They became known as the "Irreconcilables." Thirty-four of his party members were "Reservationists," torn between insisting upon major revisions or "mild" ones. The latter group could be swayed to the

Wilson camp should he offer some concessions. Lodge had also identified three Democratic Irreconcilables, whose votes meant the most to him, for their small margin could allow him to maintain that Wilson's own party defeated the Treaty. In seeking the necessary two-thirds majority, the President and Lodge would vie for the independent thinkers within the Senate: Wilson hoped to build momentum through the weight of his office and the force of his oratory; Lodge intended to throw into his path every legislative obstacle at his disposal, if not defeating the Treaty altogether then at least transforming it into something Republican. A painstaking probe of the Treaty, he figured, would only expose its flaws.

At the start of this contest, momentum seemed to be in the President's favor. "I don't see how we are ever going to defeat this proposition," said freshman Republican Senator James Watson of Indiana to Lodge. The Senate elder sighed. "Ah, my dear James," he said placatingly, "I do not propose to try to beat it by direct frontal attack, but by the indirect method of reservations." Watson would accept the strategy for a while, but in a later encounter he said, "Suppose the President accepts the treaty with your reservations. Then we are in the League." Lodge offered a paternal grin and a personal insight, explaining how much Wilson hated him. "Never under any set of circumstances in this world," he said calmly, "could he be induced to accept a treaty with Lodge reservations appended to it." Unconvinced, Watson said that was a "slender thread on which to hang so great a cause."

"A slender thread!" Lodge scoffed. "Why, it is as strong as any cable with its strands wired and twisted together."

No sooner had President Wilson delivered the Treaty than was Senator Lodge on his feet moving that it be sent to the Foreign Relations Committee, which he chaired and had packed with Irreconcilables. Thus, the document was now under his jurisdiction, and on his schedule. Within minutes it was dispatched to the Public Printer; and five hours later, *The New York Times* reported, it had been set in type, ready for distribution. But strangely, as Lodge himself noted in his memoirs, three days passed before his committee members received the text. And then, Lodge announced that he would conduct extensive public hearings—for at least a month, if not longer.

Not home even a week, Wilson already looked weary and his writing hand had stiffened yet again. He still considered touring the country to

explain the Treaty to the people. More immediately, he announced visiting hours, during which Senators might appear at the White House unannounced. When his own party leaders informed him that it would be impossible to pass the Treaty without some reservations, Wilson realized the need to develop a more aggressive strategy. In the sudden absence of Democratic leader Thomas S. Martin of Virginia, who had become terminally ill, Wilson turned to Gilbert Hitchcock of Nebraska. Although the Senator had quarreled with the President over the Federal Reserve Board, Hitchcock had become a trusty proponent of the League. He was Wilson's strongest advocate in the Senate and a worthy Minority Leader, though a somewhat dubious challenger to his Republican counterpart.

Henry Cabot Lodge closely monitored each of his committee's members as the President reminded them that this was not a partisan issue—that it was "their duty to vote for the treaty just as he had presented it to the Senate." With each step forward, Lodge introduced a new set of stalling tactics. He issued one request after another for information and documentation. And then he decided that he owed it to the country to read the entire Treaty aloud, all 264 pages, word by word, in a committee room—insisting a charter of such importance demanded as much. Committee members sometimes wandered in and out for the recitation; more often, Lodge found himself speaking to four marble walls and a scribe. His performance would kill two weeks.

At first, Wilson's private sessions proved effective—as he advanced a positive message while providing explanations for each of the Treaty's stipulations. On Friday, July 18, British liaison Sir William Wiseman found the President confident that he was winning over his opposition—including a number of those Senators who had pledged themselves to defeat the League even before they had read the Covenant. Wilson regretted that Taft was knuckling under party pressure and now leaned toward reservations. Confiding to Wiseman that he was considering some cosmetic concessions in the Treaty's language, he said yet again that he would embark on a nationwide tour only upon finding insufficient Republican support. That pleased Edith, who worried that her husband could not withstand such an ordeal, especially during the torrid summer.

Dr. Grayson shared Edith's concerns. He took to encouraging any recreation for the President whenever possible. Despite storm warnings and Wilson's experiencing an apparent case of indigestion, Grayson even

endorsed a weekend cruise to Chesapeake Bay on the *Mayflower*, just to keep him from working. Unfortunately, electrical storms struck, and so too did Wilson's gastric disorder, turning into what Grayson diagnosed as acute dysentery. At least that was what he told the press. The intense heat and strain since his return from Europe logically explained his condition; but subsequent reconsideration of the prior days' symptoms—the headaches, pallor, cramped hand, and difficulty reading and speaking—suggest a minor stroke. Whatever the case, this "transient incapacity" was likely related to some progressive cerebrovascular condition.

Back in the White House, Wilson took to his bed and canceled the next day's schedule. That did not stop Senator Lodge, who tightened the reins on his team and encouraged any disruptions to Wilson's plans. Opposition leaders leaked to the press that they were prepared to provide the President with a list of the thirty-five Senators pledged to reject the Treaty in its present form—two more than were required. Their reasons ranged from the general burdens of collective security to a specific distrust of the Japanese ever to make good on their promise to yield Shantung. Some radical Republicans simply avowed to kill the entire Treaty if their demands were not met. By Tuesday the twenty-second, the President had resumed meeting with Senators, while Lodge compiled a list of witnesses for his hearings, encouraged discussion of every sort of amendment to the Treaty, and maintained his steady demand for more documents.

Edith Wilson watched her husband achieve diminishing returns as he lobbied Senators—arguing that neither he nor they had "the moral right further to modify any Article unless every other country should be granted the same privilege." To do so would negate a half year of work and emasculate the pact. On July 28, Lodge completed his word-by-word reading of the Treaty.

After letting another three days pass, he called the first of sixty witnesses. Lodge's account of the diligence with which he and his committee had studied the Treaty masked the fact that their primary task was less to understand it than to undermine it. His goal was to ensure the Senate's dissent. The early witnesses included members of the Administration, such as Secretary of Labor William B. Wilson, who were friendly to the President but had little to offer by way of enlightenment. In thirteen days of actual testimony—stretched across the next six weeks—many of the witnesses who paraded before the panel in Room 310 of the Senate Office

Building shared one common trait—an ability to embarrass the President. The committee properly called Secretary of State Lansing to testify, and the questions targeted his dissatisfaction with the Treaty and his descriptions of having been marginalized during the Peace Conference. His circumspect hesitations spoke louder than any criticisms he could have directed toward his boss. Irish American witnesses bemoaned their cause being ignored in the Treaty. And then, allowing a plea for racial equality, the committee invited a Negro delegation, its spokesman none other than William Monroe Trotter, the only man Wilson had ever banished from the White House. Halfway through the hearings, Lodge decided his committee could make its best case by cross-examining the defendant himself. The President welcomed the opportunity, though he should have been more careful what he wished for.

Wilson was, in fact, experiencing a mental decline, which was discernible to others. On several occasions in late July and early August, he responded to queries about the Treaty with incorrect information—instances of recent actions and events that he could not recall. His once photographic memory began to blur. On August 8, 1919, he delivered to a joint session of Congress a dull address full of run-on sentences about the high cost of living.

The rest of his activities that month further reflected scattered thought and divided attention. The issues of race riots, soaring food prices, and impending railroad strikes would have challenged any President in the best of health. In his current condition, the sixty-two-year-old Wilson could only offer short shrift to every situation but the Treaty, thus salving problems without solving them. Recognizing its historical significance, Wilson performed one incidental duty to notable effect, when Secretary Newton Baker informed him that any number of official documents and communications required a name for the war they had just won. The Navy had informally adopted "the War Against Teutonic Aggression," while the commanders of the Allied armies called it "the Great War for Civilization." Great Britain chose "the War of 1914–1918." From a sampler Baker sent, Wilson selected "the World War."

As it joined the ranks of the American Revolution, the Mexican War, the Civil War, and the Spanish-American War, Upton Sinclair and Clarence Darrow urged Woodrow Wilson to consider that the World War was over and that he ought to reconsider the motives of men—most particu-

larly Eugene Debs—who had spoken their consciences and whose imprisonment for disagreeing was no longer "self-defense but a punishment undeserved." Wilson took the case to heart and wrote Socialist John Spargo that he would "deal with the matter as early and in as liberal a spirit as possible." But matters of the peace process kept intervening amid bouts of forgetfulness and fits of temper.

Senators argued the Treaty all summer—mostly Republicans expressing their distaste while Democrats proposed the least amount of compromise to make it palatable. The only fresh thought that season came from Henry Cabot Lodge himself, who reminded people that the Treaty's adherents did not have a monopoly on idealism. He tried to rival Wilson in eloquence, but he could make his case with little more than platitudes and a negation of Wilson's plan. So tired had the Treaty "debate" become, the press curtailed its coverage.

That was not the case, however, on Tuesday, August 19, 1919, when the Administration set another precedent by inviting the Foreign Relations Committee to 1600 Pennsylvania Avenue. Although the separation of powers kept the legislative branch from requiring a Chief Executive to appear before it, Woodrow Wilson embraced this opportunity. At ten o'clock, all but one of the seventeen Senators arrived and found a ring of chairs in the East Room. Wilson sat in the farthest corner, with Senator Lodge on his right and Virginia's Senator Claude A. Swanson on his left. The rest of the Senators completed the circle, which was broken by a few tables for stenographers Charles Swem from the White House pool and five others from the Senate. Neither photographers nor journalists were admitted, though much of the basement floor of the White House had been converted into a makeshift pressroom. Reporters and typists filled its main corridor and oval room, which had been rigged with tables and typewriters so the stenographers could run with the news as it broke.

After the President read a long statement expressing the need to expedite consideration of the Treaty, the Senators grilled him for the next three hours. Although not always accurate, Wilson parried any opposition, even the incisive questions from Irreconcilables Hiram Johnson and William Borah, whom Walter Lippmann had prepared with insider information. Only once did Wilson seem agitated—when first-term Ohio Senator Warren G. Harding raised a series of questions about America's moral obligations as opposed to the legal, which suggested he had not

listened to the answer Wilson had just provided. He struck the President as having "a disturbingly dull mind, and . . . it seemed impossible to get any explanation to lodge in it." Close to 1:30, Senator Lodge—who had let others speak for him—brought the proceedings to a close. The President asked his guests to remain for luncheon—a spread of melon, spring lamb, cold Virginia ham, salad, vegetables, and ices that awaited in the State Dining Room. "It will be very delightful," the courtly Wilson told his adversaries. And for the next hour, everybody tucked into what one Senator told the press was surely a five-dollar-a-plate meal. The conversation was apolitical and pleasant.

"He was nervous, but he certainly handled himself magnificently," Dr. Grayson said, calling the day "a triumph" for the President. Given that Wilson had recently suffered a cerebral incident, that was true. But objective observers judged the day a failure. The semipublic display had been more about presentation than information, and it changed nobody's heart or mind. "To those of us who just looked on and listened," noted Ike Hoover, "the President was not at his best. . . . In fact, all through this period he manifested an over-anxiety toward his guests." The transcript of the proceedings revealed as much. Talk of "national good conscience" and moral responsibilities overshadowed the specifics of the Treaty. Worst of all, perusal of the record exposed more than a dozen errors in the President's testimony—incorrect dates, erroneous assertions regarding the uncertainty of the Treaty's fate, and forgotten elements of the pact and its evolution, especially when it came to the secret treaties. As they were all apparent mental lapses, the President emerged that day as a man as compromised—physically and mentally—as his treaty.

Bernard Baruch, who saw the President regularly, knew he was not opposed to making concessions so long as the Covenant remained intact. Believing he would accept any number of Senate corollary resolutions interpreting the Treaty, Baruch discussed the matter with him, Attorney General Palmer, and War Secretary Baker. Two days after the Foreign Relations Committee met at the White House, one of Wilson's key allies, Senator Key Pittman of Nevada, introduced several "interpretative" reservations in language that suggested not only the President's blessing but even his dictation. Earlier in the week, Wilson had stood behind the clarity of the Treaty's points, but now he was granting the need for further

elucidation. To some, he was sounding more like a seasoned politico than a principled statesman.

By the end of August, Wilson realized that he was winning no converts in Washington. As opposition intensified, several Democrats urged him to play his trump card and take his case directly to the people. Wilson knew where to find the nation's most independent thinkers. Reigniting the same voters who had delivered his reelection meant going west—where greater acceptance of new ideas came with the territory. The White House's chief telegrapher, Edward Smithers, charted a four-week itinerary, which covered ten thousand miles with stops in twenty-nine cities. The President would speak in all but four of the states west of the Mississippi, half of which were represented by Irreconcilables. It would be Wilson's last opportunity to rally public opinion. Failure to wrest control of the argument would mean he had returned from Europe with nothing more than victory without peace.

While Tumulty generally considered Wilson's political fortunes paramount, in this instance, he made an exception. In a quiet moment alone with the President, he raised the subject of his health. "I know that I am at the end of my tether," Wilson said, "but my friends on the Hill say that the trip is necessary to save the Treaty, and I am willing to make whatever personal sacrifice is required, for if the Treaty should be defeated, God only knows what would happen to the world as a result of it." He acknowledged that such a trip might mean "the giving up of my life." But, he said, "I will gladly make the sacrifice to save the Treaty." Tumulty looked at the "old man" before him—grim in his determination to fight to the end, like some "old warrior." In fact, it was the young soldiers who impelled Wilson to make the trip. "If the Treaty is not ratified by the Senate," he told Edith, "the War will have been fought in vain, and the world will be thrown into chaos. I promised our soldiers, when I asked them to take up arms, that it was a war to end wars; and if I do not do all in my power to put the Treaty in effect, I will be a slacker and never able to look those boys in the eye. I must go."

A few days before his scheduled departure, Bernard Baruch called on a gaunt and pale Wilson to cancel his trip. Short of that, he asked the President to consider a brief respite during which he could compose his speeches. The President insisted he lacked the time. "Mr. President,"

Baruch asked, making his best argument, "if anything happens to you, what will we do?" Wilson replied with an unanswerable question: "What is one life in a great cause?" He had determined this was his cross to bear.

Dr. Grayson made the final appeal. Having already argued that the rigorous schedule, the inability to exercise, the constant strain of speech-making and handshaking, the discomfort of living on a train for a month—especially in the summer, when the steel cars would become ovens—could all be lethal, he visited the President in his study. Before Grayson could speak, Wilson looked up from his writing and said, "I know what you have come for. I do not want to do anything foolhardy but the League of Nations is now in its crisis, and if it fails, I hate to think what will happen to the world. You must remember that I, as Commander in Chief, was responsible for sending our soldiers to Europe. In the crucial test in the trenches they did not turn back—and I cannot turn back now. I cannot put my personal safety, my health, in the balance against my duty—I must go." Still holding his pen, Wilson rose from his desk and walked to the window, silently gazing upon the Washington Monument. Looking as though he had just signed a death warrant, he turned to his physician, who saw tears in his eyes. Grayson realized there was nothing for him to do except pack his own bags and provide the best medical attention that he could.

An unexpectedly jaunty Woodrow Wilson—in his straw boater, blue blazer, white trousers, and white shoes—strode through Washington's Union Station that Wednesday evening, September 3, 1919. The Presidential car—like the yacht, called the *Mayflower*—was attached to the rear of a Pennsylvania Railroad train and came configured with a sitting room, which doubled as a dining area, and then a bedroom for the First Lady, which connected to that of her husband; each had a single bed and a dressing table. Beyond that was an "office," with a table on which the President's typewriter sat. Finally, there was a compartment for Edith's maid and another for Dr. Grayson. Brooks, the valet, would sleep on the leather couch in the sitting room. Ahead of the *Mayflower* was a string of baggage cars, a diner, and Pullman cars to accommodate Wilson's four stenographers, seven Secret Service agents, and the largest press corps ever to make a Presidential tour. Because radio was still in its infancy, Wilson would rely upon those two dozen representatives of the media—journalists, still photographers,

newsreel photographers, and an official from the Western Union Telegraph Company—to capture him as he attempted to regain the support of the people. The train pulled away from the station a little after seven.

No President had ever gone to such lengths for a cause. Candidates in the past had campaigned for their own political fortunes; sixty-two-year-old Wilson was sallying forth across America purely for an ideal. He came prepared, having filled eight pages with thoughts and themes he intended to draw upon. The next twenty-seven days would showcase the quintessential Woodrow Wilson, who believed oratory suffused with reason, emotion, and depth of character could convert a nation.

The quest began inauspiciously the next morning at eleven, when the *Mayflower* arrived under gray skies in Columbus, Ohio. A local streetcar strike kept many away, and the morning rain doused the spirits of some who ventured downtown, but Wilson found a capacity crowd of more than four thousand waiting for him at Memorial Hall, where close to two thousand people had been turned away. Despite a headache, he touched upon most of the salient aspects of the Treaty and reminded his audience of the reason they had gone to war. This treaty, he said, sought "to punish one of the greatest wrongs ever done in history." He called the terms "severe" but "not unjust." By one o'clock the *Mayflower* was heading west.

Big crowds gathered at the small stations along the way, and Wilson stood on the rear platform to shake hands. In Richmond, Indiana, he delivered a short speech about the Treaty:

> The chief thing to notice about it . . . is that it is the first treaty ever made by great powers that was not made in their own favor. It is made for the protection of the weak peoples of the world and not for the aggrandizement of the strong. . . . The extraordinary achievement of this treaty is that it gives a free choice to people who never could have won it for themselves. It is for the first time in the history of international transactions an act of systematic justice and not an act of grabbing and seizing.

He asked his fellow citizens what difference a political party label made "when mankind is involved."

The train arrived in Indianapolis at six, and after a quick dinner, the Wilsons greeted a nonpartisan reception committee, which included the

Republican Governor, James Putnam Goodrich. An automobile parade, complete with a band, led the President to the Fair Grounds, where an audience of close to twenty thousand awaited in the Coliseum. In a slightly husky voice, Wilson attempted to reach everybody in the hall, but a few hundred people at the perimeter left in frustration. Within five minutes, Wilson had captivated those who had remained.

Nobody seemed to care that he mistakenly spoke at the outset of the assassination of the Archduke Franz Ferdinand in Sarajevo, Serbia, when he meant Bosnia. This crowd, like the others that would follow, seemed less interested in small details of the past than in Wilson's larger vision for the future. He stuck to the manner that had served him for the last decade, that of never speaking down to his audience. In so doing, he lifted their spirits and raised their aspirations. He called upon the commonsense Hoosiers to ignore the misinformation his opponents were spreading about Article X of the League Covenant and consider for themselves that "there is no compulsion upon us to take [the advice of the Council of the League] except the compulsion of our good consciences and judgment. . . . There is in that Covenant not one note of surrender of the independent judgment of the government of the United States, but an expression of it." By 10 p.m., the President was on his way to Missouri.

The *Mayflower* reached St. Louis before dawn, though the President rested on board until nine. Civic ceremonies filled the morning, and 1,500 people paid two dollars each for lunch and the privilege of hearing Wilson address the Chamber of Commerce. The Republican Mayor, Henry William Kiel, announced that most of the host committee was, in fact, Republican—opponents of the Treaty at that, as seemed to be the case with the majority of Wilson's audiences that day. He said that he was glad to hear his own phrase repeated by his adversaries—that "politics was adjourned." The President's headache persisting, Dr. Grayson was able to take him for a brisk walk in a local park, providing some exercise before his speech that night to twelve thousand people in Convention Hall. In this city with its large German American population, Wilson spoke of the need to rebuild Germany, if only so that she could pay her reparations bill. He further stated that America "went into this war to see it through to the end," but that the end had not yet come. "This is the beginning, not of the war," said Wilson, "but of the processes which are going to render a war

like this impossible." At eleven o'clock the Presidential train started across the state, arriving the next morning, Saturday, in Kansas City.

Thousands of schoolchildren, each waving an American flag, lined a five-mile parade route, as the President rode to Convention Hall. Recharged by an overflow crowd of close to twenty thousand cheering citizens, Wilson walked from the back of the hall to the stage to deliver one of the most ebullient and bare-knuckled speeches of his life. "I came back from Paris bringing one of the greatest documents of human history," he said, before spending the better part of the next hour proving as much. He clarified that the Treaty was "in spirit and essence . . . an American document," since American principles had penetrated to the hearts of the peoples of Europe and their representatives. Most significant of all, he said, was the Covenant of the League of Nations, which substituted consultation and arbitration for "the brutal processes of war." That methodology, he reminded his listeners, was the central principle of the Bryan treaties, instituted in the earliest days of Wilson's presidency. He spoke of the new power grab in Russia, where the Bolshevik government was proving itself more cruel than the Czar or even the Kaiser had been in "controlling the destinies of that great people." He warned, "If you don't want little groups of selfish men to plot the future of Europe, we must not allow little groups of selfish men to plot the future of America."

"I have come out to fight for a cause," Wilson said, leading with his chin. "That cause is greater than the Senate. It is greater than the government. It is as great as the cause of mankind, and I intend, in office or out, to fight that battle as long as I live." He explained that his ancestors were "troublesome Scotchmen," among whom were some of that nation's most stubborn and strong, the Covenanters. Upon taking his leave of the stage, Wilson said, "Here is the Covenant of the League of Nations. I am a Covenanter!"

By nightfall he was three hundred miles to the north, in Des Moines, Iowa. As in the preceding cities, the elected officials who greeted him were for the most part Republicans, which fueled Wilson's argument that the nation was looking for a unified, nonpartisan response to the Treaty. He observed that the "isolation of the United States is at an end, not because we chose to go into the politics of the world, but because . . . we have become a determining factor in the history of mankind."

On Sunday the President rested in a hotel in Des Moines. He had garnered banner headlines in the nation's newspapers his first five days on the road. Articles initially spoke of Lodge as having taken the lead in the early innings of this great debate, but now that Wilson was swinging for the fences, the shift in the country's mood was palpable. An overnight Republican survey in Missouri revealed that the President had flipped the state from anti- to pro-League. Because Wilson could dip into a $25,000 travel fund allotted the President, one Republican Congressman from Missouri proposed a resolution providing $15,000 to defray the expenses of any Senators who sought equal time on the road opposing the Treaty. Edith Wilson noticed that the waves of approval helped calm her husband's nervous energy and headaches. With friendly crowds gathering at every junction, Tumulty wanted the President to address them from the rear platform. Here Dr. Grayson put his foot down, as he anxiously knew that each appearance and each bad night's sleep depleted his patient's reserves.

At 5 a.m. on September 8, the *Mayflower* rolled into Omaha, Nebraska; and over the next week, it would zigzag north before heading west. The itinerary required as many as four speeches some days, and Wilson alone composed his material. Before retiring each night, he jotted notes for the program the next day, as he tailored each speech with an unexpected twist or inspiring phrase. He walked onto the stage of the Auditorium in Omaha with a prop—a copy of the Treaty, so that all could see it was a lot more than the few clauses that had been debated endlessly in the press. "Why, my fellow citizens," Wilson said, "this is one of the great charters of human liberty, and the man who picks flaws in it—or, rather, picks out the flaws that are in it, for there are flaws in it—forgets the magnitude of the thing, forgets the majesty of the thing, forgets that the counsels of more than twenty nations combined . . . were . . . unanimous in the adoption of this great instrument." Wilson readily conceded that this treaty created only a "presumption" that there would not be another war—because "there is no absolute guarantee against human passion." But he predicted with absolute certainty that "within another generation, there will be another world war if the nations of the world—if the League of Nations—does not prevent it by concerted action."

"Sometimes people call me an idealist," he told an audience at the Armory that night in Sioux Falls, South Dakota. "Well, that is the way I

know I am an American." Wilson's talk was not always so elevated. He said America could stay out of a society composed of the governments of the world, but that would cast suspicion on their nation. He hoped the American farmer would appreciate that "you can make more money out of men who trust you than out of men who fear you." He posited that friendship made American wheat taste better than that of Australia or Argentina, that it made American cotton better than that of India. During the night, the *Mayflower* coupled onto the Chicago & Northwestern Railroad line to Minnesota.

Wilson encountered his first political slap the next morning as his train car waited for the reception committee to arrive at the St. Paul station. Knowing the President was scheduled to address a special session of the state legislature, Governor Joseph. A. A. Burnquist—chairman of the committee and a bitter Republican opponent of the Treaty—intentionally detained the group at the Capitol for half an hour, arriving at the station with neither explanation nor apology. The President of the United States turned the other cheek. Without mentioning a single name, Wilson concluded his address with a word about the reception committees he had encountered on his tour. Most, he said, had been made up of Republicans, which gave him great pleasure—"because I should be ashamed of myself if I permitted any partisan thought to enter into this great matter. . . . Everybody knows that we are all Americans. Scratch a Democrat or a Republican, and underneath it is the same stuff."

After lunch, the President faced an enthusiastic reception on the streets of Minneapolis and then delivered a speech in the Armory. By the time he had returned to St. Paul for another speech that night, the city was abuzz over Governor Burnquist's insult that morning. Fifteen thousand Minnesotans jammed into the Auditorium and heard the President pay tribute to the soldiers who had fought in the Civil War to preserve the Union. Although he had been born and bred in the South, he said saving the Union was "the greatest thing that men had conceived up to that time." Now, Wilson said, "we come to . . . the union of great nations in conference upon the interests of peace." So rousing was Wilson, the Mayor of St. Paul leapt to the stage upon the conclusion of the address. "All those in favor of the ratification of the Treaty without a single change will vote Aye," he shouted to the crowd. And fifteen thousand shook the hall in agreement.

Each of the next five nights saw the President traveling west on the Northern Pacific Railway. And just as Wilson approached their home states, Senators Borah and Johnson launched their own nationwide opposition tour of the nation, leaving the Foreign Relations Committee with forty-five proposed amendments and four reservations to the Treaty. Because Wilson had no new themes to convey, he had to rely heavily on performance to persuade. The press removed coverage from the front pages and some days did not publicize his tour at all. Through North Dakota, Montana, Idaho, and Washington, Wilson maintained his breakneck pace nonetheless. Pounding headaches and asthma attacked him regularly, and Dr. Grayson could provide little treatment beyond propping up the President with pillows. After several nights, Wilson chose not even to bother the doctor. He simply grabbed his pillows and chair and caught what few winks of sleep he could before the next day's events.

In the meantime, four million American workers struck their jobs that year in nearly four thousand clashes between management and labor. The Amalgamated Association of Iron, Steel, and Tin Workers had attempted to organize the steel industry for decades, demanding union recognition; and in September, a national strike shut down half the industry. The violence between unionists on one hand and scabs and police on the other became so great in Gary, Indiana, the United States Army had to declare martial law. Boston faced a more difficult labor situation when much of its police force struck, prompting several nights of looting that required Governor Calvin Coolidge to unleash his State Guard. That action—calling the strikers "traitors"—transformed the Governor into a national figure representing law and order. Wilson called the strike "a crime against civilization," for the obligation of a policeman was "as sacred as the obligation of a soldier. He is a public servant, not a private employee, and . . . has no right to prefer any private advantage to the public safety." The racial violence of the Red Summer was no longer in flames but still flickering; September remained quiet until the end of the month, when disturbances broke out in Omaha and a few days later in a small town in Arkansas. Wilson expressed his "shame as an American citizen at the race riots . . . where men have forgot humanity and justice and orderly society and have run amuck." And the nation was just confronting one of the most peculiar legislative ideas ever to infringe upon American life— Prohibition, which had been ratified as the Eighteenth Amendment to

the Constitution at the start of the year. To implement that amendment, the House originated the Volstead Act that summer, and by September, Congress was preparing to send the law to the President's desk for his signature.

Elsewhere on the Hill, Senator Hitchcock submitted his minority report to the Foreign Relations Committee, urging ratification of the Treaty without amendments or reservations. Neither side found any give in this tug-of-war. Senator Lodge's hearings on the Treaty droned on, crescendoing with the appearance of William Bullitt, whose disgruntlement after his resignation from the American Peace Commission still festered. For hours—facing Lodge and five Republican colleagues—Bullitt made no effort to disguise his contempt for the Treaty of Versailles. His comments did little damage, for he was an obviously spurned minor player in the talks. But at the end of his interrogation, enjoying his moment in the sun as he cast a shadow over Wilson, he spoke about the senior members of the American diplomatic team, and how Lansing, Bliss, and White had "objected very vigorously to the numerous provisions of the treaty." Lodge commented that their objections to the Shantung provision were already known and asked if there was anything else to which they had objected. As though choreographed, Bullitt said, "I do not think that Secretary Lansing is at all enthusiastic about the League of Nations as it stands at present." With that, he produced a memorandum of a conversation he had with the Secretary on May 19. Bullitt quoted Lansing as having said, "I consider that the league of nations at present is entirely useless. The great powers have simply gone ahead and arranged the world to suit themselves. England and France in particular have gotten out of the treaty everything that they wanted, and the league of nations can do nothing to alter any of the unjust clauses of the treaty." Upon learning of Bullitt's testimony, Lansing—about to embark on a fishing trip on Lake Ontario—offered the press no comment.

The President—who heard the news from the press corps aboard the *Mayflower*—did the same, though Tumulty saw that Wilson was "incensed and distressed beyond measure." Four days later, Lansing telegraphed the President his version of what he had said to Bullitt, a feeble explanation concluding with his wish to do everything he could to promote ratification of the Treaty. He said he regretted that he ever had any conversation with "the disloyal young man who is seeking notoriety at the

expense of the respect of all honorable men." Wilson summoned Tumulty to his compartment. "Read that," he said, handing him the wire, "and tell me what you think of a man who was my associate on the other side and who confidentially expressed himself to an outsider in such a fashion?" For months in Paris, suspicions about Lansing had nagged the President. "But here in his own statement," Wilson said, "is a verification at last of everything I have suspected. Think of it! This from a man whom I raised from the level of a subordinate to the great office of Secretary of State of the United States. My God! I did not think it was possible for Lansing to act in this way." No task more pressing awaited the President's return to the White House than demanding Lansing's resignation.

The same morning that Wilson read Lansing's telegram, Dr. Grayson observed small drops of saliva at the corners of the President's mouth. His lips quivered slightly, and more spittle appeared. His face turned white. Grayson examined the rest of the itinerary, hoping to edit it.

Tumulty disagreed. He knew that the Treaty's great broker was also its most convincing speaker, and Wilson had another five thousand miles of territory to cover in which he could rally support. By the time he had reached Spokane on September 12, his voice had weakened and, the *Seattle Post-Intelligencer* reported, "there was a suggestion of a man very much fatigued in his delivery." He instinctively pumped his speeches with more emotion and vivid imagery. He spoke of the unconquerable nature of truth, even if you "blind its eyes with blood."

Before almost seven thousand in the Portland Auditorium, he brought the house down when he insisted that "peace can only be maintained by putting behind it the force of united nations determined to uphold it and prevent war." And then he revealed that he had just read them a quotation from Henry Cabot Lodge in 1915. He earned a second round of laughter and applause when he said, "I entirely concur in Senator Lodge's conclusion, and I hope I shall have his cooperation in bringing about the desired result."

Grayson insisted the President walk for half an hour before the train departed, but the staff squeezed an interview into those few minutes instead. A local reporter asked if the tremendous enthusiasm for the President was not lopsided, with the "adventurous" West leaning more favorably in his direction than the East. Wilson said the West was more demonstrative but that he believed approval of the League was just as strong

everywhere. "I am confident," he said before boarding the *Mayflower*, "that I shall not appeal in vain to the conscience of the American people."

The next leg of the trip was the longest—772 miles on the Southern Pacific Railroad to San Francisco. It allowed the President to rest his voice and enjoy the magnificent scenery, which included loyal supporters all along the route. It troubled Dr. Grayson to learn the next morning in Oakland that Wilson's head was pounding. For Tumulty, California was all-important, as the forward-thinking state of rival Hiram Johnson had scheduled more speeches than any other.

Wilson soldiered through two full days in the Bay Area. On Thursday the eighteenth, he addressed 1,500 members of the Associated Business Men's Clubs of San Francisco, 10,000 people at the outdoor Greek Theatre at the University of California, Berkeley, and more than 12,000 in the Oakland Municipal Auditorium. "I believe in divine Providence," Wilson had said at breakfast. "If I did not, I would go crazy. If I thought the direction of the disordered affairs of this world depended upon our finite endeavor, I should not know how to reason my way to sanity. But I do not believe there is any body of men, how ever they concert their power or their influence, that can defeat this great enterprise." His day finished with a six-hundred-mile ride south.

Under the California sun, support for Wilson and his treaty kept growing. Thirty thousand people awaited him in the San Diego Stadium, where he experimented with a new electrical device that Grayson called a "voice phone." On the speaker's platform at one end of the bowl stood three sides of a twenty-square-foot glass room; the "fourth wall" featured a table with megaphones, from which electrical wires carried the voice to "resonators" at various points in the stadium. Boxed in and dependent upon a mechanical contrivance, Wilson said it was the most difficult speech he ever delivered. But, except for one badly wired spot, all thirty thousand attendees could hear his seventy-minute presentation, a favorite part of which was not only the old Lodge quotation supporting a league but one from TR supporting such an organization as well. It was tempting to think that orators could thenceforth address entire coliseums at once. If only the time had come when a President could use the radio to deliver fireside chats right into people's homes, Wilson could have conducted an even more effective campaign without any of the physical duress.

After dinner that night, former President McKinley's Secretary of the

Treasury, Lyman J. Gage, a dyed-in-the-wool Republican, introduced Wilson to a much smaller assembly, assuring everybody in the room that if McKinley were still alive, he would not only endorse the President's actions but he would also say, "God bless you, Woodrow Wilson."

Two hundred thousand people greeted Wilson on the streets of Los Angeles (population: 503,812) the next day—one of the most enthusiastic demonstrations in the city's history. A capacity crowd filled the Shrine Auditorium to hear him that Saturday night, and the local press was almost unanimously supportive. Veteran newspaperman Charles H. Grasty wrote in *The New York Times*, "This is Woodrow Wilson country now, as Senator Johnson will find out when he returns." Even Harry Chandler, the fiercely Republican publisher of the *Los Angeles Times*, admitted that the majority of Southern California was pro-League, by as much as 6 to 1. More compelling, Chandler said, was that "we have come to a point where it is a question of partisanship or patriotism," and the League "is not our politics now but our religion." General consensus among the press was not just that Los Angeles had been the climax of the tour but that the President had swung the national debate in his favor.

In anticipation of the punishing itinerary home, Edith Wilson had hoped for a quiet Sunday entirely to themselves. But Woodrow had planned a nostalgic reunion. From the Presidential Suite of the Alexandria Hotel, he typed a luncheon invitation to Mary Allen Hulbert. She was living in a little house in Hollywood in reduced circumstances. Scintillating dinner parties in Bermuda, hosting the likes of Mark Twain and a Princeton president contemplating a run for public office, had become distant memories. She rode a streetcar downtown for her 1:30 engagement, and the First Lady waited at the door of the suite to greet her. "Because of the work scandalmongers had done to make an intrigue of that friendship," Edith later recorded, "I was glad to receive her, and show my disdain for such slander." In an instant Wilson and Dr. Grayson joined them, and the four withdrew for lunch and stilted small talk.

The two women sized each other up, offering faint praise for each other in their respective memoirs. Mrs. Hulbert would devote ten pages to the encounter, Mrs. Wilson fifteen lines, in which she referred to her guest as Mrs. Peck. Edith described "a faded, sweet-looking woman who was absorbed in an only son." Mary saw somebody unlike her photographs in the

newspaper—"much more junoesque, but handsome, with a charming smile that revealed her strong, white teeth." After lunch the President insisted upon hearing the details of Mary's life during the last four years. The story of her decline consumed much of the afternoon. She spoke of the President's enemies and how they had slandered her and offered exorbitant amounts of money for his letters. As both of them had survived the ordeal, they laughed; but Wilson brought the story to a close saying, "God, to think that you should have suffered because of me!"

When the President had to leave the room for a quick conference, Edith thought Mary might take that as a cue to depart, but she seemed oblivious to the preciousness of the President's time. "Poor woman," Edith recalled, "weighed down with her own problems, of course she did not understand. Darkness had fallen when she finally rose to go." Before leaving, Mary asked her old friend why he was the recipient of so much "venomous personal animosity."

"That's just it," Wilson said, with a flick of his hand. "If I had nothing to do with the League of Nations, it would go through like that." He said that Lloyd George, Clemenceau, and Orlando had all failed him. And in that moment, Mary Hulbert noted later, her personal troubles faded as she found herself looking into the face of "tragedy." Placing his hand on that of his wife, the President asked if there was anything he could do for Mary. Nothing for her, she said nobly, but he might consider helping her son. Edith walked their guest to the elevator, which the latter said "quickly dropped me out of the life of my friend Woodrow Wilson—forever." A wistful "Mrs. Peck" boarded a streetcar back to her bungalow.

A few hours later, Woodrow Wilson began his journey back to the White House, via Sacramento, across the Sierra Nevada, from one station to the next. While he was suffering from asthma and headaches, the six hundred miles of tracks that day cut through forest fires and burrowed through tunnels in which smoke mingled with train exhaust. At the other end, changes in pressure further attacked Wilson's respiratory system. By day's end, his head throbbed and his face twitched. In Reno, Nevada, he spoke for well over an hour, his remarks funneled to several remote venues through telephone receivers placed near megaphones. Then it was back onto the train for another 576 miles, stopping in Ogden, Utah, the next day for a few remarks before proceeding to Salt Lake City.

By then, Dr. Grayson considered his patient's fatigue a serious condition, which recurring headaches and coughing spells exacerbated. Throat irritation interfered with what little sleep he was getting, and the latest news from Washington was sure to ruin the rest. Senator Lodge had invited his Republican colleague Porter J. McCumber, a Mild Reservationist from North Dakota, to lunch at his house. By the time the meal ended, McCumber had agreed on a significant reservation to Article X of the Covenant, one that several Democrats came to support as well. The President fumed.

Hours before his speech that warm night in Salt Lake City, more than fifteen thousand people packed the Mormon Tabernacle, while thousands more gathered around the temple. Inside the unventilated hall, the air turned so thick that Edith Wilson took a whiff of lavender salts to keep from fainting and doused a handkerchief in the potion for her husband to take with him to the rostrum. He railed against that day's reservation, inaccurately explaining that it would mean reopening negotiations with all the nations that had been present at Versailles, including Germany. This reservation, he contended, was nothing less than taking a knife to the Treaty and cutting out "the heart of this Covenant." For ninety minutes he sermonized feverishly, and Edith saw that perspiration had soaked through his coat. Back at their hotel, Wilson changed clothes, only to saturate the fresh garment in a matter of minutes. Back on the train, Grayson spoke of a "nervous condition."

The next afternoon in Cheyenne, Wyoming, the President conceded that he was ill, but he delivered his longest speech yet, often wandering from subject to subject, sounding as tired as he looked. He reboarded the *Mayflower* to go to the next station. In their room at the Brown Palace Hotel after their late-night arrival in Denver, Edith suggested a break in the schedule for a few days of rest. "No," Woodrow replied, "I have caught the imagination of the people. They are eager to hear what the League stands for; and I should fail in my duty if I disappointed them." So obvious was Edith's dismay, he assured her, "This will soon be over, and when we get back to Washington I promise you I will take a holiday." Dr. Grayson was counting the days.

The next morning, the President delivered a rousing speech to twelve thousand people; and before lunch, the Atchison, Topeka & Santa Fe Railway was transporting him to Pueblo, a city of fifty thousand, for a

two-hour visit. As they approached the city, the President relaxed on the rear platform and asked to review that afternoon's arrangements. An aide told him he would visit the Fair Grounds, where he would greet the crowd before proceeding to the auditorium. "Who authorized such an idiotic idea?" he asked. When the aide said the visit had always been part of the day's plans, he demanded to see Tumulty and the original program. Tumulty appeared with the document, signed with Wilson's trademark "Okeh, W. W." The President snickered and said, "Any damn fool who was stupid enough to approve such a program has no business in the White House." He sent word that he would not appear at the Fair Grounds but changed his mind upon reaching Pueblo, when the reception committee informed him that ten thousand people had already assembled there. He agreed to ride around the racetrack of the fair and wave his hand. He disappointed many, especially those who had traveled from outlying towns hoping to hear him speak, but Wilson felt he had to conserve his strength for the main address in the city's new Memorial Hall.

"It seemed like we would suffocate in there," recalled one former seventh-grader who had been among the three thousand people packed into the brick building. Agent Starling accompanied the President from the car to the auditorium, and Wilson stumbled on the single step at the entrance. Starling caught him and kept his hand on his arm as he all but lifted him up a few more steps to the speaker's platform. Wilson did not object—which surprised Starling, as the President had always refused even the suggestion of physical assistance. "This will have to be a short speech," Wilson indicated to the gang of newspapermen who were about to hear variations on his themes for the fortieth time. "Aren't you fellows getting pretty sick of this?"

The big horseshoe balcony with its shiny brass rail embraced the President as he rose to speak. After a raucous welcome, he delivered a heartfelt speech, remarkable in many ways. The intimacy of the hall allowed for a more personal address, something almost conversational; and in delivering it, Wilson touched upon all the main points he had refined over the past three weeks. His weariness showed, especially in the weakness of his voice, but his frailties only enhanced the emotion of his message. For the first time, the reporters heard him falter on a line, having to restart it more than once; and unexpected pauses suggested both mental confusion as well as physical exhaustion. Starling was so concerned, he remained poised

to catch the President should he collapse. He recalled Wilson's passion on this occasion, his working himself to tears.

The effect was overpowering, as toward the end of his speech, the President struck several deeply emotional chords. He spoke of the responsibility he felt as the advocate for a special class of citizens. "My clients," he explained, "are the children; my clients are the next generation. They do not know what promises and bonds I undertook when I ordered the armies of the United States to the soil of France, but I know. And I intend to redeem my pledges to the children; they shall not be sent upon a similar errand." When the President spoke of Decoration Day at the cemetery in Suresnes, there was hope, not anger, he said, that "some men in public life who are now opposing the settlement for which these men died could visit such a spot as that. . . . I wish that they could feel the moral obligation that rests upon us not to go back on those boys, but to see the thing through." In dissociating America from the others who fought in the war, Wilson said, "There seems to me to stand between us and the rejection or qualification of this treaty the serried ranks of those boys in khaki—not only those boys who came home, but those dear ghosts that still deploy upon the fields of France." In those moments of Wilson's speech, Tumulty would later recount, "a great wave of emotion, such as I have never witnessed at a public meeting, swept through the whole amphitheatre." Not only were Edith and most of the women in tears, but he also saw several men, including the hard-boiled press corps, sneaking handkerchiefs from their pockets.

Instead of pulling out all the stops as he reached his conclusion, Wilson soft-pedaled his delivery, letting his words alone carry the message. "There is one thing that the American people always rise to and extend their hand to," he said, "and that is the truth of justice and of liberty and of peace. We have accepted that truth, and we are going to be led by it, and it is going to lead us, and, through us, the world, out into pastures of quietness and peace such as the world never dreamed of before."

Back at the train, Wilson complained again that his head ached. The pain had not stopped all day, sometimes blinding him. Dr. Grayson thought a walk might offer relief; and so, twenty miles out of Pueblo, the train stopped on the tracks, letting the Wilsons and Grayson off to stretch their legs on a country road for almost an hour. Agent Starling trailed

behind. An elderly farmer happened by and, recognizing the President, presented him with a head of cabbage and some apples, hoping they might become part of his dinner that night. Walking toward the train, Wilson saw a soldier in a private's uniform, evidently ill, sitting on the porch of a house set back from the road. The President climbed over the fence to talk to him, and the boy's parents and brothers soon joined them, visibly moved to see the President of the United States ministering to the sick soldier.

The walk did him a world of good. The pain subsided, his appetite returned, and after dinner with Grayson and Tumulty, the Wilsons prepared for bed. When the President heard that crowds were forming at each station in Colorado, he remained awake, finding five thousand people at Rocky Ford. Grayson extended Wilson's apologies to the crowd for not being able to appear, but just before the train pulled away, Wilson emerged to grasp the hands of those closest to him. He waved goodbye and then retired for the night.

Edith repaired to her room, where her maid brushed her hair and gave her a massage. At 11:30, by which time she thought her husband had fallen asleep, he knocked on their connecting door and asked to see her. She found him sitting on the side of his bed, his head pressed against the back of a chair set in front of him. The pain had grown so unbearable, he asked her to summon Grayson. The doctor arrived and found a man in the middle of a breakdown. He was nauseated; his face twitched; he gasped for air in the worst asthmatic attack of the trip. Wilson complained that the walls of the tiny compartment were closing in on him. He dressed, and they moved to the roomier "office," where nobody could offer any remedy beyond bolstering him with pillows. Duty now demanded that Grayson recommend canceling the rest of the tour, which Wilson begged him not to suggest. In the hostile political climate, he knew that his enemies would pounce upon his cessation as a sign of weakness. He told Grayson that he would be better by Wichita and that any further discussion of aborting the trip would only keep him awake the rest of the night. Sometime around 4:30, while sitting upright in his seat, Wilson fell asleep. Edith shooed Grayson off to bed, saying she would maintain the vigil.

Dr. Grayson promptly awakened Tumulty, to apprise him that continuing the trip could have fatal consequences. The two advisers conferred with

Mrs. Wilson, who had just endured what she called "the longest and most heartbreaking" night of her life. As they were all of the same mind, Grayson waited for the President to awaken, at which time he would explain their decision. But when he entered the President's compartment, he found Wilson shaving, with no intention of abandoning the schedule. Edith and Tumulty expressed their opinions, but the President would not listen. "Don't you see that if you cancel this trip," he explained, "Senator Lodge and his friends will say that I am a quitter and that the Western trip was a failure, and the Treaty will be lost." Tumulty assured him that nobody would ever consider him a quitter. Gradually, Wilson faced the truth.

"My dear boy," the President said, crumbling, "this has never happened to me before. I felt it coming on yesterday. I do not know what to do." His left arm and leg had numbed. Looking at Tumulty, he begged for a twenty-four-hour reprieve, a postponement: "I want to show them that I can still fight and that I am not afraid." Privately, Grayson argued, at last, that Wilson owed it to the country as well as to Mrs. Wilson and his children to "stop now before very serious developments should occur." He maintained that Wilson was unable to deliver another speech. Now, too exhausted even to fight back, the unhappy warrior allowed, "If you feel that way about it, I will surrender." And then, he quietly added, "This is the greatest disappointment of my life."

Grayson beckoned Tumulty back into the room. "I don't seem to realize it," Wilson told him, "but I seem to have gone to pieces. The Doctor is right. I am not in condition to go on." Unable to face anyone, he looked out the window at the flat countryside instead, as tears rolled from his eyes. "He accepted the decree of Fate as gallantly as he had fought the fight," Edith recollected; "but only he and his God knew the crucifixion that began that moment—to stretch into interminable years, during which the seal he put on his lips, never to . . . voice a syllable of self-pity or regret, remained unbroken."

Edith made her own private compact as well, one that would assume public ramifications. First light had revealed how drawn and lined her husband's face had become, suggesting interior distress even more severe. Life as she knew it "would never be the same." And from that hour forward, she decided, "I would have to wear a mask—not only to the public but to the one I loved best in the world; for he must never know how ill he was, and I must carry on."

Tumulty sprang into action, calling for a stenographer and composing a statement for the press. It said that Dr. Grayson had insisted upon the cancellation of the rest of the tour—Wichita, Oklahoma City, Little Rock, Memphis, and Louisville—despite the President's "earnest desire to complete his engagements." From the rail yard sidings in north Wichita, the newspaper correspondents raced to find telephones so that they might break the news to the world. By telegram, Wilson informed each of his daughters—Margaret visiting in New London, Jessie Sayre in Cambridge, Massachusetts, and Nell McAdoo about to arrive in Los Angeles—that he was returning to Washington and that there was nothing to be alarmed about. The reception committee in Wichita sent an emissary to the train to inform the President that 25,000 Kansans had hoped to see him; and a telegram from the committee in Oklahoma City expressed sorrow, as they had expected 100,000 people—more than inhabited the city—to welcome him. After making most of the arrangements for the direct departure back to Washington, chief clerk Thomas Brahany went to the President's compartment. He found Wilson sitting alone, slouched over, "with his head hanging and with one side of his face drooping and with saliva running out from the corner of his mouth."

Wilson remained indisposed in his stateroom and in pain. Although most of the press dealt with the news in a fair and balanced manner, several opposition newspapers—such as the New York *Sun*—suggested that the whole matter was a ruse, that the President was not really sick. Within hours, however, word had reached most of the nation; and, as Grayson wrote in his journal that day, "there was deep sorrow for the most part among those who had watched the hard fight that the President had made in carrying his side of the Treaty controversy to the people themselves." Whether one agreed with Woodrow Wilson or not, nobody disputed his dedication to his cause. More to the point, the tour was influencing Senators, as two who had been wavering had come back in line against all amendments. It looked as though the President might be able to craft a few "mild reservations or interpretations" and have his treaty approved.

At eleven o'clock that morning, the *Mayflower* pulled out from Wichita. Along the tracks, from one station to the next, crowds gathered to watch the train pass—offering no cheers, only silent respect. Railroad officials charted the fastest route home—which retraced much of the outbound trip. Sympathetic messages arrived: a batch of telegrams awaited

the President in St. Louis very early Saturday morning; cablegrams forwarded from Washington were brought on board several hours later in Indianapolis, including well-wishes from King George and Premier Clemenceau. Nothing could lift the President's spirits or ease his pain. And though time was of the essence, Grayson asked that the train slow down because the *Mayflower*, being the rearmost car, rocked wildly from side to side, which kept Wilson from sleeping. The engineers periodically sped up, but in Harrisburg, Pennsylvania, Grayson insisted the train was not to exceed twenty-five miles per hour for the rest of the trip. They lowered the shades to block onlookers, creating the air of a funeral cortege. When Wilson was not trying to rest in his bed, he sat mute in the office compartment, where Edith kept him company, knitting and attempting to divert him with small talk. But, she observed, "the air was so heavy with unspoken agony that all seemed a travesty."

The President was up and dressed at eleven o'clock that Sunday when the train finally reached Washington—exactly forty-eight hours since Wichita. Although he looked like a ghost of the man who had left Union Station twenty-five days earlier, he summoned his strength and walked unassisted and perfectly erect from the *Mayflower*. Margaret Wilson ran through the train shed to greet him and waited as he bade farewell to the railroad personnel and newspapermen. She joined Edith, Grayson, and the Secret Service as they advanced toward the motorcars waiting outside. More than a thousand people in the station cheered. With a smile and a nod, he especially acknowledged the applause of a group of wounded soldiers on a bench in the Red Cross canteen.

Within minutes the President was back in the White House. He wanted to attend church, but Grayson ordered him to bed at once. Too restless to nap and in too much pain to work, he wandered the long hall of the second floor, back and forth between his study and Edith's room. As it was a sunny early autumn day, with the first smack of cool air he had felt in months, he and Edith and Grayson took a two-hour drive through the city parks. The President dozed most of the time.

Upon their return, Admiral Grayson (as he was officially known) pulled rank. He believed Wilson needed a complete rest cure, and he imposed strict conditions. From that moment forward, he said, the President "should not be bothered with any matters of official character," especially questions of a controversial nature. He banned conferences with Cabinet

members and any other officials. "It was to be a complete rest, not partial rest," Grayson underscored, "and nothing was to be allowed to interfere with the President's restoration to health if possible."

The next day Edith invited ten of the journalists from the Western tour to tea. She hosted them alone, and they learned that the interdiction against official conferences was in effect indefinitely. The day after that, an urgent message from Sir William Wiseman of the British government arrived, requesting an audience with Wilson. Edith asked him to appear at eleven, at which time she said the President was too ill to receive him but if Wiseman would transmit the information, she would have a reply for him at two o'clock. In that interval, she mentioned the visit to her husband, who waved it off as nonessential. Grayson arranged for Wilson's ophthalmologist and a leading neurologist to examine him at the end of the week.

A shroud of secrecy descended upon the White House, which only raised suspicions. As Secretary of State Lansing saw things, the President's advocacy of the Covenant had become nothing less than "a veritable obsession," which had caused an abnormal mental state, a monomania that "excluded everything else from his thoughts." Only complete rest, he suspected, would allow him to "regain normality."

By October 1, his third day home, Wilson displayed small signs of improvement. He catnapped at night and during his daily drives, and his appetite was returning. He expressed renewed interest in his work, though Edith arranged to run motion pictures at night in the East Room to divert him. That night he felt chipper enough to play billiards for a few minutes. Later, he insisted on reading Scripture to Edith, as he had done every night during the war, and she delighted in hearing some vitality back in his voice. After his reading, Wilson wound his watch, and they talked a while before he went to his room. Minutes later, Edith noticed that Woodrow had left his timepiece on her table. When she returned it, he grumbled about losing his memory. She said that was nonsense, that she forgot such things all the time. Afterward, she felt leaving the watch behind had not worried him that much; it was simply that "he did not want to relax the tight hold he was keeping on himself."

Edith had been having troubles of her own getting through the night, as she awakened frequently in order to monitor her husband's rest. At dawn on October 2, she found him sleeping soundly, but then around

8:30, he was sitting on the side of his bed, reaching for a water bottle. As she handed it to him, she noticed his left hand had gone limp. "I have no feeling in that hand," he said. He asked her to rub it. But first, he wanted help in getting to the bathroom. She supported him as he staggered those few yards, but it required a huge effort on his part. More terrifying to her were his spasms of pain with every step. Edith asked if she could leave him alone long enough for her to telephone Dr. Grayson. He said yes; and in that split second, Edith made a curious decision.

Instead of going to the nearby bedroom phone, which connected to operators at the White House switchboard, she hastened down the hall to a private phone wired directly to the desk in the Usher's Room. Ike Hoover answered the call, and Mrs. Wilson said, "Please get Doctor Grayson, the President is very sick."

While still on the phone, Edith heard a noise from the President's apartment. Rushing back, she found her husband lying on the bathroom floor, unconscious.

16

PIETÀ

Then tooke they the body of Iesus, & wound it in
linnen clothes, with the spices, as the maner of the
Iewes is to burie . . .

—JOHN, XIX:40

Edith pulled a blanket from the Lincoln Bed and draped it over her husband's inanimate body. At last he stirred and requested a drink of water. In fetching it, Edith also grabbed a pillow, returning to elevate his head as she cradled him.

Minutes later, a White House car delivered Dr. Grayson. He hastened upstairs and rapped gently on the locked bedroom door. Ike Hoover waited in the hall as Grayson and Mrs. Wilson lifted the President into his bed. The left side of his body was immobile. After examining his patient, Dr. Grayson returned to the hall. "My God, the President is paralyzed!" he said to Hoover, whom he immediately ordered to summon both Admiral E. R. Stitt of the Naval Medical Corps and the nurse who had attended Ellen Wilson in her final illness. Within hours, an array of doctors joined them, starting with a pioneer in neurology, Francis X. Dercum, professor of nervous and mental diseases at Philadelphia's Jefferson Medical College. Edith's family physician, Sterling Ruffin, Wilson's classmate Edward P. Davis, and eye specialist George de Schweinitz followed.

Dercum examined Wilson in bed. He found his left leg

and arm in a condition of "complete flaccid paralysis," with the lower half
of the left side of the face drooping. The President was conscious but som-
nolent. His temperature, pulse, and respiration were all normal, but in
addition to his left side having lost all feeling, his left eye responded feebly
to light. He had suffered a thrombosis—an ischemic stroke—a clot in an
artery of the brain. Nothing had ruptured. Wilson's abilities to think and
speak escaped unimpaired. An air of quiet exigency filled the President's
bedroom as the medical team decided how to convert the White House
into a convalescent home. The three Wilson daughters made their way to
Washington.

Outside the bedroom, the domestic staff remained completely in the
dark. At day's end, when the furniture needed rearranging to accommodate incoming medical apparatus, Grayson allowed only Ike Hoover to
help him and the nurse move the various pieces. Hoover could not keep his
eyes off the President stretched out in the large Lincoln Bed. "He looked
as if he were dead," Hoover observed. As Edith Wilson would impart years
later, "For days life hung in the balance."

Nobody divulged as much to the public. "No details, no explanations"
were the orders of the day, recalled Ike Hoover. Outside the White House,
people knew only that the President was suffering from nervous exhaustion and that such attendant conditions as his intestinal troubles were
manifestations of the assault on his central nervous system. Only the few
within earshot of the Lincoln Bed even uttered the word "stroke." Grayson
told the press that he was confident Wilson's "reserve stamina . . . will
carry him through the crisis."

Within days, the President had emerged from danger but had entered
a twilight zone—a state of physical exhaustion, emotional turbulence, and
mental unrest. The "burning question," Edith Wilson would later explain
in her memoirs, became "how Mr. Wilson might best serve the country,
preserve his own life and if possible recover." That did not necessarily reflect the order of her priorities, as she asked the doctors for their candor.
They all asserted that Wilson's brain was "as clear as ever" and that the
immediate upturn in his condition suggested something close to a full
recovery lay ahead. But, they insisted, recovery was unattainable "unless
the President were released from every disturbing problem during these
days of Nature's effort to repair the damage done."

Edith asked how that was possible when a Chief Executive only deals

with problems. Dr. Dercum—with his bald head and walrus mustache—leaned toward her with an unexpected nostrum. "Madam," he said, "it is a grave situation, but I think you can solve it. Have everything come to you; weigh the importance of each matter, and see if it is possible by consultation with the respective heads of the Departments to solve them without the guidance of your husband. In this way you can save him a great deal." Dercum reminded her that the President's nerves were "crying out for rest" and that "every time you take him a new anxiety or problem to excite him, you are turning a knife in an open wound."

Edith suggested allowing Vice President Marshall to succeed, as the Constitution stipulated, thus granting the President the vital rest he required. Dercum disagreed. "For Mr. Wilson to resign," he explained, "would have a bad effect on the country, and a serious effect on our patient." In terms more political than medical, he noted that the President had staked his life on ratification of the Treaty. If he resigned, Dercum said, "the greatest incentive to recovery is gone." As the President's mind remained "clear as crystal," Dercum said Woodrow Wilson "can still do more with even a maimed body than any one else." Grayson had told Dercum of the President's having discussed all public affairs of the last four years privately with Edith. Knowing that, Dercum deputized her, insisting, "He has the utmost confidence in you."

"So began my stewardship," Edith would admit two decades later. In that capacity, she would determine not only what matters should come before the President but also when. More than a mere sentry, the second Mrs. Wilson took it upon herself to filter and analyze every issue that required Presidential action, executing those duties to the best of her ability. As she explained: "I studied every paper, sent from the different Secretaries or Senators, and tried to digest and present in tabloid form the things that, despite my vigilance, had to go to the President." In insisting that she never "made a single decision regarding the disposition of public affairs," Mrs. Wilson failed to acknowledge the commanding nature of her role, that in determining the daily agenda and formulating arguments thereon, she executed the physical and most of the mental duties of the office.

Edith Bolling Wilson did not become, as some have asserted, "the first female President of the United States." But she came close. She considered herself more of a lady-in-waiting to her husband than an executive; but she was in a position to act, while he could only react. Unschooled in

politics—and unskilled—she held not the least desire for any power, other than the power to heal her husband. She just wanted Woodrow to get better.

And so began the greatest conspiracy that had ever engulfed the White House. With only virtuous intent, the plot unfolded—one that was hardly a scrupulous interpretation of the Constitution, which provided for "the Case of Removal, Death, Resignation or Inability" of the President with the ascension of the Vice President "until the Disability be removed, or a President shall be elected." The devoted wife, the dedicated physician, and—soon—the devout secretary debated among themselves how to proceed, even though the legal issue ought not have been theirs to decide. But the Constitution provided neither means nor measures to determine Presidential disability, so they took the law of the land into their own hands, concluding what best served Woodrow Wilson best served the country. Their behavior tacitly acknowledged that this was a power grab, as they enshrouded the Presidency in as much secrecy as possible.

With the White House ominously dark and silent, Lansing, the most discontented Cabinet member, wanted answers. Without realizing that Wilson's illness was all that had kept him from being discharged, the Secretary of State requested a private audience with Tumulty. The Secretary came to the Cabinet Room at 11:30 on Friday, October 3, to propose that Vice President Marshall serve in a Presidential capacity. Lansing carried a volume known as Jefferson's *Manual*—parliamentary procedure for use in the Senate—from which he read aloud the Constitutional clause describing the circumstances under which the duties shall devolve upon the Vice President. Tumulty grew indignant. "Mr. Lansing," he said brusquely, "the Constitution is not a dead letter with the White House. I have read the Constitution and do not find myself in need of any tutoring at your hands." He asked Lansing just who should declare the President's disability, and Lansing said that should fall upon either Dr. Grayson or Tumulty himself.

"You may rest assured that while Woodrow Wilson is lying in the White House on the broad of his back I will not be a party to ousting him," said his first and most faithful political aide. "He has been too kind, too loyal, and too wonderful to me to receive such treatment at my hands." At that moment, Dr. Grayson appeared. Tumulty turned to him and said, "And I am sure that Doctor Grayson will never certify to this disability.

Will you, Grayson?" The doctor assured Lansing that the President's mind was "clear and acute" and that he would not be party to suggesting his incapacity. With neither willing to sign such a statement, any further suggestions of removing the President would be futile, if not faintly seditious.

Lansing believed nonetheless that the President's state was "dangerous," as was that of the government of the United States. At first he thought the Vice President should convene an emergency session of the Cabinet that weekend, but after his meeting with Tumulty he realized that it would "unduly alarm the nation." In the absence of leadership and the evident decision of the White House to bypass Marshall, Lansing felt somebody had to be in control of the executive branch. He and Tumulty agreed that he would call a meeting for the following Monday. In yielding nothing more than that to the Secretary of State, however, Tumulty officially became Mrs. Wilson's accomplice, interpreting the health of the President and that of the nation as one and the same.

Within days, newspapers reported rumors that Wilson had suffered a cerebral lesion or hemorrhage, to which Dr. Grayson issued only nondenial denials. He and the other attending physicians had agreed on a policy of not answering any questions, and that vagueness only fueled more gossip.

Cabinet members chewed on any morsel of information they could find. When David Houston ran into Newton Baker at the Shoreham Hotel on Friday, the Navy Secretary said the silence from the White House had him "scared literally to death." Two days later, again at the Shoreham, Houston happened to see the Vice President and Mrs. Marshall lunching. The Agriculture Secretary paid his respects and found Marshall deeply disturbed—not at any news that he had heard but at all that he had not heard. He felt he should be briefed, officially and immediately. Then, revealing what a ridiculous position the Vice Presidency had become, he also said that "it would be a tragedy for him to assume the duties of President, at best; and that it would be equally a tragedy for the people; that he knew many men who knew more about the affairs of the government than he did; and that it would be especially trying for him if he had to assume the duties without warnings." The first Vice President to serve two terms since 1825, he pled for any "real facts."

After a few days in which Wilson's condition was still touch and go, the co-conspirators felt obliged to prepare Thomas Marshall for the worst.

To keep from drawing attention to any possible succession, Edith agreed to a briefing through a third party. Although it meant divulging the nation's darkest secret to another person, they decided to entrust a middleman—J. Fred Essary, Washington correspondent for the Baltimore *Sun*. Upon receiving a few facts, he went to Marshall's office and, sitting next to him at his desk, privately explained the reason for his visit. As Essary reported the situation, Marshall sat speechless, staring at his clasped hands. Essary awaited some reaction but received none. He rose, approached the door, and looked back at the amiable little man from a small town in Indiana, still gazing at his hands. Not until Marshall saw Essary years later in Indiana did he apologize for his behavior that day. "I did not even have the courtesy to thank you for coming over and telling me," Marshall explained. "It was the first great shock of my life." Alice Roosevelt Longworth would later cackle over what had become Washington lore for years—that upon learning the direness of the President's situation, the Vice President had fainted.

The President's health showed incremental signs of improvement. Within days of his stroke, he was sleeping much of his days and nights. His appetite slowly returned, as did his sense of humor. Wilson had difficulty in swallowing and had to be coaxed into eating. After Mrs. Wilson was able to feed him several mouthfuls by spoon, he signaled for Grayson to draw close enough to hear something he had to say. "Doctor," he whispered,

> *A wonderful bird is the pelican*
> *His bill will hold more than his bellican.*
> *He can take in his beak*
> *Enough food for a week*
> *I wonder how in the hell-he-can.*

When Dr. Grayson focused a light on his eyes and explained he was examining his pupils, Wilson replied, "You have a large order, as I have had a great many in my day." By that weekend, Wilson asked that a stenographer be called, so he could dictate some letters. Grayson talked him out of even thinking of work by reminding him that, as a good Presbyterian, he should honor the Sabbath.

On Monday, October 6, the Cabinet convened for close to two hours.

Lansing announced that the President would not be returning to the public business for some time and that they should consider a new modus operandi. He thought the Vice President should be prevailed upon; and he asked his colleagues to consider what constituted Presidential "inability" and who was to decide it. Secretary Houston reminded the others at the table that after President James A. Garfield had been shot, he lingered in bed for two months without a declaration of inability, while the Attorney General ran the government. At Lansing's beckoning, Grayson appeared. He briefed the Secretaries to the effect that the President's mind was "not only clear but very active." He then added, with an inscrutable gaze, "The President asked me what the Cabinet wanted with me and by what authority it was meeting while he was in Washington without a call from him." He said the President was more than a little perturbed when he heard that the meeting was taking place. Lansing was taken aback. Secretary Baker suggested that Grayson tell the President that they only met "as a mark of affection," and he asked the doctor to convey their unanimous sympathy with their assurance that they were all looking out for his interests.

In a moment alone, Daniels suggested to Grayson that an honest acknowledgment of the President's condition might elicit sympathy and even greater support instead of the current "uncertainty and criticism." Grayson agreed but was clearly under orders from Mrs. Wilson, who knew her husband's desires. In truth, it seems unfathomable that either of them would have breathed a word about the Cabinet meeting to the convalescent.

The press and the public began to discuss the issue of "disability." In the cases of prior Presidents' deaths, the various departments functioned autonomously. Now some wondered what would happen if Wilson's Cabinet members disagreed about his ability to serve, whether a decision required unanimity or just a majority vote. Others were concerned about the extraordinary war powers that had been granted to the Chief Executive and whether a Cabinet member might seize the opportunity to advance his own agenda.

With any number of people assuming duties the President had once performed himself, the White House put a new mode of operation to the test on October 7. While he should not have had such matters on his mind, Wilson wanted to communicate with Josephus Daniels regarding the Navy forces in the Adriatic Sea. He called Edith to his side and dictated his message to her, which she handed to a White House stenographer.

While he transcribed the message and delivered it to the Secretary's office, she called Daniels herself to announce its impending arrival. The reply reversed the same route. Wilson had hoped to greet the participants at the opening of an industrial conference in Washington that week. In his stead, Tumulty wrote the brief welcome and asked Labor Secretary Wilson to deliver it; Samuel Gompers read a second, longer message at the conference, which Interior Secretary Lane had written. So adamant was Dr. Grayson about Wilson's adhering to his "absolute rest cure," he prohibited the President's signing anything but the most essential documents and even ordered the removal of newspapers from his bedroom, for they would only agitate him. When Colonel House returned to the United States, he solicitously wrote Edith, but she chose not even to tell her husband that he was back.

At the end of October, H.R. 6801, the Volstead Act—"to prohibit intoxicating beverages"—arrived at the White House for the President's signature. In vetoing and returning it to Congress, he enclosed his customary message of explanation for his action; but on this occasion, Tumulty wrote the justification and Secretary Houston vetted it. The House overrode the veto 175 to 55 that same day; the Senate overrode 64 to 20 the next. Within three months, the United States was under the influence of Prohibition—the first constitutional amendment ever to abridge rights of the people.

The next week Lansing submitted a Thanksgiving Proclamation for Wilson's approval, and its return the next day troubled him. Practically every other document he had ever submitted to the President came back with corrections in the schoolmaster's hand. This was unmarked, except for a disturbingly illegible signature, in pencil. Lansing could not see how Wilson could possibly "conduct the government for months to come." He told House that the President was already displeased with his having called one or two Cabinet meetings but that he intended to continue doing so, because he thought it "the proper thing to do." To the public, the mystery prevailed as to whether the President had suffered a stroke.

The charade continued. Dr. Grayson never strayed from the party line: "His body was broken," he said of the President, "but his intellect was unimpaired and his lion spirit untamed. His collapse brought no weakening of his purpose." That was not the whole truth. Ike Hoover, one of a handful of people permitted into the sickroom, saw that the President lay

there most of the time "helpless." Hoover saw improvement, but he said what most refused to admit: "There was never a moment during all that time when he was more than a shadow of his former self. He had changed from a giant to a pygmy in every wise. He was physically almost incapacitated; he could articulate but indistinctly and think but feebly." So pathetic was the sight, Hoover said the few who served him turned away from his gaze. Not Edith. So long as the government continued to function and Wilson's judgment determined its policy, she saw no reason to alter the practice of sequestering her husband and issuing documents in his name, even if it required a certain amount of extrapolation on her part. "I carried out the directions of the doctors," she would later write. "Woodrow Wilson was first my beloved husband whose life I was trying to save, fighting with my back to the wall—after that he was the President of the United States."

A month passed during which no government official, not even a secretary, saw the President of the United States. Nobody even shaved him. Once a day, somebody would hoist him from his bed and set him in a comfortable chair. After several days, Wilson tried an invalid rolling chair, but that proved ineffective because he could not sit upright in it. At last, Hoover suggested a rolling chair such as those on the boardwalk in Atlantic City. The White House rented one from a New Jersey dealer for five dollars a week, and in time, bought it outright. For months, Wilson used the chair whenever he left his bed.

Just as Wilson seemed to be improving, he suffered another setback. A troubling prostatic condition worsened, creating a urinary obstruction. One of Wilson's doctors urged the high-risk operation of an abdominal incision and the insertion of a catheter into the patient's bladder. Grayson balked, calling upon Doctor Hugh Hampton Young of the Johns Hopkins Medical School, the country's authority on the prostate gland, to join the private White House team. He believed the dangers of the operation outweighed those of waiting. Overloaded with information, Edith sided with those who would allow nature to take its course. It did, but not without sapping much of the President's strength. While it forced him to submit to more rest, it allowed him, at last, to turn a corner for the better. For a month, Woodrow Wilson had been able to perform only the most basic duties of office.

By the end of October, the White House troika of Edith, Grayson, and

Tumulty believed that Wilson was far enough out of the woods to expose the President in a few carefully managed visits. At four in the afternoon on the thirtieth, Attorney General Palmer became the first Cabinet member to see the President since his stroke. They conferred for twenty minutes about an impending coal strike, one that the Administration was challenging on grounds that it violated the Lever Act, one of those war measures that still lingered, endowing the executive branch with extraordinary powers. Palmer reported to the press that the President was alert, attentive, and had offered "suggestions of his own." He also wired the Ambassador to Japan, "Alarming rumors concerning president's condition quite unfounded. Physically weak but in every other respect in splendid shape. Doctors report him rapidly improving. He transacts public business daily."

Little more than an hour later, Wilson engaged in a more publicized private meeting. For months, King Albert and Queen Elisabeth of Belgium, and their son Prince Leopold, had planned a trip to the United States, where they were meant to be guests at the White House. They were mid-ocean when Wilson suffered his stroke. As a result, they downscaled their itinerary and turned their ceremonial visit into a less formal tour of the States, traveling largely incognito. While visiting Washington, they stayed in the private residence of an Administration diplomat, and the Thomas Marshalls entertained them.

Beyond his genuine admiration of the King and Queen, these noble survivors of German aggression making a state visit would have served Wilson well in his fight for the League. Recognizing the publicity value in the President's receiving visitors and knowing what a boost it would be for Wilson to greet them, the White House arranged an informal meeting. Edith, Jessie Sayre, and Margaret Wilson received them in the Red Room. After tea, Edith asked if she might take His Majesty to see the President. Before doing so, the Royal Couple presented Edith with a beautiful wooden box, which contained eighteen plates, each with a hand-painted representation of a historic place in Belgium, some of which had since been destroyed. Queen Elisabeth presented Edith a fan of Belgian lace, adorned with diamonds and sapphires.

Upstairs, King Albert demonstrated only "sympathy and solicitude" as he beheld the frail creature in his dressing gown and with a mustache and long white beard. While Dr. Grayson stood by, they spoke for a few

minutes, after which Albert presented the china dishes and discussed each of the scenes depicted thereon. The President, in turn, offered the King a specially bound set of his *History of the American People*, the first volume of which he had autographed. After they said their goodbyes, Edith gave the Royal Couple a tour of the White House. Just when she thought they were leaving, the Queen said she wished to see the President. Edith saw no graceful way of denying her, and by the time they had returned to the bedroom, Wilson had removed his robe and returned to bed with a favorite gray woolen sweater that he had bought years earlier in Scotland draped over his shoulders. The Queen was delighted to have come upon him studying his new plates with a large magnifying glass. When the President asked after the young prince, the Queen said he was downstairs. Grayson permitted his entry as well. Present for all three of the bedside visitations, he provided the details to the press, including the King's having told the President, "I hope that your ideas and ideals will be carried out. My feeling is that they will be."

Two weeks later, the Wilsons received the Prince of Wales, the man who would become King Edward VIII. Conversation between the President and the British media darling remained light, of little more substance than Wilson's misinforming him that his grandfather Edward VII had slept in the very bed before him when he had visited President James Buchanan in 1860.

Court intrigue accompanied the Prince of Wales's visit, as the British Ambassador, Lord Grey, had been requesting a Presidential audience for weeks, and he was deliberately not asked to accompany Edward. That was evidently the result of Grey's having invited an adjutant from England, Major Charles Kennedy Craufurd-Stuart, to be part of his delegation in America. Craufurd-Stuart, unfortunately, had a penchant for gossip, dining out on outrageous remarks. One such jape making the rounds of Washington's finest tables was his comment that when Wilson had proposed to Edith, "she was so surprised that she nearly fell out of bed."

The bedside visit between the twenty-five-year-old Prince and the sixty-two-year-old President created a lot of cheery coverage, a welcome relief from the gloomy reports emanating from the White House. It suggested Wilson's continuing recovery. Later that day, the press also reported his being wheeled to the rear porch of the White House, where he enjoyed the open air. On November 12, he called for a mirror and took a long look,

turning his head from side to side. "Doctor," he called out, before reciting one of his favorite limericks:

> *For beauty I am not a star,*
> *There are others more handsome by far,*
> *But my face I don't mind it*
> *For I am behind it,*
> *It's the folks in front that I jar.*

He received his first shave in six weeks.

In all that time, the Senate had maintained its distance from the White House, less out of respect than for political advantage. Democrats did not want to draw attention to their leader's helplessness, while Republicans happily exploited it. Lodge's intention had never been to dispose of the League altogether, merely to disguise it as a Republican plan, thereby damaging the opposition party and Wilson's reputation. Now, with the President sidelined longer than anybody had ever imagined, Lodge realized he could actually kill the entire Treaty, League and all. Lodge said he merely wanted "to Americanize the Treaty and the Covenant"—which Secretary David Houston translated as: "he would show the people that the Republicans had sufficiently rewritten the Treaty to save the situation." With the Irreconcilables in his pocket, Lodge attempted to appeal to the Mild Reservationists by appearing reasonable, knowing that the minute he suggested anything directed toward Article X, the President would be intractable.

Between the day of the President's stroke and November 6, the Senate had approved in committee a list of fifty-two modifications to the Treaty—some minor administrative paper cuts, others substantive amputations. Senator Albert B. Fall alone introduced three dozen petty proposals—such as America's sitting on commissions related to governance of the Saar Basin or sending troops to Upper Silesia or drawing the new Belgian border. Senator Lawrence Sherman of Illinois wanted to insert a phrase invoking "the gracious favor of Almighty God"; Senator Gore proposed adding an "advisory vote of the people" on top of any League decisions regarding nations resorting to war; La Follette wanted to excise the labor articles from

the Treaty; Lodge wanted to strike the Shantung provisions. Under Hitch-cock's leadership, all the President's men in the Senate had successfully defeated the amendments, prompting Lodge to spring right back with a list of what Hitchcock called "destructive reservations." These items sub-stantively reduced Lodge's objections to fifteen points. In polishing them for presentation on November 6, the Republican forces designated the first as a "preamble," so that Lodge could offer his own fourteen counterpoints. The opposition had effectively gridlocked the Treaty—to the point that anybody who had Wilson's ear over the next two weeks offered but one solution: compromise.

Gilbert Hitchcock was the first such visitor, sandwiched between the royal visits. Edith had allowed the President's initial business conference because his advocate in the Senate sought guidance in attracting his unde-cided colleagues. Granted a half hour, he had encountered an "intellectu-ally alert" but cadaverous Wilson, still with his wispy white beard. Propped up in bed, he buried his limp arm under the bedclothes. Wilson said he would accept "any compromise the friends of the treaty thought necessary to save the treaty, so long as it did not destroy the terms of the pact itself." And he made it plain that Lodge's reservations would "kill the treaty." Hitchcock insisted that without some changes, American entrance into the League would be impossible. Wilson asked how many Senators would vote for the Treaty without reservations, and Hitchcock told him "not forty-five out of ninety-six." Wilson groaned: "Is it possible, is it possible?"

Hitchcock proved to be a dogged spokesman; but, as Senator Tom Con-nally of Texas observed, he was simply "no match for the snarling growls and the biting fangs of Lodge, Borah, Johnson and Reed." As always, Lodge kept zeroing in on Article X of the Treaty, the guarantee against external aggression through collective security. Hitchcock insisted repeat-edly that any such action demanded unanimity from the League Council and Congressional approval before America could commit to engaging in League actions. Lodge paid no attention, knowing that, in politics, con-stant repetition can harden even obvious falsities into facts. He just kept saying, "The article bypassed Congress."

While Edith had feared too much politics might weaken her husband, she knew that it was his lifeblood. Still, she filtered the information that reached him, limiting incoming opinions on the Treaty to those from friends in court. Tumulty reported that his inbox was filled with messages

urging compromise. Bernard Baruch implored Wilson to accept that "half a loaf is better than no bread." Herbert Hoover wrote that, considering the reservations as a whole, "they do not seem . . . to imperil the great principle of the League of Nations to prevent war" and should be accepted at once. Even the banished Colonel House—bedridden himself, with gallstones—got involved in an intricate back-channel effort that might not only rescue the Treaty but also put him back in Wilson's good graces.

House urged Stephen Bonsal, his worldly attaché from Paris, to meet with his friend Henry Cabot Lodge. In the course of their conversation on October 28 at Lodge's house near Dupont Circle, Bonsal got the impression that the Senator was not as confident of "hamstringing" the Covenant as he appeared in public and that he was even prepared to compromise. Over two more conversations during the week, Bonsal induced Lodge to pencil right on a copy of the Treaty fifty words of "inserts," which included a few phrases that underscored Congressional authority. Bonsal persuaded Lodge to agree that those conditions were implicit within the original document, but the old Senator maintained that he had improved the Treaty, the language of which he had found unworthy. "It might get by at Princeton," he said, "but certainly not at Harvard."

Bonsal sent the Lodge-edited Treaty—which would surely have met Senate approval, if not unanimity—to House, who claimed to have forwarded it to Tumulty. Nobody knows if it ever got past his desk or if Mrs. Wilson simply dismissed it because it came from Colonel House or because she or the President saw Lodge's rewrite of Article X, which Wilson would have automatically rejected. In all likelihood, nobody ever saw it—certainly not Senator Hitchcock.

At first he thought that Lodge "merely wished to weave into the Covenant some of his great thoughts, so that this world charter would not, in the future, be regarded as a party document." Now Hitchcock realized that Lodge's "hatred of Wilson is very deep and his talking point is that, as the President did not permit any real Republicans to participate in the drafting of the Treaty," the Republicans now had "a perfectly free hand in the matter of ratification," a greater responsibility than would have been theirs had they been included during the initial drafting process. For his part, Hitchcock—like most of his Democratic colleagues—favored a ratified Treaty in almost any form, if only to "end the present disastrous anarchy that prevails in world relations." But he was obligated to honor the

President's commands. Even when the White House handed them down indirectly, the message remained clear. "I am merely told 'the President will not budge an inch,'" Hitchcock told Bonsal. "His honor is at stake. He feels he would be dishonored if he failed to live up to the pledges made to his fellow delegates in Paris."

And then, as the Senate vote approached, not even Edith Wilson could hold back any longer. "In my anxiety for the one I love best in the world," she confessed years later, "the long-drawn-out fight was eating into my very soul, and I felt nothing mattered but to get the Treaty ratified, even with those reservations." While sitting at her husband's bedside, she said, "For my sake . . . won't you accept these reservations and get this awful thing settled?"

Woodrow turned his head on the pillow and reached out to take Edith's hand. "Little girl," he said, "don't you desert me; that I cannot stand. Can't you see that I have no moral right to accept any change in a paper I have signed without giving to every other signatory, even the Germans, the right to do the same thing? It is not *I* that will not accept; it is the Nation's honour that is at stake." Almost immediately, Edith felt ashamed for having joined his "betrayers," even momentarily. "Better a thousand times to go down fighting," he said, "than to dip your colours to dishonourable compromise."

On November 17, Senator Hitchcock returned to the White House for another meeting with the President. The Senator found a different man—clean-shaven and sitting up taller—in the Lincoln Bed. Hitchcock raised the subject of the Lodge Resolution, which he had sent in advance and which Dr. Grayson had read to the President. Wilson wasted no time in expressing himself: "I consider it a nullification of the Treaty and utterly impossible," he said. Wilson maintained that the Lodge reservations cut "the very heart" out of the Treaty. "I could not stand for those changes for a moment because it would humiliate the United States before all of the allied countries," he said. Hitchcock asked the President to explain just what effect a defeat of the Treaty would have.

"The United States would suffer the contempt of the world," he said. "We will be playing into Germany's hands. Think of the humiliation we would suffer in having to ask Germany whether she would accept such and such reservation!" The President experienced a surge of energy such as he had not felt since taking to his bed. He unleashed a furious tirade over

the political situation as well as his physical inability to combat it. "If the Republicans are bent on defeating this Treaty," he said, "I want the vote of each, Republican and Democrat, recorded, because they will have to answer to the country in the future for their acts. They must answer to the people." And then, making threats an invalid could not really back, Wilson said, "I am going to debate this issue with these gentlemen in their respective states whenever they come up for re-election. . . . I shall do this even if I have to give my life to it." His spleen vented, Wilson said he held no hostility toward the Senators in opposition—only "an utter contempt." With the exception of interpretations, Wilson insisted he was as unwilling as ever to compromise on anything that would require "a recommitment to council with other nations."

Wilson spent almost another hour asking Hitchcock to walk him through the last six weeks of legislative knavery that had led to the impending vote. "I have been lying on my back and have been very weak," he said. He knew that he had been "kept in the dark" except for what Edith and Grayson had told him; and, he imparted that "they have purposely kept a good deal from me." Upon leaving, the Senator said, "Mr. President, I hope I have not weakened you by this long discussion." Wilson smiled and said, "No, Senator, you have strengthened me against the opponents." In the hall, Hitchcock said to Grayson, "I would give anything if the Democrats, in fact, all the Senate, could see the attitude that man took this morning. Think how effective it would be if they could see the picture as you and I saw it this morning!"

For the first time since his stroke, attendants rolled Wilson in his wheelchair onto the South Lawn, where his flock of Red Cross sheep continued to graze. Hitchcock returned to the Senate to make his best efforts to convince his colleagues. He drafted a letter—which he sent to Mrs. Wilson—for the President to send back, which stated his position on the upcoming vote. It urged friends and supporters of the Treaty to vote against the Lodge Resolution—"for in my opinion the resolution in that form does not provide for ratification, but rather for defeat of the treaty." Later that day, Edith read the letter to her husband, who dictated some minor changes, the most consequential of which was changing the word "defeat" to "the nullification."

At Hitchcock's direction, those Democrats who favored the Treaty caucused on the morning of November 19, 1919, to discuss the Lodge

Resolution. Senator Underwood of Alabama moved that they unite against it; and then Hitchcock drew "Wilson"'s letter from his breast pocket and read those same instructions to his most loyal supporters. Senator Ashurst asked to examine the letter and could not help noticing that the President's signature had been rubber-stamped in purple ink. At noon the Senate convened for a final debate of the Treaty. It played out as Hitchcock had predicted: the Lodge Resolution of ratification met defeat, with thirty-nine ayes against fifty-five nays—a combination of forty-two Democrats and thirteen Republicans, the Irreconcilables among them. Oscar Underwood introduced the unencumbered Treaty, exactly as Wilson had delivered it from France, and it faced an almost identical result, thirty-eight ayes to fifty-three nays. Incredulously, Henry Ashurst recorded in his diary that night that the Treaty of Versailles—a six-month labor of the world's leaders, ratified by the principal Allied and Associated Powers and even signed by the enemy—could muster the votes of only thirty-eight United States Senators. With the Senate adjourning, Lodge would declare he had done all the compromising he intended to do. Underwood and Hitchcock concurred that the Treaty was deadlocked, but not dead. Partisan politics was that day's only victor, the Treaty its victim. There would be a few months before everybody would revisit the document, during which time the President could allow the Senate to redraw the Treaty. One man held the power to break the stalemate, but he remained stuck in bed and in his unwillingness to compromise.

Fearing the effect "the fatal news" from Capitol Hill would have on her husband, Edith broke it to him gently. Silence filled the room for a moment, until Woodrow said, "All the more reason I must get well and try again to bring this country to a sense of its great opportunity and greater responsibility."

Such wishful thinking did not seem out of place in the current White House, which was awash in denial. In order to maintain strict silence, Edith had banned the public from the White House and its grounds. In the private quarters and the empty public rooms, staff members tiptoed, unaware of just how sick the patient upstairs was. Those few in the know kept up appearances, pretending everything was all right and covering for the President wherever possible. Opacity bred suspicion, and the longer this masquerade continued without the President's appearing in public, the worse the rumors became. Some said Wilson had lost his mind. His

reciting limericks was twisted into talk of his babbling nursery rhymes. Enemies whispered that bars had to be placed over the White House windows—as, in fact, people suddenly became aware of such metalwork, failing to realize that President Roosevelt had installed it years earlier to protect the glass from his rambunctious children. In truth, the President's health slowly and steadily improved; but as Ike Hoover later revealed, "If there was ever a man in bad shape, he was. He could not talk plainly, mumbled more than he articulated, was helpless and looked like a man fatally ill. Everybody tried to help him, realizing he was so dependent for everything."

Vice President Marshall showed up at the White House one day, hoping to see the President, but he could not get past Mrs. Wilson. She said she would convey news of his visit, but Marshall was never to hear from the President again. In addition to presiding over the Senate, he continued to make speeches on the after-dinner circuit. He privately believed Wilson should accept mild reservations, but he publicly stood behind the President.

While Marshall was in the middle of a speech on November 23, 1919, under the auspices of the Loyal Order of Moose of Atlanta, a prominent local stepped to his side and delivered the news that President Wilson had died. Marshall bowed his head, as did everyone else who had heard. After a moment, he faced the crowd and said, "I cannot bear the great burdens of our beloved chieftain unless I receive the assistance of everybody in this country." As men in the auditorium bowed their heads and women cried, the organist in the hall played "Nearer, My God, to Thee." Marshall hastily left the stage to telephone the Associated Press, only to learn the entire story was a hoax. Marshall would later confess to Josephus Daniels that he had been stunned, first by grief and then by "the awful responsibility that would fall upon me. I was resolved to do my duty but I can truly say that I dreaded the great task."

The incident encouraged nobody at the White House to alter the current protocol. The inner circle closed ranks. Tumulty kept the gate of the West Wing, while Edith controlled access to the bedroom and Grayson constantly observed the President. Because the public would expect a Presidential statement on the first anniversary of the Armistice, Tumulty composed it. While the three paragraphs lacked the President's eloquence, they

spoke of the need to seek peace in international councils. With the Congress set to reconvene on December 2, he also began drafting the Annual Message in the President's name. Wilson's inability to deliver (to say nothing of write) the speech himself would be a particular disappointment to the President who had reintroduced the tradition of appearing in person before the Congress. Eventually, relying on contributions of the Cabinet officers and sentences and sentiments from Wilson's Western tour, Tumulty was able to prepare a draft of Presidential stature. Wilson had the speech read to him, and he offered corrections, which his wife transcribed.

The State of the Union message—generic and bland—touched upon such issues as the need for the executive branch to submit a budget, to simplify the tax code, to achieve a better understanding between capital and labor, and to temper "the widespread condition of political restlessness in our body politic." Reaction from Congress followed party lines. Democrats praised its call to action, while Republicans issued baiting criticism. George Moses of New Hampshire said it was "a very poor piece of literary mechanics, considering its putative authorship." Fall of New Mexico said, "The President's message doesn't mean anything. I wonder when he wrote it."

The White House—presumably Tumulty—dealt with the latter issue by talking to *The New York Times*. The paper ran a page-one item detailing the marked improvement in Wilson's handwriting, even in the "extremely clear and unwavering" nature of his shorthand notes—when, in truth, the President was still incapable of writing such notes and none existed. Two months after Wilson had disappeared from public view, Congressmen were asserting that "whatever the state of his health it is time that Congress and the country should know the facts."

"The question as to whether the President is actually and generally performing his official duties and whether he is mentally and physically capable of doing so is growing more and more insistent," Robert Lansing wrote in a memorandum for his own files. He particularly questioned the authorship of the Annual Message, and was correct in assessing that "the loose stones are there but the cement is not." Seasoned politico Albert Burleson considered Tumulty's fabrication of the speech both "a fine piece of political work" and a "deception." Lansing said, "If it ever gets out it will make a fine scandal." Short of that, Republicans believed they had found

a great potential embarrassment for the President. A chorus of Senators declared that Wilson was constitutionally unable to discharge his duties. Without any substantiation, George Moses announced that Wilson had suffered a brain lesion and was unable to "transact business."

Two thousand miles away and almost ten years into Mexico's violent revolution, the Carranza government arrested an American consular official named William O. Jenkins, accusing him of staging his own kidnapping in order to discredit the current regime. The crusty and corrupt Senator from New Mexico, Albert Fall, had been complaining for weeks that the United States had no President. "We have petticoat government," he said, pounding on a table. "Wilson is not acting. Mrs. Wilson is president." And now the Senator seized the opportunity to summon Wilson not only to respond with aggressive military action but also to receive a committee, one consisting of Hitchcock and himself. At last, the Republicans would unmask the President. When Dr. Grayson presented the proposition to his patient, Wilson said he was happy to oblige.

Grayson milked the acceptance, telling Fall that the President was "undergoing a rest cure" and that he personally preferred Wilson's avoiding controversial matters . . . but that he saw no reason why the President could not "transact any business" and meet the Senate's demands. Fall called the doctor's bluff and asked when they might visit. Grayson said at 2:30 that very afternoon, a Friday. When Fall suggested the matter could wait until Monday, by which time he could consult his caucus, Grayson insisted there was no reason to delay this visit—which Wilson called "a smelling committee," one meant to ascertain whether his corpse had begun to rot.

When the two-man delegation arrived at the Executive Mansion, Senator Fall asked Grayson how long they could stay. The doctor dealt the prickly Republican Senator a "staggering blow" when he imposed no time constraints. The three men ascended to the second floor, where the Wilsons awaited in the carefully staged bedroom at the end of the hall.

The President had directed all the lights in his room turned on, to create a bright atmosphere. He remained in bed, his head only slightly elevated, his left arm buried under the covers, while papers were placed on the nightstand to his right—props with which he might demonstrate dexterity. Edith greeted the visitors, a pencil in one hand and a pad in the other—"so I would not have to shake hands with him," she later wrote of

Fall. She sat quietly through the entire meeting, taking notes in her flowery schoolgirl penmanship. "I hope you will consider me sincere," said the gentleman from New Mexico, by way of opening the meeting. "I have been praying for you, Sir."

"Which way, Senator?" the President replied, according to Edith, who also recounted Fall's laughing at the quip. And with that, for all intents and purposes, the meeting was over—as the President revealed that his wit and his wits remained intact. But the visit lasted another forty-five minutes, during which time Wilson displayed a thorough grasp of the Mexican situation, including knowledge of Fall's investments south of the border. Called to the telephone during the meeting, Grayson learned that Jenkins in Mexico, in fact, had been released the previous night. The doctor interrupted the conference to impart this information, which rendered further discussion pointless. Wilson spoke of getting on his feet again soon, so that he could visit the Capitol "and take up personally problems affecting the Government." He asked Fall to convey that sentiment to his colleague from New Hampshire, hoping Senator Moses would be "reassured." When Fall descended in the elevator, Secret Service agent Starling asked how he had found the President. "If there is something wrong with his mind," said Senator Fall, "I would like to get the same ailment." Wilson had delivered a consummate performance, conveying a vitality beyond his actual capacity.

That did not, however, put the issue of Presidential inability to rest. The public was willing to overlook Wilson's condition so long as its limitations remained abstract; but some in the Administration were less sanguine, especially the Secretary of State. While Wilson was mentally competent, Lansing wondered how long a physically incapacitated President could run the country. Fall had left the White House having failed to ascertain the extent of Wilson's paralysis, his nerves, and his overall strength. "I feel that the secrecy which has prevailed should come to an end," Lansing wrote in a memorandum intended for history's eyes only. And though he had no intention of exposing his boss, he succinctly stated what he considered a constitutional crisis, one nobody had chosen to address: "It is not Woodrow Wilson but the President of the United States who is ill. His family and his physicians have no right to shroud the whole affair in mystery as they have done."

.   .   .

"Things fall apart," William Butler Yeats wrote that year; "the centre cannot hold; / Mere anarchy is loosed upon the world." While he was pondering the dissolution of one era with dark visions of the next, he might just as well have been describing the Wilson White House. Although Wilson's physical condition continued to improve, his mind often raced ahead of his body's limitations. Post-stroke depression clouded many of his thoughts, some of which were faintly delusional. Frequently petulant because he was stuck in the world of his own mind most of the time, with few stimuli and little information beyond that which his wife and physician spoon-fed, many of Woodrow Wilson's actions after October 2, 1919, were highly questionable. Unfortunately, nobody but Edith could challenge him; and in her efforts to ensure his health, she had abdicated that responsibility. The country, like its leader, drifted.

After eleven weeks in which Edith had allowed the President to per-form the absolute minimum that his job required, the logjam of untended business brought the White House to a virtual standstill. Tumulty wrote Mrs. Wilson on December 18, 1919, listing more than a dozen items that demanded the President's attention. They were necessary not only to main-tain the steady flow of government business but also because failure to address them would highlight the President's negligence.

Washington has always relied on temporary appointees to administer the nation's bureaucracies. And at the end of 1919, the Civil Service, Fed-eral Trade, Interstate Commerce, and United States Tariff Commissions all needed positions filled; the Waterways Commission had seven vacancies. Often the bureaucracies themselves, not just the people running them, had term limits, which required Presidential attention.

The Railway Control Act of 1918, for example, had authorized the government to operate America's railroads for the duration of the war and a "reasonable time" thereafter. Railroad czar McAdoo and his successor, Walker Hines, had run the trains more effectively than private ownership. But now, a year after the Armistice, the future of the system could be de-layed no longer. Because of an inevitable drop-off in traffic as the nation retreated to a peacetime economy, a period of losses and liquidation en-sued. Many companies made claims against the government for damage to their property. Hines wrote Wilson that "widespread uncertainty" might

easily become "the basis of unfair manipulation of the prices of railroad securities," employees were pressing for increases in wages, and somebody had to take responsibility for maintaining the property currently in the hands of the Railroad Administration. Over the course of a week, the necessary paperwork—which should have required a few hours—passed through a dozen hands, always reverting to Edith and barely averting a crisis.

Equally troublesome, American foreign policy had been rudderless for months. Despite Secretary Lansing's repeated insistence, Britain's Ambassador ended his brief posting in Washington without any communication from the President. The snub was not enough to kick off an international incident, but it was an insulting misstep. In the meantime, the diplomatic corps simply floated, with at least eight countries—China, Italy, and the Netherlands among them—without an American Ambassador. In some cases, envoys had been selected but awaited final authorization from the President. One country desperately needed not only an Ambassador but the recognition that might assure its democratic future. Having deposed a military dictator, Costa Rica teetered on the brink of financial ruin and feared the return of the despot as it waited seven months for the United States to recognize its government.

As 1919 saw more changes in the world order than any year in centuries, the White House infrastructure begin to collapse. Upon the death of Virginia Senator Martin in November, Carter Glass surrendered his secretaryship to fill the seat, leaving a vacancy at the Treasury Department. The fourth Sunday into the New Year, David Houston awoke with the grippe, only to receive a call from the White House informing him that Mrs. Wilson wished to see him that afternoon. "Of course, you know that I did not ask you to take the trouble to come merely to drink tea," she said. While the President upstairs was reluctant to move Houston from the Agriculture Department, she said, "he now needs you more in the Treasury." After she delivered all her husband's arguments for his assuming the new position, Houston said, "I am in the harness until March 4, 1921, if he wishes it, and as long as I am with him, I will dig stumps, or act as Secretary of the Treasury, or assume any other task he assigns me." Edith smiled and said, "That is just what the President said you would say."

Wilson's severe mental and physical limitations forced a hurried selection of inferior appointments to his recomposed Cabinet. In discussing

Houston's replacement at Agriculture, for example, Mrs. Wilson said the President had been considering Edwin T. Meredith—a Populist Iowan with a history of newspaper and agricultural publishing and unsuccessful runs for the Senate and the governorship. Houston acknowledged that he had the right background but questioned his intellectual ability and "whether he was Cabinet size or not." Meredith received the appointment a week later, as the President simply lacked the energy to conduct a thorough search. (Meredith would leave no mark on government that could match his significant legacy in magazine publishing, especially when he changed the name of his periodical from *Fruit, Garden and Home* to *Better Homes and Gardens.*)

Interior Secretary Lane had talked of resigning for months, taking issue with the President even before the League fight, over leasing certain oil properties. The deals appeared to be legal, but Wilson—who had maintained a scandal-free administration—told Lane he wanted to study them before releasing government property to private capital. After Wilson fell ill, many such leases came to the President's desk for signature. Edith studied each such matter, put the papers in neat stacks, and carried them to the Lincoln Bed, where he signed as many documents as possible before tiring. The first time she presented one of these oil leases, however, he said, "That will not be signed, and, please, until I am able to study that situation do not bring me any more of them. It is better to let things wait than do a thing that to my uninformed judgment seems most unwise." Lane pressured Mrs. Wilson, saying the President's inaction reflected poorly on his running the Interior Department.

Even before Lane served notice, the President had sought his replacement. Mrs. Wilson told Houston that her husband preferred somebody not from the far West because most of the Department's problems stemmed from that region and "it was difficult to find a Western man who would take a sufficiently detached or national view." Within weeks, the White House had announced the appointment of Judge John B. Payne, a powerful attorney and party politician from Chicago who was also a member of the Shipping Board.

Prior to the President's stroke, Commerce Secretary Redfield had spoken of resigning, and on November 1 he returned to the private sector. Six-term Democratic Congressman Joshua W. Alexander of Missouri—a second choice, but the first in the alphabetical listing on the roster of a

Congressional Committee on Commerce—replaced him. Houston thought him "totally unfit."

And then the Cabinet almost lost Labor Secretary W. B. Wilson as a result of the first serious rupture between two department heads. Management and labor had called a ceasefire during the war, but after the Armistice, each side sought to reclaim its ground. The major struggle was between the colliers and mine operators, which sparked a dispute between Secretary Wilson and the President's old friend Harry Garfield, the acting Fuel Administrator and consumers' advocate. Miners threatened to strike if they did not receive a pay raise, and Garfield enlisted the help of Attorney General Palmer, who announced that the Cabinet unanimously supported his decision to enjoin the miners, which he said the Lever Act empowered him to do. W. B. Wilson was incensed because he had been negotiating with the miners and because the President had promised Samuel Gompers that the Lever Act would never be used to secure an injunction against labor. Only a hastily assembled bucket brigade of memos between the Cabinet Room and the Lincoln Bed could douse the ire of the Labor Secretary, as the President sided with him. More important, Josephus Daniels convinced the Labor Secretary that in those troubled times, it was "his duty to stick." He did, and Garfield resigned. "A well Wilson," Daniels later noted, "would have nipped the injunction in the bud."

A larger problem blossomed in the State Department when it became the Secretary's duty to leave. "Mr. Lansing should have retired long before," Edith would note. Like his predecessor, William Jennings Bryan, Robert Lansing realized that Wilson dictated his own foreign policy, which reduced the Secretary to little more than a facilitator. Even more humiliating, during the most challenging months in the Department's history, Wilson had always positioned Lansing behind Colonel House, often ignoring him. For his part, the President found Lansing devoid of imagination, a man of some insight but no vision. His evident displeasure with the final Treaty had demoralized Wilson at a time when he was "expending the last ounces of his strength" on its behalf. Once Wilson was confined to his bed, Lansing worked quietly but steadily to get the President to step down. As Wilson's health returned, he began to engage, at last, with the Secretary of State, but not in the way Lansing had expected.

In his series of memoranda to himself, Lansing steadily built a case against Wilson's continuance in office, and ultimately against his own. "I

don't know how I am going to stand the present state of affairs much longer," he wrote on December 10, 1919. "It has become almost intolerable."
Lansing believed Wilson was well enough to choose a successor at State
and to invalidate anything Lansing did in the interim; but he felt beholden
enough to the office not to resign until the President offered strong cause
to do so. He was correct in assuming that the President distrusted and
disliked him. "I don't care a rap about his good will," Lansing told himself,
"but I do care about his preventing me from properly conducting our foreign affairs."

Lansing never realized that his continued disappointments without
confrontation were among the reasons for Wilson's misgivings about him.
"I must continue," he recorded, ". . . though the irrascibility [sic] and tyranny of the President, whose worst qualities have come to the surface during his sickness, cannot be borne much longer." Lansing believed nobody
dared cross Wilson for fear of triggering another stroke. In the meantime,
he noted, "his violent passions and exaggerated ego have free rein." Unable
even to schedule an audience with him, Lansing went to the White House
at the turn of the new year to meet with Mrs. Wilson to stress the importance of taking action on several matters that he had already brought to
the President's attention. "The President," Edith snapped, "does not like
being told a thing twice." On January 7, 1920, Lansing told himself, "It is
only a question as to when I should send in my letter of resignation. I cannot wait much longer." He did not have to.

One month later—amid a volley of correspondence regarding Japanese
interests in Siberia and the conversion of Fiume into a free city under the
League's protection—Wilson sent Lansing a startling letter. "Is it true, as
I have been told," the President asked, "that during my illness you have
frequently called the heads of the executive departments of the Government into conference?" If that were the case, Wilson said, he felt it his
duty to remind the Secretary that under constitutional law and practice,
only the President had the right to summon the heads of the executive
departments into conference, and only he and the Congress had the right
to ask their views on public questions. The letter was the first that Lansing
had seen in months that bore the President's signature.

He felt the President's irritability had progressed to irrationality, which
he charitably assigned to his medical condition. He considered the brief
missive "brutal and offensive," especially as he considered the question

"entirely superfluous." He had no doubt that the President had known for months that he had called regular Cabinet meetings—unless, indeed, the President had become mentally imbalanced and completely forgetful. He replied that he had frequently assembled the Cabinet "to meet for informal conference," the result of the Secretaries' need to confer on interdepartmental matters. He insisted he never intended to overstep any constitutional boundaries, but if the President believed that Lansing had failed in his loyalty, he was prepared to resign. In fact, Lansing looked forward to the reprieve. "Woodrow Wilson is a tyrant," he wrote on February 9, "who even goes so far as to demand that all men shall *think* as he does or else be branded as traitors or ingrates. . . . Thank God I shall soon be a free man!"

The President's memory had not failed him. To the contrary, Wilson recalled every one of Lansing's infractions. He resented the Secretary's lack of enthusiasm for the Treaty and, even more, his expressing his opinion both privately and publicly—which had enabled Bullitt to quote Lansing before the Senate committee. These petty betrayals formed just the tip of the iceberg, as Wilson gradually realized that he had selected the wrong man for the position in the first place, a man who did not share his worldview. As Daniels observed, "Lansing was a Big Stick diplomat who believed in Dollar Diplomacy and in Force and had no part in Wilson's idealism and faith in real democracy." The last straw for Wilson came with Lansing's handling of the Jenkins affair, in which he seemed to encourage war with Mexico. Wilson's questioning Lansing about the Cabinet meetings was merely the pretext he offered for four years of untrustworthiness and attempts to steer foreign affairs from the President's path.

When Tumulty learned of the President's intention to discharge Lansing, he sat with him on the South Portico and argued that public opinion would say "it was the wrong time to do the right thing." Although still physically weak, Wilson in his "invalid chair" grabbed hold of his adviser's phrase and said, "Tumulty, it is never the wrong time to spike disloyalty. When Lansing sought to oust me, I was upon my back. I am on my feet now and I will not have disloyalty about me."

Edith implored her husband to state that his reasons for accepting the resignation went beyond the calling of meetings, that there had been "an accumulation of disloyalty." To cite only Lansing's last and most minor offense, she said, looked petty. Woodrow laughed. "Well, if I'm as big as you

think me," he said, "I can well afford to do a generous thing. If not I must take the blame." On February 11, 1920, Wilson wrote Lansing that he wished to take advantage of his "kind suggestion" to relinquish his office.

"Thank God," the Secretary of State wrote in his desk diary that day, "an intolerable situation is ended." For Lansing, perhaps; but he did not intend to let the President's letter go unanswered. The next day, instead of a one-line resignation, he sent a long letter justifying all his behavior in the last year—starting in Paris, where he had found his advice unwelcome, and proceeding to the calling of Cabinet meetings, which he believed were in the best interests of the Administration and the Republic. He insisted he had never sought to "usurp" Presidential authority. On Friday the thirteenth, Wilson accepted the resignation, effective immediately. Lansing's last act of business at the State Department was to mimeograph the final correspondence between him and the President, which he disseminated at 7:30 that evening.

"The President delivered himself into my hands and of course I took advantage of his stupidity," Lansing noted in his latest private memorandum, "for it surely was nothing less than stupidity on his part." So manifest were Wilson's "irritation and jealousy" in his letters and "so peevish" his tone, Lansing believed the President was not in his right mind. "I imagine that a pretty good-sized bomb has been exploded, which will cause a tremendous racket in this country and find an echo abroad." Lansing was right. Every newspaper in the country questioned the White House's decision.

Making matters worse was that just a few days earlier, urologist Hugh H. Young of Johns Hopkins—who was part of Wilson's medical team— had divulged details of his cerebral thrombosis. Although the doctor was quick to state that neither the vigor nor the lucidity of the President's mental processes was affected, these first details of his condition to reach the press cast suspicion over the White House. Coupled with Lansing's dismissal, the story assumed a life of its own. Appearing to be covering up, the White House had to produce other doctors to control the damage. Tumulty met with the President on Sunday, where he found the valet cutting his hair in the bathroom. "Well, Tumulty," Wilson said with a twinkle, "have I any friends left?" And Tumulty replied, "Very few." Wilson said that in a few days "what the country considers an indiscretion on my part in getting rid of Lansing will be forgotten, but when the sober,

second thought of the country begins to assert itself, what will stand out will be the disloyalty of Lansing to me."

Wilson was partially correct. The Lansing dismissal was quickly forgotten, but only because it ignited a more incendiary discussion about the President's overall competence. Newspapers invited physicians to offer their professional opinions. Dr. Arthur Dean Bevan, ex-president of the American Medical Association, took the White House to task for suggesting that the President had suffered from exhaustion when, in fact, he had suffered a paralyzing stroke. "He is evidently slowly recovering from the paralysis of his arm and leg and may recover fairly well, although never completely, the use of his limbs," said Bevan. "But the diseased arteries, which were responsible for the stroke and the damaged brain, remain and will not be recovered from." That being the case, he added, "A patient who is suffering as the President is . . . should under no circumstances be permitted to resume the work of such a strenuous position as that of President of the United States." Technically, Bevan reminded the press, the United States was still at war; and if Wilson as Commander in Chief of the Army and Navy were called before a nonpartisan medical board, "he would be at once retired as physically incapacitated to perform the duties of the position." Lansing heard that word on Capitol Hill was that the "President is crazy."

And then, in a Cabinet not known for grandstanding, one department head took advantage of the President's absence in a most aggressive, if not egregious, manner. Forty-eight-year-old Attorney General A. Mitchell Palmer was not only the youngest member of the Cabinet but also the most ambitious. With a national election less than a year away, he had his eye on the Oval Office and his hands on the issue on which he could run for election—national security.

The country had been rife with protests and growing hysteria all year. In early February 1919, the Mayor of Seattle had called for federal troops to prevent a massive workers' shutdown from becoming a subversive uprising. Later that month, while the President had been Stateside between sessions of the Peace Conference, the Secret Service had thwarted the attempts of a band of Spanish anarchists to assassinate him. In April a mail bomb arrived at the Atlanta home of Georgia's junior Senator, Thomas Hardwick, which maimed a housemaid. Identically wrapped packages, each containing a similar bomb, had been addressed to another five Senators, four Cabinet members, captains of capitalism John D. Rockefeller and J. P.

Morgan, and Supreme Court Justice Oliver Wendell Holmes, who had just ruled in the back-to-back cases that resulted in a definition of "clear and present danger" and the start of Eugene Debs's ten-year prison sentence. May Day 1919 saw protests from coast to coast that turned violent. Seeing the political havoc in Russia, some Americans became paranoid. Because there appeared to be outside agitators everywhere, xenophobia grew and "true Americans" sought to secure their borders. Anarchists, Communists, Socialists, striking union members, recent immigrants, people of color or with accents were all tarred with the same brush.

On the night of June 2, 1919—while his wife and daughter slept—Attorney General Palmer heard a car stop outside his townhouse on R Street. Carrying a suitcase, a man sprang from the car but tripped in the garden, and his bag exploded. Neighbor Franklin Roosevelt rushed across the street and learned that physical harm had come to nobody except the perpetrator, who died. At the same hour that same night, bombs at the homes of eight anti-radical judges and legislators—in Boston, New York, Pittsburgh, and Cleveland—also detonated. In all but one of those bombings, lives were spared. But back on R Street, one life got changed.

In his first days as Attorney General that spring, Palmer had been quick to recommend commutations of sentences for political prisoners, and he secured the release of five thousand enemy aliens on parole. Now he intended to vanquish "the Red Menace"—an international cabal of terrorists without borders that threatened to overthrow the American government. This war on terror was not just a political issue for the ambitious Quaker; it had become a personal vendetta.

In August 1919, Palmer enlisted a recent law graduate, J. Edgar Hoover, who was exactly half his age, to head the General Intelligence Division of the Justice Department's Bureau of Investigation. His orders were to collect enough information about radical aliens to deport them. Taking advantage of wartime sedition laws, Palmer authorized a series of pre-emptive attacks on a virtually invisible—and possibly imagined—enemy.

On November 6, 1919—the second anniversary of the Bolshevik revolution—he and the zealous Hoover unleashed an army of agents and local police forces into action in several cities. They busted into homes and meetinghouses with warrants for the arrest of more than six hundred suspected radicals. They found no bombs, but they did seize several tons of political literature. Before the end of the year, the Labor Department

deported 249 anarchists back to Russia, Emma Goldman among them. The raids were so well organized, most civilians had to admire the thoroughness of Palmer and Hoover's work. The nation's press—in which the raids were not even the lead story—generally applauded the restoration of law and order, and encouraged more such vigilance.

On January 2, 1920, Palmer delivered just that. Federal and local agents raided "centers of Red activities" in more than forty cities and towns, from Nashua, New Hampshire, to Los Angeles. For the most part, Palmer had warrants for the arrests of the suspects, largely immigrants who had sworn allegiance to the United States but then seemed bent upon overthrowing its government. He issued instructions for the conduct of the agents during the raids, which included that "violence to those apprehended should be scrupulously avoided" and that any citizen arrested as a Communist must be present while officers searched his home. Because so many different police departments were involved in the raids, it was impossible to supervise every arresting officer's behavior; and one cannot measure how much illegal behavior the federal agents overlooked as they trampled across the civil rights of many American citizens. It did become immediately apparent, however, that the local constabularies were far more severe in their arrest procedures than instructed. When Palmer tried to stop Illinois's chief law officer from conducting his own raids, the State's Attorney refused, accusing Palmer of "pussyfoot politics." Palmer and Hoover's plan had inflamed the Red Scare immeasurably, essentially encouraging fanaticism and fearmongering.

Only when the exhilaration surrounding the raids had died down did people realize the great Communist plot to usurp the United States was not as evolved as the Justice Department had suggested. The Communist Party had no great arsenal of guns and explosives; most of those arrested were not seditious, merely discontent; and their literature was not as dangerous as feared. The people realized that Palmer had ignored at least three constitutional rights—the freedom of speech, the right of the people to be secure against unreasonable searches and seizures, and citizen protection against being deprived of life, liberty, or property without due process of law. An absence of leadership created this blatant abrogation of civil rights, surely the nadir of the Wilson Administration.

A few hundred more citizens were deported. And just as the segregation of Washington had given license to other states to maintain Jim Crow

laws, so did the Palmer raids empower states and cities to impose their own standards of good citizenship, complete with loyalty oaths and witch hunts. Legionnaires and Klansmen became local vigilantes. And while the raids themselves ceased, their effects would linger through the century. Palmer, once known as a Progressive Congressman who supported labor and women's suffrage, would forever be remembered for the three months in which he abused the power of his office to an unprecedented extent. He geared up his Presidential campaign, running on a theme of "Americanism."

No evidence exists that the President had any prior knowledge of the raids, as Edith and Dr. Grayson continued to shield him from news outside the White House. Grayson said, "He is perfectly calm about everything that comes up *except* the treaty. That stirs him: makes him restless." In mid-December 1919, Wilson took his first halting steps since his collapse. A treeless Christmas and the President's sixty-third birthday passed quietly. "It has been the hardest year of your life and one that will live in history," the ever-faithful Tumulty wrote Wilson on December 28. "It may take time but you will be vindicated." Alas, Wilson strove not for vindication, but for victory.

Obsessed with the Treaty, he continued to dream up strategies to enable its passage. That month he concocted a harebrained scheme, which he asked Tumulty to draft into an open letter to the nation. He had long asserted that an overwhelming majority of the people desired its ratification, as he believed his seventeen-state tour had confirmed. Thus, with the Senate standing in the way of the people's will, the President wanted a national referendum. The Constitution providing no machinery for such a vote, he devised one. He intended to challenge more than half the nation's Senators to resign their seats and "take immediate steps to seek re-election . . . on the issue of their several records with regard to the ratification of the Treaty." If a majority of those gentlemen was reelected, Wilson promised to resign from office, as would the Vice President. Wilson had Edith ask the Attorney General to provide the legal ramifications of these mass resignations. Palmer's reply suggested the impossibility of such a phenomenon, to say nothing of the implausibility of any such mass compliance.

Kicking off the election year, the Democratic National Committee had hoped to receive a message from the President at its Jackson Day dinner.

Senator Ashurst warned Dr. Grayson that many members no longer wished to hear a demand for ratification of the Treaty without reservations, as it would further split an already divided Senate. Wilson would, of course be unable to attend the dinner, but he asked Tumulty to compose a letter to be read aloud, one that would incorporate his idea of a referendum. Tumulty obeyed, though he wondered if the President was not shooting himself in the foot. He asked Secretary Houston to vet the remarks, and he too pronounced the statement "unwise." He altered the letters in ways Wilson accepted, and the President even added a sentence of his own, stressing a moral point.

The party faithful roundly cheered the President's remarks that night, but one of the evening's guests of honor, William Jennings Bryan, neutralized their effect when he spoke of the need to come to an immediate agreement within the Senate to keep the Treaty "out of politics," for fear that it was not a winning issue for them in November. Instead, he argued for ratification of the Treaty without delay, even if that meant compromise.

The President still would not hear of it. With debate on the Treaty about to begin anew, Wilson had taken nothing from the Republican arguments except the need to dig his heels in deeper. He had released a statement that he had "no compromise or concession of any kind in mind," but intended that "the Republican leaders of the Senate shall continue to bear the undivided responsibility for the fate of the treaty and the present condition of the world in consequence of that fate." When Senator Hitchcock pressed Wilson to make peace with their chief adversary, the President snapped, "Let Lodge hold out the olive branch!"

In exasperation, several Senators from both sides of the aisle formed a bipartisan committee to produce a compromise of its own. Before they reached a final agreement, Tumulty wrote Mrs. Wilson that it behooved the White House to offer its own such document, for fear that a successful Senatorial compromise would preclude the President from having any say at all. He wrote a draft of a letter for Wilson to send to Hitchcock stating his "irreducible minimum" terms. Two days later, he wrote her again to announce that the "psychological moment" was approaching, providing the President "his great opportunity," perhaps his last. Before the bipartisan conference reached an agreement, the Republican Majority Leader threatened to strip Lodge of his leadership unless he blocked the super-

committee. Lodge told those negotiating that he would not consider further changes to his reservations.

Just when Wilson seemed as vital as he had been in months, an influenza epidemic descended upon Washington, and the President appeared to be among its victims. Dr. Grayson informed nobody other than Edith and Margaret Wilson of his condition, for fear of what the press and the President's enemies would do. That proved to be sound thinking, as within two days his flu-like virus had passed. But as had occurred in Paris after he had been similarly stricken, he suffered curious repercussions: frequent mood swings in which he experienced random moments of euphoria and depression, defiance and defeatism. But compromise remained unthinkable.

Ray Baker—who had just published a book about Wilson in Paris and had become the family's "court" historian—lunched with Edith Wilson that week. She trusted him as much as anybody outside the innermost circle. And even Baker—a true believer in the Wilsonian cause—used the opportunity to nudge her toward compromise by telling her what people outside the White House were feeling. He spoke of their wholehearted support of the spirit of the Treaty and their hope for a League, but he added that they were "profoundly disturbed" to see it bogged down in politics and semantics. For that, he suggested, people were just as inclined to blame Mr. Wilson as Mr. Lodge. "They think him stubborn," Edith declared. Baker simply reminded her how much depended on this issue, including the very existence of her husband's beloved League. "I know," she said, "but the President still has in mind the reception he got in the west, and he believes the people are with him."

Presidents traditionally speak of the isolation of the White House, but none had been as removed as Woodrow Wilson—confined for months to a bed, seeing almost nobody and hearing no direct news. "This sick man, with such enormous power, closed in from the world," Baker noted in his diary, "& yet acting so influentially upon events!" Edith seemed to be in full accord with Baker's desire for the President to offer "some great gesture" that would clear the bottleneck and allow passage of the Treaty. "Yet he hardens at any such suggestion," Baker observed: "yielding anything to the Senate seems to drive him into stubborn immovability."

"Was there ever such a situation in our history!" Baker mused on January 23, 1920. "Everything must come through one overstrained

woman!" He found himself conjuring images of "this lonely sick man, attacked from all sides" and contrasting them with the same man he had seen just the year before as he was hailed along the great boulevards of Europe. Tumulty wrote Wilson "that our forces are rapidly disintegrating." A long meeting with supportive Senators Joseph T. Robinson of Arkansas and Carter Glass convinced him that the public was demanding "immediate action," even if it meant accepting the Lodge reservations.

The next Sunday night—February 29, 1920—Tumulty joined fifteen members of the Democratic Party's power elite—Hitchcock and Glass from the Senate, Texan John Nance Garner from the House, a few governmental board chairmen, and more than half the Cabinet: resolute Wilsonians all—for dinner at the Chevy Chase Club. Party chairman Homer Cummings presided over an agenda the first item of which was how to deal with the Treaty situation. He read a letter from Frank I. Cobb, Wilson's most ardent defender in the press, who advocated acceptance of the reservations. Hitchcock seconded the opinion, expressing a willingness to prolong the fight but a preference to accept its futility.

"Well, I think we are all of one opinion, which is that the President should accept the reservations and be advised that this is our recommendation," said Carter Glass at last. "But—"; and, with that, he paused for dramatic effect. "I would like, to know," he proceeded, "in the present condition of the President's mind and his state of health, who among us will be willing to go to him and tell him that he should accept the reservations." Each man sat in silence, waiting for one of the other fifteen to speak.

Ray Baker was willing to bell the cat, and he arranged an audience with the President during his now daily outing to the South Portico. The issue arose and just as quickly fell with "sad finality," as Wilson had convinced himself that the opposition was composed of "evil men" hell-bent on destroying the League.

Carter Glass informed the President that a rewording of Article X endorsed by President Taft had proven acceptable to Lodge, the Mild Reservationists, and a host of "uncompromising friends of the Administration." Edith Wilson replied that the President felt Taft's proposed reservation was "not drawn in good faith" and that her husband believed "absolute inaction on our part is better than a mistaken initiative." When Wilson's son-in-law discussed the partisan gamesmanship in play, Wilson said,

"Mac, I am willing to compromise on anything but the Ten Commandments"—which meant that "there could be no compromise where the moral law or high principle was involved."

Spring arrived early, and the President left the White House grounds on March 3 for the first time in five months. From the rear entrance of the White House, he walked with a cane to a waiting motorcar, into which attendants assisted him. For more than an hour, he and Edith and Dr. Grayson rode along the Potomac to Capitol Hill. They passed Senator Borah, who smiled and waved. The drive proved therapeutic enough to become part of Wilson's regimen once again. He would wear a cape instead of an overcoat, because of the difficulty threading his left arm through the sleeve, and the staff would place him in the contoured front seat, where he could not slide or topple over as he did in the back. Timed with his return, Agent Starling would organize a group to stand and cheer as the car pulled through the White House gate. When the Secret Service men lifted Wilson from the car after the first of these staged welcomes, the President had tears in his eyes. "You see," he said to Edith, "they still love me!"

Realizing that the Senate was in the homestretch of its marathon debate, the President dictated one last letter to Hitchcock about the League—1,400 words full of his familiar phraseology, more fixed in his argument than ever. Over the next few days, he tinkered with the text, and his pencil markings in both shorthand and longhand revealed penmanship only slightly less readable than before his stroke and editorial skills as precise as ever. "Either we should enter the League fearlessly," he wrote, "accepting the responsibility and not fearing the role of leadership which we now enjoy, contributing our efforts towards establishing a just and permanent peace, or we should retire as gracefully as possible from the great concert of powers by which the world was saved." The White House sent the letter to Senator Hitchcock on March 8, releasing copies to the major newspapers for publication the next day.

The impending vote on the Lodge reservations would probably be the last opportunity to accept some form of the Treaty, yet Wilson was encouraging even his supporters as well as the Treaty's detractors to kill it. And the public wanted to hear no more discussion of the subject because everything had already been said. As *The New York Times* indicated, "The gulf between the President and Senator Lodge is unbridgeable"; *The Washington Post* branded the President an "affirmative irreconcilable." Even

the pro-Wilson New York *World* chastised him for not realizing that "these reservations at their worst are merely an expression of opinion on the part of a temporary majority of the Senate" and that what "a reactionary Senate under the leadership of Henry Cabot Lodge does a progressive Senate under enlightened leadership can undo." Remarked Brandegee of Connecticut, "The President has strangled his own child."

Lodge offered a minor rewrite of Article X, which afforded the President one final opportunity to compromise. Hitchcock wrote that he assumed Wilson would not accept it, and the President replied, "You are quite right." After the Senate vote, the next opportunity to consider a Treaty, if indirectly, would be in the upcoming Presidential election, in which the Republicans could run as a party of reconciliation.

Although Edith and Dr. Grayson continued to shield the President from pessimistic news, they permitted Tumulty to maintain daily visits with him on the South Portico, because sitting alone and sidelined only heightened his anxiety. A few days after the March 8 letter to Hitchcock, Tumulty found him "deeply depressed," for the inevitability of the Treaty's defeat was sinking in. After reading aloud his daily report on the situation, Tumulty stepped back from Wilson's wheeled chair and said, "Governor, you are looking very well to-day." A doleful Wilson shook his head and said, "I am very well for a man who awaits disaster." And then he lowered his gaze and wept.

On March 15 the Senate adopted Lodge's final language, but Woodrow Wilson's "ides of March" came four days later. The day dragged on with speeches until six o'clock, when a quorum call drew the Senators to the floor for an immediate vote. Forty-nine favored the Lodge version of the Treaty, while thirty-five opposed—with twelve absent Senators pairing their votes, grouped in a two-to-one ratio because of the two-thirds requirement to pass. For want of seven votes, the Treaty did not pass. Almost as many Democrats voted for ratification as those who remained loyal to the President. Wilson's dream, commented Senator Lodge with glee, was as "dead as Marley's ghost." The United States would neither ratify the Treaty Wilson had carried from Paris nor join the League of Nations. It fell upon Tumulty to break the news to his chief, who received it stoically, saying only, "They have shamed us in the eyes of the world."

In an attempt to buoy the President's spirits, Tumulty reminded him

that only the Senate had defeated him and that "the People" would vindicate his course. "Ah," said Wilson, "but our enemies have poisoned the wells of public opinion. They have made the people believe that the League of Nations is a great Juggernaut, the object of which is to bring war and not peace to the world. If I only could have remained well long enough to have convinced the people that the League of Nations was their real hope, their last chance, perhaps to save civilization!"

Grayson said the President had never truly believed the Treaty would be rejected, and it induced a depression. When Grayson encountered his patient after receiving the news, Wilson said, "I feel like going to bed and staying there." But he could not sleep, and Grayson bunked in the White House that night, stopping in the President's bedroom several times. At three o'clock in the morning, Wilson turned to him and said, "Doctor, the devil is a busy man." Moments later he asked Grayson to pick up his Bible and read from 2 Corinthians, Chapter 4, Verses 8 and 9, which he did:

> We are troubled on every side, yet not distressed; we are perplexed, but not
>   in despair;
> Persecuted, but not forsaken; cast down, but not destroyed . . .

"If I were not a Christian," Wilson said, "I think I should go mad, but my faith in God holds me to the belief that He is in some way working out His own plans through human perversities and mistakes."

Wilson stewed over this situation for the rest of his life. He believed the League of Nations represented "the birth of the spirit of the times," and its foes would be "gibbeted and occupy an unenviable position in history along with Benedict Arnold." Edith took the news just as hard, bearing her own grudge against the man bent on destroying her husband. Years later she declared her conviction that "Mr. Lodge put the world back fifty years, and that at his door lies the wreckage of human hopes and the peril to human lives that afflict mankind today." One morning in March 1920, Grayson commented on the balminess of the day. Wilson replied, "I don't know whether it is warm or cold. I feel so weak and useless. I feel that I would like to go back to bed and stay there until I either get well or die. I cannot make a move to do my work except by making a definite resolve to do so."

. . .

With another year to his term, Woodrow Wilson became the lamest duck ever to inhabit the White House, residing more than presiding for the rest of his days there. As spring arrived, he adopted the comfortable routine of a retiree. At nine o'clock every morning he exerted the greatest effort of his day, laboriously walking from his bedroom to his study, only steps away. At his desk he caught up with paperwork for an hour before an attendant wheeled him to the elevator and outside to the gardens. Around noon, he was wheeled to the East Room for his favorite indulgence—a motion picture. Douglas Fairbanks—the swashbuckling star of the silent screen and a successful film producer, who had actively participated in the Liberty Bond rallies—had sent Wilson in late 1918 a "projecting machine," hoping it might provide him some amusement. Wilson especially enjoyed Westerns starring William S. Hart.

At one o'clock, the President would lunch for an hour and then rest in bed for at least an hour. Gradually, a few afternoon appointments were permitted; but he derived the most good from a motor ride, an hour or two into Virginia or Maryland over roads that became so familiar, he and Edith made several friends along the way: two little brothers who would raise the flag when the President passed; a curly-haired tot who saluted and said, "Hi, Wilson!"; an elderly woman who knitted an afghan for the President to place over his knees. During the day's activities, Edith almost never left his side, especially toward sunset, when she would read to him, if he was not already engrossed in a detective story. Now that he was eating proper meals again, Wilson's digestion normalized, and he gained twenty pounds. After dinner, he and Edith pulled out decks of cards and played separate hands of canfield. The President was able, at last, to sleep through the night.

While Wilson evaded slipping into a "second childishness," much of his newfound happiness could be attributed to the arrival of a new friend, a daily visitor who proved to be the President's greatest diversion—his physician's two-year-old son. A precocious little boy, Gordon Grayson became the President's playmate. Taking a glass of milk in the late morning sun, Wilson would give the accompanying biscuit to his young friend; and if the toddler arrived late, the Wilsons would wait for Gordon to ask for his "tookie." During the noontime screenings, Gordon would sit on the

footrest of the President's chair and provide his own commentary. Before leaving on afternoon drives, Wilson would call for his "little partner," and Gordon became a regular passenger, as the President delighted in pointing out places of interest along the way. "His conversation with the little fellow," Dr. Grayson noted, "seems to please him and cheer him and brighten his spirits." When the Ringling Bros. and Barnum & Bailey Circus came to the capital that spring, Wilson requested that its arrival parade alter its route, detouring from Pennsylvania Avenue to Executive Avenue, behind the White House. As the animals and performers marched by, the President of the United States sat on the roof of the East Wing, with young Gordon at his side holding a yellow balloon.

Such small pleasures lifted Wilson's spirits, but the demise of the Treaty would forever weigh him down. At two o'clock in the morning of Tuesday, April 13, 1920, Wilson summoned Dr. Grayson to his bedroom. He needed to talk, which he did for the next two hours. "When I get out of office and my health has recovered," he said, "I want to devote a good deal of time to showing what a disorganization the United States Senate is." He spoke of his having "asked our boys to go overseas and to fight in the trenches for a principle," for which many gave their lives, and how the Senate rendered that fight meaningless. Henry Cabot Lodge haunted him but not as much as those lives lost in vain. "Could any self-respecting man ask our boys to go into another war? Could you expect them to make such a sacrifice," Wilson asked Grayson, "and then have a crowd in the Senate like this throw away what they had fought for?"

Wilson's health finally improved enough for him to evaluate his physical condition and consider his obligations. "My personal pride must not be allowed to stand in the way of my duty to the country," he said. "When I am well, I feel eager for work. I judge my condition because now I do not have much desire for work." Grayson suggested that Wilson call a Cabinet meeting, so that he might talk to his advisers and determine exactly how much leadership he was exerting. "If you will do this," said Grayson, "I am confident that you will find that you are doing more than you realize. You are running your office by correspondence and this naturally makes you feel greatly out of touch with things. Moreover, it gives you the impression that you are inefficient."

A little before ten o'clock the following morning, April 14, a perfectly groomed President sat at his desk in his study, awaiting the arrival of the

Cabinet for his first meeting with them since September 2. To many of the new members, Wilson did not appear sickly. His face looked full—thick and jowly even—and he exuded cheer. But each of the returning members shuddered. In a break from tradition, Ike Hoover announced each of the entrances, which bewildered them, and Wilson's failure to rise from his chair troubled them. David Houston, newly installed at Treasury, was aghast. "The President looked old, worn, and haggard," he recalled. "It was enough to make one weep to look at him.

> One of his arms was useless. In repose, his face looked very much as usual, but, when he tried to speak, there were marked evidences of his trouble. His jaw tended to drop on one side, or seemed to do so. His voice was very weak and strained.

True to form, Wilson opened the meeting with jovial banter, but Houston found it little more than a "brave front." Silence descended, and the department heads realized the President could barely initiate serious conversation.

The ranking Cabinet officer might logically have spoken up in that moment, but the Secretary of State had the least experience of anybody in the room—only three weeks on the job. Most people in the Administration had presumed Robert Lansing's Undersecretary, Frank L. Polk—who possessed the writing skills and foreign affairs experience the President sought—would have been the natural successor. Instead, Wilson had chosen a fifty-year-old New York attorney named Bainbridge Colby. Because he had little experience with international matters, the selection surprised the nominee as much as diplomatic Washington—which allowed Senate Republicans to re-question the President's capability. But Colby was hardly a man without merits. His résumé included a term in the New York State Assembly and two unsuccessful runs as a Progressive candidate for the United States Senate, anti-trust work as a special assistant to the United States Attorney General, and membership on the Shipping Board, which resulted in his participating in the 1917 Inter-Allied Conference in Paris. In his efforts to strengthen the merchant marine, Wilson had found Colby in command of his information. Above all, from the moment Colby had left the Progressive Party in 1916 to support the Democrats, Wilson had valued his loyalty. With Colby by

his side, he believed he would never have to wonder if somebody had his back.

With legal issues dominating the news, the Attorney General stepped in to direct much of the discussion that morning. Strikes had broken out across the country—involving elevator operators, truckers, and railroad workers—much of which Mitchell Palmer attributed to the Bolsheviks and the IWW. Labor Secretary Wilson blamed the unrest on economic conditions and the HCL. The two argued, largely over Assistant Secretary of Labor Louis F. Post, who had summarily dismissed most of the cases that stemmed from the Palmer raids simply because he did not believe membership in the Communist Party should mandate deportation. Palmer claimed that Post had released "alien anarchists" and ought to be relieved of his office, that his removal would be enough of a threat to end the strikes. Secretary Wilson said such action would aggravate the situation. "The President seemed at first to have some difficulty in fixing his mind on what we were discussing" and said little, David Houston observed. Indeed, this was apparently the first the President had heard of Palmer's fanatical operations with J. Edgar Hoover.

After an hour, Dr. Grayson poked his head into the study, a signal prearranged with the President to bring the meeting to a close. Wilson shook his head, indicating that he did not wish to be interrupted. Fifteen minutes later, Grayson returned, only to be dismissed a second time. At 11:30, the doctor entered with Mrs. Wilson, who said, "This is an experiment, you know." And the President adjourned the meeting. Grayson deemed the experiment a success, but one White House visitor reported that Wilson remained "a very sick man"—with a drooping jaw, vacant eyes, and a fixed scowl.

Based on the information they gathered for their psychological autopsy, William Bullitt and Sigmund Freud would later present an even bleaker picture. They pinpointed the breakdown outside Pueblo, Colorado, as the virtual death of Thomas Woodrow Wilson, because from that moment forward, he was "no longer an independent human being but a carefully coddled invalid." He was at the mercy of unpredictable, often illogical synapses, a neurological system gone haywire. "The Woodrow Wilson who lived on," they determined, "was a pathetic invalid, a querulous old man full of rage and tears, hatred and self-pity."

The President's worst moments came at night, when he was alone with

his thoughts. One evening, he again summoned Dr. Grayson and asked the nurse to leave them alone. "I have been thinking over this matter of resigning and letting the Vice-President take my place," he divulged. "It is clear that I should do this if I have not the strength to fill the office." He said that he would quit the moment he realized that his sickness was causing the country any ill effects. The declaration, of course, begged the larger question of whether a man in his mental state was in any position to judge. Even more revealing was the bathetic manner in which the rest of Wilson's scenario unspooled:

> I shall summon Congress in special session and have you arrange to get me wheeled in my chair into the House of Representatives. I shall have my address of resignation prepared and shall try to read it myself, but if my voice is not strong enough I shall ask the Speaker of the House to read it, and at its conclusion I shall be wheeled out of the room.

Wilson developed his own routine for dissolving his night frights. He kept a small flashlight on a stand by his bed, and whenever he was too distressed to sleep, he shone it upon Fred Yates's pastel portrait of Ellen. Night after night, he would stare into his late wife's eyes until he calmed down. He made plans for the following spring to visit the Lake District.

In the meantime, much of Washington continued to buzz about the second Mrs. Wilson. The cantankerous Justice McReynolds, for one, had remained friendly with Vice President Marshall, Colonel House, and Dr. Grayson, and he thought Marshall should have demanded a medical opinion under oath from the President's physicians as to his true condition and then presented that opinion to Congress, which could have declared the President disabled and spared the country several "disastrous months." Grayson also wished to let Marshall serve and said as much to McReynolds and others. But Mrs. Wilson objected. He had told the First Lady that the President had raised the subject and would have stepped aside; but Edith, more concerned with her husband's constitution than the nation's, refused to listen. "If he had resigned, the entire current of recent history might have been changed," House mused in his diary in the late spring of 1920. And even if he did not, he would have saved his treaty—"had he not been so stubborn."

Wilson never raised the subject of resignation again. He believed what Grayson considered true, "that he had the strength to administer the office capably." Reading newspapers once again, Wilson noted talk of the Senate's declaring peace on its own and wondering if he would veto such a resolution. Wilson told Grayson he would take no executive action, other than writing an excoriating message, one so distasteful that he had no doubt the Senate would try to impeach him for it. "If I were well and on my feet and they pursued such a course," he told Grayson, "I would gladly accept the challenge, because I could put them in such a light before the country that I believe the people would impeach them." Wilson the historian said the Senate had never been as unpopular as it was in that moment; and with the approach of the national conventions, he daydreamed of taking a referendum for his treaty to the people. In idle moments he drafted a series of questions for the electorate—did they wish to make use of his services as President, did they approve of the way in which the Administration conducted the war, did they wish the Treaty of Versailles ratified? Tumulty recommended to the First Lady that the President declare publicly that he would not run for a third term. He believed it would depoliticize the future of the Treaty. Wilson saw nothing to be gained from such a gesture. It would only hand the leadership of the party to William Jennings Bryan; and he felt it presumptuous to decline something that had not been offered.

There was one other factor. No President of the United States had ever defied George Washington's tradition of leaving office after two terms. But along with other talk that sounded slightly deranged, Wilson told his physician that he was considering it. Even though he said, "Everyone seems to be opposed to my running," Wilson had conjured a plot in which the Democratic Convention would find itself in a "hopeless tie-up," and, with the world in so much turmoil, the Peace Treaty with its League of Nations would become the dominant issue. Then, Wilson said, "there may be practically a universal demand for the selection of someone to lead them out of the wilderness." The only person he could envision, of course, was himself. He roughed out a new Cabinet.

Grayson was glad the President did not ask for his opinion, medical or otherwise, because he did not want to tell him the depressing truth—"that it would be impossible for him to take part in such a campaign." Nor did Grayson wish to delude him, because he feared the inevitable letdown

would affect the President physically as well as psychologically. Wilson believed that the man elected that fall would determine "whether the United States will be the leader of the world or back among the stragglers." He had no intention of backing any Democrat for the nomination. Like a broken-down fire horse, he waited for the sound of the bell.

While a hostile Congress, an inexperienced Cabinet, and his own compromised health prevented any real progress, Wilson gave the appearance of being back in action. With strikes and runaway inflation commanding most of the headlines, Wilson once again issued statements and performed the ceremonial duties of his office. Regular Cabinet meetings resumed, the President chairing his second meeting two weeks after the first. Foreign diplomats who had been queuing for months finally got to parade through the White House to present their credentials, and the President begin filling his long vacant ambassadorships. In the summer of 1920, Secretary Colby articulated America's position on Russia, reminding the world that the United States was the first government to acknowledge the validity of the revolution and recognize Russia's provisional government. Since that time, however, the rulers had ceased to govern by the will or the consent of the people.

Many in the Administration resented Colby, not only for being ill prepared but also for toadying to the President. Admiring the way he thought and wrote, Wilson made him the teacher's pet. At the President's direction, Colby wrote a note on the Polish situation that became the American doctrine toward Russia well into the next decade. He declared, "It is not possible for the Government of the United States to recognize the present rulers of Russia as a government with which the relations common to friendly government can be maintained. This conviction has nothing to do with any particular political or social structure which the Russian people themselves may see fit to embrace." In short, Colby concluded, "We cannot recognize, hold official relations with, or give friendly reception to the agent of, a government which is determined and bound to conspire against our institutions; whose diplomats will be the agitators of dangerous revolt; whose spokesmen say that they sign agreements with no intention of keeping them." An "iron curtain" was already being drawn between Russia and the non-Bolshevik world. Wilson found Colby's white paper "excellent and sufficient."

In one of the few interviews he granted a journalist that year, Wilson

said, "I do not fear Bolshevism, but it must be resisted. . . . If left alone, it will destroy itself. It cannot survive because it is wrong." In fact, he had suggested as much at his first meeting with the new Cabinet, when he buttonholed Mitchell Palmer and told him "not to let the country see red." As that was an apparent call for extra vigilance more than further violence, the Attorney General's infamous raids came to an end.

Meanwhile, an undaunted Louis Post at the Labor Department persisted in undoing the results of Palmer's recklessness, dismissing cases left and right. As a result, he became the target of a witch hunt himself—secretly investigated by Hoover at the Bureau of Investigation and publicly attacked by the House Committee on Immigration and Naturalization. Several Congressmen as well as the American Legion called for his dismissal. Strongly anti-Communist though the President was, he supported his Secretary of Labor, who backed his subordinate on constitutional grounds, praising him for resisting what would prove to be one of the most egregious miscarriages of justice in American history. "We will not deport anyone simply because he has been accused or because he is suspected of being a Red," the White House asserted. "We have no authority to do so under the law. . . . Mr. Post . . . I am satisfied ranks among the ablest and best administrative officers in the Government service."

One agitator, however, would receive no mercy from the President. Eugene V. Debs had been a thorn in Wilson's side for years now. Having served over a year in prison and with his health failing, he had more petitioners than ever pleading for lenience—not only liberal intellectuals but also labor leaders, including Samuel Gompers and Secretary Wilson. At one meeting of the Cabinet, Payne and Daniels and even Mitchell Palmer himself all advocated clemency. Tumulty agreed to meet with a committee of Socialists presenting a petition for Debs's pardon, only to read before their meeting that the National Convention of Socialists included several radical speeches favoring the Soviet form of government and attacking Wilson. At last, the President put the matter to rest. "I will never consent to the pardon of this man," he told Tumulty.

> I know that in certain quarters of the country there is a popular demand for the pardon of Debs, but it shall never be accomplished with my consent. . . . While the flower of American youth was pouring out its blood to vindicate the cause of civilization, this man, Debs, stood

behind the lines, sniping, attacking, and denouncing them. Before the war he had a perfect right to exercise his freedom of speech and to express his own opinion, but once the Congress of the United States declared war, silence on his part would have been the proper course to pursue.

Wilson knew his refusal to pardon Debs would be denounced. "They will say I am cold-blooded and indifferent," he recognized, "but it will make no impression on me. This man was a traitor to his country and he will never be pardoned during my administration."

Although many of his recent decisions seemed sclerotic in nature, Wilson had not become completely hard-hearted. That year alone, he granted stays and pardons for crimes far more serious than political dissent. Elizabeth Stroud had written Edith Wilson, pleading for the President to consider the plight of her son, Robert, a convicted murderer whose case had undergone a tortured journey through the courts. Wilson commuted his death sentence to life imprisonment in solitary confinement—first at Leavenworth and then at Alcatraz, where he became a renowned ornithologist.

Wilson also continued to demonstrate his sensitivity toward women, as the war had catalyzed a reconsideration of their role in society. That spring, he nominated Helen Hamilton Gardener—longtime activist in NAWSA— to fill a vacancy on the Civil Service Commission. Upon Senate approval, she became the first female to hold such a high federal position. Women realized that the government's glass ceilings could be shattered. In the fourteen months since the proposal to amend the Constitution and enfranchise women had passed in both houses of the Congress, Wilson had steadily lobbied state legislatures to ratify. The tally got stuck at thirty-five approvals, one short of the three-quarters necessary. Then, on August 18, 1920, the Tennessee House of Representatives came around, thereby enacting the Nineteenth Amendment. For the first time, any American over the age of twenty-one—regardless of gender or race—qualified to vote.

The election of 1920 promised to be historic in other ways as well. With Vice President Marshall having shied away from higher office, the upcoming campaign was the first since 1896 in which both the Democratic and Republican Parties would presumably nominate party leaders

who had never run on a national ticket. President Wilson, however, continued to fool himself into believing he would run for a third term, and some surrounding him nursed the delusion. So began the most surreal few weeks in the Wilson Presidency, a moment when nobody could bring himself to tell the emperor that he was not wearing any clothes.

"I saw the President the other day and found him a very old-looking tired man," the new British Ambassador, Sir Auckland Geddes, reported to Lloyd George. "He is not really able to see people and ought to be freed from all cares of office." And yet, even with a side of his body rendered useless, he was not ready to let go. Both Dr. Grayson and Edith believed another run for office would kill him, but each knew even suggesting as much reflected a disloyalty the President could not tolerate. She anxiously placated him while the doctor worked behind the scenes doing everything he could to keep the possibility of a nomination from even arising.

Mid-June—as Democrats prepared to leave for their convention in San Francisco, the first such event in the West—Carter Glass stopped by the executive offices. Dr. Grayson confided to him the President's latest scheme—that he would run for office solely to continue his fight for the Covenant and would resign upon its adoption. Grayson begged Glass "to do all possible to guard against such an untoward development." He told Grayson bluntly that he did not think the convention could be induced to nominate a man in the President's disabled condition, and that even if he were in robust health, the Democrats, to say nothing of the nation, did not seem prepared to overcome their antipathy to a third term.

Three days later, Glass met the Wilsons for tea on the South Portico of the White House. The Senator expressed regret that the President was "not in physical form to lead a great fight for the League of Nations," for the people might very well suppress their third-term aversion if things were otherwise. Neither of the Wilsons responded. Glass reengaged them when he said that he would "rather follow the President's corpse through a campaign than the live bodies of some of the men mentioned for the nomination." Wilson liked that, and they discussed the current contenders. The President dismissed every possibility with a backhanded compliment at best—most especially a run by Ohio's able and affable Governor, James M. Cox, whose candidacy, he said, would be "a fake."

"There is no man who can devise plans with more inspiration, or put them into operation with more vigor, than can Mac," Wilson had said of

his son-in-law, for whom he always felt that twinge of distrust that any boss feels for a man who marries his daughter; "but I never caught Mac reflecting." The President admitted he might be wrong, but he thought that very quality "to be essential to a successful and wise administration in the near future." McAdoo had announced just the day before that he "would not seek the nomination for the Presidency," but as Wilson and Glass realized, McAdoo had never said he would not accept it.

Grayson accompanied Glass to the train, telling him as he parted for the convention, "If anything comes up, save the life and fame of this great man from the juggling of false friends." The doctor explained that he had served three Presidents and not one had been ready to relinquish the office. To a second party operative, Robert W. Woolley, Grayson detailed Wilson's physical condition, reiterating that he must not be nominated. "No matter what others may tell you," he insisted, "no matter what you may read about the President being on the road to recovery, I tell you that he is permanently ill physically, is gradually weakening mentally and can't recover. He couldn't possibly survive the campaign." Wilson had indeed enjoyed weeklong periods of improvement, during which he transacted business with Tumulty, but setbacks ensued, usually depressions. "Cary," Woolley said, "the name of the President will receive many an ovation, his desire as to the platform will prevail, in other ways will he be honored, but his ambition to succeed himself is definitely hopeless." Said Grayson, "We must not take any chances."

Ten thousand Democrats—men and women—filled San Francisco's Civic Auditorium on June 28, 1920. Even before the speeches—when the keynoter would be paying homage to the President and his principles—the convention got off to a boisterous start. An enormous flag rose above the rostrum, and the appearance of a gigantic likeness of the President whipped the crowd into a frenzy. When a spotlight illuminated this portrait, the delegates paraded through the aisles and around the arena. All hell broke loose—except within one large area. After seven years of Wilson's Presidency, Tammany Hall and Wall Street still had not embraced him, and the New York delegation sat silent and still during this storm of adulation. Some among them expressed the fear that the parade would incite a stampede for a third term. After a few minutes, a few pro-Wilson New Yorkers could sit on their hands no longer. A fistfight broke out, and the thirty-eight-year-old Assistant Secretary of the Navy—six-foot-two-inch

Franklin Roosevelt—grabbed the state's standard from the hands of a Tammany man and joined in the parade, taking a few delegates from the Empire State along.

The convention had no decided frontrunner, though Wilson's son-in-law felt like an emotional favorite. In Washington, the President appeared indifferent, but as one ballot followed another with no candidate emerging, Wilson took increasing interest in the press reports that came over the in-house telegraph wire. He began to suffer from insomnia, asthma, and anxiety. By July 3, Governor Cox had a measurable lead over McAdoo, with Palmer a distant third. After sixteen ballots, the convention deadlocked. Grayson went to his patient's room at three o'clock that morning to deliver the latest tallies. Wilson said nothing, except that he believed Cox was "the weakest of the lot." Almost simultaneously, Bainbridge Colby, in a spur-of-the-moment gesture of loyalty to the President, sent him a telegram from San Francisco explaining that amid all the competition, the "outstanding characteristic of the convention is the unanimity and fervor of feeling for you." After monitoring the situation closely, he said an opportunity had arrived in which to move for a suspension of the rules and nominate the President by acclamation. To Colby's surprise, Wilson assented.

Colby was caught in a political riptide. The party insiders closed ranks to sink the President's plans—all feeling it would result in defeat, some knowing it might mean his death. They forced a chagrined Colby to send another telegram to the President, this time rescinding his plan— explaining that Democratic leaders did not command votes sufficient either to set aside the convention rules or to nominate him and that such a public display would only injure the party's chances in the upcoming election—as well as any hope left for the League. Wilson accepted the decision, though he suspected misconduct, especially when he heard that Burleson was supporting McAdoo and that there was serious talk among the California and New York delegations of running Bainbridge Colby.

Between the thirtieth and thirty-eighth ballots, McAdoo and Cox ran neck and neck, the former leading by a nose; but on the next roll call, Palmer, a distant third, released his delegates, and Cox pulled ahead. On the forty-third ballot he received a majority of the votes, and on the next vote the rest of the delegates jumped on the bandwagon. In November, the genial Governor of Ohio would run against his junior Senator, Warren G.

Harding, whom the Republicans had nominated weeks earlier. Harding's running mate would be the Massachusetts Governor who had shut down Boston's police strike, Calvin Coolidge. Cox would run with the fervent New Yorker who had grabbed the state standard during the opening parade—Franklin D. Roosevelt. Wilson sent congratulatory telegrams to each of the men on the Democratic ticket with "cordial" best wishes. Back in the White House, devoted stenographer Swem watched the President's moods all week. He believed Wilson had preferred Cox over McAdoo— "solely out of jealousy toward McAdoo." Either way, there was no doubt in Swem's mind the President was "a bitter man" over the Cox nomination— "not that he disliked Cox but because he didn't get it himself."

Upon the Cabinet's return to Washington, Ike Hoover observed that "they met with a cold reception from the President." A few of them earned their way back into his good graces, but he showed only the most obligatory interest in the campaign, or much else. One late morning, while Wilson was eating his crackers and milk on the South Portico, a breathless Tumulty ran up the steps waving a piece of paper. Once the butler had taken his leave, he blurted, "Governor, we've got 'em beat! Here is a paper which . . . is absolutely true, showing that Harding has negro blood in him. This country will never stand for that!" While Tumulty raved, Wilson quietly sipped his milk. "Even if that is so," the President said, "it will never be used with my consent. We cannot go into a man's genealogy; we must base our campaign on principles, not on backstairs gossip. That is not only right but good politics. So I insist you kill any such proposal."

At 10:30 on July 18, 1920, a warm Sunday morning, Cox and Roosevelt arrived at the White House for the President's blessing. They had to wait until the President had been wheeled to the South Portico. After fifteen minutes, the guests were shown outside; and, as they approached the man in the wheelchair—his left shoulder covered with a shawl to conceal his paralyzed arm—Cox murmured, "He is a very sick man."

Cox warmly greeted the President, who, in a low and weak voice, thanked the two men for coming. His frailty brought tears to Cox's eyes. But Wilson revived when he spoke of the campaign ahead, as he briefed the two hopefuls with substantial details and humorous anecdotes. He referred the nominees to the information about Harding's ancestry and was pleased to see they concurred with his decision to squelch it. When the conversation turned to the main topic, Cox assured his host, "Mr.

President, we are going to be a million percent with you, and your Administration, and that means the League of Nations." Wilson looked up and said in a barely audible voice, "I am very grateful. I am very grateful."

After close to an hour, the aspirants left the President for the executive offices to prepare statements for the press. As Roosevelt recalled, Cox just sat down at a table, asked Tumulty for paper and pencil, summoned his skills as a former newspaperman, and wrote a release committing the ticket to making the League "the paramount issue of the campaign." Franklin Roosevelt said, "It was one of the most impressive scenes I have ever witnessed."

The men returned to the President for lunch, where Mrs. Wilson, Dr. Grayson, Tumulty, and Carter Glass joined them. Wilson quickly realized that he had misjudged the quality of Cox's character, and he commented that he thought Cox would find the White House a comfortable home. The guests left by way of the White House's basement, where stenographer Swem handed them the President's statement, which assured Cox of "an absolutely united party and . . . an absolutely united nation." Confident that he would be serving alongside the next Commander in Chief, Roosevelt announced his resignation from the Navy Department. On his way out, Cox told Tumulty that "no experience of his life had ever touched him so deeply" as meeting the President. "No man could talk to President Wilson about the League of Nations and not become a crusader on its behalf," he said.

Cox and Roosevelt waged an aggressive three-month campaign. There was little the President could do beyond offering a public statement or two, which he did. On September 16, political terrorists bombed Wall Street, killing thirty-eight people and injuring four hundred, making it the deadliest act of terrorism the nation had witnessed. Wilson privately opined that a Republican victory would result in "the most terrible industrial situation in this country," which would create a breeding ground for Bolshevism. In launching his campaign, Harding attacked Wilson's earlier position on the Panama Canal, which had exempted the United States from certain tolls. Off the record, Wilson referred to Harding as shallow and voluble, dismissing him as "nothing."

On October 3, the President stated that the election had become a national referendum on the League. He asked his fellow Americans why they should "be afraid of responsibilities which we are qualified to sustain

and which the whole of our history has constituted a promise to the world we would sustain." Wilson said every nation awaited the November verdict. He was completely confident of the outcome.

The President had spent part of Election Day engaged in physical therapy—struggling with a cane to mount a few low steps. When he paused for news, he learned that Cox was trailing badly. There would be no late-night wait for results. The earliest returns foretold a landslide. Before dawn it was plain that the entire country had gone Republican, except the South—which, for the first time since Reconstruction, was not "solid." A fugitive Tennessee gave Harding thirty-seven states to Cox's eleven, an electoral count of 404 to 127. The popular vote of 16.1 million to 9.1 million (60.3 percent to 34.1 percent) marked the widest popular-vote margin in a century. Even Democratic stronghold New York City went for Harding. More than 900,000 people voted defiantly for the Socialist candidate, Eugene V. Debs, who ran from the Atlanta Federal Penitentiary. The Congressional results slapped Wilson in the face as well, yielding a Senate with fifty-nine Republicans and thirty-seven Democrats and an even more lopsided House, with its majority of 302 to 131. The victors were only too happy to embrace Wilson's premise that the election had been a referendum on his League.

Wilson admitted his disappointment to Tumulty, predicting a period of isolation that would translate into a loss of business, ultimately producing a depression.

When Tumulty suggested the Democratic loss might prove a blessing in the long run, Wilson rebuked him. "I am not thinking of the partisan side of this thing," he said. "It is the country and its future that I am thinking about. We had a chance to gain the leadership of the world. We have lost it, and soon we will be witnessing the tragedy of it all." Of Harding's victory, he could only wonder, "How can he lead when he does not know where he is going?" The day after the election, the Wilsons took their automobile ride through Washington, as though nothing had happened. In fact, Stockton Axson found his brother-in-law as serene that day as in the moments of his prior victories. "I have not lost faith in the American people," Wilson said. "They have merely been temporarily deceived. They will realize their error in a little while."

Secret Service agent Starling, who had tracked Wilson since 1914, observed that the election had, strangely, made the President more cheerful.

He could enjoy his own new freedom, as the Congress would virtually shut down until Inauguration Day, leaving Wilson only a few ceremonial duties.

An unsettling sense of purposelessness quickly replaced joy, and Wilson's feelings darkened with the approach of winter. "I hobble from one part of the house to the other and go through the motions of working every morning," he wrote daughter Jessie, "though I am afraid it is work that doesn't count very much." Foreign affairs always demanded attention, but the President followed a policy of noninterference as much as possible. He feared the new party in power might take the United States into the League but "in such a niggardly fashion" as to proceed "from prejudice and self-interest and a desire to play a lone hand and think first and only of the United States," thereby robbing the nation of dignity and influence. Dr. Grayson confirmed that Wilson's physical health improved after the election, but his nerves were on edge. "He takes it less easily, does not make light of it or joke as he did," Grayson said. "He more easily loses control of himself & when he talks is likely to break down & weep." Wilson's temper shortened. He barked at nurses, threatening to throw them all out; and he periodically did the same to Grayson, whom he summoned regularly in the middle of the night, whether something was wrong or not. He was in a near-constant state of irritation.

Nothing soothed him more than movies, and the daily matinees became essential to his well-being. One of Edith's brothers regularly brought the President copies of the latest photoplay magazines, which he studied intently, looking for films he wished to order for the coming weeks. At the end of November, they had viewed all the available Westerns, melodramas, and love stories, and they requested the Signal Corps documentary footage of his trip to Europe.

Ray Baker was there that day, and he watched the White House ushers lift the heavy red rug of the main hall and lay it aside as the sixty-three-year-old President lumbered toward him, his left arm hanging, his left leg dragging. His eyes reflected the liveliness of his mind, but Baker shook hands with a broken man—stooped, gray-faced, and white-haired. Together they walked into the East Room. The President, Mrs. Wilson, Dr. Grayson, and Baker sat quietly in the dark as the projector from Douglas Fairbanks threw flickering images onto the screen of that extraordinary week less than two years ago, when Woodrow Wilson—tall and hale and

waving his hat to the enraptured throngs—was known as "the Savior of the World." There he was sailing into the harbor at Brest . . . arriving in Paris . . . leaving Buckingham Palace . . . and everywhere flags waved and hundreds of thousands of people tossed roses and exuded so much adulation, one could almost hear their cheers emanate from the silent screen. Periodically, Wilson would comment on the scene before them, in a lifeless voice. When these glorious pictures came to an end, the audience found itself in a dim cavern of stark reality. Several attendants went to the chair of the President, who sat hunched and silent. One placed a foot against his, to brace him as he stood. Without saying another word, Wilson shuffled out of the room, to the rhythm of his cane tapping against the marble floor.

With limited energy, Wilson worked on one important document during this period, his last State of the Union message. He surely would have wished to make a final appearance before Congress, to solidify the tradition he had reestablished; but volatile as his emotions were, it was best that he did not deliver the address in person, as his appearance would surely have provoked an ovation from which he might not have recomposed himself. On Monday, December 6, 1920, the Congressional leadership came to the White House to notify the President formally that Congress had reconvened. The two Senators and three Representatives waited in the Blue Room; and as the President entered, aided by his cane, he immediately noticed Henry Cabot Lodge and said, "Gentlemen, I hope you will excuse me from going through the formality of shaking hands with you individually, but, as you see, I cannot yet dispense with my third leg." Wilson stood close enough to Senate Minority Leader Underwood to whisper, "I used the excuse of this 'third leg,' as I did not want to shake hands with Lodge." The two Democrats chuckled, and then Wilson announced that he would transmit his message to the Congress the next day. When the legislators had left, Wilson could not resist saying to Grayson, "Can you imagine what kind of a hide Lodge has got, coming up here in these circumstances and wanting to appear familiar and talk with me?"

A far cry from 1913, when Woodrow Wilson made his first dramatic appearances before joint sessions of Congress, a clerk in each chamber read the annual message as Senators and Representatives followed along reading printed copies. Except for a sentence of Abraham Lincoln's—"Let us

have faith that right makes might, and in that faith let us dare to do our duty as we understand it"—and a few Wilsonian phrases, the text lacked luster. It perfunctorily urged revision of tax laws, care for the economy, and increased veterans' benefits; and he further recommended a loan to Armenia and the independence of the Philippines. It made no mention of the Treaty, but it did ask the lawmakers to remember the purity and spiritual power of democracy: "It is surely the manifest destiny of the United States," he said, "to lead in the attempt to make this spirit prevail."

The Wilson Administration wound down, the hours growing longer and quieter. Solicitous letters from friends arrived along with occasional testimonials. One particularly generous encomium from 105 women whose names could be found in the *New York Social Register*—Eleanor Roosevelt among them—simply wanted to express the belief that "the name of Woodrow Wilson will be added to those of Washington and Lincoln as the men of vision in American history." On November 15, bells pealed in Geneva, inaugurating the League of Nations—"the first time in the history of mankind," as Edwin L. James phrased it in *The New York Times*, that "forty-one nations of the world sat together in common council." The League opened by sending a message of thanks to President Wilson with the desire that the United States would soon "take her rightful place in the League." And on December 4, 1920, Albert G. Schmedeman, the United States Ambassador to Norway, informed Wilson in a "strictly confidential" telegram that the Nobel Committee of the Norwegian Parliament intended to honor "his crucial role in establishing the League" with its prize for Peace. Woodrow Wilson became the third American to win the honor—following Theodore Roosevelt and Elihu Root, each of whom had criticized Wilson for dragging his feet before declaring war.

The better the news abroad, it seemed, the more bitter he became—ill-tempered, angry, even mean. "The President these days is much given to gratifying whatever petty prejudices he has," noted Charles Swem. He based his approvals of his final appointments upon the Senators in support of the nominees and blackballed everyone on his enemies list. Final bills went signed or unsigned because of similar prejudices. During his daily drives, he grew so intolerant of those who passed his car, he ordered the Secret Service to apprehend them for questioning; he even wrote the Attorney General to ask if the President did not also have the powers of a

magistrate, as he wished to fine the speeders a thousand dollars. When an admirer of the President had sent him a particularly bad portrait and later asked if it had been received, Wilson replied that "unfortunately" it had been "received in good shape." He managed to get one letter off to his old companion Jack Hibben, but with no friendly intent; rather, he wished the Princeton president would send him the big table in the study at Prospect, which he had purchased years earlier with his own money. His bitterest reply came when several classmates asked him to subscribe to the Princeton Endowment Fund and he refused—"because I do not believe at all in the present administration." He came to accept that part of his problem at Princeton had been in trying "to change old institutions too fast"; he muttered that the place "was bought once with Ivory Soap money."

In late January 1921, the red-baiting Attorney General himself presented Wilson with an application for pardon from Eugene V. Debs, complete with legal arguments as well as moral imperatives. "Debs is now approaching 65 years of age," Palmer wrote. "If not adequately, he has surely been severely punished." The form required only the President's signature. Wilson examined the document, grabbed his pen, and then wrote the word "Denied."

For almost two years, the Wilsons had mused about where they might live upon leaving the White House. Woodrow began rating their top five cities in terms of climate, friends, opportunities, freedom, amusements, and libraries. New York ranked highest, followed by Baltimore, Boston, and Richmond. Washington ran a distant fifth, but that was the city they chose. Although they counted few friends there and it offered "zero" freedom, other factors tipped the scales: the Library of Congress promised the best facilities for researching the book about government that Wilson proposed to write; and the city had long been Edith's home. In late 1920, she went out each morning at eight—while a valet helped Woodrow prepare for the day—to house hunt.

By mid-December she had inspected a half dozen places that interested her, including one on S Street, just off Massachusetts Avenue's Embassy Row, not far from Dupont Circle. After hearing the enthusiasm in his wife's voice as she described it, Wilson privately called upon her brother

Wilmer Bolling to work with the agent in ascertaining the price and searching the title. The day they worked out the details, as Edith recalled, he insisted that she attend a concert, a luxury she had forsaken since his stroke. When she returned to the White House, she found Woodrow sitting by a fire in the Oval Room upstairs, where he handed her the paperwork. He was purchasing the $150,000 house as a gift for her.

The sum represented more than half the money from his life savings, most of it squirreled away from his generous Presidential salary. Fortunately, the $40,000 honorarium that accompanied the Nobel Prize had just arrived. On top of that came an unexpected $100,000 windfall, when Grayson rallied ten of Wilson's dearest friends—including Cleveland Dodge, Cyrus McCormick, Jr., and Bernard Baruch—to contribute toward the house's purchase. The Wilsons would take ownership on January 31, 1921.

Since 1912, Congress had considered granting annual pensions to retired Chief Executives, but it would not enact the Former Presidents Act until 1958. Wilson felt he still had to earn a living, to say nothing of spending his time constructively. Colleagues urged him to write a history of his eight years in the White House, but he refused, thinking there was little to add to what he considered a transparent administration. Publishers invited him to write everything from an elementary history of the United States to a biography of Jesus. To the demand for his memoirs, Wilson emphatically said, "There ain't going to be none." One day Edith found Woodrow alone in his study, at his typewriter. She was thrilled to see him in his familiar place, even more so when he announced that he had written the dedication to his book on government, which he now had the leisure to compose. With that, he pulled from the machine a slip of paper. The paragraph-long dedication to "E. B. W." explained that this was a book "in which I have tried to interpret life, the life of a nation, and she has shown me the full meaning of life." The rest of the page expressed his love for her in clauses rhapsodic enough to suggest writing the dedication meant more to him than writing the book. That proved to be the case, as that was the only page he would complete.

Toward the end of February 1921, Cabinet members visited the President individually to pay their final respects. Bainbridge Colby—who had performed admirably in his position, notably during a recent trip to Latin America—spoke graciously of the honor Wilson had bestowed upon him.

Pleased with their association, the President said, "Well, Colby, what are you going to do?" The Secretary of State said that he would probably return to New York and "open a musty law office again." After his current experience, that sounded dreary, he admitted, "but I must make a living."

"Well, I, too, must make a living," Wilson said. "As I was once a lawyer, why not open an office together here in Washington?" Colby asked if he really meant that. Wilson said yes—"I can't face a life of idleness; besides, I must so something to add to my income." The next day, Edith had occasion to see Colby, who asked about the seriousness of the President's offer. She said that he had blurted it impulsively. When he asked what she thought of the prospect, she said that she was ambivalent—"that his mind must have something to feed on" but that she did not see how he could actively participate in a practice. Intrigued, Colby said he could arrange the business in such a way as to obviate any objections.

On Tuesday, March 1, 1921, the Cabinet returned to the executive offices of the West Wing for its last official meeting. David Houston had arrived early and saw the President approach, walking with great difficulty across the White House grounds. It was a "brave" endeavor, he recalled, one so tragic that he looked away and waited in a nearby room in order for Wilson to situate himself without embarrassment. The President spent the bulk of the meeting reviewing the Administration's accomplishments. After tying up loose ends, the Cabinet members asked about his prospects for the future. "I am going to try to teach ex-presidents how to behave," he said. He could not help himself from adding, "There will be one very difficult thing for me, however, to stand, and that is Mr. Harding's English."

Their business behind them, Secretary Colby expressed on behalf of his colleagues the great distinction they all felt serving him "in the most interesting and fateful times of modern history." They promised to watch his progress toward better health and pray for his complete recovery. As David Houston, one of the three Cabinet members to last the entire Administration, prepared to speak, he noticed the President struggling with emotion. His lips trembled, and in his attempts to talk, tears rolled down his cheeks. "Gentlemen," he said after a pause, "it is one of the handicaps of my physical condition that I cannot control myself as I have been accustomed to do. God bless you all." They all rose, and each shook hands

with him, saying a quiet goodbye. As a parting gift, the Cabinet members chipped in to purchase the President's chair from the government. It would join his furniture that was being pulled from storage and moved to S Street.

On March 3, the Wilsons invited the Hardings to tea. They met in the Red Room, where the President-elect sat with one of his legs slung over the arm of his chair.

The Wilsons rose early on the fourth, and by nine o'clock the Congressional leadership, Cabinet officers, and numerous aides had gathered for the arrival of the Hardings and the Coolidges. As they approached, Edith went upstairs to offer her husband any last-minute help, only to find him completely dressed in his morning coat and gray trousers. Brooks, the valet, held his top hat and gloves and handed him his cane. They took the elevator down and went to the Blue Room, arriving just as the Hardings entered. They proceeded to the porte cochere, where several cars waited— marking the first time that automobiles and not horse-drawn carriages would convey a President-elect to his inauguration. Still and motion-picture photographers captured the event.

Wilson had fully intended to observe the great traditions of the day, especially that most symbolic moment of orderly transition—accompanying his successor to the platform on the East Portico of the Capitol and watching him take the oath of office. But prior to Inauguration Day, Dr. Grayson had inspected the structure and discovered that reaching the platform would demand the President's climbing long, steep stairways, which he could not do.

Wilson and Harding drove together to the Capitol, behind a squadron of cavalry at a brisk trot, as all of Washington seemed to line the route. Wilson looked straight ahead, never acknowledging the crowds, for he insisted they had shown up to salute the new leader. The Presidential car arrived at the main entrance of the great domed building, where the fifty-five-year-old man of the hour sprang up the steps, leaving President Wilson to proceed alone to a small, private lower door around the corner— often used as a freight entrance—where an attendant with a wheelchair would take him inside. Edith, in a car right behind them, fumed over Harding's thoughtlessness. As Alice Roosevelt Longworth would later comment: "Mr. Harding was not a bad man. He was just a slob."

Dr. Grayson and Edith accompanied Wilson to an elevator that brought

them to the second floor of the Senate, where he entered the President's Room for the last time. He had more than a half hour in which he signed a few bills and received the many dignitaries who had come to pay their respects, General Pershing and the Cabinet among them. Harding arrived with Coolidge and asked if Wilson wished to enter the Senate chamber for Coolidge's swearing in, but he declined, as his continued presence would only impede the day's program.

Shortly before noon, Senator Lodge entered, and Wilson's smile dissolved. "Mr. President," he said, "as Chairman of the Joint Committee I beg to inform you that the two houses of Congress have no further business to transact and are prepared to receive any further communications you may care to make."

"Tell them I have no further communication to make. I thank you for your courtesy," he replied in his most formal tone. "Good morning, Sir."

With that, it was time to inaugurate the twenty-ninth President of the United States. Harding and Coolidge approached Wilson, the former asking in a whisper if he would remain for the swearing in. "I'm sorry, Mr. President," Wilson said, "it cannot be done." The steps still daunted him. Turning to Senator Knox, he said, "Well, the Senate threw me down before, and I don't want to fall down myself now." The dignitaries all moved toward their places for the ceremonies, and the outgoing President and his wife and doctor slipped away.

The Marine Band played "Hail to the Chief," and the eyes of the world turned to the convivial Midwesterner on the East Portico of the Capitol raising his right hand. Few saw the hobbled figure struggling into the White House limousine, which then pulled away through the dead-quiet city streets. *The New York Times* could not refrain from characterizing Wilson's unheralded exit from the public stage as "tragic." Following two policemen on motorcycles, the car sped past 1600 Pennsylvania Avenue and then veered toward Massachusetts Avenue. There was silence in the limousine until Edith, resentful of Harding's discourtesy in leaving her husband to enter the Capitol on his own, could restrain herself no longer. She criticized him with all her fury.

And as the car turned onto tranquil S Street, Woodrow Wilson laughed.

17

RESURRECTION

*. . . and loe, I am with you alway, euen vnto the end
of the world . . .*

—MATTHEW, XXVIII:20

At 12:15 the White House limousine reached 2340 S
Street NW.

Only the most faithful had come to pay homage—too
few onlookers to warrant extra police to patrol that section
of town known as Kalorama. The secluded suburban en-
clave of large gracious houses—perched above much of the
city—stood in stately silence. For the first time since his
days as a college professor, Woodrow Wilson came home to
a house that he actually owned.

Waddy Butler Wood, a popular Washington architect,
had designed the Georgian Revival house in 1915 for a
Boston businessman and lobbyist who resided there during
Congressional sessions. Edith had immediately recognized
that it "fitted to the needs of a gentleman's home"—
offering dignity without pretension and comfort without
extravagance. The red-brick edifice, trimmed in limestone,
sat back from the road and stood four stories high. A trip-
tych of huge Palladian windows on the second floor dominated the façade of the house, while a modest two-pillared
portico, crowned with a wrought-iron railing, encased the
front door. Before moving in, Edith had commissioned

Wood to modify the house to accommodate its new tenants. He added a gated automobile entrance and a side door from the driveway to provide wheelchair access. Inside, the Otis Elevator Company installed an electric elevator.

The ex-President's car pulled into the new entrance, and Secret Service agent Starling assisted him from the vehicle to his chair, which he rolled into the elevator. Wilson thanked Starling for his years of loyal service. Edith shook his hand and offered her gratitude. The chauffeur drove Starling back to the Capitol, where he immediately began serving his next President, as he would three more after that. But as the limousine pulled away, Starling would later note, "Our hearts were behind us, where we had left a great man and a great woman."

Wilson ascended to the second floor, where a new team of servants—the late Mr. Galt's family retainers, Isaac and Mary Scott, whom Edith called "the best of the old-time coloured Virginia stock"—served luncheon in the dining room. The moment the meal had ended, Grayson suggested his patient excuse himself and rest. "Mr. President—," he said, only to be interrupted by the man himself, who corrected him: "Just Woodrow Wilson."

Although Edith fretted over all the abrupt changes Woodrow had to face, her immediate concerns faded the moment he left the elevator on the third floor and stood leaning on his cane at the threshold of his bedroom. Every personal article from his room at the White House had been placed in the same relative position on S Street. Edith had ordered a bed to match the dimensions of the Lincoln Bed—eight feet six inches by six feet two inches; footrests and easy chairs and pillows and tables and lamps were all situated exactly where Wilson would expect to find them. A favorite wartime banner and a Red Cross poster adorned the walls, and the brass shell from the first American bullet fired in the World War sat on the mantel. His familiar wooden shaving stand—complete with bowl, mirror, razor, and strop—stood near the south window. Edith was especially glad to see Ruth Powderly, the Navy nurse who had been attending him in the White House. Technically no longer attached to the former Commander in Chief, she had insisted on staying with him at least until he got settled. Touched though he was by her devotion and eager to retain her, he insisted that she keep her stay brief, as the government employed her, not he.

Wilson did allow himself one government perquisite. Upon Warren Harding's becoming President, Dr. Grayson's White House detail officially

ended, subjecting him to reassignment. In an act of unexpected generosity, Harding had issued an unrequested order that Dr. Grayson be assigned to Washington, where "his services would be available to Mr. Wilson and that in no circumstances was he to be ordered elsewhere without the President's consent."

By the time Wilson had risen from his nap, Warren Gamaliel Harding's inauguration had ended. Seldom in the nation's history had the change in government swung so far in the opposite direction, as evidenced by the new President's stiff address. Twice the length of either of Wilson's inaugural addresses—and larded with "gamalielese," as H. L. Mencken referred to his pompous circumlocutions—Harding's speech exhorted Americans to "strive for normalcy" and to shun military, economic, or political commitments to any authority other than their own. The address set European ministers on edge. The venal arrogance and anti-intellectual tone appeared even starker alongside the hearty praise of Wilson that flooded the press that week. Jan Smuts of South Africa spoke for many foreign leaders in an article that ran in the *New York Evening Post* and was syndicated widely. Wilson had not failed in Paris, Smuts asserted, but humanity itself had let the world down. He maintained that the Covenant that Wilson had protected was "one of the great creative documents of human history" and that one day all nations would march behind its banner. Despite his legislative failure, Wilson had already "achieved the most enviable and enduring immortality," and future Americans "will yet proudly and gratefully rank him with Washington and Lincoln, and his fame will have a more universal significance than theirs." Smuts added that hundreds of years hence, "Wilson's name will be one of the greatest in history."

Frank I. Cobb seconded that opinion in a long panegyric in the New York *World*. "No other American has made so much world history as Woodrow Wilson," he observed. In drawing a sharp contrast to President Harding, Cobb reminded his readers that Wilson dealt almost exclusively with ideas. He cared little for party politics, and patronage bored him, as did the actual administration of government. He pronounced Wilson the most profound student of government among all the Presidents—with the exception of Madison, "the Father of the Constitution." Wilson's foreign policies had obscured the rest of his administration, he said, but his domestic policies alone guaranteed him an elevated position in American

history. Cobb called Wilson's control over Congress for six years "the most impressive triumph of mind over matter known to American politics." Wilson's words led the nation not simply into a war but into a crusade, one in which "international relations have undergone their first far-reaching moral revolution."

A little after three that afternoon, Wilson appeared at one of his third-floor windows and discovered five hundred people outside cheering. For the rest of the afternoon, a steady stream of automobiles and primitive tour buses—"rubberneck" cars, they were called, horseless wagons that could carry twenty passengers—rode into S Street. Friends and former colleagues dropped by to pay their respects, including former Attorney General Palmer and former Secretary Daniels, various Democratic Senators and Representatives, and Joe Tumulty, whose future was uncertain now that Wilson had no further need for a chief of staff.

Guests entered a generous foyer, with a floor of black marble with white inset squares. To the immediate left was what became Wilson's front office, an ample room with a fireplace. John Randolph Bolling—an inhibited, slightly hunchbacked, younger brother of Edith's—moved there to serve as Wilson's secretary and chief usher. As the actual secretarial work would require a steadily decreasing number of hours, he devoted much of his time to assembling scrapbooks, producing a detailed timeline of his brother-in-law's life. He referred to his office as his "dugout," which his sister visited each day in order to tend to some of the mail. The room also became a temporary workspace for Ray Baker, who had earlier expressed his desire to write a book about the Paris Peace Conference and in time had received carte blanche to Wilson's papers. During this transitional period, Baker became Wilson's in-house biographer, and Edith especially appreciated having somebody they both trusted on hand to spend constructive time with her husband.

Beyond the dugout was a gentlemen's cloakroom, a trunk room for storage, and, after some remodeling of servants' quarters, a billiard room. The other side of the entrance hall had a ladies' coatroom, as well as the kitchen—with its zinc sink and early General Electric refrigerator—and the servants' dining room. A mezzanine hall, which served in part as an annex for Wilson's books, was up three marble steps from the entrance, and a wide stairway carried visitors to the second-floor drawing room. It was almost six hundred square feet, furnished with a combination of

French and English pieces that Edith and Woodrow brought from their prior marriages. Because the Wilsons would seldom entertain on a grand scale, this parlor became something of a museum, housing many of the artifacts from his Presidency: a mosaic of St. Peter, a gift from Pope Benedict XV; silver-framed photographs of King George and Queen Mary; and the hand-painted plates from the King and Queen of Belgium. A black Steinway D concert grand piano sat before a huge Gobelins tapestry depicting *The Marriage of Psyche*, a gift Ambassador Jusserand had presented to Edith in 1918 on behalf of the people of France.

In the opposite corner of the second floor was a large dining room, furnished with a graceful, narrow-legged Sheraton dining set. A portrait of Edith hung over the mantelpiece. The room connected to a solarium, its glass doors opening onto a terrace that faced south, overlooking a long, brick-walled garden with several large evergreens. The sunroom and its porch connected on its eastern side to the room where the Wilsons found themselves spending most of their time—a serene wood-paneled library. Before they had moved in, Edith had requested the installation of two bookcases to accommodate much of Wilson's eight-thousand-volume library. Furnished with his Cabinet chair from the White House and the great table from Prospect (which Hibben had shipped at the university's expense), the room became the Wilsons' inner sanctum.

The first day in his new house, Wilson could not resist glancing out the window. The crowd steadily swelled into the thousands. Each glimpse of him prompted applause, which he acknowledged with a wave. When a procession of League advocates marched down S Street and stopped in front of the house, he granted an audience to a few of its leaders. Wilson received them in the drawing room, where they presented him with a huge white wicker basket filled with roses and tulips and lilacs. He shook hands, saying, "It makes me very happy to see you on this occasion. I am proud of you all." When the delegation left, a man in the crowd outside called for three cheers for Wilson, which were loud enough to bring him to an open window. He smiled, bowed, and waved a white handkerchief. The crowd quieted, as it appeared that Wilson might speak. But instead, he raised his right hand to his throat, suggesting soreness, though Edith knew he simply feared that his voice would break. He smiled and bowed a few times and then fell from sight. He spent the rest of the day in his bedroom, and stayed there for the next several weeks.

In late March, Ray Baker went upstairs to talk with his subject. He found the sixty-four-year-old propped up in bed, "looking inconceivably old, gray, worn, tired"—his hair thin, his skin parchment yellow, his face an aquiline caricature of its former looks. Only the eyes still burned, suggesting the activity of his mind. Dr. Grayson had revealed that Wilson was suffering a recurrence of trouble with his prostate, but as Baker noted in his diary, the former President was suffering from more than physical ills.

> He has been lost. . . . He seems lonelier, more cut-off than ever before. His mind still works with power, but with nothing to work upon! Only memories & regrets. He feels himself bitterly misunderstood & unjustly attacked; and being broken in health, cannot rally under it.

Homer Cummings, the former chairman of the Democratic National Committee, paid a bedside visit one month later, and found Wilson "more depressed than I had ever known him to be." In discussing foreign affairs, Wilson proved as uncompromising as ever. He had a new antagonist to curse, Harding's Secretary of State, Charles Evans Hughes. Wilson spoke of the "deplorable consequences" of America's failure to ratify the Treaty and of America's "helpless attitude" at a time when Europe was attempting to rebuild itself. He feared the military leaders occupying the Ruhr District were sowing the seeds of future discontent. He claimed that the United States had abandoned "a fruitful leadership for a barren isolation." Most chilling, Wilson told Cummings that the course of events was "leading inevitably to another world war."

Cummings assured Wilson of his own faith in the League and that he relied on all the "philosophy" he could summon to endure the humiliation he felt as an American in seeing its defeat. "If I had nothing but philosophy to comfort me," Wilson said, "I should go mad." When Cummings asked him to expound, the old man could not find the words. His voice quavered and he broke down. Cummings caught only his suggestion that they were all but small instruments in a greater divine plan.

No President had left the White House feeling so utterly depleted as Woodrow Wilson. By mid-May, he was still lying in bed most days—"too much," thought Grayson, who urged him "to get at some work that will engage, even to exhaustion, his self-consuming mind." But Wilson lacked

the spirit. He whiled away hours reading with his one good eye, mostly potboilers. He tried to remain indifferent to the news, but he could not always suppress his acrimony. Upon becoming the new Ambassador to Great Britain, Colonel George Harvey—Wilson's first important benefactor—delivered a speech that ridiculed the former President and the League. When Grayson referred to Harvey as a skunk, Wilson retorted without batting an eye, "No, no, Grayson, you are wrong: a skunk has a white streak."

Knowing her husband always responded to the call of duty, Edith fashioned an activity to get him out of bed in the morning. Stacks of mail arrived every day, and she told him that many warranted a reply. Randolph Bolling sorted them; and after Woodrow and Edith breakfasted together in the solarium—if she could get him that far—they would descend to the dugout. Wilson dictated a great number of short replies, leaving his brother-in-law to respond to those letters that did not require a personal touch. Wilson would then take his daily walk—back and forth across the vestibule. When he tired, he returned to his bedroom, where Isaac Scott had prepared his shaving stand. The one-armed exercise remained the most arduous of the day, but one he insisted upon performing himself. For the most part, Wilson remained in his dressing gown and slippers. Only the occasional guest could get him to the dining room for a formal meal. After lunch he rested for a solid hour. Bolling ushered those few with appointments to the library, where they would find Wilson in an armchair by the fire. Even when he remained in his bedroom, Wilson rigorously performed basic calisthenics to strengthen his muscles and received regular massages. So while his hair had turned white and he often replaced his trademark pince-nez with framed spectacles, Wilson's physique stayed relatively trim.

Nothing refreshed Wilson more than his motor trips around the city. He had especially liked one car in the Presidential fleet, the big black Vestibule Suburban car the government leased from Pierce-Arrow in Buffalo, New York. The six-cylinder, forty-eight-horsepower vehicle with its steering wheel on the right represented the height of luxury—eight feet high with running boards, silver-plated door handles and bud vases, German silver carriage lights, and whitewall tires—then selling for $9,250. Upon entering civilian life, he purchased the big black "used car" for

$3,000, personalizing it by having the Presidential seal on either side painted over and putting his initials in their place. He jazzed up the car with a few thin orange stripes on its body and orange accents on the spokes of the wheels. In further homage to Princeton, he replaced the Presidential hood ornament of an eagle with that of a tiger. Wherever the Wilsons drove each afternoon, the reception along the way lifted his spirits, as he invariably received cheers from the people he passed.

They always returned home by seven, so that Woodrow could change back into his dressing gown and eat dinner at a small table in the library. By the light of the fire and a dim lamp, Edith read to him until he was ready for sleep, usually around nine o'clock. While he prepared for bed, Edith and her brother would dine. Then she would visit her husband in his bedroom and read to him again until he drifted off. At that moment, he would reach for the Bible on his nightstand and read a few verses before falling asleep. The routine seldom varied, except when a local theater owner sent reels of the newest films to S Street so that Wilson could watch them in his library, employing the Douglas Fairbanks projector and a portable screen. A pianist would sometimes visit, playing the score on an upright instrument tucked in a corner of the room.

Starting in late April 1921, his favorite diversion came on Saturday nights, when the Wilsons and a few guests ritually went to Keith's Theatre on Fifteenth Street. The manager reserved seats in the last row of the theater, which not only allowed for easy access from its side door but also for Wilson to slip in without creating much of a scene. In no time his appearances had become so predictable, the public considered his presence a featured act. As Wilson entered in evening clothes, the entire audience would offer a standing ovation and the performers would present him with flowers. By the time the show ended, as many as a thousand people would swarm to the G Street entrance, where Wilson's Pierce-Arrow waited. Some of the entertainers would rush outside without taking time to remove their greasepaint. By summer, Wilson could enter the big car on his own, cheerfully doffing his hat. Sandwiches and ginger ale awaited at home, where he and Edith would stay up and review that night's songs and routines. The house was well stocked with a collection of records to which Wilson could listen on the Victrola: the latest recordings from Harry Lauder, John Philip Sousa, Nellie Melba, and Alma Gluck; Enrico Caruso's rendition of "Over There"; and the blackface comedy routines of Moran

and Mack. By fall, Wilson often propped himself up in bed with a writing board, making notes in shorthand. He even took to sitting at a desk in order to type personal letters on his Underwood with one hand.

For all the optimistic signs of his activity, Wilson's physical health had not improved much. His regimen masked the fact that his left arm and leg were still paralyzed, and his digestive tract remained as problematic as ever. Those surrounding him believed his only real salvation lay in some "systematic mental occupation," at least an hour each day. Stockton Axson, for one, hoped something might spring from the conversation Wilson had started with Bainbridge Colby about a law partnership.

Colby had not only pursued the idea but also took it upon himself to open a few doors so that Wilson would be readily admitted to the New York State Bar and that of the District of Columbia. Just before noon on June 25, the former President arrived at the District's Supreme Court, where all the justices gathered to witness Wilson taking the oath.

The following week, Colby drafted the announcement of the new partnership Wilson & Colby, "Attorneys and Counsellors at Law," with offices at 1315 F Street (in the American National Bank Building) in Washington and at 32 Nassau Street in Manhattan. Colby would man the New York office and come to Washington once a week to consult with his partner in the capital, who intended to spend an hour in the office every day. Colby proposed mailing two thousand engraved notices, but after compiling his list of contacts, Wilson suggested five thousand. On August 16, Wilson rode to F Street, where he entered the building through the rear and walked to the elevator without assistance. He met Colby in their suite, where the bookshelves remained empty and the walls bare, but the large desks and richly upholstered chairs suggested a law firm that intended to remain in business for years to come.

But, for the second time in his life, Wilson displayed his inherent lack of interest in practicing law. As with the launch of his first practice, Wilson faced a dearth of clients—though this time for different reasons. The firm faced an ethics problem—as Wilson refused to accept any case in which he felt his former official position might influence the decision in his clients' favor. He presumed his partner would follow suit. In February 1922, for example, Costa Rica approached the new firm about a border dispute with Panama. In light of America's most recent dealings with the former during Wilson's last days in office, he deemed the clients inappro-

priate. A few months later, American banks hoped the firm might smooth over a deal pending with Ecuador. Wilson feared it would contribute to new monopolies in the South American nation and felt uncomfortable associating his name with the transaction. Again, he asked Colby to "comprehend my feelings and indulge my scruple."

The most intriguing potential clients who hoped to engage Wilson & Colby were officers of the Sinclair Consolidated Oil Corporation, who sought representation in two investigations about to take place before the United States Senate. One case dealt with the fluctuating price of gasoline; the other concerned Sinclair's recent acquisition of property in Wyoming known as Teapot Dome. Through some sleight of hand endorsed by Harding, the land had come under the jurisdiction of Interior Secretary Albert B. Fall, who had, in turn, leased the vast oil field to Sinclair. Colby wrote Wilson that this promised to be "a very substantial and important employment"—a high-profile hearing with compensation in six figures. Colby also looked forward to working with ex-Senator George Sutherland of Utah as co-counsel. "Do you see any objection to accepting this employment?" he asked his partner.

Wilson did. A private oil company seeking representation from a former President whose conservation policies opposed such leases seemed highly suspect. Wilson only knew what he had read in the newspapers, which gave the impression "that some ugly business is going on in respect to the Teapot Dome," but he knew that "the oil companies are constantly attempting to invade that Reserve with or without right." Worse, Wilson considered Senator Sutherland "one of the most thick headed and impenetrable of the Senate partisans." Again, Colby deferred to Wilson's judgment. After yet another instance in which Colby had to refuse a $500,000 retainer for a case he felt sure would not compromise Wilson's integrity, he spoke to Edith. "Of course I want to go on as long as we can hold out," he said, "but day after day I sit in my office and see a procession walk through—thousands and thousands of dollars—and not one to put in our pockets. It is a sublime position on the part of your husband, and I am honoured to share it as long as we can afford it."

The Wilsons appreciated Colby's steadfastness, but Edith urged her husband to end the partnership, freeing Colby to earn a living. Wilson regretted only that he had hindered Colby more than helped him, especially as Colby had been so solicitous in his attempts to engage Wilson in

a new occupation when he clearly had little interest. Tellingly, after his first visit to the offices, Wilson never set foot in them again. His only residual from the enterprise was a distribution of $5,000, to which he felt so unentitled, he blew the money on a Rauch & Lang electric car for Edith, a newer model of the vehicle she had famously driven around Washington before their marriage.

Colby would announce the termination of the partnership in December 1922, saying that Wilson wished to redirect his energies to politics. The midterm elections that year reflected the unpopularity of the Harding Administration—halving the Republican lead in the Senate, and putting the Democrats within striking distance of recapturing the House, what with a gain of more than seventy-five Representatives. Wilson said the people regretted the verdict they had delivered in 1920, "and are preparing to render one in favor of the policies they then unwisely condemned." The party was coming back, Colby asserted, "on a tide of revived Wilsonism." Wilson himself, Colby suggested, wanted to "direct the flowing of this tide." And Colby was one of the few who knew that the former President was, in fact, considering another run for the White House.

Madness did not fuel this pipe dream so much as anger. Within Harding's first months in office, Congress introduced the highest tariffs in American history. The all-Republican government—with its protectionism and allegiance to big business—would make every attempt it could to erase Wilson's record.

On August 25, 1921, the United States signed the Treaty of Berlin, which officially ended the war with Germany. This neutered version of Wilson's Treaty of Versailles incorporated the Lodge reservations. That week, the nation also signed treaties with Austria and Hungary. The Revenue Act of 1921 dramatically reduced taxes for the very rich, which Treasury Secretary Andrew Mellon argued was necessary in order to stimulate economic growth. During his first Christmas in office, Harding commuted the sentence of Eugene V. Debs.

More than politics, White House ethics had changed. The capital buzzed with stories of the President's liquor consumption, poker games, extramarital affairs, and cronies in high places, not the least of whom were Secretary Fall and Attorney General Harry M. Daugherty, a renowned Ohio political fixer. The louche President set the tone for the rest of the nation, encouraging licentiousness. In the words of the country's new

literary sensation, F. Scott Fitzgerald, "America was going on the greatest, gaudiest spree in history"—as a lost generation ran wild in what Fitzgerald christened "the Jazz Age." To many across the nation, the priggish Woodrow Wilson had never looked more attractive.

"Never," observed Ray Baker from his desk in the dugout, "was there such a swift change of public regard for a man than for Mr. Wilson since he left the White House." This wave of admiration manifested itself in scores of ways, beyond the appreciation expressed in the press and the batches of mail. The house at 2340 S Street became a highlight of the rubberneck wagon tours of Washington, and every afternoon at three o'clock, people gathered to watch the Wilsons as they departed for their daily drive. In May, the Reverend Sylvester Beach of Princeton reported from the General Assembly of the Presbyterian Church in Indiana that the entire convocation rose to its feet and cheered for five minutes upon a Czech minister's mention of Woodrow Wilson and the League of Nations. President Alderman of the University of Virginia wrote Wilson that many of the school's students, acting upon "an independent impulse," raised money to place a bronze tablet on his former room at 31 West Range. When the boys asked Alderman for an appropriate inscription, he suggested five words from Horace—"*Justum ac tenacem propositi virum*" ("A just man who sticks to his principles"). Plaques, bridges, and streets in Wilson's name popped up around the world, from Montevideo to Bordeaux, including an avenue in Paris and a drive in Los Angeles. More than fifty Woodrow Wilson clubs sprouted on college campuses in appreciation of his "generous service to humanity." Many of the younger generation felt called to service by his "inspired leadership to establish justice and peace as the basis for a new international conception of freedom."

In the meantime, several prominent women banded to promulgate Wilson's principles. They took their idea to Cleveland Dodge; and soon more Wilson supporters, including the members of the Woodrow Wilson clubs, joined this movement to establish "a nation-wide tribute to Woodrow Wilson in appreciation of his great service for world peace." At a meeting at New York's Biltmore Hotel, several admirers developed a plan to raise $500,000 for the cause, and formed a steering committee that included Henry Morgenthau, Adolph Ochs, Bernard Baruch, Daisy Harriman, and Franklin D. Roosevelt, who served as chairman. Their initial impulse was to give several substantial prizes each year to the college

students who wrote the best papers on "international subjects related to the development of the League of Nations." This endowment became the cornerstone for the Woodrow Wilson Foundation and paved the way for future institutions that would link policy and scholarship in his name, most notably the Woodrow Wilson International Center for Scholars. Roosevelt maintained an active interest in the organization despite being struck ill in August 1921, at his summer home on Campobello Island. It left him paralyzed below the waist. By September, the Roosevelts announced that he had poliomyelitis but that it was a mild case that would have temporary effects. His unabating work on the Foundation helped conceal the actual seriousness of his condition.

On October 4, 1921, President Harding wrote Wilson of an "unusual assemblage" to take place at Arlington National Cemetery—the burial of an unknown soldier from the World War. Great Britain and France had each established a similar monument the year prior on Armistice Day; and an act of Congress in Wilson's final minutes as President authorized the exhumation of an unnamed American soldier from one of the cemeteries in France for entombment in a new marble sarcophagus at Arlington. "Undoubtedly it will be the part of the President to have a presidential party of a considerable number on that day," Harding wrote, "and I have thought it would be fine if you could find it agreeable for you and Mrs. Wilson to accept an invitation to become members thereof."

Although his disability would prevent him from visiting the grave, Wilson was determined to pay his respects to the fallen by riding in the procession that would transport the Unknown Soldier's casket from the Capitol to the cemetery. He requested an open carriage instead of a motorcar. After a series of slights on the part of the Harding White House, the Wilsons arrived at the appointed minute in their victoria, their servant Isaac Scott sitting with the coachman. No guard appeared to escort them, and when a police sergeant led them to the forming parade, they discovered that their place had already been filled. As the procession began to move down Pennsylvania Avenue, behind the flag-draped caisson, the Wilsons had to wait and then wedge themselves unceremoniously into the first available space, far behind the officials and between two phalanxes of marching veterans. Thousands lined the great boulevard, observing the passing of the Unknown Soldier in solemn stillness.

Then, as the two-horse carriage bearing the Wilsons appeared—the

former President in a dark suit and overcoat and high silk hat, and wearing a small red poppy in his lapel—whispers spread through the crowd. Slowly a ripple of applause broke out. When all the observers realized that it was Wilson himself, there was a steady wave of approbation that lasted the entire way to the White House. There Wilson detached from the procession, as he had been instructed, and retreated to S Street. He told a newspaperman that the ovation had embarrassed him "because it was given in a funeral procession."

Later that day, many found themselves drawn to S Street, spontaneously paying homage to the man some were calling "the Known Soldier." Not until Wilson appeared at his front door at three o'clock did he discover twenty thousand people had amassed in front of the house. For ten minutes they roared, offering three cheers for the League of Nations, another three cheers for Woodrow Wilson, and three more for "the greatest soldier of them all!" Leaning hard on his cane, the former President walked down the five front steps of his house in order to greet three disabled veterans in a car in his driveway. Then he went back inside, where he and Edith appeared at a window on the second floor. The crowd, not ready to disperse, again demanded his presence.

He returned to the front door, where several committees of Wilson societies had gathered. Hundreds of children waited as well, one of whom handed him a letter, which said, "Young as we are we have learned to admire you and the great principles for which you stand. . . . We, as future citizens of the United States, will do our best to perpetuate these ideals you have fought for so bravely." A member of the League of Nations Association spoke of the burial at Arlington, saying, "We haven't forgot the ideals for which we went to war and for which this soldier died." He assured Wilson that his work "shall not die."

"I wish that I had the voice to reply and to thank you for the wonderful tribute that you have paid me," Wilson told the crowd. "I can only say God bless you." Silence followed, until one man boomed, "Long live the best man in the world!" The crowd cheered once again, and tears streamed from Wilson's eyes. Trembling, he reached for Edith's hand. Like most of the crowd, she cried as well. The throng spontaneously broke into "My Country, 'Tis of Thee," and the Wilsons held on to each other as he said goodbye and kissed his wife's hand. They entered the house, but the people remained for another hour, silent and still.

The spiritual nature of the afternoon was lost on none of its witnesses. Even Senator John Sharp Williams of Mississippi, who had served in Congress since 1893, had been drawn to S Street. He found himself as inspired as all the others, who wanted nothing "political or actual to be accomplished," he wrote Wilson, "except to show good will to you for the present, faith in you for the future, and an endorsement of you in the past." The tide had definitely turned, he said, in its feelings not only toward Wilson but also his beliefs.

No less a figure than muckraker and teacher Ida Tarbell, who had been lecturing across the country, discovered that Americans were awakening to the responsibilities of foreign affairs and Wilson's approach to them. After the political denunciation he had received the year prior, she wrote an article for *Collier's* called "The Man They Cannot Forget," in which she asked why people from so many walks of life revered him. Her rhetorical answer lay in his having inspired their greatest moments through the example of his deeds as well as the power of his words. She believed the essence of Wilson's mission on earth was to elevate mankind. He made overused American catchphrases and high-minded political rhetoric real— personal and deep, "the working basis on which men may strive to liberty of soul and peaceful achievement." Above all, she wrote:

> He made them literally things to die for, lifting all of our plain, humble thousands who never knew applause or wealth or the honor of office into the ranks of those who are willing to die for an ideal—the highest plane that humans reach.

Although Wilson had never worn a military uniform, soldiers and their families held him in special regard. They felt he had sacrificed as much as they had, and they said as much in the letters that poured into S Street. An especially moving display occurred one Saturday night at Keith's Theatre, when an elderly actor came before the footlights and addressed the audience. "My only boy was killed in the war," he said, "and not in words can I express how much I miss him." He described a recent visit to Walter Reed Army Hospital, where he encountered what he called "pieces of still living men." He candidly admitted that he found comfort knowing his boy "was sleeping peacefully in France" and not among the shattered victims he had visited. "But one of the greatest casualties this war has

produced," he said, on a note of pride, "is the distinguished man who is in this audience tonight." Audience members wept openly as they rose to their feet and cheered, some leaping onto their seats and waving handkerchiefs. A girl stepped down from the stage and walked to seat U-21 to hand Woodrow Wilson a bunch of flowers.

There was a Wilson revival in the making, and his most devout follower of the last decade had to scurry to find his place in it. Not even on S Street—where Bolling performed secretarial duties, Baker advised, and Colby, Baruch, Norman Davis, and Louis Brandeis appeared for political conversation—was there a specific role for Tumulty. In November 1921, he published *Woodrow Wilson As I Know Him*, a hagiographic memoir, meant to show not only Wilson's great intellect but also his "great heart." At least one critic found the book an "incredibly vulgar, oleographic caricature," with the author basking in reflected glory. While Wilson never displayed any interest in it, the volume was just one of many that quickly appeared.

With access both to Wilson and his papers, which had no strings attached, Ray Baker published a three-volume work entitled *Woodrow Wilson and World Settlement*. It contributed enormously to Wilson's growing popularity. He allowed that Wilson's mission to Paris had failed to actualize his dreams, but he gave the public a sense of Wilson's own estimation of his work there. He had told Baker one afternoon while lying in bed, "I am not an impractical idealist, nor did I, at Paris, want everything torn up by the roots and made over according to some ideal plan." With Professor William E. Dodd of the University of Chicago—already the author of a short Wilson biography, and a future Ambassador to Germany—Baker produced six volumes of Wilson's public papers. With a healthy monthly stipend from Bernard Baruch, Baker spent another fourteen years writing an eight-volume biography to honor the former President.

Marginalized, Tumulty frantically sought ways to reenter Wilson's life. On April 5, 1922, he wrote the "Governor," as he continued to call him, that the National Democratic Club of New York City was holding its annual Jefferson banquet that week and that it would "hearten and inspire" the audience to receive a message from him. Even an expression of regret at not being able to attend would suffice, Tumulty said, as it would also extend Tumulty's credibility as an insider to the former President. Wilson refused. He felt it would be "quite meaningless" unless he offered a serious

expression of his view about the current national situation, and he did not consider this an appropriate occasion for breaking his silence.

The next morning, Tumulty called Mrs. Wilson and asked if she could not get her husband to send a letter to the dinner. Edith asked if Tumulty had not received his reply. Although he had, he fretfully stressed the importance of Wilson's writing something and beseeched her to persuade him. "No, Mr. Tumulty," Edith said, "you know him well enough to know that when he has thought a thing out and decided it there is no use to continue arguments." Then Tumulty said he had an important personal matter he needed to discuss with Wilson, and he asked if she could at least arrange for a meeting that afternoon. She respected the wish and set the meeting for three o'clock, just before the Wilsons' daily drive. An anxious Tumulty arrived early and sat in the dugout with Randolph Bolling, asking him if Mrs. Wilson had gotten Wilson to compose a message for the dinner. Bolling thought not; and because Wilson was feeling low that day, he recommended that Tumulty not even raise the matter.

Because of the "personal" nature of Tumulty's mission, Edith left the two men alone. By the time she returned from an errand, he had gone. She said to Woodrow that she hoped Tumulty had not bothered him about that message for the dinner. He said, "No, I am glad to say he had the good taste not to mention it." When she asked what he had come to discuss, it turned out to be a vague conversation about American ideals, clearly a hasty substitute for what he had hoped to talk about. Days later, the morning newspapers wrote up the speech Governor Cox had made at the Jefferson banquet . . . along with the message "from Woodrow Wilson": "Say to the Democrats of New York that I am ready to support any man who stands for the salvation of America, and the salvation of America is justice to all classes." Because Cox had addressed those very points, the audience logically interpreted the banquet as the unofficial launch of his campaign—with Wilson's endorsement. "My husband," Edith recalled a decade later, "was thunderstruck."

Wilson summoned Edith's brother and asked him to dispatch a letter to Louis Wiley of *The New York Times* expressing the former President's dismay—not only because he had never sent any message but also because of his suggested support for Cox to head the ticket again. He valued Cox as a loyal friend of the League but believed defeated teams required new captains to turn them around. Later that morning, while shaving, he told

Edith it had just occurred to him that Tumulty had been at the banquet
and that perhaps he could shed light on what had occurred. Dictating to
her, he said, "It is obviously my duty as well as my privilege to probe the
incident to the bottom."

A chagrined Tumulty hastened from New York, and after many desperate hours attempting to see Wilson in person, he sheepishly owned up
to having composed the message himself. He realized the embarrassment
he had caused his former boss and the need to rectify what he maintained
was a misunderstanding on his part. He offered a contorted explanation to
The New York Times. While he assumed responsibility for the delivery of
the fabricated message, he wrote Wilson, "I think you will hold me blame-
less for the unjust interpretations put upon it."

Tumulty knew he had not adequately apologized, and so the next day
he sent Wilson a more detailed explanation, which only dug a deeper hole
for himself. He realized he had betrayed the Governor's trust, but he presumed Wilson would take into account that since the earliest days of their
association, as he said, "I have had but one thought, but one ambition, and
that was to serve you and the great purposes which I know lay close to
your heart." Now he prostrated himself, affirming, "You will find me as a
mere private in the ranks, deferring to your unselfish leadership and de-
fending your policies at every turn of the long road which lies ahead of us."
If Wilson found it necessary to rebuke him, Tumulty said, he would not
complain, nor would he "wince under the blow nor . . . grow in the least
faint-hearted or dispirited." In all his protestations, Tumulty never simply
acknowledged that Wilson had explicitly stated he never wished to send a
message in the first place. He was shown the same door as Hibben and
House before him.

Several days later, Dr. Grayson asked Wilson whether he had had a
good night, and he said no. "I am not worrying about the Tumulty incident," he told his doctor. "If Tumulty had been my son and had acted as
he did, I would have done the same thing." But it clearly weighed on his
mind, heavily enough for Edith to suggest that Wilson air their full correspondence in the press. "No," he said, "let the unpleasant affair fade out.
Tumulty will sulk for a few days, then come like a spanked child to say
that he is sorry and wants to be forgiven." Days later, Grayson expressed
regret that Wilson had severed relations with Tumulty. Wilson snapped
that the doctor did not know what he was talking about and that it was

none of his business. During a house call a few days later, Wilson asked his wife and attendant to leave the room, so that he could discuss a private matter with Grayson. "I want to apologize for the way in which I spoke to you the other day," he said. Thereupon he showed Grayson the correspondence detailing the entire affair, which had culminated in Tumulty's evasive apology. For his part, the doctor never thought ill of his patient, always understanding his frustration. As Grayson explained one day to Axson, "He has to hate *somebody*."

Despite his mixed feelings for Tumulty, Wilson never questioned his loyalty nor forgot his service. He would even encourage New Jersey leaders to back him for the Senate because of his extensive political training. But Joseph Tumulty all but retired from politics, devoting the rest of his career to a successful law practice. Woodrow Wilson never saw him again.

In truth, more had contributed to this severance than had met the eye. Once he had moved to Kalorama, Wilson's political itch had flared up, and Tumulty's actions had encouraged it further. As was known to but a handful of people, Wilson had been preparing a white paper for months, a refreshening of progressive principles for the new decade. In June 1921, he approached the chief architect of the New Freedom, Louis Brandeis, and found him willing to collaborate on this manifesto, despite its blatantly political nature. Either out of gratitude that Wilson had elevated him to the Supreme Court or perhaps because his contributions were meant to be unofficial, he actively participated, certainly eager to advance his own progressive ideas. Wilson did not mention that he planned to offer this statement as a platform for the Democratic Presidential nominee in 1924, but as he called upon such members of his administration as Colby, Houston, Baruch, and Norman Davis, and party supporters Thomas Chadbourne and Frank I. Cobb, to help him shape a casual collection of opinions into a systematic set of issues, one could hardly imagine any other purpose for their work.

"The Document," as the collaborators called it, contained nineteen points. They included the necessity to reconstruct the progressive countries of the world and the belief that a broad-minded, liberal agenda could best provide reform. Furthermore, the policy statement demanded the immediate resumption of America's international obligations as established in the Treaty of Versailles, and it condemned the group of men who catalyzed the current "evil results as the most partisan, prejudiced, ignorant and unpatriotic group that ever misled the Senate of the United States."

Despite Republican control of the government, the Document pointed out that the Republican Party had not enacted a single piece of ameliorative legislation in the last three years. It also demanded a revision of the tax laws that would impose less upon the lower and middle classes; and it advocated a new Cabinet member, a Secretary of Transportation, who could untangle the complex skein of local and national laws to improve the flow of people and goods. "The world has been made safe for democracy," the Document read, "but democracy has not yet made the world safe against irrational revolution."

Over the next two and a half years, Wilson reworked the Document. With his longtime belief in the co-operation of government between the branches, he added a paragraph that the President and the members of his Cabinet should be accorded a place on the Congressional floor whenever the legislature was discussing affairs entrusted to the executive branch. The President should take part and be held accountable. With such matters occupying his thoughts, Wilson did nothing to suggest that he supported Cox for the 1924 nomination, because he had set his sights on his own nominee—once again, the only man who could reassert those programs that were "the best assurance for the promotion of social welfare, of justice, and of individuals and of national prosperity."

Support for his own candidacy presented itself almost every day, as the house on S Street became a mecca for liberals. In April 1922, for example, the League of Women Voters held an international conference in Baltimore to discuss world peace and social reform, gathering delegates from twenty-two nations of the Western Hemisphere. On the twenty-eighth, a thousand of them descended upon Wilson's house, merely to pay tribute to a man who had championed both peace and women's rights. Dressed in a frock coat and silk hat, he greeted them at his front door, looking especially frail that day and explaining that he was unable to make an address. He favored them instead with a limerick. The women responded with a chorus of "America," "Onward, Christian Soldiers," and a lusty cheer for the League of Nations. Throughout the spring, Wilson maintained a substantive correspondence with Cordell Hull, chairman of the Democratic National Committee, who sought his advice about mobilizing the party during the upcoming midterm elections. Even Vice President Coolidge paid homage to the League of Nations that June in a commencement ad-

dress, praising its "noble aspiration for world association and understanding," its imperfections notwithstanding.

By summer, Wilson believed the Democrats would return to power, finding themselves with "the greatest opportunity for service that has ever been accorded it." He believed the Harding Administration, with its attempt to "reestablish all the injustices of the past," had disenchanted the electorate, resisting "progress" with its chatter of getting back to normalcy. When the Council of the League of Nations confirmed the British mandate of Palestine in July, Zionist organizations remembered with gratitude Wilson's "distinguished and unselfish cooperation" on their behalf. When Supreme Court Justice John Hessin Clarke announced his retirement that September, he told Wilson that with his remaining strength, he intended to do all he could to promote American entrance into the League. "To me," he said, "it is the indispensable as well as the noblest political conception of our time and, very certainly, to have launched it as you did makes secure for you one of the highest places in history." And when Emily Newell Blair, a former suffragist and founder of the League of Women Voters, realized that women were not voting as a reliable bloc, she took it upon herself to organize them as Democrats. She did this, she wrote Wilson in October, "because of the debt the American women owe you, not only for the suffrage but for the fight you made for ideals." By autumn a Democratic sweep in the midterm elections was in the air, and with it even the growing possibility that the senior Senator from Massachusetts would be unseated.

Henry Cabot Lodge won his sixth term, eking out a victory by a few thousand votes. Wilson wrote his daughter Jessie that he hoped the election results at least "gave him a jolt which may make even him comprehend the new temper of the voters." The Democrats did not recapture either chamber, but they did enjoy considerable success—gaining five seats in the Senate and seventy-six seats in the House, putting legislative control within their reach. Members of the Farmer-Labor Party found greater kinship among Democrats, as the agrarian Midwest and the members of the American Federation of Labor no longer saw the Republican Party sensitive to their needs. Immigrants in the big cities became firmly Democratic. Two years earlier, New Yorkers had swept Governor Alfred E. Smith out of office. Now they apologized by awarding him a landslide victory over his replacement. Across the country, Democratic victories rebuked two years of

Harding and his policies—especially the tariff—and he was already being talked about as a one-term President. On the midterm Election Night, tens of thousands of people milled outside newspaper offices in Washington, and when one paper projected a picture of Woodrow Wilson on a screen, the crowd cheered lustily. Daniel C. Roper, Wilson's manager from the 1916 campaign, sent congratulations to his former candidate; and without divulging any private plans, an encouraged Wilson wired back, "Twenty four will complete the result which twenty two had begun."

Four days later, five thousand admirers flocked to S Street for what had come to be called "the annual Armistice Day pilgrimage." Wilson totemized the World War's hopes for a peaceful future, and this year such luminaries as former Ambassador Morgenthau, University of Virginia President Alderman, and former Secretary of Agriculture Meredith joined the exuberant throngs. Streetcar lines added extra cars to transport the worshipful to Kalorama. Wilson appeared, with a big malacca cane in one hand and looking healthier than he had in years. Festivities began outside his front door with a medley of Southern songs. Then Morgenthau spoke, referring to the election results as a rejection of "materialism and selfishness." A few heard Wilson exclaim, "Hear, hear!"

Hooking his cane in the upper pocket of his coat, Wilson stood on his own two feet. He spoke for several minutes, delivering his longest address since Pueblo. With all his old passion, he spoke of that "group in the United States Senate who preferred personal partisan motives to the honor of their country and the peace of the world." He reminded the crowd, "Puny persons who are now standing in the way will presently find that their weakness is no match for the strength of a moving Providence." Wilson retreated inside the house, only to reappear in a second-story window, with Edith at his side. For ten minutes the fans cheered. And then the sea of people parted, forming two long lines on either side of S Street, so that the Wilsons could ride through for their daily outing. Block after block, he acknowledged the roaring crowd, smiling and raising his hat.

Upon turning sixty-six, Wilson received two unexpected tributes. On December 27, 1922, Franklin Roosevelt informed him that in little more than a year, the organizers of the Woodrow Wilson Foundation had raised $1 million. The fund's income would be used, Roosevelt said, to prompt public welfare, democracy, and peace through justice. The next day, Wilson's birthday, he welcomed four of the Foundation's board members and

learned that most of their funding had come not from wealthy benefactors (such as Henry Ford, who had contributed $10,000) but from thousands of ordinary citizens, each of whom supported his vision with a dollar. The delegation left Wilson virtually speechless. "I wish I could have controlled my voice so I could really have expressed what I felt," he told Edith afterward; "but I could not trust myself lest I break down and cry." Despite a cold downpour that day, more than a hundred people waited in the rain, hoping for a glimpse of Wilson.

The second extraordinary gesture came from the United States Senate, an expression of "pleasure and joy" upon hearing of the former President's continued recovery to good health. "When all of us are forgotten," said Senator William J. Harris of Georgia in introducing the resolution, "the name of Woodrow Wilson will be remembered as the greatest of the century." While many of the Republicans appeared to be busy during the actual vote, there was no debate and the resolution passed with a hearty chorus of "ayes." Vice President Coolidge appended his own personal greeting in a letter that accompanied the message that was sent to S Street. Wilson told Dr. Grayson, "Think of them passing it and not meaning it. Of course, I do not mean to say that all who voted for it were not sincere, for I know many were sincere, but I feel sure some of them were not. I would much rather have had three Senators get together and draw up a resolution and have it passed with sincerity than the one that was passed today."

Wilson thought of reentering the public arena as he had entered years ago—through the written word. He conceived an ambitious book, which he was calling *The Destiny of the Republic.* It would "set forth . . . the ideals and principles which have governed my life, and which have also . . . governed the life of the nation." He tried typing with his one good hand, and when that proved too awkward, he dictated passages to Edith.

The opening lines of his text articulated the basis of what his successors would call "Wilsonianism":

Unlike the government of every other great state, ancient or modern, the government of the United States was set up for the benefit of mankind as well as for the benefit of its own people,—a most ambitious enterprise, no doubt, but undertaken with high purpose, with clear vision, and without thoughtful and deliberate unselfishness, and undertaken by men who were no amateurs but acquainted with the world

they lived in, practiced in the conduct of affairs, who set the new government up with an ordiliness [*sic*] and self-possession which marked
them as men who were proud to serve liberty with the dignity and restraint of true devotees of a great ideal.

Wilson never wrote much more than a few paragraphs of the book. As
with his prior attempts, his lavish dedication to Edith was its most realized passage.

A year passed before he could tease any of his thoughts into even a
short essay, which he did in "The Road Away from Revolution." Wilson
pecked out a thousand words on his typewriter with his right hand, arguing that the Russian Revolution had been an attack against capitalism, a
system that was not above reproach. Sometimes he worked late at night,
insisting he could not sleep until he had committed his thoughts to paper.
He said civilization could not survive materially unless it were redeemed
spiritually, that it could be saved "only by becoming permeated with the
spirit of Christ and being made free and happy by the practices which
spring out of that spirit."

Former propaganda chief George Creel had once volunteered to act as
his representative in placing any of his writing. In April 1923, Wilson
asked him to consider handling this essay. But upon reading the piece,
Creel felt the best he could do for Wilson was to suppress it. In gentle but
frank terms, he wrote Edith that its publication—what would be Wilson's
first public document since his collapse—would not live up to the people's
expectations. While strongly advising against printing it for the public, he
realized such advice would crush Wilson's confidence and might push him
back into depression.

The Wilsons could have used the money that newspaper syndication of
the article would pay, but Creel put his client's psychological needs before
the financial. He spoke to an editor friend who offered $2,000 for the
rights to publish it in *Collier's*, where it could appear with dignity and without exaggerating its importance by turning this trifle into a media event.
Creel wrote up a second letter for Edith to show her husband, a recommendation to accept the less lucrative deal because syndication would entail "a huckstering campaign that will undoubtedly have many disagreeable
reactions." Edith considered how best to approach Woodrow.

Days later, in the Pierce-Arrow, with Stockton Axson there for moral

support, she screwed up enough courage to say that somebody had read the piece and did not think it did justice to him. His temper flared—not with Edith necessarily, but with all the people who had been urging him for months to write something. "They kept after me to do this thing," he said in irritation, "and I did it." Edith tried to mollify him, telling him not to get on his "high horse about this." She simply wanted to forward the suggestion that he expand the piece by amplifying his argument. He read between the lines. "I have done all I can, and all I am going to do," Wilson insisted. "I don't want those people bothering me any more." When they returned home, Wilson went upstairs to his bedroom, and Axson sat in the dugout. After a few minutes, Axson heard a peculiar sound—Edith, in the hallway, was sobbing. He went to console her in this, one of the few times anybody ever saw her break down. "All I want to do is just to help in any way I can," she insisted. "I am not urging him to do things he doesn't want to do. I just want to help and I just don't know how to help."

Axson examined the article and suggested cutting, not lengthening—thus lessening it from a significant treatise to a simple pronouncement. Edith asked if he would present his findings to her husband, which he did. "Why, you see exactly the point," Wilson said. "Fix it." After Axson had excised a few paragraphs and retyped the article, Wilson submitted it himself to *The Atlantic Monthly*, which had published his essays in the past. Editor Ellery Sedgwick gratefully accepted the piece for $300. It reached a fraction of the audience it might have, and the author abandoned all further literary efforts.

Wilson recognized the silent strain under which Edith had functioned over the last five years. For a while he inquired about the cottages at the Grove Park Inn, a popular resort in Asheville, North Carolina, where he imagined they might spend a few months. As he never proceeded in his negotiations with the hotel proprietor, the junket met the same fate as the renewal of his law practice, the writing of his book on political theory, and his third run for the Presidency—though he did go so far as to make notes for his acceptance speech and his third inaugural address. Then, thinking his real contribution to society had been in education, not politics, Wilson contacted a former student, then at the Rockefeller Foundation, to investigate the possibility of his becoming a university president once again—only this time at a new school, one willing to accept his innovative teaching concepts. All these gauzy visions allowed him to maintain that fine line

between illusion and delusion—to imagine such exploits without having to confront the hard facts that they were beyond his capability. Indeed, for all the liveliness of Wilson's dreams, he remained prone to exhaustion and mood swings, a stroke victim with advancing arteriosclerosis who was unable to navigate a flight of stairs, a handicap then considered a fatal political liability.

Presidential incapacity became a national story once again—in the summer of 1923, when Warren Harding embarked upon a cross-country tour to the Pacific Coast. For months it had been whispered that the robust fifty-five-year-old President-elect who had bounded up the Capitol steps to his inauguration only twenty-nine months earlier had grown exceedingly tired in office as the result of heart disease. Harding showed symptoms of food poisoning in Vancouver, Canada, rushed through a speech in Seattle, and had to cancel another in Portland. On August 2, he suffered a fatal heart attack in his hotel suite in San Francisco.

The news shocked Wilson. Despite the great differences in their politics and personalities—and the fact that Wilson thought him a "fool," except for the fact that there was "nothing in his conduct that the country can laugh at with the slightest degree of enjoyment"—the two Presidents had maintained a cordial relationship. Wilson sent prompt and "profound sympathy" to Harding's widow.

By the light of a kerosene lamp at their house in rural Plymouth Notch, Vermont, Vice President Calvin Coolidge took the oath of office from his father, a notary public. The following day, Coolidge invited Wilson to participate in Harding's funeral services on Wednesday, the eighth. Wilson appreciated the honor of joining the procession, in which he hoped to include his wife and Dr. Grayson, but his lame leg, he said, made it impracticable for him to attend the exercises at the Capitol, where Harding's body was to lie in state. On the day of the services, Wilson waited in his open car outside the White House for more than an hour until the flag-covered casket was carried from the East Room to the artillery caisson. While Marines in full-dress uniforms wilted under the hot August sun, Wilson remained collected—until one dazed Colonel rushed up, wondering if he might ask a question. "Certainly," said Wilson. "Could you tell me whether Senator Lodge has arrived or not?" Wilson uttered that he could not. Then he turned to Grayson and asked "what asylum that Colonel had escaped from." For the next few minutes, the *New York Times*

reporter noticed that Wilson was visibly moved, his eyes fixed upon the coffin of his successor, nine years his junior. As Wilson's car rode down Pennsylvania Avenue, following Coolidge and the new Chief Justice, William Howard Taft—recently appointed upon the death of Edward Douglass White—hundreds of people along the sidewalks paid homage to Wilson by removing their hats. Upon reaching the Capitol, Woodrow and Edith veered back to S Street.

The ovation Wilson received at Keith's Theatre that Saturday night surpassed any he had received before. The headliner, a French soprano named Mademoiselle Diane, closed the show with a special mention of the distinguished guests. When they reached their car in the stage door alley, a double quartet surrounded his car, singing "Just a Song at Twilight." By the time the song ended, five hundred people had gathered, including that evening's entire cast. Wilson was so captivated by the reception, he asked the chanteuse to sing the "Marseillaise," and she obliged. The crowd cheered, Wilson raised his hat, and the car drove off. A man in the crowd shouted, "There's the man you can't forget."

Wilson's popularity continued to climb, especially as the Harding Administration underwent immediate and unfortunate postmortems. His controversial Interior Secretary, Albert Fall, had resigned earlier that year as the Senate began to investigate his oil leases, specifically Teapot Dome. Fall was found guilty of conspiracy and bribery and sentenced to a year in prison, becoming the first United States Cabinet member to serve time as a result of malfeasance in office. Other scandals followed, including those involving a number of mistresses Harding had entertained during his White House residency. One of them, Nan Britton, claimed he was the father of her illegitimate daughter. Because Florence Harding had not allowed an autopsy of her husband, further suspicions clung to his reputation, as people questioned whether the President had died of a heart attack, a stroke, suicide, or even poison at his wife's hand. The taciturn Calvin Coolidge proved to have a steadying influence on the nation. Despite his conservative policies, Wilson looked upon him favorably as a courteous and decent man.

Many marveled at Wilson's endurance during that especially torpid summer, though few said the same of Edith. A long profile in *The New York Times* commented on his rehabilitation and even suggested his possible reentry into politics. The journalist attributed much of his restoration

to the constant devotion of his wife, who had not left him for more than a day and a half since he had been stricken in Pueblo. After years of priding herself on her own good health, Edith recognized that she was simply worn out. Friends in the shore town of Mattapoisett, Massachusetts— Charles Sumner Hamlin, the first chairman of the Federal Reserve Board, and his wife—invited Edith to visit. Woodrow encouraged her to accept, especially after Dr. Grayson said if she did not, she would "break down completely." The doctor volunteered to stay at S Street in her absence.

Woodrow missed Edith terribly, but her week away made him realize, as he typed in one of his daily notes to her, "how completely my life is intertwined with yours." She returned in September considerably revived but could not say the same for Woodrow. For the first time, she noticed how much he had aged, not in just the last week but in the last few years. His progressive arteriosclerosis, lack of exercise, and age itself contributed to his physical malaise and mental depression. Then his good eye began to fail, the result of small retinal hemorrhages. He maintained his regimen, but he could no longer recognize people on the street, and reading became a chore. His world darkened.

Wilson's outings to Keith's and his enjoyment of moving pictures tapered off. His reading was reduced to leafing through illustrated magazines—*Country Life*, *National Geographic*, *Photoplay*, *Screenland*, *Theatre Magazine*, and *Vanity Fair*—sometimes using a magnifying glass and flashlight to study details. Edith continued to read to him, mostly old favorites—Bagehot and Sir Walter Scott. And he played thousands of hands of canfield.

For the most part, he received only those visitors whose presence guaranteed a few minutes of easy conversation. Clemenceau visited the United States for the first time in more than fifty years, and he and Wilson enjoyed what the former called an "affectionate" reunion. "We didn't discuss the future," the old Tiger later reported, "—only the occasional good moments of the old days." He said, "[We] fully forgave each other for our bitter quarrels at Versailles. That was all in the past; and both of us had lost." In October 1923, the Wilsons entertained Mr. and Mrs. David Lloyd George, and both men laid aside their past differences, as the conversation degenerated into reciting limericks. Colonel House called one afternoon and left his cards for both Mr. and Mrs. Wilson. Surely he knew he would not find Wilson at home during the hour of his ritual drive; and just as

surely Wilson could have reached House while he was in Washington—if Edith ever even mentioned the calling cards to Woodrow. Later, a number of mutual friends tried to reconnect the two old friends, but Edith never saw fit to relay their entreaties.

Visitors winnowed down to family members—Stockton Axson, Edith's mother and siblings, and, of course, Wilson's daughters. Her singing career as thin as her voice, Margaret spent years finding herself. While she was questioning her faith and searching for answers, she periodically turned up at S Street. The McAdoos visited from Los Angeles, where they were raising their two young daughters and where Mac had become general counsel to a new producing partnership of Hollywood's most important stars— Chaplin, Pickford, and Fairbanks. With his 20 percent ownership in the company, United Artists provided him an opportunity to earn some significant money and make influential contacts. McAdoo continued to plot a course to the White House, which Wilson never embraced, but Nell's sprightly appearance never failed to cheer him. And that year Jessie announced that the government of Siam had invited her husband, Frank Sayre, to take a leave from teaching law at Harvard to advise the progressive Asian nation as it opened doors to Western political thought. Wilson's heart sank at the thought of his serene daughter going so far away for so long, but he urged his son-in-law to accept what seemed to be a most interesting offer. During their farewell visit to Washington in early September, Wilson took one of his afternoon drives with his grandson Francis Junior, then eight years old. As they were driving up Massachusetts Avenue, a bystander recognized the car and shouted out, "I'm for the League!" The somewhat startled boy yelled back, "I'm for the League!" And with that, he recalled a lifetime later, "Grandfather didn't say a word. He just dissolved into tears for reasons I didn't understand, pulled me into his arm, and kissed me on the forehead."

Among Wilson's guests that autumn was Bernard Baruch's eldest daughter, Belle. She and a friend staunchly supported the League of Nations through a group they helped finance called the Nonpartisan League. They hoped to boost both their leagues by getting Wilson to speak over the radio on "The Significance of Armistice Day." Although new to broadcasting, he agreed to an Armistice Eve address. Edith noticed her husband's trepidation. Where he formerly could speak off the cuff for hours, his crippled body, his failing eyesight, and his fear of speaking into

a microphone constrained him terribly. For two weeks he fretted, as he labored over eight paragraph-long sentences. Without ever mentioning the League by name, he wrote of his country's great wrong in not bearing a responsible part in the administration of the peace after sending her soldiers to fight the war. Edith repeatedly suggested that he abandon the speech, but he insisted doing so would make him feel "like the most arrant coward."

Radio technicians arrived in the morning of November 10, 1923, and worked for hours running wires through the house to the library. Wilson spent the day in bed, suffering from a nervous headache. Just before 8:30 p.m., however, he descended in his dressing gown. He had asked to deliver the address standing because he had always spoken on his feet. Because his throbbing headache worsened his poor vision, Edith sat behind him, holding a carbon copy of the text should he need her prompting. Stations in Washington, New York, and Providence carried the speech, which reached across most of the nation. Some towns installed speakers in their civic auditoriums to simulate the collective experience of a live address. Tentative at first but finding his stride, Wilson delivered his remarks without incident—other than his discouragement over his performance. His self-criticism was harsh but understandable, for this new medium—radio—required more than a little artificiality, the demand of orating to an invisible audience. Public reaction the next day was full of praise.

Crowds, complete with banners and brass bands, began forming on S Street early that Armistice Day. Flowers, telegrams, and letters poured in. Because a short formal ceremony was planned, with Carter Glass introducing the guest of honor, Wilson decked himself out in a morning coat, gray trousers, and a silk hat. When he appeared at the front door of his house at 2:30 that afternoon, twenty thousand supporters filled the five blocks between Massachusetts and Connecticut Avenues. Journalist Raymond Clapper recalled the crowd was predominantly female, no doubt many of them mothers mourning a lost son. Many had been on their knees, praying in the street. Wilson spoke only two minutes, and the crowd interrupted him three times with overwhelming applause, moving him to tears. He asked them to transfer their homage to the men who had made the Armistice possible, especially General Pershing. Wilson said he was proud to have commanded "the most ideal army that was ever thrown together." Before leaving his admirers, he added one last thought: "I am not one of

those that have the least anxiety about the triumph of the principles I have stood for. I have seen fools resist Providence before and I have seen the destruction, as will come upon these again—utter destruction and contempt. That we shall prevail is as sure as that God reigns."

Wilson met the holidays with good cheer—enjoying family and intimate friends and a stirring Christmas Eve at Keith's, where the entire cast (including the zany comedy team of Olsen and Johnson) as well as the audience stood and sang "Auld Lang Syne." But his spirits soon plunged. Margaret, his most contemplative daughter, often sat with him in silence, at which time she felt his soul stirring. During one such "conversation" in December, he startled her by saying, "I think it was best after all that the United States did not join the League of Nations." Margaret asked why. "Because our entrance into the League at the time I returned from Europe might have been only a personal victory," he said. "Now, when the American people join the League it will be because they are convinced it is the right thing to do, and then will be the *only right* time for them to do it." With a faint smile, he added, "Perhaps God knew better than I did after all."

On December 28, 1923, Woodrow Wilson turned sixty-seven. The highlight of the celebration came at three o'clock, when the Wilsons went to the side entrance of the house for their daily excursion. In lieu of the Pierce-Arrow, a brand new Rolls-Royce Silver Ghost touring car waited in the driveway. It was a black six-passenger limousine with a narrow stripe and Wilson's initials monogrammed in Princeton orange. Other modifications included a high top and wider doors so that he could enter the car without stooping. Four friends—Cleveland Dodge and Tom Jones from his Princeton days, Bernard Baruch and Jesse H. Jones, businessmen he had engaged in government work—had privately shared the $12,782.75 cost.

Dodge and Jesse Jones also created a trust for Wilson that would provide an income of $10,000 a year for the rest of his life. With characteristic grace, Dodge wrote the former President that while they were prompted by their love and admiration for him, "the trust is in fact intended as a slight material reward for your great service to the world, and while being fully cognizant that in taking this privilege of friendship we are honoring ourselves, we are nevertheless unwilling that you deny it to us, because it is indeed a very great privilege and pleasure." On a less personal note,

Dodge and Jones drafted a memorandum explaining that they were simply providing what they thought Congress should for all retiring presidents, especially those who had lived unselfish lives and had no opportunity to lay aside sufficient savings for their retirement. Both men considered the transaction completely above board because neither had ever sought or received a single political favor from Wilson. This annuity, Wilson said, "lifted Mrs. Wilson and me out of the mists of pecuniary anxiety and placed us on firm ground of ease and confidence." He wrote Dodge, "Surely no other man was ever blessed with so true, so unselfish, so thoughtful, so helpful a friend as you are and always have been to me!"

The icing on the cake that day came from Franklin Roosevelt, who announced that the Woodrow Wilson Foundation was officially accepting nominations for its first annual prize of $25,000, to be awarded "to the individual who has rendered within the year the most unselfish public service of enduring value." Then, at its annual year-end meeting, the American Historical Association unanimously elected Wilson its president. He accepted the honor but wrote in reply, "I cannot be sure that I shall be fit for the duties that fall to the occupant of that office."

That was not false modesty. Recently asked about his health, the former President quoted one of his predecessors: "John Quincy Adams is all right, but the house he lives in is dilapidated, and it looks as if he would soon have to move out." Whenever conversation turned to the League, Wilson's eyes still shone, and he would insist, "The world is *run* by its ideals." When former student and public servant Raymond Fosdick ended a visit in January 1924, the last image he took with him from S Street was of Wilson's "tear-stained face, a set, indomitable jaw, and a faint voice whispering, 'God bless you.' With his white hair and gray, lined face, he seemed like a reincarnated Isaiah, crying to his country: 'Awake, awake, put on thy strength, O Zion; put on thy beautiful garments, O Jerusalem!' "

On the sixteenth, the Democratic National Committee concluded its meeting by adopting a resolution endorsing the Administration of Woodrow Wilson, assuring him that they were preparing for that year's Presidential campaign inspired by his administration's achievements and his high ideals. When he learned that two hundred committee members wanted to make a pilgrimage to what they called the "shrine of peace" on S Street, he agreed to receive them in his library.

On Saturday, January 26, Dr. Grayson prepared for a sorely needed

week's vacation, a shooting holiday at Bernard Baruch's Hobcaw Barony plantation in South Carolina. Before departing, he called on the Wilsons, especially Edith, just out of bed after a week with the grippe. She expressed anxiety at his leaving. Letters her husband had dictated were piling up on his table unsigned, which indicated to her that his energy was waning. Grayson said he did not share her fears. When he left, she went to Woodrow's room and found him despondent. She asked if he "felt badly," and he said, "I always feel badly now, little girl, and somehow I hate to have Grayson leave." Edith said she could still catch him, but he said, "No, that would be a selfish thing on my part. He is not well himself and needs the change." And then, very deliberately, he said the unspeakable: "It won't be very much longer, and I had hoped he would not desert me; but that I should not say, even to you."

Over the next few days, the stacks of unsigned letters rose. Edith went out to dinner on Tuesday, and her brother Randolph Bolling checked on Wilson at ten o'clock that night. The nurse asked him if Dr. Grayson was in town, because she thought the patient had become "a very sick man." When Bolling said Grayson was in South Carolina, she replied, "Oh, I wish he were here." After midnight, Edith awakened Randolph, telling him to summon the doctor home. Grayson did not receive the message until the following noon. He boarded the next train to Washington. Based on the symptoms Edith described and Wilson's medical history, he suggested it was an indigestive attack.

Examining his patient on Thursday, the thirty-first, Grayson remained unalarmed. But Edith wanted a second opinion. She called Dr. Sterling Ruffin, her internist, who concurred with the night nurse. "He is a very sick man," he told Edith, and he advised Grayson's spending the night in the house. The next morning at eight, Edith came downstairs to tell Randolph that she believed Woodrow was dying and that they should notify his children. While they were talking, Grayson entered and said that Wilson had taken a sudden turn for the worse in the early morning hours. His systems were shutting down.

Bolling telephoned Margaret in New York, telegraphed Nell in California, and cabled Jessie through the Siamese Embassy, advising them all of their father's condition. Margaret arrived that afternoon. Despite everybody's discretion, the press caught wind of the story. Grayson invited Dr. Harry A. Fowler to consult, and when he informed Wilson that he had his

two colleagues outside the sickroom ready to examine him, Wilson attempted a smile and said, "Be careful. Too many cooks spoil the broth." The next day Altrude Grayson drove over with two of their sons; the younger remained in the car with his mother while six-year-old Gordon, the President's young companion after his stroke, was invited upstairs, briefly, to look in on his old friend. Faintly, Wilson smiled.

With repeated visits from physicians and the convergence of family members upon S Street, reporters gathered outside the house for what they realized was a death vigil. They erected a small shack to shelter themselves from the winter weather. They saw Margaret arrive alone, followed by Wilson's younger brother, Josie, who was so much a stranger to Washington that few even recognized him. That night, Grayson released a statement saying that Wilson had not been allowed out of bed all day.

The next morning's headlines warned that Wilson was dying. The news, President Coolidge wrote Mrs. Wilson, had disquieted the nation. "I join in the universal prayer that there may very soon be a change for the better." Dr. Grayson telephoned the White House to inform the President that both Wilsons wanted him to know how much they had appreciated his letter. Grayson added that the former President was too weak to talk but upon having the letter read to him managed to say, "He is a fine man."

Wilson steadily declined. He ingested only a few sips of broth. With his kidneys failing came uremic poisoning. The doctors administered oxygen and morphine to ease any pain. Dr. Grayson chose his patient's final moments of lucidity, when he was fully conscious, to pronounce that his death was imminent, and Wilson did not recoil. "I am ready," he said. "I am a broken piece of machinery. When the machinery is broken——." His voice trailing off, he never completed the thought, but he recovered enough to whisper, "I am ready."

While they were not Woodrow Wilson's last words, they proved to be striking enough to resonate as such. In truth, he revived for a moment and rested his hand on Grayson's arm. "You have been good to me," he said. "You have done everything you could." Grayson turned away in tears and left the room. After composing a brief statement, he faced the hundreds standing outside in the cold, the press among them. "He knows his condition," Grayson said, choking on his words. "He is the gamest man I ever knew." And as he read in a tremulous voice from his bulletin, several in the

crowd rushed up to him, grabbing at the paper in his hand—as if stopping the announcement might prevent the inevitable.

After almost a two-year absence, Tumulty stopped by the house several times that day but did not gain admittance. He returned that night and asked for Grayson, insisting that his decade of loyal service had earned him the right to one final encounter. The doctor agreed, though he said the patient was sleeping. Edith hardly left her husband's side, and Grayson knew, of course, that she had no interest in Tumulty. By midnight, most of the crowd had dispersed, though the press corps remained. At midnight, a window on the second floor opened, and Isaac Scott poked his head out to say, "Mrs. Wilson asks you to please go away. She is trying to sleep." The house darkened, except for a faint light from her room.

By then, Wilson had slipped into unconsciousness. "Profoundly prostrated," one bulletin had reported. Grayson fought back tears with each discouraging update. All that Saturday, people dropped by—Herbert Hoover, Cordell Hull, Carter Glass; diplomats and well-wishers left their cards on the butler's silver tray; the crowd on S Street swelled; Tumulty returned. But only Wilson's wife and daughter and physician, and a few nurses, could enter the dying man's bedroom. At one point during the day, at a moment when his wife had left his side, he whispered a single word: "Edith." He hovered in a twilight state for the rest of the night.

Dawn broke on a raw Sunday, February 3, 1924. Grayson's 9 a.m. bulletin announced that Wilson remained unconscious and weak but alive. Church bells rang, producing a strange occurrence. At first dozens, and then hundreds of worshippers entered S Street and knelt before No. 2340. One could see people's lips moving in silent prayer, producing a profound stillness.

Inside the house, inexplicably, Wilson's eyes opened. Edith leaned in and held his right hand, while Margaret grasped his left. Two nurses stood at the foot of the bed. Dr. Grayson took hold of his wrist to monitor his pulse. Wilson's wife and daughter gently called to him, but he did not respond. After ten minutes, his eyes closed. At 11:15 the machinery gave out, as his pulse ebbed and then stopped.

Grayson appeared at the front door at 11:20. Reading very slowly and in a subdued voice, he announced the death, saying, "The heart muscle was so fatigued that it refused to act any longer. The end came peacefully." As he detailed the medical causes of the death—the arteriosclerosis and

hemiplegia with which Wilson had lived for years and the "digestive disturbance" that had signaled this fatal siege—he did not even attempt to keep from crying. Those in the street too far away to hear Grayson's words had only to watch him blotting his face with a handkerchief to know the end had come.

Within minutes the rest of the world knew. In Bangkok, a telegram notified Frank Sayre, who left his office that morning to break the news to Jessie, who was "heartbroken." They could do no more than attend the next day's memorial services in the local English church. Nellie McAdoo and her husband were on the California Limited, halfway across the country, with another few days before they would reach Washington. Radio programs everywhere interrupted their Sunday morning sermons to announce Wilson's death. Within minutes of hearing the news at Washington's First Congregational Church, the Coolidges left the service and drove directly to S Street. The President told Joseph Wilson and Randolph Bolling that the government awaited instructions from the family as to how it might assist with the funeral, whether it be an official state occasion or a simple private ceremony.

For his immediate part, Coolidge issued a proclamation announcing Wilson's death and directing that the flags of the White House and of the departmental buildings be displayed at half-staff for thirty days. He also ordered suitable military and naval honors for his funeral. The next day the President wrote Admiral Grayson that while he had no jurisdiction over the Capitol, he would certainly use his good offices to have Wilson's body lie in state if the family desired; and he offered Arlington National Cemetery for his interment. He placed the Departments of State, War, and Navy at the family's disposal.

Edith Wilson took charge, starting with the question of a burial place. Mindful of her husband's position in the world but in keeping with his character, she wanted to maintain as much dignity and modesty as possible. Wilson had repeatedly said that he did not wish to be buried in Arlington. Staunton, Augusta, Columbia, and Wilmington all laid legitimate claims, but Wilson had hardly returned to any of them; he had kin buried only in South Carolina, and the family plot in the churchyard was full. Princeton, where he had spent most of his life—and where Witherspoon, Jonathan Edwards, and Grover Cleveland rested in its historic cemetery—seemed appropriate were it not for the unpleasantness of his departure.

Rome, Georgia—alongside his wife of almost thirty years—was never even considered. The solution lay practically around the corner.

A mile and a half up Massachusetts Avenue, the Cathedral Church of St. Peter and St. Paul—known as the Washington National Cathedral—sat atop Mount St. Alban. It had been under construction since 1907, and would remain unfinished until 1990; but the neo-Gothic edifice—the second-largest cathedral in the United States—was operational, and its Gloria in Excelsis Tower, which would crown the structure, was destined to become the highest point in the capital. As it rose in fits and starts, its hierarchy was desperate to establish it as the Westminster Abbey of the nation, a center for spiritual ceremony and commemoration, complete with an American version of Poets' Corner. In fact, the Episcopal Bishop of Washington, James Edward Freeman, had actively solicited celebrated Americans for their burial rights. Freeman now offered Mrs. Wilson the Bethlehem Chapel of the National Cathedral, a modest but impressive sanctuary with a high vaulted ceiling and stained-glass windows, for both her husband's service and burial. The chapel could accommodate only three hundred mourners, which pleased the widow, as it provided an excuse to forgo a state funeral.

Edith decided to hold a short service at the house, followed by another at the cathedral on Wednesday, February 6. The former would be more personal, the latter adhering to Washington protocol. By handwritten note, she invited the Coolidges to both ceremonies. Upon reading in the newspapers that the Senate was suspending its business for three days and that a delegation had been assigned to attend the cathedral rites, she immediately composed a brief personal letter. "As the funeral is private and not official," she wrote Henry Cabot Lodge, "and realizing that your presence would be embarrassing to you and unwelcome to me, I write to request that you do *not* attend."

Lodge replied promptly and courteously. He explained that when the Senate committee had been appointed, he had no idea that its members were expected to attend a private service in the house or that the church service was anything but public. "You may rest assured," he wrote by hand, "that nothing could be more distasteful to me than to do anything which by any possibility could be embarrassing to you." The press would announce that Lodge withdrew from the proceedings because of a respiratory condition.

Tensions on S Street still ran high, as the circumstances elicited the worst of Edith's behavior. The McAdoos reached Washington on Monday at a particularly troubling moment in his career. Just as he was seeing a clear path to the White House, investigations of the Teapot Dome scandal revealed that one of the co-conspirators, Californian Edward L. Doheny, had paid extravagant fees to McAdoo. The association alone was enough to sully his reputation. After arriving at S Street and paying his respects, McAdoo withdrew to his father-in-law's library with a number of his supporters to discuss damage control. Finding Nellie teetering on hysteria, Edith lashed out at her for caring more about getting her husband elected President than she did about the death of her father. Margaret, who had been dabbling in Christian Science, flitted about the house, wearing a beatific smile, insisting there was no reason to lament because death was merely an illusion. Edith felt she could obtain no support from her stepdaughters, then or in the future. And the feeling was mutual.

Wednesday was cold and gray, with a passing storm periodically delivering heavy rain mixed with snow. Thunder sounded all morning, but it was, in fact, gunfire—salvos to the former President from the nearby military bases. Other salutes spread across the country. Every town and city acknowledged Wilson's death, usually with the ringing of bells or by observing moments of silence. Edith had Army trucks deliver to nearby hospitals the hundreds of flower arrangements sent in sympathy. She received in all eight thousand messages of condolence. "The names of kings and the great of the earth were on these tributes," noted Josephus Daniels, "and the names of loyal, humble friends and comrades."

At two-fifty, the President and Mrs. Coolidge arrived at 2340 S Street. Two hundred others gathered inside as well—Wilson's former Cabinet members and advisers, including Tumulty and his wife, who had not been invited until McAdoo arranged for their entry. Ike Hoover was present along with Starling from the Secret Service, a small contingent of Princetonians, and a few Woodrows, Wilsons, Axsons, and Bollings. Before the fireplace in the library sat Wilson's open black steel casket—covered with a spray of Edith's beloved orchids.

At exactly three o'clock, the Reverend James Taylor of the Central Presbyterian Church raised his voice to recite the Twenty-third Psalm— "The Lord is my shepherd." Edith stood on the landing above, her sobs threatening to drown out the preacher. The Reverend Sylvester Beach,

Wilson's pastor from Princeton, spoke next, a few sentences about Wilson's "zeal in behalf of the Parliament of Man, in which the mighty nations should be restrained and the rights of the weak maintained." Then Bishop Freeman of the National Cathedral read a few lines from Wilson's own Bible. As the clock on the landing chimed the quarter hour, eight servicemen entered the room and carried the coffin down the stairs, out the front door, and through a double line of guardsmen to the waiting hearse.

After eight years of maintaining her composure to help sustain her husband, Edith—in black and a heavy veil—wept without compunction as her brother Randolph took her arm and escorted her down to the waiting car. McAdoo followed, attending Nellie and Margaret. The Coolidges were right behind. Then the rest made their way to their cars and up Massachusetts Avenue for Wilson's final procession. Eight men in uniform accompanied the hearse, four on either side, with files of eight flanking them and with soldiers and Marines positioned along the entire route, holding back the solemn crowds on both sides of the road. Fifty thousand more waited outside the church, their umbrellas accentuating the somberness of the day. The great church bells tolled, and as the funeral caravan turned right onto the Way of Peace up to the Bethlehem Chapel, the carillon sent forth a slow rendition of "Nearer, My God, to Thee," which resounded for blocks.

Once the pallbearers had placed the casket before the altar, the three clergymen conducted the Episcopal ritual for the Burial of the Dead, beginning with the words of John: "I am the Resurrection and the life." The service, which was broadcast on radio and to the mourners outside, included readings of Psalms and the singing of one of Wilson's favorite hymns, which began: "Day is dying in the west. / Heaven is touching earth with rest." The Lord's Prayer and the Apostles' Creed followed. The Bishop closed the ceremony with his benediction, and the organ played the recessional hymn, "The Strife Is O'er, the Battle Done."

The chapel emptied, except for the family and a few intimates, and the eight servicemen guarding the casket. Workmen approached the center of the chapel and removed a marble slab and then a concrete slab, revealing the vault below. As the men lowered the heavy black casement down beams to its catacomb, a bugler from the 3rd United States Cavalry stood outside playing "Taps." That very moment, across the Potomac at Arlington National Cemetery, another bugler echoed the call.

All but one of this last group of mourners accompanied the widow back to S Street, where she would live out the rest of her days. Cary Grayson, who had promised Ellen Wilson on her deathbed that he would look after her husband, complied to the very end, remaining until the servicemen had replaced the great stone slab.

The Bethlehem Chapel did not remain Woodrow Wilson's final resting place. As construction of the cathedral proceeded, his survivors favored a more accessible shrine. In 1956—the centennial of Wilson's birth—he was re-entombed in a new limestone sarcophagus in its own bay on the south side of the nave. Its top is carved only with his name, dates, and a cross fashioned after a Crusader's sword. Eighty-five-year-old Edith Wilson had largely withdrawn from the public eye, except for occasions that honored her late husband. Naturally, she attended the reconsecration ceremonies, over which Wilson's grandson the Very Reverend Francis B. Sayre, Jr.— the boy who once exclaimed that he was "for the League!"—presided in his role as dean of Washington National Cathedral.

A little more than four years later—on January 20, 1961—Chief Justice Earl Warren administered the Presidential Oath to John F. Kennedy on the East Portico of the Capitol. Few recognized the small elderly woman in the third row on the President's Platform, or would even have believed that Mrs. Woodrow Wilson was still alive. Later that cold day, Edith rode in the inaugural parade, sharing the backseat of a convertible car with another former First Lady, Eleanor Roosevelt. On December 28, 1961—what would have been her husband's 105th birthday—Edith Wilson was meant to dedicate a new bridge across the Potomac that was being named in his honor. But, suffering from heart and lung ailments, she died in her bed on S Street that night at eighty-nine. She was interred beside her husband's tomb.

"Cathedrals do not belong to a single generation," Dean Sayre once said. "They are churches of history. They gather up the faith of a whole people and proclaim the goodly Providence which has welded that people together as they have hoped and suffered and believed across the centuries." Few, if any, figures in modern history held loftier dreams and endured greater pain and maintained deeper faith than Sayre's grandfather, especially in promoting the "ideals of public service, liberal thought, the

extension of democracy, and peace through justice," as Franklin D. Roosevelt defined his idol's vision.

And as the sun sets each day, the crepuscular light curiously illuminates a little more of the past, as the passage of each year further defines its epoch. In one decade after another, one sees that the silhouette of history that spreads across the capital city of the United States of America is not just that of its national cathedral but increasingly that of the President who is buried therein. It is the lengthening shadow of Wilson.

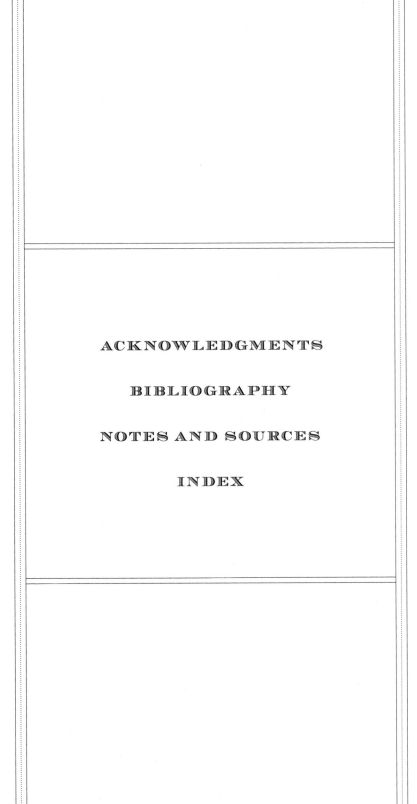

ACKNOWLEDGMENTS

BIBLIOGRAPHY

NOTES AND SOURCES

INDEX

ACKNOWLEDGMENTS

In 1965, when I was in the eleventh grade, my mother handed me a copy of Gene Smith's *When the Cheering Stopped*, which examined Woodrow Wilson's last years and Edith Wilson's role in the White House after her husband's stroke. I have been reading about Wilson ever since, but I kept feeling that I had never read a book that captured the essence of his character. From such feelings spring new biographies.

By the time I began writing this book, my subject had been dead more than seventy-five years, and there were few people alive who had known him. In 2001, however, I was fortunate enough to spend a beautiful day on Martha's Vineyard with his grandson the Very Reverend Francis B. Sayre, Jr., former Dean of the National Cathedral and, at that time, the only living person to have been born in the White House. Then in his mid-eighties, he remained a dynamic and articulate presence, who readily offered stories and observations of his mother and her sisters and their father. After Dean Sayre's death in 2008, the family discovered a mother lode of papers—hundreds of theretofore undisclosed personal letters—which Dean Sayre's son Thomas allowed me to mine for this book. Utmost thanks to Thomas H. Sayre for his trust and instant friendship.

I was also privileged to meet on several occasions with the late Cary T. Grayson, Jr., son of President Wilson's physician and as elegant a gentleman as I have ever known. He too shared not only his reminiscences and some of his family's lore but also an unexamined trove of Grayson family archives, which—like the Sayre Papers—brought countless personal details to my portrait of Wilson. I am sorry he did not live to see the book to which he contributed so generously. I am grateful as well to Cary Grayson, Jr.'s wife, Priscilla, for her gracious spirit.

In 1973 I had the good fortune to be invited to tea—"or something

out any number of issues, always with grace and aplomb. I value her friendship as much as her representation.

A number of other friends have provided great emotional support during the thirteen years it took to complete this book. Their constant vigilance, even when I was off in another century, sustained me more than they know. My heartfelt thanks to Greg Berlanti, Tony Bill, Gary Cohen, Kevin Lake, Eric Lax, Nancy Olson Livingston, John Logan, Bryan Lourd, Elsie and McKinley C. McAdoo, and Douglas Stumpf. I am sorry two friends who spurred me on for so many years departed before they could see the results: Casey Ribicoff, who never failed to ask provocative questions; and Gore Vidal, who never failed to give provocative answers, challenging almost everything Wilson had said or done. Fellow biographer David T. Michaelis has been my ideal reader for the last few decades; and his steadfast faith in this book has been a continual source of inspiration. He has long proved himself the very best of friends.

In my experience, the greatest scholars are also the most generous. That is certainly the case with Alan Brinkley, to whom many of us have turned for counsel since our undergraduate days. I am beholden to him for his critical reading of this manuscript, as he once again demonstrated that he is both a friend and historian of the highest order.

My deepest regret is that my father, Richard Berg, did not live to see this book. He was no great fan of history; but, as a motion-picture writer and producer, he loved good drama. He watched over every scene herein. My brothers—Jeffrey, Tony, and Rick—all augmented their traditional support, compensating for his absence.

In an age of great transition in the publishing industry, I continued to work with a team of people at G. P. Putnam's Sons who remain extremely dedicated to books, whatever form they take. Carole Baron, Marilyn Ducksworth, Mih-Ho Cha, and the late Dan Harvey nurtured this book at the beginning; and in recent years, I have been fortunate enough to work with Susan Petersen Kennedy, who allowed the book to progress according to its own calendar. Ivan Held has taken a deep personal interest in the work of not only the author but of all who have had a hand in the making of this book. I have had the good fortune to work once again with the same superb editorial team that I encountered fifteen years ago, with a few new additions. My greatest thanks to Neil S. Nyren for his sharp insights and his gentle humor. Thanks also to Sara Minnich, Claire Winecoff for her

meticulous care, and, most especially, Scott Auerbach. Catharine Lynch and Meredith Dros have overseen this volume's production, making the most of the very talented Claire Vaccaro's design. Kate Stark, Alexis Welby, and Kelly Welsh have cheerfully ushered the author into the twenty-first century. My friend Ian Chapman has monitored every detail of this book's British publication.

This book is dedicated with boundless love and gratitude to three people. Kevin McCormick has been my partner through four books now, but I have never relied on his devotion more than during "the Wilson administration." He has consistently offered support of every kind before I needed to ask for it; and he helped hammer out most of the thoughts in this book.

While my father got me interested in writing, my mother, Barbara Berg, got me interested in reading—especially nonfiction, specifically about the early part of the twentieth century and Woodrow Wilson. Her unceasing curiosity and indomitable energy never cease to amaze and inspire.

Phyllis Grann is the most gifted editor I know. She has perfect pitch and the rare ability to focus on details without losing sight of the big picture. Although she has left Putnam, she was the first person there with whom I discussed the idea of writing about Wilson, and she has faithfully remained this book's editor and godmother.

The moment after I had first mentioned Woodrow Wilson to her, Phyllis asked how I ever got interested in him in the first place. I told her about that book my mother had pressed into my hands when I had been in high school. Phyllis went silent for a moment . . . and then told me that in 1964, when she was a secretary at William Morrow & Company, her boss, Lawrence Hughes, had said, "Phyllis, you say you want to be an editor. Let's see what you can do with this." He set down on her desk the manuscript of *When the Cheering Stopped*.

I think Wilson would have called that Providence.

—A.S.B.
Los Angeles
April 2013

BIBLIOGRAPHY

Ackerman, Kenneth D. *Young J. Edgar: Hoover, the Red Scare, and the Assault on Civil Liberties*. New York: Carroll & Graf, 2007.

Adams, Henry. *The Education of Henry Adams*. New York: Modern Library, 1931.

Alderman, Edwin Anderson. *Woodrow Wilson: Memorial Address*. Washington, DC: Government Printing Office, 1925.

Annin, Robert Edwards. *Woodrow Wilson: A Character Study*. New York: Dodd, Mead, 1924.

Arnett, Alex Mathews. *Claude Kitchen and the Wilson War Policies*. Boston: Little, Brown, 1937.

Aucella, Frank J., and Patricia A. P. Hobbs with Frances Wright Saunders. *Ellen Axson Wilson: First Lady—Artist*. Washington, DC: Woodrow Wilson Birthplace Foundation, 1993.

Axson, Stockton. *Brother Woodrow: A Memoir of Woodrow Wilson*. Princeton, NJ: Princeton University Press, 1993.

Axtell, James. *The Making of Princeton University: From Woodrow Wilson to the Present*. Princeton, NJ: Princeton University Press, 2006.

Bagehot, Walter. *The English Constitution*. 1867. Reprint, Ithaca, NY: Cornell University Press, 1966.

———. *Physics and Politics*. New York: Cosimo Classics, 2007.

Bailey, Anne J. *War and Ruin: William T. Sherman and the Savannah Campaign*. Lanham, MD: Rowman & Littlefield, 2002.

Baker, Ray Stannard. *American Chronicle: The Autobiography of Ray Stannard Baker*. New York: Charles Scribner's Sons, 1945.

———. *Woodrow Wilson: Life and Letters*, Potomac Edition. 8 vols. New York: Charles Scribner's Sons, 1946.

Balio, Tino. *United Artists: The Company Built by the Stars*. Madison, WI: University of Wisconsin Press, 1976.

Barry, John M. *The Great Influenza: The Epic Story of the Deadliest Plague in History*. New York: Viking, 2004.

Baruch, Bernard. *Baruch: The Public Years*. New York: Holt, Rinehart and Winston, 1960.

Battey, George Magruder. *History of Rome and Floyd County*. Atlanta: Webb and Vary, 1922.

Beaty, Mary D. *A History of Davidson College*. Davidson, NC: Briarpatch, 1988.

Berkin, Carol, X. Miller, R. Cherney, and J. L. Gormly. *Making America*. Boston: Wadsworth, 2011.

Billington, Monroe Lee. *Thomas P. Gore: The Blind Senator from Oklahoma*. Lawrence, KS: University of Kansas Press, 1967.

Blight, David W. *Race and Reunion: The Civil War in American Memory*. Cambridge, MA: Belknap Press of Harvard University Press, 2001.

Blum, John Morton. *Joe Tumulty and the Wilson Era*. Boston: Houghton Mifflin, 1951.

Bonsal, Stephen. *Unfinished Business*. New York: Doubleday, Doran, 1944.

Boos, Dr. I. *Diseases of the Stomach*. Philadelphia: F. A. Davis, 1907.

Bragdon, Henry Wilkinson. *Woodrow Wilson: The Academic Years*. Cambridge, MA: Belknap Press of Harvard University Press, 1967.

Briggs, Asa. *Victorian People: A Reassessment of Persons and Themes, 1851–67.* New York: Harper Colophon Books, 1963.

Brinkley, Alan. *The Unfinished Nation: A Concise History of the American People.* New York: Alfred A. Knopf, 1993.

Brown, David J., ed. *Staunton, Virginia: A Pictorial History.* Staunton, VA: Historic Staunton Foundation, 1985.

Brown, K. L., ed. *Woodrow Wilson's Pierce-Arrow.* Staunton, VA: Woodrow Wilson Birthplace Foundation, 1990.

Brownell, Will, and Richard N. Billings. *So Close to Greatness: A Biography of William C. Bullitt.* New York: Macmillan, 1987.

Brownlow, Kevin. *Hollywood: The Pioneers.* New York: Alfred A. Knopf, 1979.

———. *The War, the West, and the Wilderness.* New York: Alfred A. Knopf, 1979.

Brownlow, Louis. *A Passion for Anonymity: The Autobiography of Louis Brownlow, Second Half.* Chicago: University of Chicago Press, 1958.

Bruce, William Cabell. *Recollections.* Baltimore: King Brothers, 1936.

Bryan, William Jennings. *The Memoirs of William Jennings Bryan.* Edited by Mary Bryan. Philadelphia: John C. Winston, 1925.

Bullock, Edna D., ed. *Short Ballot.* White Plains, NY: H. W. Wilson, 1915.

Burleigh, J. H. S. *A Church History of Scotland.* London: Oxford University Press, 1960.

Calero, Manuel. *The Mexican Policy of President Woodrow Wilson As It Appears to a Mexican.* New York: Smith & Thomson, 1916.

Calvin, John. *Institutes of the Christian Religion.* Translated by Ford Lewis Battles. Philadelphia: Westminster, 1960.

Carroll, James Robert. *The Real Woodrow Wilson: An Interview with Arthur S. Link, Editor of the Wilson Papers.* Bennington, VT: Images from the Past, 2001.

Cashin, Edward J. *General Sherman's Girl Friend and More Stories About Augusta.* Columbia, SC: Woodstone, 1992.

Chernow, Ron. *The House of Morgan: An American Banking Dynasty and the Rise of Modern Finance.* New York: Atlantic Monthly Press, 1990.

Churchill, Winston. *The World Crisis: 1911–1918.* London and New York: Thornton Butterworth and Charles Scribner's Sons, 1923.

Clapper, Raymond. *Watching the World.* New York: Whittlesey House, 1944.

Clark, Champ. *My Quarter Century of American Politics.* 2 vols. New York: Harper & Brothers, 1920.

Clements, Kendrick A. *The Presidency of Woodrow Wilson.* Lawrence, KS: University Press of Kansas, 1992.

Coben, Stanley. *A. Mitchell Palmer, Politician.* New York: Da Capo, 1972.

Coffman, Edward M. *The War to End All Wars: The American Military Experience in World War I.* New York: Oxford University Press, 1968.

Connally, Tom. *My Name Is Tom Connally.* New York: Thomas Y. Crowell, 1954.

Cooper, John Milton, Jr. *Breaking the Heart of the World: Woodrow Wilson and the Fight for the League of Nations.* Cambridge: Cambridge University Press, 2001.

Cox, James M. *Journey Through My Years.* New York: Simon & Schuster, 1946.

Creel, George. *How We Advertised America: The First Telling of the Amazing Story of the Committee on Public Information That Carried the Gospel of Americanism to Every Corner of the Globe.* New York: Harper & Brothers, 1920.

———. *Wilson and the Issues.* New York: Century, 1916.

Daniels, Josephus. *The Life of Woodrow Wilson, 1856–1924.* Philadelphia: John C. Winston, 1924.

———. *The Wilson Era.* 2 vol. Chapel Hill, NC: University of North Carolina Press, 1944.

Day, Donald, ed. *The Autobiography of Will Rogers.* Boston: Houghton Mifflin, 1949.

———. *Woodrow Wilson's Own Story.* Boston: Little, Brown, 1952.

Dos Passos, John. *U. S. A.: Nineteen Nineteen.* 1932. Boston: Houghton Mifflin, Sentry Edition, 1963.

Duiker, William. *Ho Chi Minh.* New York: Hyperion, 2003.

Eksteins, Modris. *Rites of Spring: The Great War and the Birth of the Modern Age.* Boston: Houghton Mifflin, 1989.

Elliot, Margaret Randolph Axson. *My Aunt Louisa and Woodrow Wilson*. Chapel Hill, NC: University of
     North Carolina Press, 1944.
Ellis, John. *Eye-Deep in Hell: Trench Warfare in World War I*. Baltimore: Johns Hopkins University Press,
     1976.
Esher, Viscount. *The Journals and Letters of Reginald Viscount Esher*. Edited by Maurice V. Brett. London:
     Nicholson and Watson, 1938.
Farber, Daniel, ed. *Security v. Liberty: Conflicts Between Civil Liberties and National Security in American
     History*. New York: Russell Sage Foundation, 2008.
Farwell, Byron. *Over There: The United States in the Great War, 1917–1918*. New York: W. W. Norton,
     1999.
Finch, Edith. *Carey Thomas of Bryn Mawr*. New York: Harper, 1947.
Fitzgerald, F. Scott. *This Side of Paradise*. New York: Charles Scribner's Sons, 1920.
Foner, Eric. *Reconstruction: America's Unfinished Revolution—1863–1877*. New York: Harper & Row,
     1988.
Freud, Sigmund, and William C. Bullitt. *Thomas Woodrow Wilson: A Psychological Study*. Boston:
     Houghton Mifflin, 1967.
Fussell, Paul. *The Great War and Modern Memory*. New York: Oxford University Press, 1975.
Gay, Peter. *Freud: A Life for Our Time*. New York: W. W. Norton, 1988.
Giddings, Paula J. *Ida: A Sword Among Lions*. New York: Amistad, 2008.
Glass, Carter. *An Adventure in Constructive Finance*. New York: Doubleday, Page, 1927.
Grayson, Cary T. *Woodrow Wilson: An Intimate Memoir*. Washington, DC: Potomac Books, 1977.
Grayson, David. *The Autobiography of Ray Stannard Baker*. New York: Charles Scribner's Sons, 1945.
Hagedorn, Ann. *Savage Peace: Hope and Fear in America, 1919*. New York: Simon & Schuster, 2008.
Hale, William Bayard. *Woodrow Wilson: The Story of His Life*. Garden City: Doubleday, Page, 1912.
Hanioğlu, M. Şükrü. *A Brief History of the Late Ottoman Empire*. Princeton, NJ: Princeton University
     Press, 2008.
Hatfield, Mark O., with the Senate Historical Office. *Vice Presidents of the United States, 1789–1993*.
     Washington, DC: United States Government Printing Office, 1997.
Heaton, John L. *Cobb of the World: A Leader in Liberalism*. New York: E. P. Dutton, 1924.
Hemingway, Ernest. *A Farewell to Arms*. New York: Charles Scribner's Sons, 1929.
Herman, Arthur. *How the Scots Invented the Modern World: The True Story of How Western Europe's Poorest
     Nation Created Our World and Everything in It*. New York: Crown, 2001.
Hitler, Adolf. *Mein Kampf*. Translated by James Murphy. North Charleston, SC: CreateSpace Indepen-
     dent Publishing Platform, 2011.
Hodgson, Godfrey. *Woodrow Wilson's Right Hand: The Life of Colonel Edward M. House*. New Haven, CT:
     Yale University Press, 2006.
Hoeveler, J. David, Jr. *James McCosh and the Scottish Intellectual Tradition: From Glasgow to Princeton*.
     Princeton, NJ: Princeton University Press, 1981.
Hoffman, Donald. *Mark Twain in Paradise: His Voyages to Bermuda*. Columbia, MO: University of
     Missouri Press, 2006.
Hoover, Herbert. *The Ordeal of Woodrow Wilson*. New York: McGraw-Hill, 1958.
Hoover, Irwin Hood (Ike). *Forty-Two Years in the White House*. Boston: Houghton Mifflin, 1934.
Hosford, Hester E. *The Forerunners of Woodrow Wilson*. East Orange, NJ: East Orange Record Print, 1914.
House, Edward M. *The Intimate Papers of Colonel House, Arranged as a Narrative by Charles Seymour*. 4
     vols. Boston: Houghton Mifflin, 1926.
———. *Philip Dru: Administrator*. 1912. Middlesex, England: Echo Library, 2006.
Houston, David F. *Eight Years with Wilson's Cabinet, 1913–1921*. 2 vols. Garden City: Doubleday, Page,
     1926.
Hulbert, Mary Allen. *The Story of Mrs. Peck: An Autobiography*. New York: Minton, Balch, 1933.
Hurley, Edward N. *The Bridge to France*. Philadelphia: J. B. Lippincott, 1927.
Jaffray, Elizabeth. *Secrets of the White House*. New York: Cosmopolitan Book Corporation, 1927.
Johnson, James Weldon. *Writings*. New York: Library of America, 2004.
Kandell, Jonathan. *La Capital: The Biography of Mexico City*. New York: Random House, 1988.

Karabel, Jerome. *The Chosen: The Hidden History of Admission and Exclusion at Harvard, Yale, and Princeton.* New York: Houghton Mifflin Harcourt, 2005.

Kazin, Michael. *A Godly Hero: The Life of William Jennings Bryan.* New York: Alfred A. Knopf, 2006.

Kennan, George F. *Memoirs: 1925–1950.* Boston: Little, Brown, 1967.

Keynes, John Maynard. *The Economic Consequences of the Peace.* 1919. Reprint, New York: Penguin Books, 1995.

Keyssar, Alexander. *The Right to Vote: The Contested History of Democracy in the United States.* New York: Basic Books, 2000.

Kissinger, Henry. *Diplomacy.* New York: Simon & Schuster, 1994.

Knox, John. *Letter to the Commonalty of Scotland.* Dallas: Presbyterian Heritage Publications, 1995.

Kohlsaat, H. H. *From McKinley to Harding.* New York: Charles Scribner's Sons, 1923.

Konvitz, Milton R., ed. *The Legacy of Horace M. Kallen.* Cranbury, NJ: Associated University Presses, 1987.

Lane, A. W., and L. H. Wall, eds. *Letters of Franklin K. Lane.* Boston: Houghton Mifflin, 1922.

Lansing, Robert. *War Memoirs.* Indianapolis: Bobbs-Merrill, 1935.

Lash, Joseph P. *Helen and Teacher: The Story of Helen Keller and Anne Sullivan Macy.* New York: Delacorte, 1980.

Lawrence, David. *The True Story of Woodrow Wilson.* New York: George H. Doran, 1924.

Leitch, Alexander. *A Princeton Companion.* Princeton, NJ: Princeton University Press, 1978.

Levin, Phyllis Lee. *Edith and Woodrow: The Wilson White House.* New York: Charles Scribner's Sons, 2001.

Link, Arthur S., ed. *The Papers of Woodrow Wilson.* 69 vols. Princeton, NJ: Princeton University Press, 1966–1994.

———. *The First Presbyterian Church of Princeton.* Princeton, NJ: First Presbyterian Church, 1967.

Livermore, Seward W. *Politics Is Adjourned: Woodrow Wilson and the War Congress, 1916–1918.* Middletown, CT: Wesleyan University Press, 1966.

Lodge, Henry Cabot. *The Senate and the League of Nations.* New York: Charles Scribner's Sons, 1925.

Longworth, Alice Roosevelt. *Crowded Hours.* New York: Charles Scribner's Sons, 1933.

Lucas, Marion B. *Sherman and the Burning of Columbia.* Columbia, SC: University of South Carolina Press, 2000.

MacMaster, K. Richard. *Augusta County History: 1865–1950.* Staunton, VA: Augusta County Historical Society, 1988.

MacMillan, Margaret. *Paris 1919: Six Months That Changed the World.* New York: Random House, 2001.

Marsden, George M. *The Soul of the American University: From Protestant Establishment to Established Nonbelief.* New York: Oxford University Press, 1994.

Marshall, Thomas R. *Recollections of Thomas R. Marshall: A Hoosier Salad.* Indianapolis, IN: Bobbs-Merrill, 1925.

Mayer, Arno J. *Wilson vs. Lenin: Political Origins of the New Diplomacy 1917–1918.* Cleveland and New York: Meridian Books, 1969.

McAdoo, Eleanor Wilson, ed. *The Priceless Gift: The Love Letters of Woodrow Wilson and Ellen Axson Wilson.* New York: McGraw-Hill Books, 1962.

———. *The Woodrow Wilsons.* New York: Macmillan, 1937.

McAdoo, William G. *Crowded Years.* Boston: Houghton Mifflin, 1931.

McCombs, William F. *Making Woodrow Wilson President.* New York: Fairview, 1921.

McCosh, James. *Twenty Years of Princeton College.* New York: Charles Scribner's Sons, 1888.

McWhirter, Cameron. *Red Summer: The Summer of 1919 and the Awakening of Black America.* New York: Henry Holt, 2011.

Mead, Walter Russell. *Special Providence: American Foreign Policy and How It Changed the World.* New York: Alfred A. Knopf, 2001.

Meigs, Cornelia. *What Makes a College? A History of Bryn Mawr.* New York: Macmillan, 1956.

Mencken, H. L. "Five Men at Random." In *Prejudices: Third Series.* New York: Alfred A. Knopf, 1922. First appeared in *Smart Set,* May 1920.

———. *My Life As Author and Editor.* New York: Alfred A. Knopf, 1993.

Moggridge, D. E. *Maynard Keynes: An Economist's Biography*. London and New York: Routledge, 1995.

Monnet, Jean. *Memoirs*. Translated by Richard Mayne. Garden City, NY: Doubleday, 1978.

Montgomery, Erick. *Thomas Woodrow Wilson: Family Ties and Southern Perspectives*. Augusta, GA: Historic Augusta, 2006.

Moore, John Hammond. *Columbia and Richland County: A South Carolina Community, 1740–1990*. Columbia, SC: University of South Carolina Press, 1993.

Morgenthau, Henry. *All in a Lifetime*. Garden City: Doubleday, Page, 1923.

Morris, Edmund. *Colonel Roosevelt*. New York: Random House, 2010.

Mulder, John M. "Joseph R. Wilson: Southern Presbyterian Patriarch." *Journal of Presbyterian History* 52 (1974).

Muraskin, William A. *Middle-Class Blacks in a White Society: Prince Hall Freemasonry in America*. Berkeley, CA: University of California Press, 1975.

Myers, William Starr, ed. *Woodrow Wilson: Some Princeton Memories*. Princeton, NJ: Princeton University Press, 1946.

Nasaw, David. *Andrew Carnegie*. New York: Penguin, 2006.

Nicolson, Harold. *King George the Fifth: His Life and Reign*. Garden City, NY: Doubleday, 1953.

———. *Peacemaking, 1919*. Boston: Houghton Mifflin, 1933.

Northen, William J. *Men of Mark in Georgia: A Complete and Elaborate History of the State from Its Settlement to the Present Time*. Atlanta: A. B. Caldwell, 1907–1912.

Oberdorfer, Don. *Princeton University: The First 250 Years*. Princeton, NJ: Trustees of Princeton University, 1995.

Ozment, Steven. *Protestants: The Birth of a Revolution*. New York: Doubleday, 1992.

Patton, Francis Landey. *The Inauguration of the Rev. Francis Landey Patton*. New York: Gray Bros., 1888.

Perry, Lewis. *Intellectual Life in America: A History*. New York: Franklin Watts, 1984.

Pershing, John J. *My Experiences in the World War*. New York: Frederick A. Stokes, 1931.

Pollock, Edwin T., and Paul F. Bloomhardt, compilers. *The Hatchet of the United States Ship "George Washington."* New York: J. J. Little & Ives, 1919.

Post, Louis F. *The Deportations Delirium of 1920: A Personal Narrative of an Historic Official Experience*. Chicago: C. H. Kerr, 1923.

Poucher, William A. *Perfumes, Cosmetics & Soaps, with Especial Reference to Synthetics*. New York: D. Van Nostrand, 1927.

Preston, Diana. *Lusitania: An Epic Tragedy*. New York: Walker, 2002.

Prior, James. *Life of the Right Honourable Edmund Burke*. London: Henry G. Bohn, 1854.

Reid, Edith Gittings. *Woodrow Wilson: The Caricature, the Myth, and the Man*. New York: Oxford University Press, 1934.

Rhinehart, Raymond P. *Princeton University*. New York: Princeton Architectural Press, 1999.

Roosevelt, Theodore. *Letters and Speeches*. New York: Library of America, 2004.

———. *Newer Roosevelt Messages*. Edited by William Griffith. New York: Current Literature, 1919.

Sayre, Francis Bowes. *Glad Adventure*. New York: Macmillan, 1957.

Schickel, Richard. *D. W. Griffith: An American Life*. New York: Simon and Schuster, 1984.

Schneer, Jonathan. *The Balfour Declaration: The Origins of the Arab-Israeli Conflict*. New York: Random House, 2010.

Seale, William. *The President's House: A History*. Washington, DC: White House Historical Association, 1986.

———. *The White House: The History of an American Idea*. Washington, DC: American Institute of Architects Press, 1992.

Selden, William K. *Club Life at Princeton*. Princeton, NJ: Princeton Prospect Foundation, n.d.

Seymour, Charles. *Woodrow Wilson and the World War: A Chronicle of Our Own Times*. New Haven, CT: Yale University Press, 1921.

Short, Philip. *Mao: A Life*. New York: Henry Holt, 2000.

Smith, Gene. *When the Cheering Stopped: The Last Years of Woodrow Wilson*. New York: William Morrow, 1964.

Sragow, Michael. *Victor Fleming: An American Movie Master*. New York: Pantheon Books, 2008.

Stalker, James. *John Knox: His Ideas and Ideals*. New York: A. C. Armstrong & Son, 1905.

Starling, Edmund W., and Thomas Sugrue. *Starling of the White House: The Story of the Man Whose Secret Service Detail Guarded Five Presidents from Woodrow Wilson to Franklin D. Roosevelt*. New York: Simon & Schuster, 1946.

Startt, James D. *Woodrow Wilson and the Press: Prelude to the Presidency*. New York: Palgrave Macmillan, 2004.

Steel, Ronald. *Walter Lippmann and the American Century*. Boston: Little, Brown, 1980.

Stoddard, Henry L. *As I Knew Them: Presidents and Politics from Grant to Coolidge*. New York: Harper & Brothers, 1922.

Stone, Geoffrey R. *Perilous Times: Free Speech in Wartime, from the Sedition Act of 1798 to the War on Terrorism*. New York: W. W. Norton, 2004.

Teachout, Terry. *The Skeptic: A Life of H. L. Mencken*. New York: HarperCollins, 2002.

Thomas, Charles M. *Thomas Riley Marshall, Hoosier Statesman*. Oxford, OH: Mississippi Valley Press, 1939.

Thorp, Willard, Minor Myers, Jr., and Jeremiah Stanton Finch. *The Princeton Graduate School: A History*. Princeton, NJ: Association of Princeton Graduate Alumni, 2000.

Trask, David F. *Captains and Cabinets: Anglo-American Naval Relations, 1917–1918*. Columbia, MO: University of Missouri Press, 1973.

Tribble, Edwin, ed. *A President in Love: The Courtship Letters of Woodrow Wilson and Edith Bolling Galt*. Boston: Houghton Mifflin, 1981.

Truman, Margaret, ed. *Where the Buck Stops: The Personal and Private Writings of Harry S. Truman*. New York: Warner Books, 1989.

Tuchman, Barbara. *The Guns of August*. New York: Macmillan, 1962.

———. *The Zimmermann Telegram*. New York: Macmillan, 1958.

Tumulty, Joseph P. *Woodrow Wilson As I Know Him*. Garden City, NY: Doubleday, Page, 1921.

Urofsky, Melvin I. *Louis D. Brandeis: A Life*. New York: Pantheon Books, 2009.

Vansittart, Peter, ed. *Voices from the Great War*. London: Pimlico, 1998.

Waddell, Joseph Addison. *Annals of Augusta County, Virginia*. Richmond, VA: William Ellis Jones, 1886.

Watkins, Mel, ed. *African American Humor: The Best Black Comedy from Slavery to Today*. Chicago: Lawrence Hill Books, 2002.

Watson, James E. *As I Knew Them*. Indianapolis: Bobbs-Merrill, 1936.

Weinstein, Edwin A. *Woodrow Wilson: A Medical and Psychological Biography*. Princeton, NJ: Princeton University Press, 1981.

Weisman, Steven R. *The Great Tax Wars: Lincoln to Wilson, the Fierce Battles over Money and Power That Transformed the Nation*. New York: Simon & Schuster, 2002.

Wheeler, W. Reginald, ed. *A Book of Verse of the Great War*. New Haven, CT: Yale University Press, 1917.

Whitcomb, John, and Claire Whitcomb. *Real Life at the White House: Two Hundred Years of Daily Life at America's Most Famous Residence*. New York: Routledge, 2000.

White, William Allen. *Woodrow Wilson: The Man, His Times, and His Task*. Boston: Houghton Mifflin, 1924.

Williams, Wythe W. *The Tiger of France: Conversations with Clemenceau*. New York: Duell, Sloan & Pearce, 1949.

Wilson, Andrew. *A President's Love Affair with the Lake District: Woodrow Wilson's "Second Home."* Windermere, Cumbria: Lakeland Press Agency, 1966.

Wilson, Edith Bolling. *My Memoir*. Indianapolis: Bobbs-Merrill, 1938.

Wilson, Woodrow. *Congressional Government: A Study in American Politics*. Boston: Houghton Mifflin, 1885.

———. *Division and Reunion: 1829–1899*. New York: Longmans, Green, 1902.

———. *George Washington*. New York: Harper & Brothers, 1897.

———. *A History of the American People*. 5 vols. New York: Harper & Brothers, 1902.

———. *Mere Literature and Other Essays*. Boston: Houghton Mifflin, 1896.

———. *An Old Master and Other Political Essays*. New York: Charles Scribner's Sons, 1893.

———. *The State: Elements of Historical and Practical Politics*. Boston: D. C. Heath, 1889.

———. *When a Man Comes to Himself*. New York: Harper & Brothers, 1901.

NOTES

AND SOURCES

Most of the documents cited below appear in *The Papers of Woodrow Wilson*, sixty-nine volumes edited and annotated by Arthur S. Link and a team of scholars. The books were published between 1966 and 1994. Those documents that appear in this "comprehensive edition of the documentary record of the life and thought of the twenty-eighth President of the United States" are referenced at the end of each notation with Arabic numerals indicating the volume and page number in which they appear.

Wilson's archives are housed primarily in either the Library of Congress or the Seeley G. Mudd Manuscript Library of the Princeton University Library; and many documents—including those from heretofore unseen collections recently made public by the families of Dr. Cary T. Grayson and Jessie Wilson Sayre—reside in the Woodrow Wilson Presidential Library in Staunton, Virginia.

In a few instances, information was obtained through interviews; those citations are designated with (I). Stray documents and newspaper clippings are identified as much as possible, though sometimes they are without sources (n.s.) or dates (n.d.) or page numbers (n.p.). Publishing data for references listed only by an author's name or initials followed by page numbers can be found in the Bibliography.

ABBREVIATIONS

(A)	Address
ASB	A. Scott Berg
ASL	Arthur S. Link
CD	Cleveland Dodge
CG	*Congressional Government* (by WW)
CTG	Dr. Cary Travers Grayson
(D)	Diary
EAW	Ellen Axson Wilson (WW's first wife)
EBW	Edith Bolling Galt Wilson (WW's second wife)
EMH	Edward Mandell House

EWM   Eleanor ("Nell" or "Nellie") Wilson McAdoo (WW's daughter)
FDR   Franklin Delano Roosevelt
HCL   Henry Cabot Lodge
JD   Josephus Daniels
JPT   Joseph Patrick Tumulty
JRW   Joseph Ruggles Wilson (WW's father)
JWS   Jessie Woodrow Wilson Sayre (WW's daughter)
JWW   Janet "Jeanie" Woodrow Wilson (WW's mother)
(M)   Memorandum
MAH   Mary Allen Hulbert (Peck)
(N)   Notes
NYT   *New York Times*
PUL   Princeton University Library
(R)   Remarks
RL   Robert Lansing
RSB   Ray Stannard Baker
(S)   Speech
SA   Stockton Axson
(T)   Telegram
TR   Theodore Roosevelt
(U)   Unpublished
WGM   William Gibbs McAdoo
WJB   William Jennings Bryan
WW   Woodrow Wilson (W alone signifies Wilson)
WWPL   Woodrow Wilson Presidential Library

1 ASCENSION

DECEMBER 4, 1918—WW LEAVING HOBOKEN: CTG (D), Dec. 4, 1918, 53: 313–6; "President Starts Abroad," *NYT*, Dec. 5, 1918, 1–2; Pollock, 221–9; EBW, 172–3; Starling, 117–21.

WW CHARACTERIZATIONS: Cecil Harmsworth to Colonel David Flynn, Mar. 18, 1927, n.s.; Lawrence, 13, 360; Freud, 129; Evalyn Walsh McLean (U-N, privately held), n.d.; Tribble, xvii; Carroll, 41; R. B. Fosdick (D), Dec. 11, 1918, 53: 366; EAW, "Personal" (description of WW), July 28, 1912, 24: 573; EMH (D), June 10, 1919, 60: 373; George F. Kennan, "The Legacy of Woodrow Wilson," *Princeton Alumni Weekly*, Oct. 1, 1974, 11; Alderman, 19, 32; WW (A), "Importance of Bible Study," (privately published); Francis B. Sayre, Jr., to ASB (I), Sep. 30, 2001; Nancy Toy (D), Jan. 3, 1915, 32: 8; Frank I. Cobb, "WW: An Interpretation," Mar. 4, 1921, 64: 216–29; RSB, IV: 55; CTG (press conference), Dec. 19, 1918, 53: 447; Ida Tarbell (I), c. Oct. 3, 1916, 38: 325; Walter Lippmann, "The 14 Points and the League of Nations," Cambridge, MA (Harvard

University): League of Free Nations Association, 1919 (digitized 2008); WW to Samuel Thompson, Jr., Dec. 31, 1923, 68: 515; Keynes, 38; Nicolson, *Peacemaking,* 79; CTG (D), May 2, 1919, 58: 332; Kissinger, 52; Clements, ix; Truman, 16; WW to D. R. Stuart, Jan. 30, 1921, 67: 105; RSB (D), Mar. 21, 1919, 56: 128.

THE CROSSING: "With the Country's Good Wishes," *NYT*, Dec. 5, 1918, 12; R. B. Fosdick (D), cited in Hodgson, 194; W. C. Bullitt (D), Dec. 9 [10], 11, 1918, 53: 350–53n2, 367; EBW, 172–3, 174–5; CTG (D), Dec. 7, 8; R. B. Fosdick (D), Dec. 8, 12, 1918, 53: 340, 371, 384–5; "President Spends Sunday Evening in Old Navy Fashion," *The Hatchet*, Pollock, 213; Clive Day to Elizabeth Day, Dec. 10, 1918, 53: 349; Isaiah Bowman (M), Dec. 10, 1918, 53: 353–6; Sragow, 65–74; EBW to family, Dec. 15, 1918, 53: 397.

RECEPTIONS IN BREST AND PARIS: CTG (D), Dec. 13, 14, 15, 19, 21, 22, 24, 25, 1918, 53: 378–9, 382–4, 391, 439, 458–9, 467, 488–9, 502–5; EBW, 175–83, 185–8; I. Hoover, 77; "Meester Veelson," as quoted in Dos Passos, 208–214; RSB, article draft, Nov. 29, 1920, 66: 439;

EMH (D), Dec. 14, 15, 19, 21, 1918, 53: 390, 400–1, 448, 466; H. Hoover, 68–9; T. N. Page to WW, Dec. 24, 1918, 53: 494–6; E. Benham (D), Dec. 10, 21, 1918, 53: 357–8, 459–61; News report of WW (I), Dec. 18, 1918, 53: 422–30; R. B. Fosdick (D), Dec. 14, 1918, 53: 384; WW (S), Dec. 21, 1918, 53: 461–3; EBW to family, Dec. 24, 1918, 53: 499–501; WW (R), Dec. 25, 1918, 53: 505–7.

RECEPTIONS IN LONDON AND CARLISLE: CTG (D), Dec. 26, 27, 29, 1918, 53: 508–12, 519–22, 537–41; EBW, 191–206; EBW to family, Jan. 2, 1919, 53: 591–5; "Buckingham Palace Banquet," program, Dec. 27, 1918; WW (two S), Dec. 28 and 29, 1918, 53: 531–3, 541; Kennan, "The Legacy of Woodrow Wilson," *Princeton Alumni Weekly*, Oct. 1, 1974, 11; H. Hoover, 68.

2 PROVIDENCE

WW ANCESTRY AND BIRTH: W family Bible (at WWPL), 1: 3; Ozment, ix; Calvin, 926; Knox, quoted in Burleigh, 154; Stalker, 243; Herman, quoting Sir Walter Scott on p. viii; Hale, 16–20; "W Visits Grandfather's Church," *NYT*, Dec. 30, 1918, 2; Thomas Woodrow to Robert Williamson, Feb. 23, 1836 [Boyhood Home of President WW, Augusta, GA]; *Minutes of the Synod of South Carolina*, Spartanburg, SC: Band & White, 1907, 69–78; RSB, I: 6–14; WW, "After-dinner Remarks," Mar. 17, 1909, 19: 103; D. J. Brown, 9–15, 24, 34; MacMaster, 22; WW to C. A. Talcott (referring to "the uncle after whom I am named"), Sep. 22, 1881, 2: 81.

STAUNTON; AUGUSTA: Waddell, 275–80; JWW to Thomas Woodrow, Apr. 27, 1857, [PUL: WW Papers, Project Records, Folder 7]; Montgomery, 19–82; WW (S), Feb. 12, 1909, 19: 33; WW, *DR*, 208–9, 212; JRW, "Mutual Relations of Masters and Slaves As Taught in the Bible" (Augusta, GA: Steam Press of Chronicle & Sentinel, 1861)," Jan. 6, 1861; Henry Ward Beecher, "Peace, Be Still," Jan. 4, 1861 (*American Sermons: The Pilgrims to Martin Luther King, Jr.*, New York: Library of America, 1999, 645–64); R. L. Dabney, *Discussions Evangelical and Theological* (Harrisonburg, VA: Sprinkle Publications, 1962, IV: 180; Henry Louis Gates, Jr., and John Stauffer, "A Pragmatic Precedent," *NYT*, Jan. 19, 2009, A25; RSB, I: 30, 31, 33, 36, 38–9, 42–7, 51–2; Jefferson Davis recalled in JD (D), Apr. 30, 1917, 42: 168; Bailey, 80; ASL, "W's Imaginary World," 1: 20–2; WW to L. I. M. Wylie (re: Uncle Remus), Dec. 15, 1916, 40: 169; Weinstein, 15–9;

WW (S), Oct. 24, 1914, 31: 222; CTG (D), May 27, 1919, 59: 528; Helen Bones to RSB, July 2, 1915 [RSB Papers: PUL]; Jessie Bones Brower to RSB, May 9, 1926 [RSB Papers: PUL]; Samuel G. Blythe, "A Talk with the President," *Saturday Evening Post*, Jan. 9, 1915 [Dec. 5, 1914], 31: 395–6; WW, Talk to Washington Y. M. C. A., Jan. 26, 1915, 32: 126; WW (R), Apr. 21, 1915, 33: 49–50; WW to EAW, Apr. 19, 1888, 5: 719; WW to W. J. Hampton, Sep. 15, 1917, 44: 199; Freud, 10, 12, 66; WW (S, re: Robert E. Lee), Jan. 19, 1909, 18: 631–5; Northen, 354; WW (A), Dec. 10, 1915, 35: 329–36.

COLUMBIA: Lucas, 83–94; Moore, 203–4, 224; WW, *DR*, 252, 268, 278; WW, *History*, V: 46–9; Foner, xix–xxii, 461–9; Mencken, 171–6; Brinkley, 413–6; n.a., *WW Family Home Interpretation Supplement*, Historic Columbia Foundation, June 6, 2005, 1–9; RSB, I: 59–60, 64, 66–7, 71; WW, *When a Man*, 1, 2, 37; Jessie W. Bones, cited in RSB, I: 57; parsing Webster: CTG (D), May 27, 1919, 59: 528; ASL (N), 1: 20–2; Mulder, 255.

DAVIDSON: *Davidson College Catalogue: 1874–1875*; WW (N), c. Sep. 29, 1873, 1: 30–31; Minutes of Eumenean Society, November 7 and 21, 1873, Jan. 3, Mar. 27, 1874, 1: 35 and 36–7, 39–40, 42; WW, *When a Man*, 2–3; Beaty, 86–7, 128–37, 233–4; "in the service of the Devil," cited in Henry W. Bragdon, "The WW Collection," *Princeton University Library Chronicle*, Nov. 1945 (VII: 1), 8; Walter L. Lingle, "WW at Davidson College," *Davidson College Bulletin*, Dec. 15, 1933, n.p.; JWW to WW, May 20, 1874, 1: 50.

WILMINGTON: JWS and EWM to RSB (re: McCosh), cited in RSB, I: 84; White, 58–67; WW, "Rules and Regulations," ca. July 1, 1874, 1: 54–56; John Bellamy to RSB, cited in RSB, I: 79; David Bryant to RSB, cited in RSB I: 78; RSB, I: 23.

3 EDEN

PRINCETON HISTORY: Perry, 134–8; WW, "Princeton Sesquicentennial," *NY Tribune*, 10: 9–10; "Princeton in the Nation's Service" (S), Oct. 21, 1896, 10: 11–31; Link, 8; Oberdorfer, 22–35, 43, 58; Rhinehart, 4–7, 35–7; Leitch, 301–4, 425; WW, "The Personal Factor in Education," Sep. 12, 1907, 17: 325–33; Bragdon, 19; Hoeveler, 233–43; RSB, 1: 83.

WW'S ARRIVAL AT PRINCETON; FIRST YEAR: Hoeveler, 29, 263; *Catalogue of the College of New Jersey for the Academical Year 1875–'76*, 18–22; WW to Hiram Woods, Jr., Aug. 10,

1876, 1: 175n1; Robert McCarter, quoted in Bragdon, 21–2; RSB, I: 82, 86–8; WW, *ML*, 68, 113; Briggs, 197–202; Edmund Burke, quoted in Prior, 142–3; WW, "Notebooks," c. Jan. 1, 1876, 1: 76; WW to EAW, Apr. 22, 1884, 3: 144; WW, "My Journal" (shorthand D), June 3, 1876, 1: 130–2, 134, 140, 142, 145–9, 153, 166, 221; WW, "Index Rerum," 1: 87–127.

SUMMER, 1876; THRIVING AT PRINCETON: WW, "A Christian Statesman," Sep. 1, 1876, 1: 188–9; WW, "My Journal," 1: 157, 190–1, 193, 217, 400–1; ASL (N), 1: 441n1; WW, "The Ideal Statesman," 1: 241–5; WW, "Bismarck," 1: 325–8; RSB, I: 94; WW, articles in *The Princetonian*, 1: 336–7, 402–405, 460, 461–3, 467; WW's voice described by Robert Bridges, "A Personal Tribute," *Fifty Years of the Class of 1879*, Princeton, NJ: (privately printed) Princeton University Press, 1931, 1; WW, "Constitution of the Liberal Debating Club," 1: 245–9; C. A. Talcott, Minutes of Liberal Debating Club, Mar. 31, 1877, 1: 255; Leitch, 380; Bragdon, 35–41 (McCarter, quoted on page 35); JWW to WW, Nov. 20, 1878, 1: 435; WW to JRW, May 23, 1877, 1: 265–6; JRW to WW, Jan. 14, 1878, 1: 340–1; JWW to WW, Jan. 22, 1878, 1: 342; JRW to WW, Jan. 25, 1878, 1: 345–6.

PRINCETON—"WITHERSPOON GANG" AND UPPERCLASS YEARS: JWW to WW, Feb. 16, 1877, 1: 250; Rhinehart, 25–6; WW, quoted in "Function of Universities," *Boston Evening Transcript*, Jan. 3, 1903, n.p.; WW to EAW, Oct. 30, 1883, 1: 499–505; Bridges, *op. cit.*, 3, 6; JRW to WW, Dec. 10, 1878, 1: 441; Leitch, 146; McCarter, quoted in Bragdon, 40; WW, "Review of Green's 'A History of the English People,'" May 2, 1878, 1: 373–5; RSB, I: 196; WW, "My Journal," Nov. 6, 1876, 1: 221; WW, *DR*, 283–7; C. A. Talcott, Minutes of Liberal Debating Club, Apr. 5, 1877, 1: 255–7; ASL (N), "Cabinet Government in the United States," 1: 492–3; WW's grades recorded in WW (N), 1: 444n1; WW to W. M. Sloane (draft of letter), c. Dec. 5, 1883, 2: 566–9; WW, "Cabinet Government in the United States," *International Review*, VI (Aug. 1879), 1: 493–510; JRW to WW, Feb. 25 and Mar. 11, 1879, 1: 459–60 and 464; WW (N), "Wordsworth," May 14, 1879, 1: 481–4; WW, editorials, 1: 467–71.

COMMENCEMENT: ASL (N) re: Lynde Debate, 1: 145; JRW to WW, Mar. 20 and Apr. 17, 1879, 1: 466 and 477; WW, Notebook, June 19, 1876, 1: 143; C. A. Talcott to WW, May 21, 1879, 1: 484; JWW to WW, May 13, 1879, 1: 479–80;

WW to C. A. Talcott, July 7, 1879, 1: 487–8; "business card" described by Mary Hoyt, quoted in RSB, I: 104.

4 SINAI

WILMINGTON; CHARLOTTESVILLE: WW, *When a Man*, 7–9; WW to Robert Bridges, July 30, Sep. 4, and Nov. 7, 1879, 1: 489–90, 539–42, and 580–3; WW, "Self-Government in France," Sep. 11, 1879, 1: 515–39; WW to EAW, Oct. 30, 1883, 2: 500; WW (N), Marginalia, re: Minor on slavery, c. Nov. 10, 1879, 1: 583; Hiram Woods, Jr., to WW, Oct. 28, 1879, 1: 580; "Collegiana," *Virginia University Magazine, XIX* (Dec. 1879), 190–5, 1: 588; RSB I: 112–3, 119; Minutes of Jefferson Society, Mar. 6, 1880, 1: 608; WW, "John Bright," *Virginia University Magazine* (Mar. 1880), 354–70, 1: 608–21; WW, "Mr. Gladstone, A Character Sketch," *Virginia University Magazine* (Apr. 1880), 401–26, 1: 624–42; "Collegiana," *ibid.*, 643–6; J. W. Mallet to J. F. B. Beckwith, May 3, 1880, 1: 651; Bruce, 80; ASL (N), "W's Debate with William Cabell Bruce," 1: 652; JRW to WW, May 6, June 5 and 7, Oct. 5, 1880, 1: 654, 658 and 659–60, 682; WW to C. A. Talcott, Dec. 13, 1879, and May 20, 1880, 1: 591–3 and 1: 655–8; WW to Robert Bridges, Sep. 4, 1879, Aug. 22, and Sep. 18, 1880, 1: 539–42, 671–4, and 675–8; WW to Harriet Woodrow, c. Apr. 14 and Oct. 5, 1880, 1: 647–50 and 678–82; JWW to WW, June 5 and Aug. 23, 1880, 1: 659 and 674; Marion Bones to WW, June 14, 1880, 1: 660; WW, "Constitution and By-Laws of the Jefferson Society," Dec. 4, 1880, 1: 688–99; JWW and JRW to WW, Dec. 14, 1880, 1: 701; ASL (N), "W's Withdrawal from the University of Virginia," 1: 704.

RETURN TO WILMINGTON; PROPOSES TO HARRIET WOODROW: WW to Robert Bridges, Jan. 1, 1881, 2: 9–11; WW to Harriet Woodrow, Jan. 15–19, Sep. 25, and 26, 1881, 2: 12–7, 83, and 84–9; WW to R. H. Dabney, Feb. 1, 1881, 2: 17–9; RSB I: 130; Helen Welles Thackwell, "WW and My Mother," *Princeton University Library Chronicle* (Autumn 1950), v. 12, 6–18.

ATLANTA: WW to Robert Bridges, Aug. 22, 1881, and Mar. 15, Aug. 25, Oct. 28, 1882, and Jan. 4 and May 13, 1883, 2: 75–9 and 106–10, 136–8, 147–8 and 280–1 and 354–9; WW to C. A. Talcott, Sep. 22–Oct. 1, 1881, 2: 80–3; James Bones to WW, Mar. 21, 1882, 2: 111–3; E. I. Renick to WW, Jan. 15, 1882, 2: 96–7; WW, "Account of Personal Expenditures," May–June,

1882, 2: 129–30; SA, 35; JRW to WW, Aug. 20, 1882, and Feb. 13, 1883, 2: 135–6 and 303–4; WW to R. H. Dabney, Jan. 11 and May 11, 1883, 2: 284–7 and 350–4; WW (N), "Opposing the Protective Tariff," c. Sep. 23, 1882, 2: 139; WW, "Testimony," Sep. 23, 1882, 2: 140–3; WW, "Draft of a Constitution for Georgia House of Commons," c. Jan. 11, 1883, 2: 288–91; ASL (N), "W's Practice of Law," 2: 144–5; RSB I: 148; Thomas W. Thrash, "Apprenticeship at the Bar: The Atlanta Law Practice of WW," *Georgia State Bar Journal*, v. 28, no. 3 (Feb. 1992), 149; ASL (N), "Government by Debate," 2: 152–7; WW, "Government by Debate," c. Dec. 4, 1882, 2: 159–275; WW to Hiram Woods, Jr., Apr. 25, 1883, 2: 340–2; WW, "Culture and Education at the South," Mar. 29, 1883, 2: 326–32; RSB, I: 150; George C. Osborn, "WW As a Young Lawyer," *Georgia Historical Quarterly 41* (June 1957), 126–42; George Howe, Jr., to WW, May 31, 1882, 2: 131–2.

COURTING EAW: WW to EAW, July 16, 30, Sep. 18, 27, 29, Oct. 11, 18, 30, 1883, 2: 387–90, 395–9, 427–8, 442–5, 445–7, 465–9, 480–3, 499–505; RSB I: 161; EWM, *PG*, 3–4; Aucella, et al., 5–6; WW to Robert Bridges, July 26, 1883, 2: 393–4; ASL (N), "W and His Caligraph," 2: 366–8; Jessie Bones Brower to WW, July 15, 1883, 2: 386–7; JWW to WW, June 7 and 12, 1883, 2: 365 and 368–9; Battey, 36, 292; George C. Osborn, "Romance of WW and Ellen Axson," *North Carolina Historical Review 39* (Winter 1962), 32–57; ASL (N), "The Engagement," 2: 426–7; WW, *When a Man*, 10; WW to S. E. Axson, Sep. 19 and 24, 1883, 2: 430–1 and 436; SA, 91.

BALTIMORE AND JOHNS HOPKINS: D. C. Gilman, "Inaugural Address," Feb. 22, 1876; WW, "Application," Johns Hopkins University, Sep. 18, 1883, 2: 429–30; WW to EAW, Sep. 29, Oct. 2, 16, 30, Nov. 11, 13, 20, 27, 1883, Jan. 1, 4, 16, 31, Apr. 20, June 3, 5, 25, 29, July 1, 3, 13, Oct. 7, Nov. 27, 30, Dec. 6, 7, 15, 18, 1884, Jan. 29, 1885, 2: 435–7, 445–8, 449–50, 478–80, 499–505, 523–5, 527–30, 550–3, 641–4, 644–8, 657–60, 667–8, 3: 137–9, 203–5, 208–9, 215–6, 221–3, 225, 228–30, 243–4, 337, 489–92, 498–500, 517–8, 521–25, 541–4, 552–3, 4: 196–7; WW to R. H. Dabney, May 11, 1883, and Feb. 17, 1884, Feb. 14, Oct. 28, 1885, 2: 350–4 and 3: 25–8, 4: 247–50, 5: 37–8; Bragdon, 104–5; Minutes of the Seminary of Historical and Political Science, May 8, 1884, 3: 172; WW to Robert Bridges, Dec. 15, 1883, Nov. 19, 1884, Feb. 27, 1886, 2: 585–6, 3: 464–6, 5: 26–7; John Dewey to H. W.

Bragdon, July 14, 1940, quoted in Bragdon, *op.cit.*, 111; WW, "Adam Smith" (lecture draft), c. Nov. 20, 1883, 2: 542–4, 541; WW, *CG*, Dedication page, and text: 5: 34–5, 132–3, 174, 179; JRW to WW, Sep. 25, 1883, Oct. 4, Nov. 6, 1883, 2: 441–2, 454–5, 519–20; EAW to WW, Jan. 28, 1884, Apr. 7, Nov. 28, 1884, 2: 664–6, 3: 115–8, 494–5; JWW to WW, Dec. 4, 1883, 2: 563–4; WW to Houghton Mifflin & Co., Apr. 4, 1884, 3: 111–2; Houghton Mifflin & Co. to WW, Apr. 28 and Nov. 26, 1884, 3: 149 and 486; SA, 91, 103; M. W. Kennedy to WW, Apr. 15, 1884, 3: 130–1; ASL (N), "Ellen's Visit to Wilmington and Her Trip with Woodrow to Washington and New York," 3: 329–30; WW to Albert Shaw, Feb. 21, 1885, 4: 274–6.

CONGRESSIONAL GOVERNMENT; JOB OFFERS: WW to EAW, Apr. 27, Nov. 8, Dec. 10, 1884, Jan. 24, Feb. 20, June 16, 1885, 3: 414–5, 529–30, 4: 3–5, 271–2, 532, 719; WW, *CG*, Dedication page; JRW to WW, Jan. 30, Mar. 17, 1885, 4: 208, 377; JWW to WW, Mar. 17, 1885, 4: 376; Bragdon, 135–7; Albert Shaw, "CG," *Minneapolis Daily Tribune*, Feb. 15, 1885, 4: 284–6; RSB, I: 236.

WW-EAW WEDDING AND HONEYMOON: WW to EAW (confessing "my heart's . . . deepest secret"), Feb. 24, 1885, and June 21, 1885, 4: 286–8 and 733–5; EAW to WW, Mar. 28, 1885, 4: 424–6; EWM, *PG*, 147; Margaret Godley, "Cousins Recall Wedding of WW and 'Miss Ellie Lou' Here," *Savannah Evening Press*, Sep. 4, 194, n.p.; JRW to WW, July 27, 1885, 5: 7; RSB, I: 239.

BRYN MAWR, SETTLING IN: Addie C. Wildgoss to WW, July 30, 1885, 5: 9–10; WW to EAW, May 9, 1885, May 30, June 7, 1886, Oct. 8, 1887, 4: 574–6, 5: 269–70, 294–5, 612–3; Finch, 164–5; J. E. Rhoads to WW, Feb. 11, 1885, 4: 236; Meigs, 42–7; James E. Rhoades, "Address at the Inauguration of Bryn Mawr College," Philadelphia: Sherman and Co., 1886; WW (N), c. Sep. 24, Oct. 1, c. Oct. 15–c. Dec. 1, 1885, 5: 18–23, 23–25, 27–35; RSB, I: 260–4, 290; Bragdon, 148–53; WW to J. B. Angell, Nov. 7, 1887, 5: 625–7; WW, "Copy of Bryn Mawr Catalogue," c. Feb. 1, 1888, 5: 659–63; ASL (N), "W's Desire for a Literary Life," 5: 474–5; EWM, *PG*, 148, 159–60; WW to H. B. Adams, Apr. 2, 1886, 5: 150–1; H. B. Adams to WW, Apr. 7, 1886, 5: 154–5; JRW to WW, Apr. 5, 1886, 5: 152.

EAW GIVES BIRTH; WW'S PH.D.: WW to EAW, Apr. 1, 16, 24, May 29, 1886, 5: 156–7,

157–8, 169–70, 267; L. C. H. Brown to WW, Apr. 16, 1886, 5: 158–9; WW to Robert Bridges, Apr. 19, 1886, 5: 163–4; A. L. Lowell, "Ministerial Responsibility and the Constitution," *Atlantic Monthly, LVII*, Feb. 1886, 180–93; WW, "Responsible Government under the Constitution," c. Feb. 10, 1886, 5: 107–24; H. W. Bragdon, "WW and Lawrence Lowell," *Harvard Alumni Bulletin, XLV* (May 22, 1943), 595; SA, 35–6; Robert Ewing to WW, May 28, 1887, 5: 508; EWM, *PG,* 159–60; Thomas Dixon, Jr., to WW, June 7, 1887, 5: 515–6; JRW to WW, June 11, 1877, 5: 517; RSB, I: 275; WW to R. H. Dabney, Nov. 7, 1887, 5: 500–1.

RETURNING TO BRYN MAWR, AND DEPARTING: JRW to WW, Apr. 30, 1887, 5: 500–1; WW to EAW, Apr. 17, 18, 19, 20, 1888, 5: 718–20; WW to R. H. Dabney, May 16, 1888, 5: 726; SA, 58; C. K. Adams to WW, Mar. 12, 1885, Oct. 13 and 22, 1886; 4: 357–8, 5: 351 and 357; WW, "The Study of Administration," c. Nov. 1, 1886; 5: 359–80; Johns Hopkins University Trustees Minutes, Jan. 17, 1887, 5: 431; H. B. Adams to WW, Jan. 21 and 25, 1887, 5: 431–2 and 435–6; Bragdon, 188; "Agreement Between Trustees of Bryn Mawr College and WW, Ph. D.," Mar. 14, 1887, 5: 468–9; WW to Robert Bridges, Nov. 30, 1887, and Aug. 26, 1888 ("hungry . . . for a class of *men*"), 5: 632–3 and 763–5; WW to president and trustees of Bryn Mawr College, June 29, 1888, 5: 743–7; J. E. Rhoads to M. C. Thomas, June 30 and July 6, 1888, 5: 748, 749; ASL (N), "W's First Failure at Public Speaking," 5:134–7; ASL (N), "W's Lectures on Administration at the Johns Hopkins, 1892," 7: 381; Robert Bridges to WW, Nov. 5, 1889, 6: 410–1.

WESLEYAN: "Wesleyan's Gift," *Hartford Evening Post,* Dec. 17, 1889, 6: 453–4; WW to Robert Bridges, Nov. 27, 1888, 6: 25; SA, 37–8, 60–4, 65, 259–60n24; WW, "History and Political Economy," *Wesleyan Catalogue: 1888–1889,* 6: 26–7; RSB, I: 299–301, 315–7; EAW to WW, May 22, 1886, 5: 249–51; EWM, *PG,* 164, 171; WW, "Constitution for Wesleyan House of Commons," c. Jan. 5, 1889, 6: 39–45; "Wesleyan House of Commons," *Wesleyan Argus,* Jan. 18, 1889, 6: 45–7; Carl Price, (Wesleyan) *Alumnus,* Mar. 1924, cited in RSB, I: 305; F. J. Turner to Caroline Mae Sherwood, Jan. 21, 1889, 6: 58; WW, *TS,* xxxiv, 29, 660; WW to R. H. Dabney, Oct. 31, 1889, 6: 408–9; R. H. Dabney to WW, Mar. 1, 1890, 6: 536–7; F. J. Turner to WW, Jan. 23, 1890, 6: 478–9; D. M. Means, "W's 'The

State,'" *The Nation,* Dec. 26, 1889, 6: 458–62; WW to W. W. Thompson, June 28, 1915, cited in RSB, I: 324; JRW to WW, May 9 and Oct. 30, 1889, 6: 217–8 and 408; WW to EAW, Mar. 9, 1889, 6: 139–40; M. W. Kennedy to WW, Oct. 12, 1889, 6: 402; A. B. Hart to WW, Apr. 23 and May 10, 1889, 6: 174–5 and 218–9; WW to A. B. Hart, May 13, 1889, 6: 240; WW to F. J. Turner, Aug. 23, 1889, 6: 368–71.

PRINCETON OPPORTUNITY: WW to Robert Bridges, July 23, Aug. 9, 1889, and Jan. 27, 1890, 6: 356–7, 363–4, and 480–1; Robert Bridges to WW, July 15 and 30, 1889, 6: 330 and 359–61; RSB, II: 5; F. L. Patton to WW, Feb. 18, 1890, 6: 526–8; WW (D), Feb. 13, 1890, 6: 523; Horace Elisha Scudder to WW, Dec. 20, 1889, 6: 424–5.

5 REFORMATION

RETURN TO PRINCETON: McCosh, 61–8; Thorp, 46–8; Bragdon, 203–6, 209, 213, 272; Hoeveler, 335–7; Rhinehart, 26–7; "The Favor of a University," *NYT,* Feb. 11, 1887, 3; Patton, 17–9, 24, 42–3; Axtell, 42, 65; SA, 222; WW to A. W. Howe, Apr. 21, 1895, 9: 247; ASL, "W's Teaching at Princeton," 7: 5–7; WW, anecdote of the town drunk, related in *Princeton Alumni Weekly, IV* (Apr. 23, 1904), 466–7, 15: 272–3; WW, lecture (N), July 2–10, 1894, 8: 597–608; Raymond Fosdick to RSB, n.d., RSB, II: 10, 12; Myers, 38; WW to R. H. Dabney, July 1, 1891, 7: 233; Princeton Faculty Minutes, Oct. 24, 1890, Apr. 24 and Nov. 6, 1891, Jan. 18, 1893, 7: 51, 195, 322, 8: 79; "Caledonian Games," *The Princetonian, XVI,* June 6, 1891, 7: 219; WW to *The Princetonian* editors, Jan. 8, 1892, 7: 374; C. B. Newton to WW, Nov. 9, 1891, 7: 342; Leitch, 488–9; Bliss Perry to RSB, quoted in RSB, II: 16–7; Mark Bernstein, "Shirt Cuff and Other Artifacts of Student Life," *Princeton Alumni Weekly,* Oct. 7, 2009, n.p.

PERSONAL LIFE—HIBBEN AND FAMILY: Reid, 63; Freud, 103, 130; Bliss Perry to RSB, n.d., in RSB, II: 53; SA, 28–9; EWM, *TWW,* 13–5; EAW to WW, Feb. 16, 1895, 9: 202; WW to C. W. Kent, June 29, 1893, 8: 273; WW to EAW, Feb. 6, 1894, Feb. 18, 1895, 8: 460, 9: 206.

WW LITERARY LIFE: ASL (N), "W's *Division and Reunion,* 8: 147; WW, *DR,* x, 299; Frederic Bancroft, review of *DR, Political Science Quarterly, VIII* (Sep. 1893), 533–5, 8: 345; F. J. Turner to WW, July 16, 1893, and Dec. 24, 1894, 8: 279 and 9: 118; ASL (N), "W's *Short History of the*

United States," 8: 279–81; Harper & Bros. to WW, May 5, 1896, 9: 500; WW to Harper & Bros., May 16, 1890, 9: 504–5; WW to EAW, Jan. 29 and 30, July 29 and 30, 1894, 8: 442, 632 and 634.

LIBRARY PLACE: EMW, *TWW*, 18; E. S. Child to WW, Jan. 14, 16, May 7, 1895; 9: 121–2, 123, 252; WW to Child & de Goll, Architects, Jan. 19, 1895, 9: 123; EWM, *PG*, 201; E. S. Child to EAW, Feb. 18, 1895, 9: 207; WW to EAW, Jan. 25, 1895, 9: 126; EAW to F. J. Turner, Dec. 15, 1896, 10: 80.

CEREBRAL INCIDENT; TRIP TO BRITAIN: WW to A. B. Hart, Aug. 21, 1891, 7: 274; EWM, *PG*, 201–2; Weinstein, 141; Bragdon, 220; WW to EAW, June 28 and 29, July 9, Aug. 24, 1896, 9: 528, 529, 537–8, 575; Andrew Wilson, 6–7.

SESQUICENTENNIAL ("Princeton in the Nation's Service"): Theodore J. Ziolkowski, "Princeton in *Whose* Service?," Jan. 23, 1991, appears in J. I. Merritt (ed.), *The Best of PAW* (Princeton, NJ: Princeton Alumni Weekly, 2000), 53–8; Oberdorfer, 98; Leitch, 438–40, RSB, II: 33–6; *NY Tribune*, Oct. 22, 1896, 10: 9–11; WW, "Princeton in the Nation's Service," Oct. 21, 1896, 10: 11–31; ASL (N), 10: 11–12n1; "Oration by Professor Wilson," *NYT*, Oct. 22, 1896, 2; SA, 42–3, 97; EAW to Mary Hoyt, Oct. 27, 1896, 10: 37–8; EWM, *PG*, 207.

WW'S POLITICS AND PUBLIC ADDRESSES: SA, 42–3, 73, 264; "University School," *Bridgeport* (CT) *Evening Post*, May 25, 1898, 10: 534; WW, "What Ought We to Do," c. Aug. 1, 1898, 10: 574–6; "Our Obligations," *Waterbury* (CT) *American*, Dec. 14, 1899, 11: 297–300; "Philadelphian Society," *Daily Princetonian*, May 19, 1899, 11: 119; "Liberty and Its Uses," *Brooklyn Daily Eagle*, Jan. 14, 1900, 11: 374–5; WW, "Ideals of America" (S), Dec. 26, 1901, appeared in *Atlantic Monthly, XC* (Dec. 1902), 721–34, 12: 208–27; WW, "Leaderless Government" (S), Aug. 5, 1897, 10: 288–304; WW, "American Constitutional Law," Mar. 2, 1894, 8: 563; "Address by WW," *Poughkeepsie Daily Eagle*, May 3, 1902, 12: 362.

PRINCETON POLITICS AND WW'S ASCENT: C. E. Green to WW, Mar. 27 and 28, 1897, 10: 195 and 197; WW to F. L. Patton, Mar. 28, 1897, 10: 196; SA, 262; WW (D), Jan. 21, 1897, 10: 120; WW to EAW, Feb. 27, 1896, Jan. 29 and Feb. 16, 1897, 9: 457, 10: 123 and 164; F. L. Patton to C. H. McCormick, Apr. 4, 1898, 10: 497–9; WW to F. J. Turner, Mar. 31, 1897, 10: 201; News item, *Princeton Press*, Feb. 19, 1898, and

Nov. 24, 1900, 10: 402 and 12: 35; WW to Jenny Hibben, June 26, 1899, 11: 136; Bragdon, 225; JRW to WW, Jan. 3, 1897, 10: 95; G. W. Miles to WW, Apr. 7, 1898, 10: 501–2; H. M. Alden to WW, Jan. 8, 1901, 12: 69; D. C. Gilman to WW, Mar. 16, 1901, 12: 108; J. E. Webb to WW, Mar. 11, 1901, 12: 106; W. P. Johnston to WW, June 16, 1898, 10: 557; *Princeton Alumni Weekly, II* (Oct. 26, 1901), 67–8; "Pres. Remsen Is Inaugurated," Baltimore *Sun*, Feb. 23, 1902, 12: 282; F. L Patton to C. H. McCormick, Apr. 4, 1898, 10: 496–9; C. C. Cuyler to WW, Mar. 28, May 16, Dec. 23, 1898, 10: 485, 529–30, 11: 91.

WW RETURNS TO BRITAIN; LITERARY SURGE: Andrew Wilson, 8; WW to EAW, July 2, 7, and Aug. 20, 1899, 11: 142–3, 155, and 234–6; SA, 84–9; WW, *ML*, 73–4, 197, 201; "Old-Fashioned Democrat" to Editor of *Indianapolis News*, May 1, 1902, 12: 356–8; WW to R. W. Gilder, Jan. 28, 1901, 12: 84; WW, "Robert E. Lee" (S), Jan. 19, 1909, 18: 639.

WW BECOMES PRESIDENT OF PRINCETON: M. T. Pyne to A. F. West, Oct. 16, Nov. 27, Dec. 14, 1900, cited in Thorp, 67–8; ASL (N), "The Crisis in Presidential Leadership," 12: 292; SA, 117–8, 271; C. C. Cuyler to C. H. McCormick, July 2, 1902, 12: 473–4; WW to EAW, June 1, 1902, 12: 390–1; S. B. Dod to WW, June 25, 1902, 12: 457; EWM, *PG*, 225; J. G. Hibben to RSB, cited in RSB II: 131; *Princeton Alumni Weekly, II* (June 14, 1902), 133–4, 12: 421–2; "WW," *NYT*, June 11, 1902, quoted in RSB II: 131; M. T. Pyne to WW, June 19, 1902, and TR to Grover Cleveland, June 17, 1902, both cited 12: 441; WW to F. J. Turner, Jan. 21, 1902, 12: 240.

WW'S INSTALLATION; DEATH OF JRW: WW to EAW, July 19, 1902, 14: 27; EWM, *TWW*, 61–5, 68; EAW to WW, July 24, 1902, 14:43; "WW Installed at Princeton," *NYT*, Oct., 26, 1902, 1; "WW Inauguration," *Princeton Alumni Weekly, III* (Nov. 1, 1902), 83–6, 14: 191–5; WW, "Princeton for the Nation's Service" (S), Oct. 25, 1902, 14: 170–85; EWM, *PG*, 230; RSB, II: 142; "Rev. Joseph R. Wilson, D. D.," *Princeton Press*, Jan. 24, 1903, 14: 330; "Funeral Services of the Late JRW" and "JRW," Columbia (SC) *State*, Jan. 24, 1903, 14: 331 and 331–3.

WW'S INNOVATIONS: E. G. Reid, 98; WW to Board of Trustees, Oct. 21, 1902, and Dec. 10, 1903, 14: 150–61 and 15: 69–75; Neil Rudenstine, "WW: Ideas and Goals for United States Higher Education," *WW at Princeton: Perspectives from University Presidents*, Princeton, NJ:

WW School, 2006, 28; WW (M), "Departmental Organization," c. Nov. 20, 1903, 15: 55–6; WW, "College and Methods of Instruction" (S), 15: 79–98; WW, "Report to Faculty," Apr. 16, 1904, 15: 252–63; ASL (N), "The New Princeton Course of Study," 15: 277–92; E. S. Corwin, "Departmental Colleague," in Myers, 22; WW (S) to Princeton Alumni of NY, Dec. 9, 1902, 14: 273; News items, *Princeton Alumni Weekly, III* (Nov. 8, 1902, and Mar. 7, 1903), 116 and 355, 14: 203 and 383; Mary Hoyt to RSB, quoted in RSB, II: 152; Axtell, 55; EAW to WW, May, 1903, 14: 440–1; "Faculty Song," 1903 Campus Songs, n.d., 14: 441; Finance Committee Report, Oct. 14, 1902, 14: 144.

WW AND EAW TO EUROPE; DEATH OF EDWARD AXSON: WW, "Record of a European Trip," July 10–Sep. 22, 1903, 14: 521–43; EAW to WW, May 25, 1904, 15: 348; WW to Robert Bridges, Apr. 28, 1905, 16: 86; EWM, *PG*, 240.

PRINCETON'S EXPANSION: Weinstein, 162, 163; WW (S), to Princeton Alumni of NY, Dec. 9, 1902, 14: 269; Minutes of Princeton Board, Dec. 8, 1904, 15: 569–70; News item, *Princeton Alumni Weekly, IV* (June 18, 1904), 600–1 and (Jan. 7, 1905), 213, 15: 390 and 577; WW to J. H. Reed, c. Jan. 13, 1904, 15: 124–6; M. T. Pyne to WW, July 30, 1904, 15: 424–6; C. W. McAlpin to WW, Jan. 13, 1906, 16: 282; Nasaw, 612; WW to Andrew Carnegie, Apr. 17, 1903, 14: 411–5; "Princeton Lake," *Princeton Press*, Dec. 5, 1903, 15: 66–7; "Pres. W Convalescing," *Daily Princetonian*, Jan. 7, 1905, 15: 577; WW to W. B. Pritchard, July 5, 1990, 11: 553–4; WW, "Baccalaureate Address," June 11, 1905, 16: 125; RSB II: 153; WW, "Report to Board of Trustees," Dec. 13, 1906, 16: 516; John DeWitt to WW, Oct. 29, 1904, 15: 531; R. K. Root, "Wilson and the Preceptors," Edward S. Corwin, "Departmental Colleague," Luther P. Eisenhart, "The Far-Seeing Wilson," E. G. Conklin, "As a Scientist Saw Him," J. Duncan Spaeth, "As I Knew Him and View Him Now," all in Myers, 13–16, 19 and 28, 64, 55–6 and 59, 87; "Army and Navy Crowd," *Daily Princetonian*, Dec. 4, 1905, 16: 242–3; WW (N), Oct. 28, 1905, 16: 208; "Two College Presidents Spoke," *Providence Journal*, Feb. 10, 1906, 16: 309–12.

LOTOS CLUB SPEECH: F. R. Lawrence, quoted in *NYT*, Feb. 4, 1906, 16: 293; WW (S) at Lotos Club, Feb. 3, 1906, 16: 292–9; G. B. M. Harvey (S), Feb. 3, 1906, 16: 299–301; WW to G. B. M. Harvey, Feb. 3, 1906, 16: 301; SA, 151.

6 ADVENT

FIRST POLITICAL FLIRTATION: WW to St. Clair McKelway, Mar. 11, 1906, 16: 330; WW, "Address on Thomas Jefferson," Apr. 16, 1906, 16: 362–9; "The Jefferson Celebration," *Brooklyn Daily Eagle*, Apr. 17, 1906, 16: 373n3; "Head of Princeton Defines Education," *Cleveland Leader*, May 19, 1906, 16: 396–7; James Mathers, "Annual Convention of the Western Association of Princeton Clubs," *Princeton Alumni Weekly, VI* (May 26 and June 2, 1906), 632, 651–5, 16: 405–11.

SUDDEN ILLNESS; RECUPERATION IN ENGLAND: EAW to Mary Hoyt, June 12, 1906, 16: 423; Weinstein, 149, 165–6; SA, 44–6; EWM, *TWW*, 93, 94–6; ASL (N), 16: 412n1; WW to N. M. Butler, June 1, 1906, 16: 413; WW to C. W. McAlpin, July 19, 1906, 16: 431; Minutes, Princeton Board of Trustees, June 11, 1906, 16: 422; WW to Annie W. Howe, Aug. 2, 1906, 16: 432; WW to EAW, Aug. 27 and Sep. 2, 1906, 16: 441 and 445–6; Andrew Wilson, 19; EWM, *PG*, 241–2; WW to Robert Bridges, Sep. 6, 1906, 16: 451; EAW to Florence Hoyt, June 27, 1906, 16: 429–30.

PLANS FOR PRINCETON'S SOCIAL REFORM: WW to CD, Sep. 16, 1906, 16: 453–4; "WW's Stand," NY *Evening Post*, Oct. 2, 1906, 16: 454–5; "WW's Position," NY *Evening Post*, Oct. 15, 1906, 16: 456–7; n.t., *Princeton Alumni Weekly, VI* (June 9, 1906), 673–4, 16: 419; WW, "Report on Social Coordination of the University," *Princeton Alumni Weekly, VI* (June 12, 1907), 606–15, cited in Day, 80; WW to H. B. Brougham, Feb. 1, 1910, 20: 70; WW, "Supplementary Report to Board of Trustees," c. Dec. 13, 1906, 16: 519–25.

MINORITIES AT PRINCETON: WW to J. R. Williams, Sep. 2, 1904; 15: 462n; G. M. Sullivan to WW, Nov. 20, 1909, 19: 529; WW to G. M. Sullivan (draft), c. Dec. 3, 1909, 19: 550; C. W. McAlpin to G. W. Sullivan, Dec. 6, 1909, 19: 558; J. C. Hemphill to WW, Jan. 22, 1906, 16: 286; "The Conservatism of the South," Charleston (SC) *News and Courier*, Jan. 22, 1906, 16: 286–8; WW to J. C. Hemphill, Jan. 26, 1906, 16: 288; J. F. Jameson to WW, Nov. 18, 1889, 6: 427; WW (N), June 30, 1904, 15: 400; WW, "The Making of the Nation," *Atlantic Monthly, LXXX* (July 1897), 1–14, 10: 230; ASL (N), 19: 462n2; WW

(N), Feb. 26, 1909, 19: 69; Mary Yates (D), July 31, 1908, 18: 386–7; Karabel, 71; L. M. Levy to WW, c. June 25, 1907, 17: 223; J. R. Wright to WW, Sep. 16, 1904, 15: 471; Konvitz, 17.

ANDREW FLEMING WEST AND GRADUATE COLLEGE: Andrew Fleming West, *Proposed Graduate College of Princeton University*, (Princeton: 1903), cited in 16: 414n2; Thorp, 77, 107; W. M. Sloane, et al., to Board of Trustees of Princeton University, Oct. 15, 1906, 16: 458; S. H. Thompson, Jr., to WW, Feb. 7, 1910, 20: 84–5; SA, "Princeton Controversy" (M), Feb. 1925, RSB Papers, cited in Bragdon, 468n10; WW, "A Resolution," c. Oct. 20, 1906, 16: 467; Thorp, 109.

WW TO BERMUDA: EWM, *PG*, 243; WW to EAW, Jan. 14–16, 22, 30, 1907, 17: 3–7, 10–12, 25–7; WW to MAH, Feb. 6 and 20, 1907, 17: 29 and 48; ASL (N), 17: 29–30; Hulbert, 158–63; Bragdon, 220; EAW, quoted in Florence Hoyt to RSB, RSB Papers, cited in Weinstein, 188.

QUAD FIGHT: NY *Evening Post*, quoted in EAW to Anne Harris, Feb. 12, 1907, 17: 35; WW to CD, Feb. 20 and July 1, 1907, 17: 47–8 and 240–1; CD to WW, Dec. 19, 1906, July 2 and Aug. 6, 1907, 16: 534–5, 17: 243 and 341; D. B. Jones to WW, May 15, 1907, 17: 147–8, Franklin Murphy, Jr., to WW, June 7 and 18, 1907, 17: 187 and 216; WW, "Baccalaureate," June 9, 1907, 17: 187–96; WW, "Address to Trustees," June 10, 1907, 17: 199–206; RSB, II: 231; WW (N), June 11, 1907, 17: 209; Henry van Dyke to WW, July 5, 1907, 17: 260; Henry van Dyke to W. A. White, May 17, 1924, quoted in 17: 260n1; A. F. West to WW, July 10, 1907, 17: 270–1; John Grier Hibben to WW, July 8, 1907, 17: 262–4; WW, "The Author and Signers of the Declaration of Independence," July 4, 1907, 17: 248–59; WW to J. G. Hibben, July 10, 1907, 17: 268–9; SA, 204–206; WW, "The Personal Factor in Education," c. Aug. 1, 1907, 17: 325–33; WW, "Politics," c. July 31, 1917, 17: 309–25; WW, "Address at Harvard," June 26, 1907, 17: 226; Elliot, 230; H. B. Thompson to CD, Sep. 10, 1907, 17: 379–81; "Opening Exercises," *Daily Princetonian*, Sep. 20, 1907, 17: 394–5; Minutes, Princeton Board meeting, quoted in RSB, II: 256–7; Minutes of Faculty, Sep. 26, 1907, 17: 402; EAW to JWS, Sep. 27, 1907 [PUL: JWS Papers, MC 216, Box 2]; W. S. Myers (D), Sep. 30 and Oct. 7, 1907, 17: 408–9 and 424; "The 'Quad' System," *Daily Princetonian*, Oct. 2, 1907, 17: 411–13; P. van Dyke to Editor of *Princeton Alumni Weekly*, *Princeton Alumni Weekly*, VIII (Oct. 2, 1907), 20–1, 17: 413–4; WW (N), Oct. 7, 1907, 17: 420–1; T. W. Hunt to WW, Oct. 7, 1907, 17: 424–5; WW to D. B. Jones, Sep. 27, 1907, 17: 401; A. H. Joline to editor of *Princeton Alumni Weekly*, VIII (Oct. 9, 1907), 36–8, 17: 428–31; H. B. Thompson to CD, Oct. 15, 1907, 17: 434–5; H. B. Fine to SA, quoted in RSB, II: 245; Minutes, Board of Trustees of Princeton University, Oct. 17, 1907, 17: 441–3; "Princeton's Quad," NY *Evening Sun*, Oct. 18, 1907, 17: 444–5; WW to Board of Trustees, Oct. 17, 1907 (unsent), 17: 443–4; WW to M. W. Jacobus, Oct. 23, 1907, 17: 450–1; M. T. Pyne to A. C. Imbrie, Oct. 23, 1907, 17: 453–4; WW (N), Oct. 24, 1907, 17: 454; WW to JWS, Oct. 21, 1907 [PUL: JWS Papers, MC216, Box 2].

WW'S HEALTH; RECUPERATION IN BERMUDA: ASL (N), 17: 550n1; Freud, 130; James Kerney (N), Oct. 29, 1923 [PUL: MC169]; SA, 205–6; Minutes, Princeton Board of Trustees, Jan. 9, 1908, 17: 594; EWM, *PG*, 256; WW to EAW, Feb. 4, 1908, 17: 611–3; Hulbert, 163–72; Hoffman, 96.

POLITICS—PRINCETON AND THE NATION: D. B. Jones to WW, Nov. 12, 1907, 17: 496; WW (A) to Princeton Club of Chicago, Mar. 12, 1908, 18: 18–34; WW, "Report and Recommendations Respecting Undergraduate Social Conditions at Princeton University," Apr. 8, 1908, 18: 238; WW, "The Government and Business" (A), Mar. 14, 1908, 18: 35–51; WW, "Law or Personal Power" (A), Apr. 13, 1908, 18: 263–8; WW, "Baccalaureate Address," June 7, 1908, 18: 323–33; "Faculty Song," as appears in *Carmina Princetoniana: The Songbook of Princeton University* (New York: G. Schirmer, 1968), 35; SA, 153–4; EWM, *PG*, 246.

WW RETURNS TO BRITISH ISLES: WW to EAW, June 26, 27, 29, July 1, 6, 13, Aug. 16, 1908, 18: 343–4, 345–7, 349, 351–3, 361–4, 399–401; RSB, II: 284.

W. C. PROCTER AND GRADUATE COLLEGE: Poucher, 3–99; Thorp, 113, 120–3; W. C. Procter to A. F. West, May 8, 1909, 19: 189–9; SA, 136; W. C. Procter to WW, June 7, 1909, 19: 237–8; A. F. West, "The Proposed Graduate College of Princeton University," quoted in RSB II: 292; "St. Paul's Anniversary," Concord (NH) *Evening Monitor*, June 3, 1909, 19: 226–8; WW (A), June 7, 1909, as printed in *Union College Bulletin, II* (Aug. 1909), 32–43, 19: 231–7; WW, "Baccalaureate Address," June 13, 1909, 19: 242–51; WW,

"The Spirit of Learning" (A), July 1, 1909, *Harvard Graduates' Magazine*, XVIII (Sep. 1909), 1–14, 19: 277–89.

EAW IN OLD LYME: WW to MAH, July 11 and 18, Sep. 5, 1909, 19: 307–10 and 311–14, 357–9; Aucella, et al., 5–6, 13–4; EWM, *TWW*, 104–7; RSB, II: 302.

THE PECK "AFFAIR": WW to EBW, Sep. 19 and 21, 1915, 34: 491–2 and 500; CTG, quoted in Breckinridge Long (D), Jan. 11, 1924, 68: 527; WW to EAW, June 26, 1908, 18: 372; WW to MAH, Sep. 5 and 26, 1909, 19: 357–9 and 392–4; Freud, 92, 154, 132.

GRADUATE SCHOOL BATTLE: WW to MAH, Sep. 26, Oct. 24, 1909, and Feb. 14, 1910, 19: 392, 442–4, and 20: 126; W. C. Procter to M. T. Pyne, Oct. 20, 1909, 19: 424; Minutes, Princeton Board of Trustees, Oct. 21, 1909, 19: 435–9; RSB, II: 313–4, 322–3; WW to M. T. Pyne, Dec. 22 and 25, 1909, 19: 620 and 628–31; M. T. Pyne to WW, Dec. 24, 1909, 19: 627; Wilson Farrand (N), n.d. [Selected Papers of Wilson Farrand, PUL: #CO155]; WW to H. B. Thompson, Jan. 17, 1910, quoted in RSB, II: 322; WW to Hiram Woods, Mar. 23, 1910, 20: 285–7; "Princeton," *NYT*, Feb. 3, 1910, 20: 74–6; WW to H. B. Brougham, Feb. 1, 1910, 20: 69–71; H. B. Brougham to RSB, Aug. 21, 1924, quoted in RSB, II: 328n3; G. M. Harper to Wilson Farrand, Feb. 3, 1910; CD to WW, Feb. 6, 1910, 20: 82; EWM, *PG*, 255; EAW to WW, Feb. 21, 1910, 20: 152–3; WW to EAW, Feb. 14 and 21, 1910, 20: 125–6 and 145–6; WW, "The Country and Colleges," c. Feb. 24, 1910, 20: 157–72; EWM, *TWW*, 106–7.

NJ BOSSES APPROACH WW: "James Smith, Jr. Fails in Business," *NYT*, Nov. 21, 1915, 1, 6; EWM, *PG*, 260; RSB, III: 45, 48–9; ASL (N), "Colonel Harvey's Plan for Wilson's Entry into Politics," 20: 146–8; William O. Inglis, *Collier's*, Oct. 1916, cited in RSB, III: 46–8; WW to MAH, Sep. 5, 1909, 19: 358; "Statesmanship in Banking," *NY Evening Post*, Jan. 18, 1910, n.p.; "Bankers Warned Their Narrowness Harms Country," *NY World*, Jan. 18, 1910, n.p.; "Panics Needless MacVeagh Asserts," *NYT*, Jan. 18, 1910, 3; "Wilson to Bankers," *NY Tribune*, Jan. 18, 1910, 20: 23–7; Bullock, 99; WW (A) to Short Ballot Organization, Jan. 21, 1910, 20: 32–43; WW (A) on Grover Cleveland, National Democratic Club, 20: 257–62; WW (A) to Democratic Dollar Dinner, Mar. 29, 1910, 20: 297–303.

GRADUATE SCHOOL DEFEAT: WW, "Abstract of Address to Western Association of Princeton Clubs," Mar. 26, 1910, *Princeton Alumni Weekly*, X (Mar. 30, 1910), 412–5, 20: 291–6; WW (A) to Princeton Club of NY, Apr. 7, 1910, *Princeton Alumni Weekly*, X (Apr. 13, 1910), 447–53, 20: 337–48; H. B. Thompson to CD, Apr. 15, 1910, 20: 361–2; "Disaster Forecast by Wilson," Apr. 17, 1910, *Pittsburgh Dispatch*, Apr. 17, 1910, 20: 363–5; WW, "Pittsburgh Speech," *Princeton Alumni Weekly*, X (Apr. 20, 1910), 467–71, 20: 373–6; M. T. Pyne to Bayard Henry, Apr. 20, 1910, 20: 377–8; D. B. Jones to WW, May 19, 1910, 20: 459–60; WW to E. W. Sheldon, May 16, 1910, 20: 456–7; "Gift of $10,000,000 Left to Princeton," *NYT*, May 22, 1910, 1; SA to RSB, quoted in RSB II: 346; SA, 142; J. M. Raymond and A. F. West to WW (T), May 22, 1910, 20: 464; A. F. West to M. T. Pyne, May 22, 1910, 20: 465–6; WW to Hiram Woods, May 28, 1910, 20: 482–3; WW to T. D. Jones, May 30, 1910, 20: 483–4; EWM, *TWW*, 101, 106–7; A. F. West, "Narrative of the Graduate College" [U typescript, PUL: Graduate School Records], 75–109; H. B. Thompson to E. W. Sheldon, May 31, 1910 (two letters), May 31, 1910, 20: 488–9 and 489–90; WW to MAH, June 5, 1910, 20: 500–1; WW, "Baccalaureate Sermon," June 12, 1910, 20: 520–8; ASL (N), 20: 451–2; Lawrence, 32; RSB, II: 351.

WW LEAVES FOR CONNECTICUT: EWM, *TWW*, 107; WW to G. B. Harvey (T), Jun. 25, 1910, 20: 541.

7 PAUL

WW ENTERS NEW JERSEY POLITICS: Hosford, 13–20, 31–2, 37, 49–61; EWM, *PG*, 265; WW (S), Oct. 17, 1912, 25: 428; Morgenthau, 132–3; RSB, III: 55–6; WW to D. B. Jones, June 27, 1910, 20: 544–5; EWM, *TWW*, 108–9; "Wall St. to Put Up W. Wilson for President," *NY Journal*, June 18, 1910, cited in RSB, III: 61; G. B. M. Harvey to WW, July 7 and Aug. 12 and Sep. 9, 10, 1910, 20: 563 and 21: 52 and 87–8, 88–9; ASL (N), "Lawyers' Club Conference," July 8, 1910, 20: 565–6; Hudspeth, cited in RSB, III: 63–4; WW to G. B. M. Harvey, July 14 and Aug. 3, 8, 1910, 20: 576–7 and 21: 35, 41n1; WW (S), to Princeton University Board, Oct. 20, 1910, 21: 362; WW, quoted in *Newark Evening News*, July 15, 1910, 20: 581; H. E. Alexander to WW, July 23, 1910, 21: 23; WW to James Kerney, Aug. 2, 1910, 21: 34; WW, "Proposed Democratic State Platform," Aug. 9, 1910, 21: 43–6; RSB, III: 70; WW to Edgar Williamson, Aug. 23, 1910, 21: 59–61; WW

(S), "The Lawyer and the Community," Aug. 31, 1910, 21: 64–81.

WW NOMINATED FOR GOVERNOR: Tumulty, 16–8, 19–23, 26; RSB, III: 77–9; SA, 159; WW, "Acceptance Speech," Sep. 15, 1910, 21: 91–4; EWM, *TWW*, 110–1, 120; *NY Evening Post*, Sep. 16, 1910, cited in RSB, III: 81; "Jersey Republicans Name Vivian Lewis," *NYT*, Sep. 21, 1910, 3.

RESIGNATION FROM PRINCETON: "Princeton's 164th Year," Trenton *True American*, Sep. 23, 1910, 21: 151–2; EWM, *TWW*, 111; Princeton University Board, Resolution, c. Oct. 19, 1910, 21: 353; M. T. Pyne to WW, Oct. 19, 1910, 21: 353; WW to Princeton University Board, Oct. 20, 1910, 21: 362; Wilson Farrand (M), n.d., 21: 363; WW to L. C. Woods, Oct. 27, 1910, 21: 444; C. W. McAlpin to WW, Nov. 3, 1910, 21: 536–9; WW to D. P. Foster, Oct. 29, 1910, 21: 470–1; M. T. Pyne to W. C. Procter, Oct. 25, 1910, 21: 434; "Students Give Parade for Wilson," Trenton *True American*, Oct. 11, 1915, 21: 289.

GUBERNATORIAL CAMPAIGN: WW to MAH, Sep. 25, 1910, 21: 163–4; Tumulty, 27, 28–30, 42; EWM, *PG*, 263; J. Smith, quoted in RSB, III: 83; Kerney, 62; EWM, *TWW*, 110–2, 114; SA to RSB, RSB III: 87, 93–4, 96; "Crime of Trusts," NY *World*, Sep. 18, 1910, 21: 134–6; SA, 159–61; WW (S), Sep. 28, 29, 30, and Oct. 1, 3, 5, 13, 15, 21, 25, and Nov. 2, 5, 1910, 21: 181–91, 193–8, 202–12, and 213–8, 229–38, 245–59, 310–20, 328–34, 423–33, and 508–18, 564–76; "Who WW Is," *Philadelphia Record*, Oct. 2, 1910, 21: 220–5; "W Talks Pure Politics," *Newark Evening News*, Oct. 12, 1910, 21: 301–6; "W Gets Great Reception," Trenton *True American*, Oct. 15, 1910, 21: 325–7; "W Reads a New Lesson," *Philadelphia Record*, Oct. 22, 1910, 21: 382–5; G. L. Record to WW, Oct. 17, 1910, 21: 338–47; WW to G. L. Record, Oct. 24, 1910, 21: 406–11; G. B. M. Harvey to WW, Oct. 25, 1910, 21: 433; JPT to WW (T), Oct. 25, 1910, 21: 433; "W Free of Alliances," *Philadelphia Record*, Oct. 25, 1910, 21: 413–21; "W's Last Call Greatest," *Philadelphia Record*, Nov. 5, 1910, 21: 561–4; W. H. Page to WW, Nov. 5, 1910, 21: 576.

WW ELECTED GOVERNOR OF NEW JERSEY: EWM, *TWW*, 115; RSB III: 106–7; "W Speech for Students," *Newark Evening News*, Nov. 10, 1910, 22: 3–4; T. R. Marshall to WW (T), Nov. 9, 1910, 21: 603; G. L. Record to WW, Nov. 9, 1910, 21: 596; JPT to WW (T),

Nov. 8–9, 1910, 21: 589; WW to J. Smith, Jr., Nov. 9, 1910, 21: 590.

WW AS GOVERNOR-ELECT: WW to MAH, Jan. 13, 1911, 22: 329–30; RSB, III: 108, cites Trenton *True American*, Dec. 24, 1910; CD to WW, Nov. 18, 1910, 23: 72–3; WW to J. E. Martine, Nov. 14, 1910; 22: 36–7; RSB, III: 111, 124, 132–5; M. C. Ely to WW, Nov, 23, 1910, 22: 85–6; W. W. St. John to WW, Nov. 22, 1910: 22: 81–2n1; Tumulty, 57–8, 60–2; WW to G. B. M. Harvey, Nov. 15, 1910, 22: 46–8; WW to MAH, Dec. 7 and 16, 1910, 22: 141–2n1 and 204–5; WW, "Statement," Trenton *True American*, Dec. 9, 1910, 22: 153–4; James Smith, "Statement," *Newark Evening News*, Dec. 9, 1910, 22: 166–7; WW to O. G. Villard, Jan. 2, 1911, 22: 288–9; EWM, *TWW*, 118–9.

WW INAUGURATION AND FIRST GUBERNATORIAL TEST: "Governor W Takes Office in Jersey," *NYT*, Jan. 18, 1911, 3; WW (S), Jan. 17, 1911, 22: 345–54; WW to MAH, Jan. 22 and 29, 1911, 22: 362–4 and 391–3; Tumulty, 67–71; WW, "Statement," *Newark Evening News*, Jan. 24, 1911, 22: 365; "James Smith, Jr. Fails in Business," *NYT*, Nov. 21, 1915, 1.

NEW JERSEY POLITICS: WW to MAH, Jan. 13, 15, and Mar. 26, 1911, 22: 329–30, 333–4, and 517–9; WW, "The Law and the Facts" (S), Dec. 27, 1910, 22: 264–72; WW to W. S. U'ren, Dec. 14, 1910, 22: 197; RSB, III: 131, 139–44; Tumulty, 73.

WW "ENTERS" PRESIDENTIAL CAMPAIGN: McAdoo, 114–20; Startt, 113–5; McCombs, 5–6, 32; 34–9; F. P. Stockbridge, "How WW Won His Nomination," *Current History, XX* (July 1924), 561–4; WW to MAH, Mar. 5, 13, and Apr. 2, 16, 1911, 22: 477–80, 500–1, and 531–4, 570–2; "WW Finds Opens Arms of Welcome Here," *Atlanta Journal*, Mar. 10, 1911, 22: 487–91; WW (S), Mar. 10, 1911, 22: 491–8; RSB, III: 114, 209–11, 212–3, 225, 230–2; EWM, *TWW*, 120–4; EWM, *PG*, 265–6; WJB, quoted in *Newark Evening News*, Apr. 6, 1911, quoted in James Chace, *1912: Wilson, Roosevelt, Taft & Debs—The Election That Changed the Country* (New York: Simon & Schuster, 2004), 130; Tumulty, 74–7; "An Astonishing Legislature," *Jersey Journal*, Apr. 22, 1911, quoted in August Heckscher, *Woodrow Wilson* (NY: Charles Scribener's Sons, 1981), 694n43; "W Glad to Be a Radical," *St. Paul Dispatch*, May 25, 1911, 23: 93–5.

PROGRESSIVISM; WW COMING TO TERMS WITH JEFFERSON: "People Look to

Man, Not to Party," *Indianapolis News*, Apr. 13, 1911, 23: 554–6; WW (S), Apr. 13, 1911, 22: 557–68; "Tariff Reform the Keynote at Jefferson Dinner," NY *World*, Apr. 14, 1912, 24: 330–2; WW (S), Sep. 25, 1912, 25: 250; Arthur Schlesinger, Jr. (S), "A Question of Power," Oct. 5–6, 2000 (published in *American Prospect*, Apr. 23, 2001).

WW WESTERN TOUR: "W Trusts the Public," *Kansas City Star*, May 5, 1911, 23: 3–5; WW (S), May 7, 1911, 23: 12–20; EAW to WW, May 11 and June 2, 1911, 23: 30–1 and 127–8; WW (S), May 12, 1911, 23: 32–40; "People of U.S. Should Name Senators," *Los Angeles Examiner*, May 14, 1911, 23: 50–1; "W Hailed As Political Prophet," *San Francisco Examiner*, May 16, 1911, 23: 55–8; U'Ren First Gains Gov. Wilson's Ear," *Portland Morning Oregonian*, May 18, 1911, 23: 60–3; "Press Club Is Host," *ibid.*, May 19, 1911, 23: 68–9; "W Opposes Judge's Recall," May 20, 1911, *ibid.*, 23: 73–6; "WW Welcomed on His Visit to Seattle," *Seattle Daily Times*, May 20, 1911, 23: 76–8; "Outlines His Views," Lincoln (NE) *State Journal*, May 27, 1911, 23: 96–102; T. P. Gore to H. S. Breckinridge, May 25, 1911, quoted in *NYT*, May 27, 1911, 23: 113n3.

SUMMER 1911; ENTRANCE OF WGM: RSB, III: 231, 237, 238; EWM, *TWW*, 132–3; WW to MAH, July 30, 1911, 23: 239–40; McAdoo, 109–120.

PRIMARY CAMPAIGN: Fred Williams to R. F. Pettigrew, published in *NYT*, Feb. 2, 1912, 24: 270; "Who Sought a Pension," NY *Sun*, Dec. 5, 1911, 23: 564–5; WW to *Newark Evening News*, Dec. 6, 1911, 23: 565–6; WW to H. S. Pritchett, Nov. 11, 1910, 22: 23–4n1; Lane, 84–5; WW, *History*, V: 212–4; Nicholas Pietrowski to WW, Mar. 11, 1912, 24: 241–2; WW to Nicholas Pietrowski, Mar. 13, 1912, 24: 242–3; WW to Harper & Brothers, Mar. 4, 1912, 24: 223; WW to A. H. Joline, Apr. 29, 1907, 17: 124; WW (U letter), Jan. 8, 1912, 24: 8–9; RSB, III: 247–8, 257–67; WW to MAH, Jan. 7, 14, 1912, 24: 5–6, 43–4; WW (S), Jan. 8, 1912, 24: 9–16; Morgenthau, 139–44; Tumulty, 83–8, 97; SA, 172–3; WW to G. B. M. Harvey, Dec. 21 and Jan. 11, 1911, 23: 603 and 24: 31; G. B. M. Harvey to WW, Jan. 4, 1912, 23: 652.

EMH: RSB, III: 294–309; Houston, 21–2; McAdoo, 127–8; House, 5, 107–11; Freud, 144–5; WW to MAH, Feb. 12, 1911, 22: 424–7; Hodgson, 7; SA, 207.

FINAL DAYS AS GOVERNOR; PRIMARIES: WW to MAH, Oct. 8, 1911, and Jan. 14,

May 11, June 9, 1912, 23: 424–5 and 24: 43–4, 391–2, 466–7; EWM, *TWW*, 127–8; EAW to J. G. Hibben, Feb. 10, 1912, 24: 149–50; H. D. Thompson to WW, Apr. 1, 1912, 24: 274–5; WW to H. D. Thompson, Apr. 3, 1912, 24: 284; WW (S), Jan. 9, 1912, 24: 18–25; WW to House of Assembly, Apr. 2, 1912, 24: 276–84; "Forty Vetoes Start Fight," Trenton *True American*, Apr. 12, 1912, 24: 324–8; "WW to Citizens of New Jersey," Trenton *True American*, May 24, 1912, 24: 429–34; RSB, III: 309–11, 356; McAdoo, 129–30, 156–9; WW to EMH, Oct. 24, 1911, 23: 480; Tumulty, 106–16; EWM, *PG*, 271–74; McAdoo, 137–42; *Democratic Text-Book: 1912* (New York: Isaac Goldman, 1912), 2, 115, 32; EWM, *TWW*, 158, 162, 164–5.

BALTIMORE CONVENTION, 1912; RECEIVES NOMINATION: Chace, *op. cit.*, 151; Tumulty, 120–1, 124; EAW, quoted in Baltimore *Sun*, July 3, 1912, RSB, III: 350; EWM, *PG*, 273; EWM, *TWW*, 162, 164–5; RSB, III: 356, 362; McAdoo, 156–9; "Gov. W Not Elated by Victory," *NYT*, July 2, 1912, 24: 522–8; WW to MAH, July 14, 28, 1912, 24: 550–2, 572; "W in Hiding to Write Speech," *NYT*, July 23, 1912, 24: 562–3; Luke Lea to WW, July 13, 1912, 24: 545–8; WGM to WW, July 25, 1912, 24: 570; WJB to WW, c. July 22, 1912, 24: 565; L. D. Brandeis to WW, Aug. 1, 1912, 24: 580; "W Here; Dines at a Lunch Counter," *NYT*, Aug. 4, 1912, 24: 585–9.

PRESIDENTIAL CAMPAIGN, 1912: WW (S), Aug. 7, 1912, 25: 3–18; EWM, *TWW*, 149, 154, 173–4; Dos Passos, 25–7; WW, quoted in Baltimore *Sun*, Oct. 7, 1912, cited in RSB, III: 375, 398–400; WW to MAH, Aug. 25 and Sep. 1, 29, 1912, 25: 55–6 and 66–7, 284–5; McAdoo, 163–5; M. F. Lyons to Charles Seymour, c. Oct. 29, 1947, M. F. Lyons (M), "Record of Monies That McCombs Was Personally Instrumental in Obtaining, Oct. 2, 1947," and M. F. Lyons, Minutes of Democratic National Campaign Committee, Aug. 11, 1912 [Maurice F. Lyons Collection: PUL]; Morgenthau, 150–3; Urofsky, 342–7; "Gov. W Agrees with Mr. Brandeis," *NYT*, Aug. 29, 1912, 25: 56–9; WW (two S), Sep. 2, 1912, 25: 69–79 and 80–92; WW to R. H. Dabney, Jan. 11, 1912, 24: 29; WW (speeches:, Sep. 4, 16, 17, 1912, 25: 98–109, 148, 148–56; WW (three S), Sep. 18, 1912, 25: 164–9, 169–72, 172–84; Sep. 19, 1912, 25: 186–98; Sep. 20, 1912 (2 S), 25: 198–203 and 203–12; Sep. 23, 1912, 25: 221–31; Sep. 25, 1912, 25: 234–45; Oct. 4, 8, 1912, 25: 332–8, 385–90; "Taft Meets W for Pleasant Chat," *NYT*, Sep. 26,

1912, 25: 269–71; "Gov W in Princeton Today," *Princeton Press*, Sep. 28, 1912, 25: 273; WW, "Platform of the New Jersey Democratic Party," Oct. 1, 1912, 25: 305–10; "W Sends Sympathy," *NYT*, Oct. 16, 1912, 25: 418–9; Hatfield, 325–32; "Roosevelt Stills Garden Tumult," *NYT*, Oct. 31, 1912, 1; "Garden Crowd Wild for Wilson," *NYT*, Nov. 1, 1912, 1; "Gov. W Hurt but Will Speak Despite Injury," *Trenton Evening True American*, Nov. 4, 1912, 25: 508–10; "W Laughs Over Bald Spot," *Newark Evening News*, Nov. 4, 1912, 25: 510–11; EWM, *PG*, 274; G. B. M. Harvey to WW, Nov. 4, 1912, 25: 512–3.

THE NEGRO VOTE: WW (S), Oct. 3 and 5, 1910, 21: 236 and 255; M. F. Lyons, Minutes, *op. cit.*, Aug. 11, 1912; W. M. Trotter to WW, July 18, 1912, 24: 558–9; "W and the Negro," *NY Age*, July 11, 1912, 24: 558–90; WW, quoted in *Trenton Evening News*, July 31, 1912, 24: 574; WW to Alexander Walters, Oct. 16, 1912, quoted in RSB, III: 388; WW to Alexander Walters, Oct. 21, 1912, 25: 448–9; O. G. Villard (D), Aug. 14, 1912.

ELECTION DAY, 1912: EWM, *TWW*, 180–1; EWM, *PG*, 274–5; "Mr. W Jokes While Voting," *Trenton Evening True American*, Nov. 5, 1912, 25: 517–8; "Kiss from Wife Tells W He's President-Elect," *NY World*, Nov. 6, 1912, 25: 519–20; SA, 174–5; W. H. Taft to WW (T), Nov. 5, 1912, 25: 521; TR to WW (T), Nov. 5, 1912, 25: 521; Election results, Brinkley, A–34; WW (S), Nov. 5, 1912, 25: 520–1.

8 DISCIPLES

POST-ELECTION; EMERGENCE OF EMH: EWM, *TWW*, 182, 183–5; "W Ends Talk: Takes Time to Think," *NYT*, Nov. 6, 1912, 1, 25: 523–6. McCombs, 209; Annin, 126; EMH (D), Nov. 16, 1912, 25: 550; SA (N, commenting on RSB ms, Collection #440: PUL), 197–205; Freud, 146; House, I: 93; McAdoo, 179; EAW, "Description: Personal," printed in *St. Louis Post-Dispatch*, July 28, 1912, 24: 573; Sayre, 41–3; F. B. Sayre to Jessie Wilson (U), Oct. 30, Nov. 3, 7, 13, 16, 1912 [WWPL].

FAMILY TO BERMUDA: "W Sails on Bermudian," *NYT*, Nov. 16, 1912, 5; "Gov W Enjoys His First Day at Sea," *NYT*, Nov. 17, 1912, 1; WW (R), Nov. 18, 1912, 25: 551; EWM, *TWW*, 185–8; "Tanned by Sun, W Returns in Fine Health," *Trenton Evening Times*, Dec. 16, 1912, 25: 589–90; WW to WGM, Nov. 20, 1912, 25: 552;

"W Says He Will Use Fists on Photo Man," *Trenton Evening News*, Nov. 22, 1912, 25: 556; EWM, *PG*, 276; WW to MAH, Dec. 22, 1912, 25: 615–6; "W Means to Keep Fight Up in Jersey," *Trenton Evening News*, Dec. 17, 1912, 25: 591–2.

VICTORY LAPS—NEW YORK, CHICAGO, AND VIRGINIA; FINAL BUSINESS IN NEW JERSEY: WW (A) to NY Southern Society, Dec. 17, 1912, 25: 593–603; WW (S) to Commercial Club of Chicago, June 11, 1912, Jan. 11, 1912, 27: 29–39; Rev. A. M. Fraser, quoted in RSB, III: 428; "W in the Room Where He Was Born," *NYT*, Dec. 28, 1912, 1; "W Tells Plans at Birthday Fetes," *NYT*, Dec. 29, 1912, 3; EWM *TWW*, 195; WW (A) at Mary Baldwin Seminary, Dec. 28, 1912, 25: 626–32; WW (A) to New Jersey legislature, Jan. 14, 1913, 27: 46–54; WW (S) on signing "Seven Sisters," Feb. 20, 1913, 27: 120–2; "'Seven Sisters' Bills Signed by W," *NYT*, Feb. 20, 1913, 20.

CABINET APPOINTMENTS: WW, *CG*, 257; House, I: 84, 99; Reid, 137–9; H. L. Mencken, "Bryan," Baltimore *Evening Sun*, July 27, 1925; Bryan, 188, 312–3, 318–20, 384–6; Kazin, 130; WW to WJB, Nov. 9, 1912, 25: 532–3; McAdoo, 177–8, 180–6; Annin, 162–3; EMH (D), Dec. 19, 1912, 25: 614; EMH, I: 90–2, 97, 106–7, 113; RSB, III: 45, 452–4, 447, and IV: 55; O. W. Underwood to WW, Jan. 13, 1913, 27: 44–5; WW to O. W. Underwood, Dec. 17, 1912, 25: 593; EMH (D), Jan. 8, 1913, 27: 20; JD (D), Mar. 6 and Apr. 11, 1913, 27: 157 and 290–2; JD (D), Mar. 6, 1913, 27: 157; H. L. Higginson to CD, Nov. 21, 1912 [PUL]; C. R. Crane to WW, Feb. 10, 1913, 27: 107–8; WW to WJB, Feb. 27, 1913, 27: 138; EMH (D), Feb. 14–6, 1913, 27: 112–6; A. M. Palmer to WW, Feb. 24, 1913, 27: 132; Tumulty, 138; WW (A), Jan. 11, 1913, 27: 31; W. H. Page, quoted in RSB, IV: 23; EMH (D), Feb. 21, 1913, 27: 126.

STAFF APPOINTMENTS AND AMBASSADORS: EWM, *TWW*, 196–7; Lawrence, 89–90; RSB, III: 448, 458–9, and IV: 34; EMH, I: 89, 99, 100; WW to JPT, Nov. 25, 1912, 25: 561; Freud, 147; Tumulty, 127–37; EMH (D), Jan. 15, Feb. 13, Mar. 20, 1913, 27: 57, 110, 200; McAdoo, 174; Lawrence, 35; Houston, 15; WW (M), quoted in McCombs, 228; "Pick Rich Men for Foreign Positions," *The Toronto World*, Mar. 24, 1913, 3; "The Homes of Ambassadors," *NYT*, Apr. 11, 1913, 8; EMH (D), Feb. 13, 1913, 27: 110–111; H. B. Fine to WW, Mar. 12, 1913, 27: 173–4; EMH (D), Jan. 17, 1913, 27: 63.

SAMUEL GOMPERS; NEGRO ADVO-
CATES: Samuel Gompers to Executive Council of
AFL, Dec. 21, 1912, 25: 614–5; WW to Alexander
Walters, Oct. 21, 1912, 25: 448–9; Alexander Wal-
ters to WW, Dec. 17, 1912, 25: 606–8; Giles B.
Jackson to WW, Dec. 23, 1912, 25: 619–21; WW
(A) at Mary Baldwin Seminary, Dec. 28, 1912, 25:
632; WW (A) to Commercial Club of Chicago,
Jan. 11, 1913, 27: 39; WW to O. W. Underwood,
Jan. 21, 1913, 27: 66–7; Carter Glass to WW, Jan.
27, 1913, 27: 79–80; EMH (D), Jan. 8, 1913, 27: 21.

WHITE HOUSE DOMESTIC STAFF;
LEAVING NEW JERSEY: WW to MAH, Feb.
16 and Mar. 2, 1913, 27: 116–7 and 146; WW to
W. H. Taft, Jan. 2, 1913, 27: 5; W. H. Taft to
EAW, Jan. 3, 1913, 27: 12; W. H. Taft to WW,
Jan. 6, 1913, 27: 16–8; EAW to W. H. Taft, Jan.
10, 1913, 27: 28–9; EWM, *TWW*, 198–9; WW
(A) in Staunton, Dec. 28, 1912, 25: 635; WW (A)
to NJ Senators, Jan. 28, 1913, 27: 85–90; "W
Neighbors' Farewell," *NYT*, Mar. 2, 1913, 1, 2, 27:
141–2; WW (A) to neighbors in Princeton, Mar.
1, 1913, 27: 142–4; EWM, *PG*, 276.

WW ARRIVAL IN D.C.; PRE-
INAUGURAL ACTIVITY: Lash, 389–91; Mc-
Adoo, 181–2; EWM, *TWW*, 200, 304–6; "W
Evades Vast Crowd," *NYT*, Mar. 1, 1913, 2; RSB,
IV: 16; EWM, *PG*, 277; F. Yates to family, Mar. 5,
1913, 27: 155–6; WW (A), "Princeton Smoker,"
Mar. 3, 1913, 27: 147–8; James W. Kisling (D),
Mar. 2–5, 1913 [WWPL]; I. Hoover, 49–59.

INAUGURATION DAY AND NIGHT:
WW, "Inaugural Address," Mar. 4, 1913, 27: 148–
52; EWM, *TWW*, 205, 207–8, 210; EWM, *PG*,
277; EMH (D), Mar. 4, 1913, 27: 152–3; I. Hoover,
55–9; Grayson, ix, 1; RSB, IV: 16; "W Opposes
Inaugural Ball," *Trenton Evening Times*, Jan. 17,
1913, 27: 59–60; SA (N) [PUL: 440], 324; A. W.
Halsey to WW, Mar. 5, 1913, 27: 154; WW to
A. W. Halsey, 27: 156–7.

9 BAPTISM

WASHINGTON, D.C.—HISTORY AND
DEMOGRAPHICS: Adams, 260–3; *Thirteenth
Census of the United States: 1910*, v. 4: 285–96;
EWM, *TWW*, 223; Grayson, 275.

WW'S FIRST DAYS IN THE WHITE
HOUSE: EWM, *TWW*, 223, 244; F. Yates to E. C.
M. Yates, Mar. 5, 1913, 27: 155; C. R. Crane,
quoted in RSB, IV: 13–4, 17–8; WW, "Constitu-
tional Government," Mar. 24, 1908, 18: 23; EMH
(D), Feb. 14 and Mar. 8, 1913, 27: 113–4 and

163–4; Houston, I: 37; Daniels, *Life*, 139–40;
WW, "Warning to Office-Seekers," Mar. 5, 1919,
27: 153; WW to P. C. Knox, Mar. 5, 1913, cited in
RSB, IV: 14; Alex B. Lacy, Jr., "The White House
Staff Bureaucracy," *Society* (vol. 6, no. 3), Jan. 1969,
50; A. S. Burleson to RSB, cited in RSB, IV: 43–7,
50–2; Freud, 67–9; J. R. Wilson, Jr., to WW, Jan.
27, 1913, 27: 82–3; T. P. Gore quoted by Gore Vidal to ASB (I), Jan. 28, 2004; WW to J. R. Wilson, Jr., Apr. 22, 1913, 27: 346.

HOUSE, TUMULTY, AND GRAYSON:
EMH, I: 114, 116; EMH (D), Mar. 8, 1913, 27:
164; Blum, 67; Lawrence, 89; CTG to RSB,
quoted in RSB, IV: 22; CTG, 1–4, 14–5, 80–1;
Freud, 149; Boos, 344–6; Weinstein, 20, 250–3;
WW to MAH, Aug. 10, 1913; 28: 135; WW to
Herbert Putnam, May 22, 1913, 27: 464; WW to
F. Yates, May 26, 1913, 27: 475.

MEXICO: WW, *History*, IV: 122; Kandell,
391, 397; Creel, *W and Issues*, 5, 7; V. Huerta to
WW (T), Mar. 4, 1913, 27: 152; WW to V. Huerta
(T), Mar. 7, 1913, 27: 158; Mark E. Benbow, "All
the Brains I Can Borrow," *Studies in Intelligence* (v.
51, no. 4), Dec. 2007, 3; RSB, IV: 239; Houston, I:
43–4; WW (S), "Relations with Latin America,"
Mar. 12, 1913, 27: 172–3; J. B. Moore to WW,
May 15, 1913, 27: 437–40; RSB, IV 245; JD (D),
Apr. 18, 1913, 27: 331; EWM, *PG*, 278; C. W.
Thompson to R. A. Bull, May 22, 1913, 27: 465;
CTG, 30; JPT, 146–7; JD, *Life*, 176; W. B. Hale,
"Report," June 18 and July 9, 1913, 27: 550–2 and
28: 31; WW comments regarding H. L. Wilson
written on (T) from W. B. Hale to WW, c. June
25, 1913, 28: 7; WW to WJB, July 1 and 3, 1913,
28: 17 and 22; WJB to WW, July 8, 1913, 27:
26–7; WW to EAW, July 27, 1913, 27: 85; Calero,
13–7.

CHINA; PHILIPPINES; JAPAN: "W Up-
sets China Loan Plan," *NYT*, Mar. 19, 1913, 13;
WJB to WW, Jan. 5, 1913, 27: 14; WW (S) on
Chinese Pending Loan, Mar. 18, 1913, 27: 192–4;
WJB, 361–2; Louis C. Fraina, "Imperialism in
Action" (reprinted from *The Class Struggle*, Sep.–
Oct. 1918), 4–5; JD (D), Mar. 12, 1913, 27: 174–5;
RSB, IV: 62, 454–7; WW to J. S. Williams, July
15, 1913, quoted in RSB, IV: 455; Thomas A. Bai-
ley, "California, Japan, and the Alien Land Legis-
lation of 1913," *Pacific Historical Review 1* (Mar.
1932), 36–59; "Cabinet's Open Door Amazes Old-
Timers," *NYT*, Mar. 16, 1913, 2.

PRESS CONFERENCES: "W Wins News-
papermen," *NYT*, Mar. 16, 1913, 2; ASL (N), "Introduction," 50: xiv.

TARIFF AND INCOME TAX: Lawrence, 81–4; "W Innovations Excite Washington," *NYT*, Feb. 28, 1913, 1; "President's Visit Nettles Senators," *NYT*, Apr. 8, 1913, 1, 3; "Congress Cheers Greet W," *NYT*, Apr. 9, 1913; JD (D), Apr. 8, 1913, 27: 268–9; WW (S), "Tariff Reform," Apr. 8, 1913, 27: 269–72; JD, *Life*, 158–60; WW to MAH, Apr. 8 and June 22, 1913, 27: 273 and 556; WGM, 196, 203; RSB, IV: 98–100, 112, 120–3, 170; WW, "Constitutional Government," 18: 105; Clements, 36; WW to J. C. McReynolds, Apr. 17, 1913; 27: 321; Weisman, 272; Houston, I: 50.

BANKING AND CURRENCY REFORM: WW (S), "On Banking and Currency Reform," June 23, 1913, 27: 570–3; WGM, 204–14, 229, 234; WJB, 370–3; WW to F. K. Lane, June 12, 1913, 27: 511–2; L. D. Brandeis to WW, June 14, 1913, 27: 520–1; RSB, IV: 165–9; Glass, 115–6; "Money Reform Now Is W's Demand," *NYT*, June 24, 1913, 1–2.

EAW AS FIRST LADY; PLANS FOR SUMMER 1913: EMH (D), May 11 and 25, 1913, 27: 413–4 and 227; EWM, *TWW*, 229–30, 236, 238, 250; Seale, 774–8, 784; Whitcomb, 251–2; WW to EAW (T), June 28 and Aug. 10, 1913, 28: 11 and 132–4; WW to EAW, June 29, 1911, 28: 11–2; WW to MAH, June 29 and July 27, 1913, 28: 12–4 and 86–7. WW's golfing is discussed in: CTG, 40–4, 46; Samuel G. Blythe, "A Talk with the President," Dec. 5, 1914, 31: 392; WW to Edith Reid, Aug. 15, 1913, 28: 161; Whitcomb, 258; the Dwight D. Eisenhower Memorial Commission estimated the number of holes W played: www.eisenhowermemorial.org/stories/Ike-Golf. htm; "W a Stranger in Old Yorktown," *NYT*, July 4, 1913, 1, 3.

WW AT GETTYSBURG; SEGREGATING WASHINGTON, D.C.: WW (A), July 4, 1913, 28: 23–6; "Gettysburg Cold to W's Speech," *NYT*, July 5, 1913, 1; Johnson, 462; Houston, I: 51; JD (D), Apr. 11, 1913, 27: 290–2; August Meier and Elliott Rudwick, "The Rise of Segregation in the Federal Bureaucracy, 1900–1930," *Phylon* (v. 28, no. 2), 178–84; WW, "To the Women of the South," c. Jan. 1, 1910, 27: 574; Thomas Dixon, Jr., to WW, July 27, 1913, 28: 88–9; WW to Thomas Dixon, Jr., July 29, 1913, 28: 94; WW to O. G. Villard, July 23, Aug. 21 and 29, Sep. 22, Oct. 3 and 17, 1913, 28: 65, 202 and 245–6, 316, 352 and 413; ASL (N) re: A. E. Patterson to WW, July 30, 1913, 28: 98n; Moorfield Storey and others to WW, Aug. 15, 1913, 28: 163–5; Robert N. Wood to WW, Aug. 5, 1913, 28: 115–8; Booker T.

Washington to O. G. Villard, Aug. 10, 1913, 28: 186–7; O. G. Villard to WW, Aug. 27, Sep. 29, and Oct. 14, 1913, 28: 239–40, 342–4, and 401–2; J. P. Gavit to O. G. Villard, Oct. 1, 1913, 28: 348–50; WGM to O. G. Villard, Oct. 27, 1913, 28: 453–5; Nancy Weiss, "The Negro and the New Freedom," *Political Science Quarterly*, Mar. 1969 (v. 84, no. 1), 61–79; Kathleen L. Wolgemuth, "WW and Federal Segregation," *Journal of Negro History* (v. 44, no. 2), Apr. 1959, 158–73; Henry Blumenthal, "WW and the Race Question," *Journal of Negro History*, v. 48, no. 1 (Jan. 1963), 1–21; RSB, IV: 224–5; M. C. Nerney to O. G. Villard, Sep. 30, 1913, 28: 402–10; J. S. Williams to WW, Mar. 31, 1913, 29: 387–8; WW to J. S. Williams, Apr. 2, 1914, 29: 394; WW to Champ Clark, May 4, 1914, 29: 543; W. M. Trotter to WW, Nov. 6, 1913, 28: 491–5.

WW IN CORNISH: EAW to WW, July 29, Aug. 6, and Sep. 9, 1913, 28: 96, 127, and 269; "President's Wife Shows Landscapes," *NYT*, Nov. 15, 1913, 11; "Mrs. W Earns by Art," *NYT*, Nov. 22, 1913, 1; EWM, *TWW*, 251, 253–4, 259; Sayre, 36; WW to EAW, July 27, Aug. 12, and Sep. 17, 1913, 28: 85, 145, and 279; WW to E. G. Reid, Aug. 15, 1913, 28: 160–2.

TARIFF AND BANKING BILLS: "Senate Passes Tariff," *NYT*, Sep. 10, 1913, 1–2; EWM, *TWW*, 259, 267; "W Signs New Tariff Law," *NYT*, Oct. 4, 1913, 1; WW (S), Signing Tariff Bill, Oct. 3, 1913, 28: 351–2; EAW to WW, Oct. 5, 1913, 28: 363–4; WGM, 248–9; Marshall, 242–3; WW to MAH, Sep. 28 and Oct. 12, 1913, 28: 336–8 and 395; WW to B. F. Shively, Oct. 20, 1913, 28: 418; WW to Annie Wilson Howe, Oct. 12, 1913, 28: 396–8; WW (R), re: Federal Reserve Bill, Dec. 23, 1913, 29: 63–6.

JWS MARRIED; EWM ENGAGED: EWM, *TWW*, 259–64, 271–3; Sayre, 45–8; "Miss W Bride of Francis B. Sayre," *NYT*, Nov. 26, 1913, 1, 3; WGM, 272–4; CTG, 28–9, 31; WW to JPT, Dec. 27, 1913, 29: 77n.

MEXICAN CRISIS ERUPTS: WW (A), Latin American Policy (Mobile, AL), Oct. 27, 1913, 28: 448–53; EMH (D), Oct. 30, 1913, 28: 476–7; "W Meets Lind on Ship," *NYT*, Jan. 3, 1914, 2; Kandell, 422; WW (A), Aug. 27, 1913, 28: 227–31; EWM, *TWW*, 271, 275–7; Calero, 18; Creel, *W and Issues*, 8.

EAW'S HEALTH; WGM AS FUTURE SON-IN-LAW: EWM, *PG*, 314; WW to MAH, Mar. 15, 1914, 29: 346; EWM, *TWW*, 275; WGM, 274–5; RSB, IV: 474.

TROUBLE IN VERACRUZ: Calero, 16–20, 23; JD, *Life*, 180–5; WJB to WW (T), Apr. 10, 1914, 29: 420–1; EWM, *TWW*, 277–9; EMH (D), Apr. 15, 1914, 29: 448; WW to WJB (T), Apr. 10 and 19, 1914, 29: 421 and 466; Creel, *W and Issues*, 9–11; WJB to Nelson O'Shaughnessy (T), Apr. 19, 1914, 29: 464–5; "President Before Congress," *NYT*, Apr. 21, 1914, 2; WW (A), "Mexican Crisis," Apr. 20, 1914, 29: 471–4; RSB, IV: 328; Elihu Root, *Congressional Record, 63rd Congress, 2nd Session*, v. 51, 6986–7; WW, "Memorial Address," May 11, 1914, 30: 13–5; SA (N) [PUL: 440], 303; CTG, 45; HCL, 19; Edward G. Lowry, "What the President Is Trying to Do for Mexico," *World's Work, XXVII* (Jan. 1914), 29: 94.

FORGING FOREIGN POLICY; HAY-PAUNCEFOTE TREATY: EMH (D), Apr. 15, 1914, 29: 448; WW, "Annual Message to Congress," Dec. 2, 1913, 29: 4; WJB, 386–7; JD (D), Apr. 8, 1913, 27: 267–8; JD, *Life*, 195–7; JPT, 162–8; WW (A), "Panama Canal Tolls," Mar. 5, 1914, 29: 312–3; EMH, I: 192–206, which includes W. H. Page to EMH, Aug. 28, 1914 [203–4], SA (N) [PUL: 440], 298; EWM, *TWW*, 282–3; Marshall, 420; James Viscount Bryce to WW, Mar. 6, 1914, 29: 320; Lawrence Godkin to JPT, Mar. 26, 1914, 29: 380–1.

OTHER FIRST-YEAR LEGISLATION: WW (A), "Trust Legislation," Jan. 20, 1914, 29: 153–8; L. D. Brandeis, "The Solution of the Trust Problem," *Harper's Weekly, LVIII* (Nov. 8, 1913), 18–9; F. G. Newlands to WW, Feb. 6, 1914, 29: 227; W. C. Redfield to WW, May 5, 1914, 29: 544–5; Houston, I: 195–6, 199–208; WW (S), "Rural Credits," Aug. 13, 1913, 28: 146–8; George Harvey, quoted in RSB, IV: 195; RSB, IV: 208.

EWM-WGM WEDDING: EWM, *TWW*, 285–7; WGM, 276–7; EMH (D), May 7, 1914, 30: 6–7; "Eleanor W Weds W. G. McAdoo," *NYT*, May 8, 1914, 1, 13; SA, 219, 283; WW to MAH, May 10, 1914, 30: 12–3; EWM, *PG*, 315, SA (N) [PUL: 440], 303; RSB, IV: 452.

10 ECCLESIASTES

PRINCETON REUNIONS, JUNE 1914: "President Is Just 'Tommy,'" *NYT*, June 14, 1914, 9; J. G. Hibben to WW, June 6, 1914, 30: 156; WW to J. G. Hibben, June 9, 1914, 30: 163; EMH (D), Dec. 12, 1913, 29: 33–4; WW (S), June 13, 1914, 30: 176–80.

POLITICAL TRAVAILS; EAW'S HEALTH: WW to CD, July 19, 1914, 30: 288; B. B. Lindsey

to JPT, May 16, 1914, 30: 38–9; J. P. White to WW (T), May 18, 1914, 30: 46; WW to MAH, June 7 and 21, 1914, 30: 158 and 196; CTG, 33; EWM, *TWW*, 296–7.

WAR BEGINS IN EUROPE; EAW DECLINES: Vansittart, 12–15 (Ambassador Gerard quoted, 14–5); WW to Franz Joseph I (T), June 28, 1914, 30: 222; WW to MAH, July 12, 1914, 30: 227; WW to E. P. Davis, July 28, 1914, 30: 312; SA, 283; CTG, 34–5; WW (R), at press conference, July 27, 1914, 30: 307; W. H. Page to WW, Aug. 9, 1914, 30: 366–71; press release re: WW to Heads of State, Aug. 4, 1914, 30: 342; EWM, *PG*, 315; "Mrs. W Dies in White House" and "Wife Inspired President," *NYT*, Aug. 7, 1914, 1; F. B. Sayre to Mrs. R. Sayre, Aug, 1914 [WWPL]; SA (N) [PUL: 440], 326; "Service at Capitol for Mrs. W, *NYT*, Aug. 8, 1914, 7; "Prayer at Tribute to President's Wife," *NYT*, Aug. 11, 1914, 9; "Mrs. W Buried Beside Her Parents," *NYT*, Aug. 12, 1914, 9.

WW SUFFERS THROUGH OPENING SALVOS OF WAR: CTG, 35–6; WW to MAH, Aug. 7 and 23, Sep. 6 and 20, 1914: 30: 357 and 437, 31: 3–4 and 59–60; WW to EMH, Aug. 17, 1914, 30: 390; W. H. Page to WW, July 29, 1914, 30: 316; Hitler, 135–6; RSB, IV: 161; Jacques Davignon to Emmanuel Havenith, Aug. 28, 1914, 30: 458; "President W Proclaims Our Strict Neutrality," *NYT*, Aug. 5, 1914, 7; RSB, IV: 52; WW, "Appeal to American People," Aug. 18, 1914, 30: 393–4; W. H. Page, quoted in RSB, IV: 67; C. W. Eliot to WW, Aug. 6 and 20, 1914, 30: 353–5 and 418–20; EMH (D), Aug. 30, 1914, 30: 462; WW to C. W. Eliot, Aug. 19, 1914, 30: 403; TR, quoted in JD, *Life*, 245; HCL, 26, 30; EMH to WW, Aug. 7, 1914, 30: 359; SA, 226; WW to Florence Hoyt, Oct. 2, 1914, 31: 119; CTG to EBW, Aug. 25, 1914, 31: 564.

WW IN CORNISH; CARRIES ON IN WHITE HOUSE: EMH (D), Aug. 30, Nov. 6 and 14, 1914, 30: 461–7, 31: 274 and 317–20; WW, *DR*, 211; RSB, V: 113; WW to MAH, Sep. 20, Oct. 11, Nov. 8, 1914, 31: 60, 141–2, 280–1; WW to Nancy Toy, Nov. 9 and Dec. 12, 1914, 31: 289 and 455; S. G. Blythe, "A Talk with the President," *Saturday Evening Post*, Jan. 9, 1915, 3–4, 37–8, 31: 390–403; WW to Mahlon Pitney, Sep. 10, 1914, 31: 19; Nancy Toy (D), Jan. 3, 1915, 32:9.

MIDTERM ELECTION, 1914; EARLY WARTIME FINANCIAL POLICY: JPT, 101, 126, 183; WW to F. E. Doremus, Sep. 4, 1914, 30: 475–8; WGM, 290–8, 300, 304, 309; WW (U

statement), c. Mar. 4, 1915, 32: 313–6; WW (S), Dec. 7, 1914, and Dec. 8, 1915, 31:416 and 35: 301; RSB, V: 88–91, 105; "Plan Big Loan Fund for Wool Growers," *NYT*, June 13, 1920, 99; J. P. Morgan, Jr., to WW, Sep. 4, 1914, 30: 485; WJB to WW, Aug. 10, 1914, 30: 372–3; Colville Barclay to Sir Edward Grey, Aug. 16, 1914, 30: 386; WW to J. P. Morgan, Jr., Sep. 17, 1914, 31: 39; WGM, 305; WW (S), Sep. 4, 1914, 30: 473–5; WW to W. M. Daniels, Oct. 29, 1914, 31: 247; WW to H. L Higginson, Oct. 29, 1914, 31: 247; "American Bankers May Make Loans," NY *World*, Oct. 16, 1914, 31: 153; Chernow, 186; WW to O. W. Underwood, Oct. 17, 1914, 31: 168–74; "The Democratic Peacemaker," *NYT*, Oct. 6, 1914, 10; WW to MAH, Sep. 20, 1914, 31: 59; EMH (D), Nov. 4 and 6, 1914, 31: 263–5 and 274–5; WW to Hugo Munsterberg, Nov. 7, 1914, 31: 276–8; WW to Nancy Toy, Nov. 9, 1914, 31: 289–91; Freud, 80, 156, 214.

RACE—W. M. TROTTER; *BIRTH OF A NATION*: W. M. Trotter (A) to WW, Nov. 12, 1914, 31: 298–301; WW, remarks and dialogue with W. M. Trotter, Nov. 12, 1914, 31: 301–8; "President Resents Negro's Criticism," *NYT*, Nov. 12, 1914, 1 Johnson, 608–11; O. G. Villard to JPT, Nov. 17, 1914 (with excerpts from NY *World* and NY *Evening Post* editorials of Nov. 13, 1914, 31: 328–9; WGM to WW, Nov. 28, 1914, 31: 360–1; WGM to F. I. Cobb, Nov. 26, 1914, 31: 361–3; JD to FDR, June 10, 1933, 31: 309n; Thomas Dixon, Jr., to JPT, Jan. 27, 1915, 32: 142, and May 1, 1915, cited in 32: 142n; WW to JPT, Apr. 28, 1915, and c. Apr. 22, 1918, 33:86 and 47: 388n3; Mark Calney, "D. W. Griffith and the Birth of a Monster," *American Almanac*, Jan. 11, 1993, n.p.; WW (R), on race, Dec. 15, 1914, 31: 464–5; D. W. Griffith to WW, Mar. 2, 1915, 32: 310–1; WW to D. W. Griffith, Mar. 5, 1915, 32: 325.

FOREIGN AFFAIRS—LOSING FAITH IN WJB; VENTURING BEYOND WASHINGTON: WJB to WW, Sep. 30 and Dec. 1, 1914, 31: 102 and 378–9; WW to WJB, Oct. 1, 1914, 31: 114; Sun Yat-sen to WW (T), 31: 372–3; W. H. Page to WW, Nov. 4 and 30, 1914, 31: 262 and 370–2; WW to CD, July 12, 1914, 30: 277; EMH (D), Oct. 2, Dec. 3, 1914, and Jan. 24, 1915, 31: 122, 385, and 32: 117; Nancy Toy (D), Jan. 2 and 3, 1915, 32: 8 and 9–10; Reid, 168; WW to EMH, Dec. 2, 1914, 31: 379; SA, 193–6; CTG, 49; WW to Nancy Toy, Dec. 12, 1914, 31: 456; WW to MAH, Nov. 22, 1914, Jan. 10 and 17, 1915, 31: 344, 32: 43 and 83; WW (S), Oct. 20 and Dec. 8,

1914, 31: 184–6 and 414–24; WW (S) in Indianapolis, Jan. 8, 1915, 32: 29–41; Reid, 174; F. K. Lane to WW, Jan. 9, 1915, 32: 43; EMH to WW, Jan. 9, 1915, 32: 43; RSB, V: 164.

EMH TO EUROPE; SUBMARINE WARFARE AND BLOCKADES: EMH (D), Jan. 12, 1915, 32: 61; WW, cited in Hodgson, 105; WW to EMH, Jan. 18 and 29, 1915, 32: 84–5 and 157–8; WW to EMH (T), Jan. 29, 1915, 32: 159; EMH (D), I: 352–3, 359–61, 403; RSB, V: 164, 165, 265, 275; W. H. Page to WW, Feb. 10, 1915, 32: 211–5; H. Morgenthau to WW, Nov. 10, 1914, 31: 428n; JD, *Life*, 280–1; W. H. Page to WJB, Mar. 15, 1915, 32: 378–82; WJB, 420; WGM, 322; CTG, 49; WW to MAH, Feb. 14, 1915, 23: 233; WW to JWS, Mar. 14, 1915 [WWPL].

EBW ENTERS: EBW, 1–13, 17–23, 51–4, 56–67; CTG, 50; Freud, 157; "W Hurls First Ball at Washington," *NYT*, Apr. 15, 1915, 10; WW to EBW, Apr. 30, May 4–5, 5, 6, 7 (two letters), 1915, 33: 90, 110–1, 111–2, 117–9, 124–6 and 126–7; Starling, 44; EBW to WW, May 5, 1915, 33: 108–10; WJB to WW (with enclosures), May 6, 1915, 33: 113–5; WJB to Paul Fuller, Jr., May 6, 1915, 33: 116–7; EMH to WW, May 7, 1915, 33: 121–3.

LUSITANIA SINKS; WW COURTS EBW; WJB RESIGNS: EBW to WW, May 7, 1915, 33: 127–8; ASL (N), 33: 128n1 and 129n1; "Lusitania Sunk by Submarine . . . Shocks the President," *NYT*, May 8, 1915, 1–2; HCL, 32–3; "Roosevelt Calls It an Act of Piracy," *NYT*, May 8, 1915, 1; TR, "Murder on the High Seas," statement, cited in John Whiteclay Chambers II, *The Eagle and the Dove* (Syracuse, NY: Syracuse University Press, 1991), 60–1; WJB, 420–4; Preston, 391; TR, press release, May 9, 1915, quoted in TR, *NRM*, 847–52; Herman Ridder, "Vale Lusitania," *NYT*, May 8, 1915, quoted in 33: 135n4; WJB to WW, May 9, 12 (three letters), and 13, June 9, 1915, 33: 134–5, 165–7 and 167–8 and 173, 180, 375–6; EMH to WW (T), May 9, 1914, 33: 134; Charles Swem (D), May 10, 1915, 33: 138; *Washington Post* editorial, quoted in 33: 135n1; WW to EBW, May 9, 10, 11 (two letters), June 9, 10, Aug. 13, 1915, 33: 136, 146–7, 160–1 and 162, 377–8, 381, 34: 192; EBW to WW, May 10, June 9 and 18, 1915, 33: 146, 378 and 421; WW (S—"too proud to fight"), May 10, 1915, 33: 147–50; Janet W. Wilson to WW, Nov. 15, 1876, 1: 228; JPT, 236–7; WW (S), Apr. 20, 1915, 33: 37–41; WW, press conference, May 11, 1915, 33: 153; JPT, 232–34; W. H. Taft to WW, May 10, 1915, 33: 150–1;

WW to W. H. Taft, May 13, 1915, 33: 184; WW to WJB (draft), May 11, 1915, 33: 155–8; Weinstein, 285; EMH (D), June 20 and 24, 1915, 33: 425 and 449; EBW, 62–4; "Official Translation of the German Note," *NYT*, June 1, 1915, 2; JD, *Life*, 253–4; WW, "First Draft of Second Lusitania Note," June 3, 1915, 33: 328–31.

WW EAGER TO MARRY AMID INTERNATIONAL TURMOIL: J. W. Gerard to RL, July 8, 1915, quoted in WW to RL, July 13, 1915, 33: 500n1; JD, *Life*, 255; WW to EBW, May 28 and 29, June 1, 3, 17, 18, and Sep. 11, 1915, 33: 278 and 284–5, 301–2, 334, 417, 421, and 34: 453; EMH to WW (including Lincoln Steffens to EMH, Aug. 7, 1915), Aug. 9 and Oct. 1, 1915, 34: 146–8 and 35: 3–4; RL to WW, Aug. 14, 21, and Nov. 20, 1915, 34: 196–7, 34: 280, and 35: 227–8; WW to WJB, June 2, 1915, 33: 304; Morris Sheppard to WW, July 22, 1915, 34: 13; WW to L. M. Garrison, July 21, 1915, 34: 4; L. M Garrison to WW, Sep. 17, 1915, 34: 482–5; L. M. Garrison to JPT, Nov. 1, 1915, 35: 149–50; Louis Wiley to WW, Sep. 30, 1915, 34: 452; O. G. Villard to WW, Oct. 28, 1915, 35: 120; EBW to WW, May 28, June 3, 17, 21, 29, 1915, 33: 278–9, 335, 418, 434, 458; Helen Bones to WW, May 29, 1915, 33: 285; Helen Bones to MAH (T), May 29, 1915, 33: 286; Hulbert, 244–8, 257–8; WW to MAH, May 6 and July 7, 1915, 33: 120 and 482; MAH to WW, c. June 10, 16, and 20, 1915, 33: 382, 412, 424; EMH (D), June 24, 1915, 33: 448–53; EBW, 70–4.

WW-EBW SECRET ENGAGEMENT: WW to EBW, July 20 (two letters), Aug. 6, 24, 25, 27, 28, Sep. 10 (two letters), 11, 18, 19 (7:20 a.m. and 9:10 a.m.), 1915, 33: 537–9 and 539–42, 34: 102, 301, 327–8, 346–7, 352–3, 440 and 441, 453, 489, 491–2 and 492; EBW to WW, Aug. 13, 15, 25, 26, 27, 28, Sep. 3, 18, 19, 20 (7:45 p.m.), 1915, 34: 194–5, 213, 327–8, 338, 347–9, 357, 415, 489–90, 495–6; WW to JD, July 2, 1915, 33: 465; EBW, 75–6; Margaret W. Wilson to EBW, Aug. 16, 1915, 34: 268–9; WW to Sallie White Bolling, Aug. 29, 1915, 34: 363; WW to Bertha Bolling, c. Aug. 29, 1915, 34: 364; JD, *Wilson Era*, 454; Weinstein, 290; EMH (D), Sep. 22, Dec. 15, 1915, 34: 506–8, 35: 357–60; WW to Samuel Gompers, Sep. 24, 1915, 34: 512; SA, 246–7; SA, draft of announcement, c. Oct. 2, 1915, 35: 16–7; Freud, 157–8; I. Hoover, 66–7, 70; Starling, 51–2.

WW-EBW ENGAGEMENT ANNOUNCED; INTERNATIONAL PRESSURE MOUNTS: WW, statement on suffrage, Oct. 6,

1915, 35: 28; EMH (D), Dec. 15, 1915, 35: 355–61; "W Watches Red Sox Win," *NYT*, Oct. 10, 1915, 18; EBW, 81–3; CTG to A. G. Gordon, c. Oct. 19, 1915 [WWPL]; WW to MAH, Oct. 4, 1915, 35: 23–4; MAH to WW, c. Oct. 11, 1915, 35: 53; Starling, 55–7; EBW to WW, Nov. 28, 1915, 35: 262–3n; WW to EBW (T), Dec. 1, 1915, 35: 281; W. H. Page to WW, Oct. 16, 1915, 35: 74–9; EMH to WW (enclosed: Sir Edward Grey letter, Sep. 22, 1915), Nov. 10, Dec. 1 and 16 (with Enclosure II), 1915, 35: 186–7, 279n1 and 363; WW to Haigazoun H. Topakyan, Oct. 28, 1915, 35: 119; RL to WW, Nov. 20, 1915, 35: 227–30; WW (S), Dec. 7, 1915, 35: 293–310; TR to Archibald Roosevelt, May 19, 1915, and TR to Kermit Roosevelt, Aug. 28, 1915, TR, *Letters*, 695–8; "Ford Abdicates; Sails for Home" and "Mr. Ford's Family Amazed," *NYT*, Dec. 25, 1915, 1–2; Ford, quoted in Vansittart, 87. For more on the Peace Ship, see: Burnet Hershey, *The Odyssey of Henry Ford and the Great Peace Ship* (New York: Taplinger, 1967).

WW-EBW WEDDING: EBW, 84–6; I. Hoover, 70–5; WW to EBW, Dec. 18, 1915, 35: 370; "President W Weds Mrs. Galt," Dec. 19, 1915, 1–2; Starling, 61–2.

11 DELIVERANCE

HONEYMOON: EBW, 86–8; Starling, 66; WW to L. M. Smith and M. R. Smith, Dec. 27, 1915, 35: 399; RL to WW (T), Jan. 3, 1916, 35: 422.

SUBMARINE ATTACKS; PANCHO VILLA; PREPAREDNESS POLICY: JPT, 249–50; JPT (M), Jan. 4, 1916, 35: 424; W. H. Page to WW, Jan. 15, 1916, 35: 435; EMH to WW, Jan. 15, 1916, 35: 484–6; RL to WW, Jan. 27, 1916, 35: 531; B. R. Tillman to WW, Feb. 14, 1916, 36: 173; EMH to WW, Aug. 8, 1915, and Feb. 15, 1916, 34: 133–4n and 36: 180n1–2; EMH to Edward Grey, Mar. 10, 1916, EMH, II: 220; EMH (D), Mar. 6, 1916, 36: 212; CD to WW, Jan. 14, 1916, 35: 478n1; L. M. Garrison to RSB, Nov. 12, 1928 [RSB Papers: PUL]; EBW, 93; RSB, VI: 13.

PREPAREDNESS TOUR: WW, (two S) Jan. 27, (two S) 29, 31, (two S) Feb. 3, 1916, 36: 5 and 7–16, 26–7 and 35–41, 63–73, 114–21 and 110–4; "Table 1—Urban and Rural Population: 1900 to 1990" (U.S. Census Bureau, Oct. 1995—www.census.gov/population/censusdata/urpop0090.txt) accessed Oct. 13, 2010; Lawrence, 158–61;

assassination attempt, in G. A. Gordon to CTG, Jan. 31, 1916 [WWPL].

WW-EBW DOMESTIC ROUTINE: CTG, 52; Jaffray, cited in RSB VI: 176; EBW, 89–92.

GARRISON RESIGNATION; MEXICAN EXPEDITION: Reid, 185; L. M. Garrison to RSB, Nov. 12 and 18, 1928 [RSB Papers: PUL]; L. M. Garrison to WW, Feb. 10, 1916, 36: 164; WW to L. M. Garrison, Feb. 10, 1916, 36: 164; WW to N. D. Baker (T), Mar. 5, 6, 1916, 36: 251, 259; N. D. Baker to WW (T), Mar. 6 and 31 (with enclosure J. J. Pershing to N. D. Baker, Mar. 31), 1916, 36: 259 and 397; RSB, VI: 38; WW (S), Feb. 2, 1916, 26: 104; "Night Attack on Border," NYT, Mar. 10, 1916, 1–2; F. Funston to N. D. Baker, Mar. 10, 1916, 36: 283; EMH (D), Mar. 17 and Apr. 6, 1916, 36: 335–6n1 and 424–5; N. D. Baker to Chief of Staff (M), Mar. 10, 1916, 36: 285; H. L. Scott to Adjutant General, Mar. 19, 1916, 36: 285–6; N. D. Baker to WW (M), Mar. 10 and 15 (with enclosure), 1916, 36: 286–7 and 313–4n1; WW, press release, Mar. 10, 1916, 36: 287; F. L. Polk to Associated Press (T), Mar. 17, 1916, 36: 332; D. Lawrence to WW, Mar. 14 and June 2, 1916, 36: 309n1 and 152–5; JPT to WW, Mar. 15 and June 24, 1916, 36: 317n1 and 37: 291–2; WW to RL, Mar. 30 and June 21, 1916, 36: 382n2 and 37: 277–8n; F. L. Polk to WW, Mar. 20, 1916, 36: 342–3n1; F. K. Lane to RSB, Apr. 13, 1916, cited in RSB, VI: 72; WW to EMH, June 22, 1916, 37: 281; JPT, 157–9; WW, draft of (A), June 26, 1916, 37: 302; "Cardenas's Family Saw Him Die at Bay," NYT, May 23, 1916, 5.

ARGUING INTERVENTION: German statement in WGM, 366; Billington, 70; W. J. Stone to WW, Feb. 24, 1916, 36: 209–11; WW to W. J. Stone, Feb. 24, 1916, 36: 213–4; WW to E. W. Pou, Feb. 29, 1916, 36: 231–2; WW, draft of (N), Apr. 10, 1916, 36: 452–6; H. A. Garfield to WW, Apr. 24, 1916, 36: 545n1; TR to Archibald Roosevelt, May 19, 1915, TR, Letters, 696; RL to WW, Mar. 27, 1916, 36: 372–3; EMH (D), Mar. 30, 1916, 36: 388; WW (A), Apr. 19, 1916, 36: 509–10; WW to EMH (T), Apr. 21, 1916, 36: 520; EMH to WW, Apr. 25 and May 6, 1916, EMH, II: 239 and 36: 628–9; G. v. Jagow to J. W. Gerard, May 4, 1916, 36: 621–6; WW, in a colloquy, May 8, 1916, 36: 645; American Union Against Militarism to WW (M), c. May 8, 1916, 36: 632–3.

WILL ROGERS: Day, Will Rogers, 40–3; "W at Friars' Frolic," NYT, May 31, 1916, 11.

1916 PRESIDENTIAL CAMPAIGN BEGINS: WW (S), June 29, 1916, 37: 324–8;

Democratic Text-Book: 1912, 3–43; Greg Sarris, "After the Fall," Outdoors, Los Angeles Times, Apr. 5, 2005, 5; WW to F. K. Lane, May 26, 1916, 37: 111; RSB, VI: 104, 106; Brian E. Gray, "National Park Service Act" (eNotes.com, 2010); United States Census, 1910 and 1920; WW to House of Representatives, Jan. 26, 1915, 32: 142–4; Henry Ford to WW (T), Sep. 1, 1916, 38: 125; W. S. Stone, et al., to WW, Aug. 18, 1916, 38: 48–9; WW, statement, Aug. 19, 1916, 38: 49–50; RSB, VI: 110; WW to JD, July 18, 1916, 37: 431n1.

BRANDEIS TO SUPREME COURT: WGM, 342–6; Urofsky, 438 (quotes W. H. Taft to Gus Karger, Jan. 31, 1916), 450, 749; WW to C. A. Culberson, May 5, 1916, 36: 609–11; WW to H. Morgenthau, June 5, 1916, 37: 163.

"AMERICANISM" SUMMER OF 1916: EBW, 100–2; WW, proclamation, May 30, 1916, 37: 122–3; "Hosts in Chicago on Defense Parade," NYT, June 5, 1916, 1, 14; Rotogravure section, NYT, June, 4, 1916; WW (A), May 27, 30, June 2, 13, and 14, 1916, 37: 115, 126, 147–8, 217, and 221–5; JD, Life, 268; Marshall, 336–7.

NOMINATING CONVENTIONS: WW, draft of National Democratic Platform, c. June 10, 1916, 37: 190–201; A. M. Palmer to WW, June 14, 1916, 37: 227; WW to H. S. Cummings, June 15, 1916, 37: 229; WW to Carter Glass (T), June 15, 1916, 37: 229; Carter Glass to WW (T), June 15, 1916, 37: 231; Martin H. Glynn, quoted in RSB, VI: 250–2; A. R. Longworth to ASB (I), June 5, 1973.

POST-CONVENTION, PRE-CAMPAIGN, 1916: "President Sees Dr. Grayson Wed," NYT, May 25, 1916, 13; EMH (D), May 24, 1916, 37: 106; RSB (I) with WW, May 12, 1916 [RSB Papers: PUL]; Weinstein, 305–6; Freud, 183–4; WW to JWS, Mar. 21, 1916 [WWPL]; WW (R), June 30, 1916, 37: 332–5; WW (A), July 4, 1916, 37: 353–8; H. S. Cummings (M), Aug. 7, 1916, 38: 7–8; EBW, 103–4; WW to Obadiah Gardner, Aug. 19, 1916, 38: 50–1n1; WW (S), Sep. 2, 1916, 38: 126–39.

WW CAMPAIGN OF 1916: WW (A), Sep. 4 and 8, 1916, 38: 142–5 and 161–4; EBW, 105–6, 113; Annie W. H. Cothran to WW, Mar. 23, 1917, 41: 457–8; WW to Henry Ford, Sep. 20, 1916, 38: 187n1–2; H. C. Wallace to EMH, Aug. 31, 1916, 38: 139–41; EMH (D), Nov. 26, 1916, 40: 85–6; Billington, 80–1; W. E. B. Du Bois to WW, Oct. 10, 1916, 38: 459–60; WW to JPT, Aug. 11, 1916, 38: 24n2; WW to Giles B. Jackson, Sep. 7, 1916, 38: 157n1; W. E. B. Du Bois to JPT, Oct. 24,

1916, 38: 522n1; RSB (M), May 12, 1916, 37: 37; Anna Shaw, quoted in Norman Hapgood to WW, Sep. 16, 1916, 38: 178–9; J. A. O'Leary to WW, Sep. 29, 1916, 38: 285–6; JPT, 214, JD, *Life*, 238.

REPUBLICAN CAMPAIGN OF 1916: WW (A), July 10 and Oct. 7, 1916, 37: 384 and 364; HCL, 73–4; Marshall, 336; McAdoo, 363–5; TR to Kermit Roosevelt, Aug. 28, 1915, TR, *Letters*, 698; "Roosevelt Blames W for Raids," *NYT*, Oct. 11, 1916, 6; TR (S—speaking "bombastically and carrying a big dishrag"), Oct. 19, 1916, in TR, *NRM,* 1073; JD, *Life*, 274–5; WW (I) with H. N. Hall, Oct. 31, 1916, 38: 565.

FINAL ARGUMENTS IN 1916 ELECTION: EBW to MAH (unsent D), c. Nov. 1, 1916, 38: 589; Emanuel Julius, "Eugene V. Debs, Interviewed for *Appeal*," *Appeal to Reason*, July 1, 1916, 6; Hulbert, 264; RSB VI: 290; Marshall, 336; Steel, 100, 106, and 608n11, citing Walter Lippmann, "The Case for Wilson," *The New Republic*, Oct. 14, 1916; Ida Tarbell, "A Talk with the President of the United States," *Collier's* (Oct. 28, 1916), 38: 323–34; W's resignation plan in EMH (D), Oct. 19 and Nov. 19, 1916, 38: 617–8 and 678–9, and WW to RL, Nov. 5, 1916, 38: 617–8; EBW, 113–8.

ELECTION DAY 1916 AND AWAITING RESULTS: RSB VI: 297; JPT, 216–24; TR, cited in RSB VI: 296; Reid, 186; EBW, 116; JD, *Life*, 276; Mark Grossi, "Sierra Area Had Pivotal Role in 1916," *Fresno Bee*, Nov. 10, 2000, n.p.; "W Ahead in California by Over 3,100," *NYT*, Nov. 10, 1916, 1, 2; William Hard (I) with T. P. Gore, Aug. 18, 1926 [Hard Papers—145: 2/7: PUL]; R. H. Dabney to WW, Nov. 23, 1916, 40: 61–2; C. E. Hughes to WW (T), Nov. 22, 1916, 40: 38; WW to J. R. Wilson, Jr. (T), Nov. 27, 1916, 40: 90.

WAR ABROAD AND AMERICAN DIPLOMACY: EBW, 120–1; JPT, 253; RSB, VI: 328, 374; WW, *History*, III: 192–4; WW (U), "Prolegomenon to Peace Note," c. Nov. 25, 1916, 40: 67–70; J. C. Grew to EMH, Dec. 1, 1916, 40: 160–1; EMH (D), Nov. 20 and 26, Dec. 20, 1916, Jan. 11, 1917, 40: 4–6n and 84, 304–5, 445; WW (R), Nov. 14, 1916, 38: 637–40; WW to W. J. Harris (draft), Feb. 7, 1917, 41: 146–8; WW, Peace Note (draft), c. Nov. 25, 1916, 40: 70–4; WW, "Annual Message," Dec. 5, 1916, 40: 155–9; WW, "Appeal for Statement of War Aims," Dec. 18, 1916, 40: 273–6n; Houston, I: 219; RL (S), Dec. 21, 1916, 40: 306; WW to RL, Dec. 21, 1916, 40: 307n–311; "Peace and War Talk Hit Stocks," *NYT*, Dec. 22, 1916, 1, 2; "Wall Street Relieved

by a Wave of Buying," *NYT*, Dec. 23, 1916, 1, 3; "Financial Markets," *NYT*, Dec. 23, 1916, 12.

CHRISTMAS, 1916; W FORMULATES PEACE TERMS: WW to L. M. Smith and M. R. Smith, Dec. 27, 1916, 40: 336; CD to WW, Dec. 27, 1916, 40: 338; EMH (D), Jan. 3, 1917, 40: 403–7; WW (A—"peace without victory"), Jan. 22, 1917, 40: 533–9; "W's Terms for League of Peace," *NYT*, Jan. 23, 1917, 1, 2; "President's Own Comment," *NYT*, Jan. 23, 1917, 1; "Scene in the Senate," *NYT*, Jan. 23, 1917, 2; Longworth, 242; CD to WW, Jan. 24, 1917, 41: 7; W. H. Page, (M) #5514, Jan. 20, 1917, 40: 532; EMH (D), Dec. 27, 1916, II: 423–4.

GERMANY ESCALATES SUBMARINE WARFARE; W RESPONDS: WGM, 367; JPT, 254–5; RSB, VI: 448–9; EMH (D), Feb. 1, 1917, 41: 87–8; RL to WW, Feb. 1, 1917, 41: 99; WW (A), Feb. 3, 1917, 41: 108–12; "Bernstorff Was Not Surprised," *NYT*, Feb. 4, 1917, 1, 5; WW (A—draft), Feb. 3, 1917, 41: 112n1; WW, "Bases of Peace" draft, quoted in RSB, VI: 465–6; TR to HCL, Feb. 20, 1917, TR, *Letters*, 718–9; "A Visit to the President," *Friends' Intelligencer*, Mar. 10, 1917, 41: 302–4n2.

ZIMMERMANN NOTE AND REPERCUSSIONS: "Germany Seeks an Alliance," *NYT*, Mar. 1, 1917, 1; WW (A), Feb. 26, 1917, 41: 283–7.

SECOND INAUGURATION: EBW, 130; EMH (D), Mar. 3, 1917, 41: 317–8n; WW, statement, Mar. 4, 1917, 41: 318–20; "President Inaugurated," *NYT*, Mar. 6, 1917, 1; WW, "Second Inaugural Address," Mar. 5, 1917, 41: 332–5.

12 ARMAGEDDON

POST-INAUGURAL EXHILARATION AND EXHAUSTION: "President Reviews a Parade," *NYT*, Mar. 6, 1917, 3; EMH (D), Mar. 5, 1917, 41: 340–1; EBW, 130, 116; "Take Motor Ride at Night," *NYT*, Mar. 6, 1917, 3.

WW AND CABINET RESPOND TO GERMANY: JD (D), Mar. 8 and 20, 1917, 41: 364 and 444–5; EBW, 131–2; RL (M), 41: 436–44; Houston, I: 241–4; T. W. Brahany (D), Mar. 20 and 26, 1917, 41: 445 and 473–5; EMH (D), Apr. 29, 1917, 42: 162; Heaton, 268; RSB, VI: 506.

APRIL 2, 1917—"SAFE FOR DEMOCRACY" SPEECH: T. W. Brahany (D), Apr. 2, 1917, 41: 531; EMH (D), Apr. 2, 1917, 41: 528–30; "President Holds War Conferences," *NYT*, Apr. 3, 1917, 3; RSB, VI: 508; Lansing, 238–9; "Armed

American Steamship Sunk," *NYT*, Apr. 3, 1917; "Lodge Knocks Down Pacific Assailant," *NYT*, Apr. 3, 1917, 5; "President at Golf During the Forenoon," *NYT*, Apr. 3, 1917, 10; "Must Exert All Our Power," *NYT*, Apr. 3, 1917, 1; Starling, 87; Houston, I: 253–6; EBW, 132–3; Lawrence, 208–9; WW (A), Apr. 2, 1917, 41: 519–27; "Lodge Congratulates the President," *NYT*, Apr. 3, 1917, 2; JPT, 256–9.

RESPONSE TO SPEECH; DECLARATION OF WAR: W. Lippmann to WW, Apr. 3, 1917, 41: 537; W. H. Page to WW (T), Apr. 3, 1917; Gerard, quoted in T. W. Brahany (D), Apr. 6, 1917, 41: 558; WGM to WW, Apr. 3, 1917, 41: 541; Lawrence, 210–2; "Seek to Explain Miss Rankin's 'No,'" *NYT*, Apr. 7, 1917, 4; Starling, 89; EBW, 133; Seymour, 117; WW, Last Will and Testament, May 31, 1917, 42: 426.

MOBILIZATION; BARUCH; HOOVER: "Government Acts Swiftly" and "27 Ships Taken Here," *NYT*, Apr. 7, 1917, 1–2; WW (M), Apr. 7, 1917, 42: 3; JD (D), Nov. 26, 1917, 45: 128; Samuel Gompers to WW, Aug. 2, 1917, 43: 352–4; W. G. Sharp to RL, Aug. 2, 1917, 43: 355; WW, "Appeal to American People," Apr. 15, 1917, 42: 71–5; EBW, 135–6, 160–1; Seymour, 118–29, 160, 162–70; WGM, 454–9, 464, 483–91; JPT to WW, Nov. 18, 1916, 38: 674; EMH (D), Jan. 3 and 12, Mar. 3, 1917, 40: 402 and 463, 41: 318; WW (A), Jan. 4, 1918, 45: 449; Baruch, 17, 23–5, 38–40, 55, 232; N. D. Baker to WW (includes Baruch M), May 28, 1917, 42: 411–7; JPT, 268–70; H. Hoover, 1–5, 8; WW (S), May 19, 1917, 42: 344–5; Houston, I: 256–9; "Hooverize" is defined in *Oxford English Dictionary*, VII: 374; RSB, VII: 409.

CONTROL OF IDEAS: PROPAGANDA; SEDITION: Creel, *How We Advertised*, xiii, xvii–xviii, 3, 6, 7, 10, 13, 84–7, 261–6; Stone, 113–7, 147–8, 586n32, 587n39; WW, "Annual Message," Dec. 7, 1915, 35: 306–7; WW (A), Apr. 2, 1917, 41: 526; Geoffrey Stone, "On Secrecy and Transparency" (which cites H. R. 291, tit. I § 4, 65th Congress, 1st Session, in 55 Congressional Record H1590-1 and 1695, Apr. 30 and May 2, 1917), *American Constitution Society for Law and Policy*, June, 2008, 4; A. Brisbane to WW, Apr. 20, 1917, 42: 107–8; WW to A. Brisbane, Apr. 25, 1917, 42: 129; "Canvass Forecasts Doom of Censorship," *NYT*, May 28, 1917, 4; JPT to WW, May 8, 1917, 42: 245–6; WW to E. Y. Webb, May 22, 1917, 42: 369–70; ASL (N), 42: 247; G. Creel (M), enclosed in JD to WW, Apr. 11, 1917, 42: 39–41; WW to JD, Apr. 12, 1917, 42: 43; Lawrence, 228;

H. Hoover, 13; F. C. Barnes to WW, c. Oct. 12, 1917, 44: 364; O. H. Kahn to WW, Apr. 6, 1917, 42: 7; WW to JPT, c. Apr. 7, 1917, 42: 8–9; SA (N) [PUL: 440], 314; JD, 281–2; WW to L. C. Dyer, Aug. 1, 1917, 43: 336; Brinkley, 618.

BUILDING AN ARMY; TR VOLUNTEERS: E. W. Pou to JPT, Apr. 11, 1917, 42: 42; WW to G. T. Helvering, Apr. 19, 1917, 42: 97–8; Longworth, 245–6; Morris, 486–8; JPT, 285–9; TR to WW, May 18, 1917, 42: 324; WW (S), May 18, 1917, 42: 324–6; T. W. Brahany (D), Apr. 10, 1917, 42: 31–2; EMH to WW, Apr. 10, 1917, 42: 29–30n1; JD, 284; "Drawing for Nation's Draft Army," *NYT*, July 21, 1917, 1, 6–8; Coffman, 29–31; Clements, 145–8; Seymour, 125, 129–31, 143–6, 137–40; R. H. Morris to JPT, Aug. 29, 1918, 49: 420; WW to JPT, Sep. 2, 1918, 49: 419; JD, *Life*, 285; Pershing, I: 26–8; JPT, 295–6; Lawrence, 220–2; WW (A), Aug. 11, 1917, 43: 427–31; EBW, 139–40; WW (A), Dec. 2, 1918, 53: 275.

PAPAL APPEAL; EUROPEAN ASSESSMENT OF THE WAR; WW DISPATCHES PERSHING: Pope Benedict XV's appeal, enclosed with RL to WW, Aug. 13 and 21 (enclosed with "Comments on the Pope's Peace Appeal"), 1917, 43: 438–9 and 18–22; W. H. Page to RL, Aug. 15, 1917, 43: 482–5; WW (N), "Reply to Benedict XV," c. Aug. 16, 1917, 43: 487–8; N. D. Baker to WW, Aug. 20, 1917, with W. Lippmann (M), "Reply to the Pope's Proposal," 43: 532–4; RL to W. H. Page, Aug. 27, 1917, 44: 57–9; WW, "State of the Union Address," Dec. 4, 1917, 45: 194–202; R. H. Campbell to EMH, Jan. 2, 1918, 45: 430–1; Trask, 94–5; *Congressional Record*, Oct. 21, 1939, vol. 84, 686; Churchill, 692; Coffman, 94–5; W. H. Page to WW (T), Apr. 17, 1917, 42: 82; Nicolson, *King George*, 55; D. Lloyd George to WW, Sep. 3, 1917, 44: 125–30; Seymour, 147–8; JD, *Life*, 282; G. Creel to WW, Dec. 8, 1917, 45: 246; WW to G. Creel, Dec. 10, 1917, 45: 257; W. G. Sharp to N. D. Baker, Jan. 31, 1918, attached to WW to N. D. Baker, Feb. 4, 1918, 46: 237; "W Sees End of War Only When Germany Is Beaten," *NYT*, Oct. 8, 1917, 44: 325–7; EMH (D), Oct. 24, 1917, 44: 437–9.

"THE INQUIRY"; PALESTINE: WW to EMH, July 21 and Sep. 19, 1917, 43: 238 and 44: 216–7, enclosing RL (M), 44: 217–9; EMH to WW, Sep. 20, 1917, 44: 226; H. B. Brougham to WW, Sep. 28, 1917, 44: 275–6n; A. J. Balfour to WW, Jan. 31, 1918, 46: 180–1; Lord Reading to A. J. Balfour (T), Mar. 18, 1918, 47: 63–4; Hemingway, 196; A. J. Balfour to Sir William

Phillips (D), Dec. 5, 1918 [FDR Library: Joseph P. Lash Papers, C44: 46]; WW, "State of the Union Address," Dec. 2, 1918, 53: 274–86; JD (D), Dec. 2, 1918, 53: 301; H. F. Ashurst (D), Dec. 2, 1918, 53: 305; WW to J. R. Mann, Dec. 3, 1918, and ASL (N), 53: 308; "Senators Clash over Trip," *NYT*, Dec. 4, 1918.

WW SAILS TO EUROPE; FRANCE, ENG-LAND, AND ITALY: EBW, 211–2; CTG (D), Jan. 1, 2, and 4, 1919, 53: 577–8, 589, and 605–7; Starling, 124; WW (A), Jan. 3, 1919, 53: 602–3; I. Hoover, 79; CTG, 66; WW, drafts of "Covenant," 53: 655–86; RL (M), Jan. 11, 1919, 54: 3.

DEATH OF TR: TR, quoted in J. M. Blum and A. D. Chandler (eds.), *Letters of TR* (Cambridge, MA: Harvard University Press, 1954), VIII: 1420–1; WW, proclamation, Jan. 7, 1919, 53: 635; JPT to WW (T), Jan. 6, 1919, 53: 624; N. D. Baker to WW, Jan. 1, 1919, 53: 624 and n6; WW to T. R. Marshall (T), Jan. 7, 1919, 53: 636; HCL, 134–5.

CURTAIN RISING ON PEACE TALKS: H. Hoover, 69–70; F. L. Polk to American Commissioners (M), Jan. 17, 1919, 54: 126; RSB, VIII: 577; Keynes, 4, 32–44; EBW, 233; JD, *Life*, 307; Keynes re: D. Lloyd George, quoted in Moggridge, 329; CTG to A. G. Grayson, Apr. 23–5, 1919 [WWPL]; Maurice Hankey (N: Council of Ten), Jan. 12 and 13, 1919, 54: 23–6 and 47–8; CTG (D), Jan. 12, 1919, 54: 5; Edith Benham (D), Jan. 12, 1919, 54: 34; Lord Derby to A. J. Balfour, Dec. 22, 1918, 53: 470–2; Maurice Hankey (N: Supreme War Council), Jan. 13, 1919, 54: 37–42; WW to V. E. Orlando, Jan. 13, 1919, 54: 50–1; JPT to CTG, Jan. 16, 1919, 54: 106–7n1; H. B. Swope, "Personal Cordiality Wins Colleagues to President," *NY World*, Jan. 15, 1919, n.p.; Creel, *How We Advertised*, 401.

CONFERENCE BEGINS: CTG (D), Jan. 18, 1919, 54: 126–8; "Brilliant Opening Scene" and "Bugles Greet Delegates," *NYT*, Jan. 19, 1919, 1; Protocol of Plenary Session, Jan. 18, 1919, 54: 128–32; Nicolson, *Peacemaking*, 242, 245; Lawrence, 258–9; E. Benham (D), Jan. 20, 1919, 54: 175; CTG, 70–1; "Arrest Bolsheviki Reported on the Way to Attack W," *NYT*, Jan. 19, 1919, 1; "Red Plot Reported to Assassinate W, Clemenceau and Lloyd George," *NY Tribune*, Jan. 20, 1919, 1.

NONPARTICIPANTS AND PETITIONERS: Maurice Hankey (N: C10), Jan. 21 and 22, 1919, 54: 187 and 204–6; CTG (D), Jan. 22, 1919, 54: 199; Churchill, V: 263 and "Bolshevist

Atrocities" (S), Apr. 11, 1919, quoted in W. S. Churchill (ed.), *Never Give In!* (New York: Hyperion, 2003), 77; Paul Cambon, quoted in Lord Curzon to Lord Derby, Jan. 23, 1919, 54: 235–6; Lithuanian delegation to WW, Jan. 23, 1919, attached to RSB to WW, Jan. 24, 1919 [RSB Papers: PUL]; Chaim Weizmann to WW, Jan. 24, 1919, 54: 258; E. Benham (D), Jan. 27, 1919, 54: 307; CTG (D), Jan. 28, 1919, 54: 309; WW to Boghos Nubar, Jan. 23, 1919, 54: 226; Duiker, 59–60.

SECOND PLENARY SESSION: ESTAB-LISHING LEAGUE OF NATIONS; WW VIS-ITS WAR SITES: Protocol of Plenary Session, Jan. 25, 1919, 54: 265–8; CTG (D), Jan. 25 and 26 (war sites), 1919, 54: 262–3 and 278–81; EMH to WW, Jan. 25, 1919, 54: 271; Lord Curzon to Lord Derby, Jan. 23, 1919, 54: 235–6; WW (R) to French Protestants, Jan. 27, 1919, 54: 282–3; EBW to J. R. Bolling, Jan. 27, 1919, 54: 305.

MANDATES; COMMISSION ON LEAGUE OF NATIONS: WW (R), Feb. 28, 1919, 55: 321; E. Benham (D), Jan. 18 and 21, 1919, 54: 149 and 197; Maurice Hankey (N: C10), Jan. 21, 24, 27, 28, and 30, 1919, 54: 188–9, 250–1, 291–2 and 300–1, 325–7, and 350–1 and 371; CTG (D), Jan. 28 and 30, Feb. 13, 1919, 54: 308–9 and 348, 55: 120; D. H. Miller (D), Jan. 30 and Feb. 12, 1919, 54: 379 and 55: 118; C. Seymour to his family, Jan. 30, 1919, 54: 385; EMH (D), Jan. 31, 1919, 54: 407; Minutes of Commission on the League of Nations, Feb. 10, 11, and 13, 1919, 55: 41–51, 79–80, and 121 and 136; "Covenant" of League of Nations, Feb. 3, 1919, 54: 449–58; Lord Cecil (D), Feb. 4, 1919, 55: 80.

WW PRESENTS COVENANT: EMH (D), Feb. 14, 1919, 55: 193–6; Maurice Hankey (N: C10), Jan. 30, 1919, 54: 351; Creel, *How We Advertised*, 413–4; EBW, 226–7, 236 40; Truman Talley, "Feed World and Then Talk Peace," *NY Herald*, Feb. 15, 1919, 55: 161–3; WW (A), Feb. 14, 1919, 55: 164–78; EMH to WW, Feb. 14, 1919, 55: 178; CTG (D), Jan. 22 and Feb. 14, 1919, 54: 199 and 55: 160; the junior member of the American Commission was Arthur Hornblow, Jr. (D), Feb. 14, 1919 (private collection); Maurice Hankey (N: Supreme War Council), Feb. 14, 1919, 55: 180–3.

WW LEAVES PARIS: WW to EMH (T), c. Feb. 23, 1919, 55: 230; WW to RL (T), Feb. 23, 1919, 55: 231; WW (S), Feb. 15, 1919, 55: 197; "Last Message to France," *NYT*, Feb. 16, 1919, 1, 2; EBW, 236, 240.

WW RETURNS TO U.S.: T. Talley, *op. cit.*, 55: 161–3; EBW, 233, 240–1; EMH to WW (T), c. Feb. 21, 23, 1919, 55: 223, 233; JPT to WW (T), Feb. 15 and 22, 1919, 55: 197–8, 226; CTG (D), Feb. 19, 20, 22, 24, 1919, 55: 207, 217, 224, 235–8; F. B. Sayre to WW (T), Feb. 23, 1919, 55: 234. [WW's grandchildren: After their firstborn, Francis Sayre, Jr., and before the birth of Woodrow Wilson Sayre, Francis and Jessie Wilson Sayre also had a daughter, Eleanor Axson Sayre, born Mar. 26, 1916; W. G. and Eleanor Wilson McAdoo had a daughter Ellen, born May 21, 1915; and they would have a second daughter, Mary Faith McAdoo, born Apr. 6, 1920.] RL to WW (T), Feb. 19, 1919, 55: 209; WW to JPT (T), Feb. 22 (10:41 a.m. and 4:55 p.m.), 1919, 55: 225 and 226; WW (A), Feb. 24, 1919, 55: 238–45; "Challenge to His Critics," *NYT*, Feb. 25, 1919, 1.

WW IN WHITE HOUSE; MEETS CONGRESSIONAL DELEGATION: CTG (D), Feb. 25 and Mar. 4, 1919, 55: 254 and 409–12; W. E. Rappard to Hans Sulzer, Feb. 13, 1919, 55: 151–4; JD (D), Feb. 25, 1919, 55: 266; "President Expounds League of Nations," *NYT*, Feb. 26, 1919, 55: 268–76; HCL, 100, 117, 260; WW, U statement, c. Mar. 4, 1919, 55: 408; WW (S—"A group of men . . . have . . . chosen to embarrass the administration"), Mar. 4, 1919, 55: 408–9.

REPLACING A.G. GREGORY WITH PALMER: JPT to WW (T), Jan. 12 and Feb. 1, 4, 1919, 54: 31–2 and 429, 485; WW to T. W. Gregory, Feb. 26, 1919, 55: 276; T. W. Gregory to WW, Jan. 17 and Mar. 1, 1919, 54: 125, 346–7; WW to JPT (T), Jan. 31, 1919, 54: 410; Hagedorn, 226; Coben, 200; CTG (D), Feb. 27, 1919, 55: 294; WW to A. M. Palmer, Mar. 12, 1919, 55: 482–3; WW to A. S. Burleson, Feb. 28, 1919, 55: 327.

WW RETURNS TO *GEORGE WASHINGTON*, VIA PHILA. AND NYC: WW (A), Mar. 4, 1919, 55: 413–21; CTG (D), Mar. 9–10, 11 and 12, 1919, 55: 471, 473–4, 480–1; RSB (D), Mar. 8, 1919, 55: 465–6; EMH to WW (T), Mar. 4 and 7, 1919, 55: 423 and 458–9; WW to EMH (radiogram), Mar. 10, 1919, 55: 472.

14 GETHSEMANE

FRANCE—BREST TO PARIS: CTG (D), Mar. 13 and 14, 1919, 55: 487–9 and 496–7; EBW, 245–6; EMH (D), Mar. 14, 1919, 55: 499–500; Freud, 233–4.

WW BEGINS WORK ANEW: RSB (D), Mar. 15 and 27, 1919, 55: 531 and 56: 337; EBW,

247–8; EMH to WW (T), c. Feb. 21 and 25, 1919, 55: 223 and 256–7; CTG (D), Mar. 14 and 15, 1919, 55: 497–8 and 529–31; EMH (D), Mar. 16 and 22, 1919, 55: 538 and 56: 180; Lord Cecil (D), Mar. 16, 1919, 55: 539.

SECOND ACT OF PEACE TALKS BEGINS: MIDDLE EAST; EASTERN EUROPE; RUSSIA: CTG (D), Mar. 18, 19, and 22, 1919, 56: 62, 88, and 163–5; Lord Cecil (D), Mar. 18, 1919, 56: 81; Maurice Hankey (N: C10), Jan. 27 and Mar. 20, 1919, 54: 284 and 56: 104n1, 113; Monnet, 78–81; Keynes, 83–5, 116–8, 131–2, 135, 141, 152, 161, 204; "Financial Capacity of Enemy States, Annex II, 4th Meeting," Feb. 19, 1919 [RSB Papers: Box 15, Folder 31, 5—PUL]; "Middle East" defined in *OED*, IX: 743; Nicolson, *Peacemaking*, 136, 140–3; RSB (D), Mar. 20, 1919, 56: 103; RL to WW, Mar. 20, 1919, 56: 123; H. Hoover, 133–5; Brownell, 86–9; H. Hoover to WW, Mar. 28, 1919, 56: 375–8; Ellery Sedgwick to JPT, Mar. 21, 1919, 56: 162–3.

WW REVISITS BATTLEFIELDS; CONFLICTS WITH CLEMENCEAU OVER REPARATIONS: CTG, 71–2, 85; CTG (D), Mar. 23, 25, 26, and 27, 1919, 56: 194–200, 246–9, 283–6, and 312; P. Mantoux (N: Council of Four), Mar. 24, 26, and 27, 1919, 56: 208–9, 290, and 316; EMH (D), Apr. 1, 1919, 56: 517–8; RSB (D), Apr. 1, 1919, 56: 518; WW to JPT (T), Mar. 22 and 26, 1919, 56: 191 and 310; JPT to WW (T), Apr. 4, 1919, 56: 618; "Bryan Supports League," *NYT*, Mar. 12, 1919, attached to JD to WW, Mar. 27, 1919, 56: 346n1; JD (D), Mar. 27, 1919, 56: 338; Nicolson, *Peacemaking*, 196.

SAAR VALLEY DISCUSSION: EMH (D), Mar. 28, 1919, 56: 349–50; RL (M), Mar. 28, 1919, 56: 351–2; RSB (D), Apr. 3, 1919, 56: 578; P. Mantoux (N: C4), Mar. 28 and Apr. 1, 1919, 56: 366–70 and 508; CTG (D), Mar. 28, 29, 30, Apr. 1, 1919, 56: 347, 408, 429, 490; G. L. Beer (D), Mar. 30 and Apr. 1, 1919, 56: 434 and 490; C. H. Haskins to WW (with enclosure), Apr. 1, 1919, 56: 514; EMH (D), Apr. 1 and 2, 1919, 56: 518 and 540; Freud, 245–6.

WW'S HEALTH; LOSING FAITH IN EMH: CTG (D), Apr. 3 (with ASL N), 4, 5, 6, 7, and 8, 1919; 56: 556–7 (557n2), 584, 57: 3–4, 50–2, 62–7, and 99; H. Hoover, 198–9; Weinstein, 338–9; Bert E. Park, "The Impact of W's Neurological Disease During the Paris Peace Conference," 58: 611–30; Edwin A. Weinstein, "WW's Neuropsychological Impairment and the Paris Peace Conference," 58: 630–5; James F. O'Toole,

"Some Observations on W's Neurological Illness," 58: 635–8; ASL, "Editors' Commentary," 58: 638–9; I. Hoover, 98–9; Weinstein, 340–1; RSB (D), Apr. 4 and 19, 1919, 56: 588–9 and 57: 508–9; EMH (D), Apr. 5 and May 30, 1919, 57: 34–5 and 59: 624; EBW, 248–52; Freud, 226–7; CTG to A. G. Grayson, Apr. 23–5, 1919 [WWPL]; RSB (D), Apr. 3, 1919, 56: 577–8.

SUMMONING *GEORGE WASHINGTON*: CTG (D), Apr. 6, 7 (with ASL N), and 15, 1919, 57: 50–1, 62–67 (63n1), and 351; EBW, 249; RSB, *American Chronicle*, 402; H. Hoover, 199, 202; JPT to CTG (T), Apr. 9, 1919, 57: 177; RSB (D), Apr. 7, 1919, 57: 68–70; H. White to WW, Apr. 12, 1919, 57: 301–2; H. Hoover to WW, Apr. 11, 1919, 67: 273–4.

WW LEAVES SICKBED; MARIE OF ROMANIA: Weinstein, 339; P. Mantoux (N: C4), Apr. 5, 1919, 57: 22; P. Mantoux, cited in Weinstein, 343n; Clements, 182; Park, *op. cit.*, 58: 623; RSB (D), Apr. 8, 1919, 57: 140; Minutes, League of Nations Commission, Apr. 10, 1919, 57: 218–9; EBW, 257–60; CTG (D), Apr. 10, 11, and 17, 1919, 57: 190–3, 238–9, and 426–30; E. Benham (D), Apr. 11, 1919, 57: 241–2; "Clauses Proposed for Insertion in the Treaty of Peace," attached to H. M. Robinson to WW, Mar. 24, 1919, 56: 236–8 and cf.: ASL (N), 57: 240n5; WW to P. G. Gerry, Apr. 17, 1919, 57: 446; F. P. Walsh and F. F. Dunne to WW, May 31, 1919, 59: 643; EMH (D), May 31, 1919, 59: 645; RSB (D), Apr. 11 and May 31, 1919, 57: 240–1 and 59: 646; CTG to WGM, Apr. 12, 1919, 57: 304.

ITALIAN DEMANDS: Nicolson, *Peacemaking*, 169–71; RSB (D), Apr. 18, 20, 22, and May 28, 1919, 57: 467–8, 527, 585, and 59: 575; T. N. Page to EMH, Apr. 17, 1919, 57: 434–7; CTG (D), Apr. 19, 20, and 23, 1919, 57: 477–8, 512–3, and 58: 3; Maurice Hankey (N: C4), Apr. 19, 20, and 22, 1919, 57: 482–94, 514–7, and 614; EMH (D), Apr. 20, 1919, 57: 527; N. H. Davis to WW, Apr. 18, 1919, 57: 470; WW to N. H. Davis, Apr. 19, 1919, 57: 445; H. Hoover, 206; EBW, 254–6; T. N. Page to American Mission (T: #260), Apr. 24, 1919, 58: 91–2; "Orlando Makes Protest," *NYT*, Apr. 25, 1919, 58: 97–101.

JAPANESE DEMANDS: Nicolson, *Peacemaking*, 145–7; CTG (D), Mar. 10, Apr. 25 and 30, May 1, 1919, 55: 471, 58: 110–13 and 244–5, 274–7; H. Hoover, 79, 208; Lawrence, 261; RL (M), Apr. 28, 1919, 58: 185; Seymour, 314–7; EMH, IV: 449–52; JPT to WW, Apr. 24, 1919, 58: 105; RSB (D), Apr. 25, 1919, 58: 143; RL (M), Apr. 28,

1919, 58: 185; Tasker Bliss to WW, Apr. 29, 1919, 58: 234; Tasker Bliss to E. A. Bliss, May 1, 1919, 58: 320; EMH (D), Apr. 28, 1919, 58: 185–7; RSB (D), Apr. 30, 1919, 58: 270–1n; EMH to Baron Makino, Apr. 28, 1919, EMH, IV: 453–5, including 453n2; Maurice Hankey and P. Mantoux (N: C4), May 1, 1919, 58: 277–8; Weinstein, 342n50 (N.B.: the term "ludic" was first used by Jean Piaget); Freud, 262–3; Short, 90–4.

PRESENTING THE TREATY: Confucius, *The Analects*," XI: 16; Seymour, 317–8; CTG (D), May 2, 4, 5, 7, and 8, 1919, 58: 332, 422, 430–1, 499–504, and 535–6; Churchill, "The War Is Won," Dec. 16, 1918, quoted in W. S. Churchill (ed.), *op. cit.*, 75–7; Churchill to William Griffen (editor of *NY Enquirer*), Aug. 1936, quoted in Vansittart, 162; RSB, *American Chronicle*, 416; Freud, 264; EMH (D), May 5, 7, 1919, 58: 443, 520–1; B. Baruch to WW, May 8, 1919, 58: 548–9; RSB (D), May 7, 1919, 58: 529–30; "Rantzau Proclaims Germany Unrepentant," "Treaty of Peace Is Solemnly Presented," "1871–1919," "Germans at Versailles," "Clemenceau's Speech," May 8, 1919, *American Daily Mail*, 1; Brockdorff-Rantzau (R), May 7, 1919, 58: 514–7; WW, statement, May 6, 1919, 58: 489–90; Sir R. Borden to Sir T. White (T), May 7, 1919, 58: 517–20.

WW'S HEALTH; POSSIBLE STROKE: ASL (N), 58: viii; WW (M), May 8, 1919, 58: 559; WW (R), May 9, 1919, 58: 598–600; RSB (D), May 17, 1919, 59: 245; CTG (D), May 8 and 10, 1919, 58: 536 and 59:3.

GERMANS CONSIDER TREATY: Brockdorff-Rantzau to Clemenceau, May 9, 1919, 59: 13n5; WW to Brockdorff-Rantzau, May 10, 1919, 59: 28n3; Maurice Hankey and P. Mantoux (N: C4), May 10, 1919, 59: 709; J. Smuts to WW, May 14, 1919, 59: 149–50; WW to J. Smuts, May 16, 1919, 59: 187; CTG (D), May 11, 21, and 23, 1919, 59: 39–40, 321–2, and 419–20; D. H. Miller (D), May 13, 1919, 59: 82–3.

REDRAWING MAP OF THE WORLD: E. Benham (D), May 23, 1919, 59: 420; Maurice Hankey (N: C4), June 23, 1919, 61: 88–93; F. Frankfurter to WW, May 8, 1919, 58: 555–6; H. Hoover, 224–6.

RUSSIA AND BULLITT MISSION: RSB, "Russia," n.d. [RSB Papers, 18/1, 20: PUL]; Francis P. Sempa, "William C. Bullitt: Diplomat and Prophet," *American Diplomacy* (Chapel Hill, NC: Americandiplomacy.org, 2003); Kennan, 79–80; WW (R), Feb. 28, 1919, 55: 320; Brownell, 93; W. C. Bullitt to WW, May 17, 1919, 59: 232–3;

RL to WW, May 20, 1919, 59: 314; RSB (D), May 19 and 23, 1919, 59: 287 and 447–8; Freud, 253–4; Gay, 559.

ASSESSMENTS OF TREATY: Nicolson, *Peacemaking*, 198; Keynes, 41, 226–7.

WW AT SURESNES: EBW, 260; CTG (D), May 30, 1919, 59: 605–6; WW (R), May 30, 1919, 59: 606–10; EMH to WW, May 30, 1919, 59: 610; RSB (D), May 30, 1919, 59: 621–2.

REACTION TO TREATY—IN U.S., FRANCE, ENGLAND, AND GERMANY: RSB (D), Apr. 3, May 19, 28, 31, and June 13, 1919, 56: 578, 59: 286, 574, 647, and 60: 532–3; C. Seymour to family, May 31, 1919, 59: 648; JPT, 364–5; "W, the Third Term and the Treaty," *Springfield Republican*, May 17, 1919, enclosed with WW to JPT, June 2 and 6 (T), 1919, 60: 41–2 and 247; WW, "Special Message to Congress," May 20, 1919, 59: 289–97; WW to JPT (T), May 13, 1919, 59: 120; "Suffrage Wins in Senate," *NYT*, June 5, 1919, 1; WW (R), Feb. 28, 1919, 55: 309–23; CTG (D), May 22, 29, June 2, and 15, 1919, 59: 370–2, 577, 60: 18–9, and 570; Maurice Hankey (N: C4), June 13, 1919, 60: 498; Brockdorff-Rantzau to G. Clemenceau, May 29, 1919, 59: 579–84; ASL (N), 61: 35n; Maurice Hankey and P. Mantoux (N: C4), June 2, 1919, 60: 27; WW, discussion with American delegation, June 3, 1919, 60: 67; Baruch (reporting WW telling D. Lloyd George: "You make me sick!"), 120–1; G. L. Beer (D), June 1, 1919, 60: 17; V. C. McCormick (D), June 3, 1919, 60: 72; "German Envoys Tell the Cabinet to Reject Allied Peace Treaty," *NYT*, June 19, 1919, 1–2; EBW, 26.

WILSONS VISIT BELGIUM: EBW, 261–7; CTG (D), June 18, 1919, 61: 3–8; WW (A), June 19, 1919, 61: 16–20; WW (R), June 19, 1919, 61: 21.

GERMANS READY TO SIGN TREATY; PREPARATIONS: RSB (D), June 20 and 26, 1919, 61: 34–5n1 and 231; G. A. Bauer to G. Clemenceau, June 21, 1919, 61: 72–6; CTG (D), June 23 and 24, 1919, 61: 78–9 and 118–9; RL (M), June 28, 1919, 61: 327; Tasker Bliss to E. A. Bliss, June 24, 1919, 61: 135; JPT to WW (T), June 21, 1919, 61: 66; "Knox Resolution Cannot Be Passed," *NYT*, June 21, 1919, 1; WW to T. W. Lamont, June 27, 1919, 61: 290; "Conference Officials Prepare for Signing," *NYT*, June 22, 1919, 2; EMH (D), June 21 and 23, 1919, 61: 45 and 112–5; E. Benham (D), June 24 and 26, 1919, 61: 135 and 188–9; WW to J.-J. Jusserand, June 25, 1919, 61: 173; WW (R), June 26, 1919, 61: 238.

ANALYSIS OF TREATY: Keynes, 35, 36, 56, 151; Nicolson, *Peacemaking*, 43–4; Seymour, 323–5; JD, *Life*, 312; D. Lloyd George to WW, June 26, 1919, 61: 223–5; financial costs recorded in MacMillan, 480.

SIGNING OF TREATY: CTG (D), June 28, 1919, 61: 302–6; RL (M), June 28, 1919, 61: 321–8; W. L. Westermann, June 28, 1919, 61: 328–32; EMH (D), June 28, 1919, 61: 332–3.

WILSONS LEAVE FRANCE: EMH (D), June 29, 1919, 61: 354–5; EBW, 271.

15 PASSION

VOYAGE HOME: WW (A), July 4, 1919, 61: 378; CTG (D), July 1, 2, 3, 4, 5, and 6, 1919, 61: 360–3, 369–70, 374–6, 377–8, 385, and 396; V. C. McCormick (D), July 4 and 5, 1919, 61: 383 and 385–6; JPT to CTG, July 2, 1919, 61: 372–3; WW to JPT (T—handwritten), July 3, 1919, and ASL (N), 61: 376n.

WW ARRIVES IN NJ; RETURNS TO WHITE HOUSE: CTG (D), July 8, 1919, 61: 400–1; WW (A), July 8, 1919, 61: 401–4; Longworth, 285–6; CTG (D), July 8, 1919, 61: 401; "Capital Greets W Warmly," *NYT*, July 9, 1919, 3.

POLITICAL BATTLE FOR TREATY BEGINS: WW, Report of Press Conference, July 10, 1919, 61: 417–24; "W Revises Speech on Treaty for Senate Today," *NYT*, July 10, 1919, 1, 3; "Offers Bill to Keep Presidents Home," *NYT*, July 10, 1919, 3; "Insist Majority Can Amend Treaty," *NYT*, July 11, 1919, 1–2; CTG (D), July 10, 1919, 61: 416–7; "Ovation to the President," *NYT*, July 11, 1919, 1–2; WW (A), July 10, 1919, 61: 426–36; H. F. Ashurst (D), July 11, 1919, 61: 445–6; ASL (N), 61: 446n; "W Greets Callers," *NYT*, July 11, 1919, 1–2; "Comments Divide on Party Line," *NYT*, July 11, 1919, 1, 3; "17,000 Boo and Hiss President W at Sinn Fein Rally," *NYT*, July 11, 1919, 1, 7; Houston, II: 5–6; FDR to RSB, Feb. 20, 1922 [RSB Papers: PUL]; Berkin, 581–2; E. J. Howenstone, Jr., "The High-Cost-of-Living Problem after World War I," *Southern Economic Journal*, v. 10, no. 3 (Jan. 1944), 222; "Foods Drop As Everybody Aims Smash at H. C. L.," *Chicago Daily Tribune*, Aug. 16, 1919.

"RED SUMMER" OF 1919—STATE OF THE NATION: "Negroes Again Riot in Washington," *NYT*, July 23, 1919, 1–2; "Gov. Bilbo Blames French Reception and Negro Press," *Jones County* (MS) *News*, July 8, 1919, 1, cited in McWhirter, 71; Johnson, 658–9; "Urban and Rural

Population: 1900–1990" (Washington, D.C.: United States Census Bureau, 1995); Fitzgerald, 304; "U. S. Business Cycle Expansions and Contractions" (Cambridge, MA: National Bureau of Economic Research, Aug. 10, 2011).

HCL: Adams, 419–20; HCL, 2–3, 23, 160, 163–5, 224–6; WW, "Cabinet Government," 1: 505, 509; HCL to TR, Mar. 1, 1915, cited in John A. Garrity, *Henry Cabot Lodge* (New York: Alfred A. Knopf, 1968), 312; WW, "Constitutional Government," 18: 60; "Insist Majority Can Amend Treaty," *NYT*, July 11, 1919, 1–2.

WW COURTS SENATORS; MEDICAL ISSUES: Sir William Wiseman to A. J. Balfour, July 18, 1919, 61: 541–3; WW to T. W. Lamont, July 19, 1919, 61: 544n; HCL, 56–60; "W Invites Senators," *NYT*, July 15, 1919, 1–2; "Committee Finds Treaty Readings," *NYT*, July 29, 1919, 1, 3; "W to Consult Congress Members," *NYT*, July 14, 1919, 2; "W Frankness Getting Results," *NYT*, July 19, 1919, 2; "Wilsons on Cruise Despite the Storm," *Washington Post*, July 20, 1919, 61: 562–3; "President W Returns Ill," *NYT*, July 21, 1919, 61: 569–70; "W Stays in Bed," *Washington Post*, July 22, 1919, 61: 578–9; Park, *op. cit.*, 62: 629; "35 to Block League," *Washington Post*, July 20, 1919, 61: 563–5; "W Says He Decided Shantung," *NYT*, July 22, 1919, 61: 593–5; "Deny W Power," *Washington Post*, July 23, 1919, 61: 596–8; WW to HCL, July 25 and Aug. 14 (draft), 15, 1919, 61: 623 and 62: 278–81, 310; I. Hoover, "Memoir," 63: 632; EBW, 273; N. H. Davis to WW, July 26, 1919, 62: 7; CTG to A. G. Grayson, July 29 and 30, 1919 [WWPL]; WW (M), Sep. 3, 1919, 62: 621; JPT to WW, Aug. 15, 1919, 62: 309; HCL to WW, Aug. 14, 1919, 62: 275; ASL, "Introduction," 62: viii; WW (A), Aug. 8, 1919, 62: 209–19 (especially 209n1).

NAMING THE WAR; RECONSIDERATION OF DEBS: N. D. Baker to WW, July 23, 1919, 61: 611; WW to N. D. Baker, July 31, 1919, 62: 69; C. S. Darrow to WW, July 29, 1919, 62: 58–9; WW to John Spargo, Aug. 29, 1919, 62: 559.

LEAGUE FIGHT: HCL HEARINGS; FOREIGN RELATIONS COMMITTEE AT WHITE HOUSE: Cooper, 136–7; *Congressional Record, 66th Congress, 1st Session*, Aug. 12, 1919, 3778–84; "Jovial Luncheon After Conference," *NYT*, Aug. 20, 1919, 1–2; JPT, 422–5, 435; Steel, 163; "President Defends Treaty to Senators," *NYT*, Aug. 19, 1919, 62: 535–6; Houston, II: 14–7; CTG to A. G. Grayson, Aug. 19 and 22, 1919 [WWPL]; I. Hoover,

"Memoir," 63: 632; WW, "Conference with Foreign Relations Committee" (transcript), Aug. 19, 1919, 62: 339–411; "Offer a Compromise," *Washington Post*, Aug. 21, 1919, 62: 429–32n3; Baruch, 135–6; "Itinerary—Tour of the President to the Pacific Coast" (private collection), Sep. 3–30, 191; EBW, 274; CTG, 95–6.

WESTERN TOUR—FIRST PHASE: EBW, 274–5; "W Begins Tour for Treaty," *NYT*, Sep. 4, 1919, 1–2; ASL (N), "W's Speeches on His Western Tour," 63: 5–6; "W Defends Treaty and League As Tour Begins," *NYT*, Sep. 5, 1919, 1–2; WW (A—Columbus), Sep. 4, 1919, 63: 7–18; WW (R), Sep. 4, 1919, 63: 18–9; CTG (D), Sep. 4, 5, 6, 8, 9, 1919, 63: 3–5, 31–3, 63–6, 93–6, 122–4; WW (A—Indianapolis), 63: 19–29; WW (two A—St. Louis), Sep. 5, 1919, 63: 33–42 and 43–51; WW (A—Kansas City), Sep. 6, 1919, 63: 66–75; "W Likens Treaty Obstructionists to Bolsheviks," *NYT*, Sep. 7, 1919, 1–2; WW (A—Des Moines), 63: 76–88; "W Gaining Support," *NYT*, Sep. 7, 1919, 1, 2; "Wants Senate Trailers Paid," *NYT*, Sep. 4, 1919, 2; WW (A—Omaha), 63: 97–107; WW (A—Sioux Falls), Sep. 8, 1919, 63: 107–17; WW (A—St. Paul), Sep. 9, 1919, 63: 125–31; WW (A—Minneapolis), Sep. 9, 1919, 63: 131–8; WW (A—St. Paul), Sep. 9, 1919, 63: 138–48.

REACHING THE NORTHWEST; NATIONAL CONCERNS; BULLITT TESTIMONY; RL DISLOYALTY: CTG (D), Sep. 25, 1919, 63: 489; Samuel Gompers, et al., to WW (T), Sep. 4, 1919, 63: 30n1; WW (A—Helena), Sep. 11, 1919, 63: 196; W. J. H. Cochran to JPT, Sep. 11, 1919, 63: 198–200n; RL to WW, Sep. 17, 1919, 63: 337–340n; Brownell, 97–8; "Bullitt Asserts Lansing Expected Treaty to Fail," *NYT*, Sep. 13, 1919, 1, 2; JPT, 441–3.

MEDICAL CONCERNS AS TOUR CONTINUES: Breckinridge Long, "Memoir" (U), 1924, quoted in 63: 339n4; CTG (D), Sep. 12, 18, 19, 20, 21, 1919, 63: 210–11 (211n5 cites *Seattle Post-Intelligencer*, Sep. 13, 1919), 340–1n, 369–70, 396–7, 423–4; WW (A—Helena), Sep. 11, 1919, 63: 195; WW (A—Portland), Sep. 15, 1919, 63: 281; WW (A—Portland Auditorium), Sep. 15, 1919, 63: 284–5; WW, quoted in (I) for *Oregon Daily Journal*, Sep. 16, 1919, quoted in 63: 277n7; WW to B. Baruch, Sep. 17, 1919, 63: 336; "Labor Conferees Chosen," *NYT*, Sep. 18, 1919, 1–2; "Says W Has Socialization Idea," *NYT*, Sep. 18, 1919, 1; WW (A—Berkeley), Sep. 18, 1919, 63: 350; CTG, 7–9; WW (A—San Diego), Sep. 19, 1919, 63: 376; "Find W Shy Only in Private,"

NYT, Sep. 22, 1919, 1, 3; Elliot, 299; WW to MAH, Sep. 20, 1919, 63: 419; Hulbert, 267–77; EBW, 281.

WESTERN TOUR, TURNING EAST-WARD: CTG, Jr., to ASB (I), Oct. 14, 2006; CTG (D), Sep. 22, 23, 24, 25, 1919, 63: 426, 446, 467, 487–90; HCL, 183–5; Guy Mason to JPT (T), Sep. 22, 1919, 63: 445; WW (A—Salt Lake City), Sep. 23, 1919, 63: 449–63; EBW, 281–3; CTG to A. G. Grayson, Sep. 25, 1919 [WWPL].

PUEBLO AND RETURN TO WASHING-TON: Starling, 151–3; Peter Roper, "Remember-ing W in Pueblo," *Pueblo Chieftain*, Sep. 25, 1994, n.p.; WW (A—Pueblo), Sep. 25, 1919, 63: 500–13; EBW, 284–5; JPT, 446–8; CTG (D), Sep. 26, 27, 28, 1919, 63: 518–21, 526–7, 532–3; WW (A—in Los Angeles Shrine Auditorium), Sep. 20, 1919, 63: 413; WW to JWS (T), Sep. 26, 1919; T. W. Brahany (I), Aug. 19, 1926 [Hard Archives, VIII: PUL]; A. S. Burleson to WW, Sep. 29, 1919, 63: 534–5; "W Returns to Washington Worn and Shaken," *NYT*, Sep. 29, 1919, 1, 3.

WHITE HOUSE RECUPERATION AND COLLAPSE: EBW, 286–7; "W Sleeping Better and Improving," *NYT*, Sep. 30, 1919, 63: 536–7; CTG to H. A. Garfield, Oct. 1, 1919, 63: 538–9; RL to F. L. Polk, Oct. 1, 1919, 63: 539–40; "Presi-dent Is Again Jaded After Another Restless Night," *NYT*, Oct. 2, 1919, 1; CTG 100; I. Hoover, 100–1.

16 PIETÀ

WW'S INVALIDISM: EBW, 288–9; CTG, 100, 109; " 'Very Sick Man,' Says Grayson," *Wash-ington Post*, Oct. 3, 1919, 63: 543–5; F. X. Dercum to CTG, "Dr. Dercum's Memoranda," Oct. 20, 1919, 64: 500–7; I. Hoover, 100–3; JD, *Life*, 339.

GOVERNMENT DURING WW'S AB-SENCE: *Constitution of the United States*, Article 2, Section 1; JPT, 442–5; Houston, II: 36–40; RL (D), Oct. 3, 1919, 63: 547n; "Rumor Busy about W," *NYT*, Oct. 13, 1919, 63: 564–7; Thomas, 204, 225–7, 236; "More Encouraging Day," *NYT*, Oct. 5, 1919, 63: 550–1; CTG, 108; JD (D), Oct. 5, 6, 7, 1919, 63: 552, 555, 557; "W Has a Good Day," *Washington Post*, Oct. 6, 1919, 63: 552–3; Breckin-ridge Long (D), Oct. 7, 1919, 63: 558–9; CTG (M), Oct. 6, 1919, 64: 496; JD, *Wilson Era*, II: 511–3; Weinstein, 360; "President Needs Long Rest," *NYT*, Oct. 12, 1919, 63: 561; "Reports W Suffered Shock," *NYT*, Oct. 11, 1919, 63: 561–4; "W Still Gains," *Washington Post*, Oct. 7, 1919, 63: 555–6;

EBW to JD (M), Oct. 7, 1919, 63: 556–7; JD to EBW, Oct. 7, 1919, 63: 557; JPT to W. B. Wilson, Oct. 6, 1919, 63: 554; F. K. Lane to WW, Oct. 19, 1919, 63: 582–3; "WW," statement to industrial conference, Oct. 20, 1919, 63: 584–5; EMH to EBW, Oct. 22, 1919, 63: 587–8; "WW," veto mes-sage, Oct. 27, 1919, 63: 601–2; RL (M), Nov. 5, 1919, 63: 618–9; I. Hoover, 103–4; CTG 101, EBW, 290–2; "Spent Restless Day," *Washington Post*, Oct. 15, 1919, 63: 572–3; "President Im-proves after a Setback," *NYT*, Oct. 18, 1919, 63: 577–9; B. E. Park, "WW's Stroke of Oct. 2, 1919," 63: 644–6; RSB (D), Nov. 5, 1919, 63: 622; Freud, 291.

EBW, CTG, JPT PERMIT VISITS, IN-CLUDING TWO ROYAL PARTIES: ASL (N) to JD (D), Nov. 4, 1919, 63: 613n; A. M. Palmer to R. S. Morris, Nov. 3, 1919, 63: 608n; EBW, 292–6; CTG, misc. (N), n.d., 64: 489; "Belgian Royalties See the President," *NYT*, Oct. 30, 1919, 63: 602–6; [N.B.: The Belgian Royals stayed at the home of Breckinridge Long]; EMH (D), Dec. 22, 1919, 64: 217; Levin, 399–401; Smith, 116–7; "Presi-dent on the Porch in a Wheeled Chair," *NYT*, Nov. 15, 1919, 1, 64: 32–3; "Prince Sees Wilson," *Washington Post*, Nov. 14, 1919, 64: 31–2.

WW CONDUCTS BUSINESS; HITCH-COCK VISITS, TRIES TO RALLY SENATE SUPPORT: Cooper, 661n17; "Lodge Forces Win Opening Skirmish," *NYT*, Nov. 8, 1919, 1–2; CTG (M), Nov. 17, 1919, 64: 43–5; G. M. Hitch-cock, "W's Place in History," 64: 45n1; William Hard, "Amendments" [PUL: Hard, 145, 3/15, x.3]; Connally, 101; G. M. Hitchcock to EBW, Nov. 15, 1919, 64: 37–8; EBW, 296–7; H. Hoover, 282–3; Bonsal, 274–80, CTG (M), Nov. 17, 1919, 64: 43–5; "President Will Pocket Treaty" and "Presi-dent Out on the Lawn," *NYT*, Nov. 18, 1919, 64: 45–50; "President Outdoors Again," *NYT*, Nov. 19, 1919, 64: 57; G. M. Hitchcock to EBW, Nov. 17, 1919, enclosing Hitchcock's draft of letter for "WW to G. M. Hitchcock," Nov. 17, 1919, 64: 51.

NOVEMBER 19, 1919, SENATE VOTE; STRANGENESS WITHIN WHITE HOUSE; T. R. MARSHALL: H. F. Ashurst (D), Nov. 19, 1919, 64: 62–4; "Lodge Resolution Beaten," *NYT*, Nov. 20, 1919, 1–2; "Lodge Declares for Political Fight on Peace Treaty," *NYT*, Nov. 22, 1919, 2; O. W. Underwood to WW, Nov. 21, 1919, 64: 69–70; EBW, 297–8, 300; Smith, 111; I. Hoover, 104–5; Thomas, 211–2, 227–8; "False Telephone Report of President's Death," *NYT*, Nov. 24, 1919, 1.

WW'S ABSENCE AROUSES SUSPICIONS; "SMELLING COMMITTEE": JPT to EBW, Nov. 17, 1919, 64: 42; "WW," statement, Nov. 11, 1919, 64: 7; WW, "State of the Union Address," Dec. 2, 1919, 64: 106–16n; "Congress Comment Divides," NYT, Dec. 3, 1919, 2; "President's Health Shows Steady Improvement," NYT, Dec. 3, 1919, 1; RL (M), Dec. 4, 1919, 64: 123–5; "President Jests on Moses Story," Dec. 5, 1919, 64: 132–3; CTG (M), Dec. 5, 1919, 64: 135–9; JD, Wilson Era, II: 513; Houston, II: 140–1; "W to See Senators," NYT, Dec. 5, 1919, 1; EBW, 298–9; Smith, 133; Starling, 155; RL (M), Dec. 5, 1919, 64: 139–40.

GOVERNMENT IN DISARRAY: William Butler Yeats, "The Second Coming"; JPT to EBW, Dec. 18, 1919, and c. Feb. 3, 1920, 64: 204–5 and 355, including ASL (N), 356–7; Clements, 210–1; McAdoo, 505–9; W. D. Hines to WW, Dec. 15, 1919, 64: 188–9; A. M. Palmer to WW, Dec. 23, 1919 (with enclosures: W. D. Hines to WW, Dec. 23, 1919, and WW proclamation, Dec. 24, 1919), 64: 222–7; JPT, statement, Dec. 24, 1919, 64: 228; RL to JPT, Nov. 26 and Dec. 15, 1919, 64: 95 and 187–8; F. L. Polk to JPT, Dec. 26, 1919, 64: 229–30; RL (D), Dec. 29, 1919, 64: 235; L. S. Rowe to JPT, Jan. 3, 1920, 64: 245; B. F. Chase to N. H. Davis, July 8, 1920, 65: 505–6; B. Colby to WW, July 31, 1920, 65: 571; Houston, II: 60–2; EBW, 301–2; Rudolph Forster to JPT (T), Sep. 5, 1919, 63: 52n4; EMH (D), Dec. 12, 1919, and Mar. 2, 1920, 64: 185 and 65: 41; JD, Wilson Era, 546–8; JD (D), Dec. 5 and 9, 1919, 64: 141 and 166; "President Makes Proposal to Coal Miners," NYT, Dec. 7, 1919, 64: 142–5; WW to Harry Garfield, Dec. 13, 1919, 64: 185; Harry Garfield to WW, Dec. 13, 1919, 64: 186.

RL DEPARTURE: RL (M), Dec. 4, 5, 10, 1919, Jan. 7, Feb. 9, 13, 1920, 64: 123–5, 139–40, 179, 255–6, 385–6, 415–9; RSB (D), Jan. 23, 1920, 64: 320; EMH (D), Jan. 3, 1920, 64: 243; N. D. Baker to WW, Feb. 7, 1920, 64: 389–90; RL to WW, Feb. 9 (two letters), 12, 1920, 64: 388–9 and 390–1, 408–10; WW to RL, Feb. 7 and 11, 1920, 64: 383 and 404; JD, Wilson Era, II: 519, 521–3; JPT, 445; EBW, 301; RL (D), Feb. 11 and 14, 1920, 64: 405 and 428; Bert E. Park, "The Aftermath of W's Stroke," 64: 527; "Sees President Near Recovery," NYT, Feb. 11, 1920, 64: 394–6; "President Will Never Recover" and "Doctor Dercum Declares Mind of President W Is Keen," Philadelphia Press, Feb. 15, 1920, 64: 432–4.

SEDITION; RED SCARE; PALMER RAIDS: WW to A. M. Palmer, Mar. 12, 1919, 55: 482–3; WW to A. S. Burleson, Feb. 28, 1919, 55: 327; Ackerman, 20, CTG (D), June 4, 1919, 60: 114–5; "200 Caught in New York," NYT, Nov. 8, 1919, 1, 2; Stone, 223; "Raid from Coast to Coast," NYT, Jan. 3, 1920, 1, 2; "Raiders Ordered to Make Cleanup Thorough," NYT, Jan. 3, 1920, 1; "Raids on 13 Centres Here," NYT, Jan. 3, 1920, 1, 2; "Reds Plotted Country-Wide Strike," NYT, Jan. 4, 1920, 1, 2; RSB (D), June 23, 1920, 64: 320; "W Walks," Washington Post, Dec. 14, 1919, 64: 187; "W Reported Much Better," NYT, Dec. 21, 1919, 64: 211; JPT to WW, Dec. 28, 1919, 64: 233.

WW PLOTS NEW STRATEGY FOR TREATY PASSAGE: WW, to "My Fellow Countrymen," c. Dec. 17, 1919, 64: 199–202; A. M. Palmer to WW, Dec. 22, 1919, 64: 214–5; WW, redraft of Jackson Day message, Jan. 7, 1920, 64: 252–5; Houston, II: 47–9; JPT, draft of Jackson Day message, Jan. 6, 1920, 64: 247–250; D. Houston (N), Jan. 7, 1920, 64: 250–2; "Clash at Jackson Dinner," NYT, Jan. 9, 1920, 1; "W Will Make No Offer," NYT, Dec. 15, 1919, 1, 2; JPT to EBW, Jan. 15 and 17, 1920, 64: 276–7n and 287; Cooper, 302–10; RSB (D), Jan. 23, 1920, 64: 320–1; CTG to SA, Jan. 24, 1920, 64: 324–6; JPT to WW, Feb. 27, 1920, 64: 479; JPT, 429; H. S. Cummings (D), Feb. 29, 1920, 65: 24; Hurley, 243–5; RSB, American Chronicle, 474; B. Long to JPT, Sep. 22, 1919, 63: 444; EBW to Carter Glass (draft), Feb. 11, 1920, 64: 405; Carter Glass to WW, Feb. 9 and 12, 1920, 64: 387 and 410–1; WGM, 514–5.

WW'S RENEWED STRENGTH; FINAL ATTEMPT AT TREATY PASSAGE: "W Has a Ride," NYT, Mar. 4, 1920, 65: 42; I. Hoover, 106; Starling, 156–7; WW to G. M. Hitchcock, Mar. 5 and 8, 1920; 65: 54 and 67–71; newspapers citing gulf between WW and HCL, quoted in ASL (N), 65: 71–2; Watson, 198; G. M. Hitchcock to WW, c. Mar. 11, 1920, 65: 80; Louis Seibold, "Visit to White House," June 17, 1920, 65: 403; JPT, 455–6; "Senate Adopts Curb by Lodge on Article X," NYT, Mar. 16, 1920, 1, 3; "Lack 7 Votes to Ratify," NYT, Mar. 20, 1920, 1–2; JD, Wilson Era, 464; EBW, 303, CTG (D), Mar. 31, 1920, 65: 149.

WW AS "LAMEST DUCK": H. S. Cummings (D), May 31, 1920, 65: 348; L. Seibold, op. cit., 65: 401–15; WW to JPT, Oct. 29, 1918, 51: 485; WW to Douglas Fairbanks, Jan. 13, 1919, 54: 53; CTG to CD, May 29, 1920, 65: 341–3; EBW, 304–5; Smith, 157; CTG (M), c. Mar. 22, 1920, 65: 111; "W Hails Colors in a Circus Parade," NYT, May 18, 1920, 65: 290–1; CTG (M), Apr. 13, 1920, 65: 179–80.

WW RESUMES CABINET MEETINGS; COLBY: CTG, 112–4; Houston, II: 68–70; JD, *Wilson Era*, II: 527–8; Smith, 147–8; CTG (M), Apr. 14, 1920, 65: 186; JD (D), Apr. 14, 1920, 65: 186–8; RL (D), Apr. 14 and May 29, 1920, 65: 188 and 343; Freud, 292; CTG, 114; CTG (N), n.d., 64: 490; WW to Joe Cowperthwaite, Sep. 3, 1920, 66: 92.

WW CONSIDERS RESIGNATION: EMH (D), Jun. 10, 1920, 65: 384; RSB (D), Feb. 4, 1920, 64: 362–3n1; WW (N), c. June 10, 1920, 65: 382; JPT to EBW (asking WW to declare he would not run for third term), Mar. 23, 1920, 65: 117–9; CTG, 116–7; JD, *Wilson Era*, 557; Marc Peter to Giuseppe Motta, May 28, 1920, 65: 338–40 (N. B.: 338n2); B. Colby to WW, Aug. 9, 1920 (with enclosed N), 66: 19–25; W. W. Hawkins (UI), Sep. 27, 1920, 66: 153–8; JD, *Wilson Era*, II: 545–6; H. Hoover, 150; Post, 275–7; Norman Hapgood to WW, Nov. 9, 1920, 66: 343; Samuel Gompers, to WW Dec. 15, 1920, 66: 515–6; W. B. Wilson to WW, Dec. 18, 1920, 66: 533; JPT to WW, May 12, 1920, 65: 276; JPT, 505; John Roberts to WW, Sep. 21, 1920, 66: 132; Helen H. Gardener, Mar. 22, 1920, 65: 115–6.

WW CONSIDERS THIRD TERM; 1920 DEMOCRATIC CONVENTION: Sir Auckland Geddes to D. Lloyd George, June 4, 1920, 65: 369–72; Carter Glass (M), June 16 and 19, 1920, 65: 400 and 435–6; SA, 197; JD, *Wilson Era*, II: 553, 555–7; Smith, 161–2; "Opening Session Spirited," *NYT*, June 29, 1920, 1, 2; H. S. Cummings to WW (T), June 28 and July 3, 1920, 65: 470–1n and 492–3; CTG (D), July 2 and 3, 1920, 65: 488 and 491; JPT to EAW, July 4, 1920, 65: 493–5; WW to H. S. Cummings, July 2, 1920 65: 489; B. Colby to WW, July 2 and 4, 1920, 65: 490 and 496; Charles Swem (D), c. July 6, 1920, 65: 498–9; WW to J. M. Cox (T), July 6, 1920, and ASL (N), 65: 499n1; Starling 157.

ELECTION OF 1920; COX AND FDR VISIT WW: I. Hoover, 106–7; EBW, 305–7; Cox, 241–4; CTG, 119; JPT, 499–502. W. W. Hawkins (UI), Sep. 27, 1920, 66: 156–7; WW to J. Cox, Oct. 29, 1920; JPT to WW, Sep. 24 and Oct. 10, 1920, 66: 141n and 214–6; WW, statement, Oct. 3, 1920, 66: 181–3; SA, 198–9; RSB, draft of article, Nov. 29, 1920, 66: 440; Charles Swem (D), Nov. 3, 1920, 66: 306–7; RSB 485; SA to JWS, Nov. 4, 1920, 66: 319–20; Starling, 612.

WW'S FINAL DAYS IN WHITE HOUSE: WW to JWS, Oct. 25, 1920, 66: 266–7; WW to L. C. Woods, Dec. 1, 1920, 66: 447; RSB (D),

Nov. 28 and Dec. 1, 1920, 66: 435–6 and 451; RSB, draft of article, Nov. 29, 1920, 66: 438–52; CTG (M), Dec. 6, 1920, 66: 479; WW, "State of the Union Address," Dec. 7, 1920, 66: 484–90; "W Urges Nation to Lead Democracy," *NYT*, Dec. 8, 1920, 1, 2; Eleanor Roosevelt, et al., to WW, c. Feb. 14, 1921; 67: 135–6; "League Assembly Opens, Hails W," *NYT*, Nov. 16, 1920, 1, 2; A. G. Schmedeman to WW (re: Nobel Prize) (T), Dec. 4, 1920, 66: 477–8.

PARTING SHOTS: N. H. Davis to WW, Dec. 8, 1920, 66: 492–3; RSB (D), Jan. 22, 1921, 67: 82; Charles Swem (D), Sep. 9, 1920, Jan. 15, 30, and Feb. 17, 1921, 66: 103, 67: 67–8, 103–4, and 143; Starling, 157; WW to R. B. Fosdick, Oct. 22 and Nov. 28, 1923, 68: 451n2 and 493–4; R. B. Fosdick to RSB, June 23, 1916 [RSB Papers, Box 108: PUL]; WW to J. G. Hibben, Dec. 22, 1919, 64: 213; WW to W. R. Wilder, May 3, 1920, 65: 246; A. M. Palmer to WW (re: Debs pardon), June, 29, 1921, 67: 98–102.

POST–WHITE HOUSE PLANS: EBW, 307–12, 314–8, 326–7; WW to C. Z. Klauder, Dec. 16, 1920, 66: 518–9n; CD to CTG, Feb. 14, 1921, 67: 136–7n; G. Creel to EBW, Feb. 15, 1921, 67: 141–2; Houston, II: 147–9; WW to C. E. Bacon, Oct. 18, 1920, 66: 242; WW to Curtis Brown, Sep. 17, 1920, 66: 121; J. R. Bolling to Macmillan Co., Apr. 15, 1921, 67: 259n.

INAUGURATION DAY 1921: CTG, 121; Longworth, 325; EBW, 317–9; "W's Exit Is Tragic," *NYT*, Mar. 5, 1921, 67: 205–14.

17 RESURRECTION

MOVING INTO 2340 S STREET: "W's Exit Is Tragic," *NYT*, Mar. 5, 1921, 5; "WW House—Reduced Copies of Measured Drawings,"lcweb2.loc.gov/pnp/habshaer/dc/dc0100/dc0104/data/dc0104data.pdf, accessed Feb. 19, 2013; Starling, 163–4; EBW, 320–2; WW to CTG, Mar. 2, 1921, 67: 185; "Harding Kept Grayson Within Wilson's Call," *NYT*, Aug. 3, 1923, 68: 398–9; "W Kills 4 Bills in Last Day in Office," *NYT*, Mar. 5, 1921, 8; W. B. Wilson to WW, Mar. 1, 1921, 67: 178–80; WW, veto message, Mar. 3, 1921; 67: 191–4; J. Smuts, "WW's Place in History," syndicated article, Mar. 3–4, 1921, 67: 27n; F. I. Cobb to WW, with "WW—An Interpretation," Mar. 4, 1921, 67: 216–9; EBW, 322–5; ASL (N) appending RSB (D), Mar. 20, 1921, 67: 236n; J. G. Hibben to WW, Jan. 6, 1920, 64: 246.

WW'S NEW ROUTINE: RSB (D), Mar. 22, May 25, 1921, 67: 237–8, 288–9; H. S. Cummings (M), Apr. 25, 1921, 67: 268–70; EBW, 324–6; L. C. Probert, "W Stricken 2 Years Ago, Now Puts in Healthy Day," *NY Tribune,* Sep. 26, 1921, 67: 395–8; "WW's Pierce-Arrow," K. L. Brown (ed.) (Staunton, VA: WW Birthplace Foundation, 1990); "W Attends the Theatre," *NYT,* Apr. 23, 1921, 67: 268; Smith, 218, "W Is Cheered by Theatre Crowd," *NYT,* Aug. 27, 1921, 67: 380–2; WW to E. G. Reid, Oct. 16, 1921, 67: 423; WW to B. Colby, Oct. 24, 1921, 67: 430.

WILSON & COLBY: SA to J. G. Hibben, June 11, 1921, 67: 310; EBW, 327–9; B. Colby to WW, Mar. 29, Apr. 18, 1921, 67: 248, 261; "W Goes to Court to Be Admitted to Bar," *NYT,* June 26, 1921, 67: 328–9; J. R. Bolling to B. Colby, July 4, 1921, 67: 343–4; RSB (D), July 29, 1921, 67: 361; B. Colby to J. R. Bolling, July 1, 1921, 67: 337–8; "W at His Law Office for First Time," *NYT,* Aug. 17, 1921, 1; WW to B. Colby, Feb. 17, May 19, June 10, Aug. 22, and 23 (unsent), 1922, 67: 548, 68: 56–7, 74, 119–20, and 120–1; B. Colby to WW, Dec. 5, 1921, 67: 472–3; J. R. Bolling to B. Colby, Dec. 6, 1921, 67: 475; "W Concentrates on Politics," *Washington Evening Star,* Dec. 13, 1922, 68: 235n.

HARDING ADMINISTRATION: W. B. Wilson to WW, Mar. 1, 1921, 67: 178–80; WW, veto message, Mar. 3, 1921, 67: 191–4; Day, *Rogers,* 117, 121; F. Scott Fitzgerald, "Early Success," *The Crack-Up* (New York: New Directions, 1945), 87.

INCREASED ADMIRATION FOR WW: RSB (D), Mar. 20 and May 27, 1921, 67: 237 and 295; S. W. Beach to WW (T), May 21, 1921, 67: 287; E. A. Alderman to WW, Dec. 29, 1921, 67: 498–9; J. H. Westcott to WW, Dec. 11, 1921, 67: 482; R. C. Stuart, Jr., to WW (T), Apr. 7 and 28, 1921, 67: 253 and 273–4; ASL (N), [re: WW Foundation], appended to R. C. Stuart, Jr., to J. R. Bolling, Apr. 27, 1921, 67: 272–3; WW to FDR, July 4, 1921, Jan. 5, and Apr. 30, 1922, 67: 341–2, 504, and 68: 39; J. R. Bolling to FDR, Sep. 3, 1921, 67: 386 and ASL (n2—re: FDR's polio); WW to E. Roosevelt, Nov. 9, 1921, 67: 448–9.

BURIAL OF UNKNOWN SOLDIER AND REACTION: W. G. Harding to WW, Oct. 4 and Nov. 8, 1921, 67: 400–1 and 445–6; J. R. Bolling to W. Lassiter, Oct. 25, 1921, 67: 432; WW to W. G. Harding, Nov. 8, 1921, 67: 444–5; WW to Louis Seibold, Nov. 12, 1921, 67: 453–4n; "W in Tears As 20,000 Acclaim Him World's Hero," *NY World,* Nov. 12, 1921, 67: 449–53;

"Ovation for W in Line and at Home," *NYT,* Nov. 12, 1921, 1, 2; EBW, 331; JD, *Life,* 17; J. S. Williams to WW, Nov. 12, 1921, 67: 454–5; WW to Ida Tarbell, Feb. 26, 1922, 67: 557–8n, includes excerpt of Tarbell, "The Man They Cannot Forget," *Collier's, LXIX* (Feb. 18, 1922), 14; CTG (M), c. Dec. 28, 1922, 68: 251; R. V. Oulahan, "W, Stronger Physically, Turning Again to Politics," *NYT,* June 10, 1923, 68: 382.

JPT, MARGINALIZED: JPT, xii; "Tumulty and W," *NYT,* Mar. 16, 1922, 4; RSB, *American Chronicle,* 495–8, 503, 515; JPT to WW, Apr. 5, 12, and 13, 1922; 67: 602, 68: 14–5, and 20–23; WW to JPT, Apr. 6 and 10, 1922, 67: 602 and 68: 10; B. Colby to WW, Apr. 6, 1922, 67: 602–3; J. R. Bolling to B. Colby, Apr. 7, 1922, 67: 604; EBW, 333–40; J. R. Bolling to Louis Wiley, Apr. 10, 1922, 68: 11; "Doubt Is Cast on W 'Message' to the Cox Dinner," *NYT,* Apr. 11, 1922, 68: 11–12; WW to editor of *NYT,* Apr. 12, 1922, 68: 14; Blum, 264; "Tumulty Regrets the Misunderstanding," *NYT,* Apr. 14, 1922, 3; CTG (M), May 22, 1922, 68: 60; SA (N) [PUL: 440], 316, 443; WW to James Kerney, Oct. 30, 1923, 68: 592.

"THE DOCUMENT": WW to L. D. Brandeis, June 20, 1921, and Apr. 9, 1922 (with enclosed "Confidential Document"), 67: 319–20n and 68: 4–5 (68: 5–9); WW to N. D. Baker, June 20, 1924, 68: 534–5; WW, addition to the Document, Aug. 7, 1922, 68: 105–6.

MORE TRIBUTES: "1,000 Women Cheer at Wilson's Home," *NYT,* Apr. 29, 1922, 68: 36–9; Cordell Hull to WW, May 27, 1922, 68: 70–1; WW to Calvin Coolidge, June 14, 1922, 68: 76n [quotes Coolidge (R) at American University, June 8, 1922]; WW to Cordell Hull, June 27, 1922, 68: 86; H. S. Cummings (M), June 28, 1922, 68: 90; L. Lipsky to WW (T), July 24, 1922, 68: 100n2; J. H. Clarke to WW, Sep. 9, 1922, 68: 131–2; E. J. N. Blair to WW, Oct. 17, 1922, 68: 156; WW to JWS, Nov. 9, 1922, 68: 180; ASL (N), 68: 180n1, appended to D. C. Roper to WW (T), Nov. 8, 1922, 68: 179; "Gloom at Capital," *NYT,* Nov. 8, 1922, 1, 5; WW to D. C. Roper, Nov. 8, 1922, 68: 180; "W Sees Nation Moving Forward," *NYT,* Nov. 12, 1922, 68: 185–8; FDR to WW (T), Dec. 27, (10 p.m. and 11:13 p.m.), and 28, 1922 (T), 12:54 a.m., 68: 245–6; RSB (D), Apr. 4, 1922, 67: 585; Family of F. M. Thompson to JD (copy of T), Jan. 14, 1922, 68: 266; EBW, 341–2; "Senate Felicitates W on Birthday," *NYT,* Dec. 29, 1922, 68: 247–8.

WW'S LITERARY EFFORTS: CTG, 131, WW to editor of *Washington Post,* c. Apr. 15, 1922,

68: 24; RSB (D), Apr. 4, 1922, 67: 585; WW, "Plans and Notes for Books," c. May 1, 1922, 68: 138–42; WW to J. F. Jameson, May 11, 1922, 68: 52; EBW, 347–8; WW, "The Road Away from Revolution" (draft), c. Apr. 8, 1923, 68: 322–4, final version, c. July 27, 1923, *Atlantic Monthly,* CXXXII (Aug. 1923), 145–6, 68: 393–5; WW to G. Creel, Apr. 9, 1923, 68: 325–6; G. Creel to EBW, Apr. 19 and 24, May 1, 1923, 68: 342–4 and 347–9n, 353–4; EBW to G. Creel, Apr. 20, 1923, 68: 344–5; WW to Ellery Sedgwick, May 2, 1923, 68: 354; CTG (M), May 22, 1922, 68: 58–9n.

DEATH OF HARDING: CTG, 136; WW to CD, Aug. 15, 1922, 68: 113; WW to Florence Harding (T), Aug. 3, 1923, 68: 398; Calvin Coolidge to WW, Aug. 4, 1923, 68: 399; "Ordeal for W to Attend Funeral," *NYT,* Aug. 9, 1923, 68: 402–3; "Washington Crowd Gives W Ovation," *NYT,* Aug. 12, 1923, 68: 404; White House Staff to Calvin Coolidge (M), Feb. 2, 1924, 68: 553.

EBW HOLIDAY; WW'S DIMINUTION: R. V. Oulahan, *op. cit.,* June 10, 1923, 68: 375–83; EBW, 351–2; WW to EBW, Aug. 29, 1923, 68: 412; EBW to WW, Aug. 31, 1923, 68: 415; CTG, 138–9; WW (N) for third inaugural address, c. Jan. 21, 1924, 68: 542; WW to R. B. Fosdick, Oct. 22 and Nov. 28, 1923, 68: 451n2 and 493–4; R. B. Fosdick to WW, Nov. 27, 1923, 68: 492–3; RSB (D), Jan. 22, 1921, 67: 82; R. B. Fosdick to RSB, June 23, 1926 [PUL: RSB Papers, box 108].

WW'S LIFE QUIETS: WW to Moore-Cottrell Subscription Agencies, Oct. 13, 1923, 68: 449–50; EBW, 346–7; "Tiger and W Recall Old Times in Cordial Reunion," *NYT,* Dec. 7, 1922, 68: 226–8; Williams, 234; "Col. House Calls, W Not at Home," *NYT,* Oct. 14, 1921, 67: 419; C. H. McCormick, Jr., to EBW, Jan. 13, 1924, 68: 528–9; EBW to C. H. McCormick, Jr., Jan. 13, 1924, 68: 529–30; SA (N) [PUL: 440], 316; JWS to WW, Apr. 18, 1923, 68: 338; WW to JWS, Apr. 28, 1923, 68: 351–2, Francis B. Sayre, Jr., to ASB (I), Sep. 30, 2001.

ARMISTICE DAY ADDRESS, 1923: EBW, 352–5; WW, radio address, Nov. 10, 1923, 68: 466–7; Clapper, 312–3; "W Overcome Greeting Pilgrims, Predicts Triumph," *NYT,* Nov. 12, 1923, 467–71.

HOLIDAYS AND BIRTHDAY, 1923; HONORS: Smith, 232–3; Reid, 236; EBW, 357; CD and J. H. Jones to WW, Oct. 1, 1923, 68: 441; CD to WW, Oct. 2, 1923, 68: 441–2; CD to EBW, Oct. 2, 1923 (two letters), 68: 442–3 and 444; WW to CD, Oct. 4 and Dec. 30, 1923, 68: 445 and 513; WW to CD, et al., Jan. 20, 1924, 68: 534; "W Is Honored on 67th Birthday: Friends Give Auto," *NYT,* Dec. 29, 1923, 68: 509–10; J. S. Bassett to WW, Dec. 30, 1923, 68: 514; WW to J. S. Bassett, Jan. 2, 1924, 68: 516; Smith, 234–5; "W Receives Party Committee," *NYT,* Jan. 17, 1924, 68: 531–2; WW (N) for third inaugural, c. Jan. 21, 1924, 68: 543; J. R. Bolling to J. W. Gerard, Jan. 31, 1924, 68: 551.

CTG LEAVES FOR HOLIDAY; WW FATALLY ILL: EBW, 358–60; J. R. Bolling (M), n. d., 68: 548–50; CTG, 110, 139; "Ex-President WW Dying," *NYT,* Feb. 2, 1924; 68: 553–60; CTG, Jr., to ASB (I), Oct. 14, 2006; Calvin Coolidge to EBW, Feb. 1, 1924, 68: 552; White House Staff to Calvin Coolidge, Feb. 2, 1924, 68: 553; Smith, 240; "WW's Life Slowly Ebbs As Night Passes," *NYT,* Feb. 3, 1924, 68: 561–6; "Throng in Prayer at W Home," Feb. 4, 1924, 68: 570–3; "WW Passes Away in Sleep," *NYT,* Feb. 4, 1924, 68: 566–70.

OBSEQUIES: Sayre, 95; Calvin Coolidge, proclamation, Feb. 3, 1924, appears in Alderman, iii; Calvin Coolidge to CTG, Feb. 4, 1924, 68: 573; Margaret Wilson to JWS, Feb. 8, 1924 [WWPL]; EBW to Calvin Coolidge, Feb. 4, 1924, 68: 574; EBW to HCL, Feb. 4, 1924, 68: 574 and 574n; HCL to EBW, n.d., quoted in Smith, 250; Robert Cullinane to ASB (I), Dec. 6, 2007; Smith, 250–1, 253–7; JD, *Life,* 363–9; "Simplicity Marks Service in the Home," Feb. 6, 1924, 68: 575–9; "W Buried in Cathedral Crypt with Simple Rites As Nation Mourns," *NYT,* Feb. 7, 1924, 68: 579–84.

POSTSCRIPT: "Artisans at Work on W's Tomb," *NYT,* June 4, 1956, 31; "Diagram of Seating on President's Platform," Jan. 20, 1961 [JFK Library]; Photograph AR6280–1M [JFK Library]; Dean F. B. Sayre, Jr., Washington National Cathedral, "Cathedral Staff," http://www.nationalcathedral.org/staff/francisSayre.shtml, accessed May 30, 2010; FDR, CD, and Hamilton Holt to WW (T), Apr. 6, 1922, 67: 603.

INDEX

A NOTE ABOUT THE TYPE

The text of this book is set in
Garamond 3 LT Std. and
Adobe Garamond Pro.
The display is set in
Chevalier Com Stripes Caps.